P9-AEZ-147

IOACHIM'S
LYMPH NODE PATHOLOGY

Dear Terry,
Thank you for sharing your teaching, your wisdom, and your friendship. Please accept this book as a token of my appreciation for the many things that you have contributed to make me a better pathologist and a better person.

Howard
2002

IOACHIM'S LYMPH NODE PATHOLOGY

THIRD EDITION

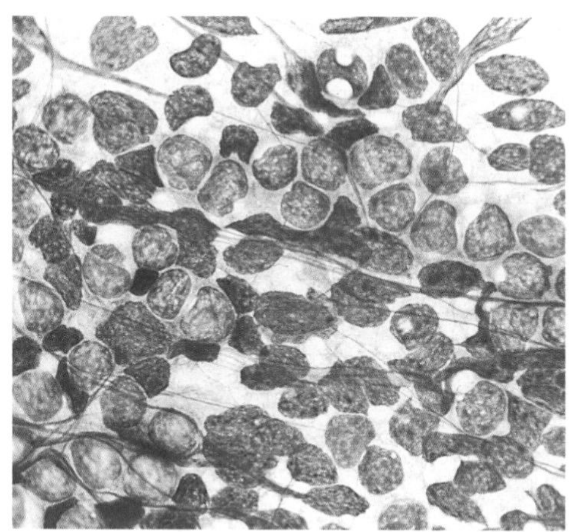

HARRY L. IOACHIM, M.D.

Professor of Pathology
New York University
Adjunct Professor of Pathology
College of Physicians and Surgeons
Columbia University
Cornell University Medical College
Chairman
Department of Pathology
Lenox Hill Hospital
New York, New York

HOWARD RATECH, M.D.

Professor of Pathology
Albert Einstein College of Medicine
Director of Hematopathology
Director of Molecular Pathology Laboratory
Montefiore Medical Center
Bronx, New York

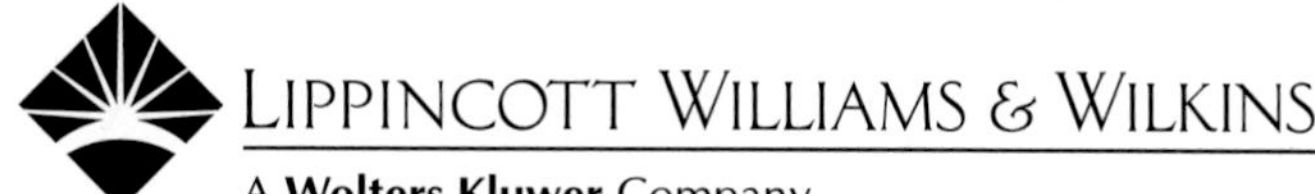

Philadelphia • Baltimore • New York • London
Buenos Aires • Hong Kong • Sydney • Tokyo

Acquisitions Editor: Ruth W. Weinberg
Managing Editor: Keith Donnellan
Production Editor: Rosemary Palumbo
Manufacturing Manager: Tim Reynolds
Cover Designer: Christine Jenny
Compositor: Maryland Composition Company, Inc.

530 Walnut Street
Philadelphia, PA 19106 USA
LWW.com

Printed in China

Library of Congress Cataloging-in-Publication Data

Ioachim, Harry L., 1924–
Ioachim's lymph node pathology / Harry L. Ioachim, Howard Ratech.–3rd ed.
p. ; cm.
Rev. ed. of: Lymph node pathology. 2nd ed. c1994.
Includes bibliographical references and index.
ISBN 0-7817-2202-0
1. Lymph nodes–Biopsy. 2. Lymph nodes–Diseases–Diagnosis. 3. Lymphomas–Diagnosis. I. Title: Lymph node pathology. II. Ratech, Howard. III. Ioachim, Harry L., 1924– Lymph node pathology. IV. Title.
[DNLM: 1. Lymph Nodes–pathology. 2. Lymphatic Diseases–diagnosis. WH 700 I635i 2002]
RC646 .I58 2002
616.4'20758–dc21 2001038788

Care has been taken to confirm the accuracy of the information presented and to describe generally accepted practices. However, the authors and publisher are not responsible for errors or omissions or for any consequences from application of the information in this book and make no warranty, expressed or implied, with respect to the currency, completeness, or accuracy of the contents of the publication. Application of this information in a particular situation remains the professional responsibility of the practitioner.

The authors and publisher have exerted every effort to ensure that drug selection and dosage set forth in this text are in accordance with current recommendations and practice at the time of publication. However, in view of ongoing research, changes in government regulations, and the constant flow of information relating to drug therapy and drug reactions, the reader is urged to check the package insert for each drug for any change in indications and dosage and for added warnings and precautions. This is particularly important when the recommended agent is a new or infrequently employed drug.

Some drugs and medical devices presented in this publication have Food and Drug Administration (FDA) clearance for limited use in restricted research settings. It is the responsibility of the health care provider to ascertain the FDA status of each drug or device planned for use in their clinical practice.

10 9 8 7 6 5 4 3 2 1

To the memory of my parents.
The strongest support and encouragement for this effort as always came from my family—
Noemi, Laura, Jackie, and Martin.

H.L.I.

To my parents, Harry and Estelle Ratech,
to my wife and best friend, Hideko Kamino
and to my teachers, Henry Rappaport,
Jerome S. Burke, and Bharat N. Nathwani.

H.R.

CONTENTS

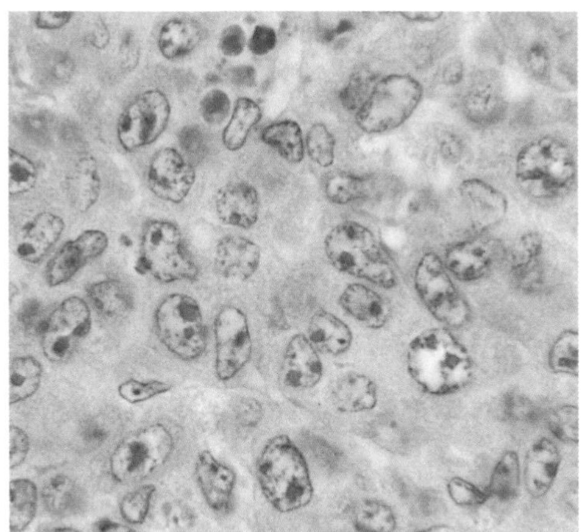

PART VII: LYMPHOPROLIFERATIVE DISORDERS ASSOCIATED WITH IMMUNE DEFICIENCY

PART VIII: SPINDLE CELL NEOPLASMS OF LYMPH NODES

PART IX: VASCULAR NEOPLASMS OF LYMPH NODES

PART X: METASTATIC TUMORS IN LYMPH NODES

PREFACE

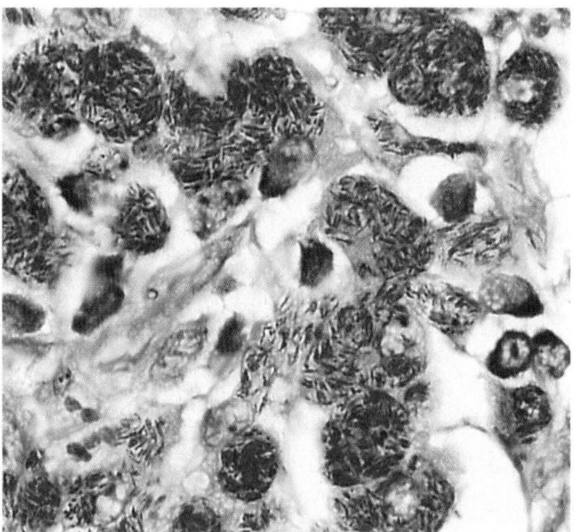

The preface of a book, often passed over by a busy reader, provides an important function. In stating the author's goals for the book, it defines the measures of comparison by which to evaluate its success or failure. In describing the structure of the book, the preface will help the reader to better use and understand it. The more personal style of the preface gives the reader an opportunity to share the thoughts of the author, hopefully establishing a rapport between writer and reader otherwise not always possible, particularly in a science book.

The first edition of this book was published in 1982, during a substantially different era in the field of pathology. At that time, there were no monoclonal antibodies, immunohistochemistry, or DNA analysis; AIDS and its complications, and at least a dozen neoplastic and nonneoplastic syndromes affecting the lymphatic system were still unknown; and textbooks dedicated to the lesions of lymph nodes were not available. The 10-year battle over the classification and nomenclature of lymphomas had just ended like most battles with a compromise: the Working Formulation, published later that same year.

Lymph Node Biopsy was an attempt to assist the practicing pathologist by providing a comprehensive source of information on the pathology of lymph nodes. It was practically oriented because it considered the pathology of lymph nodes from the point of view of their biopsy, and, for the first time, brought together the description of lymphomas with that of the more frequent nonmalignant lesions encountered in everyday practice. The book seemed to have achieved its goals and became widely used in this and many other countries.

A second edition of this book was published in 1995. Because of the rapid progress in this field achieved in the intervening 14 years, the second edition, titled *Lymph Node Pathology*, was substantially larger, included many new entities, and was thoroughly updated and illustrated in color. Even more changes in the field followed in the ensuing years. The lymphatic system by its nature was best suited for the applications of the breakthroughs in immunology and molecular biology that have occurred during the past decade. The methodology was further developed by the continuous production of monoclonal antibodies with new specificities, the expanded role of flow cytometry and the introduction of polymerase chain reaction in hematopathologic diagnosis. The unprecedented growth of hematopathology was accompanied by the development of a specialized supply industry and the continuous increase in the number of publications and journals dedicated to this specialty. The practicing pathologist, facing the challenge of keeping up with this rapidly changing field finds it difficult to cull out the needed information from the ever-expanding and widely scattered literature. Definitions of new entities and novel concepts of lymphomas led to the creation of the new World Health Organization (WHO) classification. This time an interval of only seven years marked enough changes in the field to necessitate a new edition of *Lymph Node Pathology*.

For this endeavor I was fortunate to enlist as my associate Dr. Howard Ratech, an expert and experienced hematopathologist. In the third edition, we have preserved the text's original goal: to address the needs of the practicing pathologist. The format has been maintained; we continue to treat all entities in an encyclopedic fashion as individual chapters with standard headings for easy reference and checklists for quick review. Part II, Diagnostic Methods, has been expanded, including separate chapters on Cytology, Immunohistochemistry, Flow Cytometry, and Molecular Diagnosis. The individual chapters on lymphomas follow the new WHO classification and are described in accordance with its concepts.

This third edition of *Lymph Node Pathology* contains additional chapters and has more color illustrations. In contradistinction to the textbooks on lymphoid neoplasms, this text is comprehensive, including all forms of lymphadenitides, lymphadenopathies, and lymph node metastases. The increase in volume is due to the inclusion of new entities and to the incorporation of new information into each chapter relating not only to immunohistochemistry, molecular pathology, and differential diagnosis, but also to epidemiology, pathogenesis, and clinical syndromes. References have been expanded and updated to 2001. In this way, we believe this book may be used as a workbench reference in the formulation of a diagnosis, as well as a source of information in the composition of a case presentation.

Striking a proper balance is important in producing a book. Writing exhaustively on every subject is better left to the large multiauthored tomes; writing too concisely is prone to misunderstanding and misuse. Hopefully, *Ioachim's Lymph Node Pathology* brings together the background information, the morphologic descriptions, the recommended procedures, the supportive illustrations, and the interpretation of results necessary for the reader to make the correct diagnosis. It reflects our experience and ideas resulting from many years of practice in the field. The highest reward for this endeavor, undoubtedly, will be to know that other practicing pathologists have found it useful.

Harry L. Ioachim, M.D.
May 2001

PREFACE TO THE FIRST EDITION

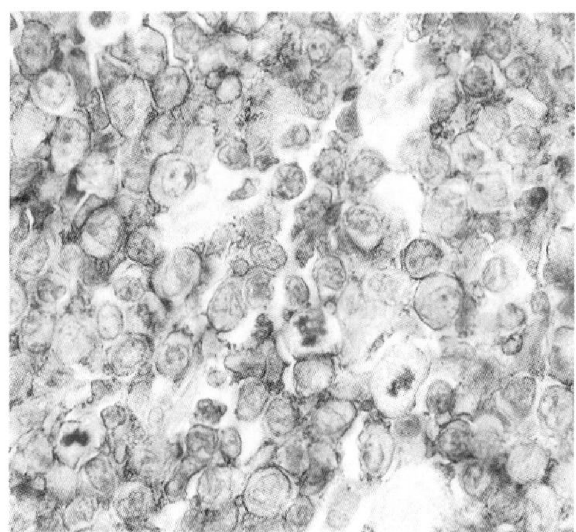

Lymph nodes are among the organs most commonly biopsied for diagnostic purposes. Their frequent involvement in regional and systemic diseases and their easy accessibility make the morphologic study of lymph nodes a permanent activity of the pathologist. Yet there appears to be less agreement between initial and review diagnosis in this field than in any other, and the rates of misdiagnosis reported by various studies are higher for lymph nodes than for other organs.

Certainly inherent difficulties exist in the interpretation of lymph node lesions. These difficulties have been compounded lately by major conceptual changes in this field. In recent years, several basic discoveries related to the origins, functions, and interrelationships of lymphocytes have been made, causing important changes in the understanding of their pathology. The application of immunologic methods to the study of normal and neoplastic lymphoid cells, a collective achievement of many investigators, has resulted in the revision of earlier histogenetic theories and in the development of new concepts, terminologies, and classifications. The nomenclature and the classification of non-Hodgkin lymphomas have become two of the most debated topics in medical literature. A lack of agreement among leading experts has led to the use of at least seven different classifications in clinical trials, routine practice, and laboratory investigations. The immunologic methods requiring technical and interpretational expertise, as well as the profusion and complexity of terminology, have contributed to projecting a forbidding image to the field of lymphomas that not infrequently has discouraged their study.

A contributing factor to the difficulty of diagnosing lymph node biopsies is the lack of specialized textbooks that could assist the practicing pathologist. There is a surprising contrast between the books available, some of excellent quality, that are devoted to other organs and tissues, and the virtual absence of books on the pathology of lymph nodes. The non-neoplastic lesions of lymph nodes comprise multiple entities that often raise difficult problems of differential diagnosis. However, these lesions have been only occasionally described, often in the form of case reports, and the pertinent information is scattered through the medical literature. The metastatic tumors in lymph nodes, another group of lesions commonly evaluated by biopsy, similarly have not all been described in available textbooks.

The literature on lymphomas, by contrast has had the benefit of two authoritative textbooks and of several excellent review articles by well recognized experts in this field. Henry Rappaport's book *Tumors of the Hematopoietic System*, published in 1966 in the

Armed Forces Institute of Pathology's *Atlas of Tumor Pathology* series, eminently written and amply illustrated, is the classic text on the subject and has been accepted and used worldwide. The book is now out of print, however, and a new edition comprising the recent changes of methods and concepts has not been published. Lennert and Mohri's book is an impressive, scholarly treatise on lymphomas, but it is not organized as a practical reference manual and uses nomenclature unfamiliar in this country.

It appears that a need exists for a comprehensive source of information on the pathology of lymph nodes. To be of assistance to practicing pathologists who must evaluate lymph node biopsies, such a book must be inclusive, practically oriented, and well illustrated. This book was conceived with these objectives in mind. It comprises 65 different pathologic entities in an attempt to include in a single source all the various kinds of lymphadenitides, lymphadenopathies, lymphomas, and metastatic tumors. To serve as a reference book, the pathologic entities are treated in encyclopedic fashion, each chapter including sections on definition, clinical syndrome, histopathology, differential diagnosis, bibliography, and, when applicable, on etiology, cytochemistry, electron microscopy, and immunopathology. To increase its usefulness as a practical manual, each chapter includes a checklist that enumerates the characteristic features supporting the diagnosis. All lesions mentioned are illustrated, with a total of 268 photographs, predominantly of light microscopy, supplemented, when contributory, by pictures of electron microscopy and immunopathology.

The sources of this book are in the specialized literature and in my own experience, which was accumulated slowly over 20 years of activity in the Departments of Pathology of Francis Delafield Hospital, Lennox Hill Hospital, and the College of Physicians and Surgeons of Columbia University. The material used in this book comes from the same departments. My indoctrination in the art of surgical pathology was through my pathology teachers in Europe, a fortunate training with Arthur Purdy Stout, a long association with Sheldon C. Sommers, and the invaluable daily cooperation of many distinguished pathologists in Bucharest, Paris, and New York. The parallel study of leukemias and lymphomas in experimental systems, also begun 20 years ago under the guidance of the late Jacob Furth and continued to present, helped me considerably in understanding the intricacies of this field.

This book, like all books, has its origin in other writings. During the past 15 years, the literature on hematopathology has been enriched by an astonishing amount of information and by new basic concepts. Rappaport, Lukes, Lennert, Kaplan, Collins, Berard, Dorfman, Seligman, Aisenberg, Bennett, Butler, their many associates, and numerous other investigators have made creative and often essential contributions that have fundamentally changed this field. To witness these changes has been exciting. To include them in this book and give the reader a balanced view of various opinions has not been easy. A textbook must generally reflect the contemporary state of the art. A reference manual should present the information available in an accessible form and in one applicable to the specialized use. In this sense, I hope that this book will be useful to the practicing pathologist for whom it was primarily written.

Harry L. Ioachim, M.D.
April 1982

ACKNOWLEDGMENTS

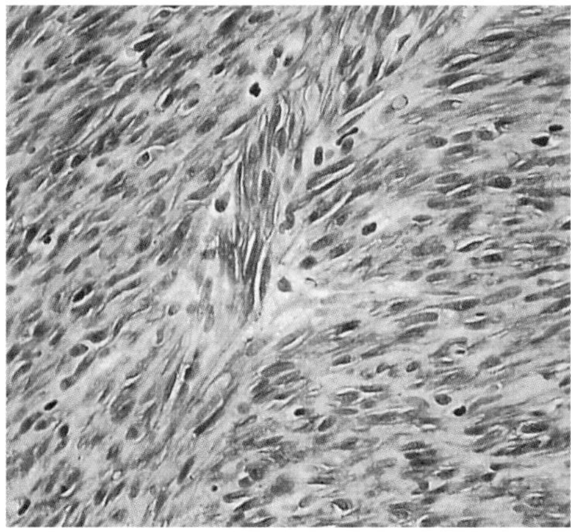

There are many who contributed directly or indirectly to the making of this book, and to whom I am very grateful. Among them are my associates at Lenox Hill Hospital, physicians, researchers, and technicians with whom I shared the satisfaction of my daily activity for the past 30 years. Most of all, I thank Tove Bamburger, who prepared all editions of this book with outstanding competence and dedication, and Brent Dorsett, who lent his talent to so many of my research projects. Keith Donnellan, Managing Editor; Rosemary Palumbo, Supervising Editor; Ruth Weinberg, Senior Editor; and their highly professional staff at Lippincott Williams & Wilkins provided expert and friendly editorial assistance.

Many physicians contributed to the illustration of this book by lending tissue sections and photographs or by permitting the reproduction of their published material. I greatly appreciate their courtesy.

PART

I

THE NORMAL LYMPH NODE

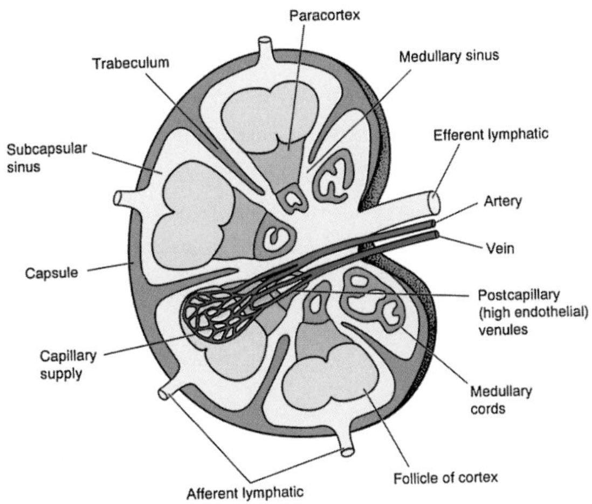

The lymph nodes are major components of the lymphatic system clustered in small groups or chains at strategic locations, where they drain the lymphatic vessels of various anatomic regions. The drainage involves not only the mechanical filtration of the foreign bodies in the lymph but also the recognition and processing of antigens. The lymph nodes exhibit a complex architecture in which a variety of cell populations are arranged in distinct interfacing compartments. This provides a favorable environment in which the various cellular components can process antigens, interact, and generate the immune response.

1

THE NORMAL LYMPH NODE

ANATOMY

In the lymphatic pathway, lymph nodes are peripheral lymphoid organs connected to the circulation by afferent and efferent lymphatics (Fig. 1.1). These ovoid, round, or bean-shaped nodular formations, composed of dense accumulations of lymphoid tissue, vary in size from 2 to 20 mm and average 15 mm in longitudinal diameter (1,2) (Fig. 1.2). Normally, lymph nodes are not palpable. They become detectable as a result of intense immune reactions or tumor metastasis. The cut surface is gray–pink, soft, and homogeneous. A diameter larger than 3 cm, a firm consistency, and a white and nodular cut surface are features suggestive of neoplasia. The characteristics of each group of lymph nodes vary in relation to age and site in the body; for example, mesenteric nodes have wider medullary cords and sinuses, whereas peripheral nodes, particularly those draining areas of active antigenic stimulation, such as the neck and abdomen, have larger and more numerous germinal centers. Peripheral nodes are also more numerous in younger than in older persons and are absent in newborns (3).

FUNCTIONS

The major functions of lymph nodes are lymphopoiesis, filtration of lymph, and processing of antigens. The immune response takes place in an integrated lymphoid system that includes the lymph nodes, spleen, and *m*ucosa-*a*ssociated *l*ymphoid *t*issues (MALT). All lymphoid cells originate in the bone marrow; B cells mature in the bone marrow, whereas T cells migrate to the thymus, where they undergo further differentiation. From these primary lymphoid organs, B and T cells colonize the secondary lymphoid organs: the lymph nodes, where they respond to antigens in body tissues; the spleen, where they monitor antigens in the circulating blood; and the MALT, where they act as a defense against antigens in the mucosae and skin (4).

STRUCTURE

Cortical Area

The cortical area, or *superficial cortex* (Fig. 1.3), includes the lymphoid follicles with their germinal centers. The cortical area represents the bursa-dependent, B-cell area of the lymph node, associated mainly with mechanisms of humoral immunity. The primary lymphoid follicles are round nodules, averaging 1 mm in diameter; the longer axis of each is oriented at a right angle to the lymph node capsule (5). The secondary or reactive lymphoid follicles comprise a peripheral area or mantle of closely packed, small lymphocytes and the centrally located germinal centers. The latter include a population of lymphoid cells in various stages of maturation, supportive reticulum cells, dendritic reticulum cells (DRCs), and histiocytes that often exhibit active phagocytosis. The germinal centers vary in size, enlarging substantially under conditions of antigenic stimulation (Fig. 1.4). The primary follicles are composed of a homogeneous cell population of small, darkly staining, inactive lymphocytes. They become secondary follicles when stimulated by antigens and include well-developed germinal centers composed of paler-staining, heterogeneous populations of cells. These predominantly include B lymphocytes, small and large, cleaved and noncleaved, in addition to a few scattered T lymphocytes (Fig. 1.5). The lymphocytes of the mantle zones are all of the B-cell type. The outer layers of the mantle zone are less tightly packed, and the cells, still of the B-cell type, have more cytoplasm, and form the marginal zone. This zone, which appears distinct in the reactive follicles of the spleen, is not well formed in the lymph nodes, where it is often indistinguishable from the mantle zone. The secondary follicles include in their reactive germinal centers the following types of cells: centroblasts, centrocytes, small lymphocytes, tingible-body macrophages, and DRCs. In their reactive phase, the germinal centers exhibit a light zone oriented toward the periphery of the lymph node that is composed predominantly of centrocytes and a dark zone oriented toward the center of the lymph node that is composed predominantly of centroblasts (Figs. 1.6 and 1.7). The zonation and orientation of follicles is not always noticeable,

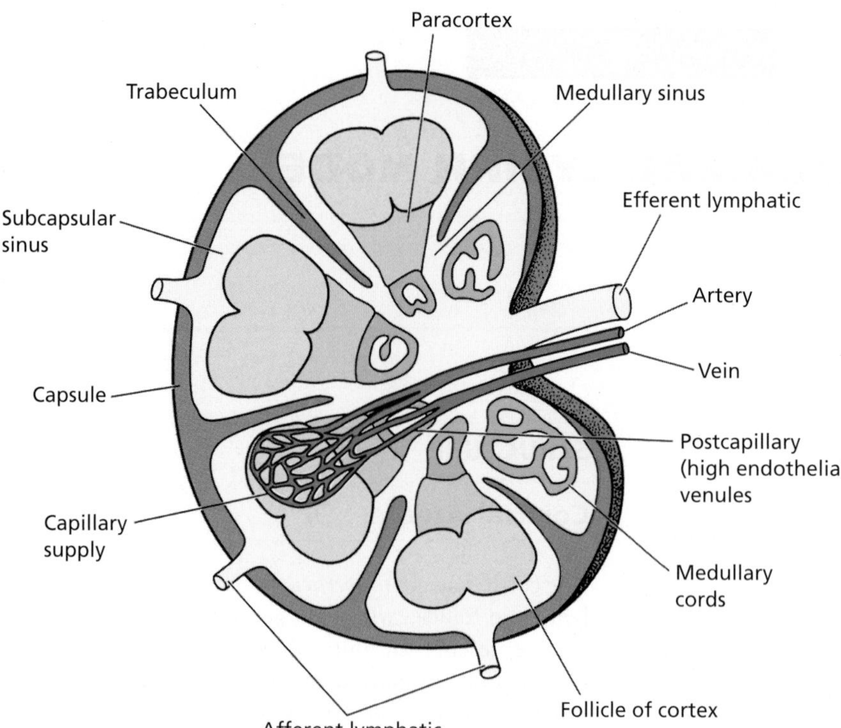

FIGURE 1.1. The structure of the lymph node. (From Stevens A, Lowe J. Lymph nodes. In: Stevens A, Lowe J. Histology. London: Gower Medical Publications, 1992:90–95, with permission.)

being dependent on the phase of immune reaction and on the sectioning of the lymph node (6).

Paracortical Area

The paracortical area, or *deep cortex* (Fig. 1.8), is the densely cellular area beneath the cortex that extends between the lymphoid follicles, forming regular interdigitations from the capsule to the corticomedullary junction. It includes lymphoid cells and postcapillary venules. The paracortex represents the thymus-dependent area, and the lymphoid cells are predominantly of T-cell types (7–12). They may be small or large but are mainly noncleaved and frequently in mitosis, representing various stages of cellular transformation in response to antigenic stimulation (Fig. 1.9). Like B lymphocytes, activated T lymphocytes change into immunoblasts, undergo active proliferation, or enter the pool of circulating lymphocytes. In addition to T cells, the paracortex contains the interdigitating cells (IDCs), which initially present antigens to lymphoid cells and thus

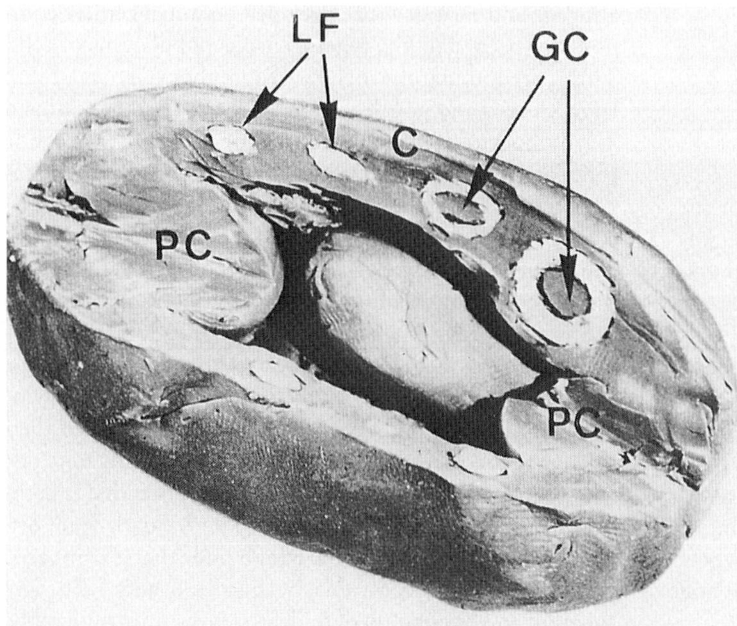

FIGURE 1.2. Tridimensional model of lymph node topography. *C,* cortical area; *PC,* paracortical area; *LF,* lymphoid follicles; *GC,* germinal center. Central area is the medulla. (From Cottier H, Turk J, Sobin L. A proposal for a standardized system of reporting human lymph node morphology in relation to immunological function. Bull World Health Organ 1972;47:375–408, with permission.)

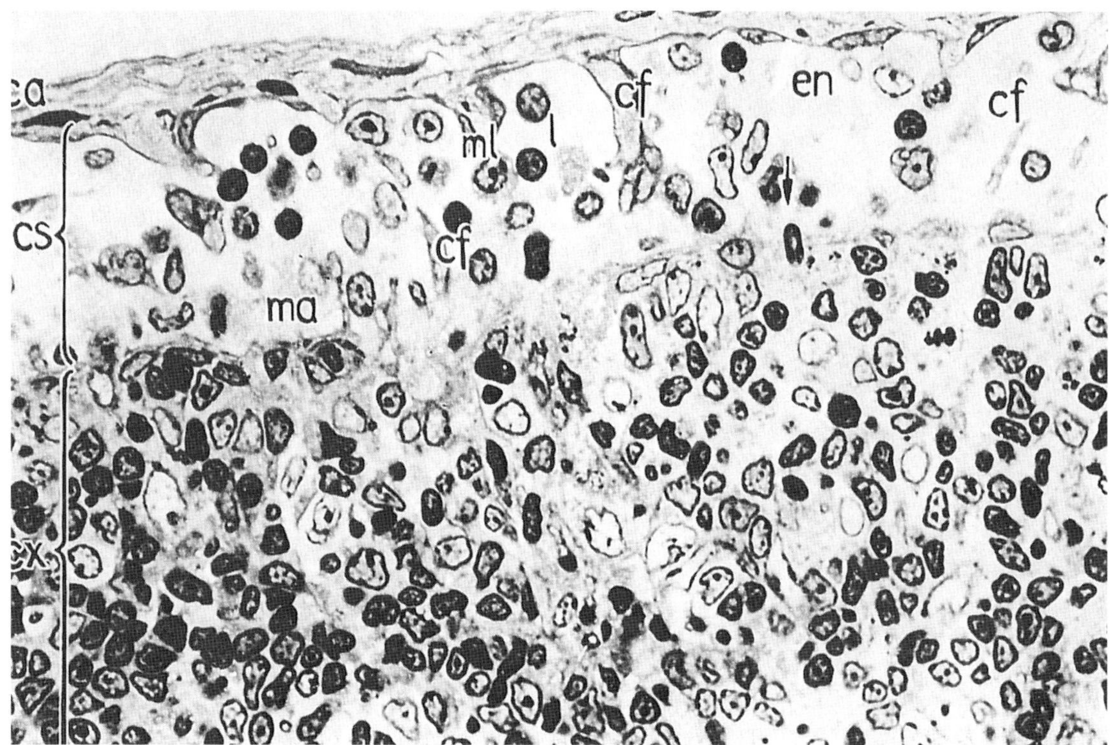

FIGURE 1.3. Capsule (*ca*), marginal sinus (*SCS*), and cortical area (*cx*) of lymph node. Sinus endothelium (*en*) is continuous at capsular side and interrupted on parenchymal side where lymphocytes (*arrow*) pass through. *cf,* reticular fibers; *ma,* macrophages; *l,* small; *ml,* large lymphocytes. (From Olah I, Röhlich P, Törö I. Lymph node. In: Ultrastructure of lymphoid organs. Philadelphia: JB Lippincott Co, 1975:216–255, with permission.)

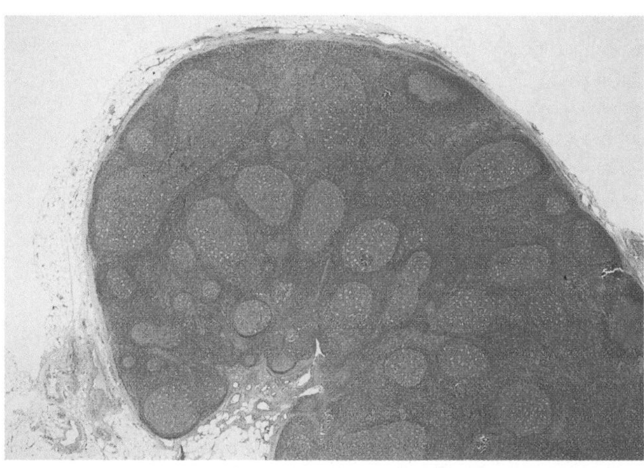

FIGURE 1.4. Reactive lymph node with enlarged, irregularly shaped follicles and germinal centers. Hematoxylin, phloxine, and saffron stain.

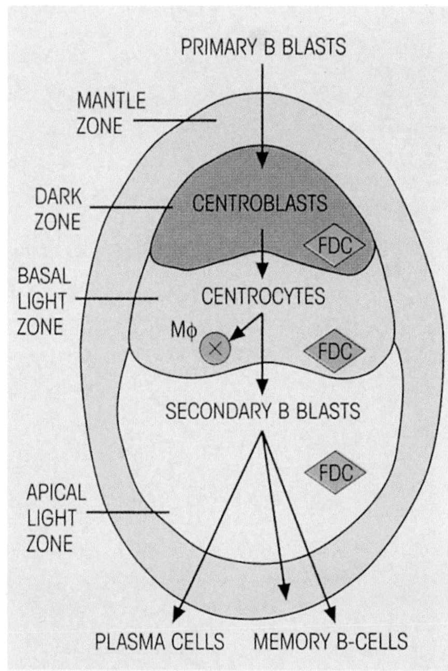

FIGURE 1.5. The structure of a lymphoid follicle indicating the differentiation of B cells during their passage through the germinal center. (From Roitt I. The anatomy of the immune response. In: Essential immunology. London: Blackwell Science, 1997:152–167, with permission.)

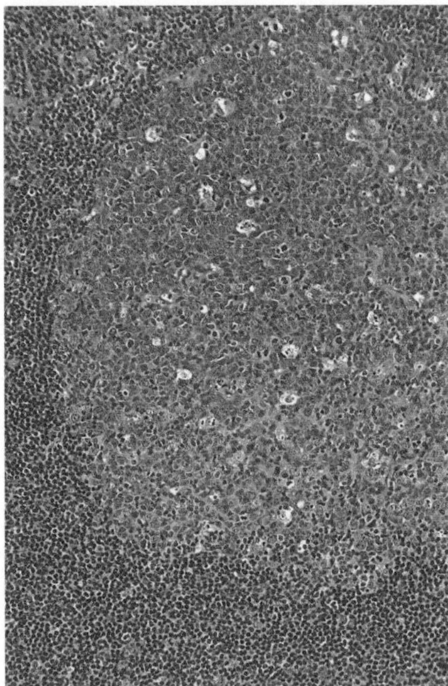

FIGURE 1.6. Lymphoid follicle with germinal center. Dark zone of centroblasts (*top*) and light zone of centrocytes (*bottom*). Mantle zone. Hematoxylin, phloxine, and saffron stain.

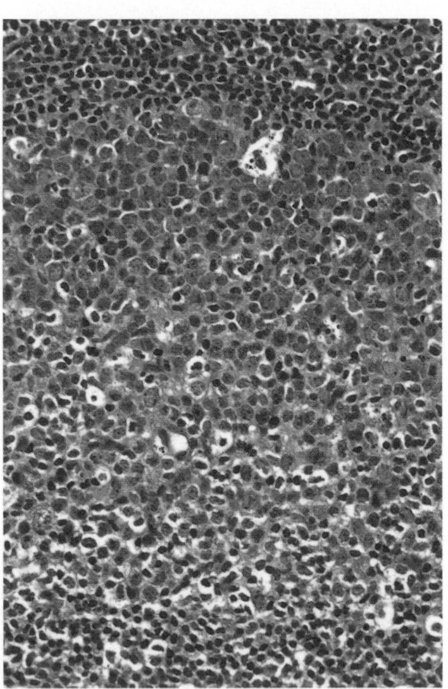

FIGURE 1.7. Same section as in Fig. 1.6. Dark zone of centroblasts (*top*), light zone of centrocytes (*bottom*). Small lymphocytes of mantle zone at upper edge. Hematoxylin, phloxine, and saffron stain.

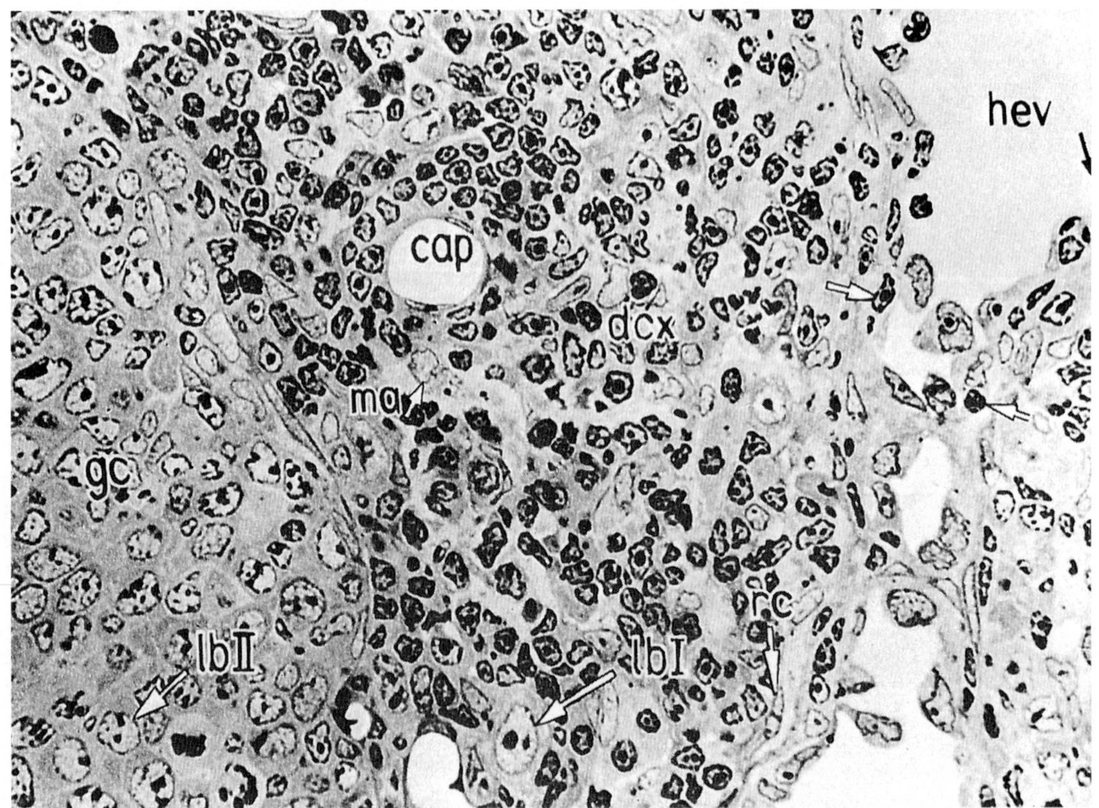

FIGURE 1.8. Cortical area with germinal center (*gc*) and paracortical area (*dcx*) of lymph node. *cap,* capillary; *hev,* venule; *lb,* large lymphocytes; *rc,* reticular cell; *ma,* macrophage. *Arrows* indicate lymphocytes migrating through endothelium. ×1,100. (From Olah I, Röhlich P, Törö I. Lymph node. In: Ultrastructure of lymphoid organs. Philadelphia: JB Lippincott Co, 1975:216–255, with permission.)

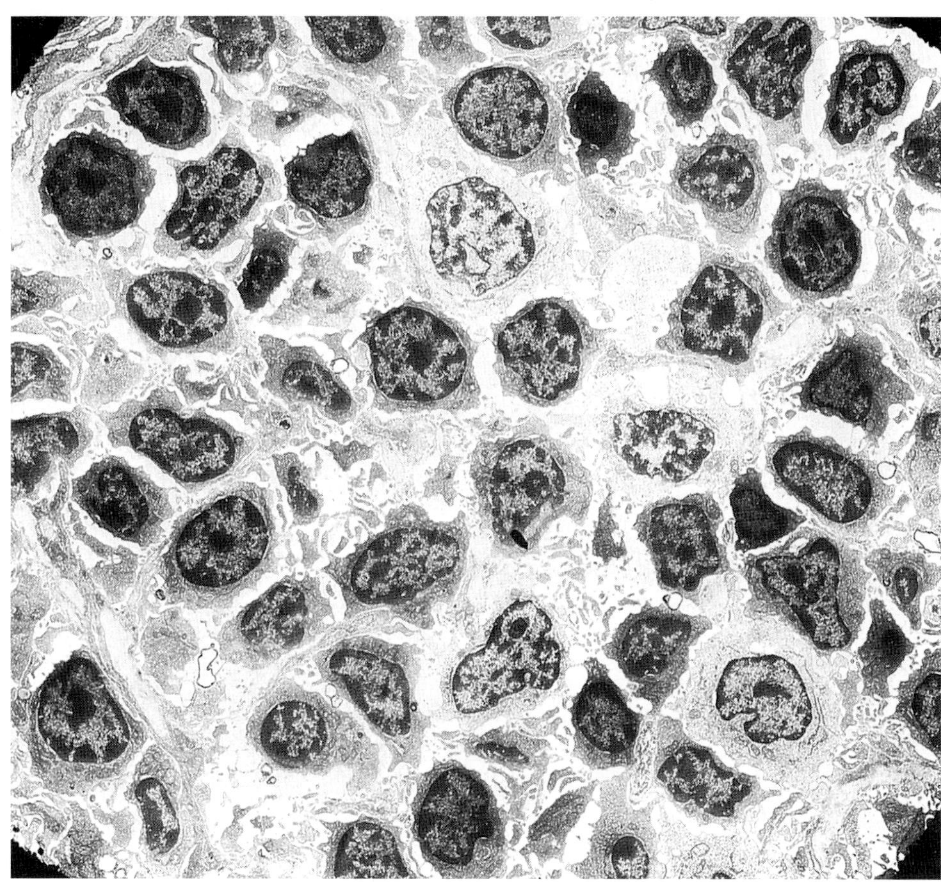

FIGURE 1.9. Section of cervical lymph node with architecture and normal cytologic appearance. Small, nonactivated lymphocytes; medium-sized and large, activated lymphocytes; and a few histiocytes are admixed in various proportions. ×3,300.

play an essential role in initiating the immune response (4,6). When the IDCs are present in large numbers, the mixture of these larger, paler cells with the smaller, darker lymphocytes results in the typical mottled aspect of the reactive paracortical areas (Fig. 1.10).

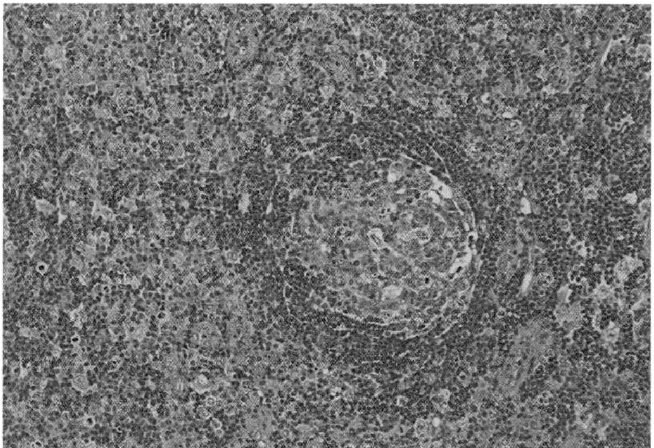

FIGURE 1.10. Paracortical area in stimulated lymph node with admixture of small dark lymphocytes and larger, paler interdigitating cells around a reactive follicle resulting in mottled aspect. Hematoxylin, phloxine, and saffron stain.

Medullary Area

The *medulla* (Fig. 1.11) is the main site of plasma cell proliferation, differentiation, and production of antibodies. It is composed of cords of cells that include lymphocytes, plasmacytoid lymphocytes, plasmablasts, and mature plasma cells in various proportions. Under intense antigenic stimulation, the medullary cords may extend deep into the cortex.

The plasma cells lose their CD20 surface markers and synthesize antibodies that are carried by lymph into the general circulation. They contain intracytoplasmic immunoglobulins of various classes, with κ and λ light chains in a ratio of approximately 2:1 (6). The cords of plasma cells and their precursors are separated by wide medullary sinuses, which, in addition to the percolating lymph, also contain numerous monocytes, plasma cells, macrophages, and mast cells.

CELLS

Lymphoid Cells

The lymph node parenchyma includes different populations of lymphoid cells in various stages of differentiation and activation lying on or moving through the supporting frame-

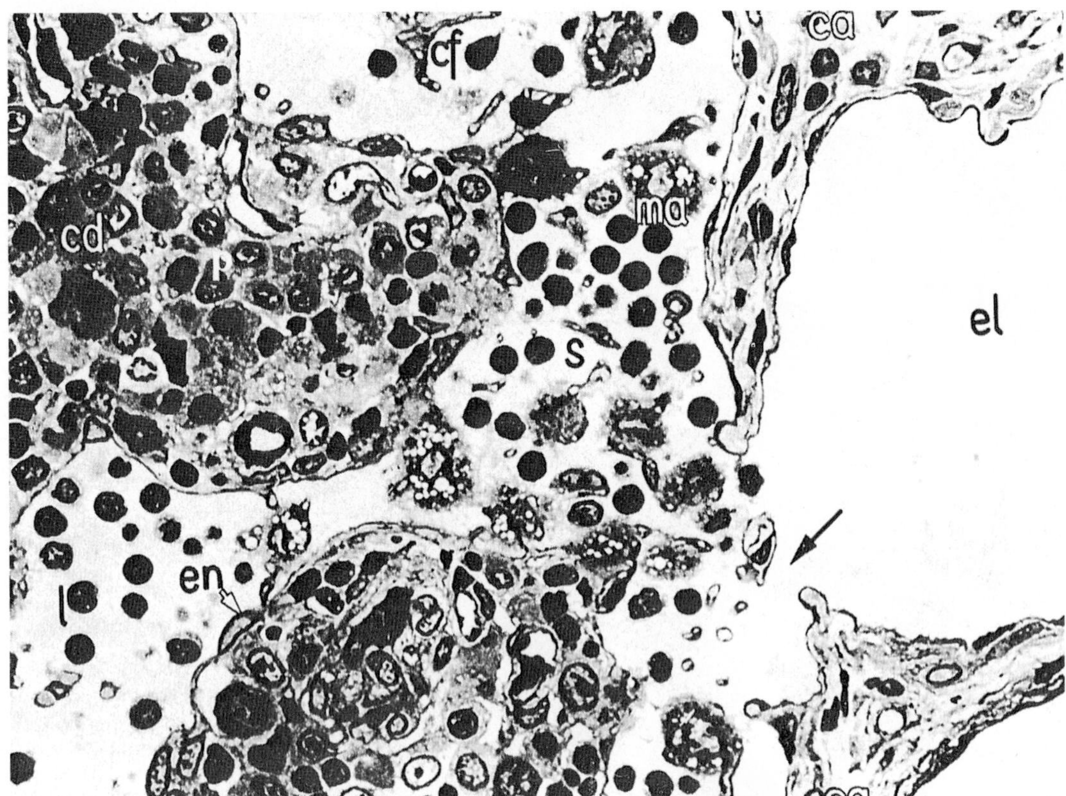

FIGURE 1.11. Medullary area (*ma*) of lymph node. Medullary cords (*cd*) with mature plasma cells (*p*); medullary sinus (*s*) in continuation with efferent lymphatic vessel (*el*). *ca*, capsule; *cf*, reticular fibers; *en*, sinus endothelium; *l*, lymphocytes. ×1,100. (From Olah I, Röhlich P, Törö I. Lymph node. In: Ultrastructure of lymphoid organs. Philadelphia: JB Lippincott Co, 1975:216–255, with permission.)

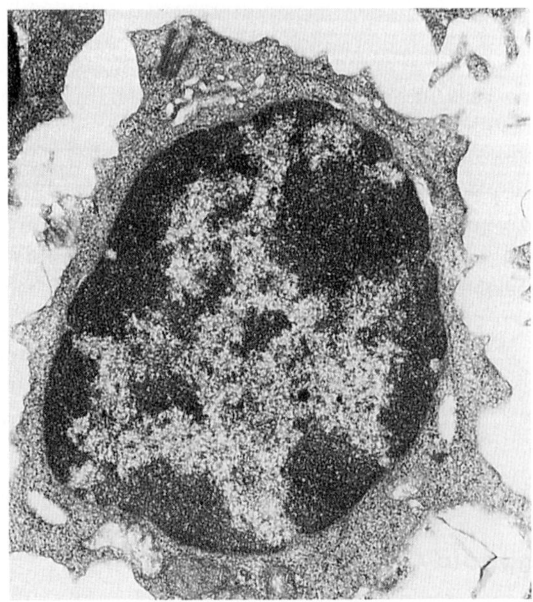

FIGURE 1.12. Small, nonactivated lymphocyte, 4 to 5 μm in diameter, with microvilli, small amount of cytoplasm, sparse organelles, and nucleus with heterochromatin. ×13,800.

work of the stroma. They comprise the main populations of B cells, T cells, and plasma cells, each with multiple subpopulations. The lymphoid cells include small, medium-sized, and large lymphocytes in various proportions (3). *Small lymphocytes,* also designated as *mature* or *circulating lymphocytes,* are nonactivated cells; after entering the lymph node through the postcapillary venules, if they do not become activated, they reenter the general circulation within a matter of hours via the efferent lymphatics (5) (Fig. 1.12). The cell diameter averages 6 μm and the diameter of the round nucleus is about 5 μm, so that the nuclear–cytoplasmic ratio is very high (1). Under light microscopy, the nucleus is dense and appears structureless, and the cytoplasm is just a thin, perinuclear rim. Under the electron microscope, the nucleus is formed almost entirely of highly condensed heterochromatin; the cytoplasm contains a large number of single ribosomes, a small Golgi body, several mitochondria, and few strands of endoplasmic reticulum (13–15). The surface shows shallow indentations and occasional short microvilli. *Large lymphocytes* have a greater amount of cytoplasm containing polyribosomes (14), a moderately large Golgi apparatus, multiple mitochondria, and a large nucleus with prominent nucleoli (Fig. 1.13).*Medium-sized lymphocytes* reflect the transition between nonactivated and activated lymphocytes. The B cells display on their surface

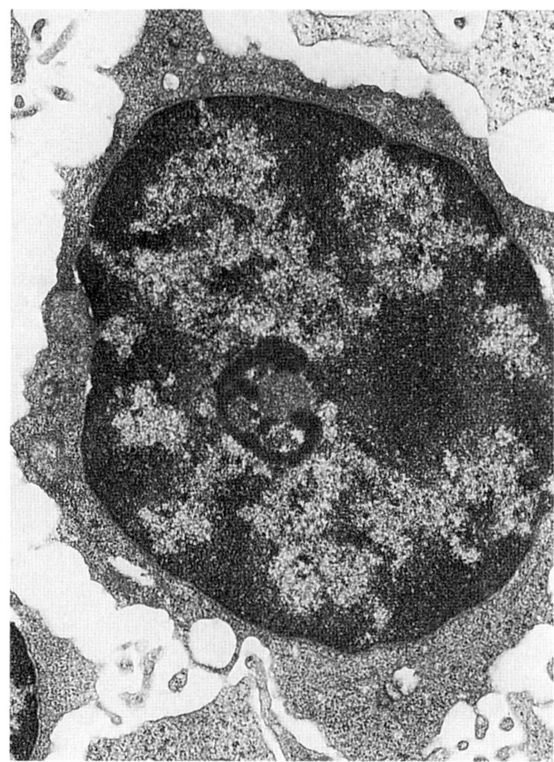

FIGURE 1.13. Medium-sized, activated lymphocyte, 10 to 12 μm in diameter, with microvilli, more abundant cytoplasm and organelles, and nucleus with prominent nucleolus. ×13,800.

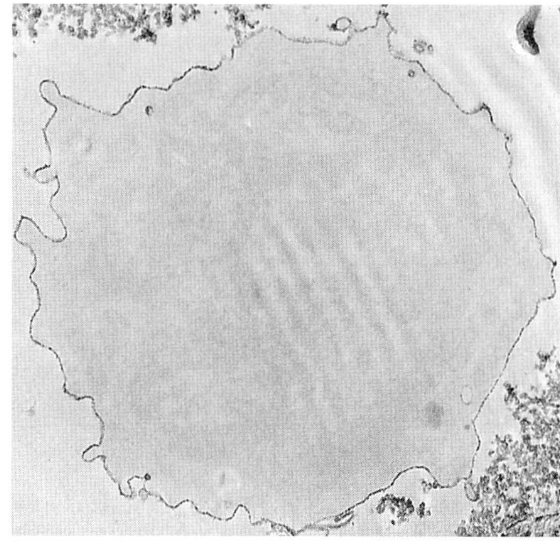

FIGURE 1.15. B lymphocyte with fine, continuous surface deposition of peroxidase after immunostaining with anti-IgG antibody, which indicates the presence of membrane immunoglobulins. ×8,400.

membrane immunoglobulins that can be visualized by staining with fluorescein-labeled (Fig. 1.14) or peroxidase-labeled (Fig. 1.15) antihuman immunoglobulin antisera, in addition to strong complement (C3) receptors (7–10).

The *primary follicle* contains mainly small and medium-sized B cells that represent resting, inactivated lymphocytes. The *secondary follicle* is characterized by its germinal center and contains B cells in various stages of reaction to antigens (Fig. 1.16). In the dark zones, the centroblasts, which express a small amount of IgM on their surface, enter a phase of a high degree of mitotic activity and differentiate into centrocytes, which begin secreting immunoglobulins and move to the opposite pole of the germinal centers to form the light zones (4,11,12) (Figs. 1.5–1.7). Among the many reacting cells in germinal centers, the ones that are best fitted to the particular antigens are selected for proliferation, whereas the others are promptly destroyed. As a result, the reacting germinal centers contain numerous cells in mitosis next to large numbers of cells in apoptosis. In the process of cell selection through apoptosis, the bcl-2 gene product is essential. As an inhibitor of apoptosis, bcl-2 is shut off in the reactive germinal center to permit the elimination of cells unfit for the immune response (Fig. 1.17). The extensive cell death releases numerous DNA nuclear fragments, which constitute the tingible bodies that are then picked up by

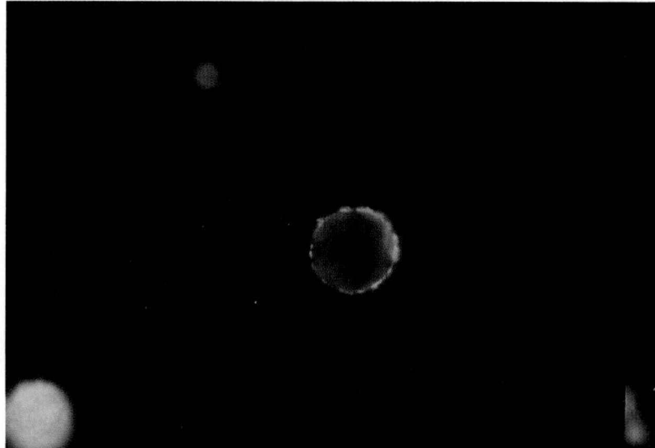

FIGURE 1.14. B lymphocyte with membrane IgG in immunofluorescence. Ring-shaped granular membrane fluorescence after staining with fluorescein isothiocyanate-labeled goat antihuman IgG antiserum.

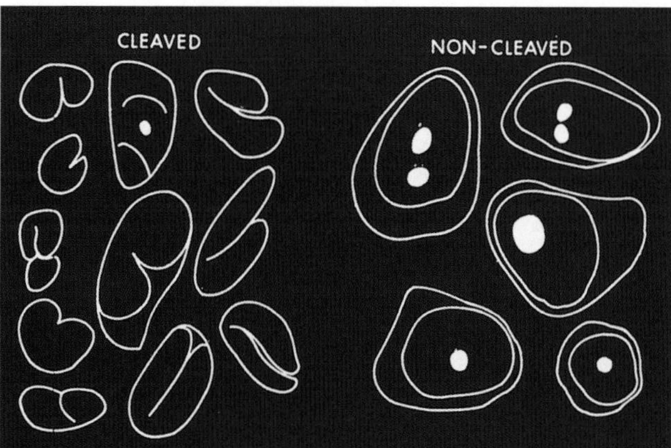

FIGURE 1.16. Small and large cleaved (centrocytes) and noncleaved (centroblasts) lymphoid cells of germinal centers.(From Lukes RJ, Collins RD. New approaches to the classification of the lymphomata. Br J Cancer 1975;31[Suppl II]:1–28, with permission.)

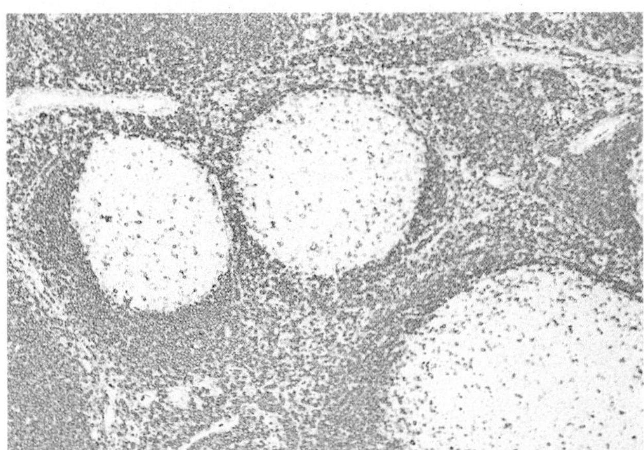

FIGURE 1.17. Lymph node with reactive follicular hyperplasia shows absence of bcl-2 activity in the proliferating cells of the germinal center. Bcl-2 /peroxidase stain.

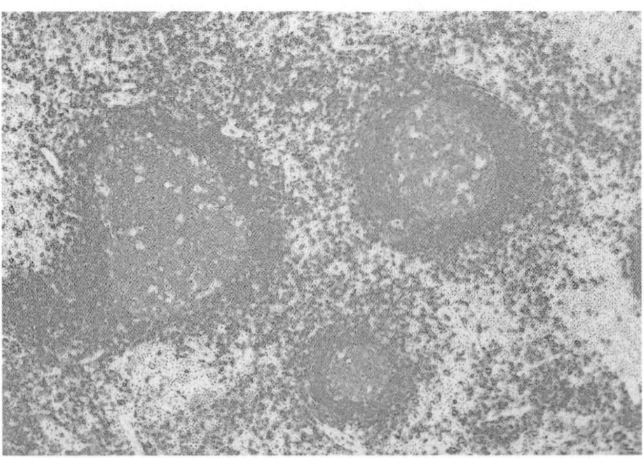

FIGURE 1.19. Lymph node B cells highlighted by immunostaining for CD20 pan-B-cell marker. Follicular germinal centers, mantle zones, and scattered B cells in perifollicular areas. L26/peroxidase stain.

phagocytic histiocytes (Fig. 1.18). In contrast, in lymphoma, bcl-2 activity present in the center of follicles prevents apoptosis and favors uncontrolled proliferation.

The selected centroblasts continue to undergo mitosis at high rates and develop cell clones that differentiate into centrocytes, up-regulate the formation of membrane immunoglobulins, and aggregate in the light zone of the center. From here, some of these cells become memory B cells, which reside in the mantle zone of the follicle; another part of the cell population differentiates further into plasmablasts and plasma cells and migrates in the medullary area of the lymph node (4) (Fig. 1.19). Thus, naïve B cells, once activated by antigen, mature and proliferate to produce an expanded population of identical plasma cells that recognize the same antigen. Normal lymph nodes contain 20% to 35% immunoglobulin-bearing cells in a cell suspension (Fig. 1.8), a proportion that may increase to 80% in some types of reactive follicular hyperplasia and to 100% in monoclonal B-cell lymphomas.

T cells also enter the lymph nodes via the high endothelial venules, and unless activated, they leave it after 6 to 8 hours through the efferent lymphatics. A small number of small, inactive T cells are scattered within the follicles. Most T cells are confined to the paracortical areas, which represent the T-cell territory (Fig. 1.20). Most of the cells are small T lymphocytes, which, depending on their cell membrane glycoprotein markers, belong to one of three major cell populations: CD4+ helper T cells, CD8+ suppressor T cells, and NK+ natural killer cells. The T-cell types can be identified with specific anti-CD (cluster of differentiation) monoclonal antibodies. Like B cells, T cells in lymph nodes may become activated, forming T immunoblasts. Once ac-

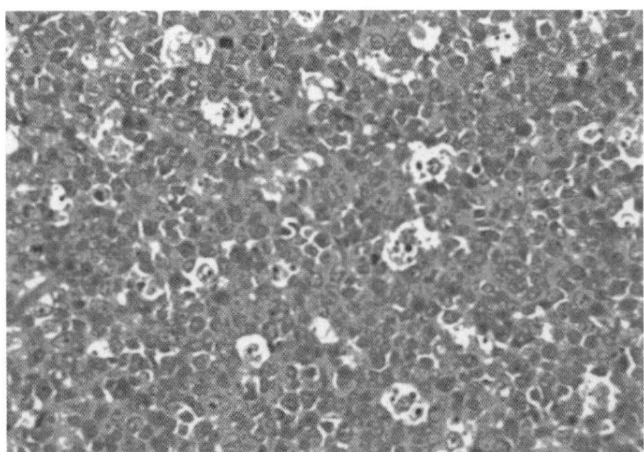

FIGURE 1.18. Lymph node with follicular hyperplasia. Multiple tingible-body macrophages in the reactive germinal center result in the starry sky appearance. Hematoxylin, phloxine, and saffron stain.

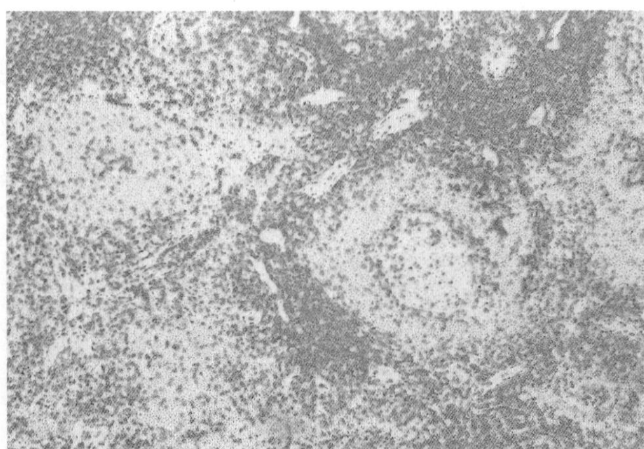

FIGURE 1.20. Lymph node T cells highlighted by immunostaining for CD3 pan-T-cell marker. Perifollicular areas, scattered T cells in germinal centers, and their absence in the mantle zones. CD3/peroxidase stain.

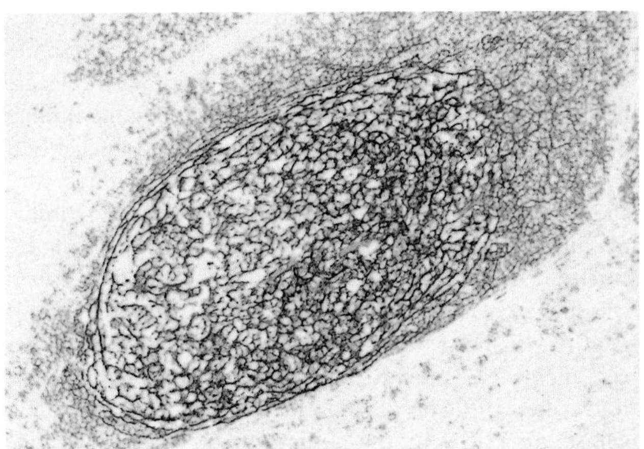

FIGURE 1.21. Lymphoid follicle with dendritic reticulum cell network. Interconnecting cell processes outlined by selective CD21 immunostaining. CD21/peroxidase stain.

tivated, they enlarge, proliferate, and expand to produce a clone that disseminates through the general circulation to peripheral sites, where most of their activity takes place (5). They resemble the B immunoblasts, having more cytoplasm than inactive T cells and a larger, round nucleus with one central nucleolus or an irregularly shaped nucleus with two to three marginal nucleoli. Most mature T cells express the $\alpha\beta$ chains of the T-cell receptor (TCR), whereas a small number of T cells express the $\gamma\delta$ chains of the TCR.

Accessory Cells

Immunologic accessory cells consist of a variety of monocytic/histiocytic cells that are part of the mononuclear phagocyte system (16) (Fig. 1.9). They originate in the bone marrow and migrate to peripheral tissues, from which they reach the lymph nodes through lymph and blood. Among the accessory cells, DRCs and interdigitating reticulum cells (IRCs) play important roles in processing antigens and presenting them to lymphocytes. *Dendritic reticulum cells* are present in germinal centers and interact with B lymphocytes (Fig. 1.21). Their role is to trap circulating antigens, process or modulate them, and present them to the B lymphocytes within the follicle (17). Because they retain the antigens on their surface, they provide a long-lasting reaction to the antigen that is relevant to the immune memory (6). DRCs are difficult to recognize under the light microscope. The cytoplasm is not discernible, but the cell processes are visible with immunohistochemical staining. The nucleus is large and irregular or elongated with an inconspicuous nucleolus. The cell processes are linked with those of other DRCs by desmosomes that form networks on which the lymphocytes are located (6). Their immunophenotype is CD21+, HLA-DR+, CD1a (Leu-6)+, and protein S100+ (16–19). *Interdigitating reticulum cells* are present mostly in the paracortex and interact with T lymphocytes. These cells are large, with a nucleus that has deep clefts and folds and inconspicuous nucleoli. The cytoplasm is abundant, pale, and ill-defined. When present in large numbers, the IDCs produce the mottled aspect of the paracortical area (6). Like the Langerhans cells of the dermis, from which they appear to originate, the IRCs contain intracytoplasmic Birbeck granules that are visible under the electron microscope. Their immunophenotype is HLA-DR+, CD1a (Leu-6)+, and protein S100+ (20,21).

Histiocytes, derived from circulating monocytes, may under stimulatory conditions accumulate in the lymph node sinuses or diffusely infiltrate the paracortical area. They are large cells with indistinct borders; the cytoplasm, neither strongly basophilic nor pyroninophilic, helps in distinguishing histiocytes from large lymphoid cells (3). Their irregular shape is a consequence of pseudopodal processes that enable histiocytes to contact and engulf foreign material, thereby developing into active macrophages (22). Histiocytes resemble reticulum cells; however, they can be distinguished by electron microscopy. Histiocytes have an abundance of primary and secondary lysosomes in addition to a large Golgi complex, some mitochondria, and a few strands of endoplasmic reticulum (1) (Fig. 1.22). Depending on their reactive stage, histiocytes may include numerous phagosomes and engulf foreign material. In the germinal centers of reactive secondary follicles, histiocytes phagocytose apoptotic nuclear debris, forming characteristic tingible-body macrophages. Soluble and particulate antigenic proteins are also engulfed by lymph node histiocytes and subsequently presented to lymphoid cells for antigen identification and initi-

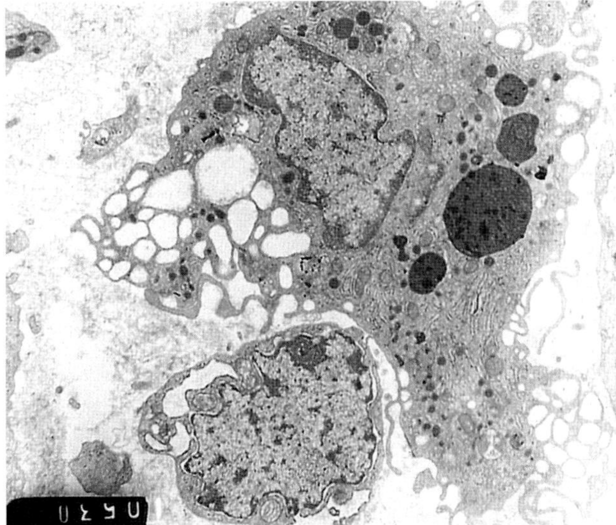

FIGURE 1.22. Histiocyte with abundant cytoplasm, lipid vacuoles, lysosomes, cell processes, and nucleus with fine euchromatin. ×14,400.

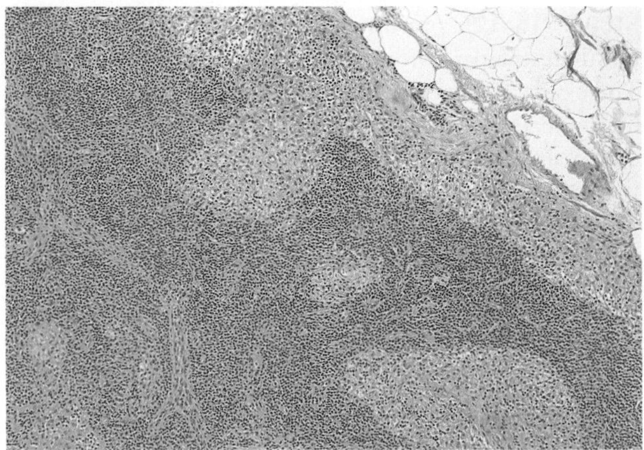

FIGURE 1.23. Reactive lymph node with markedly distended marginal and cortical sinuses. Hematoxylin, phloxine, and saffron stain.

ation of antibody production. Under specific stimulation, histiocytes may transform into epithelioid cells, acquire secretory functions, and participate in the formation of granulomas (23). Morphologically and functionally, lymph node histiocytes, like the reticulum cells (dendritic and interdigitating), belong to the mononuclear phagocyte system (16,22).

LYMPHATIC SINUSES

The *lymphatic sinuses* (Figs. 1.2, 1.3, and 1.11) carry the lymph from the afferent lymphatics on the convex surface of the lymph node through the lymphoid parenchyma into the efferent lymphatics in the lymph node hilus. They vary in size and cell composition according to functional demands (1) (Fig. 1.23). They are passages through the fine network of reticulin fibers lined by *endothelial cells* (retothelial cells, littoral cells) interconnected by desmosomes (13). According to some investigators, endothelial cells are flattened reticular cells, a concept supported by the finding of reticulin fibrils in continuation with the endothelial cells traversing the sinus lumina (2). The system of sinuses includes the marginal or subcapsular sinus, the labyrinthic medullary sinuses, and the intermediary or cortical sinuses, which are narrow sinuses connecting the first two types. The sinuses, with the exception of the larger ones, are difficult to visualize with the usual stains. The cortical sinuses have highly convoluted shapes and numerous fine extensions, whereas the lining endothelial cells are very thin and pale-staining (5). In the sinus lumina are many active macrophages (Fig. 1.24), anchored to the sinus wall, and numerous lymphocytes, plasma cells, immunoblasts, and occasional polymorphonuclear leukocytes. The phagocytic apparatus of the sinuses filters the lymph, retaining foreign bodies, and plays an important role in antigen binding. The passage of lymph and cells from one chain of lymph nodes to the next is a means by which the immune response is conveyed from the peripheral to the more central lymph nodes (2).

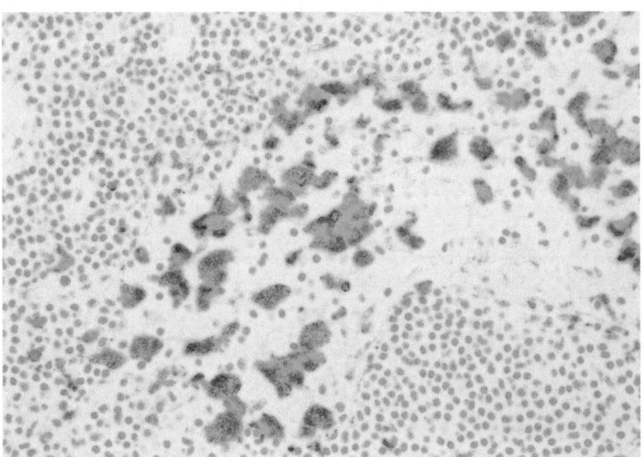

FIGURE 1.24. Reactive lymph node with distended sinuses containing numerous CD68+ macrophages. CD68/peroxidase stain.

BLOOD VESSELS

The blood supply, which is also the main route of incoming lymphocytes, is brought into the lymph node by one or more arterioles. They enter the node through the hilus and then divide into branches in the medulla, ramifying further into capillary networks in the cortex and paracortex. The blood vessels are structurally similar to those of other organs, with the exception of the postcapillary venules of the paracortical areas. These vessels are lined by tall endothelial cells that are tightly bound together by close interdigitations. The endothelial cells bear specialized lymphocyte homing receptors that are recognized by circulating lymphocytes (5). Frequently, lymphocytes are seen passing through the cytoplasm of endothelial cells (13) because the postcapillary venules are the site of lymphocyte migration from the circulating blood into the lymphoid tissue (2,5). The blood vessels of the superficial cortex and medulla are not specialized and so do not allow the exit of lymphocytes (5).

SUPPORTING FRAMEWORK, OR STROMA

The lymph node capsule (Fig. 1.2), trabeculae, and a network of reticular cells and reticulin fibers comprise the supporting framework, or stroma. Fibroblasts are the predominant cells of the capsule and trabeculae; however, these structures also include smooth muscle cells, nerves with

Schwann cells, and blood vessels with pericytes (1). The reticulin fibers are thin, delicate fibrils of type III collagen about 20 nm in diameter (5). In lymph nodes, they form the main extracellular matrix and maintain the structure by linkage to the fibrous trabeculae, and they are reinforced by fine collagen fibers. The reticulin framework supports the lymphoid cells and therefore is obscured by them on regular stainings, but it can be visualized with silver impregnation techniques (Gomori staining). The reticular (reticulum) cells have varied shapes, frequently elongated, with long dendritic processes extending for great distances between the lymphoid cells. They are intimately connected to the fine network of reticulin fibrils that originate from them.

HISTOCHEMISTRY

Histiocytes and macrophages can be identified by cytochemical stainings for nonspecific esterase (24), acid phosphatase (25), peroxidase, and other lysosomal enzymes.

IMMUNOHISTOCHEMISTRY

The various cell populations of lymph nodes can be identified with monoclonal antibodies produced to match the characteristic epitopes expressed on their membranes. Monoclonality also can be demonstrated under certain conditions with the use of immunohistochemical stainings (26,27).

Cortical Area

The lymphoid follicles, which are the main component of the cortical area, are composed of a variety of B cells that stain with the pan-B-cell antibodies CD19, CD20, and CD22 (Fig. 1.19). The centroblasts express CD10. The B cells have surface IgM and, to a much lesser degree, IgG and rarely IgA. IgD is present on mantle cells, but not on germinal center cells. The B cells also express immunoglobulin κ and λ light chains in a ratio of 2:1. Monoclonality of immunoglobulin light chains indicates the existence of neoplastic cell clones. Therefore, the demonstration of an identical light chain on all lymph node B cells is of great diagnostic importance; however, the immunohistochemical staining is reliable only on fresh, unfixed cells in flow cytometry or frozen sections (6,26,27). The bcl-2 protein is present on mantle cells but not on the centroblasts and centrocytes of the germinal centers, which undergo the normal cycle of apoptosis (Fig. 1.17). A positive stain for bcl-2 by the cells in the center of follicles indicates the suppression of apoptosis, a feature diagnostic of lymphoma (28–30). The small lymphocytes scattered throughout the follicles are T cells that stain with monoclonal antibodies for CD3, CD7, CD43, and CD4 or CD8 (Fig. 1.20). The tingible-body macrophages stain with monoclonal antibodies for CD11b, CD35, and CD68. The DRCs stain with monoclonal antibodies for CD21, CD35, C3b, and C3d (31) (Fig. 1.21).

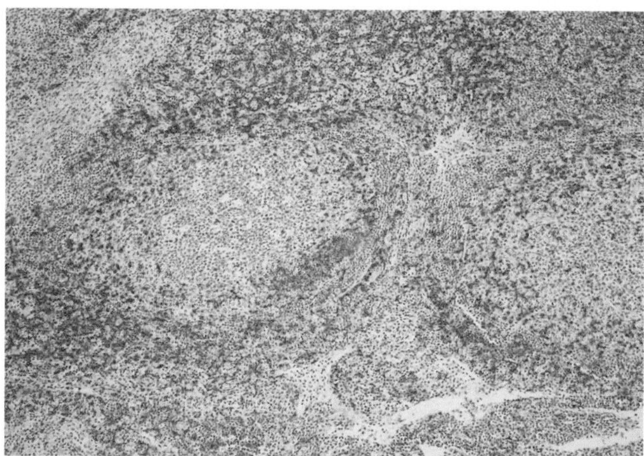

FIGURE 1.25. Reactive lymph node with predominance of CD4+ T cells in perifollicular areas. CD4/peroxidase stain.

Paracortical Area

The T cells that are the predominant cells of the paracortex are usually small lymphocytes staining with antibodies that recognize pan-T-cell markers such as CD2, CD3, CD5, CD7, CD43, and HLA-DR. The ratio of CD4+ helper cells to CD8+ suppressor cells is 3:1 (32) (Fig. 1.25). The IDCs are positive for S-100 protein, CD24, and HLA-DR (31).

Medullary Area

The B cells and plasma cells are polyclonal. Therefore, immunoglobulins synthesized on their membranes and in their cytoplasm, respectively, are of various classes, including IgM, IgG, and IgA heavy chains, but not IgD or IgE, and κ and λ light chains in a ratio of 2:1 (6,26).

Lymphatic Sinuses

The macrophages are positive for the histiocytic markers lysozyme, α_1-antitrypsin, α_1-antichymotrypsin, CD68, and S100 protein (33,34). (Fig. 1.24).

Blood Vessels

The endothelial cells of blood vessels stain with antibodies for CD31 and CD34.

Checklist

NORMAL LYMPH NODE

Framework
Capsule
Fibrous trabeculae
Reticulin network

Cortical Area
Lymphoid follicles
  Primary
  Secondary
Germinal centers
  B cells
    Centroblasts: dark zones
    Centrocytes: light zones
  T cells: small, inactivated
  Tingible-body macrophages
  Dendritic reticulum cells
Mantle zone: memory B cells
Marginal zone: monocytoid cells

Paracortical Area
T cells
  Small, inactivated
  Large, immunoblasts

Medullary Area
Plasmablasts
Plasma cells

Lymphatic Sinuses
Marginal
Cortical
Medullary

Blood Vessels
Arteries
Veins
Capillaries
High endothelial postcapillary venules

REFERENCES

1. Rhodin JAG. Lymph nodes. In: Histology. New York: Oxford University Press, 1974:378–394.
2. Olah I, Röhlich P, Törö I. Lymph node. In: Ultrastructure of lymphoid organs. Philadelphia: JB Lippincott Co, 1975:216–255.
3. Cottier H, Turk J, Sobin L. A proposal for a standardized system of reporting human lymph node morphology in relation to immunological function. Bull World Health Organ 1972;47:375–408.
4. Roitt I. The anatomy of the immune response. In: Essential immunology. London: Blackwell Science, 1997:152–167.
5. Stevens A, Lowe J. Lymph nodes. In: Stevens A, Lowe J. Histology. London: Gower Medical Publications, 1992:90–95.
6. van der Walk P, Meijer CJL. Reactive lymph nodes. In: Sternberg SS, ed. Histology for pathologists. Philadelphia: Lippincott–Raven Publishers, 1997:651–673.
7. Jaffe ES, Shevach EM, Sussman EH, et al. Membrane receptor sites for the identification of lymphoreticular cells in benign and malignant conditions. Br J Cancer 1975;31[Suppl II]:107–120.
8. Zuckerman SH, Douglas SD. The lymphocyte plasma membrane: markers, receptors and determinants. Pathobiol Annu 1976;6:119–163.
9. Lukes RJ, Taylor CR, Parker JW, et al. A morphologic and immunologic surface marker study of 299 cases of non-Hodgkin lymphomas and related leukemias. Am J Pathol 1978;90:461– 486.
10. Knowles DM. Lymphoid cell markers. Am J Surg Pathol 1985;9[Suppl]:85–108.

11. Lukes RJ, Collins RD. New approaches to the classification of the lymphomata. Br J Cancer 1975;31[Suppl II]:1–28.
12. Lennert K. Histopathology of non-Hodgkin's lymphomas based on the Kiel classification. New York: Springer-Verlag, 1981.
13. Mori Y, Lennert K. Electron microscopy atlas of lymph node cytology and pathology. New York: Springer-Verlag, 1969.
14. Tanaka Y, Goodman JR. Electron microscopy of human blood cells. New York: Harper and Row, 1972.
15. Ioachim LH. Lymph nodes and spleen. In: Johannessen JV, ed. Electron microscopy in human medicine, vol 5. New York: McGraw-Hill, 1981:385–464.
16. Van Furth R, Cohn AZ, Hirsch JG, et al. The mononuclear system: a new classification of macrophages, monocytes and their precursor cells. Bull World Health Organ 1972;46:845–852.
17. Donaldson SL, Kosco MH, Szakal AK, et al. Localization of antibody-forming cells in draining lymphoid organs during long-term maintenance of the antibody response. J Leukoc Biol 1986;40:147–157.
18. Beckstead JH. The evaluation of human lymph nodes using plastic sections and enzyme histochemistry. Am J Clin Pathol 1983;80:131–139.
19. Wood GS, Turner RR, Shiurba RA, et al. Human dendritic cells and macrophages: *in situ* immunophenotypic definition of subsets that exhibit specific morphologic and microenvironmental characteristics. Am J Pathol 1985;119:73–82.
20. Weiss LM, Beckstead JH, Warnke RA, et al. Leu-6 expressing cells in lymph nodes: dendritic cells phenotypically similar to interdigitating cells. Hum Pathol 1986;17:179–184.
21. Ralfkaier E, Stein H, Plesner T, et al. *In situ* immunological characterization of Langerhans cells with monoclonal antibodies: comparison with other dendritic cells in skin and lymph nodes. Virchows Arch A Pathol Anat Histopathol 1984;403: 401–412.
22. Spector WG. The macrophage: its origin and role in pathology. Pathobiol Annu 1974;4:33–64.
23. Ioachim HL. Granulomatous lesions of lymph nodes. In: Pathology of granulomas. New York: Raven Press, 1983:151–189.
24. Rozenszajn LA, Leibovich M, Shoham D, et al. The esterase activity in megaloblasts, leukemic and normal haematopoetic cells. Br J Haematol 1968;14:605–610.
25. Li CY, Yam LT, Lam WK. Acid phosphatase isoenzyme in human leukocytes in normal and pathologic conditions. J Histochem Cytochem 1970;18:473–481.
26. Stein H, Bonk A, Tolksdorf G, et al. Immunohistologic analysis of the organization of normal lymphoid tissue and non-Hodgkin's lymphomas. J Histochem Cytochem 1980;28:746–760.
27. Hsu SM, Jaffe ES. Phenotypic expression of B-lymphocytes. I. Identification with monoclonal antibodies in normal lymphoid tissues. Am J Pathol 1984;114:396–402.
28. Gaulard P, d'Agay M-F, Peuchmaur M, et al. Expression of the bcl-2 gene product in follicular lymphoma. Am J Pathol 1992;140:1089–1095.
29. Sheu L-F, Chen A, Meng C-L, et al. Analysis of bcl-2 expression in normal, inflamed, dysplastic nasopharyngeal epithelia and nasopharyngeal carcinoma: association with p53 expression. Hum Pathol 1997;28:556–562.
30. Torkalovic E, Cherwitz DL, Jessurun J, et al. B-cell gene rearrangement in benign and malignant lymphoid proliferations of mucosa-associated lymphoid tissue and lymph nodes. Hum Pathol 1997;28:166–173.
31. van der Valk P, van der Loor EM, Jansen J, et al. Analysis of lymphoid and dendritic cells in human lymph node, tonsil and spleen. A study using monoclonal and heterologous antibodies. Virchows Arch B Cell Pathol Mol Pathol 1984;45: 169–185.
32. Poppema S, Bhan AK, Reinherz El, et al. Distribution of T-cell subsets in human lymph nodes. J Exp Med 1981;153:30–41.
33. Papadimitriu CS, Stein H, Papacharalampoulos NS. Presence of α1-antichymotrypsin and α1-antitrypsin in hematopoietic and lymphoid tissue cells as revealed by the immunoperoxidase method. Pathol Res Pract 1980;169:287–297.
34. Crocker J, Williams M. An enzyme histochemical study of the sinuses of reactive lymph nodes. J Pathol 1984;142:31–38.

PART II

DIAGNOSTIC METHODS

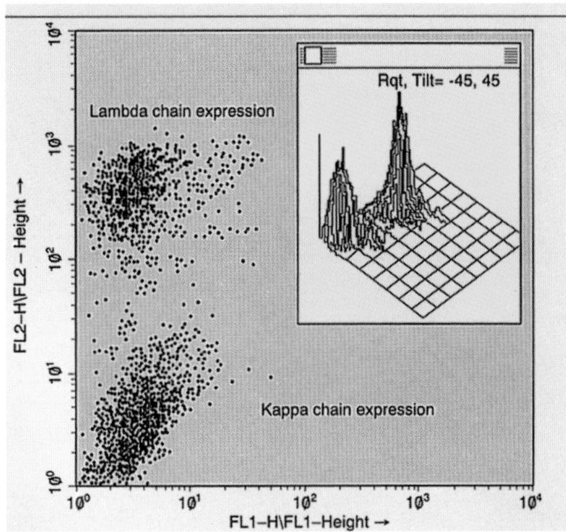

Lymph nodes are among the organs from which biopsy specimens are most commonly obtained for diagnostic purposes. Their accessibility makes them an easy target for fine needle aspiration and surgical removal. More importantly, because of the role lymph nodes play in retaining and reacting to foreign antigens, any changes therein reflect both regional and systemic disorders. The investigation of pathologic changes, previously restricted to microscopic examination, has benefited enormously from recent rapid advances in the basic sciences, in that new techniques adapted from immunology and molecular biology can be utilized.

2

THE LYMPH NODE BIOPSY

ENLARGED LYMPH NODES

In adults under normal conditions, only the inguinal lymph nodes may be palpable as several firm, 0.5- to 2-cm nodules attached to the dense fascia below the inguinal ligament. In children, small, 0.5- to 1-cm lymph nodes may be palpable in the cervical region. In both children and adults, palpable lymph nodes are commonly associated with various pathologic conditions. They may be isolated or part of a generalized lymphadenopathy, and they may occur without symptoms or during the course of systemic disease.

Localized lymphadenopathies may involve lymph nodes in various anatomic sites. Some locations are more frequently associated with certain causative agents and are therefore considered to be suggestive of the cause of lymph node enlargement. Table 2.1 lists various causes of lymphadenopathy with some of the locations most commonly affected.

The clinical and morphologic appearance of the enlarged lymph nodes depends on the causative agent, age of the patient, and status of host resistance. Biopsy specimens of enlarged lymph nodes are frequently obtained, and in 50% to 63% of cases, histologic examination leads to a positive diagnosis (1,2). The established diagnoses include specific lymphadenopathies (e.g., sarcoidosis; see Chapter 39), various lymphadenitides of known cause (e.g., infectious mononucleosis; see Chapter 9), metastatic tumors, and lymphomas (Fig. 2.1).

LYMPH NODE IMAGING AND LAPAROSCOPIC SAMPLING

Magnetic resonance imaging helps localize cervicothoracic lesions in infants and children; the most frequently identified mass is lymphangioma (3). In adults, Doppler color flow ultrasonography images the intranodal vessel architecture (4). Cervical lymph node metastases can be separated from lymphadenitis based on peripheral perfusion or diffuse blood flow patterns in metastases, but not by traditional ultrasonographic parameters such as size, homogeneity, shape, and brightness (5). Neck masses should be sampled if they are enlarging or unchanging, asymmetric, supraclavicular, or isolated, or if they are accompanied by fever or an enlarging liver, spleen, or Waldeyer ring (6). Contrast-enhanced computed tomography maps tuberculous and lymphomatous lymph nodes to somewhat different but frequently overlapping distributions. For example, disseminated and nondisseminated tuberculosis tends to involve lesser omental, mesenteric, anterior pararenal, and upper paraaortic lymph nodes; on the other hand, Hodgkin and non-Hodgkin lymphomas more often affect lower paraaortic lymph nodes (7). Lymph node enhancement on computed tomography with a peripheral, multilocular appearance suggests tuberculous lymphadenopathy, whereas homogenous attenuation typifies lymphoma (7). Laparoscopically guided biopsy successfully confirmed a suspected diagnosis of abdominal lymphoma in 24 of 51 (47%) consecutive patients (8). Although technically difficult, laparoscopic biopsies can retrieve enough tissue to determine the exact stage of Hodgkin lymphoma involving liver, spleen, and lymph nodes (9).

NONDIAGNOSTIC LYMPHADENOPATHIES

In 37% to 53% of sampled lymph nodes, a definitive diagnosis is not reached (2,10,11). Most of the diagnoses in this group are various forms of nonspecific reactive lymphoid hyperplasia (see Chapters 33–35); only about 3% of all lymph node biopsies are classified as atypical lymphoid hyperplasia (12). In several studies, patients with nondiagnostic lymph node hyperplasia were followed from 2 to 20 years to ascertain the eventual outcome of their disease (1,2,11, 12). Of 100 lymph node biopsies in children 9 months to 13 years old, 37 were classified as reactive hyperplasia, and 74% of these children were alive and well 20 years later (11). In two reviews of adults, about half of all lymph node biopsies remained without a specific diagnosis, and a disease related to the enlarged lymph nodes subsequently developed in 25% to 53% of the patients (2,12). In most cases, a definitive diagnosis became evident within 8 months to 1 year after the original biopsy, and in 17% to 20% of cases, it was a form of lymphoma (2,12). When cases of atypical

TABLE 2.1. CORRELATIONS BETWEEN LOCATION AND ETIOLOGY IN LYMPH NODE PATHOLOGY

Involved nodes	Etiology
Occipital	Scalp infections; in children, insect bites, ringworm; very rarely lymphoma or metastatic tumors
Posterior auricular	Rubella (24)
Anterior auricular	Infections of eyelids and conjunctivae; epidemic keratoconjunctivitis
Posterior cervical	Toxoplasmosis (25)
Posterior cervical and submental	Scalp infections; dental infections; tuberculosis
Anterior cervical	Infections of oral cavity and pharynx
Cervical (suppurative)	Tuberculosis
Supraclavicular (hard and fixed)	Metastases from intrathoracic or intraabdominal carcinoma; rarely infections
Axillary	Infections of upper extremities; cat-scratch disease; brucellosis; sporotrichosis; non-Hodgkin lymphomas
Epitrochlear	
Unilateral	Infections of hands
Bilateral	Viral diseases in children; sarcoidosis; tularemia
Inguinal	
Unilateral	Lymphogranuloma venereum; syphilis
Bilateral	Gonococcal, herpetic venereal infections; mycoplasmal infection; urethritis
Progressively enlarged without infection	Lymphoma; metastatic carcinoma
Pulmonary hilar	
Unilateral	Metastatic lung carcinoma
Bilateral	Sarcoidosis; tuberculosis; histoplasmosis; occidioidomycosis (26)
Mediastinal, asymmetric	Hodgkin lymphoma, nodular sclerosis; non-Hodgkin lymphoma
Intraabdominal and retroperitoneal, palpable or displacing viscera	Lymphoma; metastatic carcinoma; tuberculosis in mesenteric lymph nodes may form large masses, suppurate, rupture, or calcify (27)
Regional involvement in systemic infections	Infectious mononucleosis; viral hepatitis; cytomegalovirus disease; rubella; influenza
Generalized lymphadenopathy	Sarcoidosis; hyperthyroidism; autoimmune hemolytic anemia (28); lymphoma

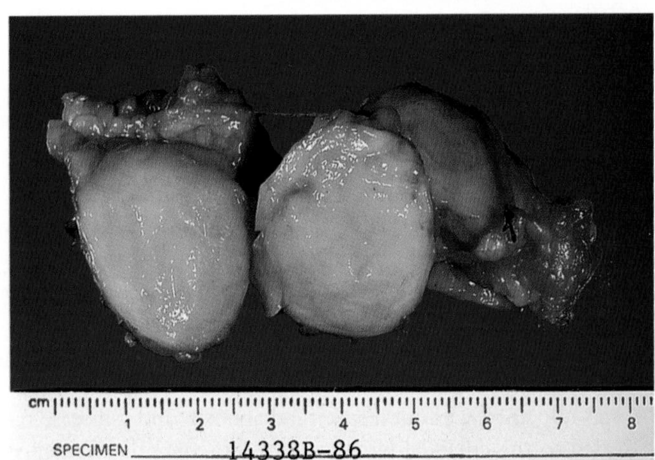

FIGURE 2.1. Enlarged inguinal lymph node with large cell non-Hodgkin lymphoma.

lymphoid hyperplasia were considered separately, the prevalence of lymphoma increased to 37% (12).

CAUSES OF MISDIAGNOSIS

In biopsies of lymph nodes, more than in those of any other organ, disparity between the original diagnosis and that made at the time of review studies appears to be common. In a series of 600 cases of lymphadenopathy initially diagnosed as Hodgkin disease, this interpretation was confirmed on subsequent review in only 53% of them by Symmers (13); the remaining 47% were considered to be mistakenly diagnosed and to represent, in most cases, nonspecific lymphadenitis. Reviewing 226 lymph node biopsies referred for a second histologic opinion after an initial diagnosis of reticulum cell sarcoma, the same author confirmed the original interpretation in only 73% of cases (14).

The causes of misdiagnosis in lymph node pathology are numerous. Some can be traced to the surgical procedure, some to the technical processing of the biopsy material, and some to the interpretation of the lesions. In the first category, Butler (15) lists poor selection of the biopsy site, poor selection of the lymph node to be sampled, and improper removal of the lymph node. In two studies comprising a total of 312 lymph node biopsies, the supraclavicular (64% to 85%) and the cervical (46% to 64%) lymph nodes yielded the highest number of diagnostic lesions, whereas the axillary (27% to 53%) and inguinal (22% to 71%) lymph nodes produced fewer identifiable lesions (1,2). Within a single group of lymph nodes, the largest accessible lymph node should be sampled because it is most likely to show specific abnormalities. If not cautioned, the surgeon may remove the most accessible lymph node, which is often too small to represent the disease process adequately (15). Special care should also be taken to excise the entire node in one piece, including the capsule and, if possible, a rim of pericapsular fibrofatty tissue, which often provide important clues to lymph node disease.

The single most important source of diagnostic errors may be improper processing of lymph nodes. The accuracy of histologic diagnosis is directly proportional to the quality of the histologic sections (15–18). Of the technical factors, fixation is irreversible and therefore the most important (15). Improper fixation leads to thick sections, poor stainings, and distorted specimens. Various authors recommend guidelines for correct handling of lymph nodes (15,17–21) (Fig. 2.2).

The essential requirements are even fixation, thin sectioning, and fine staining. To achieve these objectives, it is recommended that lymph nodes be cut with a razor blade across the longest diameter in slices 0.5 to 1 cm thick and prefixed in large amounts of fixatives. A few hours later, the slices should be recut at a thickness of about 3 mm and fixed overnight in fresh fixative. Many laboratories specializing in hematopathology have adopted the B5 fixative based on mercuric chloride; however, similar results can be obtained with Bouin or Zenker fixative or even buffered formaldehyde. Ideally, the sections should be cut at 3 mm and the hematoxylin staining properly balanced to reveal fine nuclear structural details.

FROZEN SECTION DIAGNOSIS

The indications for frozen section diagnosis in lymph node biopsies may be different from those in biopsies of other or-

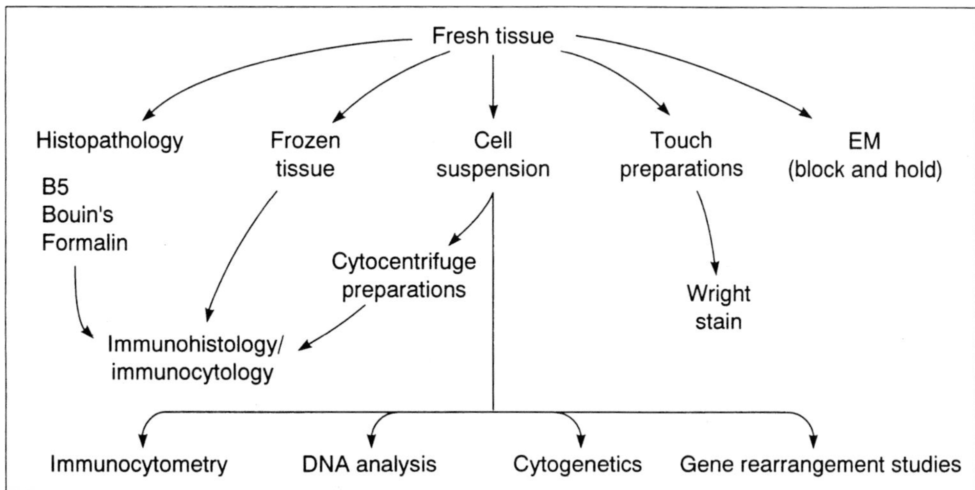

FIGURE 2.2. Processing protocol for lymph node biopsy specimen. (Adapted from Tubbs RR, Sheibani K. Immunohistology of lymphoproliferative disorders. Semin Diagn Pathol 1984; 1: 272–284, with permission.)

gans. The most important determination to be made from the frozen section of a lymph node is the presence or absence of pathologic changes. A negative result on the frozen section tells the surgeon that the diagnostic procedure is not yet complete and that perhaps an additional lymph node should be sampled. A positive result may specifically identify the lesion or at least establish that a lesion is present, even if its precise nature cannot be ascertained before permanent sections are examined.

The presence or absence of metastatic tumor in the sampled lymph nodes is important information for the surgeon. This can usually be established on frozen sections and represents the major indication for this procedure. In contrast, distinguishing between some forms of reactive lymphoid hyperplasia, particularly atypical lymphoid hyperplasia, and various Hodgkin or non-Hodgkin lymphomas can be extremely difficult and must not be attempted on frozen section specimens. This important decision is of no consequence at the time of surgery and should be deferred so that it can be made under the best circumstances—on multiple permanent sections of superior quality and with the aid of special diagnostic methods. Because the element of urgency is then removed, adjuvant technology can be used and consultation sought whenever needed. In the case of lymphomas, aiming for a definitive diagnosis or precise classification on a frozen section of a lymph node is generally hazardous and most of the time unnecessary.

Frozen Sections of Infectious Tissues

Frozen sections of specimens potentially infected by HIV (see Chapter 15), *Mycobacterium tuberculosis* (see Chapter 23), or another infectious agent should be immersed in fixatives for variable periods of time before being processed for permanent sections. This option is not available for frozen section diagnosis, which presents special risks of infection because fresh tissues must be handled (22).

Frozen section carries risks for splashes, sticks, and cuts during the preparatory dissection and microtome sectioning of potentially contaminated tissues. In addition to the possibility of such direct infection, indirect infection through contamination of the cryostat is also a possibility.

Personnel performing frozen section should follow the same universal precautions used in handling all surgical specimens and should wear a gown, apron, and gloves. The equipment must be decontaminated according to the technique recommended by the Centers for Disease Control and Prevention (23). Instruments must be immersed in 95% ethanol and work areas cleaned with 95% ethanol or 0.5% sodium hypochlorite, as HIV survives both freezing and drying. Because of potential risks, the role of frozen sections of tissues of patients with AIDS, tuberculosis, and other infections should be limited. In most cases, the lesions likely to be diagnosed in these patients may be more accurately identified on permanent than on frozen sections. An alternative method is a tentative diagnosis of imprints of intraoperative specimens, to be supplemented within the next 24 hours by diagnosis on permanent sections (22).

LYMPH NODE TRIAGE AND APPORTIONMENT

We suggest that each lymph node biopsy specimen be evaluated individually because numerous adjuvant methods are available. Ultimately, selecting tissue portions for studies beyond traditional morphology should be based on the diagnostic accuracy and specificity potentially gained with answers to infectious, immunophenotypic, molecular, or cytogenetic questions. To achieve these goals, try to begin formulating a differential diagnosis as soon as the fresh lymph node arrives in the laboratory. Consider the patient's age and sex, the relevant clinical, physical examination, and laboratory findings (including hemogram data), and anatomic biopsy site. Study the gross lymph node cut section and make a rapid touch imprint. Of course, each pathology group must establish its own minimum standards, but classifying lymphomas according to modern nomenclature often requires both morphologic and immunologic evaluation. Although molecular and cytogenetic testing significantly enhances the workup, it is absolutely necessary in only a very few cases for today's treatment protocols.

REFERENCES

1. Saltzstein SL. The fate of patients with nondiagnostic lymph node biopsies. CA Cancer J Clin 1966;16:115–116.
2. Sinclair S, Beckman E, Ellman L. Biopsy of enlarged, superficial lymph nodes. JAMA 1974;228:602–603.
3. Castellote A, Vazquez E, Vera J, et al. Cervicothoracic lesions in infants and children. Radiographics 1999;19:583–600.
4. Tschammler A, Ott G, Schang T, et al. Lymphadenopathy: differentiation of benign from malignant disease—color Doppler US assessment of intranodal angioarchitecture. Radiology 1998; 208:117–123.
5. Issing PR, Kettling T, Kempf HG, et al. Ultrasound evaluation of characteristics of cervical lymph nodes with special reference to color Doppler ultrasound. A contribution to differentiating reactive from metastatic lymph node involvement in the neck. Laryngorhinootologie 1999;78:566–572.
6. McGuirt WF. The neck mass. Med Clin North Am 1999;83: 219–234.
7. Yang ZG, Min PQ, Sone S, et al. Tuberculosis versus lymphomas in the abdominal lymph nodes: evaluation with contrast-enhanced CT. AJR Am J Roentgenol 1999;172:619–623.
8. Strickler JG, Donohue JH, Porter LE, et al. Laparoscopic biopsy for suspected abdominal lymphoma. Mod Pathol 1998;11:831–836.
9. Johna S, Lefor AT. Laparoscopic evaluation of lymphoma. Semin Surg Oncol 1998;15:176–182.
10. Moore RD, Weisberger AS, Ellman L. Biopsy of enlarged superficial lymph nodes. JAMA 1957; 228:659–662.

11. Kissane JM, Gephardt GN. Lymphadenopathy in childhood: long-term follow-up in patients with nondiagnostic lymph node biopsies. Hum Pathol 1974;5:431–439.
12. Schroer KR, Franssila KO. Atypical hyperplasia of lymph nodes: a follow-up study. Cancer 1979;44:1155–1163.
13. Symmers WS Sr. Survey of the eventual diagnosis in 600 cases referred for a second histological opinion after an initial biopsy diagnosis of Hodgkin's disease. J Clin Pathol 1968;21:650–653.
14. Symmers WS Sr. Survey of the eventual diagnosis in 226 cases referred for a second histological opinion after an initial biopsy diagnosis of reticulum cell sarcoma. J Clin Pathol 1968;21:654– 655.
15. Butler JJ. Non-neoplastic lesions of lymph nodes of man to be differentiated from lymphomas. NCI Monogr 1969;32:233–255.
16. Cottier H, Turk J, Sobin L. A proposal for a standardized system of reporting human lymph node morphology in relation to immunological function. Bull World Health Organ 1972;47:375– 417.
17. Banks PM. Technical aspects of specimen preparation and special studies. In: Jaffe ES, ed. Surgical pathology of the lymph nodes and related organs. Philadelphia: WB Saunders, 1985:1–21.
18. Stansfeld AG. Indications, technique and applications for lymph node biopsy. In: Stansfeld AG, ed. Lymph node biopsy interpretation. New York: Churchill Livingstone, 1985:26–31.
19. Berard WC, Bowling MD. Overcoming technical errors in the histologic preparation of lymph nodes. Chicago: American Society of Clinical Pathology, 1975 (Professional Educators Series).
20. Bowling MC. Achieving technical excellence. Lab Med 1979;10:467–476.
21. Tubbs RR, Sheibani K. Immunohistology of lymphoproliferative disorders. Semin Diagn Pathol 1984;1:272–284.
22. Ioachim HL. Frozen sections and the risk of HIV infection. CAP Today 1992;6:16–17.
23. Swisher BL, Ewing EP Jr. Frozen section technique for tissues infected by the AIDS virus. J Histotechnol 1986;9:26.
24. Kalmansohn RB. Rubella: observations on an epidemic with particular reference to lymphadenopathy. N Engl J Med 1952;247: 428–429.
25. Gray GF Jr, Kimball AC, Kean BH. The posterior cervical lymph node in toxoplasmosis. Am J Pathol 1972; 69:349–358.
26. Winterbauer RH, Belic N, Moores KD. Clinical interpretation of bilateral hilar adenopathy. Ann Intern Med 1973;78:65–71.
27. Studley HO. Intra-abdominal rupture of retroperitoneal tuberculous lymph node. Ann Surg 1942;115:477.
28. Zuelzer WW, Mastrangelo R, Stulberg CS, et al. Autoimmune hemolytic anemia. Natural history and viral–immunologic interactions in childhood. Am J Med 1970;49:80–93.

3

CYTOPATHOLOGY

THE ROLE OF CYTOPATHOLOGY IN LYMPH NODE DIAGNOSIS

The cytologic study of lymph node lesions, particularly lymphomas, contributes much to understanding and, implicitly, diagnosing them. This is best achieved by observing thin sections under the oil immersion objective and by examining lymph node imprints and smears. These are easily prepared from unfixed lymph nodes received in the laboratory for frozen section or as soon as possible after excision. The cytoplasmic and, particularly, the nuclear details revealed by a Giemsa or Wright stain of lymph node imprints are of great help in differentiating benign from malignant lesions, in recognizing the uniform morphology of lymphomas, and in ascertaining their cytologic variants. In this respect, Koo, Rappaport, and their collaborators (1) made an important contribution in a cytologic study of 212 lymphomas, accompanied by an atlas, that illustrates all types of non-Hodgkin lymphoma (NHL) in Giemsa-stained imprints. It must be realized, however, that cytologic diagnostic criteria are different from those applied to tissue sections, and that the study of lymph node imprints must be performed routinely to gain experience and achieve proficiency.

TOUCH IMPRINTS

Technique

Successful lymph node touch imprints should display a large, cellular monolayer that yields both architectural and cytologic information (1). To achieve this, use a perpendicular motion while lightly pressing a freshly sliced lymph node against a clean, uncoated glass slide. Alternatively, smoothly roll a glass slide, at constant speed and without pulling at the end, over a cut, firmly held lymph node (2) (Fig. 3.1). Sideways shearing disrupts fragile cells, exploding the lymphocytes into a streak of "blue spaghetti" (elongated bare nuclei). Before contacting the slide, carefully blot or wipe excess blood or serum from the cut tissue. Make several touch imprints using different pressures to find an optimal preparation, especially for lymph nodes with sticky, watery, or excessively dry surfaces (2). Touch imprints should be air-dried before staining. In general, we prefer Romanowsky-based stains (Wright-Giemsa or Diff-Quik) to hematoxylin and eosin because they provide superior nuclear detail and the ability to resolve cytoplasmic granules (Figs. 3.2 and 3.3).

Diagnostic Value

Lymph node touch imprints are suitable for analysis of immunophenotype (3,4), morphometry (5,6), and DNA ploidy (7). However, touch imprints (in comparison with cytocentrifuge smears) introduce selective bias by underrepresenting large lymphoid cells, revealing fewer nuclear irregularities, and poorly preserving cytoplasmic borders (8). Nevertheless, because of their ease of preparation and reasonably good morphologic preservation, touch imprints are still valuable for rapid intraoperative diagnosis (9). In Nigeria, pathologists without access to quick histology evaluated lymph nodes by touch imprint; they could accurately classify Burkitt lymphoma, Hodgkin lymphoma (HL), and metastatic carcinoma (sensitivity, 85% to 100%), but not other types of NHL, chronic lymphadenitis, or tuberculosis (sensitivity, 31% to 50%) (10).

FINE NEEDLE ASPIRATION BIOPSY

Indications

When is fine needle aspiration biopsy (FNAB) of lymph nodes indicated? Frable stated, ". . . unless a clinical problem is significant enough to warrant consideration of open surgical biopsy, aspiration biopsy should not be considered either" (11). In general, its diagnostic accuracy is lower for lymphomas than for metastatic tumors (12); FNAB of metastatic carcinoma in lymph nodes achieves a sensitivity of more than 90% in large series (13,14) because the tumor cells are usually abundant and their morphology is entirely dissimilar to that of normal or hyperplastic lymph node (11) (Fig. 3.4). In the past, aspiration biopsy of lymphoproliferative disorders was limited to the diagnosis of recurrent disease, staging, or obtaining additional material for immunophenotyping. The increasing acceptance of FNAB as

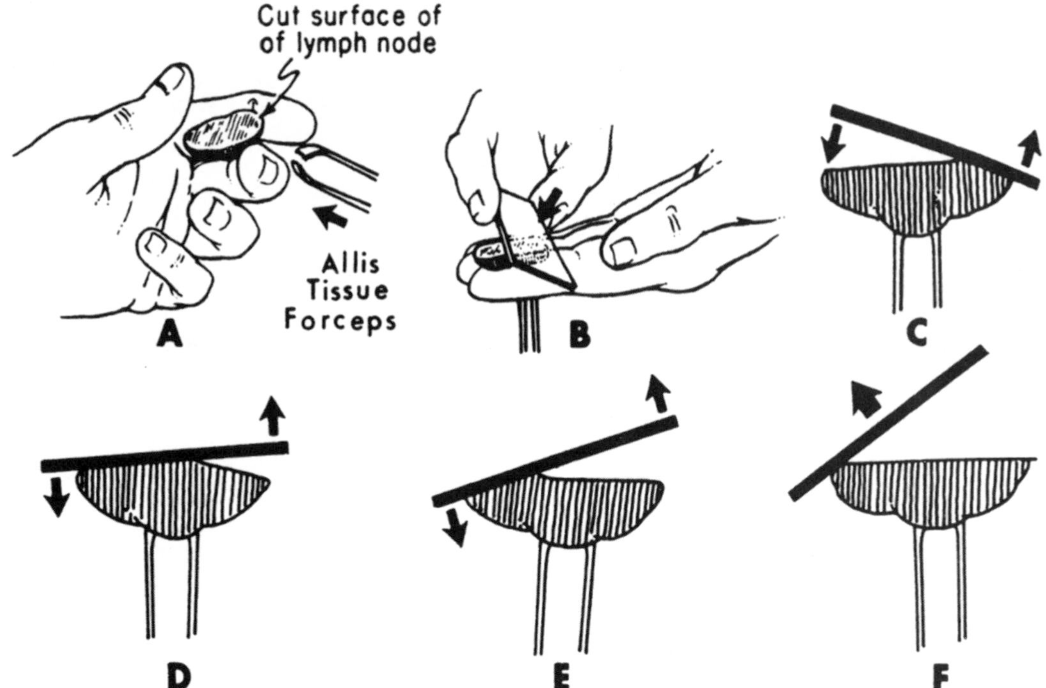

FIGURE 3.1. A–F: Technique for preparing an imprint. Lightly touch one edge of the cut surface of the node with a glass slide and at constant speed roll it over the surface of the lymph node until the surface of the glass slide touches the opposite edge, then lift it off. (From Tanapatchaiyapong P. A modification of the lymph node imprint technic. Am J Clin Pathol 1972;58:431–433, with permission.)

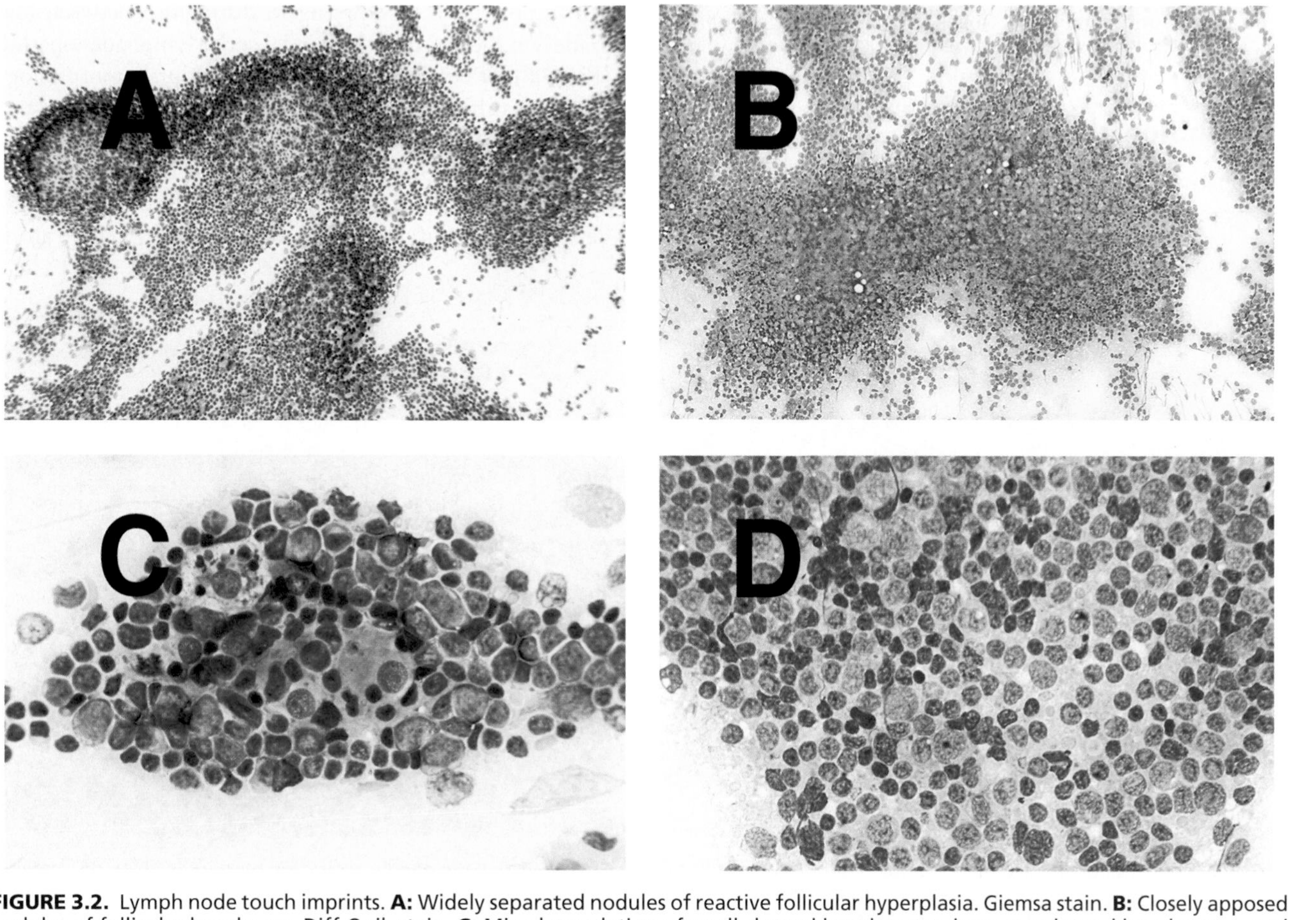

FIGURE 3.2. Lymph node touch imprints. **A:** Widely separated nodules of reactive follicular hyperplasia. Giemsa stain. **B:** Closely apposed nodules of follicular lymphoma. Diff-Quik stain. **C:** Mixed population of small cleaved lymphocytes, large noncleaved lymphocytes, and tingible-body macrophages in reactive follicular hyperplasia. Diff-Quik stain. **D:** Monotonous population of small cleaved lymphocytes without tingible-body macrophages in follicular lymphoma. Diff-Quik stain.

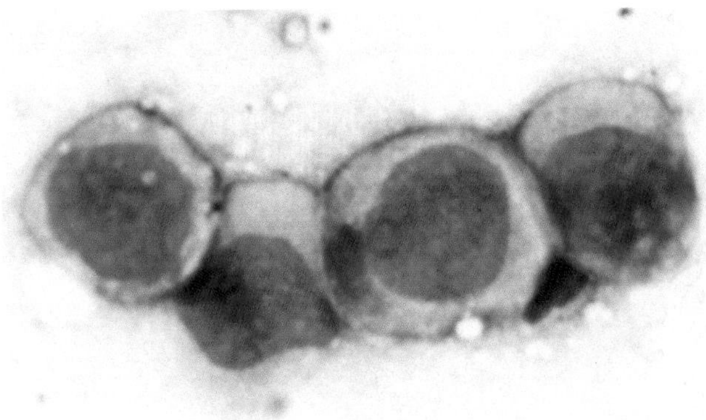

FIGURE 3.3. Lymph node touch imprint showing granulocytic sarcoma. Large blasts without granules or Auer rods can be mistaken for diffuse large cell lymphoma. Diff-Quik stain.

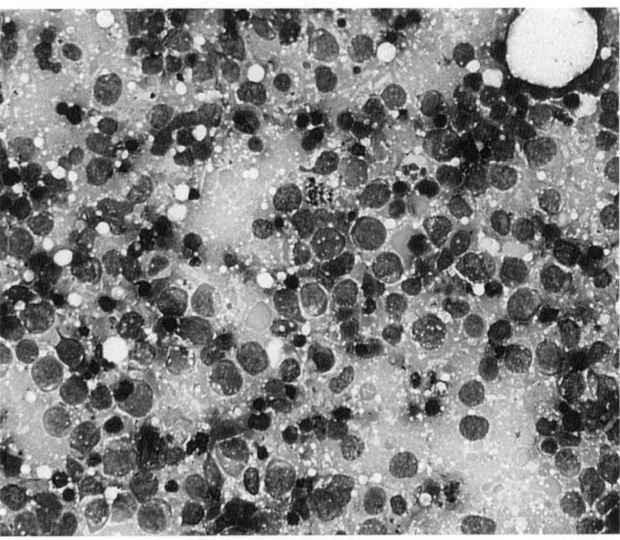

FIGURE 3.5. Fine needle aspiration biopsy specimen of a cervical lymph node with follicular lymphoma, grade 1. Homogeneous population of lymphoid cells with minimal nuclear variation in size, shape, and staining properties. Giemsa stain.

an alternate method for the diagnosis of lymph node lesions is a strong incentive for a renewed interest in cytopathology. In fact, an aspiration smear is similar to a touch preparation made from a bisected lymph node and provides excellent cytologic material that can be studied by a variety of methods. Fewer than 10% of previously aspirated lymph nodes show morphologic sequelae such as a linear tract, hemorrhage, organization, and rarely myofibroblastic proliferation or infarction (15).

Morphologic Caveats

Cytoplasmic fragments (so-called lymphoglandular bodies) occur more abundantly in smears of benign and malignant lymphoid disorders than in smears of nonlymphoid round cell tumors (16). Attempting to distinguish between low-grade lymphomas (Fig. 3.5) and reactive lymphadenopathies (Fig. 3.6), or between HL and NHL on purely morphologic criteria is difficult and sometimes unreliable (11,17,18). In the first case, reactive lymphadenopathy is favored in the presence of a mixture of cell types, including tingible-body macrophages (17,19); in the second case, the diagnosis of HL depends on identifying typical Reed-Sternberg cells in an ap-

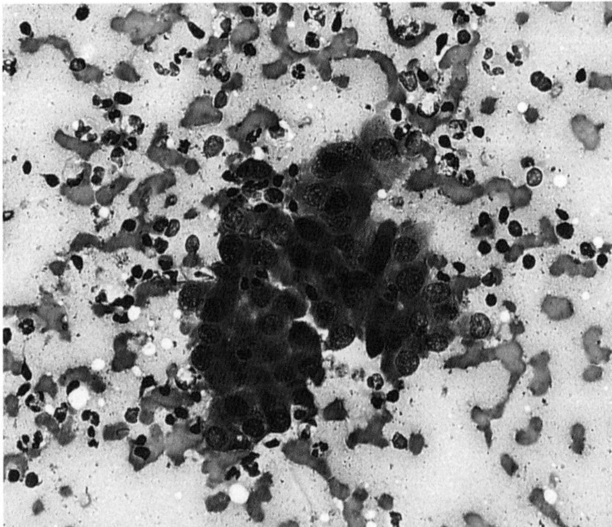

FIGURE 3.4. Fine needle aspiration biopsy specimen of axillary lymph node shows large aggregates of cells of epithelial morphology among lymphocytes and erythrocytes, an indication of metastatic breast carcinoma. Giemsa stain.

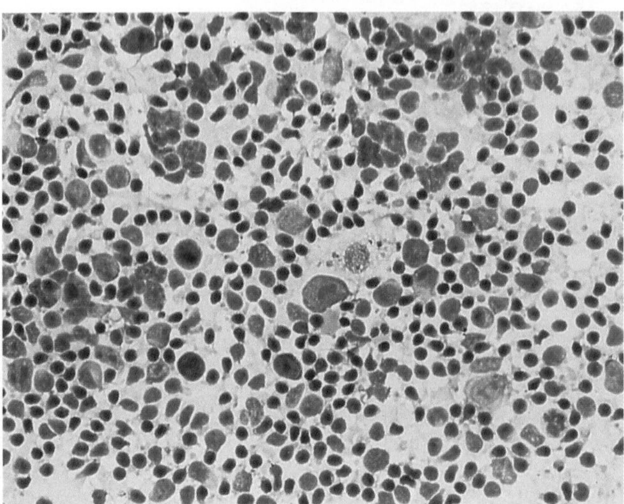

FIGURE 3.6. Fine needle aspiration biopsy specimen of a cervical lymph node with reactive lymphoid hyperplasia. Admixture of lymphoid cells with great variation in nuclear size, shape, and staining properties. Giemsa stain.

propriate cellular background (11). Several interpretive caveats routinely apply to aspiration biopsy of lymphoproliferative disorders (20): distinguishing between nodular (follicular) and diffuse NHL patterns is impossible (21–24); mixed, small cleaved and large cell NHL is often mistaken for another lymphoma category or for reactive lymphoid hyperplasia (24); without the use of immunophenotyping, low-grade NHL may be indistinguishable from reactive lymphoid hyperplasia (12); large cell lymphoma can mimic metastatic tumors (25); HL can be confused with a variety of conditions, including NHL (26), infectious mononucleosis (22), undifferentiated carcinoma (27), fat necrosis (27), or reactive lymphoid hyperplasia (26,28); HL, suppurative type (29), can appear identical to neutrophil-rich, Ki-1+ anaplastic large cell lymphoma (30); HL cannot be accurately subtyped on smears (23) (Fig. 3.7); T cell-rich B-cell lymphoma mimics reactive lymphoid hyperplasia, cytologically and immunologically (31); acute inflammation with necrosis obscures malignant lymphoma (32) and other neoplasms (33).

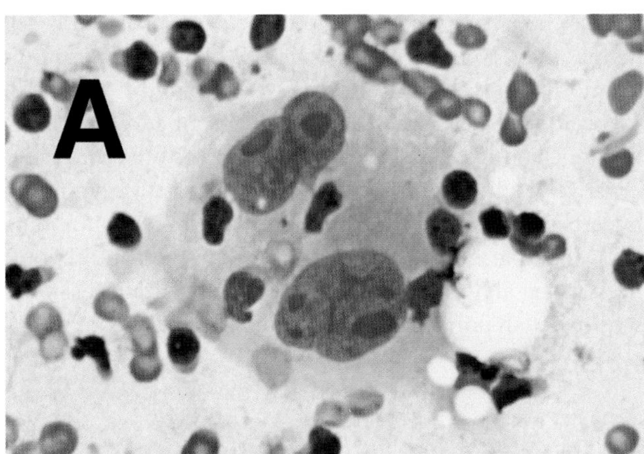

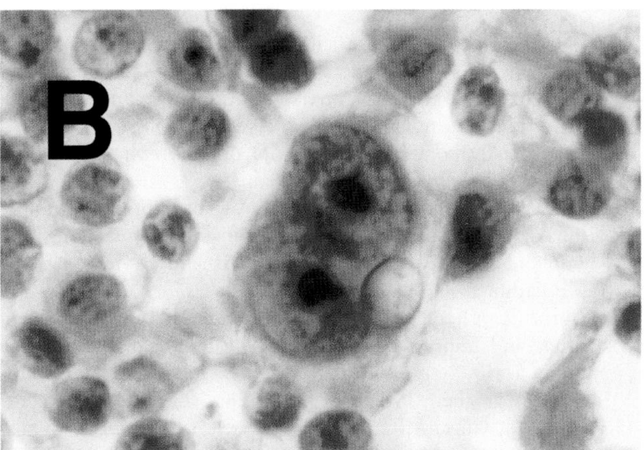

FIGURE 3.7. Fine needle aspiration biopsy specimen of Hodgkin lymphoma. **A:** Multinucleated Reed-Sternberg cell surrounded by small lymphocytes. Giemsa stain. **B:** Binucleated Reed-Sternberg cell surrounded by small lymphocytes. Papanicolaou stain. (Courtesy of Antony Cajigas, M.D.)

Reliability and Limitations

Questions have been raised concerning the reliability and limitations of lymph node diagnosis based on FNAB specimens (21,31,34–36). To assess the role of aspiration biopsy in lymphoproliferative disorders, Suhrland and Wieczorek (24) reviewed the experiences from five medical centers (17,22,24,26,28). One group had a very low rate of lymph node biopsy follow-up, only 29 of 118 (26%) cases (24,28). If these outlying data are excluded, 402 of 562 (72%) biopsy-proven cases remain (24). Their combined sensitivity, defined as "(cytology-positive plus cytology-suspicious) divided by biopsy-proven lymphomas," ranges between 81% and 88% (24). In good agreement with these figures, Das et al. (37) reported a diagnostic sensitivity of 132 of 153 (86%) biopsy-proven lymphoma cases. Lymphoma subtyping based on FNAB correlates with traditional histology in most cases: Rappaport classification and Working Formulation, 51 of 60 (85%) (38); Working Formulation, 55 of 64 (86%) (23) and 110 of 163 (68%) (37), and Kiel classification, 44 of 53 (83%) (39). Because the cytologically based Kiel classification yields similar results to the others, diagnostic accuracy in lymphoma subtyping does not appear to depend on a particular morphologic scheme. To improve the reliability of smears for a primary lymphoma diagnosis, a variety of adjunct techniques have been proposed, including cytochemistry (11,19), immunocytochemistry (18,40), flow cytometry (41), and molecular diagnosis (42). The FNAB specimens can be prepared in different ways, including smear, cytospin (8), membrane filter, and cell block preparations (40).

IMMUNOCYTOCHEMISTRY

Immunocytochemistry can be easily applied to FNAB specimens to distinguish between reactive lymphoid hyperplasia and low-grade lymphoma, and to improve lymphoma subtyping (18,20,40). The whole range of monoclonal antibodies commonly used against the various lymphoid cell markers in tissue sections (43) can be applied with comparative results on cytospin preparations (35,44–46) (Fig. 3.8). The determination of monoclonality for the diagnosis of B-cell lymphomas can be safely made when the ratio of κ to λ light chains is greater than 6:1; ratios below 3:1 indicate reactive lymphoid hyperplasias (18). However, some reactive lymphoid hyperplasias express a skewed κ-to-λ ratio, simulating monoclonality (47,48). Polyclonality suggests benign lymphadenopathies but does not exclude T-cell lymphoma (49) or HL, which requires a lymph node biopsy with histopathologic examination for confirmation.

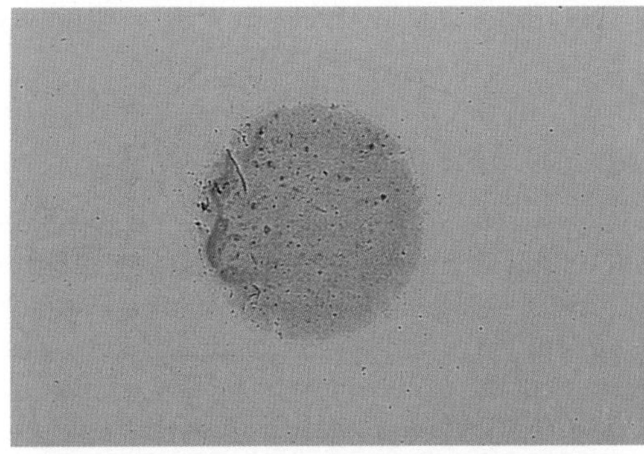

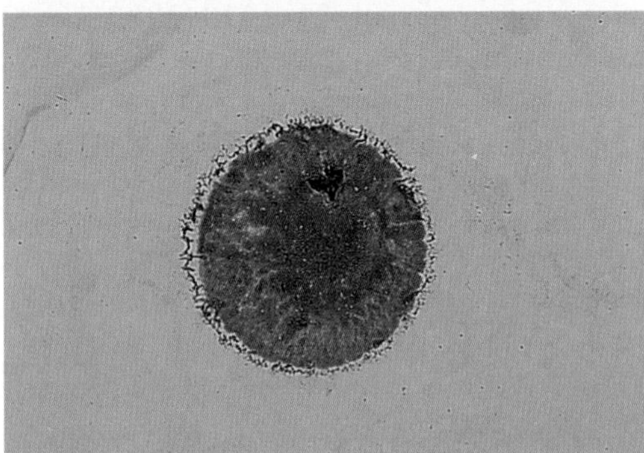

FIGURE 3.8. Cytospin preparations of lymph node fine needle aspiration biopsy specimen immunostained for anti-λ (*top*) and anti-κ (*bottom*). The diagnosis of monoclonal κ B-cell lymphoma is based on positive staining for κ and negative staining for λ. Immunoperoxidase stain. (Courtesy of A. Gritsman, M.D.)

FLOW CYTOMETRY

To overcome the limitations of smears, a minority of laboratories routinely perform flow cytometry when evaluating lymph node aspiration biopsy specimens (50). This practice may endanger a chief virtue of FNAB, its relatively low cost (14,51). If the flow cytometry data do not eliminate the need for an excisional lymph node biopsy, and if the clinician is not prepared to institute therapy based only on the combined cytologic and immunologic results, can the extra expense be justified? On the other hand, if an excisional lymph node biopsy from a deep anatomic site threatens to produce intolerable morbidity, combining FNAB with flow cytometry (52) or another adjunct technique (23,53) may be essential to making a specific diagnosis.

The concordance between dual parameter flow cytometry and cytospin immunocytochemistry for the phenotypic analysis of lymph node aspirates is good (54). Although many prefer to correlate morphology and immunophenotype on cytospins directly, flow cytometry offers greater objectivity through automation, speed, a larger sample size, and, in newer instruments, simultaneous collection of six parameters for each cell: two types of light scatter plus four fluorescent colors. Flow cytometry detects surface immunoglobulin light chain restriction, as an indicator of monoclonality, in 81% (55) to 85% (56) of B-cell lymphomas. Analyzing populations on the basis of cell size can help identify minor B-cell clones (56). The antibody panel for each sample depends on the number of cells harvested and the differential diagnosis, as revealed by smears (57). Antibodies to CD5, CD10, and CD23 facilitate subtyping neoplastic small B cells (41,56). Sampling error, the coexistence of benign and neoplastic lymphoid cells, or the absence of immunoglobulin expression can lead to false-negative results (41). The diagnosis most often missed by flow cytometry is HL (58).

MOLECULAR DIAGNOSIS

Clonality in lymph node aspirates can be determined by several molecular techniques; Southern blot (59–63) and polymerase chain reaction assays (64,65) detect immunoglobulin heavy chain gene rearrangements from extracted DNA, and *in situ* hybridization detects immunoglobulin light chain messenger RNA on cytospins (66,67). In the study of Stewart et al. (67), *in situ* hybridization was superior to polymerase chain reaction in diagnosing monoclonality in B-cell lymphomas, 16 of 24 (67%) versus 9 of 18 (50%), and in diagnosing polyclonality in reactive lymphoid hyperplasia, 31 of 36 (86%) versus 19 of 26 (73%). In addition, polymerase chain reaction yielded more false-positive and false-negative results, "monoclonal bands" in reactive lymphoid hyperplasia and "polyclonal patterns" in B-cell lymphoma (67). Comparing the two techniques in paraffin sections, McNicol et al. (68) agreed that *in situ* hybridization is more sensitive than polymerase chain reaction for detecting B-cell clonality.

REFERENCES

1. Koo CH, Rappaport H, Sheibani K, et al. Imprint cytology of non-Hodgkin's lymphomas based on a study of 212 immunologically characterized cases: correlation of touch imprints with tissue sections. Hum Pathol 1989;20:1–137.
2. Tanapatchaiyapong P. A modification of the lymph node imprint technic. Am J Clin Pathol 1972;58:431–433.
3. Banks PM, Caron BL, Morgan TW. Use of imprints for monoclonal antibody studies: suitability of air-dried preparations from lymphoid tissues with an immunohistochemical method. Am J Clin Pathol 1983;79:438–442.
4. Giorno R. Characterization of mononuclear cells in cytocentrifuge and imprint preparations using monoclonal antibodies and an avidin–biotin immunoperoxidase staining system. J Histochem Cytochem 1983;31:1326–1328.
5. Crocker J, Curran RC. A study of nuclear diameters in lymph node imprints using the Zeiss Microvideomat. J Clin Pathol 1979;32:670–674.
6. Ball PJ, van der Valk P, Kurver PH, et al. Large cell lymphoma. II. Differential diagnosis of centroblastic and B-immunoblastic subtypes by morphometry on cytologic preparations. Cancer 1985;55:486–492.
7. Van Vloten WA, Scheffer E, Meijer CJ. DNA-cytophotometry of

lymph node imprints from patients with mycosis fungoides. J Invest Dermatol 1979;73:275–277.
8. Stevens MW, Fazzalari NL, Crisp DJ. Lymph node cellular morphology: comparative study of imprints and cytocentrifuge smears. J Clin Pathol 1987;40:751–755.
9. Clarke MR, Landreneau RJ, Borochovitz D. Intraoperative imprint cytology for evaluation of mediastinal lymphadenopathy. Ann Thorac Surg 1994;57:1206–1210.
10. Ademiluyi SA, Akinyanju OO, Mordi VP. Evaluation of lymph node imprint in rapid diagnosis of lymph node biopsy specimens. J Clin Pathol 1986;39:688–689.
11. Frable WJ. Fine-needle aspiration biopsy: a review. Hum Pathol 1983;14:9–28.
12. Steel BL, Schwartz MR, Ramzy I. Fine needle aspiration biopsy in the diagnosis of lymphadenopathy in 1,103 patients. Role, limitations and analysis of diagnostic pitfalls. Acta Cytol 1995;39: 76–81.
13. Frable WJ, Frable MA. Thin-needle aspiration biopsy: the diagnosis of head and neck tumors revisited. Cancer 1979;43:1541–1548.
14. Smith TJ, Safaii H, Foster EA, et al. Accuracy and cost-effectiveness of fine needle aspiration biopsy. Am J Surg 1985;149:540–545.
15. Tsang WY, Chan JK. Spectrum of morphologic changes in lymph nodes attributable to fine needle aspiration. Hum Pathol 1992;23:562–565.
16. Francis IM, Das DK, al-Rubah NA, et al. Lymphoglandular bodies in lymphoid lesions and non-lymphoid round cell tumors: a quantitative assessment. Diagn Cytopathol 1994;11:23–27.
17. Kline TS, Kannan V, Kline IK. Lymphadenopathy and aspiration biopsy cytology. Review of 376 superficial nodes. Cancer 1984;54:1076–1081.
18. Sneige N, Dekmezian RH, Katz RL, et al. Morphologic and immunocytochemical evaluation of 220 fine needle aspirates of malignant lymphoma and lymphoid hyperplasia. Acta Cytol 1990; 34:311–322.
19. Pitts WC, Weiss LM. Fine needle aspiration biopsy of lymph nodes. Pathol Annu 1988;23:329–360.
20. Wakely PE Jr. Fine needle aspiration cytopathology of malignant lymphoma. Clin Lab Med 1998;18:541–559, vi–vii.
21. Pontifex AH, Klimo P. Application of aspiration biopsy cytology to lymphomas. Cancer 1984;53:553–556.
22. Qizilbash AH, Elavathil LJ, Chen V, et al. Aspiration biopsy cytology of lymph nodes in malignant lymphoma. Diagn Cytopathol 1985;1:18–22.
23. Cafferty LL, Katz RL, Ordonez NG, et al. Fine needle aspiration diagnosis of intraabdominal and retroperitoneal lymphomas by a morphologic and immunocytochemical approach. Cancer 1990; 65:72–77.
24. Suhrland MJ, Wieczorek R. Fine needle aspiration biopsy in the diagnosis of lymphoma. Cancer Invest 1991;9:61–68.
25. Koss LG. The lymph nodes. In: Koss LG, ed. Diagnostic cytology and its histopathologic bases. Philadelphia: JB Lippincott Co, 1992:1279–1293.
26. Friedman M, Kim U, Shimaoka K, et al. Appraisal of aspiration cytology in management of Hodgkin's disease. Cancer 1980;45: 1653–1663.
27. Kardos TF, Vinson JH, Behm FG, et al. Hodgkin's disease: diagnosis by fine-needle aspiration biopsy. Analysis of cytologic criteria from a selected series. Am J Clin Pathol 1986;86: 286–291.
28. Bottles K, McPhaul LW, Volberding P. Fine-needle aspiration biopsy of patients with acquired immunodeficiency syndrome (AIDS): experience in an outpatient clinic. Ann Intern Med 1988;108:42–45.
29. Tani E, Ersoz C, Svedmyr E, et al. Fine-needle aspiration cytology and immunocytochemistry of Hodgkin's disease, suppurative type. Diagn Cytopathol 1998;18:437–440.
30. Mann KP, Hall B, Kamino H, et al. Neutrophil-rich, Ki-1-positive anaplastic large-cell malignant lymphoma [see Comments]. Am J Surg Pathol 1995;19:407–416.
31. Galindo LM, Havlioglu N, Grosso LE. Cytologic findings in a case of T-cell-rich B-cell lymphoma: potential diagnostic pitfall in FNA of lymph nodes. Diagn Cytopathol 1996;14:253–257; discussion 257–258.
32. Dunphy CH, Ramos R. Combining fine-needle aspiration and flow cytometric immunophenotyping in evaluation of nodal and extranodal sites for possible lymphoma: a retrospective review. Diagn Cytopathol 1997;16:200–206.
33. Pontifex AH, Roberts FJ. Fine needle aspiration biopsy cytology in the diagnosis of inflammatory lesions. Acta Cytol 1985;29: 979–982.
34. Hajdu SI, Melamed MR. Limitations of aspiration cytology in the diagnosis of primary neoplasms. Acta Cytol 1984;28:337–345.
35. Tani EM, Christensson B, Porwit A, et al. Immunocytochemical analysis and cytomorphologic diagnosis on fine needle aspirates of lymphoproliferative disease. Acta Cytol 1988;32:209–215.
36. Hanson CA. Fine-needle aspiration and immunophenotyping. A role in diagnostic hematopathology? [Editorial; Comment]. Am J Clin Pathol 1994;101:555–556.
37. Das DK, Gupta SK, Datta BN, et al. FNA cytodiagnosis of non-Hodgkin's lymphoma and its subtyping under working formulation of 175 cases. Diagn Cytopathol 1991;7:487–498.
38. Carter TR, Feldman PS, Innes DJ Jr, et al. The role of fine needle aspiration cytology in the diagnosis of lymphoma [published erratum appears in Acta Cytol 1989;33:951]. Acta Cytol 1988; 32:848–853.
39. Orell SR, Skinner JM. The typing of non-Hodgkin's lymphomas using fine needle aspiration cytology. Pathology 1982;14:389–394.
40. Kung IT, Chan SK, Lo ES. Application of the immunoperoxidase technique to cell block preparations from fine needle aspirates. Acta Cytol 1990;34:297–303.
41. Young NA, Al-Saleem TI, Ehya H, et al. Utilization of fine-needle aspiration cytology and flow cytometry in the diagnosis and subclassification of primary and recurrent lymphoma. Cancer 1998;84:252–261.
42. Aiello A, Delia D, Giardini R, et al. PCR analysis of IgH and BCL2 gene rearrangement in the diagnosis of follicular lymphoma in lymph node fine-needle aspiration. A critical appraisal. Diagn Mol Pathol 1997;6:154–160.
43. Picker LJ, Weiss LM, Medeiros LJ, et al. Immunophenotypic criteria for the diagnosis of non-Hodgkin's lymphoma. Am J Pathol 1987;128:181–201.
44. Martin SE, Zhang HZ, Magyarosy E, et al. Immunologic methods in cytology: definitive diagnosis of non-Hodgkin's lymphomas using immunologic markers for T- and B-cells. Am J Clin Pathol 1984;82:666–673.
45. Levitt S, Cheng L, DuPuis MH, et al. Fine needle aspiration diagnosis of malignant lymphoma with confirmation by immunoperoxidase staining. Acta Cytol 1985;29:895–902.
46. Tani E, Liliemark J, Svedmyr E, et al. Cytomorphology and immunocytochemistry of fine needle aspirates from blastic non-Hodgkin's lymphomas. Acta Cytol 1989;33:363–371.
47. Palutke M, Schnitzer B, Mirchandani I, et al. Increased numbers of lymphocytes with single class surface immunoglobulins in reactive hyperplasia of lymphoid tissue. Am J Clin Pathol 1982;78: 316–323.
48. Levy N, Nelson J, Meyer P, et al. Reactive lymphoid hyperplasia with single class (monoclonal) surface immunoglobulin. Am J Clin Pathol 1983;80:300–308.
49. Katz RL, Gritsman A, Cabanillas F, et al. Fine-needle aspiration cytology of peripheral T-cell lymphoma. A cytologic, immuno-

logic, and cytometric study. Am J Clin Pathol 1989;91:120–131.
50. Cousar JB. Surgical pathology examination of lymph nodes. Practice survey by American Society of Clinical Pathologists. Am J Clin Pathol 1995;104:126–132.
51. Frable MA, Frable WJ. Fine-needle aspiration biopsy revisited. Laryngoscope 1982;92:1414–1418.
52. Ketai L, Chauncey J, Duque R. Combination of flow cytometry and transbronchial needle aspiration in the diagnosis of mediastinal lymphoma [Letter]. Chest 1985;88:936.
53. Daskalopoulou D, Harhalakis N, Maouni N, et al. Fine needle aspiration cytology of non-Hodgkin's lymphomas. A morphologic and immunophenotypic study. Acta Cytol 1995;39:180–186.
54. Robins DB, Katz RL, Swan F Jr, et al. Immunotyping of lymphoma by fine-needle aspiration. A comparative study of cytospin preparations and flow cytometry [see Comments]. Am J Clin Pathol 1994;101:569–576.
55. Zander DS, Iturraspe JA, Everett ET, et al. Flow cytometry. *In vitro* assessment of its potential application for diagnosis and classification of lymphoid processes in cytologic preparations from fine-needle aspirates. Am J Clin Pathol 1994;101:577–586.
56. Jeffers MD, Milton J, Herriot R, et al. Fine needle aspiration cytology in the investigation on non-Hodgkin's lymphoma [see Comments]. J Clin Pathol 1998;51:189–196.
57. Saddik M, el Dabbagh L, Mourad WA. *Ex vivo* fine-needle aspiration cytology and flow cytometric phenotyping in the diagnosis of lymphoproliferative disorders: a proposed algorithm for maximum resource utilization. Diagn Cytopathol 1997;16:126–131.
58. Tarantino DR, McHenry CR, Strickland T, et al. The role of fine-needle aspiration biopsy and flow cytometry in the evaluation of persistent neck adenopathy. Am J Surg 1998;176:413–417.
59. Hu E, Horning S, Flynn S, et al. Diagnosis of B cell lymphoma by analysis of immunoglobulin gene rearrangements in biopsy specimens obtained by fine needle aspiration. J Clin Oncol 1986;4:278–283.
60. Lubinski J, Chosia M, Huebner K. Molecular genetic analysis in the diagnosis of lymphoma in fine needle aspiration biopsies. I. Lymphomas versus benign lymphoproliferative disorders. Anal Quant Cytol Histol 1988;10:391–398.
61. Williams ME, Frierson HF Jr, Tabbarah S, et al. Fine-needle aspiration of non-Hodgkin's lymphoma. Southern blot analysis for antigen receptor, bcl-2, and c-myc gene rearrangements. Am J Clin Pathol 1990;93:754–759.
62. Katz RL, Hirsch-Ginsberg C, Childs C, et al. The role of gene rearrangements for antigen receptors in the diagnosis of lymphoma obtained by fine-needle aspiration. A study of 63 cases with concomitant immunophenotyping. Am J Clin Pathol 1991;96:479–490.
63. Cartagena N Jr, Katz RL, Hirsch-Ginsberg C, et al. Accuracy of diagnosis of malignant lymphoma by combining fine-needle aspiration cytomorphology with immunocytochemistry and in selected cases, Southern blotting of aspirated cells: a tissue-controlled study of 86 patients. Diagn Cytopathol 1992;8:456–464.
64. Wan JH, Sykes PJ, Orell SR, et al. Rapid method for detecting monoclonality in B cell lymphoma in lymph node aspirates using the polymerase chain reaction [published erratum appears in J Clin Pathol 1992;45:1124]. J Clin Pathol 1992;45:420–423.
65. Jeffers MD, McCorriston J, Farquharson MA, et al. Analysis of clonality in cytologic material using the polymerase chain reaction (PCR). Cytopathology 1997;8:114–121.
66. Stewart CJ, Farquharson MA, Kerr T, et al. Immunoglobulin light chain mRNA detected by *in situ* hybridisation in diagnostic fine needle aspiration cytology specimens. J Clin Pathol 1996;49:749–754.
67. Stewart CJ, Duncan JA, Farquharson M, et al. Fine needle aspiration cytology diagnosis of malignant lymphoma and reactive lymphoid hyperplasia. J Clin Pathol 1998;51:197–203.
68. McNicol AM, Farquharson MA, Lee FD, et al. Comparison of *in situ* hybridisation and polymerase chain reaction in the diagnosis of B cell lymphoma. J Clin Pathol 1998;51:229–233.

4

ELECTRON MICROSCOPY

It is easy and inexpensive to fix small samples of lymph node routinely in glutaraldehyde at the time of initial processing and decide later if they should be embedded for electron microscopic processing or discarded. In most cases, the glutaraldehyde-fixed tissue will not be needed because electron microscopy contributes little to diagnosing typical lymph node lesions. Ultrastructural examination can enhance the diagnosis in less common disorders, such as Gaucher disease, mycosis fungoides, granulocytic sarcoma, lymphoblastic lymphoma with convoluted nuclei, amyloidosis, and others (1–3). Even more important, electron microscopic examination may decide the difficult diagnosis of some metastatic tumors—identifying, for example, melanosomes or premelanosomes in metastatic melanoma (4), tonofilaments and various specialized desmosome-like or other types of intercellular junctions in metastatic carcinomas, abundant glycogen deposits in metastatic Ewing sarcoma (5), and neurosecretory granules in metastatic neuroblastoma, islet cell tumors, and small cell carcinomas (6).

Immunoelectron microscopy can be used for the study of cell membranes, including surface immunoglobulins (Ig) and various cell markers. This is achieved by applying peroxidase-labeled antibodies to suspensions of live, unfixed cells or to fixed sections and visualizing them under the electron microscope (Fig. 4.1).

NON-HODGKIN B-CELL LYMPHOMAS

Various B-cell malignant lymphomas have a unique ultrastructure. In chronic lymphocytic leukemia, Ig light chains are synthesized in excess over heavy chains. Ultrastructural immunoperoxidase study reveals Ig light chains in both perinuclear space lumina and rough endoplasmic reticulum, whereas heavy chains are limited to rough endoplasmic reticulum (7). After stimulation with pokeweed mitogen, the Ig heavy and light chain production appears balanced (7). Although a signet ring light microscopic appearance is most common in adenocarcinoma, several lymphoma variants occur; B-cell lymphomas of the lymphoplasmacytic type are characterized by an accumulation of Ig-containing rough endoplasmic reticulum cisternae (8), and the vacuolar type, seen in both B- and T-cell lymphomas, consists of a large, membrane-limited vacuole containing giant multivesicular bodies (9) (see Chapter 61). The ultrastructural features of mantle cell lymphoma with the translocation t(11;14)(q13;q32) include nuclear clefts or indentations and evenly dispersed heterochromatin, absent or inconspicuous nucleoli, abundant mitochondria, and a Golgi zone that can be distinguished from that of follicular lymphoma, prolymphocytic leukemia, and chronic lymphocytic leukemia (10).

Follicular lymphoma with abundant periodic acid–Schiff-positive extracellular material composed of membranous structures, membrane-bound vesicles, and electron-dense bodies probably accumulates by a process of deregulated and excessive cell membrane synthesis (11). Rarely, B-lymphoma cells engulfed by macrophages appear to be undergoing emperipolesis (12). Human herpesvirus 8 has been ultrastructurally demonstrated in a clinical sample of AIDS-related body cavity-based lymphoma (13). Ultrastructural morphometry of non-Hodgkin lymphomas has identified the interchromatic (matrix) nuclear contents as contributing the most to nuclear volume (14).

Diffuse large cell B-cell lymphomas are characterized by large cells with a high nuclear–cytoplasmic ratio. The scarce cytoplasm contains few, poorly developed organelles, including a small number of mitochondria. The large nuclei have marginated blocks of chromatin (Fig. 4.2). The immunoblastic variant is characterized by the single, prominent nucleolus (Fig. 4.3).

NON-HODGKIN T-CELL LYMPHOMAS

Lymphoblastic lymphoma under the electron microscope shows mostly round cells with a high nuclear-to-cytoplasmic ratio, a smooth surface, and no processes. The nuclei, which have been described as convoluted, have deep indentations, fine chromatin, and peripheral nucleoli (15) (Fig. 4.4).

Peripheral T-cell lymphomas are ultrastructurally heterogeneous. So-called Lennert lymphoma has a high content of non-neoplastic epithelioid histiocytes (16). Immunologic and ultrastructural study of T-cell immunoblastic sarcomas reveals that most of the neoplastic cells express a helper/inducer T-cell phenotype (17). Angioimmunoblastic-like T-cell lymphoma includes a mixed population of small,

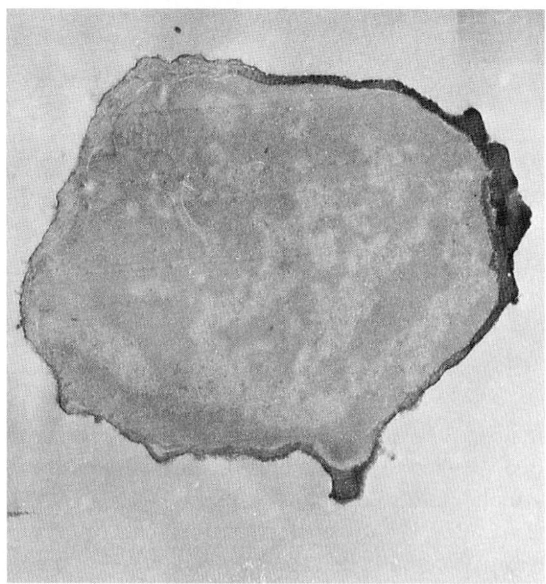

FIGURE 4.1. Non-Hodgkin lymphoma B cell. Deposition of peroxidase reveals the presence of immunoglobulin M (IgM) on the cell membrane. Anti-IgM/peroxidase stain; ×10,000.

medium, and large neoplastic lymphoid cells, often with multiple nuclear indentations, speckled heterochromatin, and prominent nucleoli (18). Large endothelial cells and a multilayered basement membrane, similar to those seen in angioimmunoblastic lymphadenopathy, line the blood vessels in angioimmunoblastic-like T-cell lymphoma (18). Polylobate lymphoma of T- and B-cell phenotypes has been reported (19–21). Human T-cell leukemia virus type 1, the etiologic agent of adult T-cell leukemia/lymphoma, has been demonstrated after *in vitro* culture of adult leukemia/lymphoma T cells, but it is only rarely observed in primary tissue samples (22). Hepatosplenic γδ T-cell lymphomas with natural killer cell-associated antigens (CD11c, CD16, or CD56) and cytotoxic effector proteins (perforin, granzyme B, TIA-1, and Fas ligand) contain cytoplasmic dense-core granules, consistent with type 1 cytolytic granules (23). Although recent lymphoma classifications include only the T-cell anaplastic large cell lymphomas (ALCLs) under the heading of Ki-1 ALCL, no electron microscopic feature separates T-cell, B-cell, and null varieties of ALCL (24).

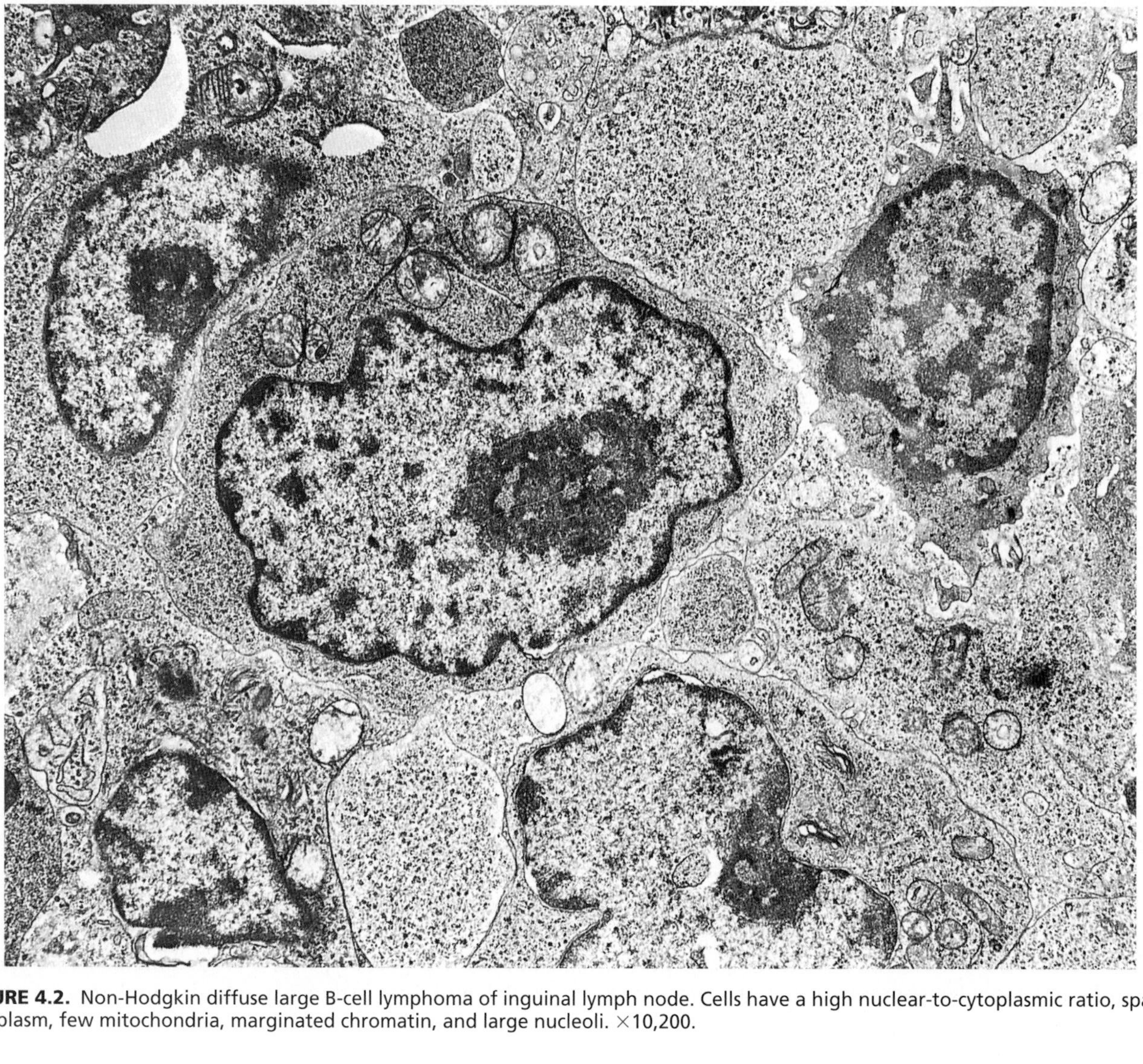

FIGURE 4.2. Non-Hodgkin diffuse large B-cell lymphoma of inguinal lymph node. Cells have a high nuclear-to-cytoplasmic ratio, sparse cytoplasm, few mitochondria, marginated chromatin, and large nucleoli. ×10,200.

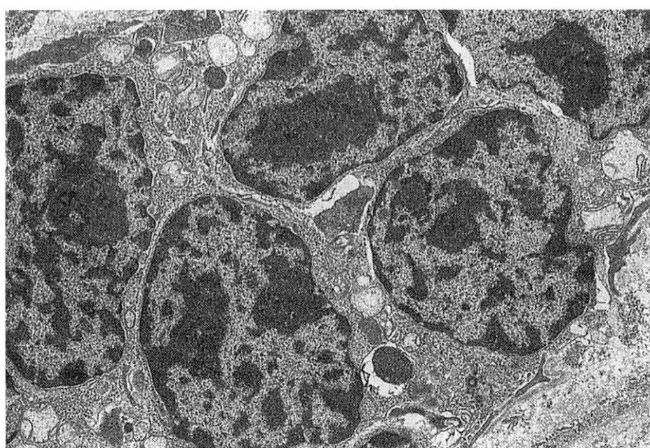

FIGURE 4.3. Non-Hodgkin diffuse large B-cell lymphoma, immunoblastic variant. Cells have large noncleaved nuclei, heterochromatin, and centrally prominent nucleoli. ×9,600.

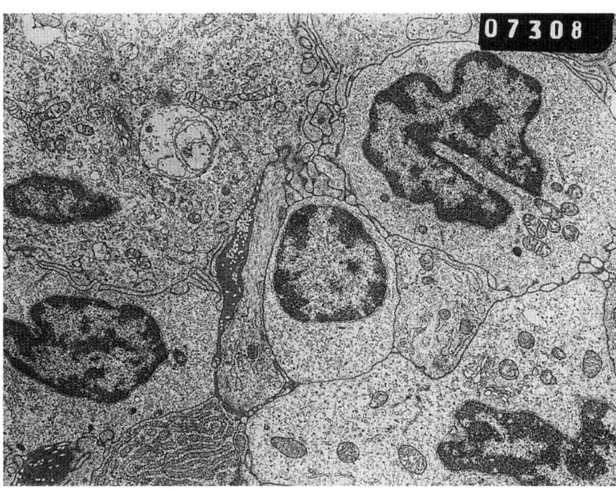

FIGURE 4.5. Hodgkin lymphoma, classic type, mixed cellularity subtype, showing various lymphoid cells and one Reed-Sternberg cell with a deeply indented nucleus. ×8,800.

HODGKIN LYMPHOMAS

The characteristic cells of classic Hodgkin lymphoma are the Hodgkin cells and the Reed-Sternberg cells, which are the mononuclear and multinuclear variants of the same cell type. Studies of single cells isolated by micromanipulation have demonstrated that the neoplastic cells of classic Hodgkin lymphoma are in fact activated B cells originating in the germinal centers of lymphoid follicles (see Chapter 57).

Ultrastructurally, the Hodgkin cells are large and mostly rounded, although occasional indentations can be noted. The cell membrane is sharply delineated, and the cytoplasm contains numerous mitochondria and polysomes but a poorly developed Golgi area and endoplasmic reticulum. The nuclei are very large and round. The abundant heterochromatin is condensed around the nuclear membrane and also irregularly distributed in clumps. The nucleolus is huge and nonhomogeneous. The general appearance resembles that of neoplastic immunoblasts of follicular center origin (Fig. 57.13).

The Reed-Sternberg cell is significantly larger and irregularly shaped; abundant cytoplasm contains numerous mitochondria, some rod-shaped, polysomes, and dense bodies. Profiles of endoplasmic reticulum are rare. The nucleus is multilobate and irregularly shaped; sometimes, thin bridges (inapparent in the plane of section) link the nuclear lobes. More euchromatin is seen in the nuclear mass with marginated heterochromatin (3) and huge, dense, reticulated nucleoli. Electron microscopic images demonstrate that the Reed-Sternberg cell is not a multinucleated cell but rather a cell with a deeply indented nucleus; the multiple nuclear lobes are connected by thin bridges that are not always visible in the planes of section. (Figs. 4.5 and 4.6; see also Figs. 57.24 and 57.25).

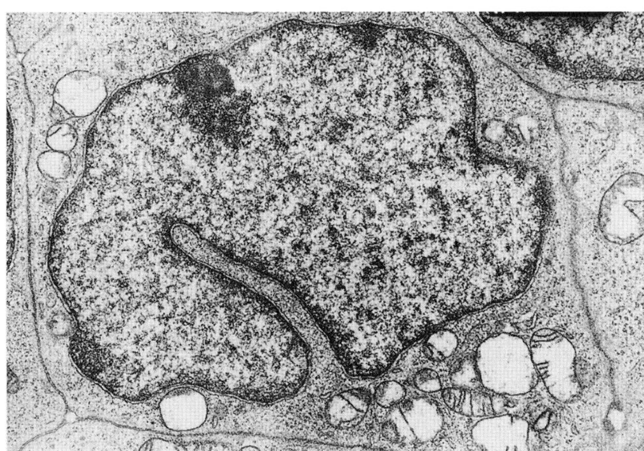

FIGURE 4.4. Non-Hodgkin lymphoblastic lymphoma, T-cell type. Cells have a small amount of cytoplasm, few organelles, and deeply indented (convoluted) nuclei with small peripheral nucleoli. ×14,000.

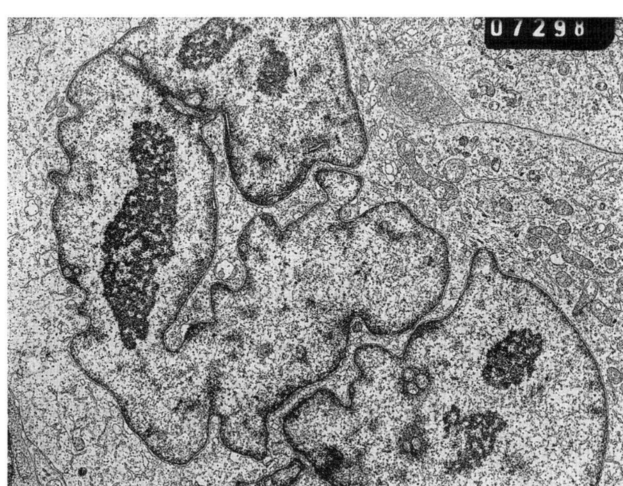

FIGURE 4.6. Reed-Sternberg cell in nodular sclerosis Hodgkin lymphoma. Multiple nuclear lobes are connected by thin bridges and huge, prominent nucleoli. ×12,000.

REFERENCES

1. Mori Y, Lennert K. Electron microscopic atlas of lymph node cytology and pathology. New York: Springer-Verlag, 1969:xi, 309.
2. Ioachim HI. Lymph nodes and spleen. In: Johannessen JV, ed. Electron microscopy in human medicine, vol 5. New York: McGraw-Hill, 1981:385–464.
3. Johannessen JV, Sobrinho-Simões M. Diagnostic electron microscopy. Washington, DC: Hemisphere Publishing, 1982:vii, 210.
4. Mazur MT, Katzenstein AL. Metastatic melanoma: the spectrum of ultrastructural morphology. Ultrastruct Pathol 1980;1:337–356.
5. Llombart-Bosch A, Blache R, Peydro-Olaya A. Ultrastructural study of 28 cases of Ewing's sarcoma: typical and atypical forms. Cancer 1978;41:1362–1373.
6. Gould VE. Neuroendocrinomas and neuroendocrine carcinomas: APUD cell system neoplasms and their aberrant secretory activities. Pathol Annu 1977;12:33–62.
7. Newell DG, Harris AH, Smith JL. The ultrastructural localization of immunoglobulin in chronic lymphocytic lymphoma cells: changes in light and heavy chain distribution induced by mitogen stimulation. Blood 1983;61:511–519.
8. Kim H, Dorfman RF, Rappaport H. Signet ring cell lymphoma. Am J Surg Pathol 1978;2:119–132.
9. Eyden BP, Cross PA, Harris M. The ultrastructure of signet-ring cell non-Hodgkin's lymphoma. Virchows Arch A Pathol Anat Histopathol 1990;417:395–404.
10. Resnitzky P, Matutes E, Hedges M, et al. The ultrastructure of mantle cell lymphoma and other B-cell disorders with translocation t(11;14)(q13;q32). Br J Haematol 1996;94:352–361.
11. Chittal SM, Caveriviere P, Voigt JJ, et al. Follicular lymphoma with abundant PAS-positive extracellular material. Immunohistochemical and ultrastructural observations. Am J Surg Pathol 1987;11:618–624.
12. Takeya M, Takahashi K. Emperipolesis in a case of malignant lymphoma: electron microscopic and immunohistochemical investigation. Ultrastruct Pathol 1988;12:651–658.
13. Hsi ED, Foreman KE, Duggan J, et al. Molecular and pathologic characterization of an AIDS-related body cavity-based lymphoma, including ultrastructural demonstration of human herpesvirus-8: a case report [published erratum appears in Am J Surg Pathol 1998;22:910]. Am J Surg Pathol 1998;22: 493–499.
14. Dardick I, Dardick AM, Caldwell DR, et al. Non-Hodgkin's lymphoma classification: ultrastructural morphometric studies for the quantification of nuclear compartments *in situ.* Hum Pathol 1985;16:1047–1060.
15. Ioachim HL, Finkbeiner JA. Pseudonodular patterns of T-cell lymphoma. Cancer 1980;45:1370–1378.
16. Bedetti CD, Ollapally E. Malignant lymphoma with a high content of epithelioid histiocytes (so-called Lennert's lymphoma). Immunocytochemical and ultrastructural observations. Virchows Arch A Pathol Anat Histopathol 1983;399:255–264.
17. Said JW, Shintaku IP, Chien K, et al. Peripheral T cell lymphoma (immunoblastic sarcoma of T cell type): an immuno-ultrastructural study. Hum Pathol 1984;15:324–329.
18. Caulet S, Audouin J, le Tourneau A, et al. Angio-immunoblastic lymphadenopathy (AIL) or T-cell malignant lymphoma of AIL-type. A histopathological, immunohistochemical and ultrastructural study of 8 cases. Pathol Res Pract 1988;183:724–734.
19. Pinkus GS, Said JW, Hargreaves H. Malignant lymphoma, T-cell type. A distinct morphologic variant with large multilobated nuclei, with a report of four cases. Am J Clin Pathol 1979;72:540–550.
20. Weiss RL, Ashwood ER, Kjeldsberg CR. Multilobated B-cell lymphoma. A clinicopathologic study of 24 cases. Arch Pathol Lab Med 1990;114:28–33.
21. Friedman HD, Hutchison RE, Smith JR, et al. CD8+ polylobated T-cell leukemia/lymphoma. A case report with immunophenotypic, ultrastructural, gene rearrangement, karyotypic, and DNA content analysis and autopsy description. Arch Pathol Lab Med 1994;118:722–727.
22. Vital C, Vital A, Moynet D, et al. The presence of particles resembling human T-cell leukemia virus type I at ultrastructural examination of lymphomatous cells in a case of T-cell leukemia/lymphoma. Cancer 1993;71:2227–2232.
23. Salhany KE, Feldman M, Kahn MJ, et al. Hepatosplenic gammadelta T-cell lymphoma: ultrastructural, immunophenotypic, and functional evidence for cytotoxic T lymphocyte differentiation. Hum Pathol 1997;28:674–685.
24. Hansmann ML, Fellbaum C, Bohm A. Large cell anaplastic lymphoma: evaluation of immunophenotype on paraffin and frozen sections in comparison with ultrastructural features. Virchows Arch A Pathol Anat Histopathol 1991;418:427–433.

5

CYTOCHEMISTRY

Special stains and cytochemical techniques are particularly useful as adjuvants in the diagnosis of lymph node lesions by identifying various biochemical and enzymatic cell markers (Table 5.1).

PERIODIC ACID–SCHIFF STAIN

Periodic acid–Schiff (PAS) stains glycogen (1) as blocklike, intracytoplasmic aggregates in some acute lymphoblastic leukemia cells or as a chunklike necklace in erythroleukemia cells. Adding diastase (or amylase) removes glycogen. PAS with diastase identifies the carbohydrate portion of intracytoplasmic immunoglobulins in plasma cells and plasmacytoid lymphocytes (2). Immunoglobulin A (IgA) myeloma cells are intensely red because IgA contains a higher percentage of carbohydrate than either IgM or IgG; they are called *flame cells.* PAS with diastase (or amylase) also strongly stains immunoglobulin deposits, such as Russell bodies and Dutcher bodies, and an interstitial amorphous substance (frequently containing immunoglobulin) that is found in some types of lymphomas and angioimmunoblastic lymphadenopathy with dysproteinemia. PAS with diastase is useful in differentiating intensely red-staining megakaryocytes from negative Reed-Sternberg cells (3).

METHYL GREEN PYRONINE STAIN

Methyl green pyronine stain can be used in the differential diagnosis of lymphoma versus plasmacytoma/multiple myeloma. Plasma cells and plasmacytoid cells secreting immunoglobulin and immunoblasts contain more RNA (intracytoplasmic pyroninophilic material) than mature B-lymphoma cells expressing surface immunoglobulin (4) (Fig. 5.1). Methyl green pyronin is also useful in distinguishing Burkitt lymphoma (abundant RNA) from lymphoblastic lymphoma (scant RNA) (5). Acid decalcification, incomplete fixation, or tissue necrosis can degrade RNA.

RETICULIN STAINING BY SILVER IMPREGNATION

Several methods of reticulin staining by silver impregnation are available (6). The reticulin fibrillar framework of lymphoid tissues becomes apparent and serves as a useful criterion to distinguish large cell (histiocytic) lymphomas from metastatic undifferentiated carcinomas or melanomas. A well-developed, fine, branching reticulin network with pericellular fibrils is generally characteristic of lymphomas, whereas thick reticulin and collagen fibers with an alveolar pattern surrounding nests and cords of cells are indicative of metastatic nonlymphoid tumors.

SUDAN BLACK B

Sudan black B (SBB) is useful in differentiating acute myeloid, lymphoid, and myelomonocytic leukemias (7). Sudan black B staining parallels peroxidase activity; it is strong in myeloid cells and eosinophils, faint in monocytes, and absent in normoblasts and lymphocytes, although rare lymphoblasts contain SBB-positive granules (8). Myeloid cells, from myeloblasts to neutrophils, show increasing sudanophilia as the number of granules increases (Fig. 5.2). Auer bodies are intensely sudanophilic. In contrast to peroxidase enzyme activity, staining with SBB does not diminish in granules in older, light-exposed smears (9).

PEROXIDASE REACTION

Peroxidase reaction is positive in neutrophilic and eosinophilic series (10) and faintly positive in monocytes (11). It can be used to differentiate these from peroxidase-negative lymphoid and erythroid cells (7) (Fig. 5.3).

NONSPECIFIC ESTERASES

Nonspecific esterases are enzymes characteristic of monocytes/histiocytes (7,12,13) (see Chapter 77). When sub-

TABLE 5.1. CELL IDENTIFICATION BY CYTOCHEMISTRY.

Cytochemical reaction	Cell types
Nonspecific esterase	Myeloid cells, monocytes, megakaryocytes, T lymphocytes (dotlike staining)
Chloroacetate esterase	Myeloid cells, mast cells
Peroxidase	Myeloid cells, eosinophils, monocytes
Sudan black B	Myeloid cells, monocytes
Methyl green pyronine	Plasma cells, immunoblasts
Periodic acid–Schiff with diastase	Plasma cells
Tartrate-resistant acid phosphatase	Hairy cell leukemia

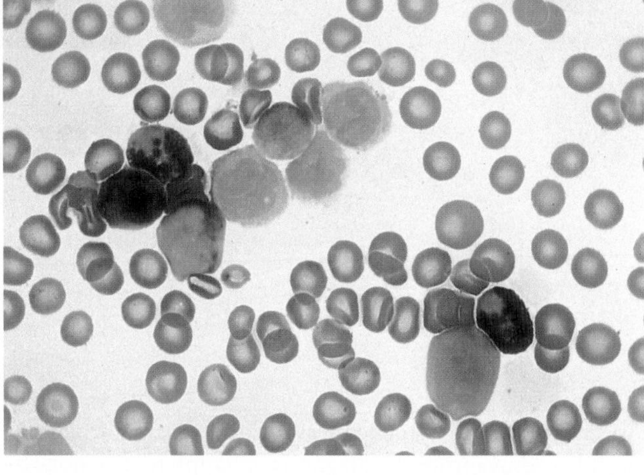

FIGURE 5.3. Peroxidase-positive cells of acute myeloid leukemia. Peroxidase stain.

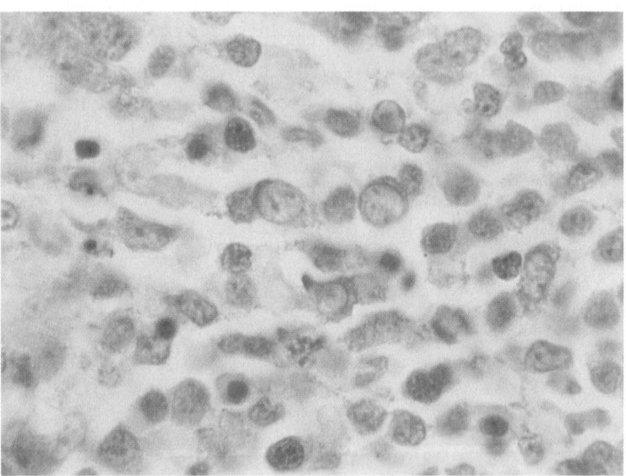

FIGURE 5.1. Pyronine staining of cytoplasm in plasmacytoid lymphoma cells. Methyl green pyronine stain.

strates such as α-naphthyl acetate (ANA) or α-naphthyl butyrate (ANB) are used, monocyte/histiocyte esterases show a strong, diffuse, orange–brown staining (Fig. 5.4). The ANA esterase reaction is inhibited by sodium fluoride in monocytes/histiocytes but not in myeloid cells, which have a fluoride-resistant isoenzyme. They may also react positively with megakaryocytes and platelets when the ANA, but not the ANB substrate, is used (14). T lymphocytes exhibit a dotlike ANA esterase staining pattern (15).

SPECIFIC NAPHTHOL AS-D CHLOROACETATE ESTERASE

Specific naphthol AS-D chloroacetate esterase is characteristically positive in myeloid and mast cells and negative in histiocytes and monocytes (7,12,16). The substrate used is

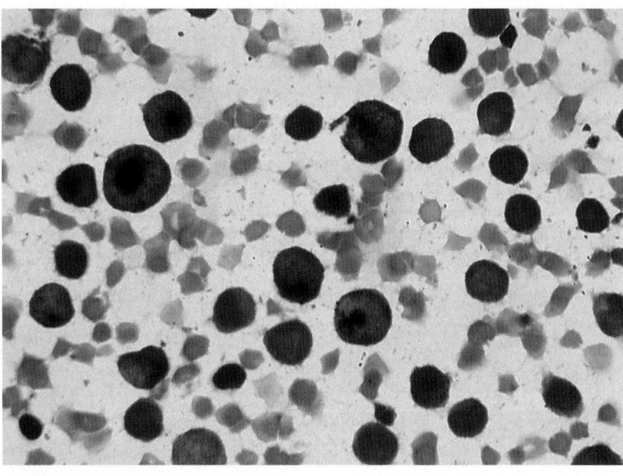

FIGURE 5.2. Sudan black B stains myelomonocytic leukemia cells. Sudan black B stain.

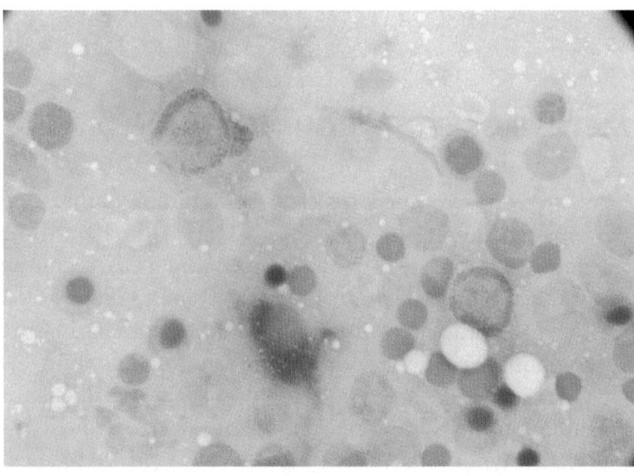

FIGURE 5.4. Nonspecific esterase staining of histiocytes. α-Naphthyl acetate substrate.

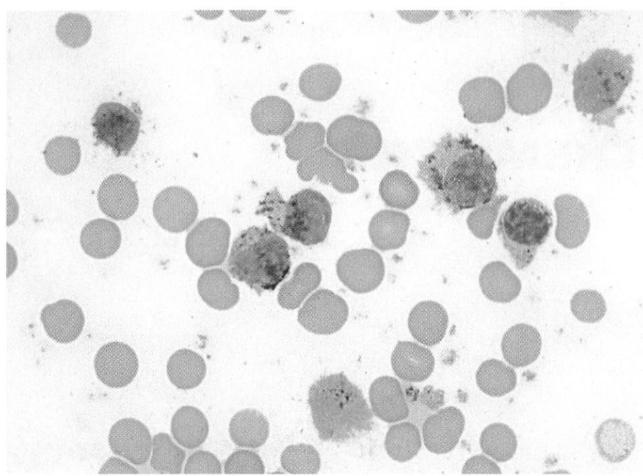

FIGURE 5.5. Tartrate-resistant acid phosphatase staining of cytoplasmic granules in hairy cell leukemia.

naphthol AS-D chloroacetate (17); the reaction product is a red intracytoplasmic precipitate. It generally parallels the SBB and peroxidase reactions; however, it has the advantage of also being applicable to paraffin-embedded sections (16) and can be useful in diagnosing granulocytic sarcoma (18) (see Chapter 76).

TARTRATE-RESISTANT ACID PHOSPHATASE

This isoenzyme is present almost exclusively in hairy cell leukemia (Fig. 5.5) but absent from other lymphocytic lymphomas and leukemias (19) (see Chapter 62).

REFERENCES

1. Wislocki GB, Rheingold JM, Dempsey EW. The occurrence of the periodic acid–Schiff reaction in various normal cells of blood and connective tissue. Blood 1949;4:562–568.
2. Gaffney E. Carbohydrates. In: Prophet EB, Mills B, Arrington JB, et al., eds. Laboratory methods in histotechnology. Washington, DC: American Registry of Pathology, 1992:149–153.
3. Hayhoe FGJ. Acute leukemia: cellular morphology, cytochemistry, and fine structure. Clin Haematol 1972;1:49–94.
4. d'Ablaing G, Rogers ER, Parker JW, et al. A simplified and modified methyl green pyronine stain. Am J Clin Pathol 1970;54: 667–669.
5. Perkins SL, Segal GH, Kjeldsberg CR. Classification of non-Hodgkin's lymphomas in children. Semin Diagn Pathol 1995; 12:303–313.
6. McElroy DA. Connective tissue. In: Prophet EB, Mills B, Arrington JB, et al., eds. Laboratory methods in histotechnology. Washington, DC: American Registry of Pathology, 1992:137–142.
7. Kass L. Cytochemistry of leukemic cells. Leukemia cytology and cytochemistry. Philadelphia: JB Lippincott Co, 1982:245–272.
8. Sheehan HL, Storey GW. An improved method of staining leucocyte granules with Sudan black B. J Pathol 1947;59:336–337.
9. Lillie RD, Burtner HJ. Stable sudanophilia of human neutrophil leukocytes in relation to peroxidase and oxidase. J Histochem Cytochem 1953;1:8–26.
10. Bainton DF. Neutrophilic granules. Br J Haematol 1975;29:17–22.
11. Nichols BA, Bainton D, Faraquhar M. Differentiation of monocytes. Origin, nature, and fate of their azurophilic granules. J Cell Biol 1971;50:498–515.
12. Yam LT, Li CY, Crosby WH. Cytochemical identification of monocytes and granulocytes. Am J Clin Pathol 1971;55:283–290.
13. Li CY, Lam KW, Yam LT. Esterases in human leukocytes. J Histochem Cytochem 1973;21:1–12.
14. Koike T. Megakaryoblastic leukemia: the characterization and identification of megakaryoblasts. Blood 1984;64:683–692.
15. Knowles DM, Hoffman T, Ferrarini M, et al. The demonstration of acid alpha-naphthyl acetate esterase activity in human lymphocytes: usefulness as a T-cell marker. Cell Immunol 1978;35: 112–123.
16. Leder LD. The selective enzymocytochemical demonstration of neutrophil myeloid cells and tissue mast cells in paraffin sections [in German]. Klin Wochenschr 1964;42:553.
17. Moloney WC, McPherson K, Fliegelman L. Esterase activity in leukocytes demonstrated by the use of naphthol AS-D chloroacetate substrate. J Histochem Cytochem 1960;8:200–207.
18. Traweek ST, Arber DA, Rappaport H, et al. Extramedullary myeloid cell tumors. An immunohistochemical and morphologic study of 28 cases. Am J Surg Pathol 1993;17:1011–1019.
19. Yam LT, Li CY, Lam KW. Tartrate-resistant acid phosphatase isoenzyme in the reticulum cells of leukemic reticuloendotheliosis. N Engl J Med 1971;284:357–360.

6

IMMUNOHISTOCHEMISTRY

TISSUE SECTION IMMUNOHISTOCHEMISTRY

Applying the Revised European American Lymphoma (REAL) or the World Health Organization (WHO) lymphoma classification schemes requires integrating immunophenotypic data with architectural patterns (1,2). Tissue section immunohistochemistry and flow cytometry (see Chapter 7) detect equally well the immunophenotype of lymph node diseases with a diffuse histologic pattern (e.g., acute or chronic leukemias, indolent or aggressive diffuse lymphomas). Tissue section immunohistochemical staining (3) is of additional value in diagnosing lymph node disorders with a nodular histologic pattern (e.g., follicular lymphoma, mantle zone lymphoma) or a small number of neoplastic cells (e.g., Hodgkin lymphoma, T cell-rich B-cell lymphoma), or in which lymph nodes are partially involved. In this chapter, we review the most useful markers for revealing immunologic architecture and sparse malignant lymphoid cells in lymph node tissue sections.

CLUSTER OF DIFFERENTIATION

Diagnostic immunohistochemistry relies on a large collection of monoclonal antibodies (Mabs) that bind to surface molecules involved in communication, adhesion, or signaling on B cells, T cells, histiocytes, and their subsets (4). Each antigen may have multiple epitopes. Each epitope is a small molecular region determining three-dimensional interaction with the antigen-binding site in the antibody variable region. The abbreviation *CD* (cluster of differentiation) refers to a group of Mabs made in laboratories around the world that recognize the same or different epitopes on a particular cell surface molecule. The study of data from several international workshops comparing Mab reactivities against cell line panels has yielded a consensus on white cell differentiation antigens (5). Many of these cell surface molecules have been cloned and characterized (6). Fortunately, the pathologist can choose diagnostically informative anti-CD Mabs from several different manufacturers. Although frozen tissue sections can be stained with the greatest variety of antibodies, a significant number of reagents suitable for fixed, paraffin-embedded tissues are now available.

ANTIBODY PANELS

The twin virtues of immunohistochemical tissue staining are that it reveals cell specificity and microenvironment topology. To achieve meaningful results consistently, we recommend focusing the differential diagnosis by using antibody panels. An ideal multi-antibody strategy should detect all relevant immunologic subsets with a minimal number of reagents, reveal both positive and negative internal controls, and improve quality assurance. We recommend simultaneously staining an external control tissue, such as tonsil. Although the widest variety of antibodies stain frozen tissue (7) (Fig. 6.1), many reagents produce good results in paraffin sections after epitope retrieval (8) (Fig. 6.2). Antigen preservation can vary depending on autolysis and necrosis (9).

B-CELL CLONALITY

Surface membrane immunoglobulin (sIg) characterizes circulating, mature B lymphocytes and most B cells in reactive lymph nodes. Ninety percent of B cells express sIgM (Fig. 6.1), with or without sIgD (Fig. 6.2), and the remaining 10% make sIgG or sIgA. Each mature B cell carries either κ or λ (but not both) Ig light chains. A normal, polyclonal B-lymphocyte population includes many cells expressing κ or λ sIg, the former about two to three times as numerous as the latter. Monoclonal, mature B-cell lymphomas exclusively express a single Ig light chain because they arise from a single cell (10). sIg light chains identify the B-cell nature of the lymphocyte population and determine its clonality, information that is useful in evaluating neoplasia. Tissue section immunohistochemistry can be superior to flow cytometry in detecting partial lymph node involvement by a monoclonal B-cell population because in cell suspension studies, abundant reactive polyclonal B cells may dilute and obscure a few neoplastic monoclonal B cells.

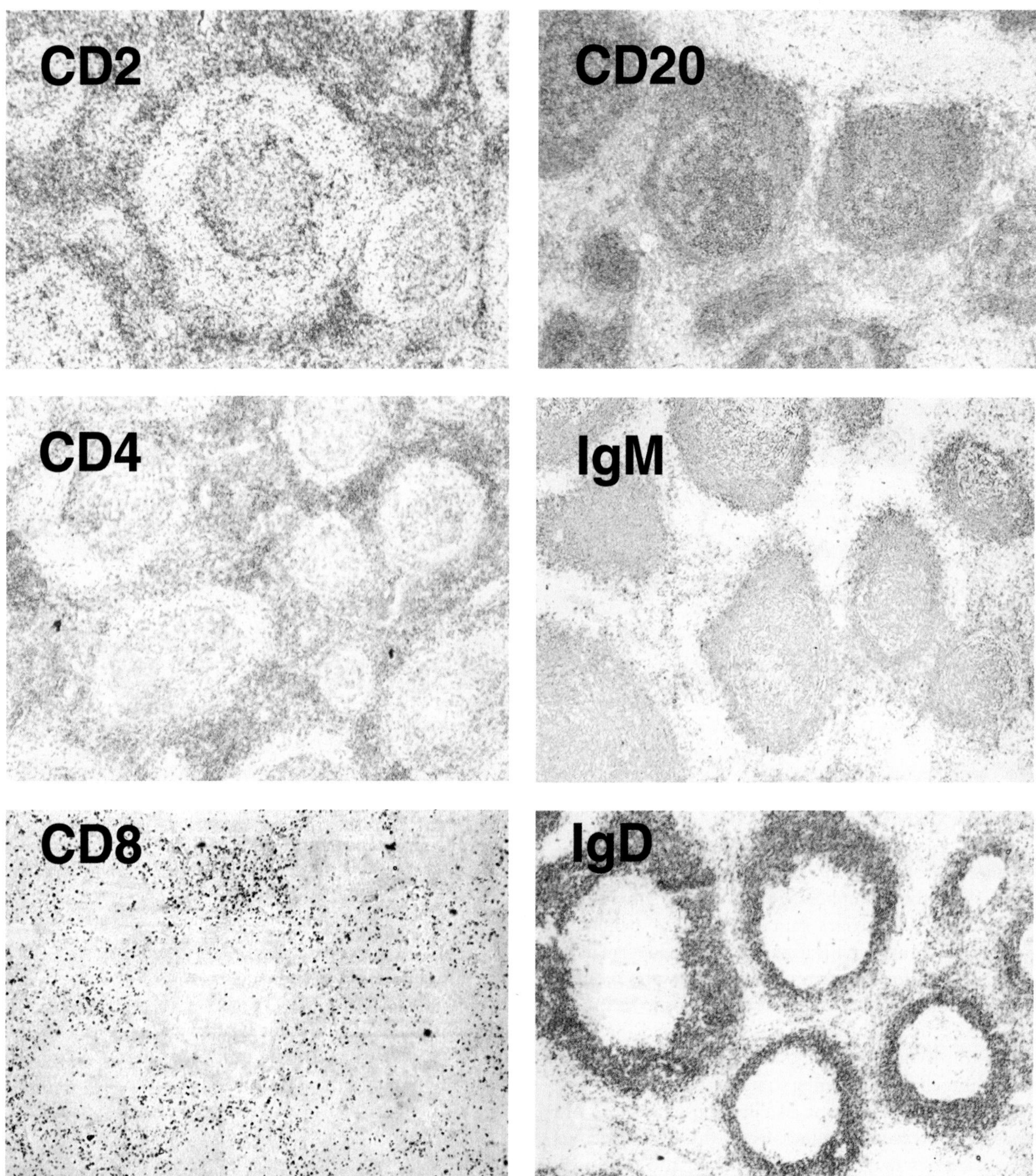

FIGURE 6.1. Frozen tissue section immunohistochemistry, reactive lymphoid hyperplasia. **Left column:** CD2 stains almost all T cells in the interfollicular zone and in the germinal center. CD4+ helper/inducer T cells, a major T-cell subset, localize to the interfollicular zone and germinal center. CD8+ suppressor/cytotoxic T cells, a minor T-cell subset, are found mostly in the interfollicular zone. **Right column:** CD20 stains almost all B cells in the mantle zone, germinal center, and interfollicular area. Both mantle zone B cells and germinal center B cells express membrane IgM. Only mantle zone B cells express IgD. Peroxidase/antiperoxidase method. Color reagent: aminoethyl carbazol. No counterstain.

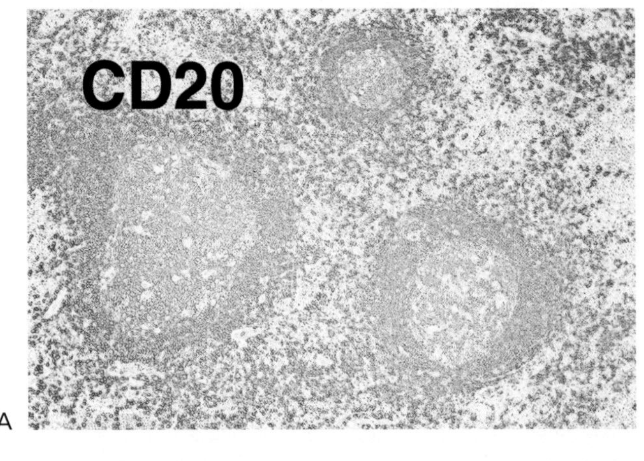

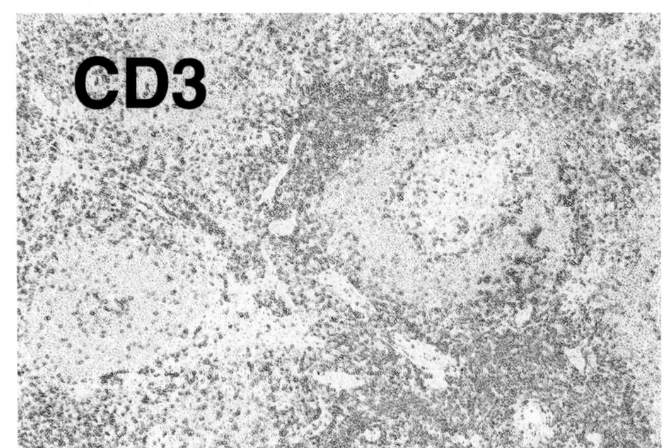

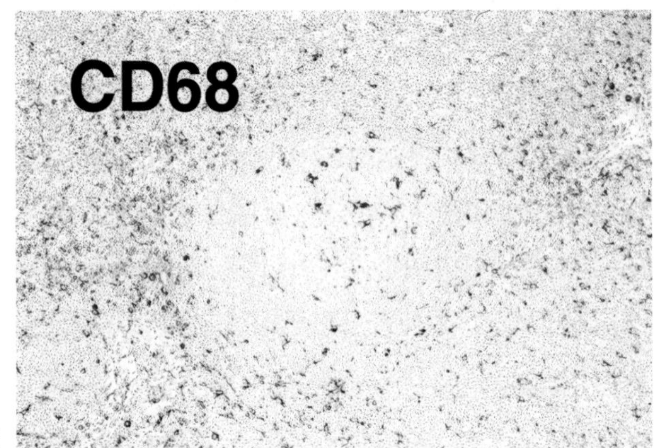

FIGURE 6.2. Paraffin section immunohistochemistry, reactive lymphoid hyperplasia. **A:** B cells expressing CD20 localize mainly to the mantle zone and germinal center; fewer B cells are found in the interfollicular zone. **B:** T cells expressing CD3 occur mostly in the interfollicular zone but also in the germinal center. **C:** Histiocytes expressing CD68 are numerous in the interfollicular zone and germinal center. Avidin–biotin complex method. Color reagent: diaminobenzidine. Light hematoxylin counterstain.

SURFACE IMMUNOGLOBULIN

To demonstrate mature B-cell sIg clonality in tissue sections, fresh, unfixed lymphoid tissues must be submitted to the laboratory. Fixed tissues stain unreliably for membrane-bound sIg, although archival paraffin-embedded material can be used to localize cytoplasmic Ig in plasma cells. Demonstrating sIg on lymphoid cells in tissue sections is best achieved by snap-freezing tissue in isopentane/liquid nitrogen (or dry ice) or acetone/dry ice baths. A variety of immunohistochemical staining strategies use conjugated enzymes, such as peroxidase or alkaline phosphatase, to produce a colored reaction product. Even with fresh frozen tissues, difficulties may be encountered in the reading of specific sIg staining as a consequence of thick sectioning, suboptimal antibody titer, excess serum Ig, necrosis, or variability of antigenic sites (11). Occasionally, because of equivocal results, diagnosing light chain clonality may be impossible, and molecular studies should be performed on the frozen tissue remainder. Intracytoplasmic Igs in plasmacytoid B cells, immunoblasts, and plasma cells withstand fixation and can be stained on paraffin-embedded tissues (12). Whereas cell viability is necessary for demonstrating sIg, killing cells by fixation facilitates the penetration of cytoplasm by labeled reagents to stain intracellular Ig. A reticular staining pattern in germinal centers for IgM, IgG, IgA, and IgE is common in reactive lymph nodes; IgE is not specific for Kimura disease or angiolymphoid hyperplasia with eosinophilia (13).

B-CELL MARKERS

In addition to Igs, B cells exhibit a large variety of other molecules that can be used to identify function and degree of differentiation. B cells, both immature and mature, express the human major histocompatability class II antigen (HLA-DR). HLA-DR can also be found on activated T cells, some monocytes, macrophages, and immature myeloid cells (14). Mature B cells also express Fc receptors (FcR) and complement receptors (e.g., CD21). CD19 is the most broadly expressed and specific marker for B cells; it appears at the earliest stages of B-cell differentiation and persists throughout B-cell maturation until the plasma cell stage, when it is down-regulated (15,16). CD20 antigen (Figs. 6.1 and 6.2) appears later in B-cell maturation and persists until the plasma cell stage (15). CD21 and CD22 are also B cell-restricted antigens but are expressed at later stages of maturation (15,16). CD23, the low-affinity IgE receptor, is found on follicular dendritic reticulum cells, sIgM/sIgD double-positive B cells, and small lymphocytic lymphoma (17). CD79a (B-cell receptor-associated protein) forms heterodimers with CD79b to anchor membrane sIg in mature B cells; CD79a begins on B-precursor cells before CD19 and stops before plasma cells (18). In contrast, CD10, or common acute lymphoblastic leukemia antigen (CALLA), is expressed on pre-B cells and again on germinal center cells in addition to neutrophils, pre-B ALL, Burkitt lymphoma, and follicular lymphoma (19–22). Small lymphocytic lymphoma and mantle cell lymphoma are B-cell disorders expressing CD5 (23). Low-grade B-cell lymphomas, except follicular lymphoma, express CD43 (24). CD38 and CD138 (syndecan 1) (25) detect plasma cells, which do not express CD19, CD20, CD45, HLA-DR, or sIg (26). CD34 and TdT (terminal deoxynucleotidyl transferase) identify very immature cells. It is possible to determine the B-cell phenotype and maturation stage of most B-cell leukemias/lymphomas by using an Mab panel that includes CD10 (CALLA), CD19, CD20, CD22, CD34, HLA-DR, TdT, and membrane plus cytoplasmic Igs (27). The B-cell lymphomas composed of small lymphocytes [small lymphocytic lymphoma, mantle cell lymphoma, follicular lymphoma, lymphoplasmacytoid lymphoma (immunocytoma), and marginal zone lymphoma (monocytoid lymphoma)] can be classified by using CD5, CD10, CD20, CD23, CD43, and cyclin D1 antibodies in frozen tissue (24) or in paraffin-embedded sections (28,29).

T-CELL MARKERS

The sheep erythrocyte rosette (Fig. 6.3) cell marker characteristic of T cells can be detected with the anti-CD2 Mab (Fig. 6.1). Mabs specific for various CD antigens present on T lymphocytes provide the means to immunophenotype T-cell leukemias and lymphomas fully. CD7 is a pan-T-cell antigen present on the majority of T cells and is very useful for identifying T-cell neoplasms when other T-cell antigens are absent. T lymphocyte-specific Mabs identify three stages of T-cell differentiation (30). In early stage I, cortical thymocytes express nuclear TdT, CD2, CD5, CD7, CD38, and CD71 (transferrin receptor) (16,30). These cells divide rapidly and enter stage II of the common thymocytes, where they lose CD71 and acquire CD1, CD4, and CD8 antigens. In stage III, medullary thymocytes lose CD1 and express CD3 (T-cell antigen receptor) for the first time and either CD4 or CD8 (but not both) (16,30). Post-thymic T cells entering the peripheral circulation lose CD38 and retain CD2, CD3, CD5, CD7, and either CD4 or CD8 (16,30). Peripheral T-cell lymphomas are immunophenotypically heterogeneous (31–33). However, most have a mature phenotype and express either CD4 or CD8 accompanied by a pan-T-cell antigen such as CD2. Peripheral T-cell lymphomas often lose one or more pan-T-cell antigens in comparison with normal T cells (32,34,35). Of these, CD5 and CD7 are absent more often than CD2 or CD3 (16). Peripheral T-cell lymphomas usually express the CD4 (helper) phenotype and uncommonly express the CD8 (suppressor) phenotype, whereas coexpression of both CD4 and CD8 is very rare (32,34). Although not T cell-restricted, the UCHL-1 Mab identifies most T cells in paraffin tissue sections. UCHL-1 reacts with a low-molecular-weight isoform of leukocyte common antigen (CD45RO), which is expressed by most T lymphocytes, macrophages, mature myeloid cells, and even some B cells (36). CD43 (Leu-22, MT-1) identifies T cells (Fig. 6.4), many neoplastic B cells

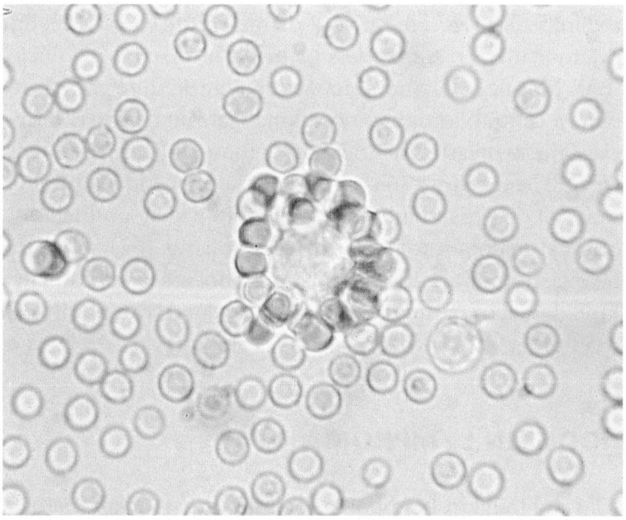

FIGURE 6.3. T lymphocyte spontaneously forming rosette with sheep erythrocytes.

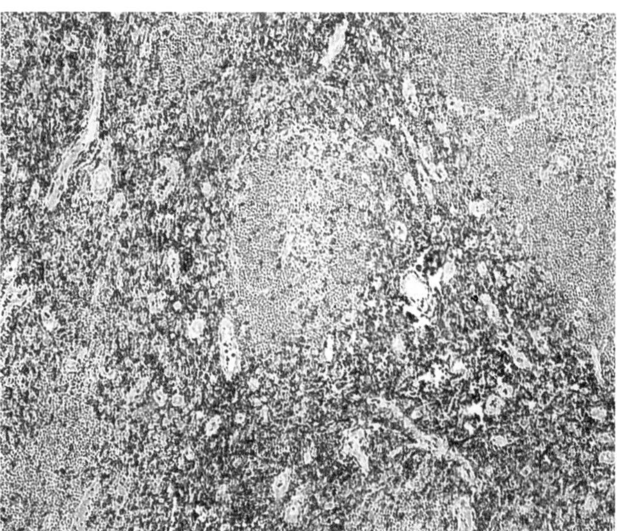

FIGURE 6.4. Normal non-neoplastic T cells (*stained*) between the neoplastic nodules of a follicular lymphoma (*unstained*). Paraffin section, anti-CD43 monoclonal antibody, peroxidase/antiperoxidase.

(but not normal B cells) (12), plus other neoplastic hematopoietic cell types, such as granulocytic sarcoma (37). Immature T lymphocytes in lymphoblastic lymphoma (MLLB) express nuclear TdT. MLLB express, in decreasing frequency, CD5, CD3 and CD7, and CD2 (38). Some MLLB express CD10 (CALLA) and HLA-DR (39). CD7 is one of the earliest surface antigens found on primitive T cells, even preceding the rearrangement of the T-cell antigen receptor genes (16). CD99 (MIC2, O13) identifies Ewing sarcoma and MLLB in routine paraffin tissue sections (40,41). Other T-cell markers detectable in fixed, paraffin-embedded tissue include CD2, CD3 (Fig. 6.2), CD4, and CD5 (42).

MONONUCLEAR PHAGOCYTE MARKERS

The mononuclear phagocyte system (MPS) is phenotypically heterogeneous, although its members have a common bone marrow origin. Macrophages are involved in host protection against microbial invasion and against the development and spread of neoplasia. In addition, a major function of MPS cells is regulation of the induction and expression of the immune response. The MPS includes cell populations that differ in morphology, immune expression, and functions, for which a variety of Mabs have been developed. CD11b (OKM1) and CD36 (OKM5) react with the majority of large, adherent, peripheral blood monocytes, which also express HLA-DR (43). CD11b, but not CD36, reacts with smaller, nonadherent, HLA-DR-negative peripheral blood monocytes. CD11b reacts with granulocytes, but not with platelets, whereas CD36 reacts with platelets but not with granulocytes (43). Anti-CD68 (KP1) (44) or antilysozyme antibodies help to identify histiocytes and macrophages in paraffin sections (Fig. 6.2). Follicular dendritic reticulum cells located in germinal centers interact with B lymphocytes and have an immunophenotype that is positive for CD21 and HLA-DR but negative for CD1a and S100 protein (45). Interdigitating reticulum cells are found mostly in the paracortex and interact with T lymphocytes. They express HLA-DR, CD1a (Leu-6), and S100 protein (45,46).

REACTIVE FOLLICULAR IMMUNOARCHITECTURE

Three main cell types cooperate to create B-cell follicles: B cells, T cells, and nonlymphoid, nonphagocytic cells known as *follicular dendritic reticulum cells* (DRCs) (47,48). A typical reactive secondary lymphoid follicle contains a germinal center surrounded by a sharply defined mantle zone. The normal reactive follicle contains several different B-cell phenotypes (49). The mantle zone contains resting, naïve CD5−, sIgM+, sIgD+ B cells (Fig. 6.1), similar to those composing primary lymphoid follicles (50), plus rare CD5+ B cells. Proliferating germinal center B cells improve antibody affinity maturation by randomly mutating the antigen-binding site in the Ig hypervariable region. Follicular DRCs express CD11b, CD14, CD21, CD23, CD35, and HLA-DR (51). A dense follicular DRC meshwork presents antigen to B cells and helps organize the germinal center (48,52). Follicular DRCs extend from the spherical network of the germinal center into the mantle zone (45,53). Follicular DRCs retain extracellular immune complexes in the outer zone of the germinal center. A small number of CD4+ helper/inducer T cells (54–56) (Fig. 6.1), some coexpressing CD57 (57), localize within the germinal center; they are essential for forming secondary follicles and promoting Ig class switching. The mantle zone contains many T lymphocytes; CD4+ T cells are more numerous than CD8+ T cells (54–56) (Fig. 6.1). In tonsils, germinal centers polarize into dark and light zones, but in lymph nodes the germinal centers often appear less sharply demarcated. The bcl-2 protein inhibits cell death. The germinal center B cells do not express bcl-2 protein, but the mantle zone B cells and most of the T cells are positive for bcl-2 protein.

NEOPLASTIC FOLLICULAR IMMUNOARCHITECTURE

Neoplastic follicles contain the same three cell types as reactive follicles: B cells, T cells, and follicular DRCs. The sharply circumscribed follicles of follicular center lymphoma closely recapitulate the immunoarchitecture of reactive secondary lymphoid follicles (51,58) except that the B cells are monoclonal (59) and overexpress bcl-2 protein (60). Even the T-cell subsets in follicular lymphomas are similar to those of non-neoplastic lymph nodes (61). In follicular center lymphoma and reactive follicular hyperplasia, the follicular DRC meshwork diameters are equal (62), but the follicular DRCs are less plentiful in neoplastic follicles (63). Mantle cell lymphoma with a mantle zone pattern retains a central, atrophic, polyclonal germinal center. However, the neoplastic mantles have a loose, ill-defined follicular DRC meshwork (64). In small lymphocytic lymphoma, some of the pseudonodules (pseudofollicular proliferation centers) maintain follicular DRC remnants (62). Even the neoplastic nodules of nodular lymphocyte predominance Hodgkin lymphoma contain a follicular DRC meshwork (65,66).

HODGKIN LYMPHOMA

Classic Hodgkin lymphoma includes the nodular sclerosis, lymphocyte-rich, mixed cellularity, and lymphocyte depletion subtypes (1,2,67). CD15 and CD30 (but not CD45), stain most Reed-Sternberg cells and variants. Reed-Sternberg cells variably express the B-lineage marker CD20 in approximately one-fourth of cases (68). Reed-Sternberg cells also express the intermediate filaments fascin (69) and restin (70) in addition to the activation markers HLA-DR, CD25, and CD71. In contrast, the lymphocytic and histiocytic (L&H) cells of nodular lymphocyte predominance Hodgkin lymphoma demonstrate a clear B-cell immunophenotype that includes CD20, CD79a, and CD45RB but not classic Reed-Sternberg cell markers such as CD15 and CD30. CD57+ cells surround (L&H) variants in a nodular B-cell background (71).

REFERENCES

1. Harris NL, Jaffe ES, Stein H, et al. A revised European-American classification of lymphoid neoplasms: a proposal from the International Lymphoma Study Group [see Comments]. Blood 1994;84:1361–1392.
2. Harris NL, Jaffe ES, Diebold J, et al. World Health Organization classification of neoplastic diseases of the hematopoietic and lymphoid tissues: report of the Clinical Advisory Committee meeting–Airlie House, Virginia, November 1997. J Clin Oncol 1999;17:3835–3849.
3. Jaffe ES. The role of immunophenotypic markers in the classification of non-Hodgkin's lymphomas. Semin Oncol 1990;17:11–19.
4. Moller P, Eichelmann A, Moldenhauer G. Surface molecules involved in B lymphocyte function. Virchows Arch A Pathol Anat Histopathol 1991;419:365–372.
5. Kishimoto T. Leucocyte typing VI: white cell differentiation antigens. Proceedings of the sixth international workshop and conference held in Kobe, Japan, November 10–14, 1996. New York: Garland, 1998:xxxiv, 1342.
6. Barclay AN, Brown MH, Law SKA, et al. The leukocyte antigen facts book. New York: Academic Press, 1997:613.
7. Sheibani K, Winberg CD, Van de Velde S, et al. Detection of lymphocyte antigens in tissues placed in transport medium. Comparison with cryostat fresh-frozen section technic. An immunologic study of 56 cases. Am J Clin Pathol 1986;85:297–304.
8. Chu PG, Chang KL, Arber DA, et al. Practical applications of immunohistochemistry in hematolymphoid neoplasms. Ann Diagn Pathol 1999;3:104–133.
9. Pelstring RJ, Allred DC, Esther RJ, et al. Differential antigen preservation during tissue autolysis. Hum Pathol 1991;22:237–241.
10. Levy R, Warnke R, Dorfman RF, et al. The monoclonality of human B-cell lymphomas. J Exp Med 1977;145:1014–1028.
11. Tetu B, Manning JT Jr, Ordonez NG. Comparison of monoclonal and polyclonal antibodies directed against immunoglobulin light and heavy chains in non-Hodgkin's lymphoma. Am J Clin Pathol 1986;85:25–31.
12. Gelb AB, Rouse RV, Dorfman RF, et al. Detection of immunophenotypic abnormalities in paraffin-embedded B-lineage non-Hodgkin's lymphomas. Am J Clin Pathol 1994;102:825–834.
13. Sundaresan M, Rhodes T, Akosa AB. Immunoglobulin heavy chain patterns in reactive lymphadenopathy. J Clin Pathol 1991;44:753–755.
14. Winchester RJ, Kunkel HG. The human Ia system. Adv Immunol 1979;28:221–292.
15. Anderson KC, Bates MP, Slaughenhoupt BL, et al. Expression of human B cell-associated antigens on leukemias and lymphomas: a model of human B cell differentiation. Blood 1984;63:1424–1433.
16. Deegan MJ. Membrane antigen analysis in the diagnosis of lymphoid leukemias and lymphomas. Differential diagnosis, prognosis as related to immunophenotype, and recommendations for testing. Arch Pathol Lab Med 1989;113:606–618.
17. Kumar S, Green GA, Teruya-Feldstein J, et al. Use of CD23 (BU38) on paraffin sections in the diagnosis of small lymphocytic lymphoma and mantle cell lymphoma. Mod Pathol 1996;9:925–929.
18. Dworzak MN, Fritsch G, Froschl G, et al. Four-color flow cytometric investigation of terminal deoxynucleotidyl transferase-positive lymphoid precursors in pediatric bone marrow: CD79a expression precedes CD19 in early B-cell ontogeny. Blood 1998;92:3203–3209.
19. Garcia CF, Weiss LM, Warnke RA. Small noncleaved cell lymphoma: an immunophenotypic study of 18 cases and comparison with large cell lymphoma. Hum Pathol 1986;17:454–461.
20. Payne CM, Grogan TM, Cromey DW, et al. An ultrastructural morphometric and immunophenotypic evaluation of Burkitt's and Burkitt's-like lymphomas. Lab Invest 1987;57:200–218.
21. McIntosh GG, Lodge AJ, Watson P, et al. NCL-CD10-270: a new monoclonal antibody recognizing CD10 in paraffin-embedded tissue. Am J Pathol 1999;154:77–82.
22. Kaufmann O, Flath B, Spath-Schwalbe E, et al. Immunohistochemical detection of CD10 with monoclonal antibody 56C6 on paraffin sections. Am J Clin Pathol 1999;111:117–122.
23. Spier CM, Grogan TM, Fielder K, et al. Immunophenotypes in "well-differentiated" lymphoproliferative disorders, with emphasis on small lymphocytic lymphoma. Hum Pathol 1986;17:1126–1136.
24. Zukerberg LR, Medeiros LJ, Ferry JA, et al. Diffuse low-grade B-cell lymphomas. Four clinically distinct subtypes defined by a combination of morphologic and immunophenotypic features [see Comments]. Am J Clin Pathol 1993;100:373–385.
25. Sebestyen A, Berczi L, Mihalik R, et al. Syndecan-1 (CD138) expression in human non-Hodgkin lymphomas. Br J Haematol 1999;104:412–419.
26. Harris NL, Bhan AK. B-cell neoplasms of the lymphocytic, lymphoplasmacytoid, and plasma cell types: immunohistologic analysis and clinical correlation. Hum Pathol 1985;16:829–837.
27. Jennings CD, Foon KA. Recent advances in flow cytometry: application to the diagnosis of hematologic malignancy. Blood 1997;90:2863–2892.
28. Kaufmann O, Flath B, Spath-Schwalbe E, et al. Immunohistochemical detection of CD5 with monoclonal antibody 4C7 on paraffin sections. Am J Clin Pathol 1997;108:669–673.
29. de Leon ED, Alkan S, Huang JC, et al. Usefulness of an immunohistochemical panel in paraffin-embedded tissues for the differentiation of B-cell non-Hodgkin's lymphomas of small lymphocytes. Mod Pathol 1998;11:1046–1051.
30. Royer HD, Reinherz EL. T lymphocytes: ontogeny, function, and relevance to clinical disorders. N Engl J Med 1987;317:1136–1142.
31. Grogan TM, Fielder K, Rangel C, et al. Peripheral T-cell lymphoma: aggressive disease with heterogeneous immunotypes. Am J Clin Pathol 1985;83:279–288.
32. Weiss LM, Crabtree GS, Rouse RV, et al. Morphologic and immunologic characterization of 50 peripheral T-cell lymphomas. Am J Pathol 1985;118:316–324.
33. Chott A, Augustin I, Wrba F, et al. Peripheral T-cell lymphomas: a clinicopathologic study of 75 cases. Hum Pathol 1990;21:1117–1125.

34. Borowitz MJ, Reichert TA, Brynes RK, et al. The phenotypic diversity of peripheral T-cell lymphomas: the Southeastern Cancer Study Group experience. Hum Pathol 1986;17:567–574.
35. Picker LJ, Weiss LM, Medeiros LJ, et al. Immunophenotypic criteria for the diagnosis of non-Hodgkin's lymphoma. Am J Pathol 1987;128:181–201.
36. Norton AJ, Ramsay AD, Smith SH, et al. Monoclonal antibody (UCHL1) that recognises normal and neoplastic T cells in routinely fixed tissues. J Clin Pathol 1986;39:399–405.
37. Segal GH, Stoler MH, Tubbs RR. The "CD43 only" phenotype. An aberrant, nonspecific immunophenotype requiring comprehensive analysis for lineage resolution. Am J Clin Pathol 1992;97: 861–865.
38. Weiss LM, Bindl JM, Picozzi VJ, et al. Lymphoblastic lymphoma: an immunophenotype study of 26 cases with comparison to T cell acute lymphoblastic leukemia. Blood 1986;67:474–478.
39. Cossman J, Chused TM, Fisher RI, et al. Diversity of immunological phenotypes of lymphoblastic lymphoma. Cancer Res 1983;43:4486–4490.
40. Perlman EJ, Dickman PS, Askin FB, et al. Ewing's sarcoma—routine diagnostic utilization of MIC2 analysis: a Pediatric Oncology Group/Children's Cancer Group Intergroup Study. Hum Pathol 1994;25:304–307.
41. Soslow RA, Bhargava V, Warnke RA. MIC2, TdT, bcl-2, and CD34 expression in paraffin-embedded high-grade lymphoma/acute lymphoblastic leukemia distinguishes between distinct clinicopathologic entities. Hum Pathol 1997;28:1158–1165.
42. Malisius R, Merz H, Heinz B, et al. Constant detection of CD2, CD3, CD4, and CD5 in fixed and paraffin-embedded tissue using the peroxidase-mediated deposition of biotin-tyramide. J Histochem Cytochem 1997;45:1665–1672.
43. Talle MA, Rao PE, Westberg E, et al. Patterns of antigenic expression on human monocytes as defined by monoclonal antibodies. Cell Immunol 1983;78:83–99.
44. Pulford KA, Rigney EM, Micklem KJ, et al. KP1: a new monoclonal antibody that detects a monocyte/macrophage-associated antigen in routinely processed tissue sections. J Clin Pathol 1989;42:414–421.
45. Wood GS, Turner RR, Shiurba RA, et al. Human dendritic cells and macrophages. *In situ* immunophenotypic definition of subsets that exhibit specific morphologic and microenvironmental characteristics. Am J Pathol 1985;119:73–82.
46. Weiss LM, Beckstead JH, Warnke RA, et al. Leu-6-expressing cells in lymph nodes: dendritic cells phenotypically similar to interdigitating cells. Hum Pathol 1986;17:179–184.
47. Stein H, Bonk A, Tolksdorf G, et al. Immunohistologic analysis of the organization of normal lymphoid tissue and non-Hodgkin's lymphomas. J Histochem Cytochem 1980;28:746–760.
48. Gerdes J, Stein H, Mason DY, et al. Human dendritic reticulum cells of lymphoid follicles: their antigenic profile and their identification as multinucleated giant cells. Virchows Arch B Cell Pathol Mol Pathol 1983;42:161–172.
49. Hofman FM, Yanagihara E, Byrne B, et al. Analysis of B-cell antigens in normal reactive lymphoid tissue using four B-cell monoclonal antibodies. Blood 1983;62:775–783.
50. Bailey DJ, Rainey M, Habeshaw JA. Immunoperoxidase analysis of B and T cell populations in human lymphoid follicles. Adv Exp Med Biol 1982;149:809–816.
51. Petrasch S, Stein H, Kosco MH, et al. Follicular dendritic cells in non-Hodgkin lymphomas: localisation, characterisation and pathophysiological aspects. Eur J Cancer 1991;27:1052–1056.
52. Parwaresch MR, Radzun HJ, Hansmann ML, et al. Monoclonal antibody Ki-M4 specifically recognizes human dendritic reticulum cells (follicular dendritic cells) and their possible precursor in blood. Blood 1983;62:585–590.
53. Stein H, Gerdes J, Mason DY. The normal and malignant germinal centre. Clin Haematol 1982;11:531–559.
54. Rouse RV, Weissman IL, Ledbetter JA, et al. Expression of T cell antigens by cells in mouse and human primary and secondary follicles. Adv Exp Med Biol 1982;149:751–756.
55. Si L, Roscoe G, Whiteside TL. Selective distribution and quantitation of T-lymphocyte subsets in germinal centers of human tonsils. Definition by use of monoclonal antibodies. Arch Pathol Lab Med 1983;107:228–231.
56. Hsu SM, Cossman J, Jaffe ES. Lymphocyte subsets in normal human lymphoid tissues. Am J Clin Pathol 1983;80:21–30.
57. Velardi A, Tilden AB, Millo R, et al. Isolation and characterization of Leu 7+ germinal-center cells with the T helper-cell phenotype and granular lymphocyte morphology. J Clin Immunol 1986;6:205–215.
58. Scoazec JY, Berger F, Magaud JP, et al. The dendritic reticulum cell pattern in B cell lymphomas of the small cleaved, mixed, and large cell types: an immunohistochemical study of 48 cases. Hum Pathol 1989;20:124–131.
59. Harris NL, Data RE. The distribution of neoplastic and normal B-lymphoid cells in nodular lymphomas: use of an immunoperoxidase technique on frozen sections. Hum Pathol 1982;13:610–617.
60. Ngan BY, Chen-Levy Z, Weiss LM, et al. Expression in non-Hodgkin's lymphoma of the bcl-2 protein associated with the t(14;18) chromosomal translocation. N Engl J Med 1988;318: 1638–1644.
61. Dvoretsky P, Wood GS, Levy R, et al. T-lymphocyte subsets in follicular lymphomas compared with those in non-neoplastic lymph nodes and tonsils. Hum Pathol 1982;13:618–625.
62. Ratech H, Sheibani K, Nathwani BN, et al. Immunoarchitecture of the "pseudofollicles" of well-differentiated (small) lymphocytic lymphoma: a comparison with true follicles [published erratum appears in Hum Pathol 1988;19:495]. Hum Pathol 1988;19: 89–94.
63. Peters JP, Rademakers LH, Roelofs JM, et al. Distribution of dendritic reticulum cells in follicular lymphoma and reactive hyperplasia. Light microscopic identification and general morphology. Virchows Arch B Cell Pathol Mol Pathol 1984;46:215–228.
64. Carbone A, Poletti A, Manconi R, et al. Heterogeneous *in situ* immunophenotyping of follicular dendritic reticulum cells in malignant lymphomas of B-cell origin. Cancer 1987;60:2919–2926.
65. Burns BF, Colby TV, Dorfman RF. Differential diagnostic features of nodular L & H Hodgkin's disease, including progressive transformation of germinal centers. Am J Surg Pathol 1984;8: 253–261.
66. Dorfman DM, Shahsafaei A. Dendritic reticulum cell immunoreactivity for low-affinity nerve growth factor receptor in malignant lymphomas. Mod Pathol 1996;9:959–965.
67. Said JW. The immunohistochemistry of Hodgkin's disease. Semin Diagn Pathol 1992;9:265–271.
68. Chang KL, Arber DA, Weiss LM. CD20: a review. Appl Immunohistochem 1996;4:1–15.
69. Pinkus GS, Pinkus JL, Langhoff E, et al. Fascin, a sensitive new marker for Reed–Sternberg cells of Hodgkin's disease. Evidence for a dendritic or B cell derivation? Am J Pathol 1997;150:543–562.
70. Delabie J, Bilbe G, Bruggen J, et al. Restin in Hodgkin's disease and anaplastic large cell lymphoma. Leuk Lymphoma 1993;12: 21–26.
71. Kamel OW, Gelb AB, Shibuya RB, et al. Leu 7 (CD57) reactivity distinguishes nodular lymphocyte predominance Hodgkin's disease from nodular sclerosing Hodgkin's disease, T-cell- rich B-cell lymphoma and follicular lymphoma. Am J Pathol 1993;142: 541–546.

7

FLOW CYTOMETRY

FLOW CYTOMETRY OF LYMPH NODES

The most important indicator of B-cell neoplasia, immunoglobulin light chain restriction, is more sensitively evaluated by flow cytometry of cell suspensions than by immunoperoxidase staining of frozen tissue sections (1,2). Flow cytometry can reveal complex lymphoma phenotypes by simultaneously measuring light scatter and multiple antigens on each cell (3). Typical lymphoma panels contain between 10 and 20 antibodies (4) (Table 7.1). However, few laboratories establish their own lymph node reference ranges (5) because a well-designed antibody panel creates an array of positive and negative internal controls from mutually exclusive cell populations. Flow cytometry for lymphoma immunophenotyping requires attention to the many details of specimen collection and storage, clones of antibodies, immunofluorescence staining, instrumentation, data analysis and interpretation (6), reporting (7), and quality assurance (8,9). Because flow cytometry necessarily destroys tissue architecture, it introduces a risk for sampling error (10). Examining a cytospin or smear prepared from the lymph node cell suspension helps confirm that the sample is appropriate, but in fibrotic or necrotic samples, histologic sections are more informative.

B-CELL CLONALITY

To recognize foreign antigens, mature B cells must express membrane-bound cell surface immunoglobulin (sIg) molecules containing both heavy and light chains (11). An individual B cell exclusively synthesizes either κ or λ light chains. Because the normal κ/λ ratio is approximately 3:1, marked skewing of this ratio implies an excessively proliferating single B cell yielding a monoclonal population. Multicolor flow cytometry improves the accuracy of the measurement of the κ/λ ratio. Measuring sIg on cells simultaneously expressing a pan-B-cell marker (CD19 or CD20) improves the background by eliminating monocytes, which can nonspecifically bind sIg via their Fc receptors, and T cells (Fig. 7.1). Visually inspecting one-dimensional histograms or two-dimensional plots or calculating simple κ/λ ratios (12) usually suffices to diagnose polyclonal versus monoclonal B-cell populations. By transforming all κ/λ ratios to maximum ratios—that is, $R_{max} = \max(\kappa/\lambda, \lambda/\kappa)$—so that all resulting ratios have a value of at least 1, sIg light chain restriction data can be used to establish a laboratory range for improving quality assurance and comparing results between laboratories (13) (Fig. 7.2). The Kolmogorov-Smirnov statistical test helps determine B-cell clonality by analyzing differences in κ and λ fluorescence curve shape and peak position (14). It is extremely sensitive but may yield too many false-positive results.

LOW-GRADE B-CELL LYMPHOMAS/CHRONIC LEUKEMIAS

Low-grade non-Hodgkin lymphomas and chronic leukemias were historically separated because their presumed lymph node and bone marrow origins were thought to predict unique biological behavior. However, flow cytometry reveals immunophenotypic identity between low-grade lymphoma cells circulating in peripheral blood and equivalent chronic leukemia cells infiltrating lymph node (15,16). The sIg level plus specific B-cell antigens distinguish B-cell small lymphocytic lymphoma/chronic lymphocytic leukemia (SLL/CLL), mantle cell lymphoma (MCL), follicle center lymphoma (FL), lymphoplasmacytoid lymphoma (LYP), marginal zone (monocytoid) lymphoma (MZL), prolymphocytic leukemia (PLL), and hairy cell leukemia (HCL) (17,18).

During physiologic B-cell maturation, the sIg density changes. The hypermutator mechanism, which enhances antibody affinity by introducing single nucleotide exchanges in the Ig variable region, operates when B cells pass through the germinal center. Results of somatic mutational analysis of the variable region of B-cell lymphoma antigen receptor DNA sequences correlate with the sIg level in pregerminal center versus postgerminal center B cells (11). Levels of sIg in developing normal B cells generally parallel those in equivalent B-cell lymphomas/chronic leukemias: negative to dim sIg, post-bone marrow, early B cells correspond to SLL/CLL; intermediate sIg, antigen-inexperienced B cells (located in primary follicles and secondary follicle

TABLE 7.1. CLUSTERS OF DIFFERENTIATION

Cluster of differentiation	Distribution	Antigen/Function	MW × 10^{-3}
CD1a	Cortical thymocytes, Langerhans cells, interdigitating cells, B subset	Associated with β_2 microglobulin	49
CD2	T cells, NK subset	CD58 receptor	50
CD3	Thymocytes and mature T cells	T-cell antigen receptor complex	20–30
CD4	Helper/inducer T cells, monocytes	Binds MHC class II antigen/HIV-1 receptor	55
CD5	T cells, B-cell subset, B CLL		67
CD6	Medullary thymocytes, mature T cells, B-cell subset, brain	CD166 receptor	120
CD7	Earliest T-lineage marker, most T cells, NK cells, ALL, 10% AML		40
CD8	Suppressor/cytotoxic T cells, NK subsets	Binds MHC class 1 antigen	32
CD9	Pre-B cells, monocytes, platelets	Associates with CD63, CD81, and CD29 integrins	24
CD10	Early B and T precursors, pre-B ALL, granulocytes, kidney epithelium	Neutral endopeptidase, CALLA	100
CD11a	Lymphocytes, granulocytes, monocytes	Combines with CD 18 (LFA-1) to bind CD50, CD54, and CD102 ligands	180
CD11b	Myeloid, NK cells	Combines with CD18 (Mac-1): Complement receptor 3	155
CD11c	Monocytes/myeloid, NK, T subset	Complement receptor 4	150
CD13	Monocytes, myeloid	Aminopeptidase N Coronavirus receptor	150
CD14	Monocytes, langerhans cells, myeloid (low)	LPS complex receptor	55
CD15	Granulocytes, Reed-Sternberg cells, carcinoma	Lewis X (Le^x)	CH0
CD16	NK, granulocytes, macrophages, mast cells, Fetal thymocytes	IgG receptor III (p60)	50–70
CD18	Leukocytes (platelets negative)	β_2 integrin subunit	95
CD19	B-lineage cells (but not plasma cells)	CD19/CD21/CD81/Leu-13 signaling complex	95
CD20	B cells		37/32
CD21	Mature B cells, follicular dendritic cells	Complement receptor 2 Epstein-Barr virus receptor	140
CD22	B cells (not plasma cells)	Binds to sialoglycoconjugates	135
CD23	B cells, monocytes, and other leukocytes	Fc ε receptor II: receptor for IgE (Fc portion), CD21, CD11b, CD11c	45
CD24	B cells (not plasma cells), granulocytes	Sialoglycoprotein	41/38
CD25	T and B subsets, activated T cells	IL-2 receptor (p55)	55
CD26	Thymocytes, T subset, epithelial cells	Dipeptidyl peptidase IV Adenosine deaminase binding protein	110
CD29a	Leucocytes, platelets	Heterodimerizes with α-integrin subunit	130
CD30	Activated B and T cells, Reed-Sternberg cells	Binds to CD153	120
CD32	Monocytes, neutrophils, B cells, platelets	Binds aggregated IgG (FcRII)	40
CD33	Myelomonocytic lineage (not stem cells or neutrophils)	Binds to sialoglycoconjugates	67
CD34	Progenitor cell, endothelial cells	Binds to selectins CD62L and CD62E	105–120
CD35	B cells, T subset, monocytes, granulocytes, RBCs	Complement receptor 1 (CR1)	220
CD37	Mature B cells (not pre-B or plasma cells)	Associates with MHC class 11, CD19, CD21	40–52

continues

TABLE 7.1. CONTINUED

Cluster of differentiation	Distribution	Antigen/Function	MW × 10^{-3}
CD38	NK, B, T subsets, plasma cells	Cyclic ADP–ribose synthesis and hydrolysis	45
CD40	Mature B cells (not plasma cells)	TNFR superfamily member, binds to CD154 Germinal center formation	48
CD41	Megakaryocytes, platelets	Integrin αIIb subunit of gpIIb/IIIa complex	120
CD42a	Megakaryocytes, platelets	gpIX	23
CD43	T cells, neutrophils, activated B cells	Leukosialin (mucinlike extracellular domain)	95
CD44	Hematopoietic and nonhematopoietic cells	Lymphocyte homing receptor, Hermes antigen	80–95
CD45	All hematopoietic cells except RBCs	Leukocyte common antigen, multiple isoforms	180–220
CD45RA	Most T, B, NK cells	High-molecular-weight CD45 isoform(s)	205–220
CD45RO	Activated/memory T cells	Low-molecular-weight CD45 isoform	180
CD54	Activated B and T, macrophages, other cells	CD11a/18 (LFA-1) ligand, Rhinovirus receptor	85
CD56	NK, T subset	Neural cell adhesion molecule (NCAM)	140–220
CD57	NK, T subsets	Oligosaccharide; binds to L- and P-selectins	CHO
CD61	Megakaryocytes, platelets, monocytes	Integrin β_3 subunit, gpIIIa	110
CD62L	Most B and naive T cells, monocytes, NK	Lymphocyte homing to lymph nodes/Peyer patches	150
CD69	Activated lymphocytes		28/32
CD71	Proliferating cells	Transferrin receptor	90
CD79a,b	Pre-B and mature B cells (not plasma cells)	B-cell antigen receptor (mIg) complex	33/40
CD95	Activated lymphocytes, Monocytes, Neutrophils	Fas, Apo-1, apoptotic cells	42
CD103	Intraepithelial lymphocytes, thymus, spleen	Integrin αE subunit, HML-1 antigen Associates with Ig heavy chains	150–25
CD117	Hematopoietic precursors mast cells	c-kit, stem cell factor	145
CD138	Plasma cells (not mature B cells)	Extracellular matrix receptor, syndecan-1	20

NK, natural killer; MHC, major histocompatibility complex; B CLL, B-cell chronic lymphocytic leukemia; ALL, acute lymphoblastic leukemia; AML, acute myeloblastic leukemia; CALLA, common acute lymphoblastic leukemia antigen; RBC, red blood cell; ADP, adenosine diphosphate; LPS, lipopolysaccharide; CHO, carbohydrate; TNFR, tumor necrosis factor receptor.

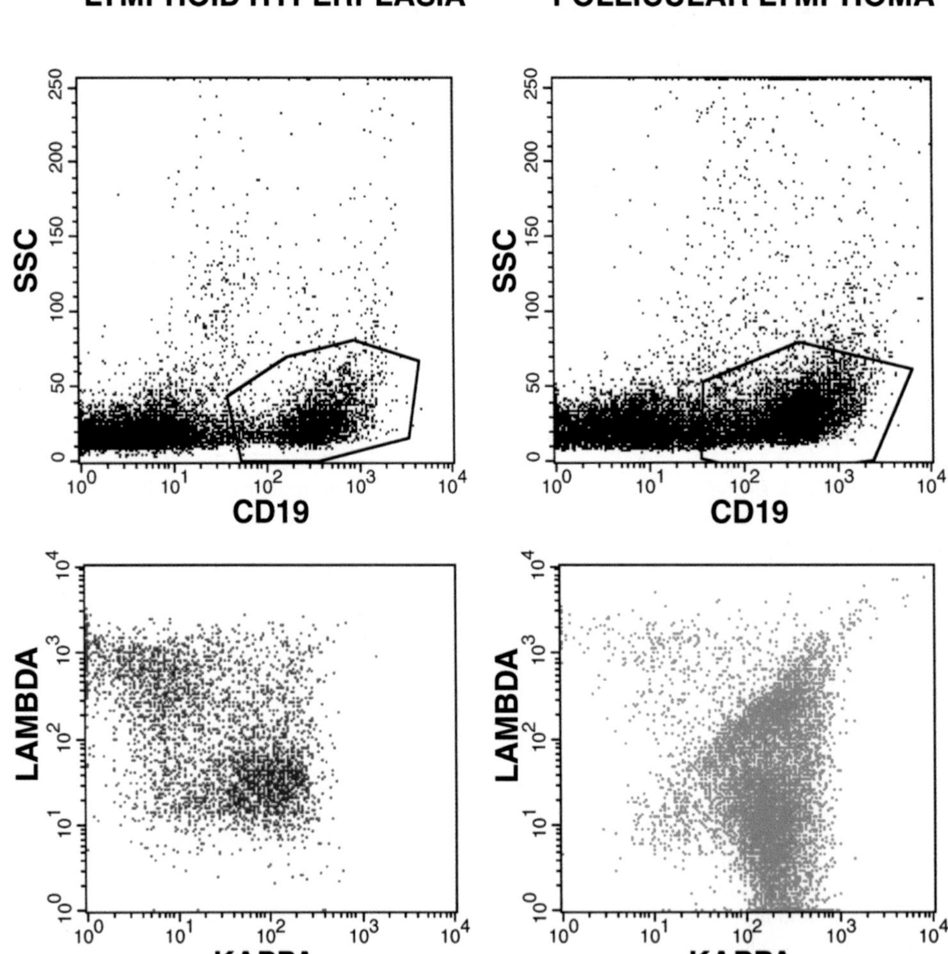

FIGURE 7.1. Lymphoid hyperplasia (LH) versus follicular lymphoma (FL). In LH, gating the CD19+ B cells (*upper left*) reveals a polyclonal population of κ+ and λ+ cells (*lower left*). In FL, gating the CD19+ B cells (*upper right*) reveals a monoclonal population of κ+ cells (*lower right*). A prominent diagonal population probably represents serum immunoglobulin (κ+ and λ+) nonspecifically bound by Fc receptors on FL B cells (*lower right*). *SSC,* side scatter (right angle light scatter).

mantle zones) correspond to MCL; postgerminal center, memory B cells with bright sIg correspond to PLL; mature B cells or preplasma cells with negative, dim, or bright sIg and variable cytoplasmic Ig correspond to LYP, MZL, and HCL. Paradoxically, reactive germinal centers express dim sIg, but FL expresses bright sIg.

Specific B-cell antigens (Table 7.1) further refine the flow cytometric analysis of the low-grade B-cell lymphomas/chronic leukemias (Fig. 7.3):CD5+ (SLL/CLL and MCL); CD10+ (FL); bright CD11c+ (PLL and HCL); CD23+ (SLL/CLL); CD25+ (HCL); CD103+ (HCL); bright FMC7+ (PLL and HCL) (17–21). CLL/SLL expresses low levels of CD20 but high levels of CD19 (Fig. 7.3); most other B-cell lymphomas express high levels of CD20 (22). FMC7 intensity may be a surrogate CD20 indicator (21). The presence of CD23 in CD5+ B-cell lymphoproliferative disorders discriminates SLL/CLL (CD23+) from MCL (CD23−) (23). About one-third of FLs produce both CD10 and CD23 (24). Because no single marker is 100% specific, a low level of antigen expression should be interpreted in the context of a full antibody panel with particular attention to lymphocyte gating (25).

PERIPHERAL T-CELL LYMPHOMA

Unfortunately, flow cytometry cannot determine T-cell clonality as it does B-cell clonality. The numerous T-cell antigen receptor (TCR) αβ or γδ gene combinations would require a panel of anti-TCR reagents unmanageably large for a clinical

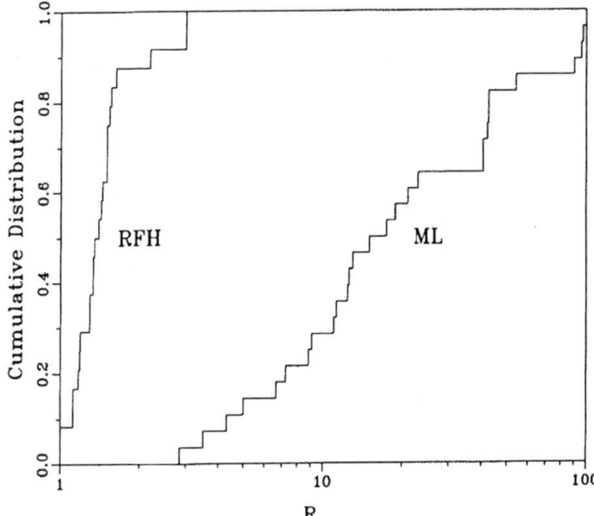

FIGURE 7.2. Cumulative distribution of R_{max} values of reactive follicular hyperplasia (*RFH*) and B-cell malignant lymphoma (*ML*). This is a statistic for evaluating surface immunoglobulin light chain restriction by transforming all κ/λ ratios to maximum ratios—that is, R_{max} = max (κ/λ, λ/κ). All resulting ratios have a value of at least 1. (From Ratech H, Litwin S. Surface immunoglobulin light chain restriction in B-cell non-Hodgkin malignant lymphomas. Am J Clin Pathol 1989;91:583–586, with permission.)

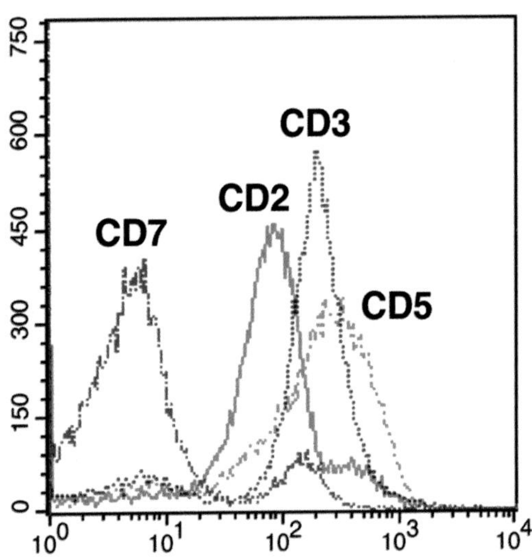

FIGURE 7.4. Pan-T-cell markers in peripheral T-cell lymphoma. Nearly complete expression of CD2, CD3, and CD5, but CD7 is essentially absent. Very dim CD7 fluorescence overlaps negative control region defined by using an irrelevant antibody (not shown). See Table 7.1 for a description of the cell surface markers.

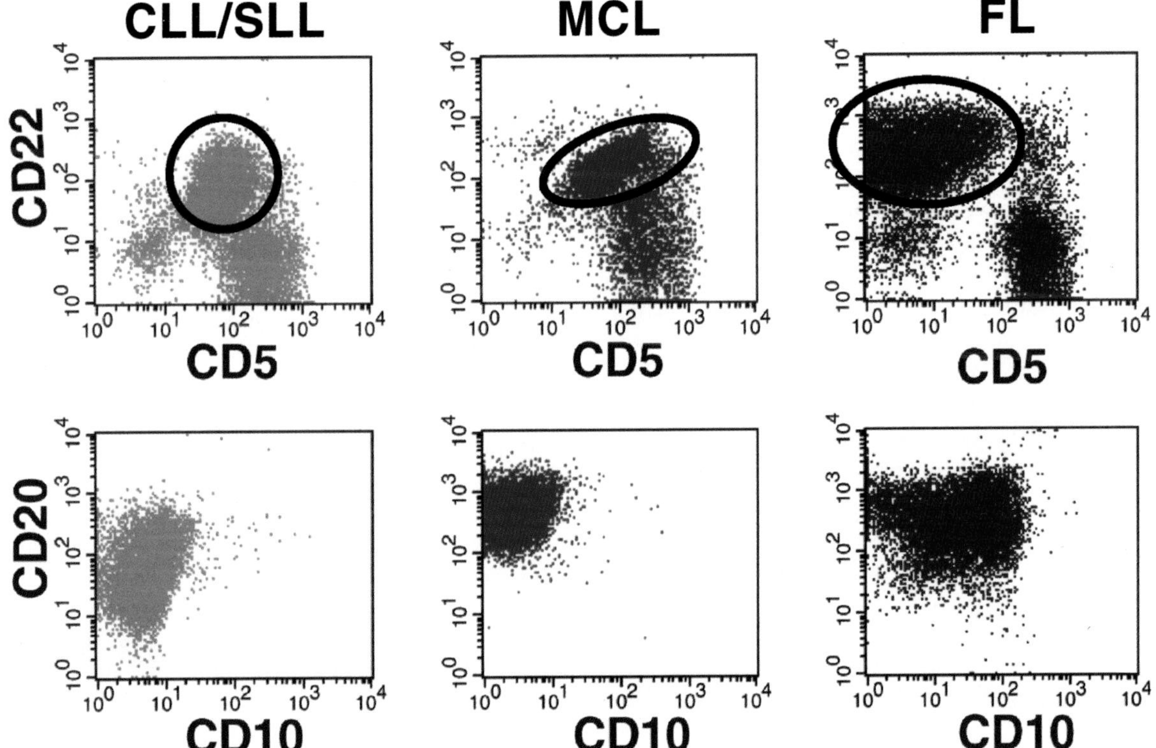

FIGURE 7.3. Immunophenotypic differences in three B-cell lymphomas with small cell morphology: B-cell chronic lymphocytic leukemia/small lymphocytic lymphoma (*CLL/SLL*) versus mantle cell lymphoma (*MCL*) versus follicular lymphoma (*FL*). The lymph node samples in the upper panel were gated in the lymphocyte region based on forward scatter versus side scatter light properties; they include B cells, T cells, and monocytes. Neoplastic B cells are identified within ellipses in the upper panels. Both CLL/SLL and MCL express CD5, but FL does not (*upper panels*). Normal T cells express CD5 but do not express CD22 (*upper panels*). CD22+ B-cell CLL/SLL expresses dimmer CD5 than do CD22− non-neoplastic T cells (*upper left*). The lymph node samples in the lower panel were gated in the B-cell region based on CD19+ fluorescence versus low side scatter; they include only B cells. FL expresses CD10, but neither CLL/SLL nor MCL does (*lower panels*). CLL/SLL expresses CD20 and CD22 less brightly than either MCL or FL. See Table 7.1 for a description of the cell surface markers.

laboratory. For this reason, the phenotypic diagnosis of T-cell neoplasia relies indirectly on aberrant T-cell antigen expression: unusual combinations; loss of pan-T-cell marker(s) (CD2, CD3, CD5, or CD7) (Fig. 7.4); markedly skewed ratios of helper (CD4+) to suppressor (CD8+) cells; activation markers (CD25, CD30, HLA-DR) (17,26).

ACUTE LEUKEMIA

Enlarged lymph nodes infiltrated by acute leukemia are occasionally submitted for a "lymphoma workup," particularly in patients without a diagnosis and without circulating blasts (i.e., aleukemic leukemia). If the major cell population expresses few or no lymphoid markers, then one may suspect acute myeloblastic leukemia (AML) infiltrating lymph node because standard non-Hodgkin lymphoma flow cytometry antibody panels do not recognize granulocytic, monocytic, erythrocytic, or megakaryocytic progenitors. Clues to acute lymphoblastic leukemia (ALL) infiltrating lymph node include positive B-cell antigens without sIg, which suggest B-precursor or pre-B ALL, and positive pan-T-cell antigens without surface CD3 or simultaneous CD4 and CD8, which suggest T-cell ALL. The differential diagnosis also includes non-Hodgkin lymphoma without sIg (about 10% of low-grade and 18% of high-grade B-cell lymphomas) (27) and peripheral T-cell lymphoma. The phenotypic discrimination of ALL from non-Hodgkin lymphoma often requires an analysis of the earliest maturation markers, such as terminal deoxynucleotidyl transferase (TdT) and CD34 (28).

If unstained lymph node cells have been saved, then an acute leukemia antibody screen can supplement the initial analysis (16,29). However, residual small lymphocytes tend to overlap with blasts in the traditional gating strategy based on forward angle light scatter (FALS; size) versus right angle light scatter (RALS; granularity or complexity). Adding anti-CD45 antibody to each tube as the third (or fourth) color, and using RALS (linear scale) versus CD45 fluorescence (logarithmic scale), improve blast identification (30). Originally described for bone marrow, this method works for lymph node too; the normal lymphocytes expressing bright CD45 and the blasts (or lymphoma cells) expressing dim CD45 resolve well (31). Nonhematopoietic tumors and some ALLs lack CD45 (32). Myelocytic and monocytic cells typically deflect more light perpendicular to the direction of the laser beam (RALS) than do lymphocytes or blasts without granules. Exceptionally, acute promyelocytic leukemia scatters abundant right angle light.

To overcome less than 100% specificity and sensitivity for most antibodies, an ideal acute leukemia panel should contain at least two antibodies per cell lineage. AMLs express the most specific myeloid markers, CD33 and CD13, in 85% to 90% and 75% of cases, respectively (33,34). More than 90% of AMLs express CD13, CD33, or both. Add antimyeloperoxidase (requiring cell permeation) (35) or anti-CD117 (c-kit receptor) antibodies to classify AML with no or minimal differentiation accurately. Sixty-seven percent of AMLs but only 4% of ALLs express CD117 (36). AMLs, French–American–British classification (FAB) M1 or M2, do not usually express monocyte-associated markers CD11b, CD14, or CD36, except for CD14 in a minority of cases (37). In both classic and hypogranular variants of acute promyelocytic leukemia, FAB M3, the promyelocytes phenotypically resemble normal promyelocytes, which lack HLA-DR (38,39). However, 10% of non-M3 AMLs do not express HLA-DR either. Monocytic leukemias, FAB M4 or M5, often express myeloid markers CD13, CD15, and CD33 in addition to monocyte-associated markers CD11b, CD11c, CD14, and CD36. Erythroleukemia, FAB M6, expresses the transferrin receptor CD71, but so do other AMLs and some ALLs (40). Morphologically recognizable basophilic erythroblasts express glycophorin A (41). Acute megakaryoblastic leukemia, FAB M7, expresses megakaryocyte/platelet glycoproteins (gp) IIb/IIIa, composed of integrin αIIb subunit (CD41) and integrin β^3 subunit (CD61), and gpIb (CD42) (42,43). Correlating cytospins or smears with flow cytometry data helps eliminate false-positive results caused by platelets adhering to blasts (44).

Leukemia markers originally thought to be highly specific may react with more than one cell lineage. For example, antibody My4 (CD14) stains the myelomonocytic lineage and a number of B-cell non-Hodgkin lymphomas (45). CD56, neural cell adhesion molecule (NCAM), detects natural killer cells and a minimal differentiation AML subtype expressing CD33 and CD56 only. CD38 is found on early thymocytes, activated T cells, plasma cells, and AML. CD4, major histocompatibility class II antigen receptor, occurs on helper T lymphocytes, monocytes, and monocytic leukemia. CD7, pan-T-cell marker, resides on 10% to 20% of AMLs of all subtypes, but M7 has a relatively high proportion of CD7+ cases (46,47).

During normal lymphopoiesis, fetal and adult bone marrow B cells sequentially acquire various surface, nuclear, and cytoplasmic markers. The physiologic B-cell developmental stages correspond to some, but not all, of the numerous B-lineage ALL phenotypes (48,49). For practical purposes, hematopathologists classify B-lineage ALL as B-precursor, pre-B, or B-cell (Burkitt type) (16). The most diagnostically useful surface antigens, from early to late expression, include HLA-DR, CD34, CD19, CD10, CD20, and CD22. Nuclear TdT (50), cytoplasmic CD22 (35), and cytoplasmic Ig μ heavy chain (51) are also useful markers. B-precursor ALL, equivalent to the earliest B cells, expresses TdT, CD34, or both; pre-B ALL, an intermediate stage, synthesizes cytoplasmic Ig μ heavy chain; B-cell ALL (Burkitt type), the most mature phenotype, expresses surface Ig heavy and light chains (16).

Almost all T-ALLs express CD2, CD5, and CD7 (52–54). The other T-cell antigens help define thymic stages but do not contribute additional prognostic or diagnostic information. Fewer than one-third of T-ALLs expresses surface CD3 (54–56), an important subunit of the TCR. However, more than 95% of T-ALLs or lymphoblastic lymphomas synthesize cytoplasmic CD3 (35,57,58). Cytoplasmic CD3 is produced before CD3 appears on the cell surface and before the TCR genes productively rearrange (59–62). Misinterpreting the significance of cytoplasmic CD3 led some early investigators to conclude that T-ALL is phenotypically more immature than lymphoblastic lymphoma (58,63). CD7 may be the earliest T-cell antigen, but it is also expressed in 5% to 10% of AMLs (46,47). Similarly, CD2 may be found in 5% of AMLs (64). T-ALL can also express so-called myeloid associated markers CD11b, CD11c, and CD15 (20% to 60% of cases), CD10 (CALLA) and/or HLA-DR (10% to 40% of cases), and CD34 (10% to 20% of cases) (52,65–67). T-ALLs express either the α/β TCR (95%) or the γ/δ TCR (5%) (68–70), which is similar to the TCR subtypes found in normal peripheral blood T cells.

DNA PLOIDY AND CELL CYCLE

Flow cytometric DNA ploidy and cell cycle analysis with use of an argon laser depends on double-stranded DNA stoichiometrically binding the fluorescent dye propidium iodide. The fluorescence of the G0/G1 phase of the cell cycle is one-half as bright as that of the G2+M phase, reflecting the linear difference between 2N versus 4N, where 1N equals haploid DNA content. During normal DNA synthesis, the S phase spans values between 2N and 4N. The DNA index, a measure of DNA ploidy, compares an abnormal, neoplastic G0/G1 DNA peak with a normal G0/G1 DNA peak derived from either an internal standard (non-neoplastic lymphocytes in the sample) or an external standard (chicken or trout cells added to the sample).

The S-phase measurement of proliferative activity correlates with lymphoma grade (71–74) and has been reported to predict clinical outcome (75–78). However, neither S phase nor aneuploidy added any additional prognostic information to the International Index (79) in a large flow cytometric study of 242 uniformly staged and treated patients with diffuse, aggressive non-Hodgkin lymphoma (80). Apoptotic cells can also be enumerated with flow cytometry after free DNA ends have been labeled with fluorescent nucleotides (81). Although apoptosis also correlates with histologic grade (82), it does not predict survival (83). The clinical relevance of aneuploidy remains unclear, although it is more frequent in intermediate- and high-grade than in low-grade lymphomas (84–87) and more common in B-cell than in T-cell non-Hodgkin lymphomas (88–90).

REFERENCES

1. Witzig TE, Banks PM, Stenson MJ, et al. Rapid immunotyping of B-cell non-Hodgkin's lymphomas by flow cytometry. A comparison with the standard frozen-section method. Am J Clin Pathol 1990;94:280–286.
2. Biesemier KW, Dent GA, Pryzwansky KB, et al. A comparative study of frozen-section immunoperoxidase and flow cytometry for immunophenotypic analysis of lymph node biopsies. Clin Diagn Lab Immunol 1994;1:299–303.
3. Ichinohasama R, DeCoteau JF, Myers J, et al. Three-color flow cytometry in the diagnosis of malignant lymphoma based on the comparative cell morphology of lymphoma cells and reactive lymphocytes. Leukemia 1997;11:1891–1903.
4. Hassett J, Parker J. Laboratory practices in reporting flow cytometry phenotyping results for leukemia/lymphoma specimens: results of a survey. Cytometry 1995;22:264–281; discussion 330.
5. McCoy JP Jr, Overton WR. A survey of current practices in clinical flow cytometry. Am J Clin Pathol 1996;106:82–86.
6. Borowitz MJ, Bray R, Gascoyne R, et al. U.S.–Canadian consensus recommendations on the immunophenotypic analysis of hematologic neoplasia by flow cytometry: data analysis and interpretation. Cytometry 1997;30:236–244.
7. Braylan RC, Atwater SK, Diamond L, et al. U.S.–Canadian consensus recommendations on the immunophenotypic analysis of hematologic neoplasia by flow cytometry: data reporting. Cytometry 1997;30:245–248.
8. Rothe G, Schmitz G. Consensus protocol for the flow cytometric immunophenotyping of hematopoietic malignancies. Working Group on Flow Cytometry and Image Analysis. Leukemia 1996;10:877–895.
9. National Committee for Clinical Laboratory Standards. Clinical applications of flow cytometry: quality assurance and immunophenotyping of lymphocytes; approved guideline, vol. 18. Wayne, PA: National Committee for Clinical Laboratory Standards, 1998:62.
10. Hanson CA. Immunophenotyping of hematologic malignant conditions: to flow or not to flow? [Editorial]. Am J Clin Pathol 1991;96:295–298.
11. Kuppers R, Klein U, Hansmann ML, et al. Cellular origin of human B-cell lymphomas. N Engl J Med 1999;341:1520–1529.
12. Geary WA, Frierson HF, Innes DJ, et al. Quantitative criteria for clonality in the diagnosis of B-cell non-Hodgkin's lymphoma by flow cytometry. Mod Pathol 1993;6:155–161.
13. Ratech H, Litwin S. Surface immunoglobulin light chain restriction in B-cell non-Hodgkin's malignant lymphomas [published erratum appears in Am J Clin Pathol 1989;92:560]. Am J Clin Pathol 1989;91:583–586.
14. Weinberg DS, Pinkus GS, Ault KA. Cytofluorometric detection of B cell clonal excess: a new approach to the diagnosis of B cell lymphoma. Blood 1984;63:1080–1087.
15. Harris NL, Jaffe ES, Stein H, et al. A revised European–American classification of lymphoid neoplasms: a proposal from the International Lymphoma Study Group [see Comments]. Blood 1994;84:1361–1392.
16. Jennings CD, Foon KA. Recent advances in flow cytometry: application to the diagnosis of hematologic malignancy. Blood 1997;90:2863–2892.
17. Tbakhi A, Edinger M, Myles J, et al. Flow cytometric immunophenotyping of non-Hodgkin's lymphomas and related disorders. Cytometry 1996;25:113–124.
18. Tworek JA, Singleton TP, Schnitzer B, et al. Flow cytometric and immunohistochemical analysis of small lymphocytic lymphoma, mantle cell lymphoma, and plasmacytoid small lymphocytic lymphoma. Am J Clin Pathol 1998;110:582–589.

19. Huh YO, Pugh WC, Kantarjian HM, et al. Detection of subgroups of chronic B-cell leukemias by FMC7 monoclonal antibody. Am J Clin Pathol 1994;101:283–289.
20. Almasri NM, Iturraspe JA, Braylan RC. CD10 expression in follicular lymphoma and large cell lymphoma is different from that of reactive lymph node follicles. Arch Pathol Lab Med 1998;122:539–544.
21. Hubl W, Iturraspe J, Braylan RC. FMC7 antigen expression on normal and malignant B-cells can be predicted by expression of CD20 [see Comments]. Cytometry 1998;34:71–74.
22. Almasri NM, Duque RE, Iturraspe J, et al. Reduced expression of CD20 antigen as a characteristic marker for chronic lymphocytic leukemia. Am J Hematol 1992;40:259–263.
23. Kilo MN, Dorfman DM. The utility of flow cytometric immunophenotypic analysis in the distinction of small lymphocytic lymphoma/chronic lymphocytic leukemia from mantle cell lymphoma. Am J Clin Pathol 1996;105:451–457.
24. Kaleem Z, White G, Vollmer RT. Critical analysis and diagnostic usefulness of limited immunophenotyping of B-cell non-Hodgkin lymphomas by flow cytometry. Am J Clin Pathol 2001;115:136–142.
25. Hoffkes HG, Schmidtke G, Schmucker U, et al. Lymphocyte gating of peripheral blood in patients with leukemic low-grade non-Hodgkin's lymphoma by multiparametric flow cytometry. Eur J Med Res 1996;1:215–222.
26. Little JV, Foucar K, Horvath A, et al. Flow cytometric analysis of lymphoma and lymphoma-like disorders [published erratum appears in Semin Diagn Pathol 1989;6:313]. Semin Diagn Pathol 1989;6:37–54.
27. de Martini RM, Turner RR, Boone DC, et al. Lymphocyte immunophenotyping of B-cell lymphomas: a flow cytometric analysis of neoplastic and nonneoplastic cells in 271 cases. Clin Immunol Immunopathol 1988;49:365–379.
28. Diamond LW, Nguyen DT, Andreeff M, et al. A knowledge-based system for the interpretation of flow cytometry data in leukemias and lymphomas. Cytometry 1994;17:266–273.
29. General Haematology Task Force of BCSH. Immunophenotyping in the diagnosis of acute leukaemias. J Clin Pathol 1994;47:777–781.
30. Borowitz MJ, Guenther KL, Shults KE, et al. Immunophenotyping of acute leukemia by flow cytometric analysis. Use of CD45 and right-angle light scatter to gate on leukemic blasts in three-color analysis. Am J Clin Pathol 1993;100:534–540.
31. Sun T, Sangaline R, Ryder J, et al. Gating strategy for immunophenotyping of leukemia and lymphoma. Am J Clin Pathol 1997;108:152–157.
32. Rainer RO, Hodges L, Seltzer GT. CD 45 gating correlates with bone marrow differential. Cytometry 1995;22:139–145.
33. Griffin JD, Davis R, Nelson DA, et al. Use of surface marker analysis to predict outcome of adult acute myeloblastic leukemia. Blood 1986;68:1232–1241.
34. Griffin JD, Linch D, Sabbath K, et al. A monoclonal antibody reactive with normal and leukemic human myeloid progenitor cells. Leuk Res 1984;8:521–534.
35. Drach D, Drach J, Glassl H, et al. Flow cytometric detection of cytoplasmic antigens in acute leukemias: implications for lineage assignment. Leuk Res 1993;17:455–461.
36. Bene MC, Bernier M, Casasnovas RO, et al. The reliability and specificity of c-kit for the diagnosis of acute myeloid leukemias and undifferentiated leukemias. The European Group for the Immunological Classification of Leukemias (EGIL). Blood 1998;92:596–599.
37. Matutes E, Rodriguez B, Polli N, et al. Characterization of myeloid leukemias with monoclonal antibodies 3C5 and MY9. Hematol Oncol 1985;3:179–186.
38. Griffin JD, Mayer RJ, Weinstein HJ, et al. Surface marker analysis of acute myeloblastic leukemia: identification of differentiation-associated phenotypes. Blood 1983;62:557–563.
39. van der Reijden HJ, van Rhenen DJ, Lansdorp PM, et al. A comparison of surface marker analysis and FAB classification in acute myeloid leukemia. Blood 1983;61:443–448.
40. Goding JW, Burns GF. Monoclonal antibody OKT-9 recognizes the receptor for transferrin on human acute lymphocytic leukemia cells. J Immunol 1981;127:1256–1258.
41. Greaves MF, Sieff C, Edwards PA. Monoclonal antiglycophorin as a probe for erythroleukemias. Blood 1983;61:645–651.
42. Newman PJ, Allen RW, Kahn RA, et al. Quantitation of membrane glycoprotein IIIa on intact human platelets using the monoclonal antibody, AP-3. Blood 1985;65:227–232.
43. Barclay AN, Brown MH, Law SKA, et al. The leukocyte antigen facts book. San Diego: Academic Press, 1997:613.
44. Betz AL. An overview of the multiple functions of the blood–brain barrier. NIDA Res Monogr 1992;120:54–72.
45. Medeiros LJ, Herrington RD, Gonzalez CL, et al. My4 antibody staining of non-Hodgkin's lymphomas. Am J Clin Pathol 1991;95:363–368.
46. Ben-Ezra J, Winberg CD, Wu A, et al. Leu-9 (CD 7) positivity in acute leukemias: a marker of T-cell lineage? Hematol Pathol 1987;1:147–156.
47. Kurtzberg J, Waldmann TA, Davey MP, et al. CD7+, CD4-, CD8- acute leukemia: a syndrome of malignant pluripotent lymphohematopoietic cells. Blood 1989;73:381–390.
48. Nadler LM, Korsmeyer SJ, Anderson KC, et al. B cell origin of non-T cell acute lymphoblastic leukemia. A model for discrete stages of neoplastic and normal pre-B cell differentiation. J Clin Invest 1984;74:332–340.
49. Loken MR, Shah VO, Dattilio KL, et al. Flow cytometric analysis of human bone marrow. II. Normal B lymphocyte development. Blood 1987;70:1316–1324.
50. Roma AO, Kutok JL, Shaheen G, et al. A novel, rapid, multiparametric approach for flow cytometric analysis of intranuclear terminal deoxynucleotidyl transferase. Am J Clin Pathol 1999; 112:343–348.
51. Crist W, Boyett J, Jackson J, et al. Prognostic importance of the pre-B-cell immunophenotype and other presenting features in B-lineage childhood acute lymphoblastic leukemia: a Pediatric Oncology Group study. Blood 1989;74:1252–1259.
52. Greaves MF, Rao J, Hariri G, et al. Phenotypic heterogeneity and cellular origins of T cell malignancies. Leuk Res 1981;5:281–299.
53. Link M, Warnke R, Finlay J, et al. A single monoclonal antibody identifies T-cell lineage of childhood lymphoid malignancies. Blood 1983;62:722–728.
54. Knowles DMD. The human T-cell leukemias: clinical, cytomorphologic, immunophenotypic, and genotypic characteristics. Hum Pathol 1986;17:14–33.
55. Reinherz EL, Kung PC, Goldstein G, et al. Discrete stages of human intrathymic differentiation: analysis of normal thymocytes and leukemic lymphoblasts of T-cell lineage. Proc Natl Acad Sci U S A 1980;77:1588–1592.
56. Roper M, Crist WM, Metzgar R, et al. Monoclonal antibody characterization of surface antigens in childhood T-cell lymphoid malignancies. Blood 1983;61:830–837.
57. Link MP, Stewart SJ, Warnke RA, et al. Discordance between surface and cytoplasmic expression of the Leu-4 (T3) antigen in thymocytes and in blast cells from childhood T lymphoblastic malignancies. J Clin Invest 1985;76:248–253.
58. Weiss LM, Bindl JM, Picozzi VJ, et al. Lymphoblastic lymphoma: an immunophenotype study of 26 cases with comparison to T cell acute lymphoblastic leukemia. Blood 1986;67:474–478.
59. Meuer SC, Acuto O, Hussey RE, et al. Evidence for the T3-associated 90K heterodimer as the T-cell antigen receptor. Nature 1983;303:808–810.

60. Royer HD, Acuto O, Fabbi M, et al. Genes encoding the Ti beta subunit of the antigen/MHC receptor undergo rearrangement during intrathymic ontogeny prior to surface T3-Ti expression. Cell 1984;39:261–266.
61. Furley AJ, Mizutani S, Weilbaecher K, et al. Developmentally regulated rearrangement and expression of genes encoding the T cell receptor–T3 complex. Cell 1986;46:75–87.
62. Gonzalez-Sarmiento R, LeBien TW, Bradley JG, et al. Acute leukemia expressing the gamma gene product of the putative second T cell receptor. J Clin Invest 1987;79:1281–1284.
63. Bernard A, Boumsell L, Reinherz EL, et al. Cell surface characterization of malignant T cells from lymphoblastic lymphoma using monoclonal antibodies: evidence for phenotypic differences between malignant T cells from patients with acute lymphoblastic leukemia and lymphoblastic lymphoma. Blood 1981;57: 1105–1110.
64. Cross AH, Goorha RM, Nuss R, et al. Acute myeloid leukemia with T-lymphoid features: a distinct biologic and clinical entity. Blood 1988;72:579–587.
65. Ross CW, Stoolman LM, Schnitzer B, et al. Immunophenotypic aberrancy in adult acute lymphoblastic leukemia. Am J Clin Pathol 1990;94:590–599.
66. Ritz J, Nadler LM, Bhan AK, et al. Expression of common acute lymphoblastic leukemia antigen (CALLA) by lymphomas of B-cell and T-cell lineage. Blood 1981;58:648–652.
67. Sobol RE, Royston I, LeBien TW, et al. Adult acute lymphoblastic leukemia phenotypes defined by monoclonal antibodies. Blood 1985;65:730–735.
68. Triebel F, Hercend T. Subpopulations of human peripheral T gamma delta lymphocytes [see Comments]. Immunol Today 1989;10:186–188.
69. Itohara S, Nakanishi N, Kanagawa O, et al. Monoclonal antibodies specific to native murine T-cell receptor gamma delta: analysis of gamma delta T cells during thymic ontogeny and in peripheral lymphoid organs. Proc Natl Acad Sci U S A 1989; 86:5094–5098.
70. Inghirami G, Zhu BY, Chess L, et al. Flow cytometric and immunohistochemical characterization of the gamma/delta T-lymphocyte population in normal human lymphoid tissue and peripheral blood. Am J Pathol 1990;136:357–367.
71. Braylan RC, Benson NA, Nourse VA. Cellular DNA of human neoplastic B-cells measured by flow cytometry. Cancer Res 1984;44:5010–5016.
72. Srigley J, Barlogie B, Butler JJ, et al. Heterogeneity of non-Hodgkin's lymphoma probed by nucleic acid cytometry. Blood 1985;65:1090–1096.
73. Joensuu H, Klemi PJ, Soderstrom KO, et al. Comparison of S-phase fraction, working formulation, and Kiel classification in non-Hodgkin's lymphoma. Cancer 1991;68:1564–1571.
74. Vuckovic J, Forenpoher G, Marusic M, et al. Prognostic relevance of non-Hodgkin's lymphomas cell cycle data. Neoplasma 1998;45:332–335.
75. Christensson B, Lindemalm C, Johansson B, et al. Flow cytometric DNA analysis: a prognostic tool in non-Hodgkin's lymphoma. Leuk Res 1989;13:307–314.
76. Rehn S, Glimelius B, Strang P, et al. Prognostic significance of flow cytometry studies in B-cell non-Hodgkin lymphoma. Hematol Oncol 1990;8:1–12.
77. Macartney JC, Camplejohn RS, Morris R, et al. DNA flow cytometry of follicular non-Hodgkin's lymphoma. J Clin Pathol 1991;44:215–218.
78. Duque RE, Andreeff M, Braylan RC, et al. Consensus review of the clinical utility of DNA flow cytometry in neoplastic hematopathology. Cytometry 1993;14:492–496.
79. A predictive model for aggressive non-Hodgkin's lymphoma. The International Non-Hodgkin's Lymphoma Prognostic Factors Project [see Comments]. N Engl J Med 1993;329:987–994.
80. Winter JN, Andersen J, Variakojis D, et al. Prognostic implications of ploidy and proliferative activity in the diffuse, aggressive non-Hodgkin's lymphomas. Blood 1996;88:3919–3925.
81. Gorczyca W, Bigman K, Mittelman A, et al. Induction of DNA strand breaks associated with apoptosis during treatment of leukemias. Leukemia 1993;7:659–670.
82. Leoncini L, Del Vecchio MT, Megha T, et al. Correlations between apoptotic and proliferative indices in malignant non-Hodgkin's lymphomas. Am J Pathol 1993;142:755–763.
83. Stokke T, Smeland EB, Kvaloy S, et al. Tumour cell proliferation, but not apoptosis, predicts survival in B-cell non-Hodgkin's lymphomas. Br J Cancer 1998;77:1839–1841.
84. Diamond LW, Nathwani BN, Rappaport H. Flow cytometry in the diagnosis and classification of malignant lymphoma and leukemia. Cancer 1982;50:1122–1135.
85. Juneja SK, Cooper IA, Hodgson GS, et al. DNA ploidy patterns and cytokinetics of non-Hodgkin's lymphoma. J Clin Pathol 1986;39:987–992.
86. Morgan DR, Williamson JM, Quirke P, et al. DNA content and prognosis of non-Hodgkin's lymphoma. Br J Cancer 1986;54:643–649.
87. Cavalli C, Danova M, Gobbi PG, et al. Ploidy and proliferative activity measurement by flow cytometry in non-Hodgkin's lymphomas. Do speculative aspects prevail over clinical ones? Eur J Cancer Clin Oncol 1989;25:1755–1763.
88. Shackney SE, Levine AM, Fisher RI, et al. The biology of tumor growth in the non-Hodgkin's lymphomas. A dual parameter flow cytometry study of 220 cases. J Clin Invest 1984;73:1201–1214.
89. Wain SL, Braylan RC, Borowitz MJ. Correlation of monoclonal antibody phenotyping and cellular DNA content in non-Hodgkin's lymphoma. The Southeastern Cancer Study Group experience. Cancer 1987;60:2403–2411.
90. O'Brien CJ, Holgate C, Quirke P, et al. Correlation of morphology, immunophenotype, and flow cytometry with remission induction and survival in high-grade non-Hodgkin's lymphoma. J Pathol 1989;158:31–39.

8

MOLECULAR DIAGNOSIS

New insights during the last decade have catapulted genetic studies of malignant lymphomas from a research tool to a routine laboratory test. Unlike flow cytometry or immunohistochemistry, which depend on protein expression, molecular diagnosis directly analyzes the DNA of genes encoding immunoglobulins (Igs), T-cell receptors (TCRs), and oncogenes (1–4). To provide a framework for readers with different backgrounds, this chapter emphasizes both the theory and practice of useful strategies for the molecular diagnosis of antigen receptor gene rearrangements and chromosomal translocations involving oncogenes. We also compare the pros and cons of Southern blot, polymerase chain reaction (PCR), and cytogenetics and fluorescence *in situ* hybridization (FISH).

GENOME SIZE AND ORGANIZATION

A healthy human immune system recognizes an almost unlimited variety of foreign antigens. Because Igs and TCRs are proteins, and because genes encode proteins, the information for these molecules must be stored in the DNA. Paradoxically, although millions of complete antigen receptor molecules are manufactured, the entire human germline DNA contains no more than 100,000 different genes. The discovery of introns in 1977, which overturned the "one gene encoding one protein" hypothesis (5,6), paved the way for our current understanding of the modular genetic organization of the immune system. By shuffling and recombining a few hundred discontinuous gene segments belonging to the Ig and TCR gene families, each of us can theoretically produce more than 100 million complete antigen receptor molecules (7).

SUPERGENE FAMILY

Because Ig and TCR genes belong to the same supergene family, it is not surprising that they are structurally and functionally similar; corresponding Ig and TCR gene segments share homologous size and DNA sequence. Ig and TCR genes also utilize similar heptamer–nonamer consensus DNA sequences and the same recombinase enzymes to facilitate rearrangement (8,9). However, theoretically multiplying the known variable (V), joining (J), diversity (D), and constant (C) gene segments severely underestimates the actual immune repertoire.

GENERATION OF DIVERSITY

At least six molecular mechanisms, operating at different stages of lymphoid differentiation, act synergistically to generate the enormous antigen-recognizing capacity of the immune system: (a) the presence of noncoding DNA sequences, called *introns,* which separate the protein-coding DNA sequences, called *exons,* of the V, D, J, and C antigen receptor gene segments; (b) somatic recombination; (c) sharing of junctional nucleotides donated from contiguously rearranged gene segments (e.g., part V and part J) to create a new hybrid codon, which can alter the amino acid sequence; (d) somatic mutation; (e) derivation of multiple proteins from a single gene, either with multiple transcriptional promoters or with different exons that can be alternatively spliced into or out of the messenger RNA; (f) combinatorial association of polypeptide subunits.

SOMATIC RECOMBINATION

Somatic recombination, a step-by-step process of deleting and joining discontinuous gene segments, creates a new linear genetic code that differs substantially from the original embryonic, or germline, DNA in the same region (Fig. 8.1). Heptamer–nonamer sequences flanking the gene segments and active recombinase enzymes RAG1 and RAG2 are required. Because the probability of two cells rearranging identically is low, the DNA of each lymphocyte is marked uniquely before antigen exposure. Imprecise gene segment alignment further diversifies the immune repertoire. Deleting nucleotides via exonucleases and inserting non–template-dependent nucleotides (N insertion) via terminal deoxynucleotidyl transferase (TdT), especially at the

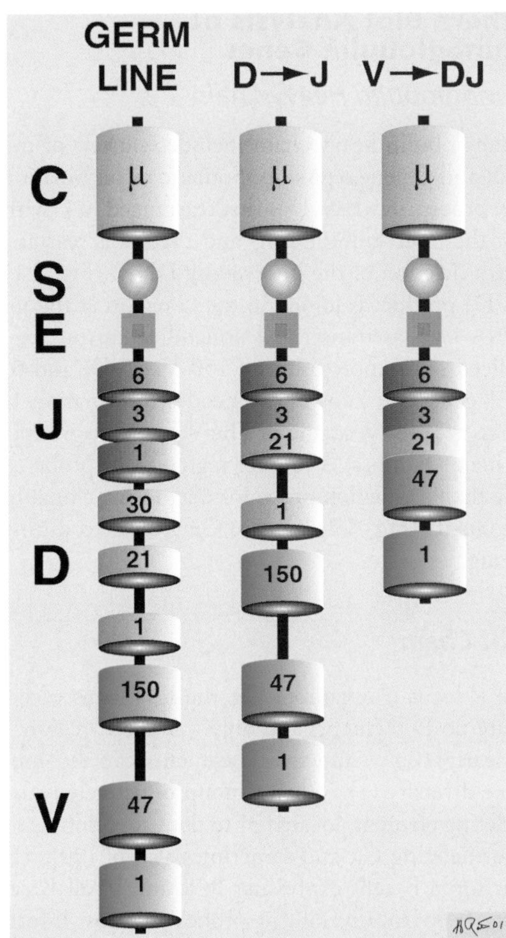

FIGURE 8.1. Somatic recombination. Immunoglobulin heavy chain gene segments rearrange stepwise from germline (*left*), to D-J (*center*), to V-DJ (*right*). The combinatorial possibilities of 150 Vs, 30 Ds, and 6 Js are suggested by an example. D-21 moves adjacent to J-3, deleting DNA sandwiched between (*center*). Then, V-47 links to D-21, removing any connecting DNA (*right*) and completing a unique VDJ recombination. *C*, constant; *S*, switch region; *E*, enhancer; *J*, joining; *D*, diversity; *V*, variable.

immunoglobulin heavy chain (IgH) D junctions, generates further diversity.

COMPLEMENTARITY-DETERMINING REGION

Junctional alterations help refine the specificity of the antigen-binding domain, also called the complementarity-determining region 3 (CDR-3), by producing hypervariable DNA sequences at V-D-J (IgH) and V-J (κ and λ) joints. At a later stage of maturation, antigen-stimulated germinal center memory B cells hypermutate their complementarity-determining regions to produce high-affinity antibodies. In contrast, T-cell antigen receptors rarely mutate, so that the accidental generation of autoreactive T-cell clones is prevented. These genetic mechanisms irreversibly alter the DNA to produce a molecular signature for each B cell and T cell.

IN-FRAME ALIGNMENT OF GENE SEGMENTS

Exact, in-frame alignment of several widely separated exons is required for successful Ig gene rearrangement. Failure occurs often. In particular, faulty gene segment joints can disrupt the DNA coding sequence and lead to improperly located stop codons or missense codons. For example, instead of a full-length functional Ig, mistakes will create either an abnormally short protein or an incorrect amino acid sequence. Only about one-third of V to J light chain gene segments rearrange correctly in-frame. This agrees with predictions based on genetic code syntax because a nucleotide triplet determines each amino acid. Even fewer heavy chains align in-frame because they depend on two consecutive events: V to D followed by VD to J rearrangement. An interesting difference between Ig and TCR is that IgH D gene segments have only one open reading frame, whereas TCRδ D gene segments are readable in all three frames.

GENETIC HIERARCHY

During early, antigen-independent lymphoid differentiation, normal B-cell and T-cell precursors hierarchically recombine discontinuous antigen receptor gene segments to produce functional antigen receptors. The usual early to late rearrangement order for B cells is IgH, κ, λ Ig genes; for T cells, it is δ, γ, β, α TCR genes (10,11).

ALLELIC EXCLUSION

As immature T cells transit from cortical to medullary thymic epithelium, positive and negative selection determines T-cell survival and exportation to the peripheral lymphoid organs. The expression of the TCR plays a central role; clones detecting a single antigen–major histocompatability complex interaction live, and clones recognizing self-antigens die. Individual mature T cells express either TCR αβ (95% of T cells) or TCR γδ (5% of T cells), but not both. TCR polypeptide chains are encoded by just one of the two parental alleles; the other is excluded from producing a protein.

Allelic exclusion also operates for B cells. Ig molecules have a basic heterodimeric structure: Ig heavy chain plus Ig light chain. Depending on the Ig heavy chain class, these heterodimers then form dimers (IgG) or oligomers (IgM) to produce a fully functional Ig antigen receptor. If one IgH allele rearranges its gene segments in such a fashion as to preclude encoding a complete Ig heavy chain (referred to as a *nonproductive gene rearrangement*), then the other IgH allele attempts to rearrange. A similar rule applies to the Ig light chain loci, with the additional requirement for κ to precede λ rearrangement. In a normal B cell, only one of the two IgH alleles and one of the four possible Ig light chain loci (two κ and two λ) may contribute to a functional Ig molecule. However, all the productive and all the nonproductive gene rearrangement attempts are permanently recorded in the DNA and can be detected with Southern blot analysis. In the most extreme case (e.g., an IgM λ-bearing B cell), both IgH alleles, both κ alleles, and both λ alleles could rearrange before yielding a functional Ig molecule.

MULTIPLE CONSTANT REGIONS AND CLASS SWITCHING

The VDJ (or VJ) DNA regions encoding the antigen-binding portion of the IgH, TCR γ, and TCR β antigen receptors may recombine with more than one C region. For IgH, reexposure to antigen in the germinal centers of secondary follicles leads to class switching by deleting Cμ and rearranging VDJ next to one of the other Ig heavy chains (e.g., Cγ or Cα). No switch region is adjacent to Cδ.

MOLECULAR DIAGNOSIS OF CLONALITY

Molecular testing is the gold standard for diagnosing B-cell or T-cell clonality (12). The clinical laboratory routinely determines lymphocytic clonality either by restriction fragment length polymorphism (RFLP) analysis with Southern blot (1) or by antigen receptor VDJ (or VJ) recombination analysis with PCR (13,14). Although molecular diagnostic testing for clonal antigen receptor gene rearrangements is highly specific, a variety of biological and technical factors limit sensitivity; true natural killer cell lymphomas maintain their antigen receptor gene segments in a germline DNA configuration (although natural killer-like T-cell lymphomas do not), some lymphomas delete previously rearranged antigen receptor genes, and others may lose large pieces or entire chromosomes containing the relevant loci. An important caveat is that a variety of reactive lymphoid lesions may contain detectable clones (15–18). Because clonality is not synonymous with malignancy, molecular tests should be correlated with clinical, morphologic, and immunophenotypic data.

Southern blot analysis of antigen receptor gene rearrangements requires high-molecular-weight genomic DNA as starting material. Traditionally, this meant freezing and storing fresh lymph node tissue at extremely cold temperatures. Recently, a new lysing, storage, and transportation (LST) buffer promises to facilitate tissue processing by preserving lymph node samples up to 4 weeks at room temperature for genomic DNA Southern blotting or PCR analysis (19).

Southern Blot Analysis of Immunoglobulin Genes

Immunoglobulin Heavy Chain

Immunoglobulin heavy chain includes clusters of multiple V, J, D, and C gene segments. Somatic recombination is an orderly process in which D is first rearranged to J (with deletion of the intervening DNA) and then V is rearranged to DJ (with deletion of the intervening DNA) (Fig. 8.1). The final VDJ product is joined to the C region at the messenger RNA level as transcribed noncoding intron sequences are spliced out. Approximately 150 V, 30 D, and 6 functional J genes are known. C encodes information for the IgH classes: μ, δ, γ, α, and ϵ. The V genes are grouped into seven major families. A joining region (JH) probe is more reliable than a C region probe for diagnosing clonal IgH rearrangements (Fig. 8.2) because Cμ is deleted during class switching.

κ Light Chain

The Ig κ locus is organized like the IgH locus except that there are no D segments and only a single C region. However, nearly 100 V and five J segments can recombine to produce diversity (1). When κ nonproductively rearranges, a κ-deleting element, located 3′ to the Cκ region, is responsible for deleting Cκ and sometimes also Jκ (20). This occurs in some B cells expressing Ig κ and in all B cells expressing Ig λ (1). Overall, Jκ probes are most informative when this region is analyzed.

λ Light Chain

The arrangement of the Ig λ locus is slightly different from that of the other Igs: Jλ and Cλ regions occur in tandem. Because of polymorphisms, the number of JλCλ tandem genes can vary between 6 and 9 (21,22). Because it is difficult to distinguish between many germline bands and a true clonal rearrangement, Ig λ is not usually evaluated by Southern blot analysis. Although about 10% of T-cell malignancies rearrange IgH, the Ig κ and λ light chain genes remain germline (23).

Southern Blot Analysis of T-cell Receptor Genes

TCR β

Southern blot analysis detects TCR β rearrangements in 90% to 95% of peripheral T-cell lymphomas and T-cell acute lymphoblastic leukemias/lymphoblastic lymphomas. A single Cβ probe detects rearrangements involving almost identical Cβ1 and Cβ2 constant regions. The locations of an *Eco*RI site between Jβ2 and Cβ2 and a *Hind*III site between Jβ1 and Cβ2 renders rearrangements involving Jβ2

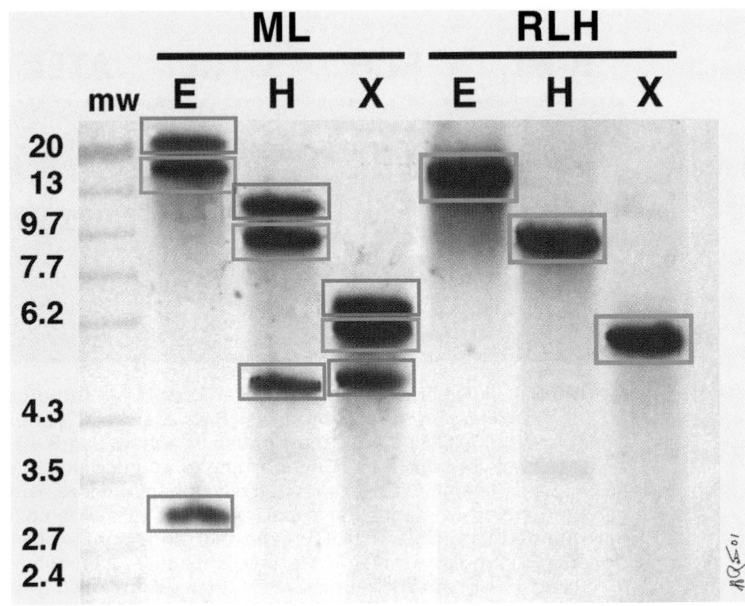

FIGURE 8.2. Southern blot analysis, immunoglobulin heavy chain (*IgH*). A radioactively labeled JH probe detects germline bands (*green boxes*) in B-cell malignant lymphoma (*ML*) and reactive lymphoid hyperplasia (*RLH*). Only ML has novel, nongermline, rearranged bands (*red boxes*), which indicate a clonally rearranged IgH. *mw,* molecular-weight markers in kilobases. Restriction endonucleases: *E,* EcoRI; *H, Hind*III; *X, Xba*I.

undetectable in *Eco*RI-digested DNA, and rearrangements involving Jβ1 undetectable in *Hind*III-digested DNA. As an alternative strategy, a mixture of Jβ1 and Jβ2 probes can be used. However, a single Cβ probe is usually preferred because it both determines T-cell clonality and estimates the percentage of polyclonal T-cells. In *Eco*RI-digested DNA, the intensity of the 12-kb Cβ1 germline band diminishes proportionally to the percentage of polyclonal T cells in the sample (Fig. 8.3); each polyclonal T cell has a unique Cβ1 rearrangement that usually migrates differently according to a log-linear relationship of molecular mass versus gel distance. In contrast, Cβ2 is not diminished in intensity, in comparison with the germline band, when either Cβ1 or Cβ2 is rearranged because the *Eco*RI site is 5′ to the Cβ2 allele (2).

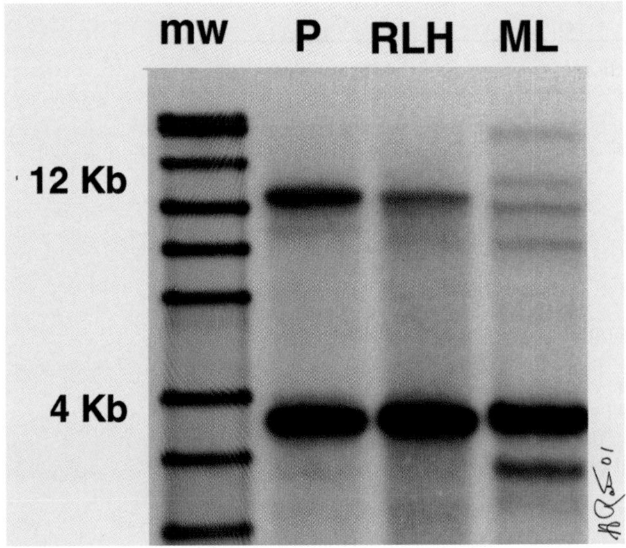

FIGURE 8.3. Southern blot analysis, T-cell receptor (TCR) β. The DNA was digested with restriction endonuclease EcoRI and a radioactively labeled Cβ probe was used. The intensity of the 12-kb Cβ1 germline band (*P*) diminishes proportionally to the percentage of polyclonal T cells (*RLH*) or monoclonal T cells that have rearranged this DNA region (*ML*) in the sample. *mw,* molecular-weight markers in kilobases; *P,* placenta; *RLH,* reactive lymphoid hyperplasia; *ML,* T-cell malignant lymphoma.

TCR α

The complexity and size of the TCR α locus is not suitable for standard Southern blot analysis. The Jα region (80 kb) is approximately three to four times the size of the largest DNA fragment (20 to 25 kb) routinely studied, and the numerous (approximately 50) Jα gene segments require multiple probes (1,2). However, this region can be evaluated in a research environment with the use of pulsed-field gel electrophoresis, which is capable of resolving extremely large DNA fragments.

TCR δ

The TCR δ locus is flanked by TCR α V and J gene segments. During normal αβ T-cell maturation, Vα to Jα gene rearrangement deletes all intervening DNA sequences, including the TCR δ region. Analysis of the recovered DNA circles indicates that most TCR δ genes are in a germline configuration before deletion. Clonal TCR δ gene rearrangements can be detected in acute lymphoblastic leukemia/lymphoblastic lymphomas corresponding to the earliest stages of lymphoid differentiation (i.e., after TCR δ but before TCR α gene rearrangements) and also in T-cell lymphoproliferative disorders expressing TCR γδ (24).

TCR γ

TCR γ rearrangements are retained in nearly all normal and neoplastic T cells expressing TCR αβ protein, including the majority of peripheral T-cell lymphomas and cutaneous T-cell lymphomas. Some investigators initially suggested that Hodgkin disease might be a clonal T-cell disorder based on TCR γ gene rearrangements (25), but this was not confirmed. Because of the limited number of possible Vγ–Jγ gene rearrangements, Southern blot detects discrete bands in polyclonal T cells, and mixed monoclonal and polyclonal T-cell populations have complex and confusing band patterns (26). Because of these pitfalls, molecular diagnosis of this region with Southern blot is not recommended. However, TCR γ gene rearrangements are commonly analyzed with PCR.

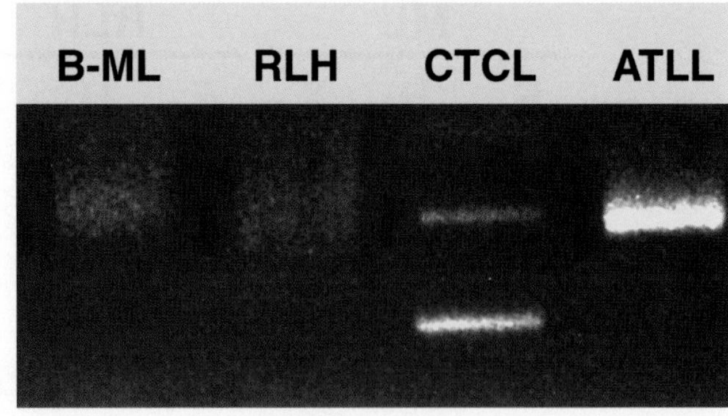

FIGURE 8.4. Polymerase chain reaction analysis, T-cell receptor (TCR) γ. Polyclonal T cells in B-ML and RLH show smears. Monoclonal T cells in CTCL and ATLL show one or two sharp bands. Although B-ML contains a clonally rearranged immunoglobulin heavy chain gene, the TCR γ genes in the lymphoma cells remain germline; however, background reactive T cells in this sample have numerous different TCR γ gene rearrangements (polyclonal) appearing as a smear. *B-ML,* B-cell malignant lymphoma; *RLH,* reactive lymphoid hyperplasia; *CTCL,* cutaneous T-cell lymphoma; *ATLL,* adult T-cell lymphoma/leukemia.

Polymerase Chain Reaction

Polymerase Chain Reaction and Southern Blot

Polymerase chain reaction is rapidly replacing Southern blot analysis for evaluating B-cell or T-cell antigen receptor gene rearrangements (27) (Fig. 8.4). Even small, formalin-fixed, paraffin-embedded tissues, including biopsy specimens of skin or gastrointestinal tract, are routinely assayed (28–30). Because the turn-around time is quick, many laboratories advocate the use of PCR as an initial screen. However, a negative PCR result should be followed by Southern blot analysis, which remains the gold standard (Table 8.1).

Polymerase Chain Reaction Basics

Polymerase chain reaction is a versatile molecular technique for assessing clonality, chromosomal translocations, minimal residual disease, gene mutations, and viruses. The

TABLE 8.1. CLONAL DETECTION: POLYMERASE CHAIN REACTION VERSUS SOUTHERN BLOT

	Polymerase chain reaction	Southern blot
DNA amount	1 μg or less	30 μg minimum per probe used
DNA quality/size	Can be severely degraded, 100–300 bp	High-quality, high-molecular-weight DNA needed, at least 20 kb
DNA source	Fresh or frozen tissue, LST buffer, or paraffin blocks	Fresh or frozen tissue, or LST buffer
Restriction enzyme digestion	Not needed	Essential
Gel electrophoresis	Usually polyacrylamide, single-strand conformation polymorphism (SSCP) or denaturing gradient gel electrophoresis (DGGE), but other methods without gels possible	Agarose gel required
Time to completion	1 to 2 days	1 to 2 weeks
Single-copy gene detection methods	Fluorescent dyes, silver stain, chemiluminescence, radioactivity	Usually radioactivity, less often chemiluminescence
Clonal sensitivity	1 cell per 10^4 to 10^6 cells	1–5% of total DNA
Clonal specificity	60–80% B cells; 90–95% T cells, if sufficient number of primer pairs used	More than 95% B cells or T cells

LST, lysing, storage, and transportation.

lymph node sample can be fresh, frozen, stored in LST buffer, or formalin-fixed. The target molecule can be either genomic DNA (standard PCR) or messenger RNA, which is enzymatically converted to complementary DNA before standard PCR is used [reverse-transcriptase PCR (RT-PCR)]. Repetitively altering the reaction temperature during heat denaturation, primer annealing, and extension geometrically amplifies the template DNA sequence 2^N times, where N equals the number of cycles (14).

Primer Design

In clinical PCR applications, the DNA target usually spans 2,000 bp or less. Prior knowledge of the sequences at the upstream (5′) and downstream (3′) extremities is required to synthesize short (20 to 30 bp) matching oligonucleotides, also called *primers* or *amplimers.* The primers specifically anneal to the template DNA and provide the initial sequences for *Taq* DNA polymerase extension. Selecting optimal sequences for both 5′ and 3′ primers often involves compromise; the desire for equivalent guanine and cytosine (G+C) content, which affects melting temperature, must be balanced against the need to avoid complementarity between the 3′ ends, which promotes wasteful primer–dimer formation instead of amplifying the template (31–33).

Clonality

Most DNA-based PCR strategies detect Ig or TCR clonality by exploiting the proximity of V and J DNA sequences after successful rearrangement of VDJ (Fig. 8.1) or VJ antigen receptor genes. In contrast, multigene families of germline V, D, and J gene segments are too widely dispersed to generate significant PCR products (Fig. 8.1). Upstream and downstream consensus primers are designed to recognize homologous DNA sequences of V genes, such as the framework regions or leader sequence, and the 5′ end of J genes. The PCR product (also called the *amplicon*) of the hypervariable region, for either Ig or TCR analysis, undergoes electrophoresis through a high-resolution polyacrylamide gel. Clonal populations yielding one or two overrepresented homogeneous PCR species appear as sharp bands (Fig. 8.4); polyclonal populations yielding many heterogeneous PCR species, each differing in length by a few base pairs, appear as a smear (27,30,34) (Fig. 8.4). Unfortunately, interpretation is not always straightforward; sometimes a sharp band superimposed on a smear of similar size and intensity cannot be clearly resolved. Alternative gel systems, either single-stranded conformation polymorphism (SSCP) gel electrophoresis or denaturing gradient gel electrophoresis (DGGE) (35), can be used to detect clonality. In these systems, the PCR product nucleotide sequence determines gel mobility by affecting secondary or tertiary DNA structure.

False-Positive and False-Negative Results

Because of the high sensitivity of PCR assays, one must avoid the pitfall of over-interpreting faint bands as significant neoplastic clones when they may represent just a slightly expanded background population of no clinical relevance. Clinicopathologic correlation is required.

The TCR γ PCR assay is useful for diagnosing clonality in most T-cell lymphomas expressing either $\alpha\beta$ or $\gamma\delta$ TCRs (Fig. 8.4). In contrast, the false-negative rate for detecting IgH VDJ rearrangement in B-cell lymphomas is high because of poor matches between the consensus V primer and its DNA target; there are multiple V families, and some B-cell lymphomas hypermutate the V primer binding region. To improve sensitivity, multiple primer sets have been suggested (31–33,36).

Multiplex Polymerase Chain Reaction

Multiplex PCR strategies for detecting clonality mix primers with similar sequences (e.g., several V and J sequences) in a single tube. Although this saves time and reagents by reducing the number of separate PCR reactions and gel lanes, it may potentially yield false-negative results. For example, a polymorphism or mutation within the target DNA sequence of a clone could prevent successful binding of the best matching primer in the multiplex mixture. If the complementary sequences of the DNA target and the primer cannot bind to one another, the PCR reaction fails, so that the clone remains unamplified and goes undetected. However, the other oligonucleotides in the multiplex mixture amplify the background DNA sequences to yield a smear (Fig. 8.4). Because a smear pattern usually indicates polyclonality, a false-negative interpretation may be made despite the presence of a true clone in the sample.

Inhibitors and Fixatives

If PCR is attempted on fixed tissue, heavy metal-based fixatives should be avoided because they inhibit *Taq* polymerase. DNA extracted from especially bloody samples should be treated with a metal chelator because heme is also a PCR inhibitor. Processing tissue with B5, Zenker, or Bouin fixative yields excessively degraded DNA (37).

Chromosomal Translocations

In malignant lymphomas, chromosomal translocations juxtapose an oncogene either to an Ig or TCR gene or to a non-antigen receptor gene. Common examples of the former include IgH partnering with c-myc in Burkitt lymphoma (Fig. 8.5), bcl-1 in mantle cell lymphoma (Fig. 8.6), and bcl-2 in follicular lymphoma (Fig. 8.7). An example of the latter involves translocating the nucleophosmin (NPM) gene adjacent to the anaplastic lymphoma kinase (ALK) gene in Ki-

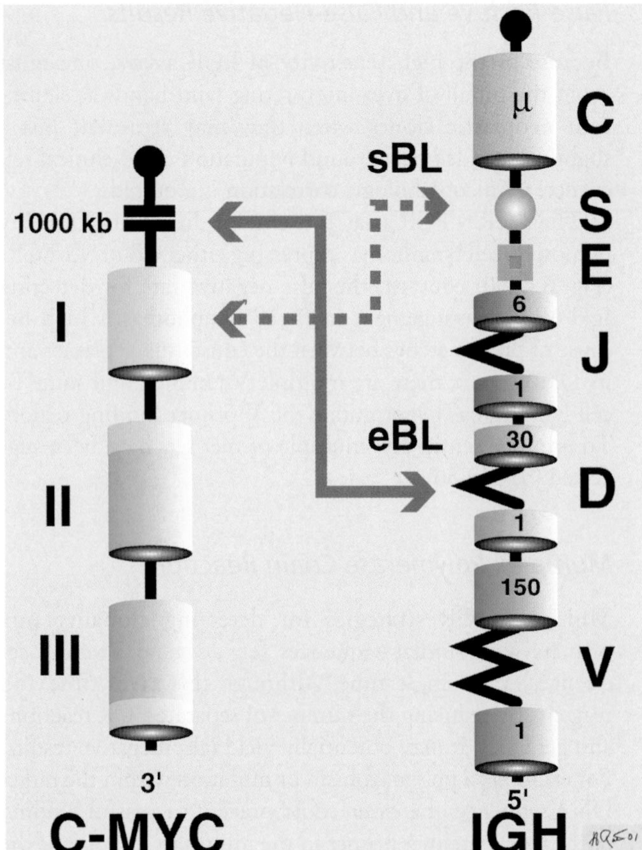

FIGURE 8.5. Translocation of c-myc, t(8q24;14q32). In the majority of cases, reciprocal chromosomal translocations involve the c-myc protooncogene on 8q24 and the immunoglobulin heavy chain (IgH) locus on 14q32. Endemic Burkitt lymphoma (*eBL*), arising in equatorial Africa, tends to have breakpoints outside c-myc. Sporadic Burkitt lymphoma (*sBL*), arising in Europe and North America, tends to have breakpoints within or close to c-myc. *Roman numerals* designate c-myc exons: *blue,* coding regions; *yellow,* untranslated regions. *IgH,* zigzag lines represent germline configuration. *C,* constant; *S,* switch region; *E,* enhancer; *J,* joining; *D,* diversity; *V,* variable.

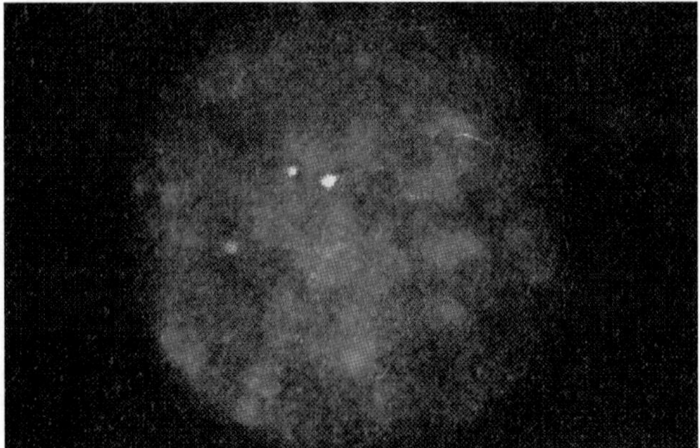

FIGURE 8.6. Translocation of bcl-1, t(11;14)(q13;q32). Interphase fluorescence *in situ* hybridization with the use of cosmid panels for a 450- to 750-kb region symmetrically localized around the major translocation cluster (MTC) of the bcl1 locus at 11q13. Cells from a patient carrying t(11;14)(q13;q32). One cosmid panel, centromeric of the MTC, was labeled with tetrarhodamine isothiocyanate (*red*), and the other cosmid panel, telomeric to the MTC, was labeled with fluorescein isothiocyanate (*green*). Co-localization at one allele results in a yellow signal, indicating an intact, normal chromosome. Segregation at the other allele gives rise to one green and one red signal, indicating a chromosomal break. (From Coignet LJA, Schuuring E, Kibbelaar RE, et al. Detection of 11q13 rearrangements in hematologic neoplasia by double-color fluorescence *in situ* hybridization. Blood 1996;87:1512–1509.)

1+ anaplastic large cell lymphoma. Although incompletely understood, the same molecular mechanisms responsible for physiologic VDJ recombination and IgH class switching may sometimes generate pathologic chromosomal translocations (38) and bizarre IgH V–TCR Cα hybrid genes (39).

DNA-based PCR is useful for diagnosing chromosomal translocations if the DNA sequences surrounding the breakpoint are known, if the breakpoints tend to cluster in a small region, and if only two chromosomes participate. These three criteria are satisfied best by t(14;18) involving IgH (Fig. 8.1) and bcl-2 at the major breakpoint cluster region (Fig. 8.7). Only c-myc translocations in sporadic Burkitt lymphoma involving the Cμ switch region, and none in endemic Burkitt lymphoma, can be analyzed by routine PCR owing to large distances between c-myc and IgH (40) (Fig. 8.5). The potential chromosomal partners for bcl-6 are numerous (41). Translocations of bcl-1 are identified by PCR in only about one-third to one-half of cases without karyotypic analysis (42–46). ALK translocations involving t(2;5) require long-range genomic DNA PCR for diagnosis because of variable breakpoints between cases (47,48).

Minimal Residual Disease

The largest number of B-cell lymphoma cases analyzed for minimal residual disease have relied on DNA-based PCR to

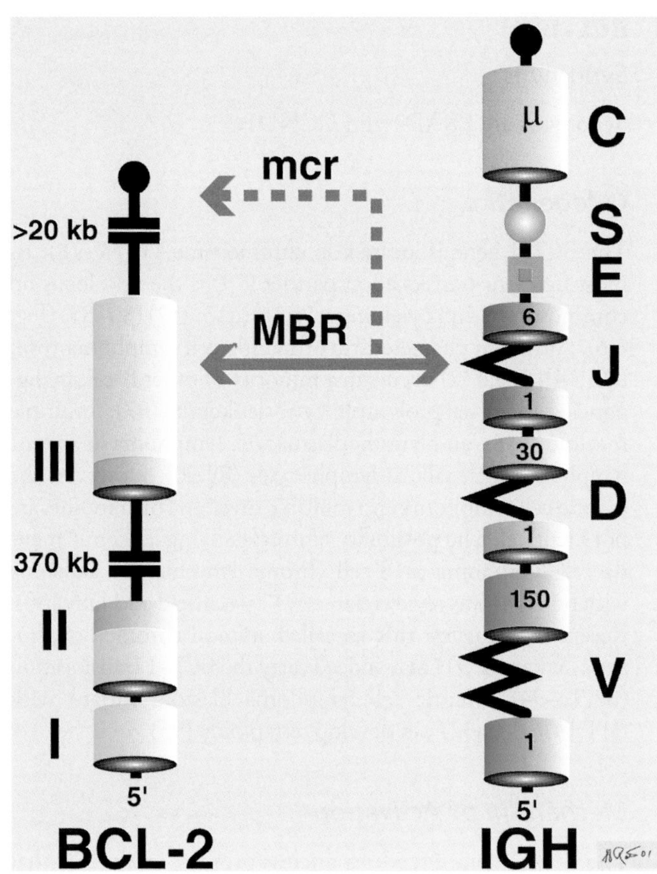

FIGURE 8.7. Translocation of bcl-2, t(14;18)(q32;q21). Chromosome 18 breaks involving bcl-2 occur in the major breakpoint region (*MBR, solid red line*) in the majority of cases and in the minor cluster breakpoint region (*mcr, dotted red line*) in the minority of cases. Even fewer variant breaks are located 5′ to bcl-2 (not shown). The J region of the immunoglobulin heavy chain (IgH) locus is almost always involved. *Roman numerals* designate bcl-2 exons: *blue,* coding regions; *yellow,* untranslated regions. *IgH,* zigzag lines represent germline configuration. *C,* constant; *S,* switch region; *E,* enhancer; *J,* joining; *D,* diversity; *V,* variable.

detect t(14;18) (Fig. 8.7). However, only a subset of lymphomas has this chromosomal translocation. Few studies take advantage of the unique IgH VDJ DNA sequence because it must be laboriously obtained for each new patient (49). Nevertheless, RNA-based PCR strategies for detecting minimal residual disease in lymphomas, called *anchored PCR* or *rapid amplification of cDNA ends* (RACE), can yield the entire nucleotide sequence of any productive IgH VDJ rearrangement transcribing messenger RNA (50,51).

Cytogenetics and Fluorescence *In Situ* Hybridization

Classic cytogenetics is a valuable technique for global chromosome analysis. It has provided the initial raw data for cloning most of the oncogenes involved in recurring chromosomal translocations. If several chromosomal partners are possible or if the breakpoint region is variable, cytogenetics can detect chromosomal translocations missed by Southern blot or PCR. The *Atlas of Genetics and Cytogenetics in Oncology and Hematology* (URL: *http://www.infobiogen.fr/services/chromcancer*) concisely catalogues many lymphoma and leukemia chromosomal aberrations. However, the resolution of the banding patterns in Giemsa-stained metaphase spreads is limiting; various microscopic chromosomal deletions, insertions, or inversions may be invisible.

Fluorescence *in situ* hybridization is a useful technique for localizing and enumerating two, or a few, specific genetic loci in interphase nuclei. Each gene can be analyzed with a unique DNA probe conjugated to a fluorochrome of a different color (e.g., oncogene = red; IgH = green). If a nucleus contains a chromosomal translocation juxtaposing the oncogene and the IgH loci, three signals will be obtained: one red non-translocated oncogene, one green non-translocated IgH, and one red + green = yellow translocated oncogene juxtaposed to translocated IgH. Normal nuclei have two red non-translocated oncogenes, two green non-translocated IgH, and no yellow signals. For an alternative FISH strategy, see Fig. 8.6. The three-dimensional geometry of the nucleus precludes seeing all signals in all cells, rendering FISH too insensitive for detecting minimal residual disease.

SPECIFIC ONCOGENES IN MOLECULAR DIAGNOSIS

C-MYC

Cytogenetics

The C-MYC gene is located on the long arm of chromosome 8 in the region translocated in Burkitt lymphoma: 8q24 (52,53). The C-MYC gene breaks most often in its 5′ region to juxtapose IgH on chromosome 14, t(8q24;14q32). In less common variants, fragments of chromosomes 2 or 22, carrying the Ig κ or λ light chain gene, translocate to the 3′ region of c-myc retained on chromosome 8: t(2q12;8q24) or t(8q24;22q11) (54). The C-MYC translocation occurs in Burkitt lymphoma/acute lymphoblastic leukemia, L3 type (40% to 100% of cases), intermediate- to high-grade B-cell non-Hodgkin lymphoma (approximately 15% of cases), and blastic transformation of low-grade B-cell lymphoma (55–58).

Mechanism of Activation

The C-MYC phosphoprotein, a DNA-binding transcription factor (59–61), associates with its partner, max, to regulate cell proliferation and apoptosis (62–64). Deregulated c-myc expression depends on translocating C-MYC to one of the Ig genes (54,65). The IgH, κ, and λ loci each can contribute at least three regulatory elements essential to overexpression of C-MYC: two positionally independent transcriptional enhancers and a matrix attachment region capable of organizing chromatin structure (66–71). The c-myc translocation yields high-level transcription of the translocated c-myc gene and silencing of the normal allele, intron 1/exon 1 structural alterations (especially in sporadic Burkitt lymphoma), shifting from the usual P1 promoter to the P2 promoter, and removal of the RNA elongation block.

Molecular Diagnosis

Translocations of C-MYC are classified according to the location of the chromosomal breakpoint relative to the c-myc gene on chromosome 8 (Fig. 8.5): class I, within intron 1/exon 1; class II, immediately upstream of C-MYC; and class III, distant from C-MYC. Sporadic Burkitt lymphoma and AIDS-related lymphoma most often have class I or II translocations. Endemic African Burkitt lymphomas typically have breakpoints ranging over a 300-kb region far upstream from the C-MYC gene (65,72–75) (Fig. 8.5). In t(8;14), chromosome 14 breaks between the V and C gene segments of IgH affecting diversity or joining segments in endemic Burkitt lymphoma, or within or near the μ switch region in sporadic and AIDS-related Burkitt lymphoma (40,76) (Fig. 8.5). Based on the normal hierarchical order of IgH DNA gene rearrangements, translocations involving D or J segments occur earlier in B-cell development than do those involving switch regions. Translocations of C-MYC are detectable by Southern blot analysis with the C-MYC exon 3 probe in sporadic but not in endemic Burkitt lymphoma because of the great distance separating class I and II versus class III breakpoints. This limitation has been overcome by a two-color interphase FISH assay in which cosmid clones spanning c-myc and IgH are used (77).

BCL-1

Synonyms

Synonyms are PRAD1 and CCND1.

Cytogenetics

The BCL-1 gene is located on chromosome 11q13 (78). Its most frequent translocation partner (79) is the IgH locus on chromosome 14q32 yielding t(11;14)(q13;q32) (80–85) (Fig. 8.6). Although characteristic of mantle cell lymphoma (86), t(11;14)(q13;q32) occurs in a minority of other B-cell malignancies, such as prolymphocytic leukemia (87), multiple myeloma (88), and lymphoplasmacytic lymphoma or splenic lymphoma with villous lymphocytes (89,90). However, the mantle cell lymphoma and multiple myeloma breakpoints are not identical. The possibility of misclassifying leukemic mantle cell lymphoma as B-cell chronic lymphocytic leukemia with t(11;14) was reviewed in 1991 by Raffield and Jaffe (80). Recent data suggest that so-called atypical chronic lymphocytic leukemia (91) may indeed carry the BCL-1 translocation (87,92–94). Mantle cell lymphoma blastoid variant with t(11;14)(q13;q32) can develop tetraploidy (95).

Mechanism of Activation

The BCL-1 gene encodes a nuclear protein, cyclin D1, that normally interacts with cyclin-dependent kinases (CDKs) (96), usually CDK4 (97), during the cell cycle transition from G1 to S (98–100). Unphosphorylated retinoblastoma protein with bound E2F acts as a brake to the cell cycle (101). After mitogenic activation, the cyclin D1–CDK complex is responsible for phosphorylating retinoblastoma protein and liberating E2F (102). E2F is then free to induce DNA-replicating gene products required in S (103,104). Normal lymphoid tissues express little or no cyclin D1 (105,106). In malignant lymphomas, juxtaposing the BCL-1 gene to the IgH enhancer via chromosomal translocation t(11;14)(q13;q32) inappropriately produces cyclin D1 protein to deregulate the cell cycle (107). In carcinomas, BCL-1 gene amplification yields cyclin D1 overexpression (108).

Molecular Diagnosis

Cyclin D1 activation results from the reciprocal chromosomal translocation of the BCL-1 gene locus, 11q13, and the IgH locus, 14q32 (109–111). The 11q13 breakpoints associated with inappropriate activation of BCL-1 tend to occur in the major translocation cluster (MTC) located 5′ of the BCL-1 gene. In cases with 11q13 breaks centromeric to BCL-1, in a postulated negative control region, cyclin D1 is not overexpressed (112). This suggests that translocation to the IgH locus on chromosome 14 may release the BCL-1 gene from potential silencing elements so that cyclin D1 protein is inappropriately produced. In mantle cell lymphomas with known t(11;14)(q13;q32), the MTC breakpoint was diagnosed in 13 of 18 cases (72%) by Southern blot analysis and in 10 of 12 cases (83%) by PCR (113). In other series of mantle cell lymphomas, usually without karyotypic confirmation, the MTC breakpoint was detected in only 34% to 48% of cases by Southern blot and in 33% to 50% of cases by PCR (42–46). The majority of MTC breakpoints revealed by Southern blot were also identified by PCR (110,114). Because multiple probes are required to detect bcl1 rearrangement by Southern blot analysis, interphase FISH may be more sensitive (Fig. 8.6).

BCL-2

Cytogenetics

The BCL-2 gene, on chromosome 18q21 (115–118), juxtaposes the IgH locus on chromosome 14q32 as a reciprocal translocation in most follicular lymphomas and in approximately 20% of diffuse large B-cell lymphomas (119–124) (Fig. 8.7). About half of the diffuse large B-cell lymphomas with t(14;18)(q32;q21) have evolved from follicular lymphomas (121,125).

Mechanism of Activation

The t(14;18) translocation places the BCL-2 gene under the regulatory control of IgH elements to yield constitutive overexpression (126,127). Overexpression of BCL-2 protein blocks programmed cell death (128,129) but does not lead to cellular proliferation. In addition, BCL-2 prevents apoptosis even if growth factors normally required for survival are withheld (129). Although all the details have not been precisely worked out, it has been proposed that BCL-2 promotes cell survival by opposing the action of cysteine proteases responsible for initiating the apoptotic pathway (130).

Molecular Diagnosis

The IgH breakpoint almost always involves the J region (Fig. 8.7), the translocation probably occurring at the pre-B-cell stage during active recombination. In contrast, some variability on chromosome 18 is seen; the major breakpoint cluster region (MBR) spans a short 150 bp in the untranslated 3′ region of BCL-2 but includes a half to two-thirds of follicular lymphomas (Fig. 8.7); the minor breakpoint cluster region (mbr) (131), located 20 to 30 kb 3′ to BCL-2, is the site of about one-fourth of follicular lymphomas (Fig. 8.7); the variant cluster region 5′ to BCL-2, plus additional 3′ sites, encompass the remainder. Southern blot and PCR methods detect the t(14;18) breakpoint in most molecular lesions involving either MBR or mbr (132). The remaining BCL-2 translocations are undetectable by standard assays. Nevertheless, in most patients, the DNA-based PCR assay can be used to identify minimal residual disease. One caveat is that highly sensitive, nested PCR assays do detect BCL-2–IgH translocations in normal lymphoid tissue (133,134). If necessary, the breakpoint junction can be DNA-sequenced to confirm identity between the residual disease and the original lymphoma.

ALK

Cytogenetics

Immunostaining of T-cell or null cell phenotype anaplastic large cell lymphomas (135,136) with ALK-specific antibodies reveals either of two patterns: nucleolar/nuclear/cytoplasmic or cytoplasmic restricted (137). Anaplastic large cell lymphomas expressing the former ALK pattern typically possess the t(2;5)(p23;q35) recurrent reciprocal translocation joining NPM (also known as *B23* or *numatrin*) on 5q35 with ALK on 2p23 to create a hybrid fusion gene, NPM-ALK (138,139). CD30+ anaplastic large cell lymphomas with t(2;5)(p23;q35) occur more often nodally than extranodally (140). A minority of anaplastic large cell lymphomas expressing cytoplasmic restricted ALK protein juxtapose the ALK gene and a putative alternative non-NPM fusion partner, such as nonmuscular tropomyosin (TPM3): t(1;2)(q25;p23) (141,142), or an unknown gene: inv(2)(p23q35) (143,144).

Mechanism of Activation

NPM-ALK links the N terminus of NPM with the truncated cytoplasmic enzymatic portion of the neural-specific receptor tyrosine kinase ALK (145,146). The normal NPM gene encodes a highly conserved nucleolar phosphoprotein (147) participating in ribosomal assembly and nucleolar/cytoplasmic transport (148,149). NPM contributes a strong constitutive promoter for expressing the NPM-ALK fusion gene (138). Some of the hybrid NPM-ALK protein shuttles into the nucleolus/nucleus, probably by attaching to the N-terminal oligomerization domain of wild-type NPM (150). Non-oligomerized NPM-ALK cannot enter the nucleus because the DNA sequence encoding the NPM nuclear localizing motif is not retained in the fusion gene (138). Oligomerization through the NPM portion of NPM-ALK also simulates ligand binding and cross-linking to activate ALK activity (150). Aberrant ALK tyrosine kinase activity may hyperphosphorylate inappropriate substrates to trigger lymphomagenesis (151). Truncated ALK, juxtaposed to N-terminus partners other than NPM, still maintains transforming ability without nucleolar/nuclear localization (150,152).

Molecular Diagnosis

Polymerase chain reaction strategies to detect t(2;5) in anaplastic large cell lymphomas include RT-PCR (138), which generates the same size product for all cases, and long-range genomic DNA PCR (47,48), which produces different size products reflecting variability in the breakpoint between cases. The DNA PCR assay appears advantageous because DNA is less labile than RNA; also, contamination can be monitored because the PCR product size varies. However, PCR strategies designed to detect t(2;5) necessarily miss variants such as t(1;2) and inv(2). The presence of numerous NPM pseudogenes (153) complicates Southern blot analysis with NPM probes (47,154). In addition to anaplastic large cell lymphoma, the t(2;5) has been detected in other varieties of large cell lymphoma (155). Although a small number of investigators initially reported the NPM-ALK translocation in Hodgkin lymphoma based on Southern blot (156) and RT-PCR analyses (157,158), the data accumulated during the study of more than 100 cases of Hodgkin lymphoma with RT-PCR (155,159–164), genomic DNA PCR (165,166), Southern blot (167), and FISH (168,169) convincingly demonstrate that t(2;5) rarely if ever occurs in this disorder. In addition, ALK protein was absent from both Hodgkin lymphoma and "Hodgkin-like" anaplastic large cell lymphoma (170). A genomic DNA PCR assay did not detect the t(2;5) in lymphomatoid papulosis (164,165) or in CD30+ primary cutaneous lymphoma (164). In contrast, Beylot-Barry et al. (171) detected NPM-ALK transcripts with RT-PCR in 1 of 11 cases of lymphomatoid papulosis and 7 of 15 cases of CD30+ primary cutaneous T-cell lymphoma, but ALK protein was rarely expressed. Although cutaneous T-cell lymphoma may transform into an aggressive T-cell lymphoma with numerous CD30+ anaplastic cells, the t(2;5) does not accompany histologic progression.

REFERENCES

1. Cossman J, Uppenkamp M, Sundeen J, et al. Molecular genetics and the diagnosis of lymphoma. Arch Pathol Lab Med 1988;112:117–127.
2. Knowles DM. Immunophenotypic and antigen receptor gene rearrangement analysis in T cell neoplasia. Am J Pathol 1989; 134:761–785.
3. Ratech H. The uses of molecular biology in hematopathology. Oncogenes as diagnostic markers in non-Hodgkin's malignant lymphoma. Am J Clin Pathol 1993;99:381–384.
4. Kirsch IR, Kuehl WM. Gene rearrangements in lymphoid cells. In: Stamatoyannopoulos G, Nienhuis AW, Majerus PW, et al., eds. The molecular basis of blood diseases. Philadelphia: WB Saunders, 1994:xix, 986.
5. Breathnach R, Mandel JL, Chambon P. Ovalbumin gene is split in chicken DNA. Nature 1977;270:314–319.
6. Jeffreys AJ, Flavell RA. The rabbit beta-globin gene contains a large large insert in the coding sequence. Cell 1977;12:1097–1108.
7. Tonegawa S. Somatic generation of antibody diversity. Nature 1983;302:575–581.
8. Schatz DG, Oettinger MA, Baltimore D. The V(D)J recombination activating gene, RAG-1. Cell 1989;59:1035–1048.
9. Oettinger MA, Schatz DG, Gorka C, et al. RAG-1 and RAG-2, adjacent genes that synergistically activate V(D)J recombination. Science 1990;248:1517–1523.
10. Korsmeyer SJ, Hieter PA, Ravetch JV, et al. Developmental hierarchy of immunoglobulin gene rearrangements in human leukemic pre-B-cells. Proc Natl Acad Sci U S A 1981;78:7096–7100.
11. de Villartay JP, Hockett RD, Coran D, et al. Deletion of the human T-cell receptor delta-gene by a site-specific recombination. Nature 1988;335:170–174.
12. Cossman J, Zehnbauer B, Garrett CT, et al. Gene rearrangements in the diagnosis of lymphoma/leukemia. Guidelines for use based on a multiinstitutional study [see Comments]. Am J Clin Pathol 1991;95:347–354.
13. Eisenstein BI. The polymerase chain reaction. A new method of using molecular genetics for medical diagnosis. N Engl J Med 1990;322:178–183.
14. Templeton NS. The polymerase chain reaction. History, methods, and applications. Diagn Mol Pathol 1992;1:58–72.
15. Lipford EH, Smith HR, Pittaluga S, et al. Clonality of angioimmunoblastic lymphadenopathy and implications for its evolution to malignant lymphoma. J Clin Invest 1987;79: 637–642.
16. Fishleder A, Tubbs R, Hesse B, et al. Uniform detection of immunoglobulin-gene rearrangement in benign lymphoepithelial lesions. N Engl J Med 1987;316:1118–1121.
17. Locker J, Nalesnik M. Molecular genetic analysis of lymphoid tumors arising after organ transplantation. Am J Pathol 1989;135:977–987.
18. Soulier J, Grollet L, Oksenhendler E, et al. Molecular analysis of clonality in Castleman's disease. Blood 1995;86:1131–1138.
19. Schultz CL, Akker Y, Du J, et al. A lysis, storage, and transportation buffer for long-term, room-temperature preservation of human clinical lymphoid tissue samples yielding high molecular weight genomic DNA suitable for molecular diagnosis. Am J Clin Pathol 1999;111:748–752.
20. Hieter PA, Korsmeyer SJ, Waldmann TA, et al. Human immunoglobulin kappa light-chain genes are deleted or rearranged in lambda-producing B cells. Nature 1981;290:368–372.
21. Taub RA, Hollis GF, Hieter PA, et al. Variable amplification of immunoglobulin lambda light-chain genes in human populations. Nature 1983;304:172–174.
22. Hieter PA, Hollis GF, Korsmeyer SJ, et al. Clustered arrangement of immunoglobulin lambda constant region genes in man. Nature 1981;294:536–540.
23. Pelicci PG, Knowles DM 2nd, Dalla Favera R. Lymphoid tumors displaying rearrangements of both immunoglobulin and T cell receptor genes. J Exp Med 1985;162:1015–1024.
24. de Villartay JP, Pullman AB, Andrade R, et al. Gamma/delta lineage relationship within a consecutive series of human precursor T-cell neoplasms. Blood 1989;74:2508–2518.
25. Griesser H, Feller A, Lennert K, et al. The structure of the T cell gamma chain gene in lymphoproliferative disorders and lymphoma cell lines [published erratum appears in Blood 1987; 69:368]. Blood 1986;68:592–594.
26. Uppenkamp M, Andrade R, Sundeen J, et al. Diagnostic interpretation of T gamma gene rearrangement: effect of polyclonal T cells. Hematol Pathol 1988;2:15–24.
27. Lehman CM, Sarago C, Nasim S, et al. Comparison of PCR with Southern hybridization for the routine detection of immunoglobulin heavy chain gene rearrangements. Am J Clin Pathol 1995;103:171–176.
28. Kuppers R, Zhao M, Rajewsky K, et al. Detection of clonal B cell populations in paraffin-embedded tissues by polymerase chain reaction. Am J Pathol 1993;143:230–239.

29. Lorenzen J, Jux G, Zhao-Hohn M, et al. Detection of T-cell clonality in paraffin-embedded tissues. Diagn Mol Pathol 1994;3:93–99.
30. Ilyas M, Jalal H, Linton C, et al. The use of the polymerase chain reaction in the diagnosis of B-cell lymphomas from formalin-fixed paraffin-embedded tissue. Histopathology 1995; 26:333–338.
31. Diss TC, Peng H, Wotherspoon AC, et al. Detection of monoclonality in low-grade B-cell lymphomas using the polymerase chain reaction is dependent on primer selection and lymphoma type. J Pathol 1993;169:291–295.
32. Segal GH, Jorgensen T, Masih AS, et al. Optimal primer selection for clonality assessment by polymerase chain reaction analysis: I. Low-grade B-cell lymphoproliferative disorders of nonfollicular center cell type [see Comments]. Hum Pathol 1994; 25:1269–1275.
33. Segal GH, Jorgensen T, Scott M, et al. Optimal primer selection for clonality assessment by polymerase chain reaction analysis: II. Follicular lymphomas [see Comments]. Hum Pathol 1994;25:1276–1282.
34. Sioutos N, Bagg A, Michaud GY, et al. Polymerase chain reaction versus Southern blot hybridization. Detection of immunoglobulin heavy-chain gene rearrangements. Diagn Mol Pathol 1995;4:8–13.
35. Greiner TC, Raffeld M, Lutz C, et al. Analysis of T cell receptor-gamma gene rearrangements by denaturing gradient gel electrophoresis of GC-clamped polymerase chain reaction products. Correlation with tumor-specific sequences. Am J Pathol 1995;146:46–55.
36. Inghirami G, Szabolcs MJ, Yee HT, et al. Detection of immunoglobulin gene rearrangement of B cell non-Hodgkin's lymphomas and leukemias in fresh, unfixed and formalin-fixed, paraffin-embedded tissue by polymerase chain reaction. Lab Invest 1993;68:746–757.
37. Greer CE, Peterson SL, Kiviat NB, et al. PCR amplification from paraffin-embedded tissues. Effects of fixative and fixation time [see Comments]. Am J Clin Pathol 1991;95:117–124.
38. Wyatt RT, Rudders RA, Zelenetz A, et al. BCL2 oncogene translocation is mediated by a chi-like consensus. J Exp Med 1992;175:1575–1588.
39. Lipkowitz S, Stern MH, Kirsch IR. Hybrid T cell receptor genes formed by interlocus recombination in normal and ataxia–telangiectasis lymphocytes. J Exp Med 1990;172:409–418.
40. Shiramizu B, Magrath I. Localization of breakpoints by polymerase chain reactions in Burkitt's lymphoma with 8;14 translocations. Blood 1990;75:1848–1852.
41. Ye BH, Lista F, Lo Coco F, et al. Alterations of a zinc finger-encoding gene, BCL-6, in diffuse large-cell lymphoma. Science 1993;262:747–750.
42. Molot RJ, Meeker TC, Wittwer CT, et al. Antigen expression and polymerase chain reaction amplification of mantle cell lymphomas. Blood 1994;83:1626–1631.
43. Lim LC, Segal GH, Wittwer CT. Detection of bcl-1 gene rearrangement and B-cell clonality in mantle cell lymphoma using formalin-fixed, paraffin-embedded tissues. Am J Clin Pathol 1995;104:689–695.
44. Segal GH, Maiese RL. Mantle cell lymphoma. Rapid polymerase chain reaction-based genotyping of a morphologically heterogeneous entity. Arch Pathol Lab Med 1996;120:835–841.
45. Lasota J, Franssila K, Koo CH, et al. Molecular diagnosis of mantle cell lymphoma in paraffin-embedded tissue. Mod Pathol 1996;9:361–366.
46. Ott MM, Helbing A, Ott G, et al. bcl-1 rearrangement and cyclin D1 protein expression in mantle cell lymphoma. J Pathol 1996;179:238–242.
47. Waggott W, Lo YM, Bastard C, et al. Detection of NPM-ALK DNA rearrangement in CD30 positive anaplastic large cell lymphoma. Br J Haematol 1995;89:905–907.
48. Ladanyi M, Cavalchire G. Detection of the NPM-ALK genomic rearrangement of Ki-1 lymphoma and isolation of the involved NPM and ALK introns. Diagn Mol Pathol 1996;5:154–158.
49. Yamada M, Hudson S, Tournay O, et al. Detection of minimal disease in hematopoietic malignancies of the B-cell lineage by using third-complementarity-determining region (CDR-III)-specific probes. Proc Natl Acad Sci U S A 1989;86:5123–5127.
50. Ratech H, Masih A. Sensitive detection of clonal antigen receptor gene rearrangements in non-Hodgkin's malignant lymphoma with an anchored polymerase chain reaction-based strategy. Am J Clin Pathol 1993;100:527–533.
51. Doenecke A, Winnacker EL, Hallek M. Rapid amplification of cDNA ends (RACE) improves the PCR-based isolation of immunoglobulin variable region genes from murine and human lymphoma cells and cell lines. Leukemia 1997;11:1787–1792.
52. Dalla-Favera R, Bregni M, Erikson J, et al. Human c-myc onc gene is located on the region of chromosome 8 that is translocated in Burkitt lymphoma cells. Proc Natl Acad Sci U S A 1982;79:7824–7827.
53. Neel BG, Jhanwar SC, Chaganti RS, et al. Two human c-onc genes are located on the long arm of chromosome 8. Proc Natl Acad Sci U S A 1982;79:7842–7846.
54. Magrath I. The pathogenesis of Burkitt's lymphoma. Adv Cancer Res 1990;55:133–270.
55. Offit K, Chaganti RS. Chromosomal aberrations in non-Hodgkin's lymphoma. Biologic and clinical correlations. Hematol Oncol Clin North Am 1991;5:853–869.
56. Offit K. Chromosome analysis in the management of patients with non-Hodgkin's lymphoma. Leuk Lymphoma 1992;7: 275–282.
57. Johansson B, Mertens F, Mitelman F. Cytogenetic evolution patterns in non-Hodgkin's lymphoma. Blood 1995;86:3905–3914.
58. De Jong D, Voetdijk BM, Beverstock GC, et al. Activation of the c-myc oncogene in a precursor-B-cell blast crisis of follicular lymphoma, presenting as composite lymphoma. N Engl J Med 1988;318:1373–1378.
59. Stone J, de Lange T, Ramsay G, et al. Definition of regions in human c-myc that are involved in transformation and nuclear localization. Mol Cell Biol 1987;7:1697–1709.
60. Blackwell TK, Kretzner L, Blackwood EM, et al. Sequence-specific DNA binding by the c-myc protein. Science 1990;250: 1149–1151.
61. Marcu KB, Bossone SA, Patel AJ. myc function and regulation. Annu Rev Biochem 1992;61:809–860.
62. Amati B, Dalton S, Brooks MW, et al. Transcriptional activation by the human c-myc oncoprotein in yeast requires interaction with Max. Nature 1992;359:423–426.
63. Milner AE, Grand RJ, Waters CM, et al. Apoptosis in Burkitt lymphoma cells is driven by c-myc. Oncogene 1993;8:3385–3391.
64. Hanson KD, Shichiri M, Follansbee MR, et al. Effects of c-myc expression on cell cycle progression. Mol Cell Biol 1994;14: 5748–5755.
65. Cory S. Activation of cellular oncogenes in hemopoietic cells by chromosome translocation. Adv Cancer Res 1986;47:189–234.
66. Hayday AC, Gillies SD, Saito H, et al. Activation of a translocated human c-myc gene by an enhancer in the immunoglobulin heavy-chain locus. Nature 1984;307:334–340.
67. Madisen L, Groudine M. Identification of a locus control region in the immunoglobulin heavy-chain locus that deregulates c-myc expression in plasmacytoma and Burkitt's lymphoma cells. Genes Dev 1994;8:2212–2226.

68. Polack A, Feederle R, Klobeck G, et al. Regulatory elements in the immunoglobulin kappa locus induce c-myc activation and the promoter shift in Burkitt's lymphoma cells. EMBO J 1993;12:3913–3920.
69. Hortnagel K, Mautner J, Strobl LJ, et al. The role of immunoglobulin kappa elements in c-myc activation. Oncogene 1995;10:1393–1401.
70. Blomberg BB, Rudin CM, Storb U. Identification and localization of an enhancer for the human lambda L chain Ig gene complex. J Immunol 1991;147:2354–2358.
71. Gerbitz A, Mautner J, Geltinger C, et al. Deregulation of the proto-oncogene c-myc through t(8;22) translocation in Burkitt's lymphoma. Oncogene 1999;18:1745–1753.
72. Pelicci PG, Knowles DMD, Magrath I, et al. Chromosomal breakpoints and structural alterations of the c-myc locus differ in endemic and sporadic forms of Burkitt lymphoma. Proc Natl Acad Sci U S A 1986;83:2984–2988.
73. Shiramizu B, Barriga F, Neequaye J, et al. Patterns of chromosomal breakpoint locations in Burkitt's lymphoma: relevance to geography and Epstein-Barr virus association. Blood 1991;77: 1516–1526.
74. Joos S, Falk MH, Lichter P, et al. Variable breakpoints in Burkitt lymphoma cells with chromosomal t(8;14) translocation separate c-myc and the IgH locus up to several hundred kb. Hum Mol Genet 1992;1:625–632.
75. Joos S, Haluska FG, Falk MH, et al. Mapping chromosomal breakpoints of Burkitt's t(8;14) translocations far upstream of c-myc. Cancer Res 1992;52:6547–6552.
76. Neri A, Barriga F, Knowles DM, et al. Different regions of the immunoglobulin heavy-chain locus are involved in chromosomal translocations in distinct pathogenetic forms of Burkitt lymphoma. Proc Natl Acad Sci U S A 1988;85:2748–2752.
77. Siebert R, Matthiesen P, Harder S, et al. Application of interphase fluorescence *in situ* hybridization for the detection of the Burkitt translocation t(8;14)(q24;q32) in B-cell lymphomas. Blood 1998;91:984–990.
78. Rosenberg CL, Wong E, Petty EM, et al. PRAD1, a candidate BCL1 oncogene: mapping and expression in centrocytic lymphoma. Proc Natl Acad Sci U S A 1991;88:9638–9642.
79. Tsujimoto Y, Yunis J, Onorato-Showe L, et al. Molecular cloning of the chromosomal breakpoint of B-cell lymphomas and leukemias with the t(11;14) chromosome translocation. Science 1984;224:1403–1406.
80. Raffeld M, Jaffe ES. bcl-1, t(11;14), and mantle cell-derived lymphomas [Editorial]. Blood 1991;78:259–263.
81. Banks PM, Chan J, Cleary ML, et al. Mantle cell lymphoma. A proposal for unification of morphologic, immunologic, and molecular data [see Comments]. Am J Surg Pathol 1992;16: 637–640.
82. Rimokh R, Berger F, Cornillet P, et al. Break in the BCL1 locus is closely associated with intermediate lymphocytic lymphoma subtype. Genes Chromosomes Cancer 1990;2:223–226.
83. Leroux D, Le Marc'Hadour F, Gressin R, et al. Non-Hodgkin's lymphomas with t(11;14)(q13;q32): a subset of mantle zone/intermediate lymphocytic lymphoma? Br J Haematol 1991;77: 346–353.
84. Williams ME, Swerdlow SH, Rosenberg CL, et al. Chromosome 11 translocation breakpoints at the PRAD1/cyclin D1 gene locus in centrocytic lymphoma. Leukemia 1993;7:241–245.
85. Vandenberghe E, De Wolf Peeters C, Wlodarska I, et al. Chromosome 11q rearrangements in B non-Hodgkin's lymphoma. Br J Haematol 1992;81:212–217.
86. Kurtin PJ. Mantle cell lymphoma. Adv Anat Pathol 1998;5: 376–398.
87. Brito-Babapulle V, Ellis J, Matutes E, et al. Translocation t(11; 14)(q13;q32) in chronic lymphoid disorders. Genes Chromosomes Cancer 1992;5:158–165.
88. Fiedler W, Weh HJ, Hossfeld DK. Comparison of chromosome analysis and BCL-1 rearrangement in a series of patients with multiple myeloma. Br J Haematol 1992;81:58–61.
89. Jadayel D, Matutes E, Dyer MJ, et al. Splenic lymphoma with villous lymphocytes: analysis of BCL-1 rearrangements and expression of the cyclin D1 gene. Blood 1994;83:3664–3671.
90. Troussard X, Mauvieux L, Radford-Weiss I, et al. Genetic analysis of splenic lymphoma with villous lymphocytes: a Groupe Francais d'Hématologie Cellulaire (GFHC) study. Br J Haematol 1998;101:712–721.
91. Bennett JM, Catovsky D, Daniel MT, et al. Proposals for the classification of chronic (mature) B and T lymphoid leukaemias. French–American–British (FAB) Cooperative Group. J Clin Pathol 1989;42:567–584.
92. Bosch F, Jares P, Campo E, et al. PRAD-1/cyclin D1 gene overexpression in chronic lymphoproliferative disorders: a highly specific marker of mantle cell lymphoma. Blood 1994;84:2726–2732.
93. Lishner M, Lalkin A, Klein A, et al. The BCL-1, BCL-2, and BCL-3 oncogenes are involved in chronic lymphocytic leukemia. Detection by fluorescence *in situ* hybridization. Cancer Genet Cytogenet 1995;85:118–123.
94. Cuneo A, Bigoni R, Negrini M, et al. Cytogenetic and interphase cytogenetic characterization of atypical chronic lymphocytic leukemia carrying BCL1 translocation. Cancer Res 1997; 57:1144–1150.
95. Ott G, Kalla J, Ott MM, et al. Blastoid variants of mantle cell lymphoma: frequent bcl-1 rearrangements at the major translocation cluster region and tetraploid chromosome clones. Blood 1997;89:1421–1429.
96. Hunter T, Pines J. Cyclins and cancer. II: Cyclin D and CDK inhibitors come of age [see Comments]. Cell 1994;79:573–582.
97. Konstantinidis AK, Radhakrishnan R, Gu F, et al. Purification, characterization, and kinetic mechanism of cyclin D1 CDK4, a major target for cell cycle regulation. J Biol Chem 1998;273: 26506–26515.
98. Sherr CJ. G1 phase progression: cycling on cue. Cell 1994;79: 551–555.
99. Lukas J, Jadayel D, Bartkova J, et al. BCL-1/cyclin D1 oncoprotein oscillates and subverts the G1 phase control in B-cell neoplasms carrying the t(11;14) translocation. Oncogene 1994; 9:2159–2167.
100. Lukas J, Bartkova J, Bartek J. Convergence of mitogenic signalling cascades from diverse classes of receptors at the cyclin D-cyclin-dependent kinase-pRb-controlled G1 checkpoint. Mol Cell Biol 1996;16:6917–6925.
101. Lukas J, Petersen BO, Holm K, et al. Deregulated expression of E2F family members induces S-phase entry and overcomes p16INK4A-mediated growth suppression. Mol Cell Biol 1996;16:1047–1057.
102. Wang JY, Knudsen ES, Welch PJ. The retinoblastoma tumor suppressor protein. Adv Cancer Res 1994;64:25–85.
103. Betticher DC. Cyclin D1, another molecule of the year? [Editorial]. Ann Oncol 1996;7:223–225.
104. Bates S, Peters G. Cyclin D1 as a cellular proto-oncogene. Semin Cancer Biol 1995;6:73–82.
105. Palmero I, Holder A, Sinclair AJ, et al. Cyclins D1 and D2 are differentially expressed in human B-lymphoid cell lines. Oncogene 1993;8:1049–1054.
106. Bartkova J, Lukas J, Strauss M, et al. Cell cycle-related variation and tissue-restricted expression of human cyclin D1 protein. J Pathol 1994;172:237–245.
107. Gronbaek K, Nedergaard T, Andersen MK, et al. Concurrent disruption of cell cycle associated genes in mantle cell lymphoma: a genotypic and phenotypic study of cyclin D1, p16, p15, p53 and pRb. Leukemia 1998;12:1266–1271.

108. Berenson JR, Yang J, Mickel RA. Frequent amplification of the bcl-1 locus in head and neck squamous cell carcinomas. Oncogene 1989;4:1111–1116.
109. Williams ME, Meeker TC, Swerdlow SH. Rearrangement of the chromosome 11 bcl-1 locus in centrocytic lymphoma: analysis with multiple breakpoint probes. Blood 1991;78:493–498.
110. Rimokh R, Berger F, Delsol G, et al. Detection of the chromosomal translocation t(11;14) by polymerase chain reaction in mantle cell lymphomas. Blood 1994;83:1871–1875.
111. Tsujimoto Y, Louie E, Bashir MM, et al. The reciprocal partners of both the t(14;18) and the t(11;14) translocations involved in B-cell neoplasms are rearranged by the same mechanism. Oncogene 1988;2:347–351.
112. Raynaud SD, Bekri S, Leroux D, et al. Expanded range of 11q13 breakpoints with differing patterns of cyclin D1 expression in B-cell malignancies. Genes Chromosomes Cancer 1993;8:80–87.
113. Fan H, Gulley ML, Gascoyne RD, et al. Molecular methods for detecting t(11;14) translocations in mantle-cell lymphomas. Diagn Mol Pathol 1998;7:209–214.
114. Williams ME, Swerdlow SH, Meeker TC. Chromosome t(11;14)(q13;q32) breakpoints in centrocytic lymphoma are highly localized at the bcl-1 major translocation cluster. Leukemia 1993;7:1437–1440.
115. Tsujimoto Y, Gorham J, Cossman J, et al. The t(14;18) chromosome translocations involved in B-cell neoplasms result from mistakes in VDJ joining. Science 1985;229:1390–1393.
116. Tsujimoto Y, Cossman J, Jaffe E, et al. Involvement of the bcl-2 gene in human follicular lymphoma. Science 1985;228:1440–1443.
117. Bakhshi A, Jensen JP, Goldman P, et al. Cloning the chromosomal breakpoint of t(14;18) human lymphomas: clustering around JH on chromosome 14 and near a transcriptional unit on 18. Cell 1985;41:899–906.
118. Cleary ML, Sklar J. Nucleotide sequence of a t(14;18) chromosomal breakpoint in follicular lymphoma and demonstration of a breakpoint-cluster region near a transcriptionally active locus on chromosome 18. Proc Natl Acad Sci U S A 1985;82:7439–7443.
119. Yunis JJ, Oken MM, Kaplan ME, et al. Distinctive chromosomal abnormalities in histologic subtypes of non-Hodgkin's lymphoma. N Engl J Med 1982;307:1231–1236.
120. Speaks SL, Sanger WG, Linder J, et al. Chromosomal abnormalities in indolent lymphoma. Cancer Genet Cytogenet 1987; 27:335–344.
121. Levine EG, Arthur DC, Frizzera G, et al. There are differences in cytogenetic abnormalities among histologic subtypes of the non-Hodgkin's lymphomas. Blood 1985;66:1414–1422.
122. Correlation of chromosome abnormalities with histologic and immunologic characteristics in non-Hodgkin's lymphoma and adult T cell leukemia-lymphoma. Fifth International Workshop on Chromosomes in Leukemia–Lymphoma. Blood 1987; 70:1554–1564.
123. Croce CM. Molecular biology of lymphomas. Semin Oncol 1993;20:31–46.
124. Nowell PC, Croce CM. Philip Levine award lecture. Chromosome translocations and oncogenes in human lymphoid tumors. Am J Clin Pathol 1990;94:229–237.
125. Richardson ME, Chen QG, Filippa DA, et al. Intermediate- to high-grade histology of lymphomas carrying t(14;18) is associated with additional nonrandom chromosome changes. Blood 1987;70:444–447.
126. Weiss LM, Warnke RA, Sklar J, et al. Molecular analysis of the t(14;18) chromosomal translocation in malignant lymphomas. N Engl J Med 1987;317:1185–1189.
127. Seto M, Jaeger U, Hockett RD, et al. Alternative promoters and exons, somatic mutation and deregulation of the Bcl-2-Ig fusion gene in lymphoma. EMBO J 1988;7:123–131.
128. Vaux DL, Cory S, Adams JM. Bcl-2 gene promotes haemopoietic cell survival and cooperates with c-myc to immortalize pre-B cells. Nature 1988;335:440–442.
129. Nunez G, London L, Hockenbery D, et al. Deregulated Bcl-2 gene expression selectively prolongs survival of growth factor-deprived hemopoietic cell lines. J Immunol 1990;144:3602–3610.
130. Cory S. Regulation of lymphocyte survival by the bcl-2 gene family. Annu Rev Immunol 1995;13:513–543.
131. Ngan BY, Nourse J, Cleary ML. Detection of chromosomal translocation t(14;18) within the minor cluster region of bcl-2 by polymerase chain reaction and direct genomic sequencing of the enzymatically amplified DNA in follicular lymphomas. Blood 1989;73:1759–1762.
132. Horsman DE, Gascoyne RD, Coupland RW, et al. Comparison of cytogenetic analysis, Southern analysis, and polymerase chain reaction for the detection of t(14;18) in follicular lymphoma. Am J Clin Pathol 1995;103:472–478.
133. Limpens J, de Jong D, van Krieken JH, et al. Bcl-2/JH rearrangements in benign lymphoid tissues with follicular hyperplasia. Oncogene 1991;6:2271–2276.
134. Aster JC, Kobayashi Y, Shiota M, et al. Detection of the t(14;18) at similar frequencies in hyperplastic lymphoid tissues from American and Japanese patients. Am J Pathol 1992;141: 291–299.
135. Falini B, Bigerna B, Fizzotti M, et al. ALK expression defines a distinct group of T/null lymphomas ("ALK lymphomas") with a wide morphological spectrum. Am J Pathol 1998;153:875–886.
136. Falini B, Pileri S, Zinzani PL, et al. ALK+ lymphoma: clinico-pathological findings and outcome. Blood 1999;93:2697–2706.
137. Benharroch D, Meguerian-Bedoyan Z, Lamant L, et al. ALK-positive lymphoma: a single disease with a broad spectrum of morphology. Blood 1998;91:2076–2084.
138. Morris SW, Kirstein MN, Valentine MB, et al. Fusion of a kinase gene, ALK, to a nucleolar protein gene, NPM, in non-Hodgkin's lymphoma [published erratum appears in Science 1995;267:316–317]. Science 1994;263:1281–1284.
139. Shiota M, Fujimoto J, Semba T, et al. Hyperphosphorylation of a novel 80 kDa protein-tyrosine kinase similar to Ltk in a human Ki-1 lymphoma cell line, AMS3. Oncogene 1994;9:1567–1574.
140. Ott G, Katzenberger T, Siebert R, et al. Chromosomal abnormalities in nodal and extranodal CD30+ anaplastic large cell lymphomas: infrequent detection of the t(2;5) in extranodal lymphomas. Genes Chromosomes Cancer 1998;22:114–121.
141. Pulford K, Lamant L, Morris SW, et al. Detection of anaplastic lymphoma kinase (ALK) and nucleolar protein nucleophosmin (NPM)-ALK proteins in normal and neoplastic cells with the monoclonal antibody ALK1. Blood 1997;89:1394–1404.
142. Lamant L, Dastugue N, Pulford K, et al. A new fusion gene TPM3-ALK in anaplastic large cell lymphoma created by a (1;2)(q25;p23) translocation [In Process Citation]. Blood 1999;93:3088–3095.
143. Pittaluga S, Wiodarska I, Pulford K, et al. The monoclonal antibody ALK1 identifies a distinct morphological subtype of anaplastic large cell lymphoma associated with 2p23/ALK rearrangements. Am J Pathol 1997;151:343–351.
144. Wlodarska I, De Wolf-Peeters C, Falini B, et al. The cryptic inv(2)(p23q35) defines a new molecular genetic subtype of ALK-positive anaplastic large-cell lymphoma. Blood 1998;92: 2688–2695.
145. Iwahara T, Fujimoto J, Wen D, et al. Molecular characterization of ALK, a receptor tyrosine kinase expressed specifically in the nervous system. Oncogene 1997;14:439–449.
146. Morris SW, Naeve C, Mathew P, et al. ALK, the chromosome 2 gene locus altered by the t(2;5) in non-Hodgkin's lymphoma,

encodes a novel neural receptor tyrosine kinase that is highly related to leukocyte tyrosine kinase (LTK) [published erratum appears in Oncogene 1997;15:2883]. Oncogene 1997;14:2175–2188.

147. Chan WY, Liu QR, Borjigin J, et al. Characterization of the cDNA encoding human nucleophosmin and studies of its role in normal and abnormal growth. Biochemistry 1989;28:1033–1039.
148. Schmidt-Zachmann MS, Hugle-Dorr B, Franke WW. A constitutive nucleolar protein identified as a member of the nucleoplasmin family. EMBO J 1987;6:1881–1890.
149. Borer RA, Lehner CF, Eppenberger HM, et al. Major nucleolar proteins shuttle between nucleus and cytoplasm. Cell 1989; 56:379–390.
150. Bischof D, Pulford K, Mason DY, et al. Role of the nucleophosmin (NPM) portion of the non-Hodgkin's lymphoma-associated NPM-anaplastic lymphoma kinase fusion protein in oncogenesis. Mol Cell Biol 1997;17:2312–2325.
151. Fujimoto J, Shiota M, Iwahara T, et al. Characterization of the transforming activity of p80, a hyperphosphorylated protein in a Ki-1 lymphoma cell line with chromosomal translocation t(2;5). Proc Natl Acad Sci U S A 1996;93:4181–4186.
152. Mason DY, Pulford KA, Bischof D, et al. Nucleolar localization of the nucleophosmin-anaplastic lymphoma kinase is not required for malignant transformation. Cancer Res 1998;58: 1057–1062.
153. Liu Q-R, Chan PK. Characterisation of seven processed pseudogenes of nucleophosmin/B23 in the human genome. DNA Cell Biol 1993;12:149–156.
154. Simonitsch I, Panzer-Gruemayer ER, Ghali DW, et al. NPM/ALK gene fusion transcripts identify a distinct subgroup of null type Ki-1 positive anaplastic large cell lymphomas. Br J Haematol 1996;92:866–871.
155. Downing JR, Shurtleff SA, Zielenska M, et al. Molecular detection of the (2;5) translocation of non-Hodgkin's lymphoma by reverse transcriptase-polymerase chain reaction. Blood 1995;85: 3416–3422.
156. Bullrich F, Morris SW, Hummel M, et al. Nucleophosmin (NPM) gene rearrangements in Ki-1-positive lymphomas. Cancer Res 1994;54:2873–2877.
157. Orscheschek K, Merz H, Hell J, et al. Large-cell anaplastic lymphoma-specific translocation (t[2;5] [p23;q35]) in Hodgkin's disease: indication of a common pathogenesis? [see Comments]. Lancet 1995;345:87–90.
158. Orscheschek K, Merz H, Hell J, et al. Presence of the t(2;5) in Hodgkin's disease [Letter; Comment]. Blood 1995;86:4383–4385.
159. Ladanyi M, Cavalchire G, Morris SW, et al. Reverse transcriptase polymerase chain reaction for the Ki-1 anaplastic large cell lymphoma-associated t(2;5) translocation in Hodgkin's disease [published erratum appears in Am J Pathol 1995;146:546]. Am J Pathol 1994;145:1296–1300.
160. Elmberger PG, Lozano MD, Weisenburger DD, et al. Transcripts of the npm-alk fusion gene in anaplastic large cell lymphoma, Hodgkin's disease, and reactive lymphoid lesions. Blood 1995;86:3517–3521.
161. Wellmann A, Otsuki T, Vogelbruch M, et al. Analysis of the t(2;5)(p23;q35) translocation by reverse transcription-polymerase chain reaction in CD30+ anaplastic large-cell lymphomas, in other non-Hodgkin's lymphomas of T-cell phenotype, and in Hodgkin's disease. Blood 1995;86:2321–2328.
162. Weiss LM, Lopategui JR, Sun LH, et al. Absence of the t(2;5) in Hodgkin's disease [see Comments]. Blood 1995;85:2845–2847.
163. Lamant L, Meggetto F, al Saati T, et al. High incidence of the t(2;5)(p23;q35) translocation in anaplastic large cell lymphoma and its lack of detection in Hodgkin's disease. Comparison of cytogenetic analysis, reverse transcriptase-polymerase chain reaction, and P-80 immunostaining. Blood 1996;87:284–291.
164. Wood GS, Hardman DL, Boni R, et al. Lack of the t(2;5) or other mutations resulting in expression of anaplastic lymphoma kinase catalytic domain in CD30+ primary cutaneous lymphoproliferative disorders and Hodgkin's disease. Blood 1996;88: 1765–1770.
165. Sarris AH, Luthra R, Papadimitracopoulou V, et al. Amplification of genomic DNA demonstrates the presence of the t(2;5) (p23;q35) in anaplastic large cell lymphoma, but not in other non-Hodgkin's lymphomas, Hodgkin's disease, or lymphomatoid papulosis [see Comments]. Blood 1996;88:1771–1779.
166. Waggott W, Delsol G, Jarret RF, et al. NPM-ALK gene fusion and Hodgkin's disease [Letter; Comment]. Blood 1997;90: 1712–1713.
167. Yee HT, Ponzoni M, Merson A, et al. Molecular characterization of the t(2;5) (p23;q35) translocation in anaplastic large cell lymphoma (Ki-1) and Hodgkin's disease. Blood 1996;87:1081–1088.
168. Weber-Matthiesen K, Deerberg-Wittram J, Rosenwald A, et al. Translocation t(2;5) is not a primary event in Hodgkin's disease. Simultaneous immunophenotyping and interphase cytogenetics. Am J Pathol 1996;149:463–468.
169. Mathew P, Sanger WG, Weisenburger DD, et al. Detection of the t(2;5)(p23;q35) and NPM-ALK fusion in non-Hodgkin's lymphoma by two-color fluorescence *in situ* hybridization. Blood 1997;89:1678–1685.
170. Herbst H, Anagnostopoulos J, Heinze B, et al. ALK gene products in anaplastic large cell lymphomas and Hodgkin's disease. Blood 1995;86:1694–1700.
171. Beylot-Barry M, Groppi A, Vergier B, et al. Characterization of t(2;5) reciprocal transcripts and genomic breakpoints in CD30+ cutaneous lymphoproliferations. Blood 1998;91:4668–4676.

PART III

SECTION ONE

VIRAL LYMPHADENITIDES

A variety of viruses may cause acute or chronic lymphadenitis. In some cases, the presence of viruses in the affected lymph nodes can be demonstrated by histologic, immunologic, or biochemical methods. As a result, clinicopathologic entities have been defined. These are described in the following chapters. In others, although viruses are sometimes suspected, they cannot be demonstrated. This may be the case with some lymphadenitides included in the nonspecific categories of reactive hyperplasias and probably with some lymphadenopathies of yet undetermined etiology.

9

INFECTIOUS MONONUCLEOSIS LYMPHADENITIS

DEFINITION

Acute lymphadenitis caused by infection with Epstein-Barr virus (EBV).

SYNONYM

EBV lymphadenitis.

ETIOLOGY

Infectious mononucleosis is induced by EBV, a DNA virus that is a member of the Herpesviridae family (1). EBV is an enveloped, icosahedral virus containing a double-stranded segment of DNA expressed in a linear form during active replication in the acute infection and as circular episomes in infected cells in the latent infection (2).

EPIDEMIOLOGY

Epstein-Barr virus is ubiquitous in nature; however, its spread varies in different human populations. In conditions of inadequate standards of living, EBV infection occurs early in life and is almost universal. By the age of 3, almost 100% of children have positive serology. The infection may pass unnoticed; however, more than half of the population continues to shed virus and thus disseminate the infection (3,4). In countries with better living conditions, only about 50% of persons exposed to EBV acquire the infection. This occurs as infectious mononucleosis (IM), an acute, self-limited disease that affects primarily adolescents and young adults, with a peak incidence between 15 and 20 years of age. In the United States, the incidence is 50 per 100,000, or about 100,000 cases per year (3,4).

PATHOGENESIS

Epstein-Barr virus is present in the throat of 85% of patients with IM. The virus infects susceptible lymphoid cells in the oropharynx through the C3d cell receptor for complement, and an active or latent infection results (5). Whether the epithelial cells of the oropharynx that express a similar EBV receptor are also infected by the virus is still a matter of debate (6,7). During the acute infection, replication of EBV in the activated perifollicular B cells triggers a vigorous humoral and cellular immune response. Antibodies against EBV, which are absent before the onset of IM, appear during the illness in rising titers and persist for years thereafter (3,4). They are able to contain the infection and are used in the serologic diagnosis of IM. In addition, an agglutinin to erythrocytes of sheep and horses that is produced provides the basis for the heterophil test of Paul-Bunnell, widely used as the MonoSpot diagnostic test. The cellular immune response is represented by the activation of interfollicular T cells, which appear as large, transformed immunoblasts (8–10). Both activated B and T cells may circulate in the peripheral blood as atypical lymphocytes (Downey cells). They are transformed lymphocytes (immunoblasts) with abundant, bluish, typically "pleated" cytoplasm and large nuclei with conspicuous nucleoli (Fig. 9.1). Eventually, the acute infection subsides and converts to a low-grade, latent B-cell infection that persists throughout life (11). In persons with immune deficiencies, particularly of the T-cell system, life-threatening diseases rather than self-limited IM may be the result of EBV infection. Thus, persons with the congenital X-linked lymphoproliferative syndrome may be affected by fatal IM, post-transplant lymphoproliferative disorders may develop in immunosuppressed recipients of organ transplants, and large B-cell non-Hodgkin lymphoma may develop in persons with AIDS as the result of persistent EBV infection (12).

CLINICAL SYNDROME

Infectious mononucleosis usually affects teenagers and young adults. Occasionally, elderly persons, an 80-year-old patient in one reported case (13), may be affected severely, so that a diagnosis of lymphoma is suspected.

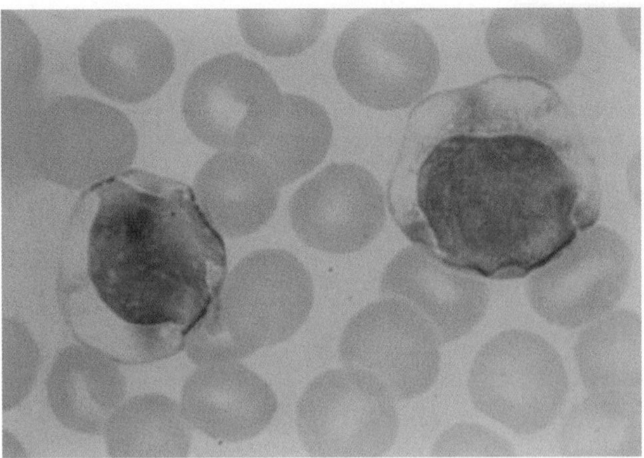

FIGURE 9.1. Atypical lymphocytes (Downey cells) in the peripheral blood of a patient with infectious mononucleosis. These are transformed lymphocytes (immunoblasts) with abundant bluish, "pleated" cytoplasm and large, nucleolated nuclei. Giemsa stain.

The incubation period is 30 to 40 days (3). The characteristic triad includes fever, pharyngitis, and cervical or generalized lymphadenopathy. Occasionally, splenomegaly, palatine petechiae, tonsillitis, and hepatomegaly are present. The peripheral leukocyte count rises to more than 10,000/mm^3 in the second week, with lymphomononuclear elements representing 60% and atypical lymphocytes 10% to 20% of the total (3). The number of circulating lymphocytes forming rosettes with sheep erythrocytes is increased, indicating that the atypical lymphoid cells in the peripheral blood are of T-cell origin (14).

Sometimes, malaise, fatigue, and palpable lymph nodes are the only manifestations. Uncommonly, complications such as hepatitis with elevated hepatic enzymes and jaundice, splenitis with splenic rupture, nephritis, encephalitis, and skin rashes may occur. Persons with congenital immune deficiencies are highly vulnerable to EBV-induced diseases. Males with the X-linked recessive lymphoproliferative syndrome, first described in six boys of the Duncan kindred, inherit a progressive combined variable immunodeficiency; if they become infected with EBV, a fatal IM (Fig. 9.2), aplastic anemia, hypogammaglobulinemia, or malignant B-cell lymphoma develops (9,15). A defect at the lymphoproliferative control locus on the X chromosome is responsible in these subjects for the inability to control the proliferation of EBV-stimulated B cells (16). Similar situations may develop in heavily immunosuppressed recipients of organ transplants, in whom the uncontrolled proliferation of EBV-transformed B cells gives rise to a broad spectrum of lymphoproliferative disorders, ranging from polyclonal B-cell hyperplasias to monoclonal B-cell lymphomas (17–20).

GROSS APPEARANCE

Involved lymph nodes are moderately enlarged and soft, but not matted. The capsule is not thickened, and the shape is generally preserved. The section appears uniform, pink–gray, and wet, with occasional foci of necrosis.

HISTOPATHOLOGY

The lymph node architecture is regionally distorted but not entirely effaced. The major changes are reactive hyperplasia

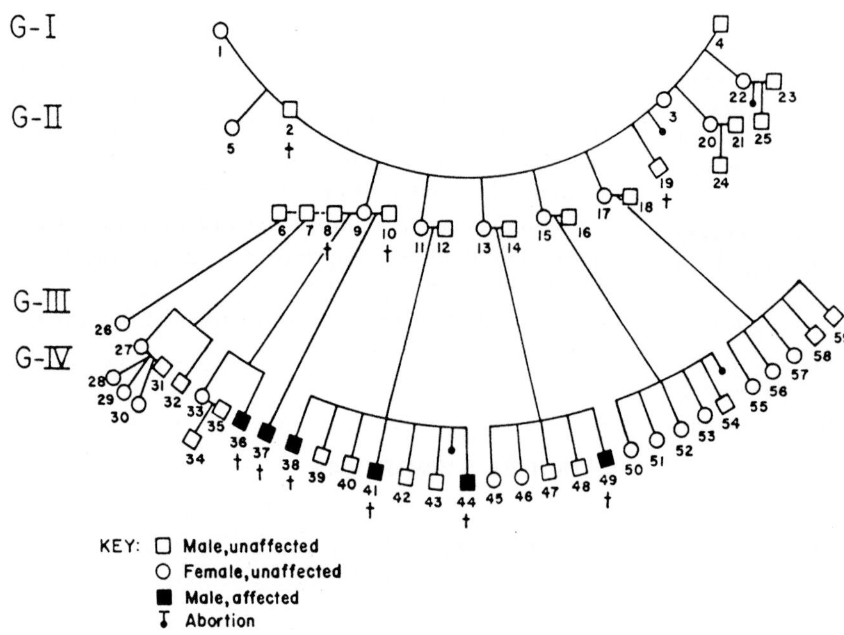

FIGURE 9.2. Pedigree of the Duncan kindred affected by the X-linked lymphoproliferative syndrome. [From Purtilo DT, Cassel C, Yang JPS, et al. X-linked recessive combined variable immunodeficiency (Duncan's disease). Lancet 1975;1:935, with permission.]

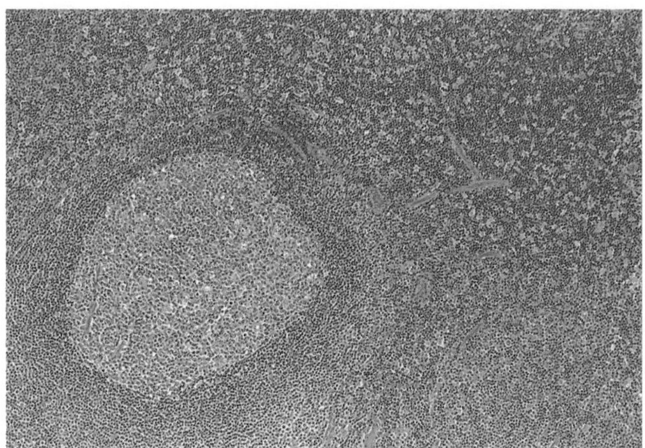

FIGURE 9.3. Infectious mononucleosis lymphadenitis. Hyperplastic, irregularly shaped follicle with reactive germinal center comprising numerous tingible-body macrophages. The interfollicular paracortex is expanded and has a mottled appearance. Hematoxylin, phloxine, and saffron stain.

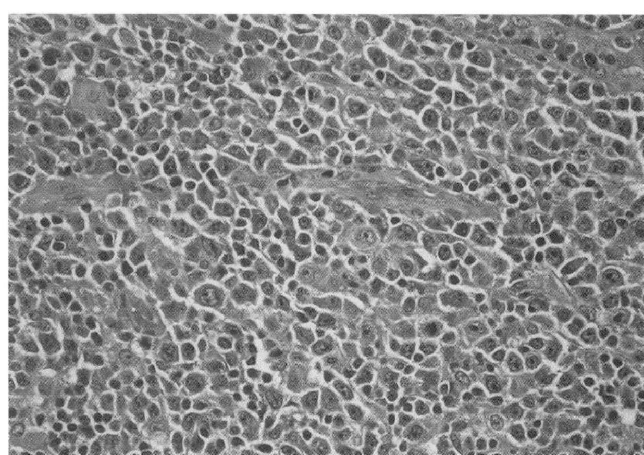

FIGURE 9.5. Infectious mononucleosis lymphadenitis. Paracortex expanded by sheets of transformed T lymphocytes (immunoblasts). Hematoxylin, phloxine, and saffron stain.

of the lymphoid follicles, expansion and distortion of the paracortex or T-cell zone, and the dilation of the sinuses (21). The involvement of these various lymph node components in the reactive process results in a mixed pattern of lymphoid hyperplasia (22). The follicles are moderately hyperplastic and irregularly shaped (15, 23) (Figs. 9.3 and 9.4). The germinal centers are enlarged and show signs of cell necrosis and regeneration. They are littered with broken nuclei and include macrophages containing nuclear debris (tingible-body macrophages) and numerous centroblasts in mitosis. A characteristic feature is the involvement of the paracortical area or the inner cortex, another indication that the T cells are the main cellular element involved in IM (14). Because of extensive proliferation of immunoblasts in the paracortical area, a mottled ("moth-eaten") aspect, not unlike that seen in other viral lymphadenitides, may result (23) (Fig. 9.3). Immunoblasts, sometimes in confluent sheets (Fig. 9.5), represent activated lymphocytes; these are three to four times larger (15 to 25 μm) than the small, resting lymphocytes and contain abundant, strongly pyroninophilic cytoplasm and vesicular nuclei that contain one or more prominent nucleoli and frequent mitoses (Fig. 9.6). On occasion, unusually large cells, mononucleated or polynucleated with prominent nucleoli, that resemble and are sometimes indistinguishable from the Hodgkin and Reed-Sternberg cells of Hodgkin lymphoma, may be present (24–26) (Fig. 9.6). In most cases, however, the nucleoli, although prominent, lack the eosinophilia and inclusion-like appearance of Hodgkin or

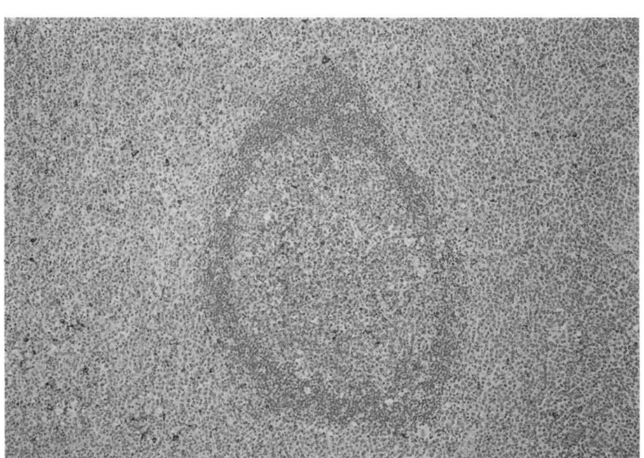

FIGURE 9.4. Same lymph node as in Fig. 9.3 with hyperplastic follicle and reactive germinal center immunostained for B-cell marker CD74. LN-2 antibody/peroxidase stain.

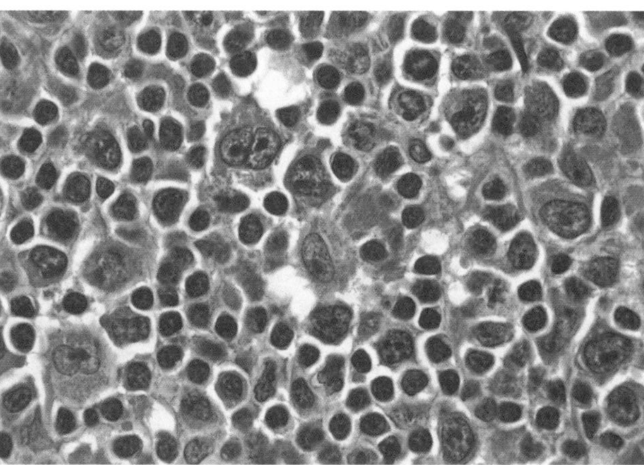

FIGURE 9.6. Same section as in Fig. 9.5. Transformed lymphocytes (immunoblasts) appear in sheets. They are four to six times larger than lymphocytes and have large nuclei and prominent nucleoli, often resembling Hodgkin cells and Reed-Sternberg cells. Hematoxylin, phloxine, and saffron stain.

Reed-Sternberg cells (21). An important differential feature is that the cells surrounding the Reed-Sternberg cells in Hodgkin lymphoma are small lymphocytes and eosinophils, whereas the cells surrounding the Reed-Sternberg-like cells in IM are immunoblasts. Circulating in the peripheral blood are activated T cells or immunoblasts, known as *atypical lymphocytes* or *Downey cells*; these are considered characteristic of IM. On blood smears, the atypical lymphocytes are larger than normal, with indented or horseshoe-shaped nuclei that are eccentrically placed. The cytoplasm is basophilic and has a characteristic "pleated" appearance (Fig. 9.1). In the lymph node, the immunoblasts are diffusely scattered throughout the interfollicular areas. Lymph node sinuses are either compressed by the expanded paracortex or dilated and filled with hyperplastic sinus histiocytes, immunoblasts, plasma cells, lymphocytes, and abundant, eosinophilic, proteinaceous fluid. Capillaries are more numerous, lined by hyperplastic endothelial cells. The lymph node capsule and perinodal fat are frequently infiltrated by immunoblasts, lymphocytes, and plasma cells (14,23). Single-cell apoptosis is common and focal necrosis is occasionally seen; extensive necrosis is the hallmark of fatal IM (9). Reticulin staining demonstrates follicular contours and preserved architecture despite an appearance of being partially overrun by immunoblasts, which creates the impression of lymphoma (21).

IMMUNOHISTOCHEMISTRY

Staining with monoclonal antibodies for B-cell markers [CD20 (L26), CD74 (LN-2; Fig.9.4), CDw75 (LN-1), CD79a] and T-cell markers (CD3, CD43, CD45RO1) (Fig. 9.7) shows the mixed nature of the immunoblasts. The Hodgkin/Reed-Sternberg-like cells of IM are negative for CD15 (Leu-M1) and CD30 markers and positive for B-cell markers; in contrast, the Hodgkin/Reed-Sternberg cells of Hodgkin lymphoma are positive for CD15 and

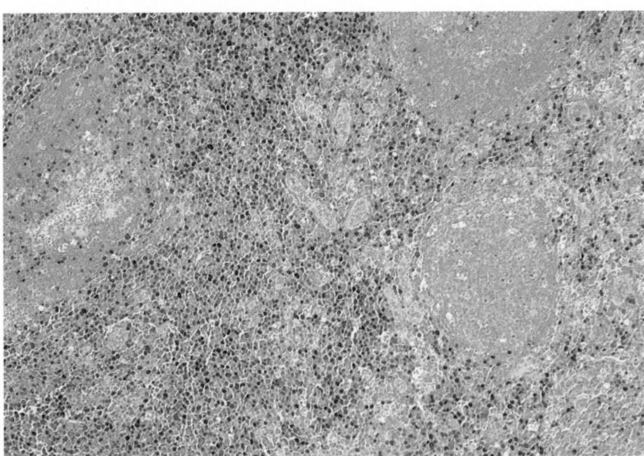

FIGURE 9.8. Infectious mononucleosis lymphadenitis. Virtually all transformed T cells (immunoblasts) are positive for the Epstein-Barr virus RNA antigen EBER. In contrast, B-cell follicles (*right*) remain unstained after *in situ* hybridization. Epstein-Barr virus *in situ* hybridization (EBER reaction).

CD30 and negative for B-cell markers (27,28). Occasionally, large immunoblasts in mononucleosis resembling the Hodgkin/Reed-Sternberg cells may stain positively with the Ki-1 (CD30) antibody, but not with the Leu-M1 (CD15) antibody (29). By immunohistochemistry and *in situ* hybridization, it can be demonstrated that both types of cells, the Hodgkin/Reed-Sternberg cells and the cells that resemble them may express the EBV antigens LMP and EBER (30) (Figs. 9.8 and 9.9).

LABORATORY TESTS

- *Hematologic changes.* Leukocyte count increased (average of 10,000/mm3), differential leukocyte count altered (lymphoid cells 50% to 60%), atypical lymphocytes (Downey cells) present in peripheral blood (10% to 20%).

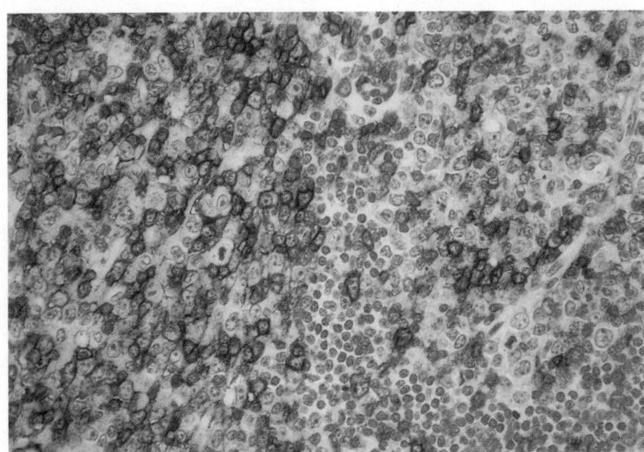

FIGURE 9.7. The transformed lymphocytes (immunoblasts) in the paracortex are positive for CD43, a T-cell marker. Anti-CD43/peroxidase.

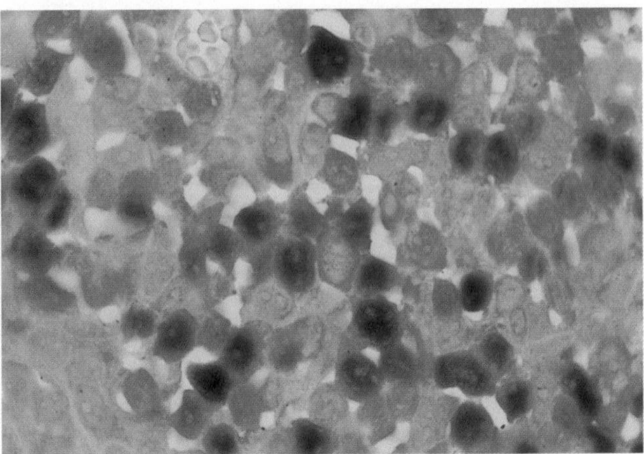

FIGURE 9.9. Same section as in Fig. 9.8 showing positive nuclear EBER hybridization (cytoplasm and nucleoli negative). Epstein-Barr virus *in situ* hybridization (EBER reaction).

Minimal morphologic criteria for the diagnosis of IM on a blood smear would be more than 50% mononuclear cells, at least 10 atypical lymphocytes per 100 leukocytes, and considerable lymphoid cell heterogeneity (10).

- *Heterophil antibodies (Paul-Bunnell test).* Based on agglutination of sheep erythrocytes by the patient's serum after absorption with guinea pig kidney. Positive in high titers in 60% of cases in the first 10 days and in 90% of cases within 1 month (3). Tests with negative results, particularly during first 2 weeks of symptoms, must therefore be repeated.
- *MonoSpot test.* This is a more sensitive assay, in which horse erythrocytes, the most specific antigen for the serologic diagnosis of IM, are used (31). Agglutinin titers for heterophil antibodies are about three times higher when horse rather than sheep erythrocytes are used. However, false-positive MonoSpot test results have occasionally been reported in patients with hepatitis and with lymphoma (32). Some patients with a clinical syndrome characteristic of IM may have persistently negative results on heterophil tests. In some of these patients, a rise in complement-fixing antibodies to cytomegalovirus is eventually demonstrated (33).
- *EBV-specific antibodies.* Viral capsid antigen (VCA)-specific immunoglobulin M (IgM), VCA-specific IgG in high titers, early antigen (EA), and Epstein-Barr nuclear antigen (EBNA) appear at various times after infection and indicate different phases in the immune response.

DIFFERENTIAL DIAGNOSIS

- Cytomegalovirus mononucleosis is characterized by lymph node enlargement and hematologic changes similar to those of IM. However, heterophil antibody test results are negative and cytomegalovirus antibody test results are positive (33).
- Other viral lymphadenitides may be similar morphologically and must be differentiated clinically and serologically.
- *Toxoplasma* lymphadenitis: Epithelioid cells singly and in clusters infiltrate the germinal centers; patches of monocytoid cells are present next to blood vessels and sinuses.
- Non-Hodgkin lymphoma, immunoblastic type is the most important and often the most difficult differential diagnosis. The large accumulations of immunoblasts with atypical nuclei and prominent nucleoli of IM may suggest immunoblastic lymphoma; however, at least focally, the features of IM are present (i.e., reactive follicles with tingible-body macrophages and mottled paracortical areas).

Checklist

INFECTIOUS MONONUCLEOSIS LYMPHADENITIS

Adolescents and young adults
Fever, pharyngitis, lymphadenopathies
Lymphocytosis
Atypical lymphocytes (Downey cells)
Partial architectural effacement
Marked follicular hyperplasia
- Irregularly shaped follicles
- Reactive germinal centers
- Apoptosis
- Tingible-body macrophages
- Frequent mitoses
- Preservation of mantle zone

Expanded paracortex (T-cell zone)
- Mottled pattern
- Polymorphous cellularity
- Immunoblasts
- Hodgkin/Reed-Sternberg-like cells

Sinus dilation
Focal necrosis, occasional
Capsular and pericapsular infiltration
Heterophil antibodies present (Paul-Bunnell test result positive)
MonoSpot test result positive
EBV-specific antigens (EA, VCA, EBNA, LMP, EBER) present

Reticulin staining shows preservation of architecture. Immunohistochemical stainings show mixed cell populations.

- Anaplastic large cell lymphoma: Large cells with highly pleomorphic or Reed-Sternberg-like nuclei are present in the paracortex and sinuses that are strongly positive for the CD30 activation antigen and stain with Ki-1 (Ber-H2) antibodies. They are positive for anaplastic lymphoma kinase (ALK) protein and epithelial membrane antigen (EMA). However, in IM, such cells are few and isolated, whereas they form solid, cohesive cords in anaplastic large cell lymphoma.
- Hodgkin lymphoma, lymphocyte predominance type: The lymphocyte population is predominantly of small lymphocytes without the follicular hyperplasia of IM. The lymphocytic and histiocytic cells lack eosinophilic, inclusion-like nucleoli.
- Hodgkin lymphoma, classic type: The Hodgkin/Reed-Sternberg cells are positive for CD15 (Leu-M1) and CD30 and negative for CD20 (L26), unlike the Hodgkin/Reed-Sternberg-like cells of IM, which are negative for CD15 and CD30 and positive for pan-B-cells. The cellular infiltrates consist of small lymphocytes, eosinophils, and plasma cells in Hodgkin lymphoma but are large, activated lymphoid cells (immunoblasts) in IM. EBV antigens are present in both and therefore are not a differential feature.

REFERENCES

1. Henle W, Henle GE, Horowitz CA. Epstein-Barr virus specific diagnostic tests in infectious mononucleosis. Hum Pathol 1974; 5:551–565.
2. Kieff E, Dambaugh T, Heller M, et al. The biology and chemistry of Epstein-Barr virus. J Infect Dis 1982;146:506–517.
3. Evans AS. Perspectives in infectious mononucleosis. In: Glade PR, ed. Infectious mononucleosis. Philadelphia: JB Lippincott Co, 1973.
4. Evans AS, Niederman JC. Epstein-Barr virus. In: Evans AE, ed. Viral infections of human. New York: Plenum Publishing, 1976.
5. Fingeroth JD, Weiss JJ, Tedder TF, et al. Epstein-Barr virus receptor of human B lymphocytes is the C3d receptor CR2. Proc Natl Acad Sci U S A 1984;81:4510.
6. Wolf H, zur Hausen H, Becker V. EB viral genomes in epithelial nasopharyngeal carcinoma cells. Nat New Biol 1973;244: 245–247.
7. Niedobitek G, Hamilton-Dutoit S, Herbst H, et al. Identification of Epstein-Barr virus-infected cells in tonsils of acute infectious mononucleosis by *in situ* hybridization. Hum Pathol 1989; 20:796–799.
8. Jondal M, Klein G. Surface markers on human B and T lymphocytes. Presence of Epstein-Barr virus receptors on B lymphocytes. J Exp Med 1973;138:1365.
9. Purtilo DT, Cassel C, Yang JPS et al. X-linked recessive combined variable immunodeficiency (Duncan's disease). Lancet 1975;1:935.
10. Strickler JG, Fedeli F, Horwitz CA, et al. Infectious mononucleosis in lymphoid tissue. Histopathology, *in situ* hybridization, and differential diagnosis. Arch Pathol Lab Med 1993;117:269–278.
11. Gaffey MJ, Weiss LM. Association of Epstein-Barr virus with human neoplasia. Pathol Annu 1992;27[Part I]:55–74.
12. Ioachim HL. Immune deficiency: opportunistic tumors. In: Encyclopedia of cancer, vol 2. New York: Academic Press, 1997: 901–915.
13. Shin SS, Berry GJ, Weiss LM. Infectious mononucleosis. Diagnosis by *in situ* hybridization in two cases with atypical features. Am J Surg Pathol 1991;15:625–631.
14. Gowing NFC. Infectious mononucleosis: histopathologic aspects. Pathol Annu 1975;10:1–20.
15. Veltri RW, Shah SH, McClung JE, et al. Epstein-Barr virus, fatal infectious mononucleosis and Hodgkin's disease in siblings. Cancer 1983;51:509–520.
16. Purtilo DT. Pathogenesis and phenotypes of an x-linked recessive lymphoproliferative syndrome. Lancet 1979:882–885.
17. Hanto DW, Frizzera G, Purtilo DT, et al. Clinical spectrum of lymphoproliferative disorders in renal transplant recipients and evidence for the role of Epstein-Barr virus. Cancer Res 1981; 41:4253–4261.
18. Davey DD, Kamat D, Laszewski M, et al. Epstein-Barr virus-related lymphoproliferative disorders following bone marrow transplantation: an immunologic and genotypic analysis. Mod Pathol 1989;2:27–34.
19. Randhawa PS, Markin RS, Starzl TE, et al. Epstein-Barr virus-associated syndromes in immunosuppressed liver transplant recipients. Am J Surg Pathol 1990;14:538–547.
20. Randhawa PS, Yousem SA, Paradis IL, et al. The clinical spectrum, pathology, and clonal analysis of Epstein-Barr-associated lymphoproliferative disorders in heart-lung transplant recipients. Am J Clin Pathol 1989;92:177–185.
21. Childs CC, Parham DM, Berard CW. Infectious mononucleosis. The spectrum of morphologic changes simulating lymphoma in lymph nodes and tonsils. Am J Surg Pathol 1987;11:122–132.
22. Dorfman RF, Warnke R. Lymphadenopathy simulating the malignant lymphomas. Hum Pathol 1974;5:519–550.
23. Salvador AH, Harrison EG, Kyle RA. Lymphadenopathy due to infectious mononucleosis, its confusion with malignant lymphoma. Cancer 1971;27:1029–1040.
24. Lukes RJ, Tindle BH, Parker JW. Reed-Sternberg-like cells in infectious mononucleosis. Lancet 1969;2:1003–1004.
25. Strum SB, Park KJ, Rappaport H. Observations of cells resembling Reed-Sternberg cells in conditions other than Hodgkin's disease. Cancer 1970;26:176–190.
26. Tindle BH, Parker JW, Lukes RJ. "Reed-Sternberg cells" in infectious mononucleosis. Am J Clin Pathol 1972;58:607–617.
27. Fellbaum C, Hansmann ML, Parwaresch MR, et al. Monoclonal antibodies Ki-B3 and Leu-M1 discriminate giant cells of infectious mononucleosis and of Hodgkin's disease. Hum Pathol 1988;19:1168–1173.
28. Isaacson PG, Schmid C, Pan LX, et al. Epstein-Barr virus latent membrane protein expression by Hodgkin and Reed-Sternberg-like cells in acute infectious mononucleosis. J Pathol 1992;167: 267.
29. Abbondanzo SL, Sato N, Straus SE, et al. Acute infectious mononucleosis. CD30 (Ki-1) antigen expression and histologic correlations. Am J Clin Pathol 1990;93:698–702.
30. Reynolds DJ, Banks PM, Gulley ML. New characterization of infectious mononucleosis and a phenotypic comparison with Hodgkin's disease. Am J Pathol 1995;146:379–388.
31. Lee CL, Davidsohn I, Panczyszyn O. Horse agglutinins in infectious mononucleosis. II. The spot test. Am J Clin Pathol 1968; 49:12–18.
32. Wolf P, Dorfman R, McClenahan J, et al. False-positive infectious mononucleosis spot test in lymphoma. Cancer 1970;25: 626–628.
33. Klemola E, von Essen R, Wager O, et al. Cytomegalovirus mononucleosis in previously healthy individuals. Ann Intern Med 1969;71:11–19.

10

CYTOMEGALOVIRUS LYMPHADENITIS

DEFINITION

Lymphadenitis caused by infection with cytomegalovirus (CMV).

SYNONYM

CMV lymphadenitis.

ETIOLOGY

Cytomegalovirus, the largest of human viruses, is a member of the family of herpesviruses and, as such, a DNA virus that replicates in the cell nucleus (1). It is characterized by its large size (110 to 130 nm in diameter) and is composed of a dense core, an icosahedral capsid, and a surrounding envelope with periodic short projections. Within a population of virions, many particles do not possess envelopes, and others have empty capsids without the internal DNA nucleoid (1,2).

EPIDEMIOLOGY

Cytomegalovirus is a ubiquitous pathogenic agent with worldwide distribution. In the United States, complement-fixing antibodies to CMV are present in 44% to 53% of males over 15 years of age. In homosexual males between 18 and 29 years of age, the presence of anti-CMV antibodies has been reported to be as high as 92% (3).

PATHOGENESIS

Cytomegalovirus may be transmitted by blood transfusion and transplacental passage and also from person to person through saliva and respiratory secretions. In homosexual males, CMV-infected semen is the main route of transmission (3). In the population at large, CMV infection occurs in childhood and is accompanied by flulike symptoms. Subsequently, the infection becomes clinically occult and the virus is undetectable by laboratory techniques because the viral genome has been integrated into the host genetic material of various cells. Thus, a latent infection may persist indefinitely and be reactivated under conditions of immune deficiency (4). In the peripheral blood, where atypical lymphocytes are present in up to 20% of cases, CMV has been identified in lymphocytes, particularly T cells, and other mononuclear cells (5). Endothelial cells in all the organs are preferential sites of CMV infection, and the reticular cells of hematolymphoid organs also appear to be a favorable location (6).

CLINICAL SYNDROME

In immunocompetent adults, CMV infection, like infectious mononucleosis, an Epstein-Barr viral (EBV) infection, may take the form of an acute, usually benign syndrome of fever, malaise, night sweats, enlarged lymph nodes, and mild hepatitis (7). Transmitted to newborns, CMV infection may result in a severe and frequently lethal syndrome that affects the central nervous system (8). Far more often, CMV affects immunosuppressed persons, such as recipients of organ transplants, patients with neoplastic diseases who are receiving chemotherapy, and particularly people with AIDS, in which a latent infection is reactivated (8,9). In these patients, widespread CMV infection involves a variety of organs, including the regional lymph nodes. Disseminated CMV infection, used by the Centers for Disease Control and Prevention as one of the criteria for the diagnosis of AIDS, most often affects the adrenals, lungs, gastrointestinal tract, eyes, and central nervous system (6,10,11).

HISTOPATHOLOGY

Lymph nodes in various locations may be involved during generalized infection with CMV, both in infants and adults. The lymph node changes are nonspecific and closely resemble those of EBV lymphadenitis. Moderate follicular hyperplasia, aggregates of monocytoid cells, and sheets of

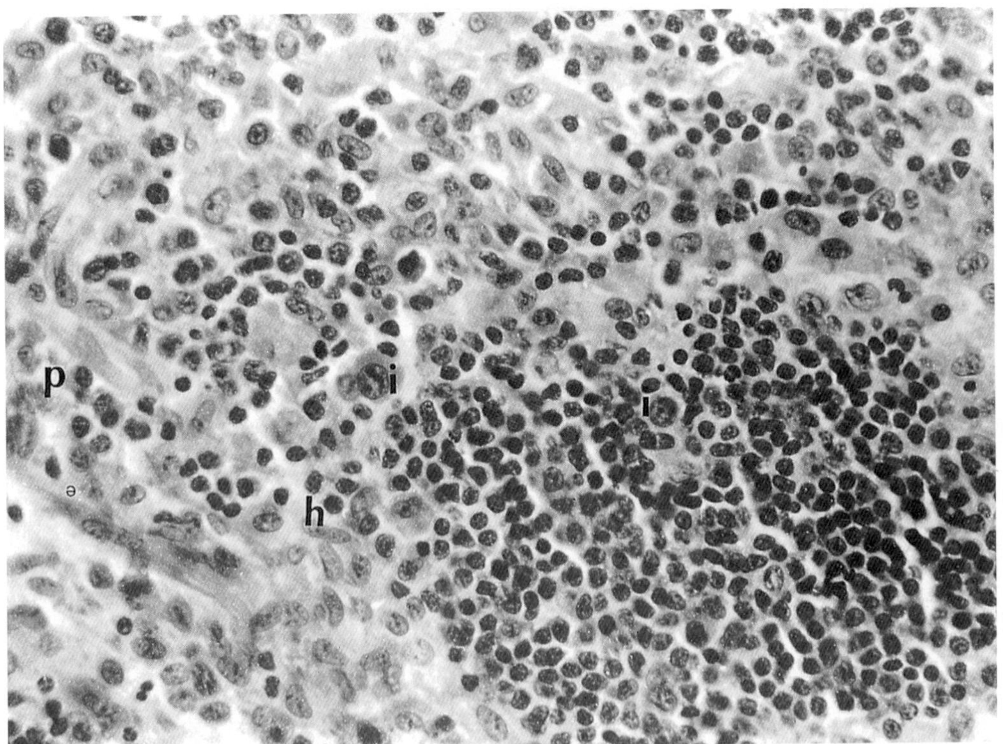

FIGURE 10.1. Axillary lymph node in cytomegalovirus disease. Numerous immunoblasts (*i*), histiocytes (*h*), and plasma cells (*p*) intermingle with and partly replace the lymphocytes. Hematoxylin, phloxine, and saffron stain.

immunoblasts admixed with small lymphocytes and polynuclear and monocytoid cells efface the architecture and produce a mottled appearance (Fig. 10.1). Occasionally, large, atypical lymphoid cells with multilobate nuclei and prominent nucleoli, resembling Reed-Sternberg cells, may be seen (Fig. 10.2). The CMV-infected cells are increased in size, and the markedly enlarged nuclei contain the characteristic "owl's eye" viral inclusions (Fig. 10.3). These inclusion bodies, the largest produced by any virus in humans, are up to 15 μm in diameter, strongly acidophilic, and surrounded by a clear vacuolar space (1). Sometimes, minute strands of eosinophilic material are present within the halo. The nucleolus is persistent in CMV-infected cells, unlike the nucleolus in cells infected by other herpesviruses, and nucleolar persis-

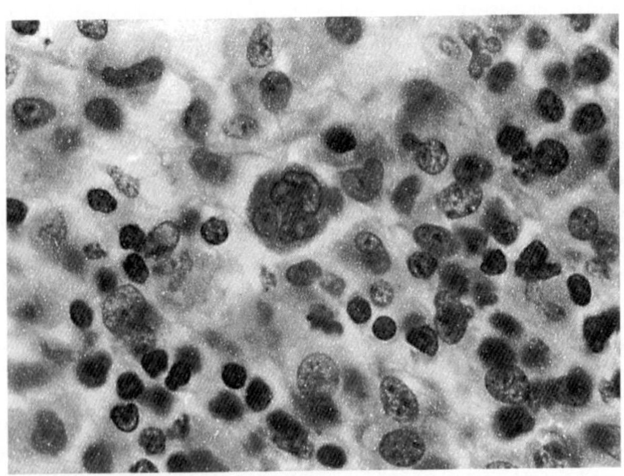

FIGURE 10.2. Reed-Sternberg-like cell with multilobate nucleus and prominent nucleoli amid mixed cell population. Hematoxylin, phloxine, and saffron stain.

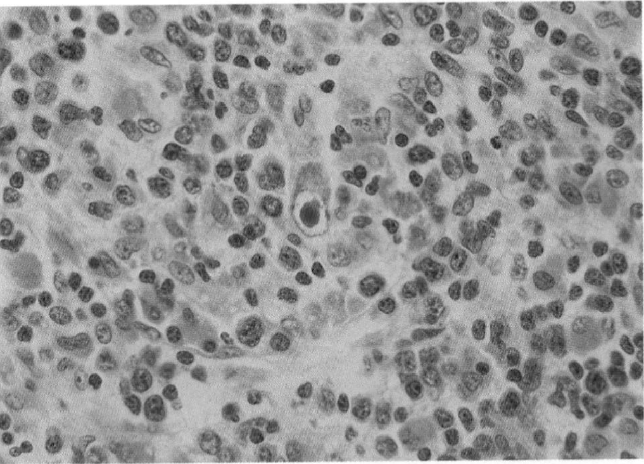

FIGURE 10.3. Cytomegalovirus lymphadenitis. Admixed with lymphocytes in the paracortex are numerous immunoblasts, including one with an intranuclear viral inclusion (*center*). Hematoxylin, phloxine, and saffron stain.

tence is a characteristic diagnostic feature (12). The cytoplasmic inclusions are less visible, smaller (2 to 4 μm in diameter), multiple (as many as 20 in a single cell), and basophilic (1). They contain DNA and polysaccharides and therefore stain with the Feulgen method and with periodic acid–Schiff stain (1). Immunohistochemical staining and *in situ* hybridization of lymph nodes for CMV show that not only the inclusion-containing cells but also numerous normal-looking cells are infected with the virus (8). Such cells are located mostly in the medulla and at the corticomedullary junction. Their mostly elongated appearance in one study led to the suggestion that the CMV-infected cells are not lymphocytes but reticular cells (8). An immunophenotypic study of a lymph node from a patient without immune compromise has shown that CMV infects only T cells, both CD4+ and CD8+ subsets, but not B cells (13). Thus, CMV infection suppresses T-cell proliferation and natural killer cell activity (5).

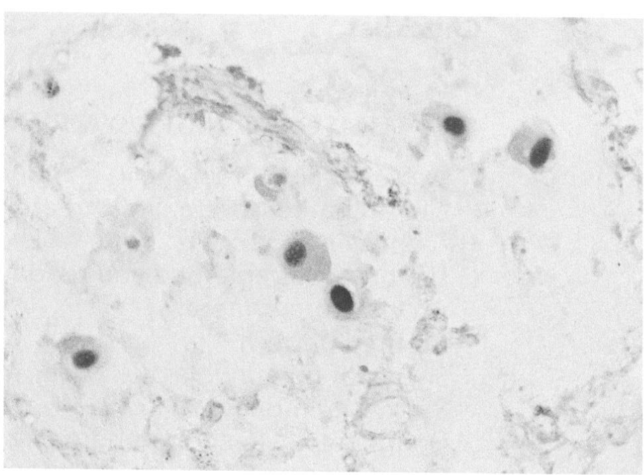

FIGURE 10.5. Intranuclear cytomegalovirus (*CMV*) inclusions in histiocytes identified by *in situ* hybridization with a CMV probe.

ELECTRON MICROSCOPY

Viral particles located in the nucleus are composed of dense DNA cores, capsids, and envelopes. Many particles are empty (lacking the internal core) or lack the surrounding envelope (2).

IMMUNOHISTOCHEMISTRY

Detection and identification of CMV in formalin-fixed, paraffin-embedded tissues is possible by immunohistochemical staining with anti-CMV antibodies (Fig. 10.4) and by *in situ* hybridization with biotinylated probes to CMV (6) (Fig. 10.5). In a comparative study, both techniques proved equally effective when the results were correlated with the results of isolation of CMV in human embryonic fibroblast cultures, the most sensitive but also the most difficult and expensive method (14,15). An interesting observation has been the staining of CMV-infected cells by Leu-M1 antibody (16). The immune reaction product is granular and located near the nucleus in the Golgi zone, as in Hodgkin and Reed-Sternberg cells, for which this antibody directed against CD15 antigen is commonly used. Hodgkin-like and Reed-Sternberg-like cells may be part of CMV and other viral lymphadenitides, and because their staining characteristics with Leu-M1 antibody are similar to those of cells infected with virus, the cell types are at times indistinguishable (16). In such cases, the identification of intranuclear inclusions by anti-CMV immunohistochemical staining or *in situ* hybridization is necessary to differentiate between CMV lymphadenitis and Hodgkin lymphoma.

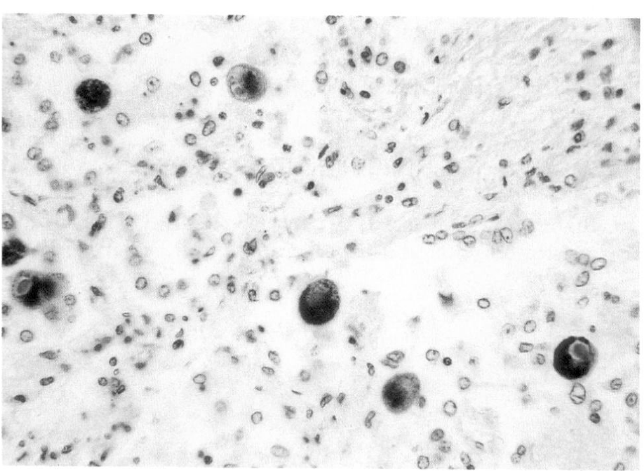

FIGURE 10.4. Cytomegalovirus (*CMV*)-infected histiocytes showing cytoplasmic and nuclear staining with anti-CMV antibody and peroxidase stain.

DIFFERENTIAL DIAGNOSIS

- Herpesvirus lymphadenitides such as EBV lymphadenitis (infectious mononucleosis) and herpes simplex lymphadenitis exhibit similar intranuclear inclusions that can be differentiated by immunohistochemical staining or *in situ* hybridization.
- Non-Hodgkin lymphomas: In diffuse non-Hodgkin lymphomas of various large cell types, the cell population is more uniform, without immunoblasts, monocytoid cells, or cells with intranuclear inclusions.
- Hodgkin lymphomas exhibit eosinophils, plasma cells, and bands of fibrosis. Leu-M1 staining is not reliable to differentiate the Hodgkin-like and Reed-Sternberg-like cells of CMV lymphadenitis, for which anti-CMV immunostaining or *in situ* hybridization should be used.

Checklist

CYTOMEGALOVIRUS LYMPHADENITIS

Acute, flulike syndrome in immunocompetent persons
Disseminated, severe, life-threatening infection in immune-deficient persons
Lymph nodes enlarged and tender
Architecture effaced
Mottled pattern
Sheets of immunoblasts
Patches of monocytoid cells
Hodgkin-like, Reed-Sternberg-like cells
Intranuclear, huge, acidophilic viral particles surrounded by clear halos
Persistence of nucleoli
Smaller, multiple intracytoplasmic viral inclusions
Dense-core DNA viral particles with capsids and envelopes or empty capsids
Leu-M1 staining of Golgi zone
CMV identified in tissue sections by anti-CMV immunohistochemical staining or *in situ* hybridization

REFERENCES

1. Davis BD, Dulbecco R, Eisen HN, et al. Cytomegalovirus. In: Microbiology. Hagerstown, MD: Harper & Row, 1980:1071–1073.
2. Smith JD, De Harven E. Herpes simplex virus and human cytomegalovirus replication in WI-38 cells. I. Sequence of viral replication. J Virol 11973;2:919–930.
3. Drew WL, Mintz L, Miner RC, et al. Prevalence of cytomegalovirus infection in homosexual men. J Infect Dis 1981; 143:188–192.
4. Myerowitz RL. Cytomegalovirus. In: The pathology of opportunistic infections. New York: Raven Press, 1983:161–176.
5. Schrier RD, Nelson JA, Oldstone MB. Detection of human cytomegalovirus in peripheral blood lymphocytes in a natural infection. Science 1985;230:1048–1051.
6. Ioachim HL. Pathology of AIDS. Textbook and atlas. Philadelphia: JB Lippincott Co, 1989.
7. Klemola E, von Essen R, Wager O, et al. Cytomegalovirus mononucleosis in previously healthy individuals. Five new cases and follow-up of 13 previously published cases. Ann Intern Med 1969;71:11–19.
8. Myerson D, Hackman RC, Nelson JA, et al. Widespread presence of histologically occult cytomegalovirus. Hum Pathol 1984;15:430–439.
9. Collier AC, Meyers JD, Corey L, et al. Cytomegalovirus infection in homosexual men. Relationship to sexual practices, antibody to human immunodeficiency virus, and cell-mediated immunity. Am J Med 1987;82:593–601.
10. Centers for Disease Control. Revision of the case definition of acquired immunodeficiency for national reporting—United States. MMWR Morb Mortal Wkly Rep 1985;34:471–475.
11. Klatt EC, Shibata D. Cytomegalovirus infection in the acquired immunodeficiency syndrome. Arch Pathol Lab Med 1988;112: 540–544.
12. Strano AJ. Cytomegalovirus pneumonia. In: Binford CH, Connor DH, eds. Pathology of tropical and extraordinary diseases. Washington, DC: Armed Forces Institute of Pathology, 1976:58.
13. Younes M, Podesta A, Helie M, et al. Infection of T but not B lymphocytes by cytomegalovirus in lymph node. An immunophenotypic study. Am J Surg Pathol 1991;15:75–80.
14. Grody WW, Lewin KJ, Naeim F. Detection of cytomegalovirus DNA in classic and epidemic Kaposi's sarcoma by *in situ* hybridization. Hum Pathol 1988;19:524–528.
15. Strickler JG, Manivel JC, Copenhaver CM, et al. Comparison of *in situ* hybridization and immunohistochemistry for detection of cytomegalovirus and herpes simplex virus. Hum Pathol 1990;21: 443–448.
16. Rushin JM, Riordan GP, Heaton RB, et al. Cytomegalovirus-infected cells express Leu-M1 antigen. Am J Pathol 1990;136: 989–995.

11

HERPES SIMPLEX VIRUS LYMPHADENITIS

DEFINITION

Lymphadenitis caused by infection with herpes simplex viruses (HSV).

SYNONYM

HSV lymphadenitis.

ETIOLOGY

Herpes simplex virus type 1 (HSV-1) and herpes simplex virus type 2 (HSV-2) belong to the human herpesvirus family, the Herpesviridae, which includes three additional members: cytomegalovirus, Epstein-Barr virus, and varicella-zoster virus. All are DNA viruses with a linear, double-stranded DNA that can assume several isomeric orientations (1). They have an ether-sensitive envelope, an icosahedral capsid, and a dense core containing the viral nucleoproteins. Despite their similarities, the herpesviruses differ significantly in biochemical and biologic properties and in the human diseases that they can cause. HSV-1 and HSV-2 have a wide host range. They possess approximately 50% sequence homology yet can be distinguished by antigen identification and restriction enzyme analysis (1).

A more recently described herpesvirus, human herpesvirus type 6 (HHV-6), has been detected in the lymph nodes of persons with benign and malignant lymphoproliferative lesions (2). In a recent study of 32 lymph node biopsy specimens, HHV-6 was detected by polymerase chain reaction and *in situ* hybridization in two cases of high-grade lymphoma, one of fatal infectious mononucleosis lymphadenitis, and two of reactive lymphadenitis (3). A new herpesvirus, HHV-8, has been identified in Kaposi sarcoma and primary effusion lymphomas, but not in other types of lymphoma (4).

CLINICAL SYNDROME

The herpesviruses are pathogens of a variety of infectious and neoplastic conditions. Herpes simplex viruses have been isolated from nearly all visceral and mucocutaneous sites (5). HSV-1 can cause gingivostomatitis, keratoconjunctivitis, and esophagitis. It can also cause systemic diseases such as acute necrotizing encephalitis in adults and hepatic and adrenal necrosis in infants (6). HSV-2 causes primarily anogenital lesions. Nevertheless, both viral subtypes can cause genital and orofacial infections, and the lesions are clinically indistinguishable. The frequency of reactivations depends on the anatomic site and type of virus. Genital HSV-2 infection recurs 8 to 10 times more often than genital HVS-1 infection, and oral and labial HSV-1 infection recurs more frequently than HVS-2 infection in that location (7). In immunosuppressed patients, particularly those with AIDS, herpetic involvement of the esophagus and lower respiratory tract may have a chronic, severe course. Patients with leukemias, lymphomas, and other hematologic malignancies are at increased risk for disseminated herpetic infection (8–10); however, in some, only a localized, self-limited lymphadenopathy may develop (11).

Herpetic lymphadenitis is uncommon, and few cases have been reported in the literature. It can be (a) disseminated, involving multiple organs (8–10,12–13); (b) a generalized lymphadenopathy associated with an erythematous rash and no other organ involvement (14–15); or (c) a localized lymphadenopathy with no other manifestations (11,16–19). The latter form may be seen particularly in the inguinal region, which is tender and affected by an erythematous or vesicular rash (20). The frequent localization to inguinal lymph nodes suggests lymphatic spread from infections of the urogenital tract (21).

HISTOPATHOLOGY

The lymph node architecture is only partially altered by enlargement of the paracortex and the presence of focal

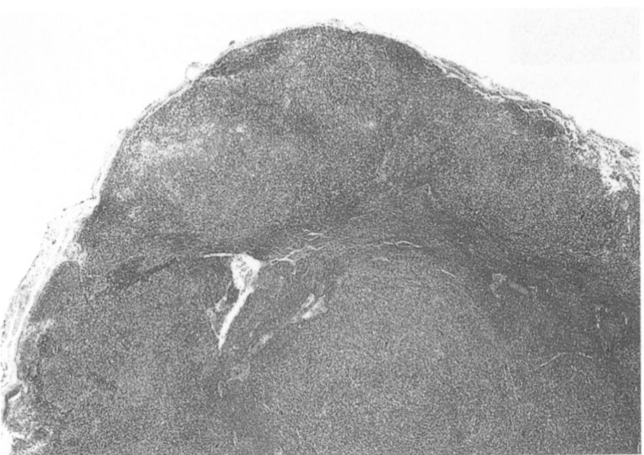

FIGURE 11.1. Herpetic lymphadenitis. Marked expansion of paracortex by proliferation of activated T cell leaving atrophic follicles and islands of small lymphocytes. (From Tamaru J-I, Mikata A, Horie H, et al. Herpes simplex lymphadenitis. Report of two cases with review of the literature. Am J Surg Pathol 1990;14:571–577, with permission. Slide courtesy of Tamura J-I, Saitama Medical School, Saitama, Japan.)

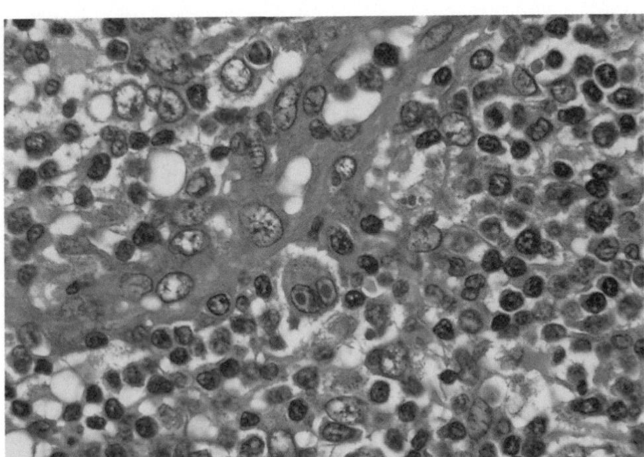

FIGURE 11.3. Herpes lymphadenitis. Mixed cell populations of small lymphocytes, immunoblasts, smudge cells, and Reed-Sternberg-like activated lymphoid cell (*center*). (From Tamaru J-I, Mikata A, Horie H, et al. Herpes simplex lymphadenitis. Report of two cases with review of the literature. Am J Surg Pathol 1990;14:571–577, with permission. Slide courtesy of Tamura J-I, Saitama Medical School, Saitama, Japan.)

necrosis. The paracortical areas appear prominent (sometimes nodular) and compress the lymphoid follicles, which are mostly atrophic (15) (Fig.11.1). These areas are composed predominantly of T-cell immunoblasts in clusters or sheets, often with atypical nuclei (Fig. 11.2). Within such areas are foci of cellular necrosis that on low-power microscopy look like infarcts or microabscesses. They are formed of nuclear debris, smudged eosinophilic remnants of cells, neutrophils, and cells with viral particles (18) (Figs. 11.3 and 11.4). The latter are located at the edge of the lesions and appear markedly enlarged and usually hyperchromatic. They comprise the typical intranuclear inclusions surrounded by clear halos. When herpetic infection occurs as a complication of leukemia/lymphoma, foci of necrosis and cells with intranuclear viral inclusions may be seen within lymphomatous lymph nodes (11). Cases of acute lymphadenitis with HHV-6 may also show large numbers of typical intranuclear herpesvirus inclusions.

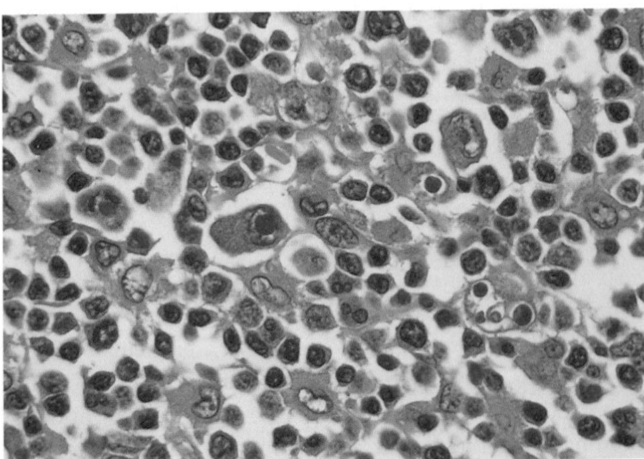

FIGURE 11.2. Herpes lymphadenitis. Numerous activated lymphocytes (immunoblasts) with abundant cytoplasm, vesicular nuclei, and intranuclear herpetic inclusions (*center*). (From Tamaru J-I, Mikata A, Horie H, et al. Herpes simplex lymphadenitis. Report of two cases with review of the literature. Am J Surg Pathol 1990;14:571–577, with permission. Slide courtesy of Tamura J-I, Saitama Medical School, Saitama, Japan.)

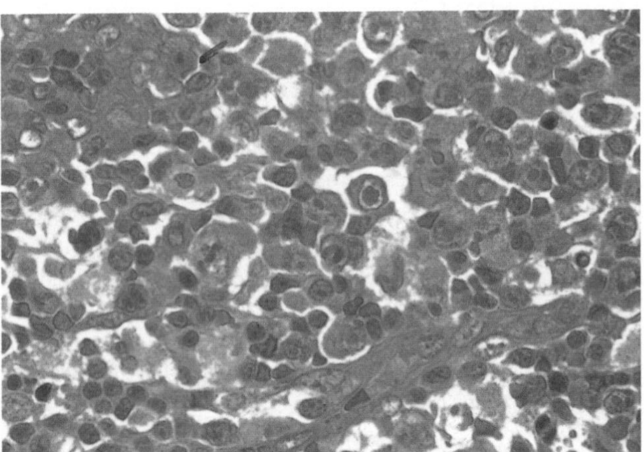

FIGURE 11.4. Herpes lymphadenitis. Paracortical sheets of activated lymphocytes (immunoblasts) with intranuclear herpetic inclusions and frequent mitoses. (From Tamaru J-I, Mikata A, Horie H, et al. Herpes simplex lymphadenitis. Report of two cases with review of the literature. Am J Surg Pathol 1990;14:571–577, with permission. Slide courtesy of Tamura J-I, Saitama Medical School, Saitama, Japan.)

Multinucleated cells with ground-glass nuclei may also be present (17). Occasionally, immunoblasts with large, folded nuclei resembling those of Hodgkin lymphoma are noted (15) (Fig. 11.3). Marked histiocytosis, sometimes with erythrophagocytosis, is also present (16). Epithelioid cells and granulomas are not seen. Perinodal tissue is infiltrated by lymphocytes and plasma cells (19).

IMMUNOHISTOCHEMISTRY

Immunoperoxidase staining with anti-HSV antibodies and *in situ* hybridization may be used to identify HSV (3,15,18,21). Such identification may be confirmed by Southern blot analysis of endonuclease fragments of DNA from the involved lymph nodes (3,18).

The identity of the cells infected by HSV has been controversial. Some authors have reported staining of HSV-infected cells with UCHL-1 and MT-1 antibodies (Fig. 11.5) and no staining with L26 antibody and so have concluded that they are T lymphocytes (15). This finding is in accordance with the earlier demonstration *in vitro* of HSV replication in human mitogen-stimulated T cells, which indicated an affinity for lymphoid cells in addition to their well-known neurotropism. Other authors, using double-labeling techniques for virus and cells, demonstrated the infected cells to be positive for vimentin but negative for LCA, Leu-22, factor VIII-related antigen, and *Ulex europaeus* lectin and therefore concluded that they could not be lymphocytes, monocytes, or endothelial cells and are probably stromal cells, possibly fibroblasts (21).

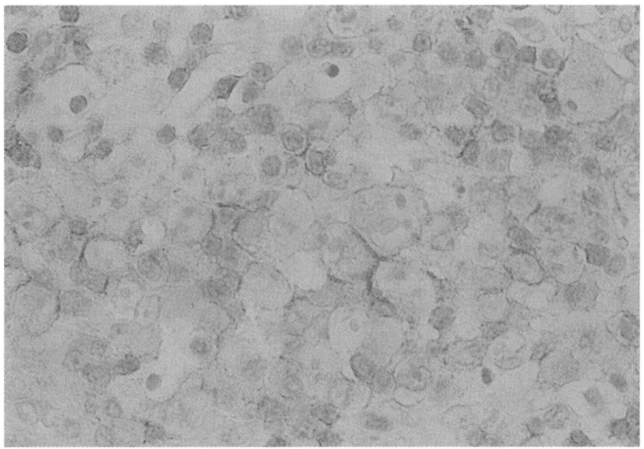

FIGURE 11.5. Herpetic lymphadenitis. Paracortical area of activated lymphocytes (immunoblasts) with membrane staining for T-cell marker (MT-1 antibody). (From Tamaru J-I, Mikata A, Horie H, et al. Herpes simplex lymphadenitis. Report of two cases with review of the literature. Am J Surg Pathol 1990;14:571–577, with permission. Slide courtesy of Tamura J-I, Saitama Medical School, Saitama, Japan.)

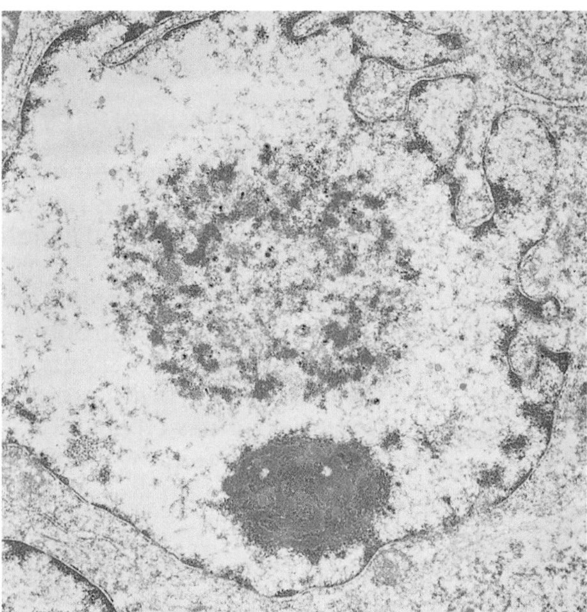

FIGURE 11.6. Nucleus of infected cell with nucleolus (*center*) and intranuclear inclusion body composed of viral particles and highly electron-dense reticular material (*bottom*). (From Tamaru J-I, Mikata A, Horie H, et al. Herpes simplex lymphadenitis. Report of two cases with review of the literature. Am J Surg Pathol 1990;14:571–577, with permission. Slide courtesy of Tamura J-I, Saitama Medical School, Saitama, Japan.)

ELECTRON MICROSCOPY

Viral particles with cores and capsids separated by clear halos or just empty capsids devoid of internal cores are seen in the nuclei (Fig. 11.6). They measure 90 to 110 nm and are most often located within the perinuclear cisternae (15,21).

DIFFERENTIAL DIAGNOSIS

- Tuberculous lymphadenitis is characterized by caseating necrosis, a granulomatous cell reaction, and acid-fast bacilli.
- Necrotizing lymphadenopathy of Kikuchi has accumulations of histiocytes, foci of necrosis, and no neutrophils.
- Necrotizing lymphadenopathy in lupus erythematosus has, in addition to necrosis, deposits of basophilic material (hematoxylin bodies) and plasma cells.
- Cat-scratch lymphadenitis also shows foci of necrosis with neutrophils but has epithelioid cells, the configuration of granulomas, and bacilli that stain with Warthin-Starry silver.

Checklist

HERPES SIMPLEX VIRUS LYMPHADENITIS

Associated with disseminated infection and rash
More common in immunosuppressed persons
Rarely appears as localized lymphadenopathy, mainly inguinal
Paracortical T-cell areas enlarged
Foci of necrosis with neutrophils
Hyperplasia, sometimes sheets of T-cell immunoblasts
Multinucleated cells with ground-glass nuclei
Intranuclear herpes-type viral particles
HSV identified *in situ* by immunohisto-chemical staining and DNA hybridization

REFERENCES

1. Rapp F. The challenge of herpesviruses. Cancer Res 1984;44: 1309–1315.
2. Salahuddin S, Ablashi D, Markham PD, et al. Isolation of a new virus, HBLV, in patients with lymphoproliferative disorders. Science 1986;234:596–601.
3. Borisch B, Ellinger K, Neipel F, et al. Lymphadenitis and lymphoproliferative lesions associated with the human herpesvirus-6 (HHV-6). Virchows Arch B Cell Pathol Mol Pathol 1991;61: 179–187.
4. Moore PS, Chang Y. Detection of herpes-like DNA sequences in Kaposi's sarcoma in patients with and those without HIV infection. N Engl J Med 1995;332:1181–1185.
5. Corey L, Spear PG. Infections with herpes simplex viruses. N Engl J Med 1986;314:749–757.
6. Nahmias JA. Disseminated herpes simplex infection. N Engl J Med 1970;282:684–685.
7. Reeves WC, Corey L, Adams HG, et al. Risk of recurrence after first episodes of genital herpes: relation to HSV type and antibody response. N Engl J Med 1981;305:315–319.
8. Rosen P, Hajdu SI. Visceral herpesvirus infections in patients with cancer. Am J Clin Pathol 1971;56:459–465.
9. Muller SA, Herrman EC Jr, Winkelmann RK. Herpes simplex infections in hematologic malignancies. Am J Med 1972;52: 102–114.
10. Pierre C, Jaubert D, Carloz E, et al. Massive necrotizing adenitis complicating a disseminated herpes simplex virus 2 infection in chronic lymphoid leukemia. Ann Pathol 1991;11: 31–35.
11. Higgins PT, Warnke RA. Herpes lymphadenitis in association with chronic lymphocytic leukemia. Cancer 1999;86:1210–1215.
12. Abraham A, Manko M. Disseminated herpes virus hominis 2 infection following drug overdose. Arch Intern Med 1977;137: 1198–1200.
13. Ramsey P, Fife K, Hackman R, et al. Herpes simplex virus pneumonia. Clinical, virologic and pathologic features in 20 patients. Ann Intern Med 1982;97:813–820.
14. Lapsley M, Kettle P, Sloan JM. Herpes simplex lymphadenitis: a case report and review of the published work. J Clin Pathol 1984; 3:1119–1122.
15. Tamaru J-I, Mikata A, Horie H, et al. Herpes simplex lymphadenitis. Report of two cases with review of the literature. Am J Surg Pathol 1990;14:571–577.
16. Audouin J, Tourneau AL, Aubert J-P, et al. Herpes simplex virus lymphadenitis mimicking tumoral relapse in a patient with Hodgkin's disease in remission. Virchows Arch A Pathol Anat Histopathol 1985;408:313–321.
17. Taxy JB, Tillawi I, Goldman PM. Herpes simplex lymphadenitis. An unusual presentation with necrosis and viral particles. Arch Pathol Lab Med 1985;109:1043–1044.
18. Epstein JI, Ambinder RF, Kuhajda FP, et al. Localized herpes simplex lymphadenitis. Am J Clin Pathol 1986;86:444–448.
19. Miliauskas JR, Leong AS-Y. Localized herpes simplex lymphadenitis: report of three case and review of the literature. Histopathology 1991;19:355–360.
20. Finberg RW, Mattia AR. A 47-year old man with inguinal lymphadenopathy and fever during preparation for bone marrow transplant. N Engl J Med 1994;331:1703–1711.
21. Gaffey MJ, Ben-Ezra JM, Weiss LM. Herpes simplex lymphadenitis. Am J Clin Pathol 1991;95:709–714.

12

VARICELLA-HERPES ZOSTER LYMPHADENITIS

DEFINITION

Lymphadenitis caused by infection with varicella or herpes zoster virus.

ETIOLOGY

The viruses isolated from patients with varicella (chickenpox) or herpes zoster (shingles) are physically and immunologically identical (1). The herpesvirus varicella-zoster (HVZ) is a DNA virus that multiplies only in the nucleus of permissive cells and has developmental stages similar to those of the herpes simplex virus (1). Herpesviruses are the etiologic agents of various afflictions, from localized lesions to severe generalized diseases; the latter develop only in persons with inadequate immunity, either congenital or acquired as a result of therapeutic immunosuppression or HIV infection. The varicella-zoster virus is relatively unstable in culture; however, the vesicle fluid from patients is highly infectious for a long time (1).

PATHOGENESIS

Varicella, the primary disease produced in a host without specific immunity, is usually a mild, self-limited illness of young children. Herpes zoster is the recurrent form of the disease, developing in adults who were previously infected with HVZ and possess circulating antibodies. It results from the reactivation of latent virus within the dorsal roots or cranial nerve ganglia and spreads centrifugally along sensory nerves (2). During the primary disease, the virus enters the respiratory tract and multiplies locally and in the regional lymph nodes; it is then disseminated to the blood, skin, and other organs. Herpes zoster results from the reactivation of latent virus in a susceptible adult with incomplete immunity by trauma, infection, various drugs, or cancer. In immune-deficient persons, the infection may spread to the spinal cord or cranial nerves and cause paralysis or fatal disease (1).

CLINICAL SYNDROME

In varicella, the onset is sudden and mild; malaise, anorexia, and slight fever are followed in 24 to 48 hours by a maculopapular eruption. The cutaneous lesions of herpes zoster resemble those of varicella but are usually limited to one or several sensory dermatomes (2). The involvement varies from a few small vesicles to massive spread of large bullae accompanied by intense pain. The rash has a centripetal distribution and is usually more extensive and severe in older patients. On rare occasions, probably as a result of immune deficiency, atypical, generalized zoster develops. The disseminated lesions are usually preceded by localized dermatomal eruptions, which in turn are preceded by an occult phase of primary viremia (3). In a 20-year-old woman presenting with a prostrating febrile illness and generalized lymphadenopathy, varicella-zoster virus was demonstrated in the lymph nodes 2 1/2 weeks before the appearance of characteristic skin lesions (3).

HISTOPATHOLOGY

Lymph nodes, more commonly cervical, supraclavicular, and axillary, are tender and persistently enlarged. The architecture, including follicles, sinuses, and capsule, is effaced by a diffuse proliferation of lymphocytes, immunoblasts, histiocytes, and occasional plasma cells, which creates a mottled appearance (Fig. 12.1). As in vaccinia and infectious mononucleosis lymphadenitis, lymphoid cells are destroyed and histiocytes proliferate and engulf nuclear debris (4–6), and numerous immunoblasts with some atypical nuclei and frequent mitoses are seen. Some of these cells are markedly enlarged and have a characteristic intranuclear inclusion body surrounded by a clear halo (Fig. 12.2).

The diffuse pattern, capsular involvement, and atypical lymphoid cells, mostly immunoblasts, may lead to a mistaken diagnosis of lymphoma (3). After the acute phase of the disease, during recovery, the diffuse lymph node hyperplasia may be replaced by follicular hyperplasia.

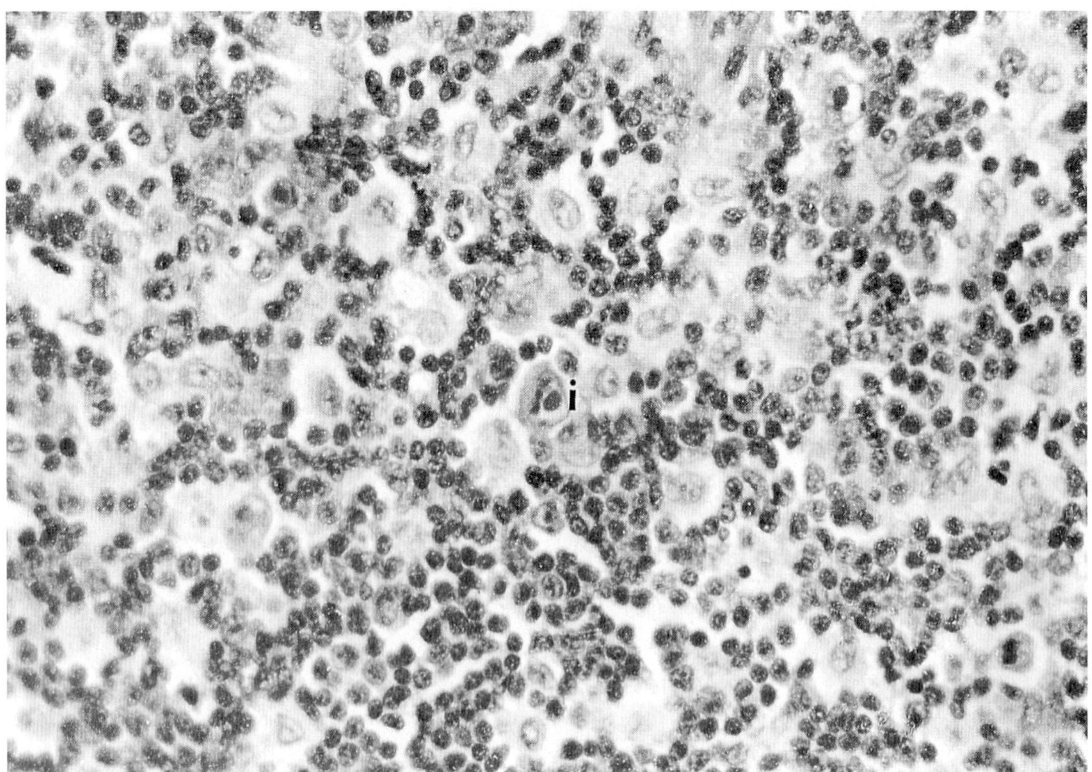

FIGURE 12.1. Varicella-herpes zoster lymphadenitis in axillary lymph node. Mottled appearance is caused by diffuse infiltration of immunoblasts and histiocytes. Inclusion body *(i)* is seen within clear vacuolar space in atypical lymphoid cell. (From Patterson SD, Larson EB, Corey L. Atypical generalized zoster with lymphadenitis mimicking lymphoma. N Engl J Med 1980;302:848–851, with permission.)

ELECTRON MICROSCOPY

An ultrastructural study of lymph nodes during the acute phase of herpes zoster observed characteristic inclusion bodies within the nuclei of 5% to 10% of the large, transformed lymphocytes (3). These were formed of multiple spherical viral particles, 90 to 105 nm in diameter, typical of herpesviruses. The intranuclear virions had a dense DNA core surrounded by an inner lucent and an outer dense capsid. Some complete, enveloped virions were seen leaving the lymphocytes, which were intact and showed no degenerative features.

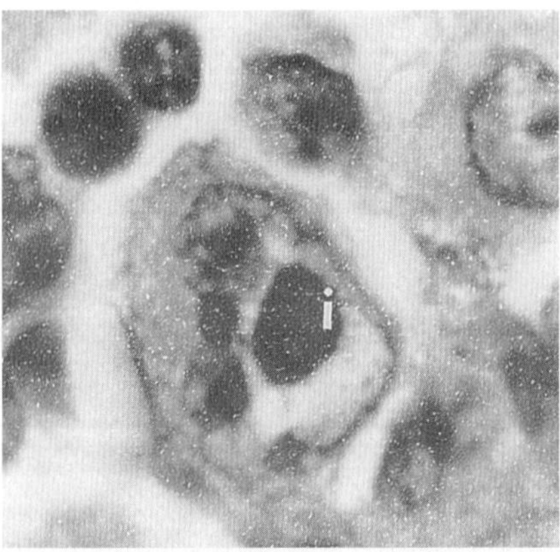

FIGURE 12.2. At higher magnification of the cell, probably an immunoblast, the large inclusion is seen within an intranuclear vacuole. (From Patterson SD, Larson EB, Corey L. Atypical generalized zoster with lymphadenitis mimicking lymphoma. N Engl J Med 1980;302:848–851, with permission.)

LABORATORY TESTS

Varicella giant cells and cells with typical inclusion bodies may be seen in smears prepared from fluid from the base of a vesicle stained with Giemsa stain (1).

Unfixed lymph node imprint preparations examined by direct immunofluorescence with the use of fluorescein-conjugated varicella-zoster antiserum exhibit strong nuclear fluorescence that can be blocked with unconjugated HVZ antibody (3). Sera against herpes simplex virus or cytomegalovirus are used as negative controls.

DIFFERENTIAL DIAGNOSIS

- Viral lymphadenitides caused by Epstein-Barr virus (infectious mononucleosis), cytomegalovirus, or human herpesvirus may be indistinguishable histologically but can be separated by serologic methods or immunofluorescence staining with fluorescein-conjugated specific antisera.

Checklist

VARICELLA-HERPES ZOSTER LYMPHADENITIS

Children with signs of varicella
Elderly patients with recurrent varicella-zoster infection
Antecedent dermatomal rash and pain
Generalized eruption
Generalized lymphadenopathy
Lymph nodes enlarged, tender
Architecture effaced
Mottled pattern
Follicular hyperplasia during recovery
Immunoblasts, plasma cells
Macrophages with tingible bodies
Intranuclear inclusion bodies surrounded by clear halos
Dense-core DNA virus particles
Fluorescence staining with specific anti-HVZ serum

- Large cell lymphomas are a potential diagnostic hazard (3,6). In these, the cell population is more uniform and the nuclear configuration more pleomorphic. Histiocytes with tingible bodies, plasma cells, and particularly the characteristic inclusion bodies are not present. In herpes zoster, clinical signs, particularly the cutaneous dermatomal eruption and pain, are strong diagnostic indications.

REFERENCES

1. Davis BD, Dulbecco R, Eisen HN, et al. Herpes viruses. In: Microbiology. Hagerstown, MD: Harper & Row, 1980:1061–1076.
2. Strano AJ. Herpes group exanthemas. In: Binford CH, Connor DH, eds. Pathology of tropical and extraordinary diseases, vol. 1. Washington, DC: Armed Forces Institute of Pathology, 1976: 68–73.
3. Patterson SD, Larson EB, Corey L. Atypical generalized zoster with lymphadenitis mimicking lymphoma. N Engl J Med 1980; 302:848–851.
4. Butler JJ. Non-neoplastic lesions of lymph nodes of man to be differentiated from lymphomas. NCI Monogr 1969;32:233–255.
5. Dorfman RF, Warnke R. Lymphadenopathy simulating the malignant lymphomas. Hum Pathol 1974;5:519–550.
6. Hartsock RJ. Reactive lesions in lymph nodes. In: Rebuck JW, Berard CW, Abell MR, eds. The reticuloendothelial system. International Academy of Pathology Monograph No. 16. Baltimore: Williams & Wilkins, 1975:153–184.

13

VACCINIA LYMPHADENITIS

DEFINITION

Lymphadenitis caused by infection with vaccinia virus.

SYNONYMS

Postvaccinial lymphadenitis, smallpox vaccination adenitis.

ETIOLOGY

Vaccinia virus infections usually do not occur naturally, being generally induced as vaccination against smallpox infection (1). Vaccinia is a poxvirus, considerably less virulent and with a broader host range than smallpox (2). The two DNA poxviruses are antigenically similar, so vaccinia virus is used to vaccinate against smallpox virus. From 1 to 3 weeks after the administration of vaccinia virus, a regional lymphadenopathy may develop in lymph nodes draining the vaccination site. The most common locations are the supraclavicular, cervical, and axillary lymph nodes. Lymphadenitis occurs in response to the vaccinia virus, usually present in the affected lymph nodes. Vaccinia lymphadenitis was experimentally reproduced in monkeys and rabbits (3). Eight days after the injection, the regional lymph nodes were diffusely hyperplastic and showed a typically mottled appearance, whereas at 15 days, the changes in the lymph nodes were characterized by follicular hyperplasia. Vaccinia virus was detected in the lymph nodes of monkeys at 8 and 10 days, and the maximal antibody response was reached at 15 days (3–5). Postvaccinial lymphadenitis is rarely seen nowadays because vaccination against smallpox is no longer required for travel to most parts of the world (6).

HISTOPATHOLOGY

The morphologic changes may be of variable intensity and are generally similar to those produced by infection with other viruses, notably herpesvirus, measles virus, and other unidentified viral agents (5). The basic architecture of lymph nodes is preserved, although marked hyperplasia is present with a follicular, diffuse, or combined follicular and diffuse pattern (4–8) (Fig. 13.1). The characteristically mottled (moth-eaten) appearance is caused by a marked proliferation of immunoblasts, which are scattered throughout the lymph node parenchyma (4). Intermingled with these cells in the parafollicular areas are mature lymphocytes, plasma cells, eosinophils, and mast cells. Proliferating vessels and distended sinuses filled with immunoblasts and plasma cells floating in abundant proteinaceous fluid are other features. Immunoblasts, which represent the predominant cell type, are two to three times larger than mature lymphocytes and have large nuclei with thick nuclear membranes, one to three prominent nucleoli, and frequent mitoses. The immunoblasts in mitosis are more numerous in the first 10 days after vaccination, whereas plasma cells become more common after the first 10 days (4). Not infrequently, very large immunoblasts with bizarre, multilobate nuclei and prominent nucleoli are present. Some of these unusual immunoblasts that are seen occasionally in other viral lymphadenitides closely resemble mononuclear Hodgkin cells or multilobate Reed-Sternberg cells and may lead to an erroneous diagnosis of Hodgkin disease (4,5,9).

DIFFERENTIAL DIAGNOSIS

- Hodgkin lymphoma, lymphocyte predominance type, is the most common misinterpretation. Nine of the first 20 cases reviewed by Hartsock (4) had been misdiagnosed as Hodgkin disease. In Hodgkin disease, the lymphocyte population consists almost entirely of the small, mature type, and immunoblasts are infrequent. In the nodular sclerosis type of Hodgkin disease, the presence of lacunar cells and fibrosis, both absent in postvaccinia lymphadenitis, indicates the differential diagnosis.
- Non-Hodgkin lymphoma that is poorly differentiated and diffuse may be a difficult differential diagnosis (9). However, in lymphoma, the nodal structure is effaced and the cellular population is homogeneous with neoplastic morphologic features.
- Infectious mononucleosis lymphadenitis must be distinguished by heterophil antibody agglutination test findings above 1:40 and the presence of atypical lymphocytes (Downey cells) in the peripheral blood smear.

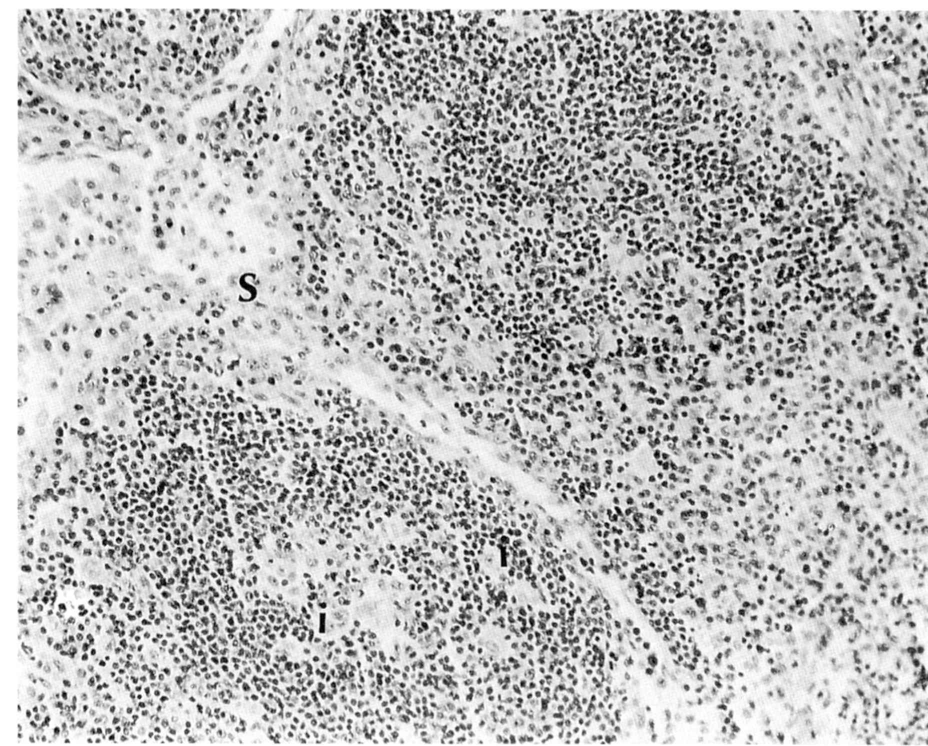

FIGURE 13.1. Axillary lymph node 6 days after vaccination. The markedly distended sinuses (*S*) and mottled appearance of the nodal parenchyma are caused by scattered infiltrates of immunoblasts (*i*). Hematoxylin and eosin stain.

Checklist

VACCINIA LYMPHADENITIS

History of recent vaccination
Cervical or axillary lymphadenopathy
Diffuse, follicular, or combined pattern
Mottled appearance
Proliferation of immunoblasts
Scattered plasma cells
Eosinophils, mast cells
Vascular proliferation
Dilated sinuses

- *Toxoplasma* lymphadenitis is distinguished by the presence of clusters of epithelioid cells in parafollicular areas and germinal centers and positive results of the Sabin-Feldman dye test or specific immunofluorescence tests.

REFERENCES

1. Ropp SL, Esposito JJ, Loparev UN. Poxviruses infecting humans. In: Murray PR, et al., eds. Manual of clinical microbiology. Washington, DC: ASM Press, 1999:1137–1144.
2. Davis BD, Dulbecco R, Eisen HN, et al. Poxviruses. In: Microbiology. Hagerstown, MD: Harper & Row, 1980:1078–1093.
3. Hartsock RJ, Bellanti JA. Comparative histologic changes of postvaccinial lymphadenitis in man, monkey and rabbit. Fed Proc 1966;25:534(abst).
4. Hartsock RJ. Postvaccinial lymphadenitis: hyperplasia of lymphoid tissue that simulates malignant lymphomas. Cancer 1968;21:632–649.
5. Hartsock RJ. Reactive lesions in lymph nodes. In: Rebuck JW, Berard CW, Abell MR, eds. The reticuloendothelial system. International Academy of Pathology Monograph No. 16. Baltimore: Williams & Wilkins, 1975:153–184.
6. Schnitzer B. Reactive lymphoid hyperplasia. In: Jaffe ES, ed. Surgical pathology of the lymph nodes and related organs. Philadelphia: WB Saunders, 1995:115.
7. Butler JJ. Non-neoplastic lesions of lymph nodes of man to be differentiated from lymphomas. NCI Monogr 1969;32:233–255.
8. Dorfman RF, Warnke R. Lymphadenopathy simulating the malignant lymphomas. Hum Pathol 1974;5:519–550.
9. Rappaport H. Tumors of the hematopoietic system. In: Atlas of tumor pathology. Washington, DC: Armed Forces Institute of Pathology, 1966: section II, fascicle 8.

14

MEASLES LYMPHADENITIS

DEFINITION

Lymphadenitis caused by infection with measles virus.

ETIOLOGY

Measles virus, a paramyxovirus, produces an acute, highly contagious, exanthematous infection in unimmunized patients. The measles virus does not have a natural reservoir other than in humans, and therefore its persistence in a community depends on the presence of unimmunized persons (1). In developed countries, measles is usually mild and causes periodic epidemics that most commonly affect children 5 to 7 years of age (1).

CLINICAL SYNDROME

In primitive communities, measles affects children less than 2 years old, whereas in the United States, older children and teenagers may acquire the infection, which in such cases tends to be more severe (1). Multiplication of the virus in macrophages and lymphocytes facilitates its dissemination to various organs. Pharyngitis, conjunctivitis, otitis, pneumonia, and in severe cases even encephalomyelitis may occur. The characteristic giant cells may be found not only in the tonsils but also in lymph nodes, intestinal Peyer patches, and appendix. Immunization against measles is achieved with formalin-inactivated virus and more effectively with attenuated live virus vaccine. Measles lymphadenitis may occur in the course of measles infection or days to weeks after vaccination with live attenuated virus (1–3). The axillary, cervical, and inguinal lymph nodes are most commonly involved.

HISTOPATHOLOGY

The lymph node architecture is partially or totally obliterated by the diffuse proliferation of immunoblasts and the relative depletion of small lymphocytes, which results in a mottled (moth-eaten) pattern (Figs. 14.1 and 14.2). In one case of severe reaction to measles vaccination, thrombosis of blood vessels and partial hemorrhagic necrosis of the regional inguinal lymph nodes were noted (4). Multinucleated giant cells, independently described by Warthin and Finkeldey, usually appear in the prodromal phase of measles in various hyperplastic lymphoid tissues, including tonsils, adenoids, lymph nodes, spleen, appendix, and thymus (1,2,5,6). They tend to disappear with the rise in antibody titers or when the cutaneous eruption is established (1). These polykaryocytes, which are large syncytia, are round or lobulated, 25 to 150 μm in diameter, with abundant acidophilic cytoplasm and from 4 to 50 darkly stained nuclei distributed in grapelike clusters (mulberry cells) in the center of cells (7,8) (Figs. 14.1 and 14.2). Cellular inclusions may be infrequently observed in the cytoplasm of giant cells (1) or endothelial cells (4). Polykaryocytes resembling the Warthin-Finkeldey giant cells associated with measles have also been seen in a variety of reactive and neoplastic lesions of lymph nodes (8,9). Morphologically indistinguishable from the Warthin-Finkeldey cells, they may be present in reactive lymphoid hyperplasia and other benign lymphadenopathies, including pattern A in the acute phase of HIV lymphadenitis (10). In lymphoma, polykaryocytes are more often noted in the lesions of the lymphocyte predominance type of Hodgkin lymphoma and in well-differentiated or poorly differentiated lymphocytic non-Hodgkin lymphomas (8,9). In general, these cells seem to be associated with lymphadenitides of viral origin and with lymphomas of low-grade malignancy (8,9).

ELECTRON MICROSCOPY

Cytoplasmic inclusions of various sizes and shapes were observed within endothelial cells in a node involved by measles that was examined ultrastructurally (4). The inclusions consist of dense granular material resembling coiled fibrils contained by a single membrane, which may represent ribonucleoproteins of the measles virus. The Warthin-Finkeldey cells account for a relatively small amount of cytoplasm and very few organelles (8). They occupy most of the space and

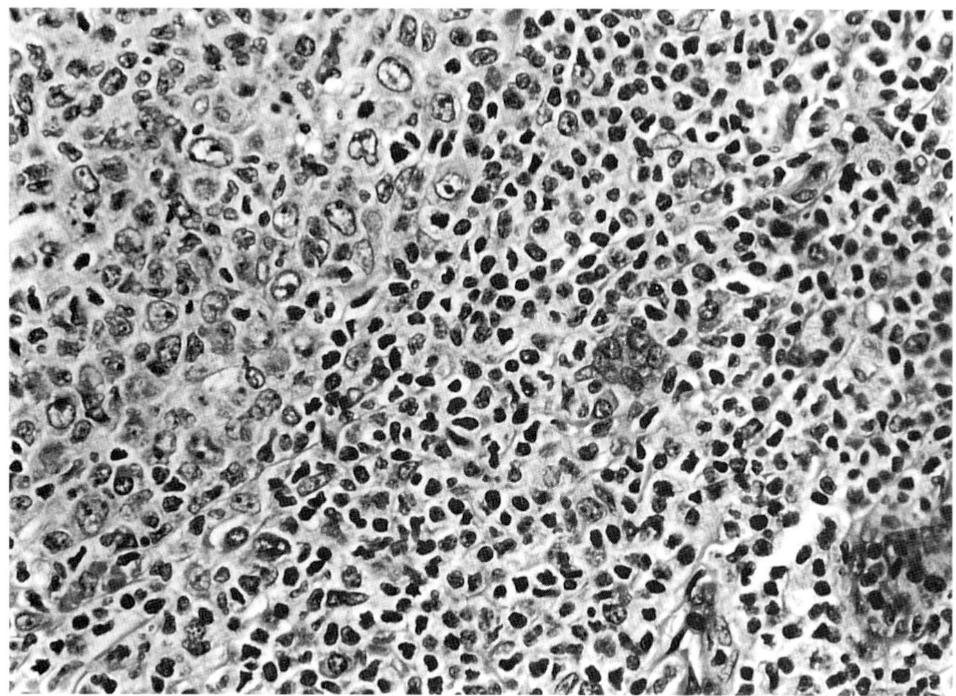

FIGURE 14.1. Cervical lymph node removed 5 days after administration of measles vaccine to a 6-year-old child. Reactive germinal center *(upper left)* and Warthin-Finkeldey multinucleated giant cells *(right)*. Hematoxylin and eosin stain.

exhibit variable shapes and nuclear molding (8,9). Virus particles have not been identified, and the origin of the cells remains unknown.

IMMUNOHISTOCHEMISTRY

The immunophenotype of the Warthin-Finkeldey cells was investigated with multiple monoclonal antibodies in three cases of various etiologies (11). Reaction of these polykaryocytes with antibodies directed against CD3, CD4, and CD43 (Leu-22) indicated them to be of helper T cell origin. A study of the Warthin-Finkeldey-type giant cells in HIV infection in which electron microscopy, immunohistochemistry, and *in situ* hybridization were used concluded that the multinucleated cells are derived from the follicular dendritic cells of the lymph nodes (12). The explanation for the discordant results of the studies may be that the Warthin-Finkeldey-type cells are in fact a heterogeneous group of cells.

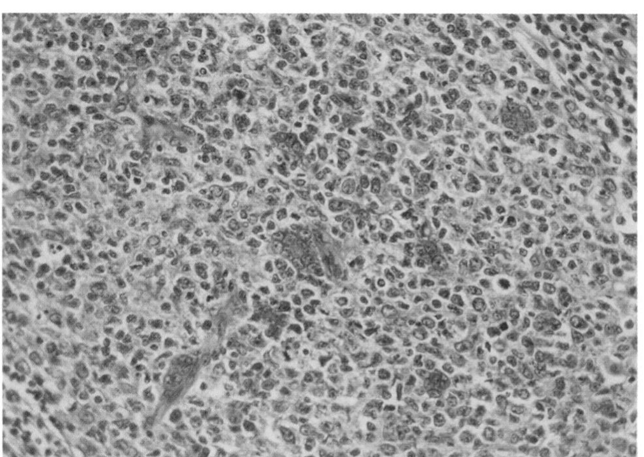

FIGURE 14.2. Measles lymphadenitis. Mixed population of lymphocytes, immunoblasts, and Warthin-Finkeldey multinucleated giant cells. Hematoxylin, phloxine, and saffron stain.

DIFFERENTIAL DIAGNOSIS

- Viral lymphadenitides of various kinds (Epstein-Barr virus, cytomegalovirus, herpes simplex virus) exhibit the mottled pattern of diffuse immunoblastic infiltration but do not usually include the Warthin-Finkeldey giant cells.
- HIV lymphadenitis in the acute phase includes giant cells resembling the Warthin-Finkeldey cells of measles; however, they are accompanied by folliculolysis and patches of monocytoid cells.
- Reactive lymphadenitides; Hodgkin lymphoma, lymphocyte predominance type; and non-Hodgkin lymphoma, low-grade types may include Warthin-Finkeldey giant cells. The diagnosis is confirmed by positive measles serology.

Checklist

MEASLES LYMPHADENITIS

Measles or history of recent vaccination
Axillary, cervical, inguinal lymph nodes affected
Mottled histologic pattern
Mild depletion of lymphocytes
Proliferation of immunoblasts
Warthin-Finkeldey giant cells

REFERENCES

1. Davis BD, Dulbecco R, Eisen HN. Paramyxoviruses. In: Microbiology, 3rd ed. Hagerstown, MD: Harper & Row, 1980:1138–1159.
2. Allen MS Jr, Talbot WH, McDonald RM. Atypical lymph node hyperplasia after administration of attenuated, live measles vaccine. N Engl J Med 1966;274:667–678.
3. Dorfman RF, Herweg JC. Live, attenuated measles virus vaccine: inguinal lymphadenopathy complicating administration. JAMA 1966;198:320–321.
4. Stejskal J. Measles lymphadenopathy. Ultrastruct Pathol 1980;1: 234–247.
5. Warthin AS. Occurrence of numerous large giant cells in tonsils and pharyngeal mucosa in the prodromal stage of measles. Arch Pathol 1931;11:864.
6. Finkeldey W. Uber Riesenzellbefunde in den Gaumenmandeln, zugleich ein Betrag zur Histopathologie der Mandelveränderungen in Maserninkubations-stadium. Virchows Arch A Pathol Anat Histopathol 1931;281:323.
7. Dorfman RF, Warnke R. Lymphadenopathy simulating the malignant lymphomas. Hum Pathol 1974;5:519–550.
8. Kjeldsberg CR, Kim H. Polykaryocytes resembling Warthin-Finkeldey giant cells in reactive and neoplastic lymphoid disorders. Hum Pathol 1981;12:267–272.
9. Delsol G, Pradere M, Voigt JJ, et al. Warthin-Finkeldey-like cells in benign and malignant lymphoid proliferations. Histopathology 1982;6:451–465.
10. Ioachim HL, Lerner CW, Tapper ML. The lymphoid lesions associated with the acquired immunodeficiency syndrome. Am J Surg Pathol 1983;7:543–553.
11. Kamel OW, LeBrun DP, Berry GJ, et al. Warthin-Finkeldey polykaryocytes demonstrate a T-cell immunophenotype. Am J Clin Pathol 1992;97:179–183.
12. Orenstein JM. The Warthin-Finkeldey-type giant cell in HIV infection, what is it? Ultrastruct Pathol 1998;22:293–303.

15

HUMAN IMMUNODEFICIENCY VIRUS LYMPHADENITIS

DEFINITION

Lymphadenitis caused by infection with human immunodeficiency virus (HIV).

SYNONYM

HIV lymphadenitis.

ETIOLOGY

HIV-1, the etiologic agent of HIV infection, is a member of the lentiviruses, which are a subfamily of retroviruses (1). The lentiviruses cause indolent, slowly progressing infections in a variety of animals; these frequently involve the nervous system and severely affect the immune system to cause immune deficiency. Unlike most retroviruses, which have only three genes, lentiviruses have a complex genome containing multiple genes (1); HIV-1 has nine genes. It has an icosahedral structure with 72 external spikes formed by two major viral envelope proteins, gp120 and gp41, and a core containing four nucleocapsid proteins, p24, p17, p9, and p7 (1) (Fig. 15.1). The core also contains two copies of the single-stranded RNA; associated with it are several enzymes, including the characteristic reverse transcriptase. Monoclonal antibodies to the various viral proteins have been produced and can be used to detect the virus in serum and tissue sections.

PATHOGENESIS

HIV manifests a strong tropism for the lymphoid tissues, particularly CD4+ T lymphocytes, monocytes, and dendritic cells. The cause of this high degree of cellular specificity is the presence on the cell membranes of CD4, a receptor molecule to which the HIV envelope protein gp120 binds avidly (1–5). In the early, acute phase of HIV infection, viremia is present at high titers and HIV infects mononuclear cells in the peripheral blood (6–8). Infected lymphocytes and monocytes migrate to lymphoid organs, causing acute reactive lymphadenitis. In the lymph nodes, follicular dendritic cells entrap HIV for presentation to immune T lymphocytes (9). While the infected T lymphocytes disseminate the virus, the macrophages in the circulation and the dendritic cells in the lymph nodes provide reservoirs for HIV, in which it can survive and replicate safely for long periods of time (10–16). HIV characteristic virus particles, HIV RNA, and membrane antigens can be detected in the germinal centers of reactive infected lymph nodes (8–14). As a result of occult yet continuous infection, the CD4+ T lymphocytes are destroyed by cytopathic mechanisms not yet fully understood and eventually become completely depleted. Similarly, the infected dendritic cells involute, so that the follicular germinal centers disappear (15). The late phase of the HIV infection, marked by depletion of CD4+ T lymphocytes, involution of lymph nodes, and resurgent viremia, is the background of AIDS and its host of opportunistic infections and tumors (4).

CLINICAL FEATURES

The acute phase of HIV infection generally lasts several weeks and manifests as a nonspecific, flulike syndrome that varies from almost unnoticeable symptoms to fever, sore throat, malaise, lymphadenopathies, and sometimes cutaneous rashes (17). The lymphadenopathies may persist during the following chronic phase of clinical latency that lasts for various periods of time (median, 10 years) (5). They are indolent and involve two or more sites. The patients are usually free of other symptoms and in fairly good health. The progression of disease parallels the continuous destruction of CD4+ T lymphocytes by the activity of virus released from lymphoid reservoirs (5). A drop in the CD4+ T-cell count to below 200/mm^3 signals the deep immune deficiency that characterizes AIDS and favors the opportunistic infections and neoplasms of this terminal stage of the disease (4). Biop-

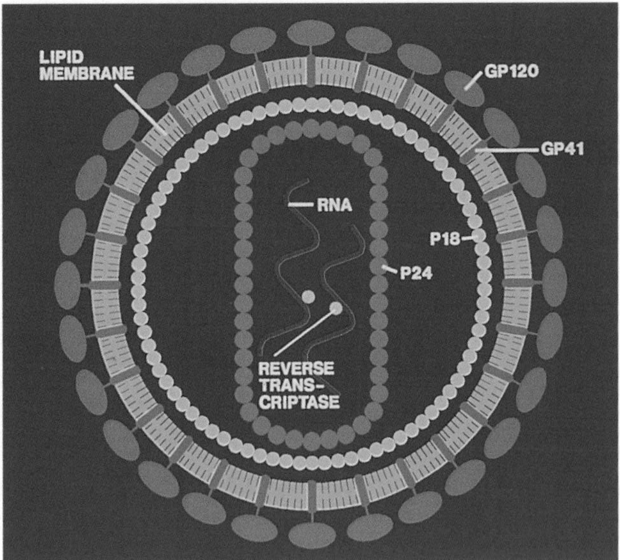

FIGURE 15.1. Schematic HIV structure showing locations of envelope glycoproteins gp120 and gp41 and of reverse transcriptase and nucleocapsid proteins p24 and p18. (From Abbott Diagnostics, Abbott Park, IL.)

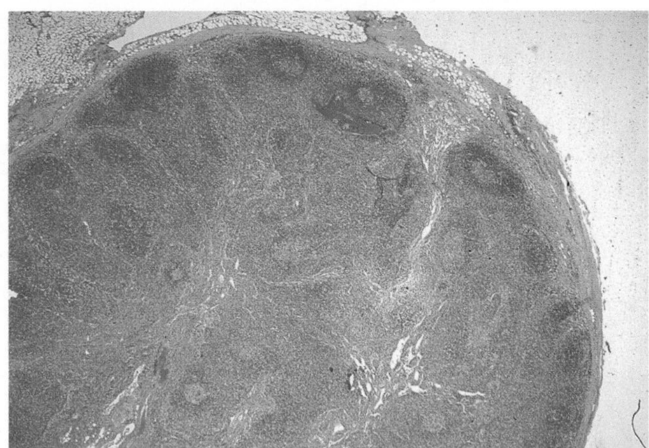

FIGURE 15.2. Acute HIV lymphadenitis, pattern A. Hyperplastic lymphoid follicles with reactive germinal centers and area of hemorrhage in axillary lymph node. Hematoxylin, phloxine, and saffron stain.

sies are frequently performed on the enlarged lymph nodes of patients with HIV lymphadenopathies, even those with known HIV serum positivity, because of the need to diagnose the many complications of AIDS that affect the lymph nodes and institute the proper treatment (18). The increasing incidence of non-Hodgkin lymphomas in long-term AIDS survivors undergoing antiretroviral treatment is a major reason for the biopsy and examination of enlarged lymph nodes in HIV-infected patients (19).

HISTOPATHOLOGY

The histopathology of HIV lymphadenitis has been considered nonspecific by some authors (20,21). In the acute phase, many of the morphologic features are indeed similar to those of other acute viral lymphadenitides. However, the histologic patterns repeatedly described by various authors are sufficiently characteristic to permit a tentative diagnosis of HIV lymphadenitis in the presence of relevant clinical and immunologic manifestations, which is confirmed subsequently by serologic testing (22–32). Three histologic patterns, A, B, and C, have been described (22,33–35) that generally correspond to clinical stages of acute, chronic, and burnout. (5).

Pattern A

Pattern A shows the general features of an acute lymphadenitis of viral origin. The lymphoid follicles are greatly enlarged, sometimes with serpiginous or hourglass shapes (Figs. 15.2 and 15.3). They comprise reactive hyperplastic germinal centers with widespread apoptosis, phagocytosis of nuclear debris by tingible-body histiocytes, and cellular regeneration with numerous centroblasts in mitosis (Fig. 15.4). The follicular mantle of small lymphocytes is diminished or absent; however, aggregates of small lymphocytes may penetrate into the germinal centers and contribute to their disruption, a process described by some authors as *folliculolysis* (29). In the interfollicular areas are focal hemorrhages (Fig. 15.2) and aggregates of monocytoid cells located next to blood vessels and sinuses (Fig. 15.5). These cells are fairly large and uniform, with distinct cellular borders, clear cytoplasm, and round, dark nuclei (Fig. 15.6). Immunohistochemical staining shows them to be transformed B lymphocytes. Clusters of polymorphonuclear neutrophils are also seen within the sinuses or patches of

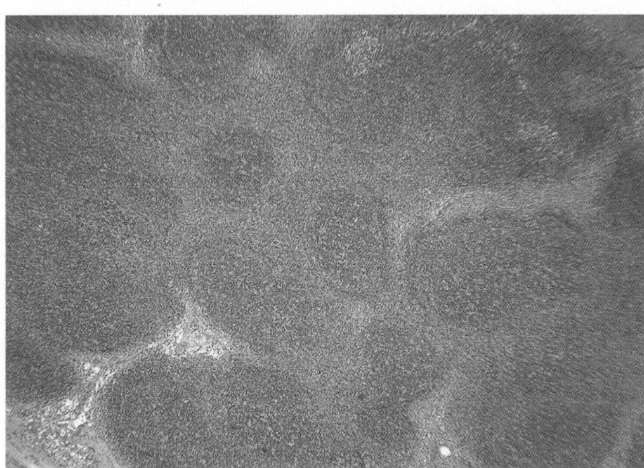

FIGURE 15.3. Acute HIV lymphadenitis, pattern A. Enlarged, coalescing lymphoid follicles in inguinal lymph node. Hematoxylin, phloxine, and saffron stain.

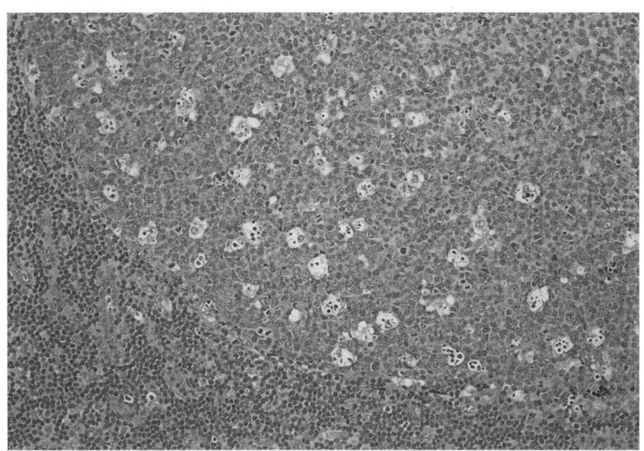

FIGURE 15.4. Acute HIV lymphadenitis, pattern A. Reactive germinal center with numerous apoptotic cells and tingible-body macrophages. Hematoxylin, phloxine, and saffron stain.

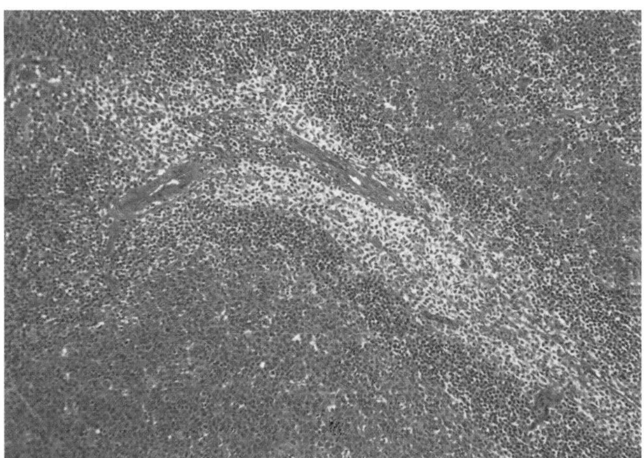

FIGURE 15.5. Acute HIV lymphadenitis, pattern A. Strip of monocytoid cells along blood vessels. Hematoxylin, phloxine, and saffron stain.

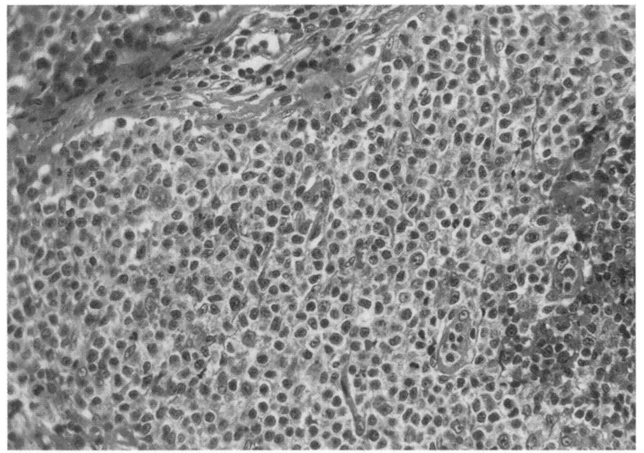

FIGURE 15.6. Acute HIV lymphadenitis, pattern A. Area of monocytoid cells with sharp cellular borders, clear cytoplasm, and small, centrally located, hyperchromatic nuclei. Hematoxylin, phloxine, and saffron stain.

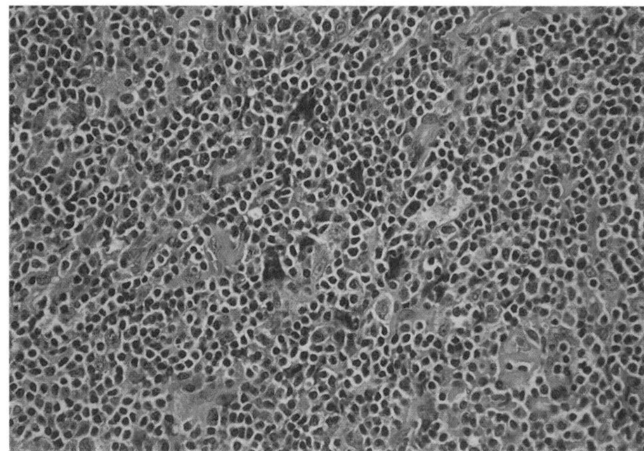

FIGURE 15.7. Acute HIV lymphadenitis, pattern A. Multinucleated hyperchromatic giant cells scattered among lymphoid cells. Hematoxylin, phloxine, and saffron stain.

monocytoid cells. Multinucleated giant cells of the Warthin-Finkeldey type, characterized by a grapelike cluster of overlapping nuclei, are often scattered at random throughout the nodal parenchyma (Figs. 15.7 and 15.8). Electron microscopy and immunohistochemistry studies showing these cells to express CD21 and CD35 markers concluded that they represent a multinucleated form of follicular dendritic cells (36).

Pattern B

Pattern B is a transition from pattern A to pattern C. It includes the effacement of follicles, disruption of dendritic cell networks, and involution of germinal centers. Depletion of lymphocytes, accumulation of plasma cells, and excessive proliferation of blood vessels in and around the lymphoid follicles are seen (Fig. 15.9). These features are suggestive of

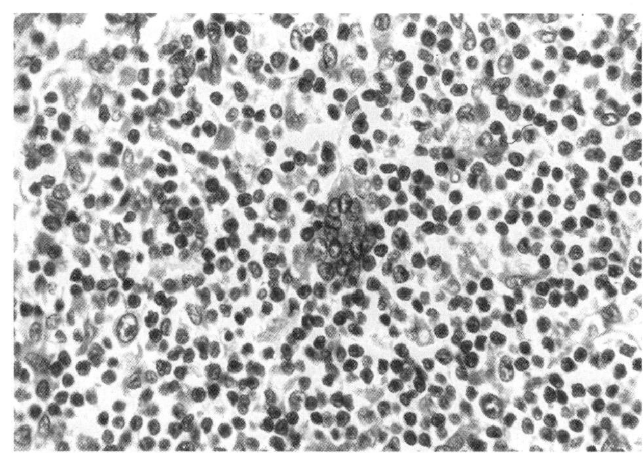

FIGURE 15.8. Acute HIV lymphadenitis, pattern A. Multinucleated giant cell (polykaryon) of Warthin-Finkeldey type with overlapping grapelike nuclei. Hematoxylin, phloxine, and saffron stain.

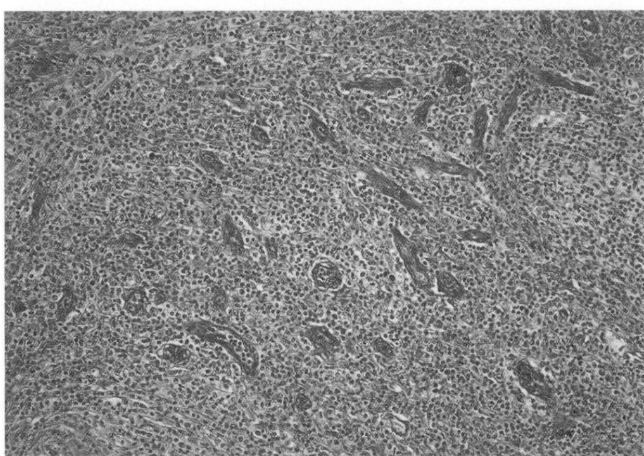

FIGURE 15.9. Subacute HIV lymphadenitis, pattern B. Effacement of lymph node architecture and excessive proliferation of blood vessels in the paracortex. Hematoxylin, phloxine, and saffron stain.

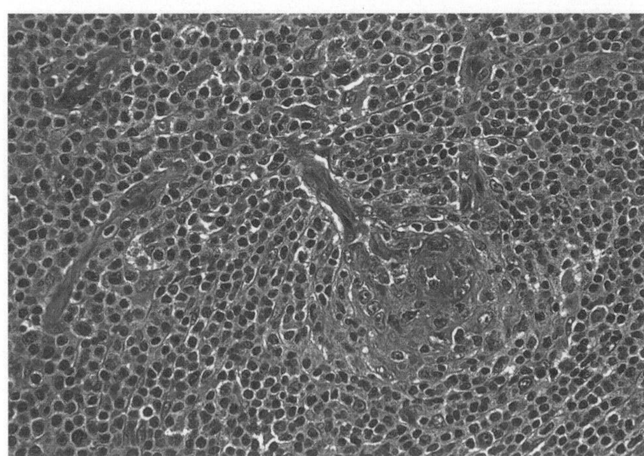

FIGURE 15.11. Chronic HIV lymphadenitis, pattern C. Hyalinized lymphoid follicle with transfixing, collagen-ensheathed arteriole ("lollipop" follicle). Hematoxylin, phloxine, and saffron stain.

subacute or chronic lymphadenitis, representing a stage in the progression of the HIV infection.

Pattern C

Pattern C shows lymph nodes with atrophic, burned-out follicles and extensive, diffuse vascular proliferation (Fig. 15.10). The follicles are small and depleted of lymphocytes, often with a central transfixing, collagen-ensheathed arteriole and deposits of periodic acid-Schiff (PAS)-positive material ("lollipop" follicle) (Fig. 15.11). In later stages, the follicles are inconspicuous and focally or entirely hyalinized. The interfollicular cortex shows a significant loss of lymphocytes and excessive vascularization. Frequent plasma cells and diffuse fibrosis are also seen. The appearance is that of an exhausted, involuted lymph node characterized by follicular atrophy, extensive angiogenesis, and fibrosis (34–36) (Figs. 15.9–15.11).

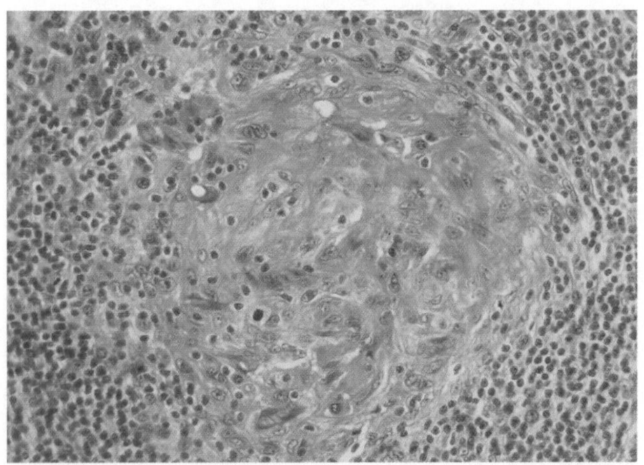

FIGURE 15.10. Chronic HIV lymphadenitis in inguinal lymph node, pattern C. Lymphoid follicle depopulated of lymphocytes and largely fibrosed. Hematoxylin, phloxine, and saffron stain.

In a study of 79 patients with HIV lymphadenitis who were followed for intervals of up to 7.2 years, the histologic patterns observed at the initial biopsy were correlated with immunologic status, course of disease, and length of survival (35). Of 31 patients who initially showed the histologic A pattern, the condition of 18 (58%) remained stationary and 13 (42%) progressed to AIDS; of 31 patients with a B pattern initially, the condition of 11 (36%) remained stationary and 20 (64%) progressed to AIDS; of 17 patients who initially had a histologic C pattern, the condition of one (6%) remained stationary and 16 (94%) progressed to AIDS. The 41 patients who died during this follow-up represented 32% of those who had a pattern A, 52% of those who had a pattern B, and 88% of those who had a pattern C at the initial lymph node biopsy. Survival curves of the three groups of patients are presented in Fig. 15.12.

The differences between the survival curves of the A and C patterns were statistically significant ($p = .001$). The histologic patterns of HIV lymphadenopathies (types A, B, and C) also correlate with lymphocyte evaluations as expressed by the total number of CD4+ T cells, CD4+/CD8+ cell ratios, and levels of antilymphocyte antibodies, as previously shown (35,37). Therefore, specifying the histologic pattern in the diagnosis of HIV lymphadenitis is clinically important because it provides information about the stage of disease and indicates the prognosis. The pathogenesis of lymph node lesions in HIV lymphadenitis and their association with AIDS are not well understood. However, the histologic patterns, by their resemblance to morphologic changes seen in other lymphadenopathies, provide some explanations. The extensive apoptosis and cytophagocytosis seen in the reactive germinal centers of pattern A are similar to those of other viral lymphadenitides, such as infectious mononucleosis and varicella, in the acute phase. The characteristic

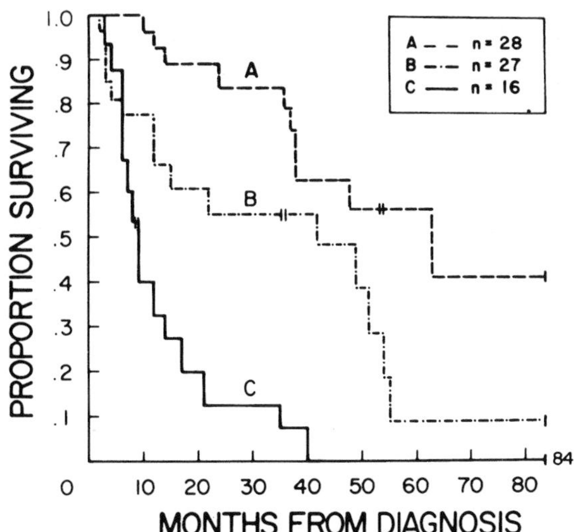

FIGURE 15.12. Survival curves for HIV lymphadenitis. Of 41 patients who died during 84 months, 32% had histologic pattern A, 52% pattern B, and 88% pattern C at initial diagnosis.

multinucleated giant cells and aggregates of monocytoid cells are also features of acute viral infections of lymph nodes. The identification of viral antigen and particles during the acute phase within dendritic cells, giant cells, and lymphocytes confirms the etiologic role of HIV in the origin of pattern A lesions. The histologic changes described in pattern C are similar to the lymphadenopathies associated with immune deficiencies. The involuted follicles with centrally penetrating "lollipop" arterioles (Fig. 15.11) and layered peripheral lymphocytes resemble Castleman lymphadenopathy, and the excessive, diffuse proliferation of blood vessels particularly affecting the T-cell territories (Fig. 15.9) may be similar to angioimmunoblastic lymphadenopathy. Kaposi sarcoma, a neoplastic proliferation of blood vessels, often arises in lymph nodes with the pattern C adenopathy of HIV infection (38–40). Thus, it appears that the histologic patterns noted in the HIV-infected lymph nodes parallel the clinical symptoms of the disease: the reactive follicles with the extensive apoptosis of pattern A in the acute stage, the progressive depletion of CD4+ T lymphocytes and disruption of dendritic networks of pattern B in the subchronic stage, and follicle involution and scarring of pattern C in the final burnout stage, which is the AIDS phase of HIV infection.

ELECTRON MICROSCOPY

Electron microscopy studies of lymph nodes from patients with AIDS-associated lymphadenopathies first demonstrated the presence and morphology of HIV (9,10,40,41). The virus-like particles are seen in the germinal centers, more commonly next to the cytoplasmic processes of the dendritic cells, but not in the interfollicular areas and deep cortex (10). They measure 100 to 120 μm in diameter and have an electron-dense core and an electron-lucent halo. The nuclear shape may be round or rectangular; often, it is a truncated cone or pyramid (10,14,41) (Fig. 15.13). The particles resemble the lentiviruses and in general have the structure of retroviruses; however, in contrast to retroviruses, budding from the plasma membrane is generally not noted (10). In addition to virus particles, virus-associated intracytoplasmic organelles are present in HIV-infected lymph nodes. Described as tubuloreticular inclusions and test tube- and ring-shaped forms, and later designated as cylindrical confronting cisternae, these structures are found in lymphocytes, macrophages, and endothelial cells (41) (Fig. 15.14). They are not specific for HIV, occasionally being noted in other viral infections, and appear to be related to the secretion of interferon (42).

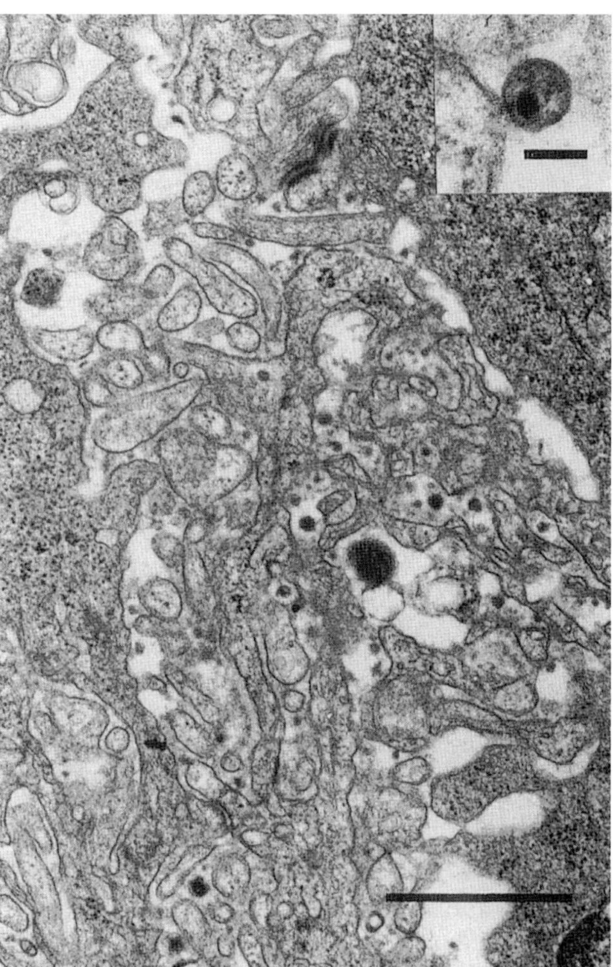

FIGURE 15.13. HIV lymphadenitis. Viral particles between the processes of follicular dendritic cells. Inset: Viral particle with eccentric cone. Original magnification ×84,000. Bar = 100 nm. (From O'Hara CJ, Groopman JE, Federman M. The ultrastructural and immunohistochemical demonstration of viral particles in lymph nodes from human immunodeficiency virus-related and non-human immunodeficiency virus-related lymphadenopathy syndromes. Hum Pathol 1988;19:545–549, with permission.)

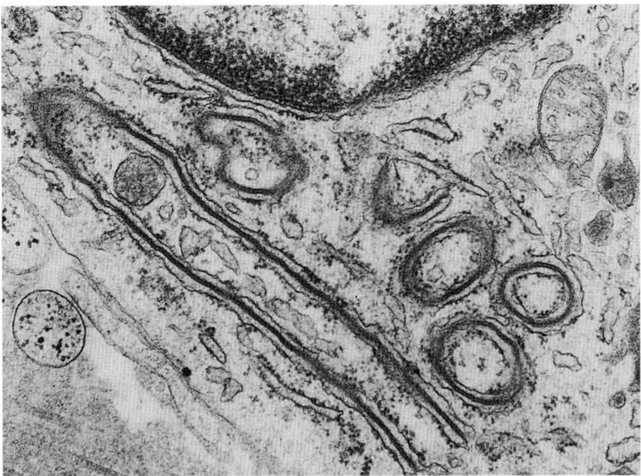

FIGURE 15.14. HIV lymphadenitis. Test tube- or ring-shaped formations in a paracortical interdigitating cell. (From Sidhu GS, Stahl ER, El-Sadr W, et al. The acquired immunodeficiency syndrome: an ultrastructural study. Hum Pathol 1985;16:377–386, with permission.)

IMMUNOHISTOCHEMISTRY

The presence of HIV in the affected lymph nodes is demonstrated with antibodies to various HIV antigens, particularly to the core protein p24. The staining for p24 is localized to the reactive germinal centers (Fig. 15.15) along the cell processes of the dendritic cells (11,12,14,43) (Fig. 15.16). This location is the same as that of the virus-like particles, which demonstrates their HIV identity (14,43). Isolated cells with morphologic and immunohistochemical features of follicular dendritic cells also express HIV core proteins p15 and p17 and envelope protein gp41 (Fig. 15.17), in addition to HIV messenger RNA (43). The presence of HIV in the lymphoid follicles of reactive lymph nodes has also been demonstrated by *in situ* hybridization (15,16) and polymerase chain reaction (5).

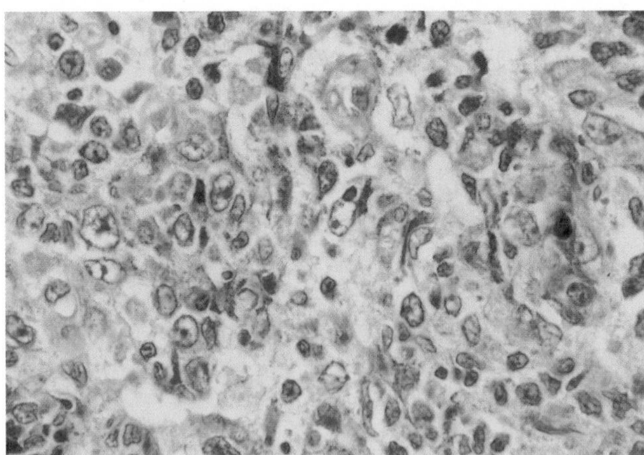

FIGURE 15.16. Acute HIV lymphadenitis p24 antigen trapped by dendritic cell processes in the germinal center. Anti-p24/peroxidase stain.

The follicular dendritic cells may be selectively immunostained with the monoclonal antibodies DRC-1 (Dako) and Ki-M4 (Behringwerke).

DIFFERENTIAL DIAGNOSIS

- Infectious mononucleosis lymphadenitis as the prototype of acute viral lymphadenitis resembles pattern A of HIV lymphadenitis, particularly in the reactive germinal centers, with abundant apoptosis and tingible-body macrophages. Serologic testing for Epstein-Barr virus and HIV antibodies is necessary for etiologic diagnosis.
- Cytomegalovirus, measles, and varicella lymphadenitides show similar germinal center changes and may be impossible to distinguish on morphologic grounds alone because cytomegalovirus inclusion bodies are rarely present, giant cells of the Warthin-Finkeldey type may be seen in both measles and HIV lymphadenitis, and the immunoblasts of varicella may not be prominent. For these

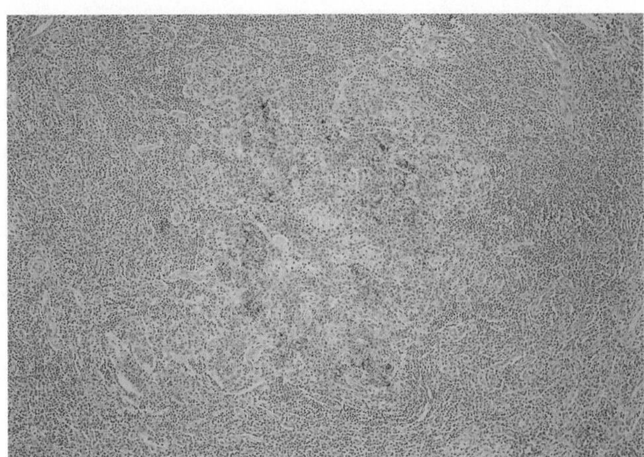

FIGURE 15.15. Acute HIV lymphadenitis in which p24-positive cells are located exclusively in the germinal center of a reactive follicle. Anti-p24/peroxidase stain.

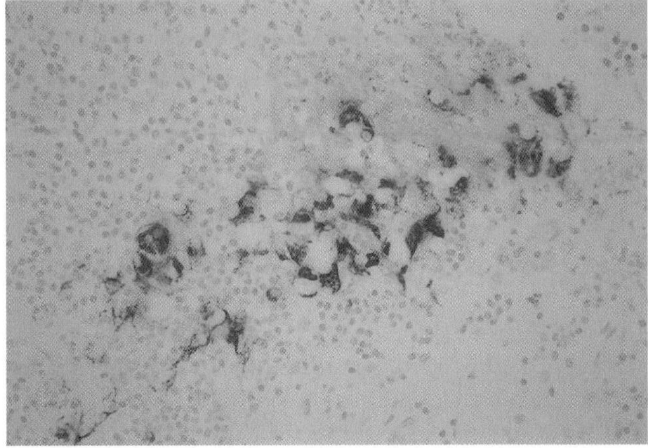

FIGURE 15.17. Acute HIV lymphadenitis of cervical lymph node. Abundant gp41 antigen is trapped by dendritic cells of the germinal center. Anti-gp41/peroxidase stain.

Checklist

HIV LYMPHADENITIS

Persons at risk for HIV infection and AIDS
Palpable lymphadenopathy at two or more sites
Absence of infection or apparent illness
Decreased number of CD4+ T cells
Reversed CD4+/CD8+ T-cell ratio
Positive results of HIV antigen or antibody tests

Pattern A (acute)
Enlarged lymph node
Hyperplastic, serpiginous follicles
Reactive germinal centers
Apoptosis, folliculolysis
Tingible-body macrophages
Disruption of dendritic network
Mitoses
Hemorrhages, polynuclear cells
Monocytoid aggregates
Warthin-Finkeldey giant cells

Pattern B (chronic)
Effacement of follicles
Involution of germinal centers
Depletion of lymphocytes
Plasma cells
Vascular hyperplasia

Pattern C (burnout)
Small or absent follicles
Hyalinized germinal centers
Transfixing, collagen-ensheathed arterioles ("lollipop" follicle)
Lymphocyte depletion
Plasma cells
Deposits that stain with periodic acid–Schiff
Extensive angiogenesis

reasons, serologic testing for specific antibodies is needed in all viral infections, including HIV infection, to confirm a tentative diagnosis.

- *Toxoplasma* lymphadenitis may show patches of monocytoid cells similar to those of HIV lymphadenitis but should also show perifollicular and intrafollicular clusters of epithelioid cells, which are not part of HIV infection.
- Castleman lymphadenopathy has in common with pattern C of HIV lymphadenitis involuted follicles with hyaline germinal centers and vascular proliferation. It lacks a general depletion of lymphocytes. HIV serum antibody testing is necessary for a definitive diagnosis.
- Angioimmunoblastic lymphadenopathy shows abundant vascular proliferation and in this respect resembles patterns B and C of HIV lymphadenitis; however, it also includes effaced follicles and abundant proliferation of immunoblasts.

HIV LYMPHADENITIS

Pattern A (acute)
- Infectious mononucleosis lymphadenitis
- Cytomegalovirus, varicella, measles lymphadenitis
- *Toxoplasma* lymphadenitis

Pattern B (chronic)
- Castleman lymphadenopathy, plasma cell type
- Angioimmunoblastic lymphadenopathy

Pattern C (burnout)
- Castleman lymphadenopathy, hyaline vascular type
- Fibrosed end-stage lymphadenitis

REFERENCES

1. Greene WC: Mechanisms of disease. N Engl J Med 1991;324: 308–317.
2. Klatzman D, Barre-Sinoussi F, Nugeyre MT, et al. Selective tropism of lymphadenopathy associated virus (LAV) for helper-inducer T lymphocytes. Science 1984;225:59–64.
3. Ho DD, Pomerantz, RJ, Kaplan J. Pathogenesis of infection with human immunodeficiency virus. N Engl J Med 1987;317:278–286.
4. Ioachim HL. Immunopathogenesis of human immunodeficiency virus infection. Cancer Res 1990;50:5612s–5617s.
5. Pantaleo G, Graziosi C, Fauci AS. The immunopathogenesis of human immunodeficiency virus infection. N Engl J Med 1993;328:327–335.
6. Daar ES, Moudgil T, Meyer RD, et al. Transient high levels of viremia in patients with primary human immunodeficiency virus type l infection. N Engl J Med 1991;324:961–964.
7. Embertson J, Zupancic M, Ribas JL, et al. Massive covert infection of helper T lymphocytes and macrophages by HIV during the incubation period of AIDS. Nature 1991;362:359–362.
8. Harper ME, Marselle LM, Gallo RC, et al. Detection of lymphocytes expressing human T-lymphotropic virus type III in lymph nodes and peripheral blood from infected individuals by *in situ* hybridization. Proc Natl Acad Sci U S A 1986;83: 772–776.
9. Armstrong JA, Horne R. Follicular dendritic cells and virus-like particles in AIDS-related lymphadenopathy. Lancet 1984;2:370–372.
10. Le Tourneau A, Audoin J, Diebold J, et al. LAV-like particles in lymph node germinal centers in patients with the persistent lymphadenopathy syndrome and the acquired immunodeficiency syndrome-related complex: an ultrastructural study of 30 cases. Hum Pathol 1986;17:1047–1053.
11. Tenner-Racz, R, Racz P, Bofill M, et al. HTLV-III/LAV viral antigen in lymph nodes of homosexual men with persistent generalized lymphadenopathy and AIDS. Am J Pathol 1986;123:9–15.
12. Baroni CD, Pezella F, Pezella M, et al. Expression of HIV in lymph node cells of LAS patients. Am J Pathol 1988;133:498–506.
13. Schuurman H-J, Krone W J-A, Broekhuizen R, et al. Expression of RNA and antigens of human immunodeficiency virus type-1 (HIV-1) in lymph nodes from HIV-1 infected individuals. Am J Pathol 1988;133:516–524.
14. O'Hara CJ, Groopman JE, Federman M. The ultrastructural and immunohistochemical demonstration of viral particles in lymph nodes from human immunodeficiency virus-related and non-human immunodeficiency virus-related lymphadenopathy syndromes. Hum Pathol 1988;19:545–549.
15. Fox CH, Tenner-Racz K, Racz P, et al. Lymphoid germinal centers are reservoirs of human immunodeficiency virus type 1 RNA. J Infect Dis 1991;164:1051–1057.
16. Spiegel H, Herbst H, Niedobitek G, et al. Follicular dendritic cells are a major reservoir for human immunodeficiency virus type 1 in lymphoid tissues facilitating infection of CD4+ T-helper cells. Am J Pathol 1992;140:15–22.
17. Steeper TA, Horwits CA, Hanson M, et al. Heterophil-negative mononucleosis-like illnesses with atypical lymphocytosis in patients undergoing seroconversions to the human immunodeficiency virus. Am J Clin Pathol 1988;89:169–174.
18. Ioachim HL. Biopsy diagnosis in human immunodeficiency virus and acquired immunodeficiency syndrome. Arch Pathol Lab Med 1990;114:284–294.
19. Ioachim HL. Immune deficiency: opportunistic tumors. In: Encyclopedia of cancer, Bertimo JD, ed. New York: Academic Press, 1997.
20. Stanley MW, Frizzera G. Diagnosis specificity of histologic features in lymph node biopsy specimens from patients at risk for the acquired immunodeficiency syndrome. Hum Pathol 1983;17: 1231–1239.
21. O'Murchada MT, Wolf BC, Neiman RS. The histologic features of hyperplastic lymphadenopathy in AIDS-related complex are nonspecific. Am J Surg Pathol 1987;11:94–99.
22. Ioachim HL, Lerner CW, Tapper ML. Lymphadenopathies in homosexual men. Relationships with the acquired immune deficiency syndrome. JAMA 1983;250:1306–1309.
23. Ioachim HL, Lerner CW, Tapper ML. The lymphoid lesions associated with the acquired immunodeficiency syndrome. Am J Surg Pathol 1983;7:543–553.
24. Metroka CE, Cunningham-Rundles S, Pollack MS, et al. Generalized lymphadenopathy in homosexual men. Ann Intern Med 1983;99:585–591.
25. Brynes RK, Chan WC, Spira TJ, et al. Value of lymph node biopsy in unexplained lymphadenopathy in homosexual men. JAMA 1983;250:1313–1317.
26. Guarda LA, Butler JJ, Mansell P, et al. Lymphadenopathy in homosexual men. Morbid anatomy with clinical and immunologic correlations. Am J Clin Pathol 1983;79:559–568.
27. Meyer PR, Yamagihara ET, Parker JW, et al. A distinctive follicular hyperplasia in the acquired immune deficiency syndrome (AIDS) and the AIDS-related complex: a prelymphomatous state for B-cell lymphoma. Hematol Oncol 1984;2:310–347.
28. Turner RR, Meyer PR, Taylor CR, et al. Immunohistology of persistent generalized lymphadenopathy. Evidence for progressive lymph node abnormalities in some patients. Am J Clin Pathol 1984;88:10–19.
29. Burns BF, Wood GS, Dorfman RFL. The varied histopathology of lymphadenopathy in the homosexual male. Am J Surg Pathol 1985;9:287–297.
30. Diebold J, Audouin J, Marche CL, et al. Aspects histopathologiques des adénopathies dans le syndrome des adénopathies persistantes (LAS) et les syndromes associés au SIDA (ARC). Ann Pathol 1986;6:266–270.
31. Farthing CF, Shanson HK, Taube M, et al. Clinical investigations of lymphadenopathy, including lymph node biopsies, in 24 homosexual men with antibodies to the human T-cell lymphotropic virus type III (HTLV-III). Br J Surg 1986;73:180–182.
32. Chadburn A, Metroka C, Mouradian J. Progressive lymph node histology and its prognostic value in patients with acquired immunodeficiency syndrome and AIDS-related complex. Hum Pathol 1989;20:579–587.
33. Wenig BM, Thompson LDR, Frankel SS, et al. Lymphoid changes of the nasopharyngeal and palatine tonsils that are indicative of human immunodeficiency virus infection. A clinicopathologic study of 12 cases. Am J Surg Pathol 1996;20:572–587.
34. Ioachim HL. Pathology of AIDS. Textbook and color atlas. Philadelphia: JB Lippincott Co, 1989.
35. Ioachim HL, Cronin W, Roy M, et al. Persistent lymphadenopathies in people at high risk for HIV infection. Am J Clin Pathol 1990;93:208–218.
36. Ioachim HL. Lymphadenopathies of HIV infection and AIDS. In: Pangalis GA, Polliack A, eds. Benign and malignant lymphadenopathies. Chur, Switzerland: Harwood Academic, 1993: 159–171.
37. Dorsett BH, Cronin W, Ioachim HL. Presence and prognostic significance of antilymphocyte antibodies in symptomatic and asymptomatic human immunodeficiency virus infection. Arch Intern Med 1990;150:1025–1028.

38. Chen KTK. Multicentric Castleman's disease and Kaposi's sarcoma. Am J Surg Pathol 1984;8:287–293.
39. Harris NL. Hypervascular follicular hyperplasia and Kaposi's sarcoma in patients at risk for AIDS. N Engl J Med 1984;310:462–463.
40. Tenner-Racz K, Racz P, Dietrich M, et al. Altered follicular dendritic cells and virus-like particles in AIDS and AIDS-related lymphadenopathy. Lancet 1985;1:105–106.
41. Sidhu GS, Stahl ER, El-Sadr W, et al. The acquired immunodeficiency syndrome: an ultrastructural study. Hum Pathol 1985;16:377–386.
42. Bockus D, Remington F, Luu J, et al. Induction of cylindrical confronting cisternae (AIDS inclusions) in Daudi lymphoblastoid cells by recombinant-interferon. Hum Pathol 1988;19:78–82.
43. Parmentier HK, Van Wichen D, Sie Go D, et al. HIV-1 infection and virus production in follicular dendritic cells in lymph nodes. Am J Pathol 1990;137:247–251.

16

HUMAN IMMUNODEFICIENCY VIRUS LYMPHADENITIS OF SALIVARY GLANDS

DEFINITION

HIV lymphadenitis of salivary gland lymph nodes causing cystic lymphoepithelial lesions.

SYNONYMS

HIV sialadenitis, HIV parotitis, Sjögren-like syndrome in AIDS.

PATHOGENESIS

Normally, lymph nodes are intimately associated with the salivary glands, particularly the parotids. Five to ten lymph nodes are embedded in the parotid gland, several lymph nodes are adjacent to the submaxillary gland, and salivary gland acini and ducts are commonly present in the medulla of upper cervical lymph nodes (1). The ratio of lymphoid to salivary tissues varies, with the former sometimes reduced to a thin shell around the parotid lobules (1). Whereas it was once believed that glandular inclusions in lymph nodes represent ectopic salivary glands, sequential studies of human embryos have shown that rudimentary lymph nodes arising in the primitive mesenchyme penetrate the salivary glands and proliferate around their ductal and acinar structures. By the thirteenth week, these formations are already in place, and their association with the salivary glands is a constant feature of normal development (2,3).

In the course of HIV infection, salivary gland lymph nodes may be a primary target for the viral infection, like any other peripheral lymph nodes that are commonly involved (4,5). In such cases, persons at risk for AIDS present with a tumor-like mass of the salivary gland, usually without any other symptoms. Because of this presentation, and particularly because of histologic similarities, the enlarged salivary glands in HIV-positive patients were formerly considered to represent AIDS-associated Sjögren syndrome (6). Sjögren syndrome, or sicca syndrome, is defined by the triad of xerophthalmia, keratoconjunctivitis, and autoimmune disorder, expressed by the presence of auto-antibodies; however, none of these symptoms were present in patients with HIV lymphadenitis of salivary glands (7). Salivary gland lymph nodes, again like lymph nodes in other locations, can also be the primary site of AIDS-related lymphomas and Kaposi sarcoma (5,8) (see Chapters 81 and 85). Three cases of non-Hodgkin lymphoma were included in a series of cases in which involvement of the salivary gland lymph nodes was reported as a complication of AIDS (5).

CLINICAL SYNDROME

The involved salivary glands, usually the parotids, present as unilateral or bilateral masses. They are nodular and generally large, reaching 4 to 7 cm in diameter (5). Surgically excised with the tentative diagnosis of salivary gland tumor, the masses are composed of multiple enlarged lymph nodes and portions of salivary gland that are not easily distinguishable on gross examination.

HISTOPATHOLOGY

Microscopically, the bulk of the excised tissues consists of lymph nodes showing excessive follicular hyperplasia. The enlarged follicles comprise markedly expanded and irregularly shaped reactive germinal centers that show the typical starry sky pattern of acute HIV lymphadenitis (Fig. 16.1). Cellular lysis, nuclear breakage, tingible-body macrophages with engulfed nuclear debris, patches of monocytoid lymphocytes, and multinucleated giant cells can be observed, as in other HIV lymphadenitides (Fig. 16.2). HIV trapped by dendritic cells, a source for the infected saliva, can be demonstrated by immune staining for HIV antigens (Fig. 16.3).

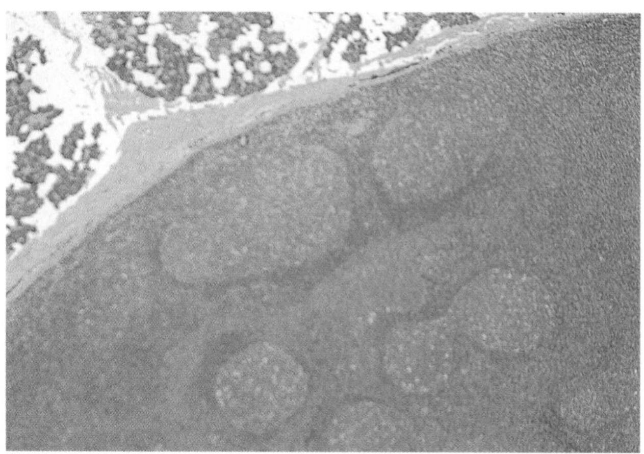

FIGURE 16.1. Enlarged salivary gland lymph node with hyperplastic coalescing follicles and reactive germinal centers. Salivary gland (*upper left*) is uninvolved. Hematoxylin, phloxine, and saffron stain.

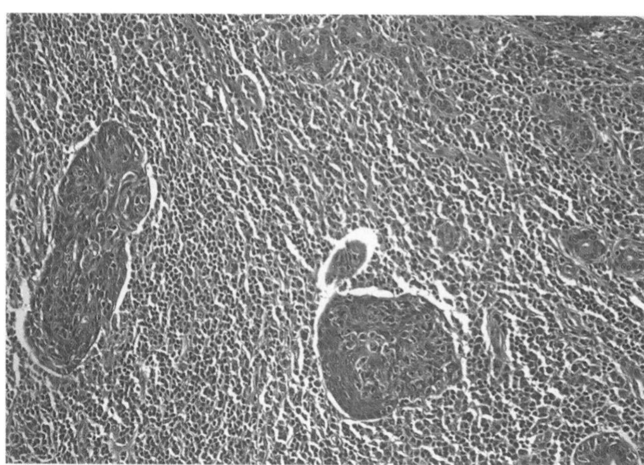

FIGURE 16.4. Epimyoepithelial islands in HIV salivary lymphadenitis. Hematoxylin, phloxine, and saffron stain.

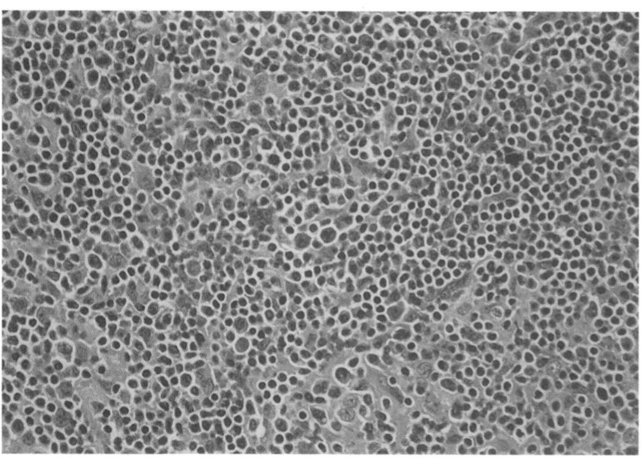

FIGURE 16.2. Salivary gland HIV lymphadenitis. Monocytoid cells and multinucleated giant cells (polykaryons). Hematoxylin, phloxine, and saffron stain.

Other morphologic changes usually seen in the chronic stages of HIV lymphadenitis (e.g., lymphocyte depletion, excessive vascular proliferation, atrophic fibrosed germinal centers) are also present. Foci of inflammation may be present in the salivary glands, particularly around the salivary ducts. The latter show cellular proliferation and squamous metaplasia with characteristic epithelial and myoepithelial aggregates that are also known as *epimyoepithelial islands* (1) (Figs. 16.4–16.6). The obliteration of ducts and accumulation of keratin produced by the newly formed squamous epithelium result in the formation of large cystic structures filled with keratin (Fig. 16.7). The leakage of keratin is accompanied by the accumulation of foreign body giant cells in addition to large amounts of neutrophils, plasma cells, and lymphocytes (4,5).

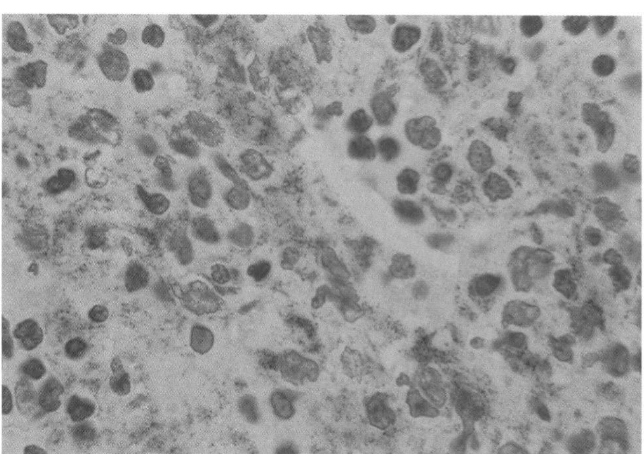

FIGURE 16.3. Reactive germinal center with deposits of p24 antigen on dendritic cells in HIV salivary lymphadenitis. Anti-p24/peroxidase stain.

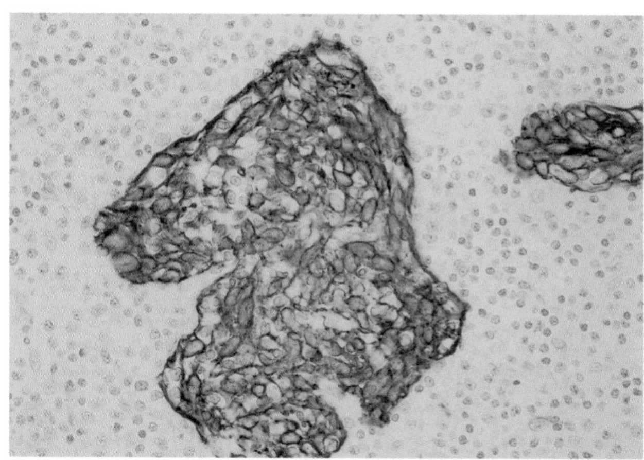

FIGURE 16.5. Epimyoepithelial island positively stained with anticytokeratin antibody. Anticytokeratin/peroxidase stain.

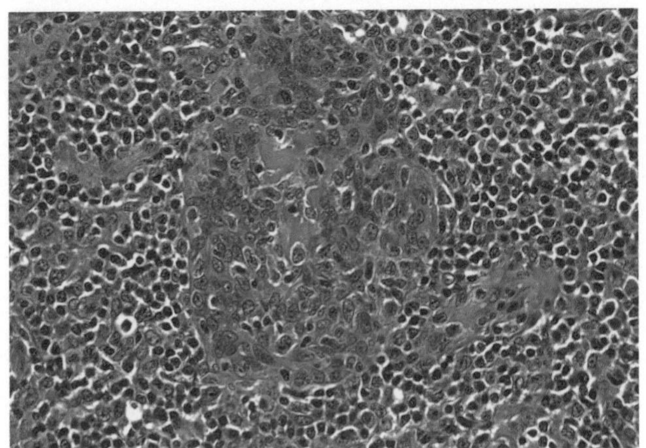

FIGURE 16.6. Characteristic epimyoepithelial lesion consisting of squamous epithelial island infiltrated by natural killer T cells in HIV salivary lymphadenitis. Hematoxylin, phloxine, and saffron stain.

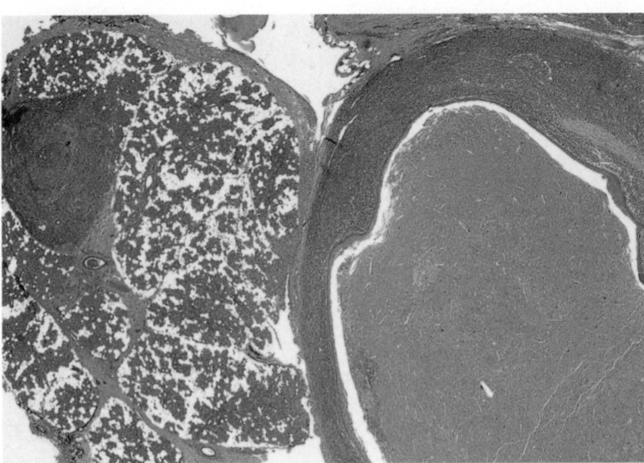

FIGURE 16.7. HIV lymphadenitis in enlarged parotid gland. Lymphoid follicle with reactive germinal center (*upper left*) within uninvolved salivary gland. Large keratin cyst (*right*) compressing the surrounding reactive lymphoid tissue. Hematoxylin, phloxine, and saffron stain.

Primary non-Hodgkin lymphoma limited to the salivary gland was reported to occur in patients with HIV lymphadenitis (5). They were high-grade, immunoblastic, and Burkitt types (9), arose in the parotid gland lymph nodes, and invaded the adjacent salivary gland (see Chapter 81).

DIFFERENTIAL DIAGNOSIS

- Sjögren syndrome and Mikulicz syndrome are characterized by lymphoepithelial lesions; however, as autoimmune disorders, these syndromes are associated with additional clinical symptoms in addition to auto-antibodies (rheumatoid factor in 84% of cases) (10).
- Warthin tumor and sialolithiasis after prolonged secondary inflammation may show destruction of gland architecture and lymphoepithelial lesions; however, in both entities, the inflammatory infiltrates affect primarily the salivary gland, and reactive germinal centers are not part of the process.

Checklist

HIV LYMPHADENITIS OF SALIVARY GLANDS

Persons with HIV infection
Absence of apparent illness
Reversed helper/suppressor T-lymphocyte ratio
Positive result of anti-HIV antibodies test
Intraparotid lymph nodes affected
Presentation as salivary gland tumor masses
Salivary gland lymphadenitis
- Enlarged lymphoid follicles
- Hyperplastic germinal centers
- Foliculolysis
- Tingible-body macrophages
- Obstructed, dilated salivary ducts
- Epimyoepithelial islands
- Keratin cysts with squamous cell lining

REFERENCES

1. Thackray AC, Lucas RB. Tumors of the major salivary glands. In: Atlas of tumor pathology. Washington, DC: Armed Forces Institute of Pathology, 1974:fascicle 10.
2. Brown RB, Gallard RA, Turner JA. The significance of aberrant or heterotopic parotid gland tissues in lymph nodes. Ann Surg 1953;138:850–856.
3. Marques B, Gay G, Jozan S, et al. Origine embryologique des inclusions salivaires dans les ganglions lymphatiques parotidiens. Bull Assoc Anat 1983;76:219–228.
4. Ryan JR, Ioachim HL, Marmer J, et al. Acquired immune deficiency syndrome-related lymphadenopathies presenting in the salivary gland lymph nodes. Arch Otolaryngol 1985;111:554–556.
5. Ioachim HL, Ryan JR, Blaugrund SM. Salivary gland lymph nodes, the site of lymphadenopathies and lymphomas associated with human immunodeficiency virus (HIV) infection. Arch Pathol Lab Med 1988;112:1224–1228.
6. Ulirsch RC, Jaffe ES. Sjögren's syndrome-like illness associated with the acquired immuno-deficiency syndrome-related complex. Hum Pathol 1987;18:1063–1069.
7. Ioachim HL, Ryan JR. Salivary gland lymphadenopathies associated with AIDS. Hum Pathol 1988;19:616–617.
8. Puterman M, Goldstein J. Primary lymph nodal Kaposi's sarcoma of the parotid gland. Head Neck Surg 1985;5:535–556.
9. Ioachim HL, Antonescu C, Giancotti F, et al. EBV-associated primary lymphomas in salivary glands of HIV-infected patients. Pathol Res Pract 1998;194: 87–95.
10. Elkon KB, Gharavi AE, Hughes ER, et al. Autoantibodies in the sicca syndrome (primary Sjögren's syndrome). Ann Rheum Dis 1984;43:243.

PART III

SECTION TWO

BACTERIAL LYMPHADENITIDES

In a broad sense, bacterial diseases include infections produced by ordinary cocci and bacilli and also by mycobacteria, rickettsiae, and spirochetes. This heterogeneous group of microorganisms can produce tissue damage in various ways and elicit different kinds of tissue reactions. Bacteria cause cell injury by secreting exotoxins or by releasing endotoxins from their cell walls when they are destroyed. Tissue reactions to bacteria may be acute and nonspecific, dominated by polymorphonuclear leukocytes, or chronic and specific, such as the formation of granulomas. Lymph nodes that drain tissues infected by bacteria may be subjected to similar damage that results in various combinations of suppurative, necrotic, proliferative, and sclerosing lesions.

17

ORDINARY BACTERIAL LYMPHADENITIS

DEFINITION

Acute, sometimes suppurative lymphadenitis caused by bacterial infection.

PATHOGENESIS

Common bacteria, more often *Staphylococcus aureus* than group A streptococci, may infect the regional lymph nodes draining a dental abscess (1), an infected wound, pleural emphysema, appendicitis, a tuboovarian abscess, or another site of pyogenic inflammation (2,3). They are more common in superficial nodes, particularly axillary and inguinal nodes, and may on rare occasions destroy the lymph node, with resulting abscess or sinus formation. In such cases, the biopsy may not show any lymphoid tissue, and therefore the evidence of acute lymphadenitis is lacking (4). Less acute and more localized suppurative lymphadenitis may also accompany other infections, such as yersiniosis (5,6), tularemia (7,8), typhoid fever (9), melioidosis (10,11), listeriosis, fungal infections (Chapters 26–29), and cat-scratch disease (4) (Chapter 18). Acute gonorrhea, particularly in men, may be accompanied by severe, rapidly developing, usually symmetric inguinal lymphadenitis (2). Generally, because of antibiotic treatment, suppurative lymphadenitides have become uncommon. Nevertheless, repeated lymph node abscesses in children caused by a catalase-positive bacterium such as *S. aureus* may be a manifestation of chronic granulomatous disease (12) or defective neutrophil chemotaxis (13).

HISTOPATHOLOGY

The lymph node involved is variably enlarged, soft, and tender, with the overlying skin reddened and edematous. In an early phase, the lymph node shows sinus catarrh, in which dilated sinuses contain a weakly eosinophilic proteinaceous fluid with numerous granulocytes and macrophages (4) (Fig. 17.1). The blood vessels are congested. The granulocytes, mostly neutrophils, eventually infiltrate the lymph node parenchyma, forming microabscesses (Fig. 17.2). Bacteria may be free or phagocytosed. Involvement of perinodal fibroadipose tissues by the inflammation may result in periadenitis (Figs. 17.3 and 17.4). In a later stage, the acute inflammatory process subsides, and polymorphonuclear leukocytes are progressively replaced by lymphocytes, plasma cells, and particularly macrophages containing ingested cellular debris. Rarely, healed, late-stage suppurative lymphadenitis appears xanthogranulomatous (14). Bacterial sepsis may lead to a severe hemophagocytic syndrome involving the liver, spleen, and lymph nodes (15).

ADJUVANT DIAGNOSTIC METHODS

- Gram's stain of paraffin-embedded sections is useful in identifying the presence and nature of bacteria.
- Bacteriologic study of smears and cultures is indispensable for specific etiologic identification. Therefore, sterile, fresh tissues from the area of suppuration must be sent immediately to the microbiology laboratory for bacterial culture and antibiogram.
- The microbiologic culture yield (30%) from the fine needle aspiration of lymph nodes is comparable with that of open biopsy (16).

DIFFERENTIAL DIAGNOSIS

- Cat-scratch lymphadenitis and lymphogranuloma venereum lymphadenitis include focal areas of necrosis with accumulations of polymorphonuclear leukocytes. However, these lesions also have a granulomatous organization and contain epithelioid and multinucleated giant cells. A neutrophil-rich variant of Ki-1 anaplastic large cell lymphoma (see Chapter 75) can contain more neutrophils than lymphoma cells, which obscure the neoplastic cells (17) (Fig. 17.5). Tissue neutrophilia is rare in other types of non-Hodgkin malignant lymphoma except during infection, when transient polymorphonuclear leukocytic infiltrates may occur (18).

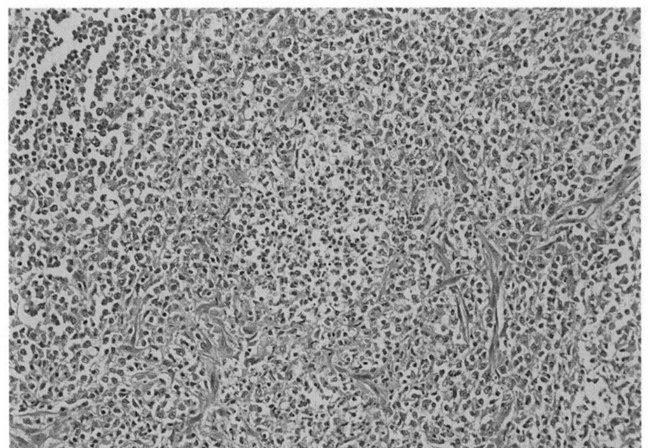

FIGURE 17.1. Bacterial lymphadenitis. Polymorphonuclear neutrophils infiltrate diffusely and form microabscess (*center*) in an axillary lymph node. Hematoxylin, phloxine, and saffron stain.

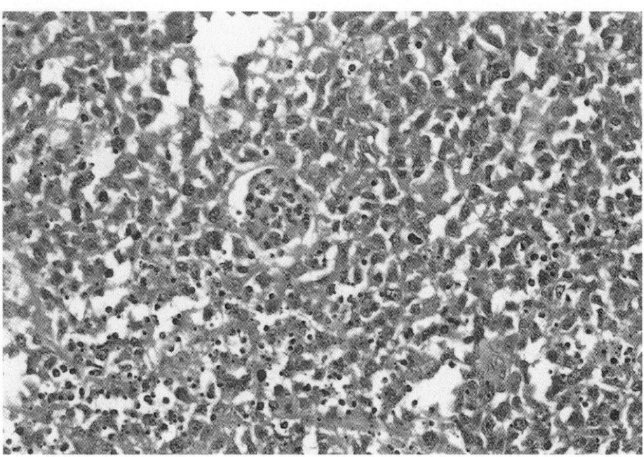

FIGURE 17.2. Same section. Diffuse apoptosis of lymphoid cells and accumulations of neutrophil leukocytes. Hematoxylin, phloxine, and saffron stain.

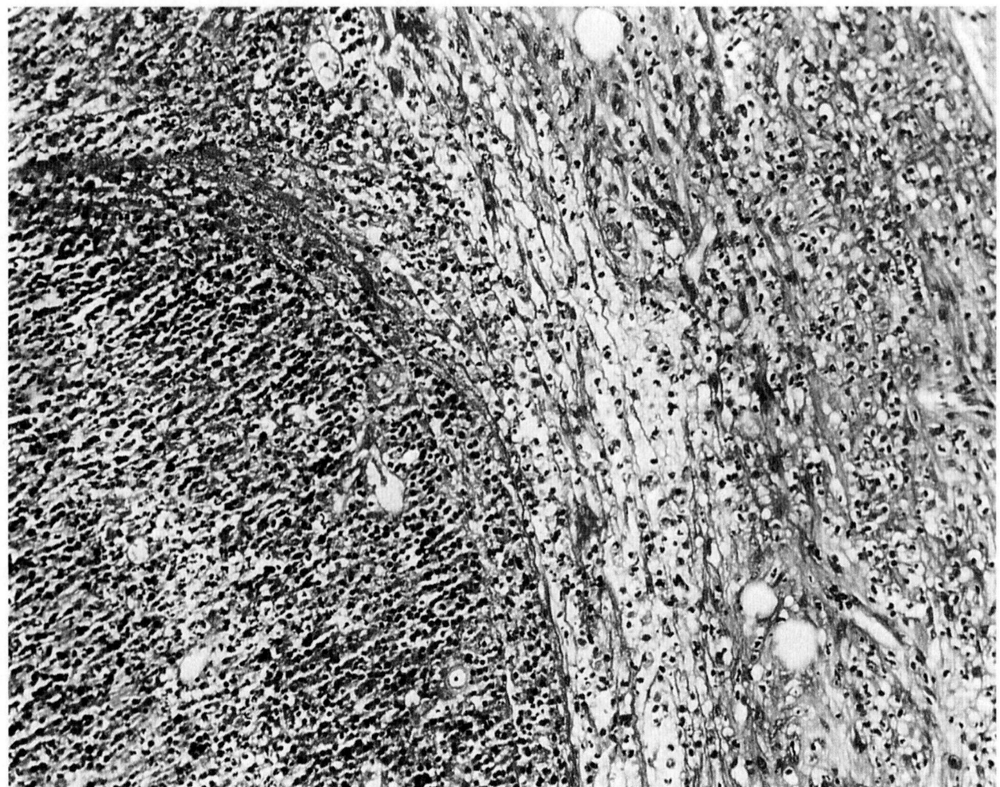

FIGURE 17.3. Acute gonococcal lymphadenitis and perilymphadenitis of inguinal lymph node. Capsule and pericapsular fibrofatty tissues with marked edema and infiltration of polymorphonuclear leukocytes. Focal suppurative necrosis in lymph node parenchyma. Hematoxylin, phloxine, and saffron stain.

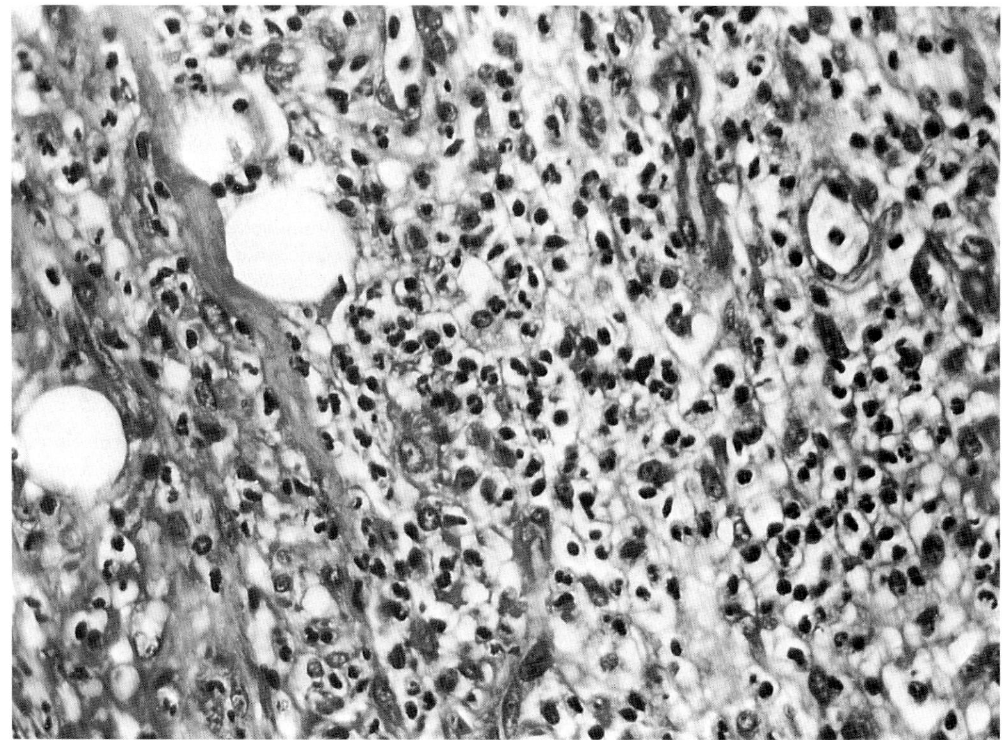

FIGURE 17.4. Same lymph node as in Fig. 17.1. Inflammatory exudate with edema and neutrophils in perinodal tissues. Hematoxylin, phloxine, and saffron stain.

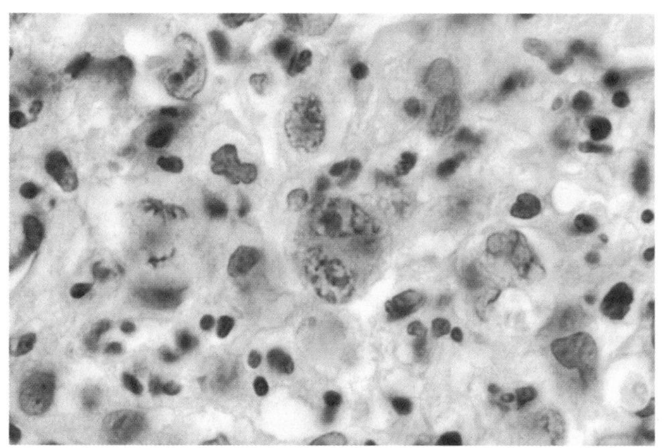

FIGURE 17.5. Neutrophil-rich variant of Ki-1 anaplastic large cell lymphoma containing more neutrophils than anaplastic lymphoma cells (*center*), so that it can be confused with an abscess. Hematoxylin and eosin stain.

REFERENCES

1. Barton LL, Feigin RD. Childhood cervical lymphadenitis: a reappraisal. J Pediatr 1974;84:846–852.
2. Symmers WSC. Infective lymphadenitis. In: Symmers WSC, ed. Systemic pathology, vol 2. Edinburgh: Churchill Livingstone, 1978:572–584.
3. Swartz MS. Lymphadenitis and lymphangitis. In: Mandell GL, Douglas RG, Bennett JE, eds. Principles and practice of infectious diseases, vol 1. New York: Churchill Livingstone, 1995: 936–944.
4. Stansfeld AG. Acute lymphadenitis. In: Stansfeld AG, ed. Lymph node biopsy interpretation. Edinburgh: Churchill Livingstone, 1985.
5. Schapers RF, Reif R, Lennert K, Knapp W. Mesenteric lymphadenitis due to *Yersinia* enterocolitica. Virchows Arch A Pathol Anat Histopathol 1981;390:127–138.

Checklist

ORDINARY BACTERIAL LYMPHADENITIS

Enlarged, soft, tender lymph nodes
Perilymphadenitis
Sinus catarrh
Neutrophil leukocytes, macrophages
Suppurative foci, microabscesses
Bacteria

6. Toshniwal R, Kocka FE, Kallick CA. Suppurative lymphadenitis with *Yersinia* enterocolitica. Eur J Clin Microbiol 1985;4:587–588.
7. Speert DP, Britt WJ, Kaplan EL. Tick-borne tularemia presenting as ulcerative lymphadenitis. Clin Pediatr (Phila) 1979;18: 239–241.
8. Sutinen S, Syrjala H. Histopathology of human lymph node tularemia caused by *Francisella tularensis* var *palaearctica.* Arch Pathol Lab Med 1986;110:42–46.
9. Naqvi SH, Thobani S, Moazam F, et al. Generalized suppurative lymphadenitis with typhoidal salmonellosis. Pediatr Infect Dis J 1988;7:882–883.
10. Yee KC, Lee MK, Chua CT, et al. Melioidosis, the great mimicker: a report of 10 cases from Malaysia. J Trop Med Hyg 1988; 91:249–254.
11. Lumbiganon P, Viengnondha S. Clinical manifestations of melioidosis in children. Pediatr Infect Dis J 1995;14:136–140.
12. Jung K, Elsner J, Emmendorffer A, et al. Severe infectious complications in a girl suffering from atopic dermatitis were found to be due to chronic granulomatous disease. Acta Derm Venereol 1993;73:433–436.
13. Hill HR, Estensen RD, Hogan NA, et al. Severe staphylococcal disease associated with allergic manifestations, hyperimmunoglobulinemia E, and defective neutrophil chemotaxis. J Lab Clin Med 1976;88:796–806.
14. Cozzutto C, Soave F. Xanthogranulomatous lymphadenitis. Virchows Arch A Pathol Anat Histopathol 1979;385:103–108.
15. Risdall RJ, Brunning RD, Hernandez JI, et al. Bacteria-associated hemophagocytic syndrome. Cancer 1984;54:2968–2972.
16. Layfield LJ, Glasgow BJ, DuPuis MH. Fine-needle aspiration of lymphadenopathy of suspected infectious etiology. Arch Pathol Lab Med 1985;109:810–812.
17. Mann KP, Hall B, Kamino H, et al. Neutrophil-rich, Ki-1-positive anaplastic large-cell malignant lymphoma. Am J Surg Pathol 1995;19:407–416.
18. Badve S, Blumstein A, Wiernik P, et al. Non-Hodgkin malignant lymphoma with tissue neutrophilia: a report of 3 cases. Arch Pathol Lab Med 2000;124:735–738.

18

CAT-SCRATCH LYMPHADENITIS

DEFINITION

Necrotizing granulomatous lymphadenitis caused by *Bartonella henselae* (formerly *Rochalimaea henselae*) (1–3). Usually, a cat scratch, bite, or lick, or rarely a dog, monkey, or thorn introduces the bacteria at the site of infection. In contrast to earlier reports (4), it is now generally believed that few, if any, cases of cat-scratch disease (CSD) are caused by *Afipia felis* (5).

EPIDEMIOLOGY

In the United States, national databases reveal an estimated incidence of 9.3 cases of CSD per 100,000 population per year; 55% of patients are 18 years of age or younger, and the distribution varies seasonally, the majority occurring between September and January (6). Patients, particularly children, report contact with a cat in 90% of cases and cat scratch or bite in three-fourths of these (7). The cats, usually young and healthy in appearance, act as a reservoir for *B. henselae* organisms (8,9).

ETIOLOGY

The bacterial pathogen of CSD, *B. henselae*, is a gram-negative pleomorphic bacillus appearing as small rods 0.3 to 1.0 μm by 0.6 to 3.0 μm, or as coccoid or *L*-shaped forms singly, in chains, or in clumps (10). They are located in foci of necrosis, vessel walls, and characteristically in the vicinity of collagen fibers (10–12). CSD bacteria are gram-negative and faintly stained by the Brown-Hopps Gram's stain but not by the Brown-Brenn Gram's stain (10,11). The best results are obtained with formalin-fixed tissues stained with the Warthin-Starry silver impregnation stain, which slightly enlarges the microorganisms by depositing silver, thus increasing their visibility (10). CSD bacilli from the lymph nodes of patients with CSD lymphadenitis have been successfully cultured, and antisera to CSD bacilli have been produced (13). *B. henselae* and *B. quintana* are both members of the α subgroup of proteobacteria (14). Although biochemical and molecular analyses implicate *B. henselae* and *B. quintana* in causing bacillary angiomatosis in the United States (15–17), only *B. quintana* 16S ribosomal DNA sequences are found in bacillary angiomatosis in Europe (3).

CLINICAL FEATURES

Cat-scratch bacilli cause a spectrum of diseases, depending on the immunocompetence of the host (10,18). In normal, immunocompetent persons, the primary lesion that may be present in 20% to 50% of cases appears as an area of erythema at the site of the cat scratch. This is followed by a papular and then a vesicular lesion that oozes fluid and eventually dries to form a scab (19,20). Most often, the upper extremities are affected, followed by the cervical and facial regions. After 1 to 3 weeks, regional lymphadenopathy appears. This is usually unilateral and involves axillary, epitrochlear, cervical, or inguinal lymph nodes. Involvement of multiple nodes is unusual. The lymphadenitis may be associated with fever, malaise, headache, or aches of bones and joints. The involved lymph nodes are enlarged, nodular, matted, and adherent to the surrounding soft tissues and skin (Fig. 18.1). The sections show focal areas of necrosis and, on occasion, formation of microabscesses (Fig. 18.2). In the general population, CSD is a benign, self-limited illness, characterized by lymphadenitis, that is most common in children (21). In contrast, in patients with AIDS, CSD may result in a systemic, severe, and sometimes life-threatening disease with involvement of multiple internal organs (22–24).

HISTOPATHOLOGY

The early lymph node changes consist of follicular hyperplasia with little distortion of the general architecture (20,25). Intense tingible-body macrophage activity and the deposition of pink, amorphous intercellular proteinaceous material are characteristic (10). Vascular proliferation and patches of clear, monocytoid cells are also seen in

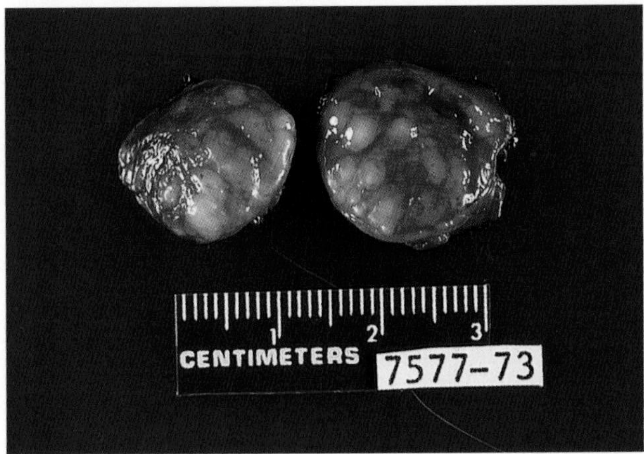

FIGURE 18.1. Inguinal lymph node with multiple abscesses in cat-scratch disease.

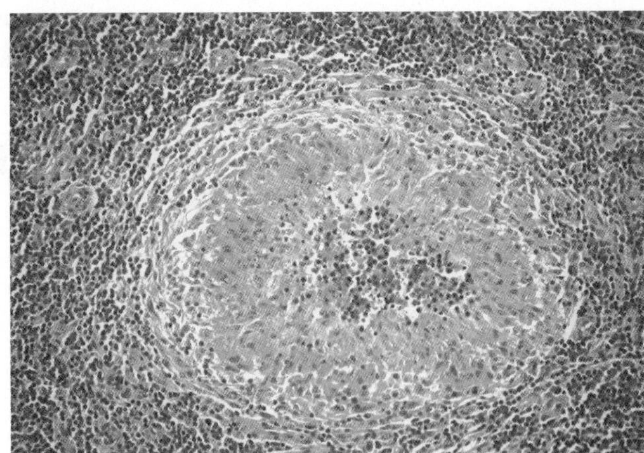

FIGURE 18.3. Cat-scratch lymphadenitis with central microabscess and peripheral area of epithelioid cells. Hematoxylin, phloxine, and saffron stain.

this early stage. Small abscesses with focal necrosis and clusters of neutrophils appear first under the subcapsular sinus, progressing then from the cortex into the medulla (11,19) (Fig. 18.2). The foci of necrosis enlarge, the neutrophils become fragmented, fibrin is deposited, and the abscesses protrude under the lymph node capsule with occasional suppuration. Finally, macrophages surround the abscess, forming a peripheral rim of epithelioid cells with rare multinucleated giant cells of Langhans type that result in the classic stellate necrotizing granulomas of CSD (Figs. 18.3 and 18.4). The silver stain shows the presence of CSD bacilli, even in the very early lesions (11) (Fig. 18.5). In a study of 516 lymph nodes with histologic features of CSD, bacilli were found in 61% (26). They were centered in areas of necrosis and were less frequent in granulomas

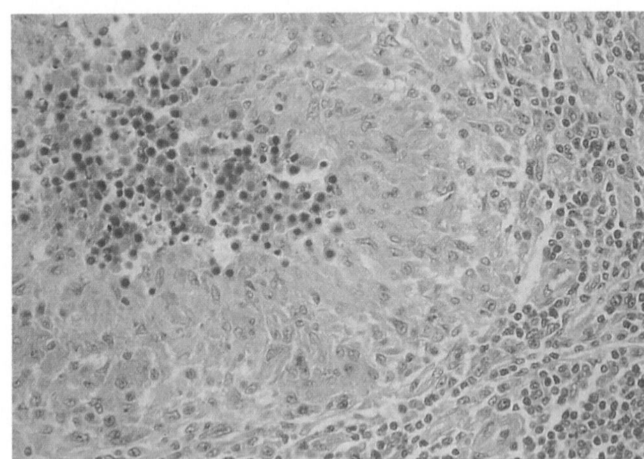

FIGURE 18.4. Microabscess with central area of necrosis and polymorphonuclear leukocytes and peripheral area of palisading epithelioid cells. Hematoxylin, phloxine, and saffron stain.

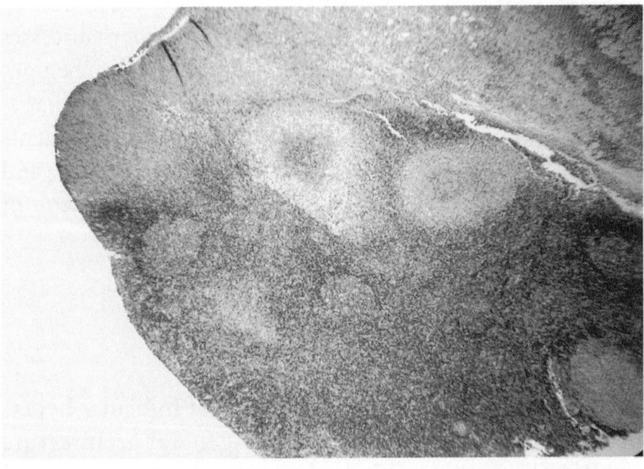

FIGURE 18.2. Same lymph node as in Fig. 18.1 shows thickened capsule and multiple cortical microabscesses. Hematoxylin, phloxine, and saffron stain.

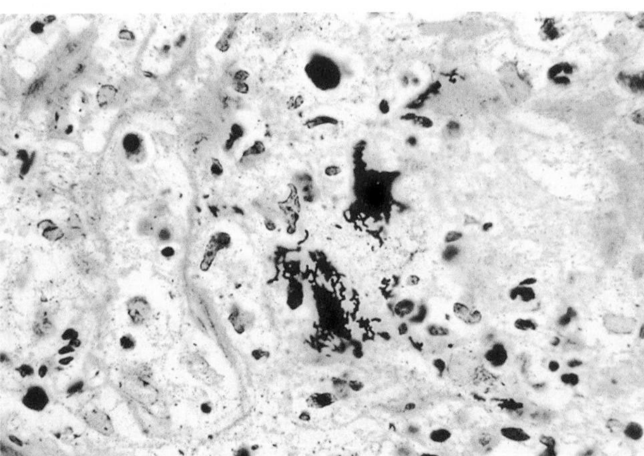

FIGURE 18.5. Clumps of silver-stained rod- and *L*-shaped bacilli in cat-scratch disease. Warthin-Starry stain.

without necrosis. Cat-scratch bacilli usually are distributed focally, with hundreds of organisms in one area and none in others (11).

ELECTRON MICROSCOPY

Most CSD bacilli are extracellular and clustered in small groups, frequently next to bundles of collagen fibrils (12) (Fig. 18.6). They are also found in the walls of capillaries and within macrophages (10). The bacterial wall shows no evidence of a membrane but rather has a thick peptidoglycan layer (Fig. 18.7), which is characteristic of gram-positive organisms and prompted some authors to suggest that the gram-negativity of CSD bacilli, indicated by the Brown-Hopps Gram's stain, is caused by alterations in the bacterial wall (12).

LABORATORY TESTS

- Staining of CSD bacilli by the Warthin-Starry silver stain can be confirmed by the Brown-Hopps Gram's stain. The former clearly stains the CSD bacilli but may similarly stain other bacteria, such as *Hemophilus ducreyi*; the latter stains the organisms that appear at the limit of microscopic resolution more faintly but has greater specificity (11).
- Immunoperoxidase staining of tissue sections can specifically identify the bacilli of CSD (13,27).
- Isolation of *B. henselae* with a blood culture system (28).
- In the cat-scratch skin test (Hangar-Rose test, introduced in 1945), aspirated pus from involved lymph nodes is used for intradermal inoculation. Although the skin test was considered highly reliable (20), it is no longer practiced, owing to unavailability of standardized preparations and the risk for transmitting other infections.
- Cultures, smears, and tissue staining for acid-fast bacilli and fungi must be performed to rule out these infections.
- Indirect fluorescent antibody and enzyme-linked immunosorbent assays for serologic diagnosis of *Bartonella*-associated illness (29,30).
- Polymerase chain reaction identifies *Bartonella* DNA sequences in aspirated pus from lymph nodes and in fresh and archival tissue samples (2,3,31).

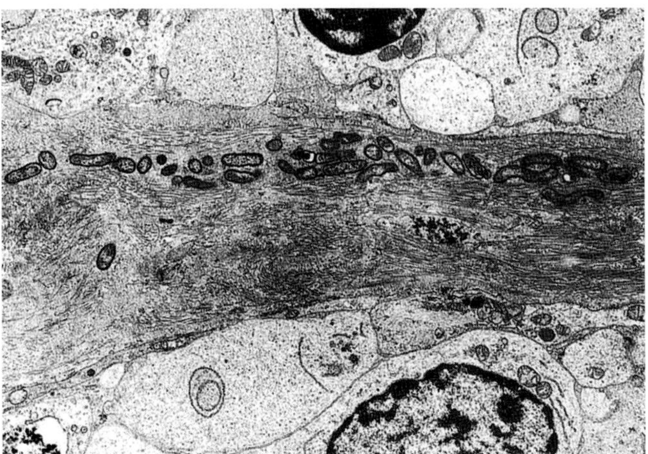

FIGURE 18.6. Extracellular bacilli located within collagen in cat-scratch lymphadenitis. (Courtesy of Dr. Bruce Mackay.)

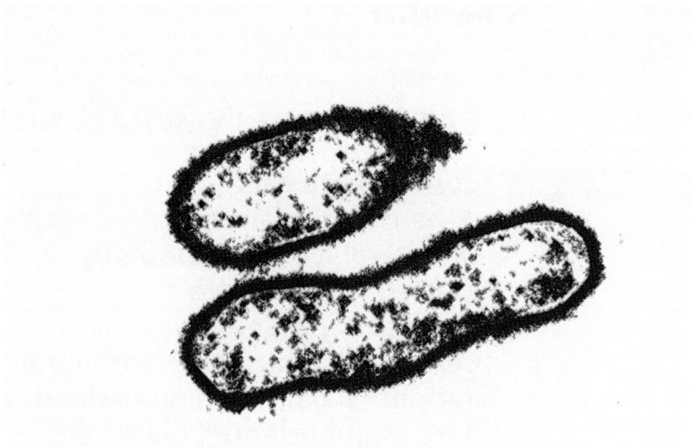

FIGURE 18.7. Thick-walled bacilli in cat-scratch lymphadenitis. (Courtesy of Dr. Bruce Mackay.)

DIFFERENTIAL DIAGNOSIS

- Suppurative lymphadenitis caused by a variety of bacteria is basically an abscess composed of neutrophils, fibrin, and necrotic tissues. Gram's stain reveals the microorganisms.
- Tuberculous lymphadenitis: The necrosis is caseous—that is, without nuclear remnants or tissue debris. Neutrophils are not present. Acid-fast staining shows bacilli.
- Fungal lymphadenitides such as cryptococcosis, histoplasmosis, and aspergillosis, frequently seen in association with AIDS, require Grocott methenamine silver staining to reveal yeasts and hyphae.
- Lymphogranuloma venereum and tularemia: Similar histologic appearance with stellate necrotizing granulomas. Often impossible to differentiate (32). Demonstration and identification of microorganisms is necessary.
- Kikuchi necrotizing lymphadenitis: Patchy necrosis with abundant nuclear debris and lack of epithelioid cells with granulomatous arrangement. Negative for Gram's stain and Warthin-Starry stain.

Checklist

CAT-SCRATCH LYMPHADENITIS

Contact with cats
B. henselae, gram-negative bacillus
Unilateral lymphadenopathy
Matted lymph nodes
Necrotizing granulomas
Central microabscesses with neutrophils
Peripheral palisaded epithelioid cells
Rare multinucleated giant cells
Capsular and perinodal involvement
Clumps of pleomorphic bacilli
Positive for Warthin-Starry silver stain
Positive for Brown-Hopps Gram's stain
Immunoperoxidase staining with anti-*B. henselae* antibody
Disseminated CSD in patients with AIDS

REFERENCES

1. Brenner DJ, O'Connor SP, Winkler HH, et al. Proposals to unify the genera *Bartonella* and *Rochalimaea,* with descriptions of *Bartonella quintana comb. nov., Bartonella vinsonii comb. nov., Bartonella henselae comb. nov.,* and *Bartonella elizabethae comb. nov.,* and to remove the family Bartonellaceae from the order Rickettsiales. Int J Syst Bacteriol 1993;43:777–786.
2. Anneke MC, Bergmans AM, Groothedde JW, et al. Etiology of cat scratch disease: comparison of polymerase chain reaction detection of *Bartonella* (formerly *Rochalimaea*) and *Afipia felis* DNA with serology and skin tests. J Infect Dis 1995;171:916–923.
3. Dauga C, Miras I, Grimont PA. Identification of *Bartonella henselae* and *B. quintana* 16s rDNA sequences by branch-, genus- and species-specific amplification. J Med Microbiol 1996;45:192–199.
4. Brenner DJ, Hollis DG, Moss CW, et al. Proposal of *Afipia gen. nov.,* with *Afipia felis sp. nov.* (formerly the cat scratch disease bacillus), *Afipia clevelandensis sp. nov.* (formerly the Cleveland Clinic Foundation strain), *Afipia broomeae sp. nov.,* and three unnamed genospecies. J Clin Microbiol 1991;29:2450–2460.
5. Giladi M, Avidor B, Kletter Y, et al. Cat scratch disease: the rare role of *Afipia felis.* J Clin Microbiol 1998;36:2499–2502.
6. Jackson LA, Perkins BA, Wenger JD. Cat scratch disease in the United States: an analysis of three national databases. Am J Public Health 1993;83:1707–1711.
7. Zangwill KM, Hamilton DH, Perkins BA, et al. Cat scratch disease in Connecticut. Epidemiology, risk factors, and evaluation of a new diagnostic test [see Comments]. N Engl J Med 1993;329:8–13.
8. Regnery R, Martin M, Olson J. Naturally occurring "Rochalimaea henselae" infection in domestic cat [Letter]. Lancet 1992;340:557–558.
9. Koehler JE, Glaser CA, Tappero JW. *Rochalimaea henselae* infection. A new zoonosis with the domestic cat as reservoir [see Comments]. JAMA 1994;271:531–535.
10. Wear DJ, Margileth AM, Hadfield TL, et al. Cat scratch disease: a bacterial infection. Science 1983;221:1403–1405.
11. Miller-Catchpole R, Variakojis D, Vardiman JW, et al. Cat scratch disease. Identification of bacteria in seven cases of lymphadenitis. Am J Surg Pathol 1986;10:276–281.
12. Osborne BM, Butler JJ, Mackay B. Ultrastructural observations in cat scratch disease. Am J Clin Pathol 1987;87:739–744.
13. English CK, Wear DJ, Margileth AM, et al. Cat-scratch disease. Isolation and culture of the bacterial agent. JAMA 1988;259: 1347–1352.
14. Relman DA, Lepp PW, Sadler KN, et al. Phylogenetic relationships among the agent of bacillary angiomatosis, *Bartonella bacilliformis,* and other alpha-proteobacteria. Mol Microbiol 1992;6:1801–1807.
15. Cockerell CJ, Tierno PM, Friedman-Kien AE, et al. Clinical, histologic, microbiologic, and biochemical characterization of the causative agent of bacillary (epithelioid) angiomatosis: a rickettsial illness with features of bartonellosis. J Invest Dermatol 1991;97:812–817.
16. Koehler JE, Quinn FD, Berger TG, et al. Isolation of *Rochalimaea* species from cutaneous and osseous lesions of bacillary angiomatosis [see Comments]. N Engl J Med 1992;327:1625–1631.
17. Regnery RL, Anderson BE, Clarridge JED, et al. Characterization of a novel *Rochalimaea* species, *R. henselae sp. nov.,* isolated from blood of a febrile, human immunodeficiency virus-positive patient. J Clin Microbiol 1992;30:265–274.
18. Margileth AM, Wear DJ, English CK. Systemic cat scratch disease: report of 23 patients with prolonged or recurrent severe bacterial infection. J Infect Dis 1987;155:390–402.
19. Winship T. Pathologic changes in so-called cat-scratch fever. Am J Clin Pathol 1953;23:1012–1018.
20. Naji AF, Carbonell F, Barker HJ. Cat scratch disease. Am J Clin Pathol 1962;38:513–521.
21. Carithers HA. Cat-scratch disease. An overview based on a study of 1,200 patients. Am J Dis Child 1985;139:1124–1133.
22. Koehler JE, LeBoit PE, Egbert BM, et al. Cutaneous vascular lesions and disseminated cat-scratch disease in patients with the acquired immunodeficiency syndrome (AIDS) and AIDS-related complex. Ann Intern Med 1988;109:449–455.
23. Pilon VA, Echols RM. Cat-scratch disease in a patient with AIDS. Am J Clin Pathol 1989;92:236–240.
24. Black JR, Herrington DA, Hadfield TL, et al. Life-threatening cat-scratch disease in an immunocompromised host. Arch Intern Med 1986;146:394–396.

25. Dorfman RF, Warnke R. Lymphadenopathy simulating the malignant lymphomas. Hum Pathol 1974;5:519–550.
26. Wear D, English C, Margileth A, et al. Histopathologic changes in the lymph nodes of over 500 patients with cat scratch disease. Lab Invest 1988;58:100A.
27. Min KW, Reed JA, Welch DF, et al. Morphologically variable bacilli of cat scratch disease are identified by immunocytochemical labeling with antibodies to *Rochalimaea henselae.* Am J Clin Pathol 1994;101:607–610.
28. Lucey D, Dolan MJ, Moss CW, et al. Relapsing illness due to *Rochalimaea henselae* in immunocompetent hosts: implication for therapy and new epidemiological associations. Clin Infect Dis 1992;14:683–688.
29. Dalton MJ, Robinson LE, Cooper J, et al. Use of *Bartonella* antigens for serologic diagnosis of cat-scratch disease at a national referral center. Arch Intern Med 1995;155:1670–1676.
30. Bergmans AM, Peeters MF, Schellekens JF, et al. Pitfalls and fallacies of cat scratch disease serology: evaluation of *Bartonella henselae*-based indirect fluorescence assay and enzyme-linked immunoassay [see Comments]. J Clin Microbiol 1997;35:1931–1937.
31. Scott MA, McCurley TL, Vnencak-Jones CL, et al. Cat scratch disease: detection of *Bartonella henselae* DNA in archival biopsies from patients with clinically, serologically, and histologically defined disease. Am J Pathol 1996;149:2161–2167.
32. Strano AJ. Cat-scratch fever. In: Binford CH, Connor DH, eds. Pathology of tropical and extraordinary diseases, vol 1. Washington, DC: Armed Forces Institute of Pathology, 1976:85–86.

19

BACILLARY ANGIOMATOSIS OF LYMPH NODES

DEFINITION

Tumor-like proliferation of small blood vessels caused by infection with *Bartonella henselae.*

SYNONYM

Epithelioid angiomatosis.

ETIOLOGY

The pathogenic agent of bacillary angiomatosis and bacillary peliosis, *B. henselae,* is a small, curved, motile, gram-negative bacillus. Because its culture and speciation are difficult, the identity of this etiologic agent was revealed only after multiple studies and name changes based on the application of molecular techniques. By amplifying through polymerase chain reaction bacterial 16S ribosomal RNA from lesions of bacillary angiomatosis and analyzing sequences of complementary DNA, a new *Rickettsia*-like microorganism closely related to *Rochalimaea quintana* was revealed (1). A similar organism was isolated from the blood of a febrile patient with HIV positivity and named *Rochalimaea henselae* (2,3). Subsequently, the two genera *Rochalimaea* and *Bartonella* were merged under the designation *Bartonella,* which now includes *B. henselae, B. quintana,* and *B. bacilliformis* (4).

EPIDEMIOLOGY

Bacillary angiomatosis has been described primarily in HIV-positive patients and a few patients with chronic lymphocytic leukemia on immunosuppressive therapy (5). Epidemiologic studies show a significant association between infection with *B. henselae* and owning or being exposed to cats, particularly young cats infested with fleas (6). Domestic cats are the major reservoir for infection with *B. henselae,* which is transmitted by fleas from cat to cat (7).

PATHOGENESIS

The transmission from cats to humans is not well understood. Cat scratches, but rarely bites, are associated with cat-scratch disease, which is caused by the same microorganism, *B. henselae.* It is believed that in bacillary angiomatosis, the infection is acquired through the skin by traumatic inoculation with flea feces, just as infection with *B. quintana,* a closely related microorganism causing trench fever, is transmitted through louse feces (8). The question still unanswered is why the same pathogenic agent, *B. henselae,* is able to cause both bacillary angiomatosis and cat-scratch disease, two entirely different clinicopathologic entities. Bacillary angiomatosis is characterized by numerous red to violaceous vascular papules and nodules that involve the skin and sometimes extend to lymph nodes and internal organs, whereas cat-scratch disease consists of a unilateral suppurative lymphadenitis rarely accompanied by other localizations. Bacillary angiomatosis occurs almost exclusively in HIV-infected patients with AIDS; cat-scratch disease affects otherwise normal, immune-competent persons. The basic lesion of the former is angiomatosis, and of the latter, necrotizing granulomas. Treatment with antibiotics, particularly erythromycin, is curative in bacillary angiomatosis and totally ineffective in cat-scratch disease (9,10). Nonetheless, in both lesions, bacilli stainable with the Warthin-Starry silver stain and identified as *B. henselae* are the only microorganisms consistently present. Furthermore, a contact with cats is usually established in both diseases. A tentative explanation for the differences between the two syndromes induced by the same agent is that the deficient cellular immunity of patients with bacillary angiomatosis is unable to mount a granulomatous response, such as occurs in cat-scratch disease, and that the vascular proliferation may be caused by the unregulated production of angiotropic cytokines in the course of HIV infection (9).

The various pathologic lesions produced by *Mycobacterium leprae* and *Mycobacterium tuberculosis* are given as an example in support of the argument that similar agents can produce a broad spectrum of pathologic responses depending on the degree of cellular immunity of the host (8). However, the mechanisms must be more complex because bacillary angiomatosis of similar appearance has been also reported in an HIV-negative immunocompetent patient (11).

CLINICAL SYNDROME

Patients with bacillary angiomatosis are with few exceptions HIV-seropositive and may belong to any of the known risk groups: homosexual men, intravenous drug abusers, and recipients of blood transfusions (12). In a series of 13 cases, 12 were men between the ages of 31 and 56 years (9). In addition, a case of an immunosuppressed cardiac transplant recipient (13) and one of a healthy, HIV-negative man (11) were reported.

The cutaneous lesions of bacillary angiomatosis consist of vascular red to violaceous dome-shaped papules and nodules. Their location may be superficial in the upper dermis with a collarette, deep in the dermis, or subcutaneous (9,12). They range in numbers from one to hundreds and show no predilection for specific sites (12). In addition to the skin, the lymph nodes (10,13,14), soft tissues (13,15), spleen (16), liver (16), and bones (9,10) may be involved. In the liver and spleen, the lesions consist of cystic, blood-filled spaces and are referred to as *peliosis hepatis* or *splenis* (16). Most skin lesions resolve spontaneously; however, in cases of systemic disease in AIDS patients, severe, occasionally fatal, complications may occur (12,17). Bacillary angiomatosis lesions generally respond to erythromycin, which induces a complete remission. Therefore, early diagnosis is of the utmost importance because it allows curative treatment with antibiotics, whereas unrecognized and untreated bacillary angiomatosis may lead to a fatal outcome.

HISTOPATHOLOGY

Lesions in the skin, which grossly resemble pyogenic granulomas, appear histologically as lobules or nodules of newly formed vessels in the upper or deep dermis and subcutis. The covering epidermis may be thinned over a polypoid protrusion or form a collarette (10). The vascular lobules are composed of small and large capillaries lined by hyperplastic endothelial cells (Fig. 19.1).

In the lymph nodes draining the involved skin, the lymphoid parenchyma is replaced by similar vascular nodules formed by blood vessels of various sizes and shapes, some round and ectatic, others small with barely visible lumina (Figs. 19.2 and 19.3). The endothelial cells lining the vessels are hyperplastic and protrude into the lumina (Figs. 19.4 and 19.5). The nuclei show slight variations in shape (Figs. 19.4 and 19.5). They include two to three fine nucleoli and three to five mitoses per high-power field (14). Solid clusters of endothelial cells without vascular formation are also seen. Poorly formed vessels and solid cell clusters are more common in lymph nodes and internal organs than in cutaneous lesions of bacillary angiomatosis lesions. Some of these lesions may be highly suggestive of malignancy (9,18). Between the vessels lies a granular material (Fig. 19.6) in

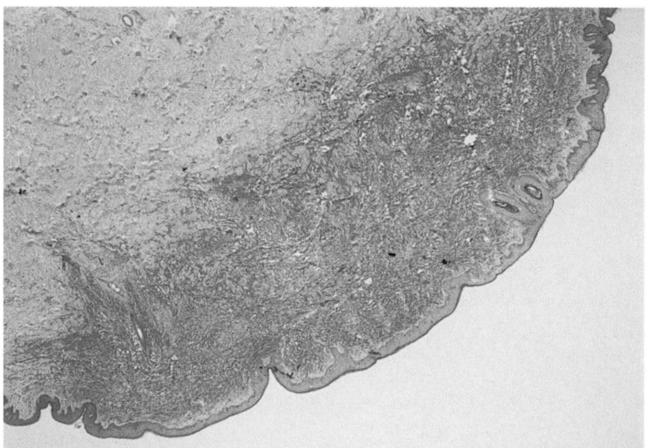

FIGURE 19.1. Bacillary angiomatosis in the skin forms a polypoid lesion with a collarette. The epidermis is raised by confluent nodules of newly formed vessels in the superficial dermis. Hematoxylin, phloxine, and saffron stain.

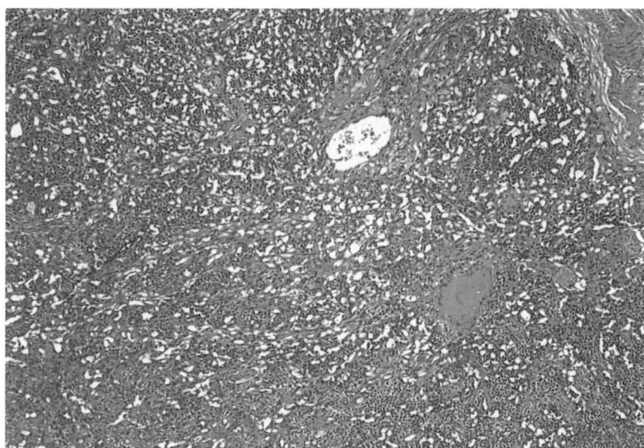

FIGURE 19.2. Bacillary angiomatosis in an inguinal lymph node. Lymphoid tissue is largely replaced by a network of capillaries. Hematoxylin, phloxine, and saffron stain.

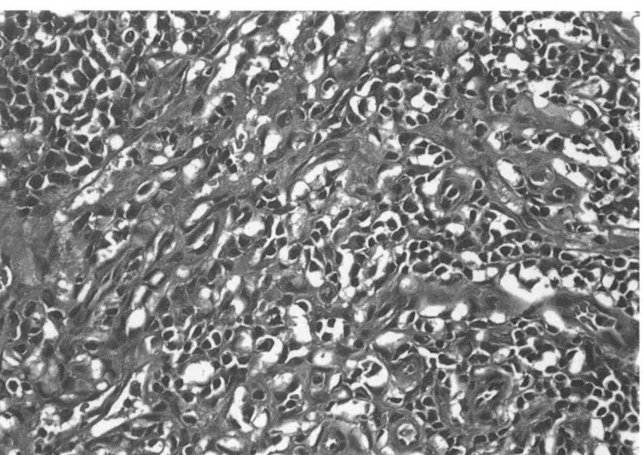

FIGURE 19.3. Specimen in Fig. 9.2 at higher magnification shows capillaries of various sizes and shapes separated by deposits of bacteria (unstained) and collagen. Hematoxylin, phloxine, and saffron stain.

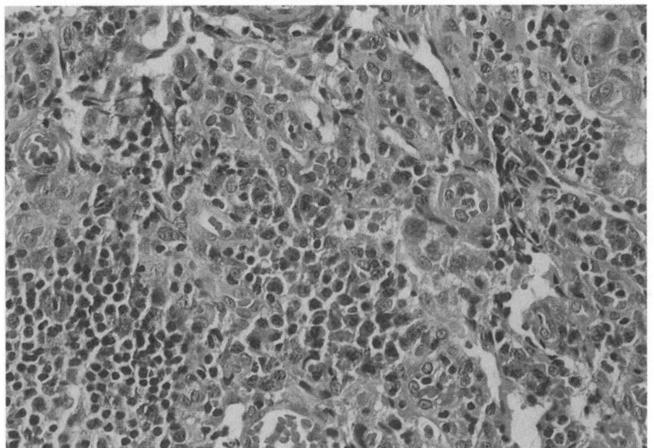

FIGURE 19.4. Bacillary angiomatosis of cervical lymph node. Blood vessels are lined by hyperplastic endothelial cells. In intervascular spaces are lymphocytes, plasma cells, and tissue debris. Hematoxylin, phloxine, and saffron stain.

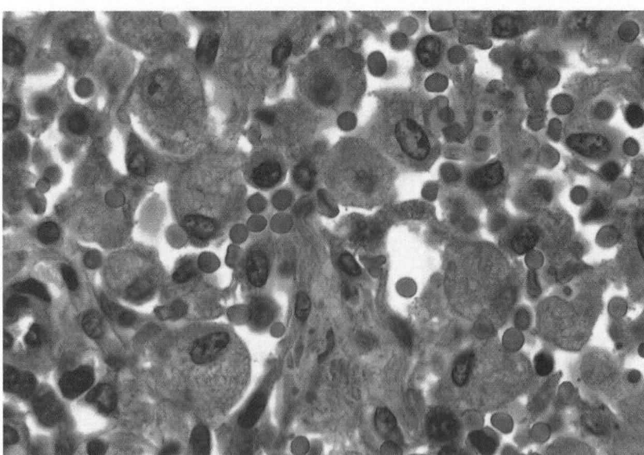

FIGURE 19.6. Capillaries containing erythrocytes are lined by hyperplastic endothelial cells separated by amorphous matrix and foamy histiocytes. Hematoxylin, phloxine, and saffron stain.

which Warthin-Starry staining reveals clumps of bacterial rods (Fig. 19.7). Admixed with them are viable and degenerated inflammatory cells, mostly neutrophils. Large numbers of erythrocytes, within vascular lumina and extravasated, are also present. The bacterial rods are always interstitial (9). These bacilli indistinguishable from those observed in cat-scratch disease, which stain with the Warthin-Starry stain, but not with the Gram's, periodic acid–Schiff, Ziehl-Neelsen, or silver methenamine stains (14). An alternative to Warthin-Starry staining is the Giemsa stain, which shows the bacilli as delicate, violaceous rods (19). The histology of lymph node lesions in bacillary angiomatosis is entirely similar to that of lesions in the skin, liver, spleen, and other involved organs (10).

ELECTRON MICROSCOPY

The organisms present in the lesions of bacillary angiomatosis are extracellular, small (0.2 to 0.3 μm), pleomorphic bacilli with trilaminar walls and characteristic ribosomal and nuclear structures (9,14,17). The endothelial cells show mitochondria and rough endoplasmic reticulum. Multiple Weibel-Palade bodies per cell are noted (9).

IMMUNOHISTOCHEMISTRY

Monoclonal antibodies and immunoperoxidase staining show the endothelial cells to express factor VIII-reacting antigen, *Ulex europaeus* antigen, and α_1-antichymotrypsin (9,12).

DIFFERENTIAL DIAGNOSIS

- Kaposi sarcoma resembles bacterial angiomatosis clinically and histologically and also occurs in immune-deficient, particularly HIV-positive, persons. However, the vessels are cleft-like and the lining endothelial cells are spindle-shaped. They

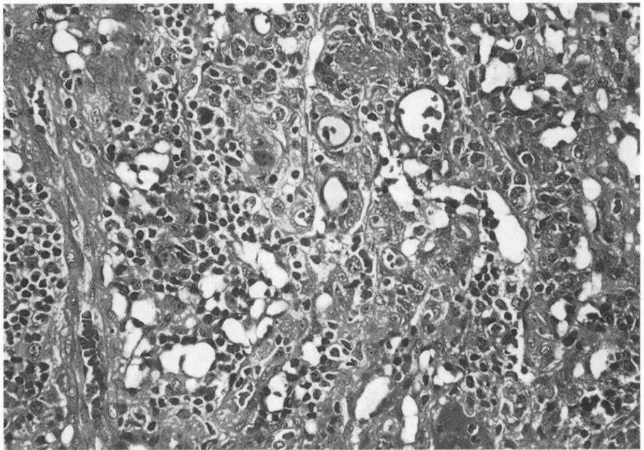

FIGURE 19.5. Newly formed capillaries of various shapes, often ectatic, contrast with blood vessels that are well-formed and have thickened fibrous walls (*bottom*). Masson stain.

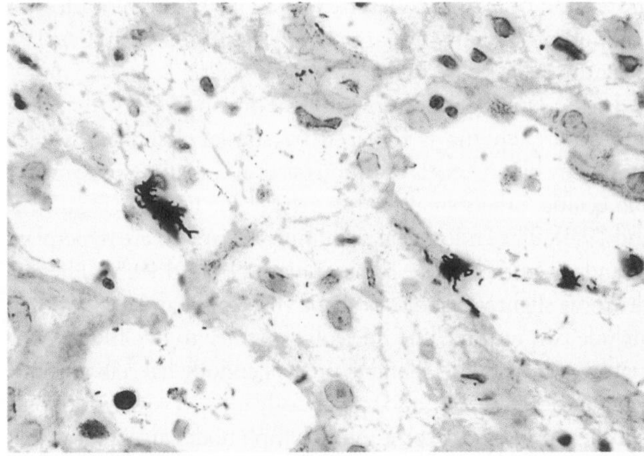

FIGURE 19.7. Clumps of silver-stained bacteria within the amorphous substance deposited between the hyperplastic capillaries. Warthin-Starry stain.

Checklist

BACILLARY ANGIOMATOSIS OF LYMPH NODES

HIV-positive persons
Cutaneous vascular lesions
Regional lymphadenopathy
Vascular nodules replacing lymphoid tissue
Admixed capillary and ectatic vessels
Extravasated erythrocytes
Interstitial eosinophilic granular material
Clumps of Warthin-Starry-positive bacilli and neutrophils
Endothelial cells with intracytoplasmic Weibel-Palade bodies
Factor VIII-reacting antigen-positive and *Ulex europaeus* antigen-positive
B. henselae, gram-negative bacillus, etiologic agent
Antibiotic (erythromycin) treatment effective
Systemic disease fatal if untreated

may be positive for *Ulex europaeus* antigen but are generally negative for factor VIII-reacting antigen. Warthin-Starry bacilli are not present. Plasma cells in Kaposi sarcoma versus neutrophils in bacillary angiomatosis accompany the lesions.

- Pyogenic granuloma: Capillaries lined by flat endothelial cells, more inflammatory cells, absence of microorganisms.
- HIV lymphadenopathy, pattern B: The vessels, although numerous, are mature and thick-walled. Lymphoid follicles are involuted.
- Castleman lymphadenopathy: Numerous mature, thick-walled vessels. Characteristic involuted follicles with hyalinized germinal centers.
- Angioimmunoblastic lymphadenopathy: Effaced architecture. Frequent, arborizing, mature blood vessels. Immunoblasts.
- Vascular transformation of sinuses: Lymph node architecture preserved. Marginal, cortical, and medullary sinuses transformed to blood-filled vascular spaces.
- Angiosarcoma: Poor tumor delineation, atypical endothelial cells with pleomorphic nuclei and frequent mitoses. Microorganisms absent.

REFERENCES

1. Relman DA, Loutit JS, Schmidt TM, et al. The agent of bacillary angiomatosis. An approach to the identification of uncultured pathogens [Editorial]. N Engl J Med 1990;323:1573–1580.
2. Regnery RL, Anderson BE, Clarridge JE, et al. Characterization of a novel *Rochalimaea* species, *R. henselae sp. nov.,* isolated from blood of a febrile, human immunodeficiency virus-positive patient. J Clin Microbiol 1992;30:265–274.
3. Koehler JE, Quinn FD, Berger TG, et al: Isolation of *Rochalimaea* species from cutaneous and osseous lesions of bacillary angiomatosis. N Engl J Med 1992;327:1625–1631.
4. Nosal JM. Bacillary angiomatosis, cat-scratch disease, and bartonellosis: what's the connection? Int J Dermatol 1997;36: 405–411.
5. Torok L, Viragh SZ, Borka I, et al. Bacillary angiomatosis in a patient with lymphocytic leukemia. Br J Dermatol 1993;130:665–668.
6. Tappero JW, Mohle-Boetani J, Koehler JE, et al. The epidemiology of bacillary angiomatosis and bacillary peliosis. JAMA 1993;269:770–775.
7. Koehler JE, Glaser CA, Tappero W. *Rochalimaea henselae* infection: a new zoonosis with the domestic cat as a reservoir. JAMA 1994;271:531–535.
8. Tompkins LS. Of cats, humans and *Bartonella.* N Engl J Med 1997;337:1916–1917.
9. LeBoit PE, Berger TG, Egbert BM, et al. Bacillary angiomatosis. The histopathology and differential diagnosis of a pseudoneoplastic infection in patients with human immunodeficiency virus disease. Am J Surg Pathol 1989;13:909–920.
10. LeBoit PE. The expanding spectrum of new disease, bacillary angiomatosis. Arch Dermatol 1990;126:808–811.
11. Cockerell CJ, Bergstresser PR, Myrie-Williams C, et al. Bacillary epithelioid angiomatosis occurring in an immunocompetent individual. Arch Dermatol 1990;126:787–790.
12. Cockerell CJ, Webster GF, Whitlow MA, et al. Epithelioid angiomatosis: a distinct vascular disorder in patients with the acquired immunodeficiency syndrome or AIDS-related complex. Lancet 1987;2:654–656.
13. Schinella RA, Greco MA. Bacillary angiomatosis presenting as a soft-tissue tumor without skin involvement. Hum Pathol 1990; 21:567–569.
14. Chan JKC, Lewin KJ, Lombard CM, et al. Histopathology of bacillary angiomatosis of lymph node. Am J Surg Pathol 1991; 15:430–437.
15. Stoler MH, Bonfiglio TA, Steigbigel RT, et al. An atypical subcutaneous infection associated with acquired immune deficiency syndrome. Am J Clin Pathol 1983;80:714–718.
16. Perkocha LA, Geaghan SM, Benedict TS, et al. Clinical and pathological features of bacillary peliosis hepatis in association with human immunodeficiency virus infection. N Engl J Med 1990;323:1581–1586.
17. Kemper CA, Lombard CM, Deresinski SC, et al. Immunocompromised host: a report of two cases. Am J Med 1990;89:216– 222.
18. Perez-Piteira J, Ariza A, Mate JL, et al. Bacillary angiomatosis: a gross mimicker of malignancy. Histopathology 1995;26:476– 478.
19. Tsang WYW, Chan JKC. Giemsa stain for histological diagnosis of bacillary angiomatosis [Letter]. Histopathology 1992;21:299.

20

LYMPHOGRANULOMA VENEREUM LYMPHADENITIS

DEFINITION

Lymphadenitis caused by the sexually transmitted bacterium *Chlamydia trachomatis.*

SYNONYM

Nicolas-Favre disease.

ETIOLOGY

C. trachomatis is an obligatory intracellular bacterium (1). About 15 serovars of *C. trachomatis* have been recognized (2–4). Of these, the serovars A, B, and C are pathogens of endemic trachoma, D through K are associated with urethritis and/or conjunctivitis, and L1, L2, and L3 cause sexually transmitted lymphogranuloma venereum (LGV) (1–4). *C. trachomatis* undergoes two developmental stages. The small, infectious elementary body with stores of adenosine triphosphate enters the cell by endocytosis; the larger, replicative, and metabolically active form, the reticulate body, divides by binary fission to fill the endosome (cytoplasmic inclusion) with infectious units and glycogen (1–4).

EPIDEMIOLOGY

Although LGV is worldwide in distribution, it is most prevalent in the tropics and subtropics (5). In the United States, infections caused by non-LGV serovars of *C. trachomatis* are the most common sexually transmitted diseases (6). LGV is most common in heterosexuals and in members of lower socioeconomic classes (7). More recently, it has become common in homosexual men, leading to proctocolitis with fistulae and strictures (8,9). The LGV lymphadenopathy is reported to be 10 to 20 times more prevalent in men than in women, a disproportion that is in part accounted for by the fact that genital lesions in women frequently go unnoticed (10).

CLINICAL SYNDROME

The first manifestation appears at the site of infection after a latent period of 7 to 12 days. It consists of a painless, herpetiform lesion, an erosion or shallow ulcer of the genitals that heals without scarring and often passes unnoticed (11,12). In women, the primary lesion is often on the cervix and therefore seldom observed (10,13). The regional lymph nodes become tender and enlarged 1 week to 2 months later. The lymphadenopathy is usually unilateral but may be bilateral in up to one-third of cases (14). It is far more frequently detectable in men because the inguinal lymph nodes are usually involved. In women, the perianal or deep pelvic lymph nodes drain the area of primary infection (15,16). If both inguinal and femoral lymph nodes enlarge, the inguinal ligament produces the characteristic LGV "groove sign" (16). The nodes are initially firm, tender, and movable, then become matted and fixed to the surrounding tissues (Fig. 20.1). Rupture of the nodes leads to chronic sinus tract formation (14), but only about one-third of buboes rupture; the rest form masses or resolve (17). In women, the involvement of pelvic and iliac nodes may lead to chronic pelvic lymphangitis and lymphatic obstruction with chronic vulvar edema and rectal strictures (16). Systemic infection with fever, myalgia, and headache was reported in 60% of patients in one study (18). LGV may also involve the anus, fallopian tubes, synovium, heart, lungs, and central nervous system (1–4,16).

HISTOPATHOLOGY

The early lesions in the lymph nodes consist of accumulations of neutrophils and small, necrotic foci. Shortly thereafter, lymphocytes and plasma cells surround the necrotic foci, which coalesce to form the typical abscesses of LGV (15,19). Their configuration is described as stellate or geographic (Fig. 20.2), and they comprise a central area of necrosis and polymorphonuclear leukocytes surrounded by a zone of palisaded epithelioid cells, macrophages, and multinucleated giant cells (15) (Figs. 20.3 and 20.4). Diagnostic

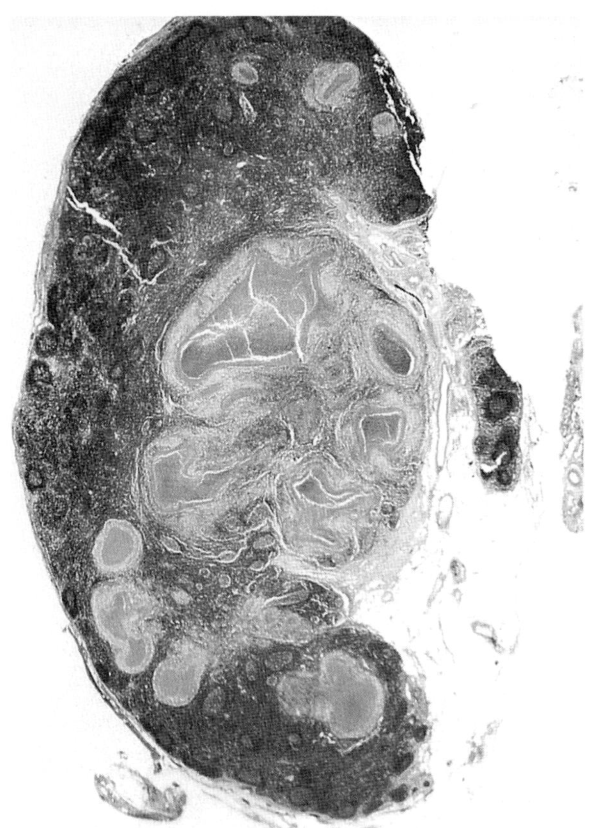

FIGURE 20.1. Lymphogranuloma venereum, late stage, with multiple abscesses showing central necrosis and peripheral hyalinization. (From Strano AJ. Lymphogranuloma venereum. In: Binford CH, Connor DH, eds. Pathology of tropical and extraordinary diseases, vol 1. Washington, DC: Armed Forces Institute of Pathology, 1976:82–85, with permission.)

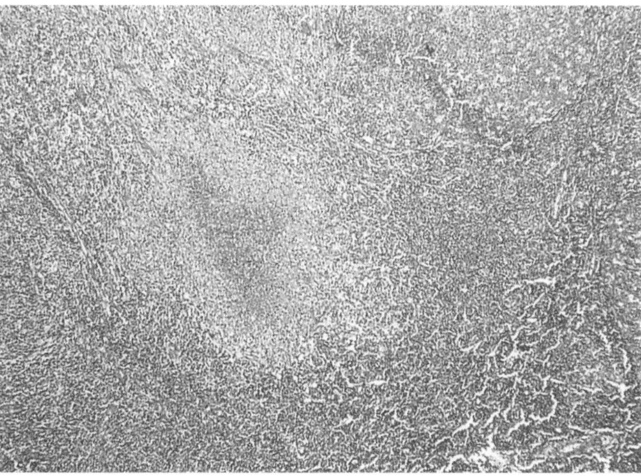

FIGURE 20.3. Stellate microabscess with central necrosis and peripheral palisading epithelioid cells. Hematoxylin, phloxine, and saffron stain.

macrophages with individual or clustered vacuoles up to 40 μm in diameter localize to necrotic and suppurative regions (20) (Fig. 20.5). Intravacuolar *C. trachomatis* bacteria measure 0.2 to 2.0 μm in diameter and form a thin peripheral rim or central clump (20) (Fig. 20.5). In tissue sections, the microorganisms stain red to violet (gram-negative, Brown-Hopp); light blue (Giemsa or hematoxylin and eosin); and black (Warthin-Starry) (20). The suppurative lesions may form sinus tracts, which often reach the skin. In other cases, the necrotic central zone is inspissated and encircled by dense bands of fibrocollagen (15). The architecture of the lymph node parenchyma that is uninvolved by abscesses is preserved; hyperplastic follicles and distended sinuses are usually seen. The intima of the blood vessels thickens progressively

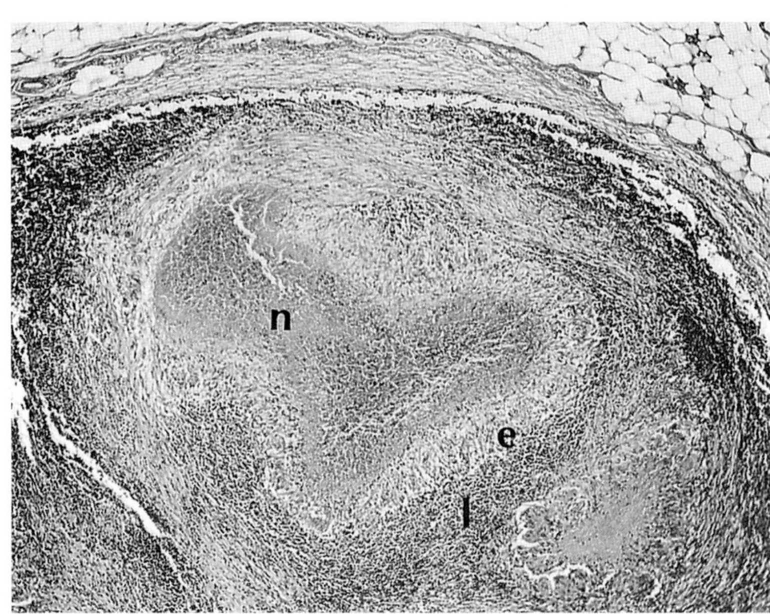

FIGURE 20.2. Lymphogranuloma venereum, early stage, with large granuloma including central area of necrosis (*n*), area of palisading epithelioid cells (*e*), and peripheral area of lymphocytes and plasma cells (*l*). (From Strano AJ. Lymphogranuloma venereum. In: Binford CH, Connor DH, eds. Pathology of tropical and extraordinary diseases, vol 1. Washington, DC: Armed Forces Institute of Pathology, 1976:82–85.)

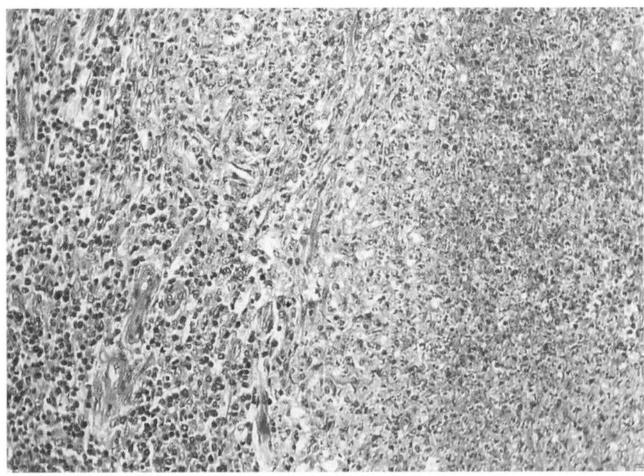

FIGURE 20.4. Central necrosis and polymorphonuclear leukocytes (*left*), epithelioid cells and macrophages (*center*), and lymphoid nodal parenchyma (*right*). Hematoxylin, phloxine, and saffron stain.

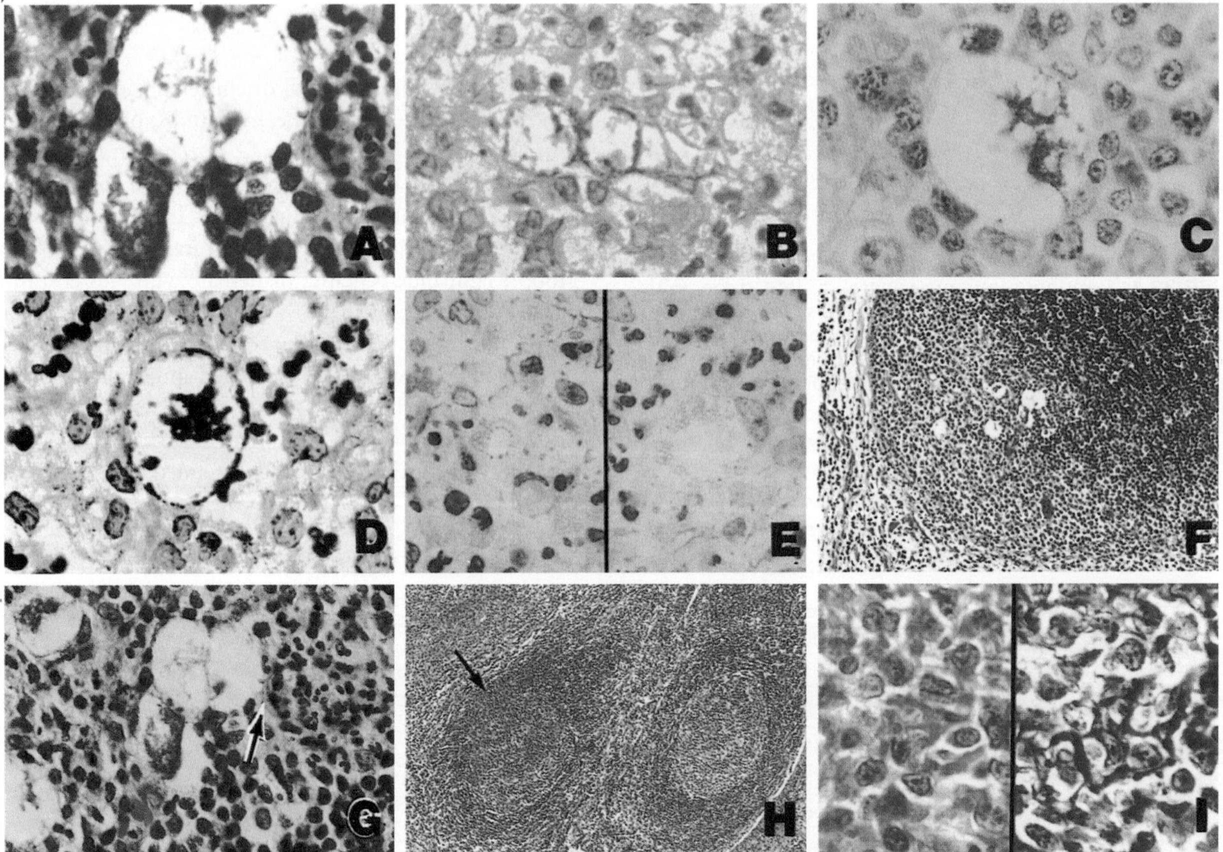

FIGURE 20.5. Inguinal lymph nodes of patients with lymphogranuloma venereum. **A:** Minute blue organisms clump in the center of two vacuoles and along the periphery of the third. Hematoxylin and eosin stain. **B:** Blue organisms line periphery of two vacuoles. Giemsa stain. **C:** Clumped organisms are gram-negative. Brown-Hopp stain. **D:** Silvered organisms line the periphery and clump in the center of vacuole. Warthin-Starry stain. **E:** Plastic-embedded semi-thin section stained with toluidine blue. On left, reticulate bodies line limiting membrane of small cytoplasmic vacuole. On right, numerous elementary bodies clump in larger vacuole. Note that larger reticulate bodies are in smaller vacuole and vacuoles are in histiocytes (*left,* nucleus to left; *right,* nucleus at upper right of vacuole). **F:** Cluster of vacuoles among subcapsular monocytoid B cells near periphery of mantle cells. **G:** Microabscess (*arrow*) at junction of vacuoles and peripheral lymphocytes of mantle zone. Hematoxylin and eosin stain. **H:** Unique pattern of eosinophilic deposits (*arrow*) obscures portion of one germinal center. Hematoxylin and eosin stain. **I:** Eosinophilic deposit is a fibrin network around germinal center cells. Hematoxylin and eosin, phosphotungstic acid hematoxylin stain. *(continued)*

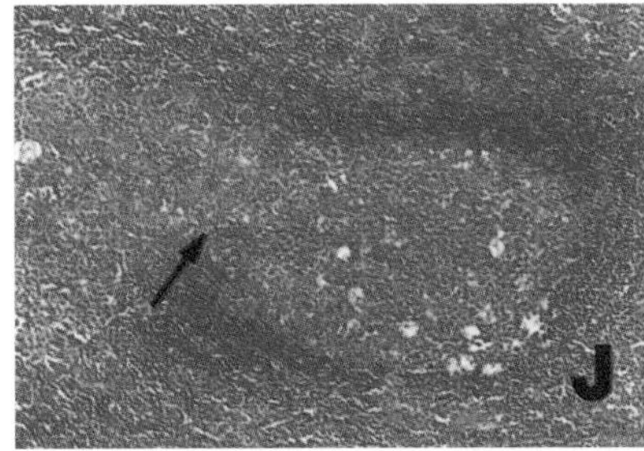

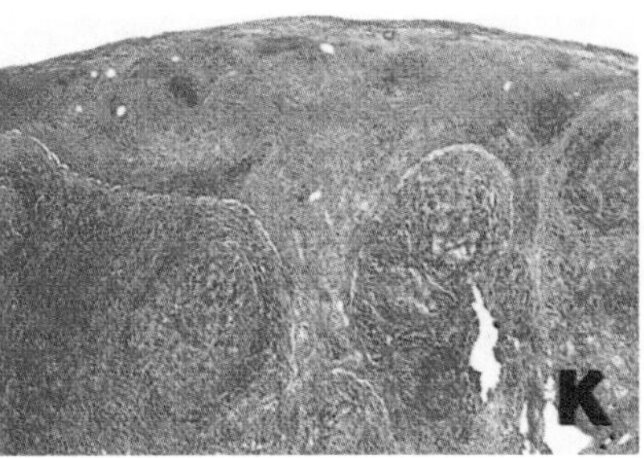

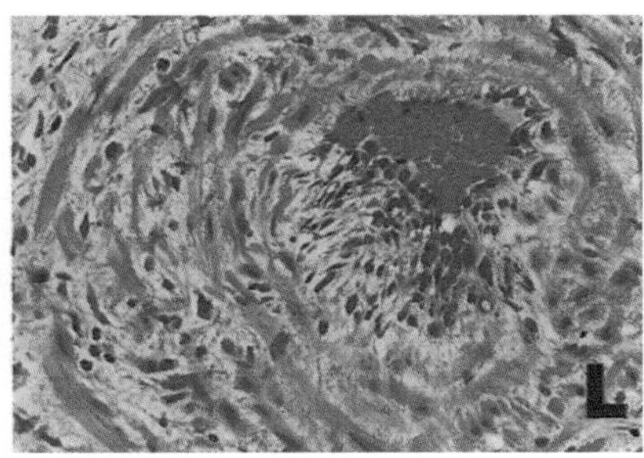

FIGURE 20.5. *Continued* **J:** Expanding abscess (*arrow*) impinges on germinal center; on left, a single vacuole with organisms; on right, numerous tingible-body macrophages in germinal center. Hematoxylin and eosin stain. **K:** Invading lymphocytes and plasma cells and fibrosis focally thicken capsule. Hematoxylin and eosin stain. **L:** Focal, eccentric proliferation of endothelial cells and inflammatory cells narrow lumen of capsular vessel. Hematoxylin and eosin stain. (From Hadfield TL, Lamy Y, Wear DJ. Demonstration of *Chlamydia trachomatis* in inguinal lymphadenitis of lymphogranuloma venereum: a light microscopy, electron microscopy and polymerase chain reaction study. Mod Pathol 1995;8:924–929, with permission.)

and often eventually obliterates the lumina. The lymph node capsule and perinodal tissues are usually extensively involved, initially by abscesses and later by fibrosis. Extensive fibrosis produces lymphangiectasia and sometimes elephantiasis.

LABORATORY TESTS

The Frei test is a delayed-type skin reaction to the inoculation of killed organisms grown in yolk sac. In positive cases, a papule 6 mm in size or larger is present at 48 or 72 hours (14). The biopsy of the Frei skin test tissue shows nodules of epithelioid cells, plasma cells, and occasionally giant cells. A positive skin test result indicates only previous exposure to *Chlamydia* antigen, and skin reactivity can last for years. False-negative reactions can occur in as many as 20% of cases (5). The Frei test is no longer in use, for lack of standardization. Instead, LGV is diagnosed by one of three serologic tests: complement fixation, microimmunofluorescence, or counterimmunoelectrophoresis (21). Of these, complement fixation is generally available as a routine test. In suspected cases of LGV, titers above 1:64 are considered significant (21). *C. trachomatis* organisms can be also isolated and grown in tissue cultures. All *Chlamydia* strains, however, must be treated as potentially infectious agents. Therefore, spreading these organisms in the laboratory by aerosols should be avoided, and all work should be done under standard biologic hoods. Polymerase chain reaction can amplify chlamydial DNA from lymph nodes (20), cervical scrapes (22), and other clinical specimens (22).

DIFFERENTIAL DIAGNOSIS

- Cat-scratch lymphadenitis may be morphologically indistinguishable from LGV lymphadenitis. The differential diagnosis must be made by identification of primary lesions and serologic tests.
- Tularemia lymphadenitis is also morphologically similar, and again, the differential diagnosis depends on clinical features, sex, sites, circumstances, and results of serologic tests.

Checklist

LYMPHOGRANULOMA VENEREUM LYMPHADENITIS

Inguinal, perianal, and pelvic lymph nodes
Often unilateral
Stellate abscesses
Central necrosis and neutrophil leukocytes
Plasma cells, lymphocytes
Palisaded epithelioid cells
Multinucleated giant cells
Fibrosis, lymphangiectasia
Vascular obliteration
Capsular involvement
Complement fixation test

REFERENCES

1. Jones RB. *Chlamydia trachomatis* (trachoma, perinatal infections, lymphogranuloma venereum, and other genital infections). In: Mandell GL, Douglas RG, Bennett JE, eds. Principles and practice of infectious diseases, vol 2. New York: Churchill Livingstone, 1995:1679–1693.
2. Schachter J. Chlamydial infections (third of three parts). N Engl J Med 1978;298:540–549.
3. Schachter J. Chlamydial infections (second of three parts). N Engl J Med 1978;298:490–495.
4. Schachter J. Chlamydial infections (first of three parts). N Engl J Med 1978;298:428–435.
5. Strano AJ. Lymphogranuloma venereum. In: Binford CH, Connor DH, eds. Pathology of tropical and extraordinary diseases, vol 1. Washington, DC: Armed Forces Institute of Pathology, 1976:82–85.
6. Centers for Disease Control and Prevention. *Chlamydia trachomatis* genital infections—United States, 1995. JAMA 1997; 277:952–953.
7. Centers for Disease Control and Prevention. Recommendations for the prevention and management of *Chlamydia trachomatis* infections, 1993. MMWR Morb Mortal Wkly Rep 1993;42:1–39.
8. Quinn TC, Goodell SE, Mkrtichian E, et al. *Chlamydia trachomatis* proctitis. N Engl J Med 1981;305:195–200.
9. Papagrigoriadis S, Rennie JA. Lymphogranuloma venereum as a cause of rectal strictures. Postgrad Med J 1998;74:168–169.
10. Brunham RC, Paavonen J, Stevens CE, et al. Mucopurulent cervicitis—the ignored counterpart in women of urethritis in men. N Engl J Med 1984;311:1–6.
11. Goens JL, Schwartz RA, De Wolf K. Mucocutaneous manifestations of chancroid, lymphogranuloma venereum and granuloma inguinale. Am Fam Physician 1994;49:415–418, 423–425.
12. Martin DH, Mroczkowski TF. Dermatologic manifestations of sexually transmitted diseases other than HIV. Infect Dis Clin North Am 1994;8:533–582.
13. Stansfeld AG. Lymphogranuloma venereum. In: Stansfeld AG, ed. Lymph node biopsy interpretation. New York: Churchill Livingstone, 1985:123–124.
14. Becker LE. Lymphogranuloma venereum. Int J Dermatol 1976;15:26–33.
15. Smith EB, Custer RB. The histopathology of lymphogranuloma venereum. J Urol 1950;63:546–563.
16. Perine PL, Osoba AO. Lymphogranuloma venereum. In: Holmes KK, Mardh P-A, Sparling PF, et al., eds. Sexually transmitted diseases. New York: McGraw-Hill, 1990:195–204.
17. D'Aunoy R, von Haam E. Venereal lymphogranuloma. Arch Pathol 1939;27:1032–1082.
18. Abrams AJ. Lymphogranuloma venereum. JAMA 1963;308: 1563–1565.
19. Dorfman RF, Warnke R. Lymphadenopathy simulating the malignant lymphomas. Hum Pathol 1974;5:519–550.
20. Hadfield TL, Lamy Y, Wear DJ. Demonstration of *Chlamydia trachomatis* in inguinal lymphadenitis of lymphogranuloma venereum: a light microscopy, electron microscopy and polymerase chain reaction study. Mod Pathol 1995;8:924–929.
21. Joseph AK, Rosen T. Laboratory techniques used in the diagnosis of chancroid, granuloma inguinale, and lymphogranuloma venereum. Dermatol Clin 1994;12:1–8.
22. Lan J, Walboomers JM, Roosendaal R, et al. Direct detection and genotyping of *Chlamydia trachomatis* in cervical scrapes by using polymerase chain reaction and restriction fragment length polymorphism analysis. J Clin Microbiol 1993;31:1060–1065.

21

SYPHILITIC LYMPHADENITIS

DEFINITION

Lymphadenitis in the course of syphilis caused by infection with *Treponema pallidum.*

SYNONYM

Luetic lymphadenitis.

EPIDEMIOLOGY

The epidemiology of syphilis has radically changed with time. After high levels in the post-World War II era, the incidence of syphilis decreased dramatically owing to the successful introduction of penicillin treatment. However, after years of quiescence, syphilis began to reemerge through the late 1980s disproportionately among male homosexuals affected by AIDS (1,2). The adoption of safer sex practices by this group led to a declining incidence of new cases. More recently, a shift toward heterosexual transmission has been recorded as more drug-addicted women contract the disease (3,4), and transmit it to their newborns.

ETIOLOGY

Syphilis is caused by a bacterial spirochete, *T. pallidum,* which can be acquired through sexual contact or intrauterine transmission from mother to fetus. *T. pallidum* is a slender, spiral organism, 5 to 15 μm long and 0.2 μm thick (5). In its natural form, the spirals are regular, with a depth of 0.5 to 1 μm (Fig. 21.1). The basic structure is that of a cylinder of protoplasm surrounded by a trilaminar membrane. Bundles of axial filaments stretch from one end to the other, maintaining the elasticity of the organism and making its movements possible (5). The surface consists of a phospholipid-rich layer with few exposed proteins, a strategy that prevents antibody attack from the host (6). To initiate infection, a minimum of approximately 50 organisms is necessary.

CLINICAL SYNDROME

The course of the disease is divided into three stages. Primary syphilis, characterized by a chancre at the site of entry, may persist from several days to 4 weeks, although in most patients the lesion disappears in 2 weeks. The treponemes spread from the chancre through lymphatics to the regional lymph nodes, which are enlarged, hard, and painless (7). Secondary syphilis, beginning 6 to 8 weeks after the onset, is manifested by symptoms including generalized lymphadenopathy, and localized or generalized skin and mucosal eruptions (7). Rashes, in the form of macules or papules, and condylomata lata in genital and anal areas are characteristic of this stage. After a period of latency lasting as long as 2 years and interrupted by occasional relapses, tertiary syphilis develops, with the formation of nodules, ulcers, and gummata affecting various organs, notably in the cardiovascular and central nervous systems.

Luetic lymphadenitis regularly accompanies primary, secondary, and possibly latent or early tertiary stages of syphilis (8). The lymphadenopathy is caused by the persistence of spirochetes in the tissues, particularly the lymph nodes, which provide continuous antigenic stimulation. The inguinal lymph nodes are most commonly involved, especially in primary syphilis. Femoral, epitrochlear, cervical, and axillary lymph nodes are sometimes affected, and generalized lymphadenopathy is often present in secondary syphilis (9).

HISTOPATHOLOGY

Histopathologic features include marked hyperplasia of the lymphoid follicles, which sometimes assume bizarre shapes and occasionally form a second row in the deep cortex that extends to the medullary region (Fig. 21.2). The secondary follicles contain scattered macrophages and a sharply defined margin formed by small lymphocytes (8). On occasion, the excessive follicular hyperplasia resembles follicular lymphoma (10–12). The lymph node capsule is substantially broadened by chronic inflammation and fibrosis (Fig. 21.3). In addition, the T zones are expanded by a mixed cel-

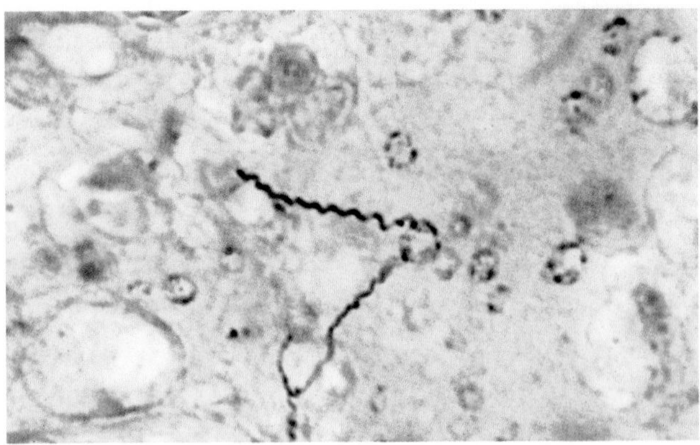

FIGURE 21.1. *T. pallidum* identified by Warthin-Starry silver stain.

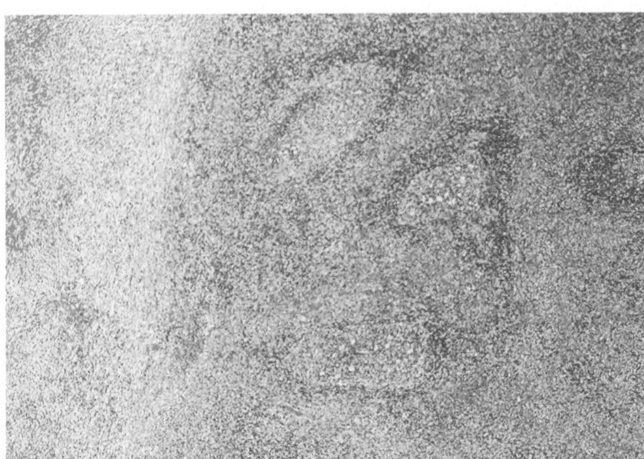

FIGURE 21.2. Inguinal lymph node involved by syphilis. Marked hyperplasia of lymphoid follicles, including a secondary row of follicles and irregularly shaped germinal centers. Hematoxylin and eosin stain.

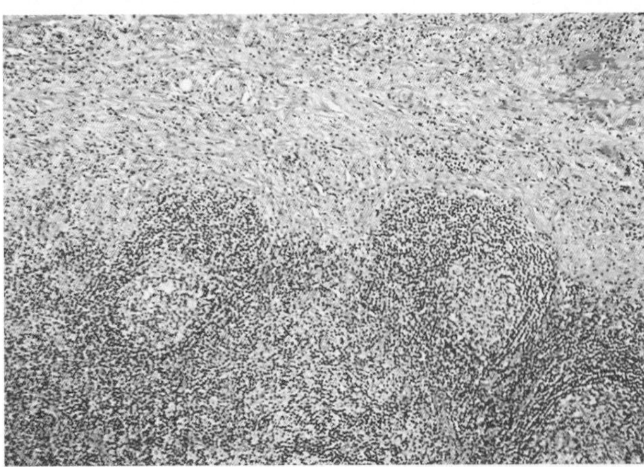

FIGURE 21.3. Same lymph node as in Fig. 21.2. Reactive germinal centers with frequent tingible-body macrophages, indicating cytolysis. Thickened, scalloped fibrous capsule (*top*). Hematoxylin and eosin stain.

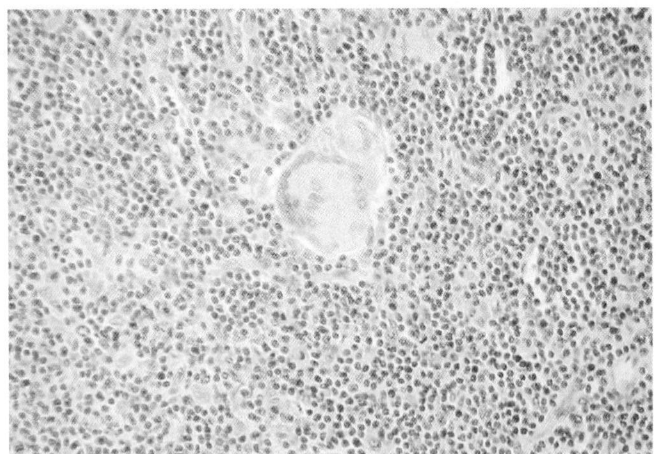

FIGURE 21.4. Paracortex with mixed cellular infiltrate, including immunoblasts and giant cells without granulomas ("naked giant cells"). Hematoxylin and eosin stain.

lular infiltrate that includes numerous immunoblasts (13) (Fig. 21.4).

Arteritis and phlebitis affect the numerous, newly formed vessels of the capsule and pericapsular tissues, which show wide, perivascular cuffs of plasma cells and lymphocytes (Fig. 21.5). Intramural lymphocytes are also present in the affected vessels. Capillaries, arterioles, and venules, capsular and parenchymatous, show marked hyperplasia of the lining endothelial cells, which protrude into and partially obliterate the lumina (Fig. 21.6).

Proliferation of plasma cells is extensive, particularly in the medulla, sometimes resulting in solid cellular sheets. Scattered, small, usually noncaseating epithelioid granulomas are sometimes present, whereas at other times single, multinucleated giant cells, completely isolated ("naked giant cells") among the lymphocytes of the parenchyma, can be seen (Fig. 21.4).

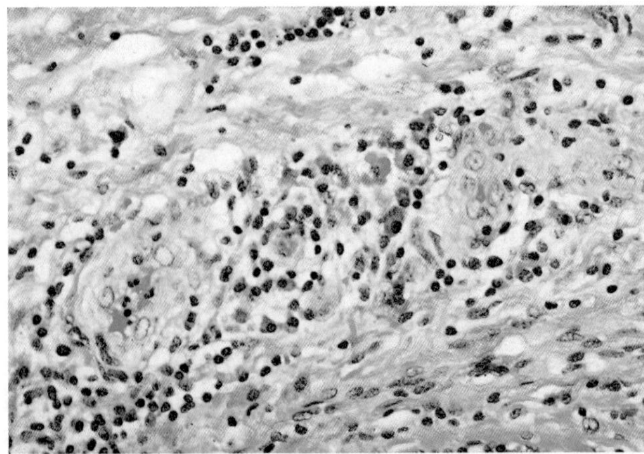

FIGURE 21.5. Markedly widened lymph node capsule with vascular proliferation, perivascular lymphoplasmacytic infiltrates, and fibrosis. Hematoxylin and eosin stain.

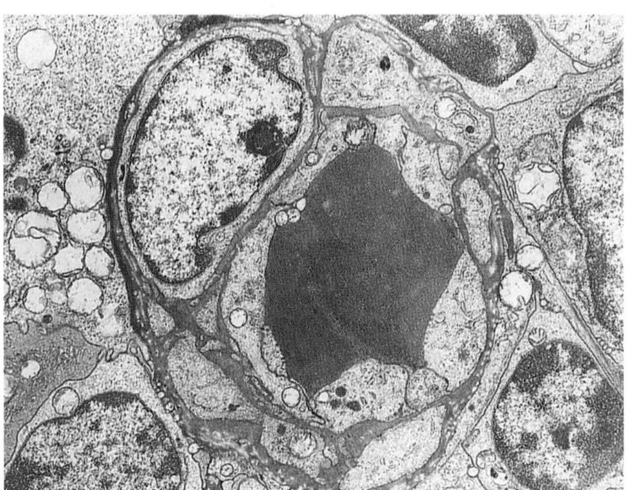

FIGURE 21.6. Postcapillary venule with hyperplastic endothelial cells bulging into the lumen. Lymphocytes and part of a plasma cell outside the vessel. ×8,400.

Silver staining with the Warthin-Starry technique or the Levaditi technique reveals the presence of spirochetes in the lymph node parenchyma and more often in the walls of postcapillary venules and capsular vessels (8) (Fig. 21.1). In 20 cases of lues, including primary, secondary, and tertiary syphilis, spirochetes were identified in sections of all lymph nodes (9). Immunofluorescent and immunoperoxidase staining with specific antisera directed against *T. pallidum* has successfully demonstrated spirochetes in both lymph node imprints (14) (Fig. 21.7) and tissue sections (15).

An unusually large amount of fibrosis is typical of chronic luetic lymphadenitis; dense bands of fibrocollagen thicken the capsule and penetrate the lymph node cortex, between the follicles, creating a characteristic scalloped capsule (Fig. 21.3). The histologic changes are the same in syphilitic lymph nodes from HIV-positive and HIV-negative patients (16).

LABORATORY TESTS

Because of the variability of syphilitic lesions and the frequency of atypical cases, a definitive diagnosis depends on serologic tests for syphilis (5). This is achieved by demonstrating *T. pallidum* in the suspected lesions or by detecting specific antibodies in the serum. The serologic tests for syphilis measure two types of antibodies: nonspecific nontreponemal reaginic antibody and specific antitreponemal antibody.

Demonstration of *T. pallidum*

- Visualization of *T. pallidum* by dark-field examination of exudate from primary lesion or a lymph node touch preparation is one of the oldest and simplest methods to identify the spirochete and is still reliable (17). Negative results do not rule out the infection because 10^3 to 10^4 microorganisms must be present per milliliter to detect a few spirochetes in the dark field. A standardized technique was published by the Centers for Disease Control and Prevention (18).
- Immunofluorescent staining of imprints and sections by the direct or indirect method with absorbed antiserum to *T. pallidum* (14,19).

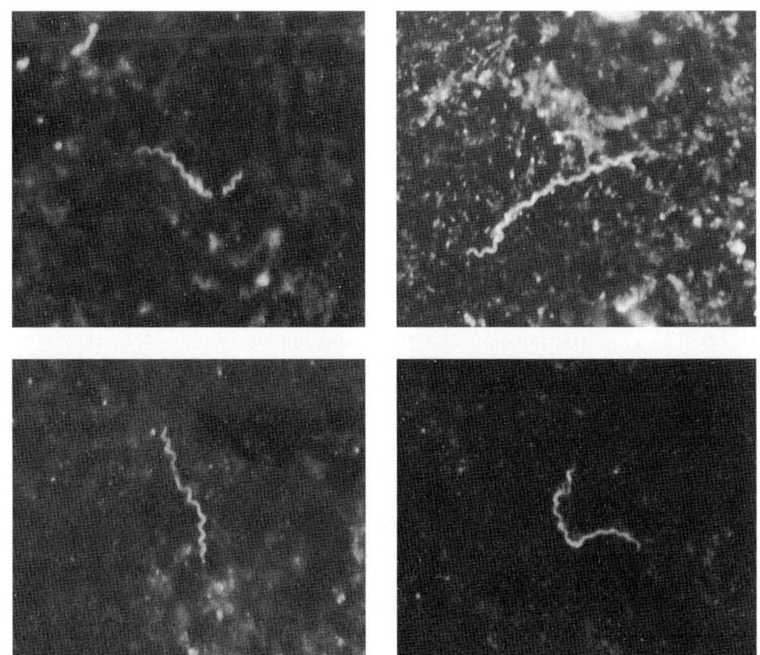

FIGURE 21.7. *T. pallidum* identified by immunofluorescent staining on imprints of lymph node tissue with the use of specific antiserum. (From Choi Y, Reiner L. Syphilitic lymphadenitis: immunofluorescent identification of spirochetes from imprints. Am J Surg Pathol 1979;3:553–555, with permission.)

Checklist

SYPHILITIC LYMPHADENITIS

Inguinal lymphadenopathy more common
Follicular hyperplasia
Arteritis and phlebitis, particularly capsular
Perivascular lymphoplasmacytic infiltrates
Capillary endothelial hyperplasia
Plasma cells in clusters and sheets
Epithelioid granulomas
Isolated multinucleated giant cells
Capsular fibrosis
Warthin-Starry staining of spirochetes
Detection of antitreponemal antibodies

- Silver impregnation of *T. pallidum* in paraffin-embedded tissues by the technique of Warthin-Starry or that of Levaditi (20).
- Polymerase chain reaction to amplify *T. pallidum* DNA sequences in tissue (21).

Detection of Nonspecific Nontreponemal Reaginic Antibodies

- Cardiolipin antibodies, which react with the lipoidal antigen generated by host interactions with *T. pallidum* or with antigen from *T. pallidum* alone, also are known as *Wasserman antibodies* or *reagin* (5). The Venereal Disease Research Laboratory (VDRL) slide test is a standard nontreponemal test in which the ability of heated serum to precipitate suspended cardiolipin–cholesterol–lecithin antigen is determined. It is helpful in following a patient's response to therapy. Routine syphilis screening depends on the rapid plasma reagin (RPR) card test or the automated reagin test (ART) (22).

Detection of Specific Treponemal Antibodies

- *T. pallidum* organisms grown in rabbit testes are used as the antigen in standard indirect immunofluorescence assays [fluorescent treponemal antibody absorption (FTA-Abs), *T. pallidum* hemagglutination (TPHA)]. Once a test result is positive, it usually remains positive indefinitely. A specific treponemal antibody test is used mostly to confirm a positive nontreponemal reaginic test result.

DIFFERENTIAL DIAGNOSIS

- Tuberculous lymphadenitis lacks vasculitis and spirochetes. Includes caseous necrosis and acid-fast bacilli.
- Sarcoidosis lacks the vasculitis and extensive infiltration with plasma cells of syphilis. Granulomas are well formed and predominant.
- Polyarteritis nodosa lacks follicular hyperplasia and spirochetes.
- Hodgkin lymphoma, in common with lues, includes plasma cells, fibrosis, and occasional epithelioid granulomas. It lacks vasculitis and contains Reed-Sternberg and Hodgkin cells.
- Nodular (follicular) lymphoma in rare cases of marked luetic follicular hyperplasia. In lymphomas, the lymph node architecture is not preserved, and vasculitis, granulomas, and plasma cells are lacking.

REFERENCES

1. Nakashima AK, Rolfs RT, Flock ML, et al. Epidemiology of syphilis in the United States, 1941–1993. Sex Transm Dis 1996;23:16–23.
2. Centers for Disease Control and Prevention. Primary and secondary syphilis—United States, 1997. JAMA 1998;280:1218–1219.
3. Ansell DA, Hu TC, Straus M, et al. HIV and syphilis seroprevalence among clients with sexually transmitted diseases attending a walk-in clinic at Cook County Hospital. Sex Transm Dis 1994; 21:93–96.
4. Siegal HA, Carlson RG, Falck R, et al. High-risk behaviors for transmission of syphilis and human immunodeficiency virus among crack cocaine-using women. A case study from the Midwest. Sex Transm Dis 1992;19:266–271.
5. Tramont EC. *Treponema pallidum* (syphilis). In: Mandell GL, Douglas RG, Bennett JE, eds. Principles and practice of infectious diseases, vol 2. New York: Churchill Livingstone, 1995: 2117–2133.
6. Radolf JD, Norgard MV, Schulz WW. Outer membrane ultrastructure explains the limited antigenicity of virulent *Treponema pallidum.* Proc Natl Acad Sci U S A 1989;86:2051–2055.
7. Singh AE, Romanowski B. Syphilis: review with emphasis on clinical, epidemiologic, and some biologic features. Clin Microbiol Rev 1999;12:187–209.

8. Turner DR, Wright DJM. Lymphadenopathy in early syphilis. J Pathol 1973;110:305–308.
9. Hartsock RJ, Halling LW, King FM. Luetic lymphadenitis: a clinical and histologic study of 20 cases. Am J Clin Pathol 1970; 53:304–314.
10. Evans N. Lymphadenitis of secondary syphilis: its resemblance to giant follicular lymphadenopathy. Arch Pathol 1944;37:175–179.
11. Goffinet DR. Secondary syphilis misdiagnosed as lymphoma. Calif Med 1970;112:22–23.
12. Dorfman RF, Warnke R. Lymphadenopathy simulating the malignant lymphomas. Hum Pathol 1974;5:519–550.
13. Stansfeld AG. Spirochaetal infections. In: Stansfeld AG, ed. Lymph node biopsy interpretation. Edinburgh: Churchill Livingstone, 1985:108–111.
14. Choi YJ, Reiner L. Syphilitic lymphadenitis: immunofluorescent identification of spirochetes from imprints. Am J Surg Pathol 1979;3:553–555.
15. Beckett JH, Bigbee JW. Immunoperoxidase localization of *Treponema pallidum*: its use in formaldehyde-fixed and paraffin-embedded tissue sections. Arch Pathol Lab Med 1979;103:135–138.
16. Farhi DC, Wells SJ, Siegel RJ. Syphilitic lymphadenopathy. Histology and human immunodeficiency virus status. Am J Clin Pathol 1999;112:330–334.
17. Wicher K, Wicher V. Syphilis. In: Sun T, ed. Sexually related infectious diseases. New York: Field, Rich, 1986:15–41.
18. Centers for Disease Control. Manual of tests for syphilis. Washington, DC: U.S. Department of Health, Education and Welfare, 1969.
19. Sun T. Syphilis. In: Sun T, ed. Sexually related infectious diseases. New York: Field, Rich, 1986:266–269.
20. Warthin-Starry method for staining spirochetes. Manual of histologic and special staining techniques. Washington, DC: Armed Forces Institute of Pathology, 1957:184–185.
21. Horowitz HW, Valsamis MP, Wicher V, et al. Brief report: cerebral syphilitic gumma confirmed by the polymerase chain reaction in a man with human immunodeficiency virus infection [see Comments]. N Engl J Med 1994;331:1488–1491.
22. Aberle-Grasse J, Orton SL, Notari Et, et al. Predictive value of past and current screening tests for syphilis in blood donors: changing from a rapid plasma reagin test to an automated specific treponemal test for screening. Transfusion 1999;39:206–211.

22

LYMPHADENITIS OF WHIPPLE DISEASE

DEFINITION

Lymphadenitis caused by infection with *Tropheryma whippelii.*

ETIOLOGY

The agent of the disease described in 1907 by George Whipple, *T. whippelii,* is a rod-shaped, silver-stained bacillus presently classified with the actinomycetes (1). All efforts to culture this organism failed, and the bacterium was finally identified only through a molecular genetic approach. Thus, the bacterial 16S ribosomal RNA sequence was amplified directly by the polymerase chain reaction from the involved tissues of patients with Whipple disease (2). Recently, *T. whippelii* isolated from the aortic valve of a patient with endocarditis was cultured and successfully passaged in a human fibroblast cell line (3). The same authors developed an immunofluorescence serologic test.

PATHOGENESIS

The unique cell wall structure of the bacillus *T. whippelii* attracts macrophages that engulf and degrade it; as a result, inclusions that stain with periodic acid–Schiff (PAS) can be seen in prepared tissues (4). Macrophages containing the diastase-resistant, PAS-positive inclusions infiltrate the lamina propria of the gastrointestinal tract in addition to the mesentery, lymph nodes, heart, central nervous system, and nearly every other organ system (2). The bacterium does not form hyphae in human tissues; however, like other actinomycetes, it is gram-positive and PAS-positive (2). Whether the infection is acquired primarily or exclusively through the gastrointestinal tract is not clear (5).

CLINICAL SYNDROME

Whipple disease is an uncommon, chronic, systemic illness. The largest study published includes 29 patients seen at the Mayo Clinic during a 30-year period (6). A male predominance was noted, and the overall mean age of the patients was 54 years. The main symptoms are fever, diarrhea, weight loss, arthralgia, and central nervous system manifestations such as headache, diplopia, and depression (6). Basically, the major syndrome is that of malabsorption, expressed by significant weight loss in 90% of patients. The usual radiographic pattern is one of prominent and edematous jejunal folds, consistent with malabsorption and extensive paraaortic and retroperitoneal lymphadenopathy. On physical examination, the most frequent abnormalities are lymphadenopathies involving predominantly the axillary and cervical lymph nodes. Hepatomegaly and generalized hyperpigmentation may also be present (6). Before the introduction of antibiotic treatment, the disease usually ended in death. A variety of antibiotics, singly or in combination, are now used, but even with proper treatment, relapses may occur. Treatment for at least a year is recommended, including antibiotics that readily cross the blood–brain barrier to prevent central nervous system complications (6). Recently, a case of chronic wasting illness accompanied by massive abdominal lymphadenopathy was reported in a veteran of the Persian Gulf war (7). A lymph node biopsy indicated a diagnosis of Whipple disease; however, the epidemiologic significance of this isolated case is unclear.

HISTOPATHOLOGY

The enlarged lymph nodes comprise large numbers of foamy mononuclear cells, singly and in loose aggregates, in the sinuses and lymphoid areas (8,9). The cells are histiocytes containing a PAS-positive, diastase-resistant mucopolysaccharide substance. Intercellular deposits of the PAS-positive substance are also seen, sometimes within cystic spaces (Fig. 22.1), at other times surrounded by a granulomatous reaction of a few epithelioid and foreign body giant cells. The PAS-positive characteristic granules are most likely degenerated bacteria (5) (Fig. 22.2). Tissue necrosis is absent, and the result of Ziehl-Neelsen acid-fast staining is negative. Similar PAS-positive foamy histiocytes infiltrate the submucosa of the small intestine, particularly the villi of the jejunum, which appear

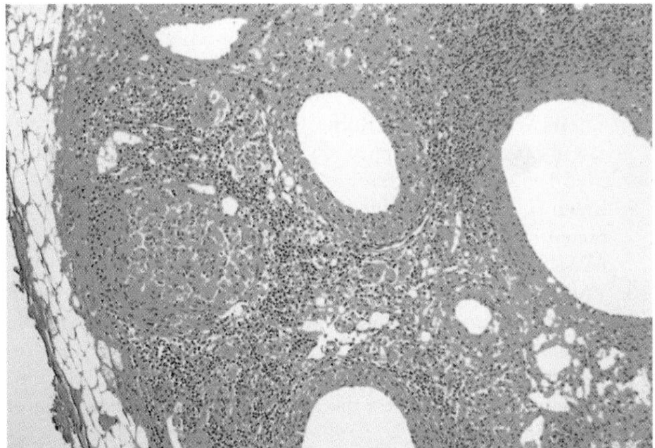

FIGURE 22.1. Lymphadenitis of Whipple disease. Cystic spaces and non-necrotizing granuloma (*right*). (From Ereno C, Lopez J, Elizalde JM, et al. A case of Whipple's disease presenting as supraclavicular lymphadenopathy. A case report. APMIS 1993;101: 865–868, with permission.)

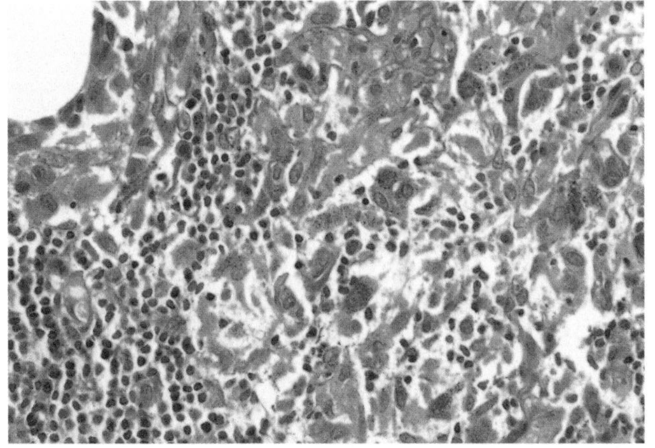

FIGURE 22.2. Histiocytes with granular, diastase-resistant, periodic acid–Schiff-positive cytoplasm. (From Ereno C, Lopez J, Elizalde JM, et al. A case of Whipple's disease presenting as supraclavicular lymphadenopathy. A case report. APMIS 1993;101: 865–868, with permission.)

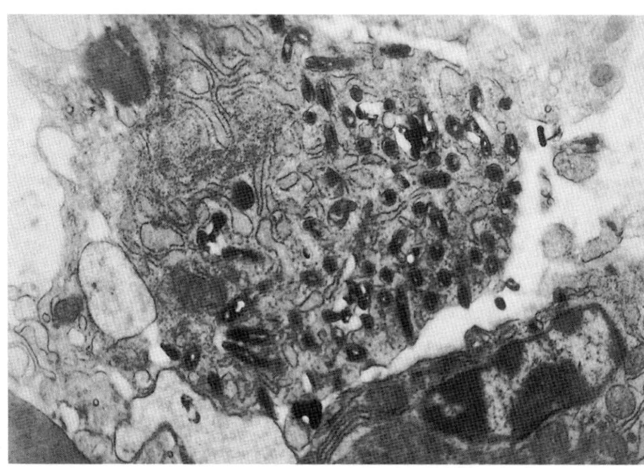

FIGURE 22.3. Histiocyte in Whipple lymphadenitis filled with intracytoplasmic bacillary bodies. (From Ereno C, Lopez J, Elizalde JM, et al. A case of Whipple's disease presenting as supraclavicular lymphadenopathy. A case report. APMIS 1993;101:865–868, with permission.)

prominent and edematous (6). In disseminated disease, the PAS-positive cells may be also seen in the endocardium, pericardium, liver, spleen, mesentery, synovium, meninges, and appendix (10). They may form vegetations on the cardiac valves and infiltrate the adrenals, muscles, and brain (11,12). The rupture of lymphatics obstructed by enlarged mesenteric lymph nodes may cause chylous ascites (6).

ELECTRON MICROSCOPY

The agent of Whipple disease under the electron microscope appears as a rod-shaped bacillary body, 1 μm long and 0.2 μm wide with a trilaminar plasma membrane, within the cytoplasm of histiocytes (6,9) (Fig. 22.3).

LABORATORY TESTS

An immunofluorescence serologic test in which monolayer cells infected with *T. whippelii* are used can identify high titers of specific immunoglobulin G (IgG) and IgM antibodies in patients with various manifestations of the disease (3).

Checklist

LYMPHADENITIS OF WHIPPLE DISEASE

Diarrhea, wasting illness
Multiple lymphadenopathies
Foamy histiocytes
Intracellular and extracellular PAS-positive deposits of degenerated bacteria
Rod-shaped bacilli with trilaminar walls

REFERENCES

1. Whipple GA. A hitherto undescribed disease characterized anatomically by deposits of fat and fatty acids in the intestinal and mesenteric lymphatic tissues. Bull Johns Hopkins Hosp 1907;18: 382–391.
2. Relman DA, Schmidt TM, MacDermott RP, et al. Identification of the uncultured bacillus of Whipple's disease. N Engl J Med 1992;327:293–301.
3. Raoult D, Birg ML, La Scola B, et al. Cultivation of the bacillus of Whipple's disease. N Engl J Med 2000;342:650–655.
4. Yardley JH, Hendrix TR. Combined electron and light microscopy in Whipple's disease: demonstration of "bacillary bodies" in the intestine. Bull Johns Hopkins Hosp 1961;109:80–98.
5. Swartz NIN. Whipple's disease—past, present and future. N Engl J Med 2000;342:648–650.
6. Fleming JL, Wiesner RH, Shorter RG. Whipple's disease: clinical, biochemical, and histopathologic features and assessment of treatment in 29 patients. Mayo Clin Proc 1988;63: 539–551.
7. Friedman HD. Two Persian Gulf veterans with lymphadenopathy. Arch Pathol Lab Med 1996;120:425.
8. Chears WC, Smith AG, Ruffin JM. Diagnosis of Whipple's disease by peripheral lymph node biopsy. Report of a case. Am J Med 1959;27:351–353.
9. Ereno C, Lopez J, Elizalde JM, et al. A case of Whipple's disease presenting as supraclavicular lymphadenopathy. A case report. APMIS 1993;101:865–868.
10. Viteri LA, Stinson JC, Barnes MC, et al. Rod-shaped organism in the liver of a patient with Whipple's disease. Dig Dis Sci 1979;24:560–564.
11. Sieracki JC, Fine G, Hom RC, et al Central nervous system involvement in Whipple's disease. J Neuropathol Exp Neurol 1960;19:70–75.
12. Johnson L, Diamond I. Cerebral Whipple's disease diagnosis by brain biopsy. Am J Clin Pathol 1980;74:486–490.

PART III

SECTION THREE

MYCOBACTERIAL LYMPHADENITIDES

Mycobacteria are aerobic, non–spore-forming, nonmotile bacilli that are essentially defined by their distinctive acid-fast staining property (1). Owing to their lipid-rich cell walls, mycobacteria are relatively impermeable to various basic dyes; however, once stained, they retain the stain with tenacity. Thus, they resist decolorization with acidified organic solvents and are therefore considered to be acid-fast. Mycobacteria range from organisms that are highly pathogenic for humans, such as *Mycobacterium tuberculosis* and *Mycobacterium leprae,* to a variety of innocuous organisms widely spread in soil and water that can become pathogenic under conditions of immunodeficiency.

REFERENCE

1. Wolinsky E. Mycobacteria. In: Davis BD, Dulbecco R, Eisen HN, et al., eds. Microbiology, 3rd ed. Hagerstown, MD: Harper & Row, 1980:723–742.

23

MYCOBACTERIUM TUBERCULOSIS LYMPHADENITIS

DEFINITION

Lymphadenitis caused by infection with *Mycobacterium tuberculosis.*

SYNONYM

Tuberculous lymphadenitis.

ETIOLOGY

M. tuberculosis var *hominis* and var *bovis* is the agent of tuberculosis in humans and other animal species. The organisms are slightly curved, slender rods that are 2 to 4 μm long. Also known as *tubercle bacilli,* they appear in stained tissues uniformly or more often beaded and can be easily cultured on specific media (1). The walls of mycobacteria have a lipid content of up to 60% attached to polysaccharides. Because of the high lipid content of their outer walls, mycobacteria are hydrophobic, impermeable to stains, acid-fast, and resistant to bactericidal substances, antibodies, and complement (1). Ziehl-Neelsen, Kinyoun, and Fite-Faraco are specific histologic stains based on the acid-fast property of mycobacteria.

EPIDEMIOLOGY

Tuberculosis was for centuries one of the most severe human diseases, and although its incidence has steadily decreased in more advanced countries, it remains a major health problem in developing nations. Among infectious diseases, tuberculosis is still the leading cause of death (2). About a third of the world's population harbors *M. tuberculosis* and is at risk for development of the disease (2). In the United States, tuberculosis had been decreasing annually by an average of 5%, remaining confined largely to elderly, institutionalized, and foreign-born persons. Since 1985, when 5,000 more cases of tuberculosis than expected were recorded, the declining trend has reversed, and annual increases in the incidence of tuberculosis are again being registered (2–5). The shift in the epidemiology of tuberculosis has been caused by the epidemics of drug abuse and HIV infection. In one inner city hospital in New York, the total number of new mycobacterial isolates increased 10-fold from 1982 to 1986. Of these patients, 80% were intravenous drug abusers, and their tuberculosis presented early and aggressively (6).

PATHOGENESIS

The broad range of lesions that can be observed in tuberculosis is the result of a continuous interaction between bacterial virulence and individual response. The latter varies from hypersensitivity, expressed by exudative, generally nonspecific lesions, to immunity, expressed by proliferative, granulomatous, specific lesions. Primary tuberculosis develops when *M. tuberculosis* var *hominis* is inhaled into the lungs or, far less frequently, when *M. tuberculosis* var *bovis* is ingested and infects the intestines.

The lymph nodes are involved in primary tuberculosis as tubercle bacilli disseminate from the initial focus of infection through the lymphatics to the tributary lymph nodes. Because the primary focus is usually in the lungs, most commonly subjacent to the pleurae of the upper lobes, the bronchopulmonary lymph nodes become involved, forming together the classic Ghon complex. With the rare primary lesions that occur in intestine, tonsil, eye, ear, or skin, regional lymph nodes may be similarly involved. Secondary tuberculosis arises in a previously sensitized person by reactivation of a primary complex, usually the lymph nodes, in which tubercle bacilli may survive for long periods of time, or by new exogenous infection. The new lesions may remain restricted to the lungs, disseminate widely in the form of miliary tuberculosis, or localize in a variety of organs with further local chronic progression. In any of these cases, the regional draining lymph nodes are affected, and chronic proliferative tuberculous lymphadenitis results. In unimmunized organisms, the tissue reaction to tubercle bacilli is essentially exudative, necrotizing, and nonspecific. As specific immunity develops, the lesions become localized, proliferative, and specific, reflected by the characteristic tuberculous granuloma. In most cases, cell-mediated specific immunity to *M. tuberculosis* develops within 2 to 6 weeks after infection. Most bacilli are killed by macrophages, and a few persist in a dormant but viable state. The only signs of the primary infection are a small, healed, calcified lesion in the lung and skin test reactivity to a purified protein derivative (PPD) of tuberculin (2). In persons with immune deficiency, whether congenital or acquired (e.g., organ transplant recipients, HIV-infected persons), the course of tuberculosis is entirely different (2,7). As cellular immunity is gradually destroyed, old, latent tuberculous lesions are reactivated, PPD reactivity is compromised, and the progress of disease is accelerated. Extrapulmonary tuberculosis, such as miliary tuberculosis, lymphadenitis, and various visceral localizations, is more common (2,7–9).

The immunization of newborns with bacille Calmette-Guérin (BCG), an attenuated form of *M. tuberculosis,* may result in enlarged lymph nodes, usually the axillary nodes. BCG-caused lymphadenopathies occur in 0.73% to 2.2% of children after a mean interval of 2.5 months and as late as 3 years after vaccination (10,11). The iliac lymph nodes may be involved when BCG is used for the intravesical treatment of bladder cancer (12). Children and adults with normal immunity recover spontaneously or after the excision of a tuberculous lymph node. However, in children with congenital immune deficiencies, such as severe combined immunodeficiency, Swiss-type hypogammaglobulinemia, or thymic alymphoplasia (13), and in patients with HIV infection and AIDS, suppurative lymphadenitides and disseminated, sometimes fatal, tuberculosis develop (11,14).

GROSS APPEARANCE

The gross features of tuberculosis are usually sufficiently distinctive that a tentative diagnosis can be made and precautions taken for avoiding infection (10). On section, the caseous necrotic areas appear as creamy white patches, becoming chalky with the deposition of calcium. The periphery is densely fibrosed. In time, some nodes may be entirely converted into radiopaque, rock-hard masses (10). The tuberculous lymph nodes are matted, and large areas may be entirely necrotic. The tracheobronchial lymph nodes commonly involved in the tuberculous primary complex may reach large proportions, particularly in children. They may spread to adjacent structures, causing abscesses or traction diverticula (15), or adhere to blood vessels. Subsequent invasion of a blood vessel results in miliary dissemination.

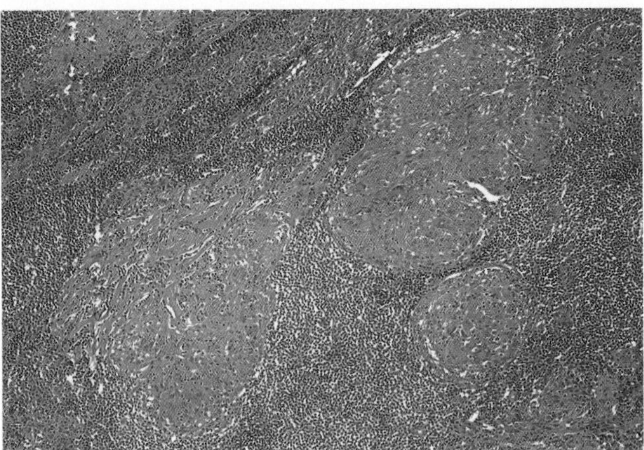

FIGURE 23.1. Tuberculous granulomas are isolated (*left*) or confluent with central area of necrosis (*right*). Hematoxylin, phloxine, and saffron stain.

HISTOPATHOLOGY

The major immune responses of the host to tuberculous infection are macrophage activation, specific T cell-mediated reactivity, and granuloma formation (12). Because of the interaction of bacterial virulence, individual hypersensitivity, and immunity to infection, a range of different lesions may result. *M. tuberculosis* is an intracellular parasite. Engulfed by the alveolar macrophages, the mycobacteria multiply within the cells and are transported to new locations (16). When macrophages laden with bacilli encounter CD4+ T cells, the T cells become activated and produce a variety of lytic enzymes that kill mycobacteria but also cause tissue necrosis. The epithelioid cells of tuberculous granulomas are highly activated macrophages that secrete various cytokines, interferon-γ, and fibroblast-stimulating factor, which eventually cause granulomatous fibrosis (17). The tuberculous granuloma is classically described as having a necrotic center and concentric areas of epithelioid cells, Langhans giant cells, and lymphocytes (Figs. 23.1–23.3). More often, how-

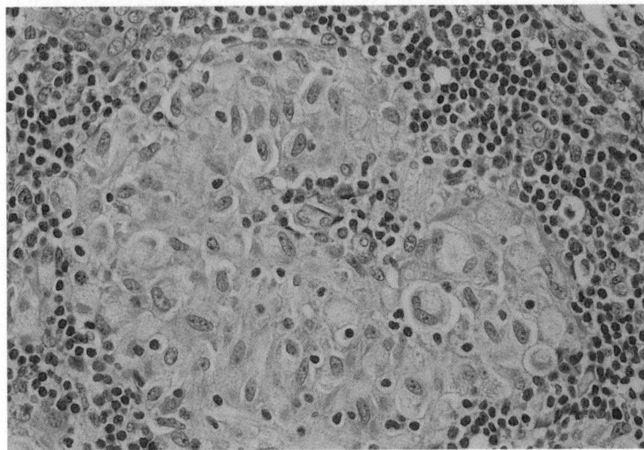

FIGURE 23.2. Same lymph node lesion showing granuloma formed of epithelioid cells and giant cells within lymphoid tissue. Hematoxylin, phloxine, and saffron stain.

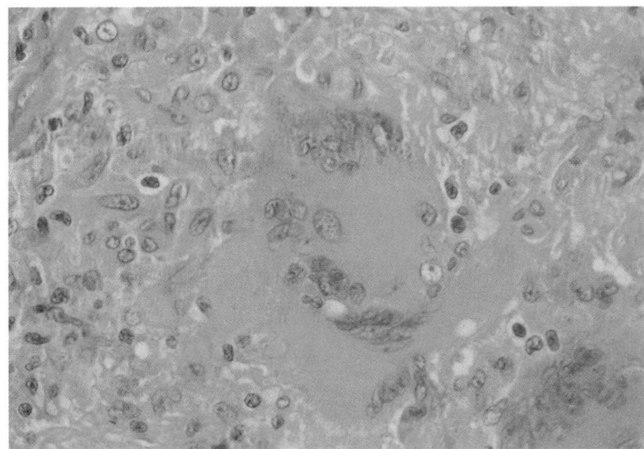

FIGURE 23.3. Multinucleated giant cell of Langhans type with nuclei arranged in a peripheral crown surrounded by epithelioid cells and lymphocytes. Hematoxylin, phloxine, and saffron stain.

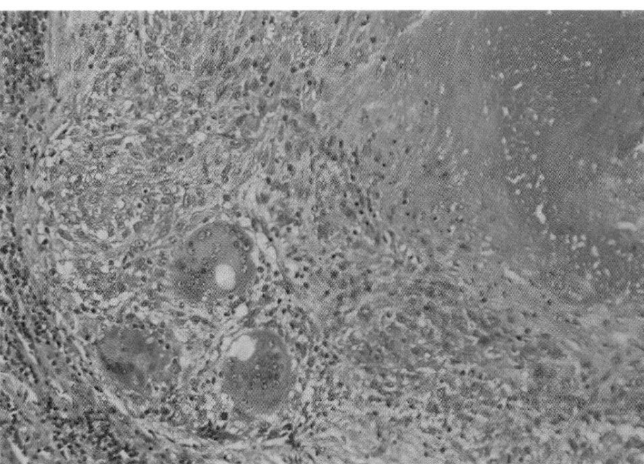

FIGURE 23.5. Same lesion at higher magnification showing epithelioid and giant cells without formation of distinct granulomas. Hematoxylin, phloxine, and saffron stain.

ever, the follicles are confluent, forming irregularly shaped areas of necrosis surrounded by epithelioid cells, occasional giant cells, lymphocytes, plasma cells, and fibroblasts (18) (Figs. 23.4 and 23.5). The lymph node parenchyma may be only partially involved, and in that case, the architecture of the unaffected areas remains unchanged. The caseous necrosis characteristic of tuberculosis is a coagulative, total necrosis that leaves no cellular traces or nuclear debris (Fig. 23.6). The Langhans giant cell has a strongly acidophilic cytoplasm and multiple, peripherally arranged nuclei (Fig. 23.3). However, multinucleated giant cells of various types can be observed. Fibrosis, hyalinization, and calcification of tuberculous lymph nodes, partial or total, are the common forms of healing, although latent bacilli can be preserved for years in such lesions (Fig. 23.7). The identification of characteristic beaded, rod-shaped, acid-fast bacilli is needed for a positive diagnosis and can be made on the special, acid-fast

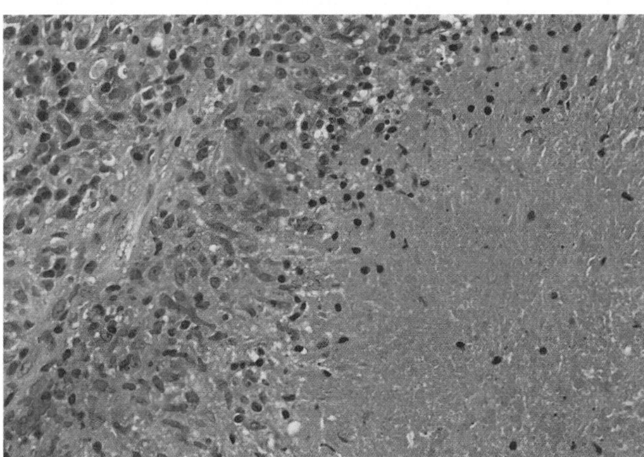

FIGURE 23.6. Area of caseous necrosis with a small amount of nuclear debris surrounded by palisading epithelioid cells and lymphocytes. Hematoxylin, phloxine, and saffron stain.

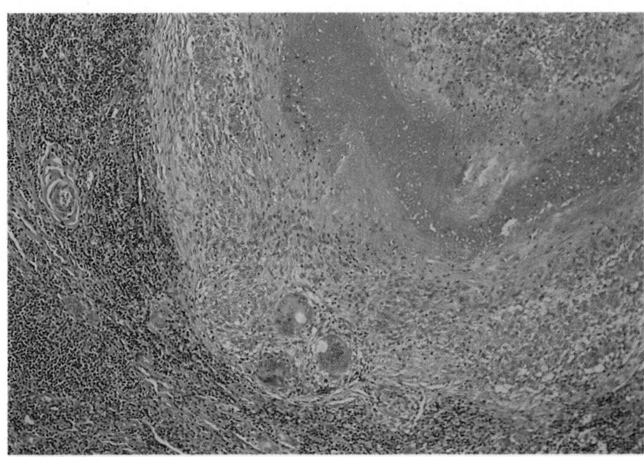

FIGURE 23.4. Confluent epithelioid granulomas with central necrosis (*red*) and fibrosis (*yellow*) Hematoxylin, phloxine, and saffron stain.

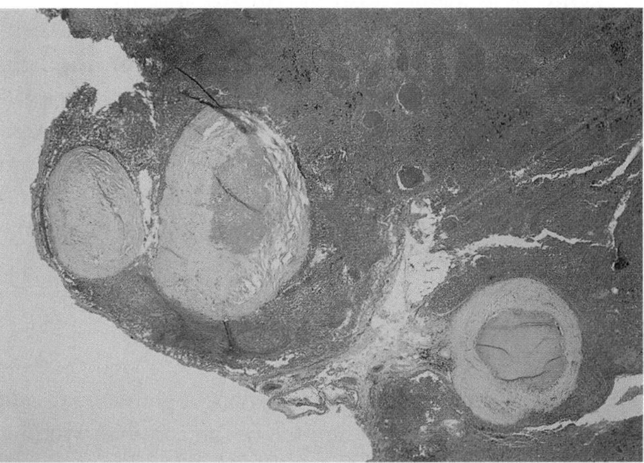

FIGURE 23.7. Peritracheal lymph nodes with metastatic squamous cell carcinoma (*upper right*) and three old tuberculous granulomas encircled by fibrosis, still with central necrosis. Hematoxylin, phloxine, and saffron stain.

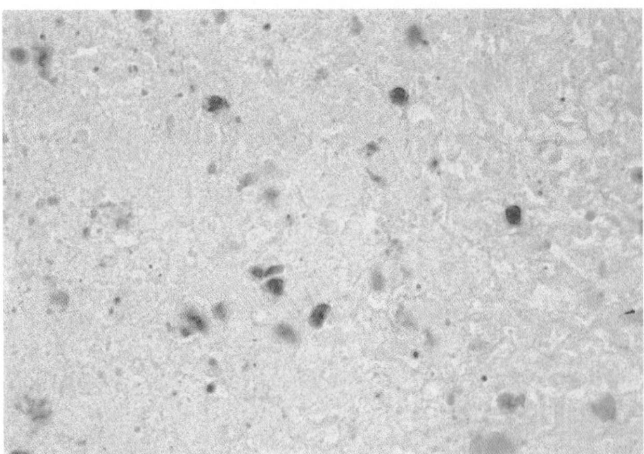

FIGURE 23.8. Few acid-fast bacilli in area of tissue necrosis. Ziehl-Neelsen stain.

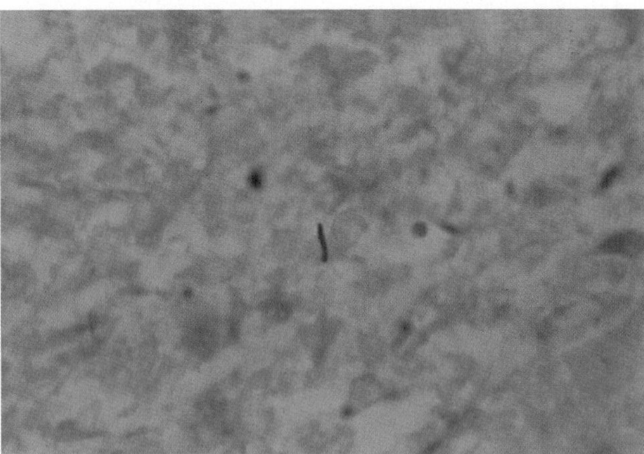

FIGURE 23.9. Single, slender, beaded, acid-fast-stained bacillus in area of caseous necrosis. Ziehl-Neelsen stain.

stainings (Fig. 23.8). Preferential locations of mycobacteria are at the periphery of necrotic areas, among the epithelioid cells, and rarely within the cytoplasm of giant cells. The number of bacilli in tuberculous lesions varies greatly, depending on local immunity, age of the lesion, and previous treatment. It has been estimated that 10,000 organisms per milligram of tissue must be present to be identified by a special acid-fast stain (19). The search for acid-fast bacilli in paraffin-embedded tissues is often disappointing, and not infrequently the search for acid-fast bacilli in lesions morphologically typical of tuberculosis is unsuccessful. In such cases, the diagnosis of tuberculosis should not be ruled out, and attempts at confirmation must be pursued by other means.

HISTOCHEMISTRY

Acid-fast bacilli can be demonstrated in smears or sections of lymph node tissues with one of the specific stainings: Ziehl-Neelsen, Kinyoun, or Fite-Faraco. The typical slender, beaded, acid-fast bacilli are brilliant red on the light blue tissue background (Fig. 23.9). They can also be visualized with the Truant stain, with which an auramine–rhodamine dye mixture and a fluorescent light source afford greater sensitivity (7). An average of more than one organism per oil immersion field is described as numerous (20).

IMMUNOHISTOCHEMISTRY

The epithelioid and giant cells of tuberculous granulomas stain strongly with anti-Leu-M1, anti-CD68, and antilysozyme antibodies (Fig. 23.10). Studies investigating the cell types in various kinds of granulomas have found that tuberculous granulomas are devoid of B lymphocytes and natural killer cells and that the ratio of CD4+ to CD8+ cells is usually greater than 2 (21,22). Mycobacterial antigens can be detected and the types identified with monoclonal antibodies and peroxidase/antiperoxidase staining (23,24). In addition to the staining of acid-fast bacilli, the immunohistochemical technique reveals clumps of antigens deposited in areas of caseous necrosis that do not stain with the Ziehl-Neelsen stain.

LABORATORY TESTS

Direct Evidence

The reference standard for the diagnosis of *M. tuberculosis* infection is culture and identification on specific media; however, incubation takes from 2 to 6 weeks, so that diagnosis and treatment are greatly delayed. Polymerase chain reaction can be successfully performed on sputum, fluid aspirates, and tissue homogenates; its sensitivity is comparable with that of culture, and it requires far less time. The technology of poly-

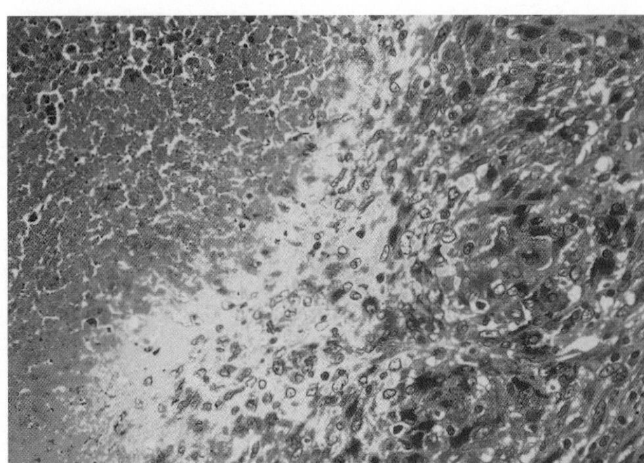

FIGURE 23.10. Tuberculous lymphadenitis with area of caseous necrosis (*right*) and epithelioid cells stained by Leu-M1 antibody (*left*). Anti-Leu-M1/alkaline phosphatase stain.

Checklist

MYCOBACTERIUM TUBERCULOSIS LYMPHADENITIS

History of tuberculosis
Positive tuberculin test
Multiple lymph nodes involved
Caseation necrosis
Coalescent lesions
Langhans giant cells
Epithelioid cells
CD4+ T cells, rare B cells
Bacilli visualized by acid-fast stainings
Antigen deposits identified by monoclonal antibodies
M. tuberculosis organisms cultured on specific media
Fibrosis, hyalinization
Occasional calcification

merase chain reaction has also been adapted to formalin-fixed, paraffin-embedded tissues, so that *M. tuberculosis* organisms can be detected in 4 to 5 hours and archival cases can be investigated (25,26). In culture, bacterial colonies of *M. tuberculosis* var *hominis* on Lowenstein-Jensen slant preparations can be seen in about 4 weeks; they appear dry, rough, and cauliflower-like (20). Their identification can be confirmed by biochemical tests. The number of positive results is substantially greater with cultures than with smears, and in one series, only 22% of culture-positive cases also had positive smears (27). In a series of 59 patients with cervical lymph node tuberculosis from Helsinki, *M. tuberculosis* organisms were isolated from 41 specimens (69%), equally often from caseating and noncaseating lesions. No mycobacteria were isolated from 10 patients who had received antituberculosis drugs before the biopsy (28). BCG lymphadenitis shows epithelioid granulomas with giant cells and restricted, centrally located necrosis with few acid fast-bacilli in immunocompetent patients, and large, stellate, caseous abscesses without giant cells and numerous bacilli in immunodeficient patients (11,29).

Indirect Evidence

Demonstration of acid-fast bacilli in sputum or gastric washings

Growth of bacilli in culture
Positive tuberculin test in children
Recent conversion of tuberculin test in adults
Diagnostic radiographic pulmonary lesions

DIFFERENTIAL DIAGNOSIS

- *Mycobacterium avium–intracellulare* lymphadenitis: Almost exclusively in AIDS patients. Sheets of phagocytic histiocytes filled with acid-fast bacilli. Granulomas and giant cells infrequent. Necrosis, focal; fibrosis, minimal; calcifications, absent.
- BCG lymphadenitis: Lymph nodes showing collections of histiocytes and extensive necrosis. Acid-fast bacilli are abundant; giant cells and granulomas are absent.
- *Histoplasma* lymphadenitis: Necrosis may be extensive and is usually associated with calcification. Grocott methenamine silver staining reveals the characteristic yeasts of *Histoplasma capsulatum.*
- Cat-scratch lymphadenitis: The stellate areas of necrosis include polymorphonuclear leukocytes. Warthin-Starry staining may identify the aggregates of bacilli.
- Sarcoidosis lymphadenopathy: Granulomas are well organized and demarcated by fibrocollagen. Necrosis is minimal or absent. Plasma cells are present. Schaumann and asteroid bodies are occasionally present. Acid-fast bacilli are absent. Kveim-Siltzbach test is positive.

REFERENCES

1. Wolinsky E. Mycobacteria. In: Davis BD, Dulbecco R, Eisen HN, et al., eds. Microbiology, 3rd ed. Hagerstown, MD: Harper & Row, 1980:723–742.
2. Bloom BR, Murray CJL. Tuberculosis: commentary on a reemergent killer. Science 1992;257:1055–1064.
3. Bass JB. The face of TB changes again. Hosp Pract 1989;(April 30):81–100.
4. Davidson PT. Tuberculosis. New views of an old disease. N Engl J Med 1985;312:1514–1516.
5. Sunderam G, McDonald RJ, Maniatis T, et al. Tuberculosis as a manifestation of the acquired immunodeficiency syndrome (AIDS). JAMA 1986;256:362–366.
6. Ramaswamy G, Rao SV, Reddy SA, et al. Mycobacterial infection and acquired immunodeficiency syndrome: a New York City hospital experience. Lab Med 1988;19:652–654.

7. Sinnott JT, Emmanuel PJ. Mycobacterial infections in the transplant patient. Semin Respir Infect 1990;5:65–73.
8. Barnes PF, Bloch AB, Davidson ED, et al. N Engl J Med 1991; 324:1644.
9. Shafer RW, Kim DS, Weiss JP, et al. Extrapulmonary tuberculosis in patients with human immunodeficiency virus infection. Medicine 1991;70:384–397.
10. Stansfeld AG. Inflammatory and reactive disorders. In: Stansfeld AG, ed. Lymph node biopsy interpretation. Edinburgh: Churchill Livingstone, 1985:85–141.
11. Al-Bhlal AL. Pathologic findings for bacille Calmette-Guérin infections in immunocompetent and immunocompromised patients. Am J Clin Pathol 2000;113:703–708.
12. El Dein AB, Nabeeh A. Tuberculous iliac lymphadenitis: a rare complication of intravesical bacillus Calmette-Guérin and cause of tumor overstaging. J Urol 1996;156:1766–1767.
13. Abramowsky C, Gonzalez B, Sorensen RU. Disseminated bacillus Calmette-Guérin infections in patients with primary immunodeficiencies. Am J Clin Pathol 1993;100:22–26.
14. Ninane J. Grymonprez A, Burtonboy G, et al. Disseminated BCG in HIV infection. Arch Dis Child 1988;63:1268–1269.
15. Wilkins EW Jr, Galdabini JJ. Esophageal diverticulum associated with a mass in the neck. N Engl J Med 1977;296:384–390.
16. Youmans GP. Mechanisms of immunity in tuberculosis. Pathobiol Annu 1979;9:137–161.
17. Slack MPE. Mycobacterial infections. In: McGee, et al., eds. Oxford textbook of pathology, vol 1. Oxford: Oxford University Press, 1992:481–484.
18. Ioachim HL. Granulomatous lesions of lymph nodes. In: Ioachim HL, ed. Pathology of granulomas. New York: Raven Press, 1983:151–187.
19. Strole WE, Compton C. A 28-year-old Cambodian immigrant woman with recent fever and abdominal distention. N Engl J Med 1986;315:952–957.
20. Bartlett JG, Mark EJ. Progressive pulmonary infiltration in a 41-year-old man. N Engl J Med 1977;297:1390–1398.
21. Van den Oord JJ, De Wolf-Peters C, Facchetti F, et al. Cellular composition of hypersensitivity-type granulomas. Immunohistochemical analysis of tuberculous and sarcoidal lymphadenitis. Hum Pathol 1984;15:559–565.
22. Brincker H, Pedersen NT. Immunological marker patterns in granulomatous lymph node lesions. Histopathology 1989;15: 495–503.
23. Humphrey DM, Weiner MH. Mycobacterial antigen detection by immunohistochemistry in pulmonary tuberculosis. Hum Pathol 1987;18:701–708.
24. Barbolini G, Bisetti A, Colizzi V, et al. Immunohistologic analysis of mycobacterial antigens by monoclonal antibodies in tuberculosis and mycobacteriosis. Hum Pathol 1989;20:1078– 1083.
25. Akcan Y, Tuncer S, Hayran M, et al. PCR on disseminated tuberculosis in bone marrow and liver biopsy specimens: correlation to histopathological and clinical diagnosis. Scand J Infect Dis 1997;29:271–274.
26. Marchetti G, Gori A, Catozzi L, et al. Evaluation of PCR in detection of *Mycobacterium tuberculosis* from formalin-fixed, paraffin-embedded tissues: comparison of four amplification assays. J Clin Microbiol 1998;36:1512–1517.
27. Boyd JC, Marr JJ. Decreasing reliability of acid-fast smear techniques for detection of tuberculosis. Ann Intern Med 1975;82: 489–492.
28. Huhti E, Brander E, Paloheimo S, et al. Tuberculosis of the cervical lymph nodes: a clinical, pathological and bacteriological study. Tubercle 1975;56:27–37.
29. Ioachim HL. Pathology of AIDS. Textbook and atlas. Philadelphia: JB Lippincott Co, 1989.

24

NONTUBERCULOUS MYCOBACTERIAL LYMPHADENITIS

A. Atypical Mycobacterial Lymphadenitis

DEFINITION

Lymphadenitides caused by nontuberculous mycobacteria.

SYNONYM

Nontuberculous mycobacterial lymphadenitides.

ETIOLOGY

A variety of mycobacteria, referred to as *nontuberculous* or *atypical,* are widely spread in nature, associated with water, soil, and vegetation. They are acid-fast, like other mycobacteria, but their culture characteristics are different, and many are resistant to streptomycin and isoniazid (1,2). They may not induce granuloma formation and under normal conditions are not pathogenic for humans. A detailed classification made by Runyon according to growth rate and pigment production includes such types as *Mycobacterium marinum, Mycobacterium fortuitum, Mycobacterium kansasii, Mycobacterium scrofulaceum,* and others (3). *Mycobacterium avium* and *Mycobacterium intracellulare* have emerged as major pathogens for persons with AIDS and are described separately in Part B of this chapter.

PATHOGENESIS

In contrast to tuberculosis, the diseases caused by atypical mycobacteria, although infectious, are not communicable (3). Atypical mycobacteria have been recognized as a cause of chronic lymphadenitis in children. In a study of 36 lymph node biopsies in children, atypical mycobacteria were recovered by culture, and bacilli were identified in tissues by acid-fast staining (4). A review of 30 cases of nontuberculous mycobacterial infections showed that 18 involved children, and 10 cases involved patients with immunosuppression or hematologic diseases (5). Swimming pool granulomas caused by *M. marinum* and localized cervical lymphadenopathies caused by various other atypical mycobacteria have been reported in children (6). *M. kansasii* is known to cause cervical lymph node infections in children. These are more often submandibular, unilateral, and associated with erythema and abscess formation (2). In adults, nontuberculous mycobacterial infections have occurred in patients whose immunity has been iatrogenically suppressed for the treatment of malignant disease or the prevention of organ transplant rejection (5). Infections caused by nontuberculous mycobacteria have been reported in kidney, heart, and liver transplant recipients (7). *M. kansasii, M. fortuitum, M. chelonae,* and *M. marinum* produced nodular lesions, more often in the skin and lungs; these generally remained localized but involved lymph nodes when the infection was able to disseminate. Atypical mycobacterial infections have been reported in 9% to 25% of cases of hairy cell leukemia; the prevalence is higher than in any other malignancy, possibly because of the monocyte deficiency associated with this neoplasm (8). The mycobacterium most often reported in infections complicating hairy cell leukemia is *M. kansasii* involving the lymph nodes and lungs (9).

HISTOPATHOLOGY

The lymph node lesions caused by atypical mycobacteria tend to be suppurative, particularly in children (2). In some cases, the histologic changes may be indistinguishable from those of tuberculosis, but in others, a dimorphic pattern of coexistent suppurative and granulomatous inflammation without caseation has been described (4) (Figs. 24.1–24.3). It is generally thought that the lesions are more acute and more exudative and contain larger amounts of acid-fast bacilli in atypical than in typical tuberculosis. This probably reflects the immunodeficiency of the host rather than the virulence of the pathogens. The presence of polymorphonuclear leukocytes in

Checklist

ATYPICAL MYCOBACTERIAL LYMPHADENITIDES

Children or immunosuppressed adults
Extensive necrosis
Polymorphonuclear leukocytes in areas of necrosis
Dimorphic (suppurative plus granulomatous) pattern
Abundant acid-fast bacilli

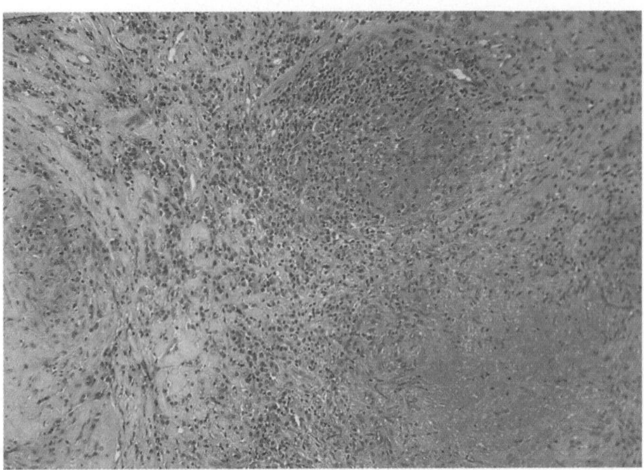

FIGURE 24.1. Paratuberculosis lymphadenitis. Cervical lymph node in a 6-year-old child. Loose granuloma with necrosis. Hematoxylin, phloxine, and saffron stain.

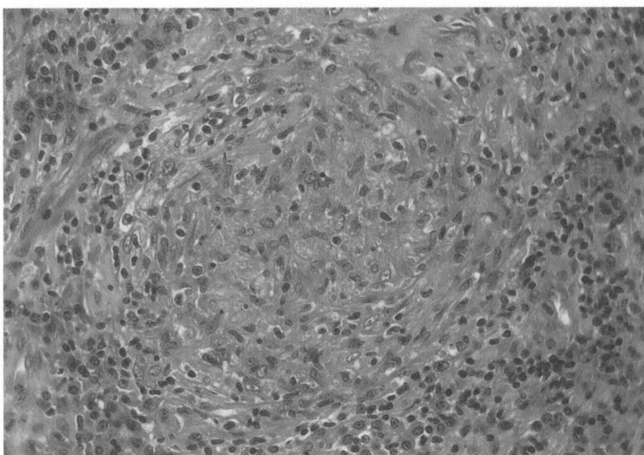

FIGURE 24.3. Same section as in Fig. 24.1. Granuloma poorly formed, lack of typical epithelioid cells and giant cells. Hematoxylin, phloxine, and saffron stain.

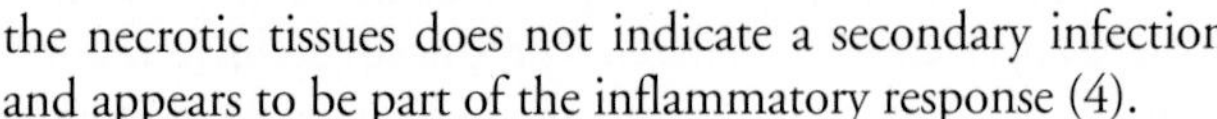

the necrotic tissues does not indicate a secondary infection and appears to be part of the inflammatory response (4).

DIFFERENTIAL DIAGNOSIS

- *Mycobacterium tuberculosis* lymphadenitis: Fewer organisms, more organized granulomas. Definitive diagnosis is possible only by culture.

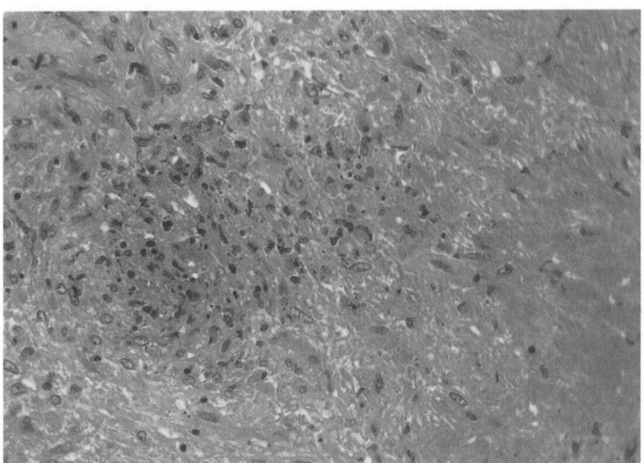

FIGURE 24.2. Same section as in Fig. 24.1. Poorly formed granuloma with spindle-shaped histiocytes, lymphocytes, and few neutrophils. Hematoxylin, phloxine, and saffron stain.

REFERENCES

1. Karlson AG. Mycobacteria of surgical interest. Surg Clin North Am 1973;53:905–917.
2. Milliard M. Tuberculosis. In: Anderson WAD, Kissane JM, eds. Pathology, vol 2. St. Louis: Mosby, 1977:1107–1124.
3. Wolinsky E. Nontuberculous mycobacteria and associated diseases. Am Rev Respir Dis 1979;119:107.
4. Reid JD, Wolinsky E. Histopathology of lymphadenitis caused by atypical mycobacteria. Am Rev Respir Dis 1969;99:8–12.
5. Chester AC, Winn WC Jr. Unusual and newly recognized patterns of nontuberculous mycobacterial infection with emphasis on the immunocompromised host. Pathol Annu 1986;21:251–271.
6. Lincoln EM, Gilbert LA. Disease in children due to mycobacteria other than *Mycobacterium tuberculosis.* Am Rev Respir Dis 1972; 105:683.
7. Patel R, Roberts GD, Keating MR, et al. Infections due to nontuberculous mycobacteria in kidney, heart and liver transplant recipients. CID 1994;19:263–273.
8. Weinstein RA, Golomb HM, Grumet G. Hairy cell leukemia: association with disseminated atypical mycobacterial infection. Cancer 1981;48:380–383.
9. Mc Loud TC, Harris NL. Case record 52-1982. N Engl J Med 1982;307:1693–1700.

24

NONTUBERCULOUS MYCOBACTERIAL LYMPHADENITIS

B. Mycobacterium Avium-Intracellulare Lymphadenitis

DEFINITION

Lymphadenitis caused by *Mycobacterium avium–intracellulare* (MAI) complex.

SYNONYM

MAI lymphadenitis.

ETIOLOGY

M. avium and *M. intracellulare* are two closely related atypical or nontuberculous *Mycobacterium* species, similar in their culture properties, that are usually referred to as the *MAI complex.*

EPIDEMIOLOGY

Mycobacteriosis, the disseminated MAI infection, is very rarely seen in normal people. The incidence in transplant patients, although low, far exceeds that in the healthy population. In transplant recipients, 25% to 40% of mycobacterial infections are caused by nontuberculous strains, in comparison with 5% to 10% of mycobacterial infections in the general population. These patients also experience a higher rate of extrapulmonary disease (1). In patients with AIDS, mycobacteriosis has emerged as one of the most critical, life-threatening opportunistic infections, with high rates of morbidity and mortality (2,3). In North American patients with AIDS, mycobacteriosis can be identified in 40% to 60% of cases in the terminal stages of the disease (4).

PATHOGENESIS

In the rare cases in which MAI organisms infect persons who do not have AIDS, they cause chronic, localized, slowly progressive pulmonary disease in the elderly and in children (2). It is only in association with AIDS that disseminated MAI infection, with multiple organ localization and frequent fatal outcome, occurs. The source of infection is the environment, where MAI organisms are ubiquitous. The reason for the selective infection of AIDS patients is unknown, but it appears to be related to specific defects in the function of macrophages, possibly failure of the depleted CD4+ T cells to activate them and their inability to secrete lymphokines (5). As a result, the macrophages are loaded with MAI organisms, which they carry from one organ to another without being able to eradicate them (6). Alternative explanations have focused on the depletion of a specific population of T lymphocytes that are particularly effective against MAI organisms (7).

HISTOPATHOLOGY

Peripheral and visceral lymph nodes are involved by mycobacteriosis. They are indolent and moderately enlarged, and biopsies are frequently performed to rule out lymphoma or metastatic tumor. The architecture is partially or totally effaced, follicles are inapparent, and lymphocytes are profoundly depleted (Fig. 24.4). The normal structures and cell populations are replaced by sheets of large, pale histiocytes with abundant striated or foamy cytoplasm and small dark nuclei without pleomorphism or mitoses (8,9). The striations and vacuoles of the cytoplasm are in fact the unstained, negative images of the MAI bacilli (Fig. 24.5). These histiocytes are different from the epithelioid cells of tuberculosis, rather resembling Gaucher cells and possibly representing histiocytes in an intermediate stage of development between an unstimulated macrophage and a well-formed epithelioid cell (7–10). The MAI histiocytes rarely form multinucleated giant cells and are not organized into granulomas (Fig. 24.6). Necrosis, calcification, and fibrosis also are not part of the picture. Aggregates of histiocytes containing MAI organisms may be found in the lymph nodes, bone marrow, spleen, liver, and gastrointestinal tract of up to 10% of AIDS patients at autopsy (7). Stainings with Ziehl-Neelsen

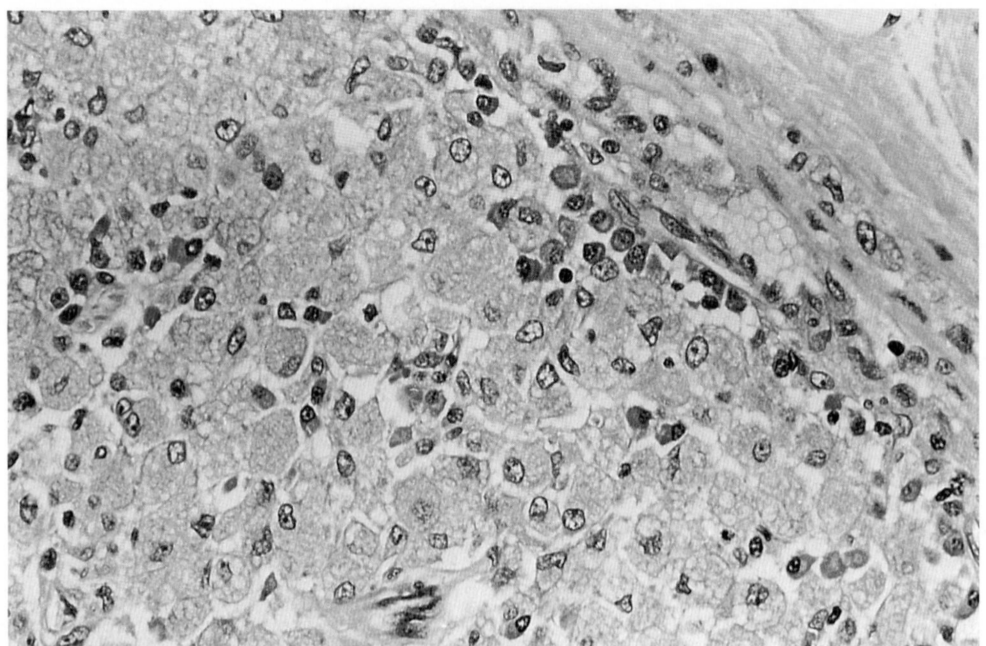

FIGURE 24.4. Lymph node cortical architecture (capsule, *upper right*) replaced by sheets of large, pale-staining, foamy histiocytes. Hematoxylin, phloxine, and saffron stain.

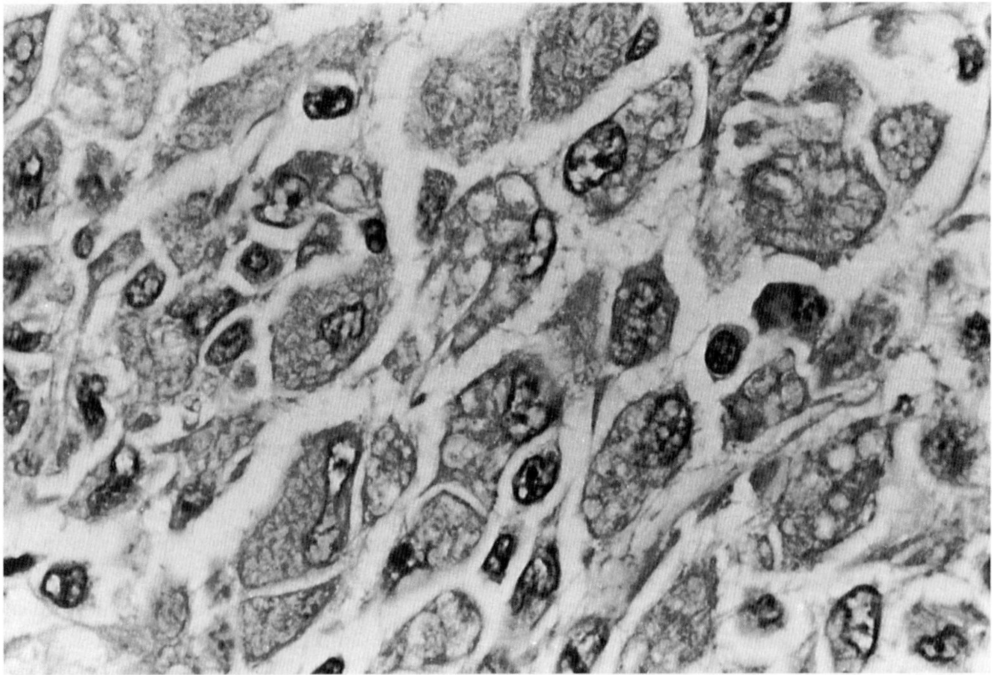

FIGURE 24.5. Histiocytes with abundant foamy cytoplasm, intracytoplasmic vacuoles, striations representing negative images of *Mycobacterium avium–intracellulare* organisms, and small, darkly stained nuclei. Hematoxylin, phloxine, and saffron stain.

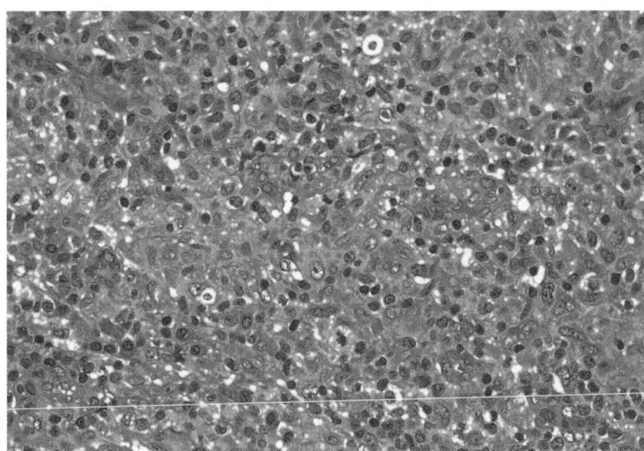

FIGURE 24.6. Lymph node infiltrated diffusely by foamy histiocytes containing *Mycobacterium avium–intracellulare* organisms. No granulomas, giant cells, necrosis, or fibrosis is present. Hematoxylin, phloxine, and saffron stain.

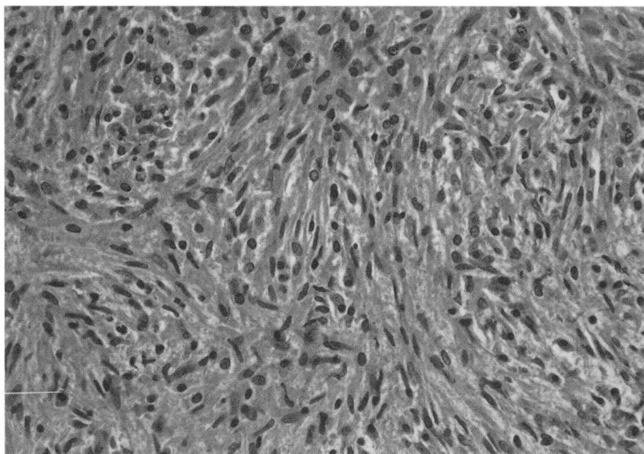

FIGURE 24.8. Histoid mycobacteriosis. Lymph node parenchyma is replaced by bundles of elongated spindle cell histiocytes containing *Mycobacterium avium–intracellulare* organisms. Hematoxylin, phloxine, and saffron stain.

or Kinyoun stain reveal large amounts of acid-fast bacilli engulfed by the distended histiocytes (Fig. 24.7). It has been observed that the number of MAI bacilli is far greater in AIDS patients with mycobacteriosis than in those who have been medically immunosuppressed (7,11).

Mycobacterial Spindle Cell Pseudotumor

A rare form of mycobacterial lymphadenopathy is the MAI spindle cell pseudotumor. In this case, for unknown reasons, the MAI-containing histiocytes are spindle-shaped, resembling fibroblasts, and arranged in bundles or whorls (Fig. 24.8). The spindle-shaped appearance of histiocytes engulfing mycobacteria was first observed in leprosy and named *histoid form* (12). A rare case of histoid cell proliferation was described in a transplant patient with *Mycobacterium tuberculosis* infection (13). Other cases of MAI spindle cell pseudotumors were seen in the lymph nodes of AIDS patients (14–18). Because of the elongated appearance of the histiocytes, these lesions resemble various spindle cell proliferations of lymph nodes, such as myofibroblastoma, inflammatory pseudotumor, Kaposi sarcoma, and even leiomyosarcoma. Kaposi sarcoma frequently involves the lymph nodes of AIDS patients and in some cases coexists with spindle-shaped MAI lymphadenitis; it is extremely important to differentiate the two. As reported, both lesions, sometimes in the same lymph node, form bundles of spindle-shaped cells and can be distinguished from each other by the erythrocyte-containing slitlike spaces of Kaposi sarcoma and the bacilli-containing striated histiocytes of mycobacteriosis (18). Histochemical and immunohistochemical stainings are necessary to confirm the diagnosis, which in both instances significantly affects management. The histiocytes stain for the specific markers CD68, lysozyme (19), α-antichymotrypsin (17), and vimentin. Interestingly, stainings for desmin and actin have also been reported (16) (Fig. 24.9),

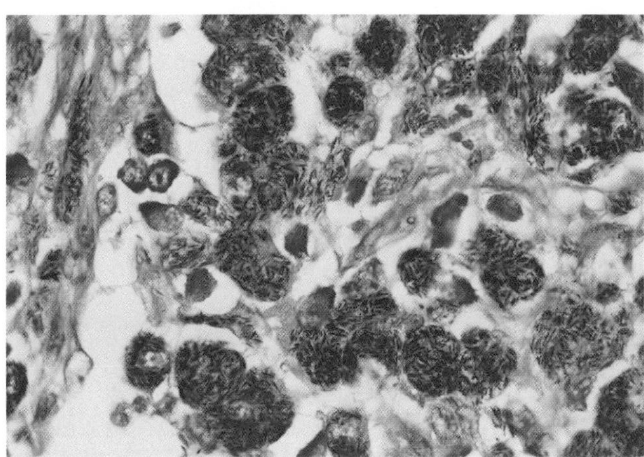

FIGURE 24.7. Foamy histiocytes filled with huge numbers of acid-fast mycobacteria. Ziehl-Neelsen stain.

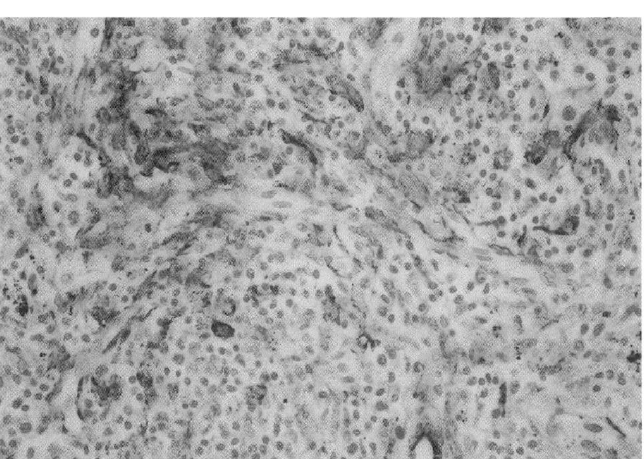

FIGURE 24.9. Histoid mycobacteriosis. Spindle-shaped histiocytes containing *Mycobacterium avium–intracellulare* organisms that stain with actin. Anti-actin/peroxidase stain.

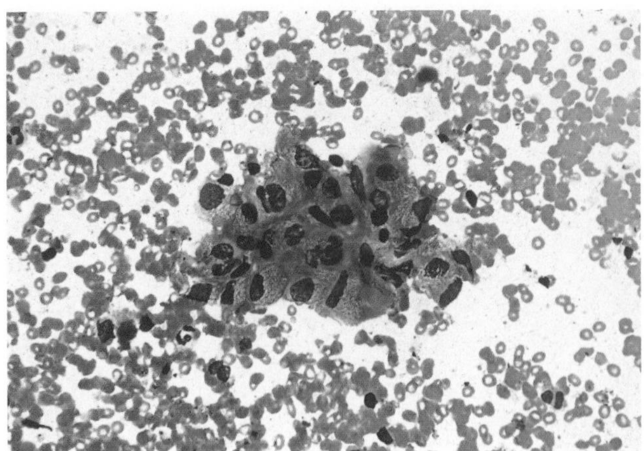

FIGURE 24.10. Fine needle aspiration of retroperitoneal tumor. Large cells with irregularly shaped nuclei suspected of being a malignant neoplasm. Giemsa stain.

which in the case of spindle-shaped mycobacterial lymphadenopathy may raise difficult problems of differential diagnosis with leiomyomas or sarcomas until an acid-fast stain may provide the answer. It appears that actin-like material is also present in other microorganisms, such as *Pseudomonas* (20) and *Mycoplasma* (21), which explains the similar positive staining for actin in the MAI-containing spindle-shaped histiocytes (16).

CYTOPATHOLOGY

Touch imprint preparations to evaluate MAI-infected lymph nodes can be used successfully for intraoperative diagnosis (19) (Figs. 24.10 and 24.11). Touch imprints of lymph nodes, spleen, and bone marrow, stained with Diff-Quik or Wright-Giemsa stain and air-dried, reveal the typical histiocytes with negative images of bacilli arranged in parallel or crisscross bundles at surgery or autopsy. Acid-fast stains, immunostains, or both can also be applied.

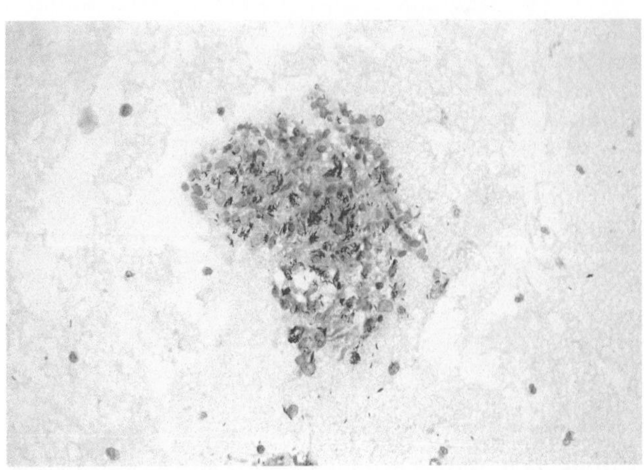

FIGURE 24.11. Same cells show abundant intracellular *Mycobacterium avium–intracellulare* organisms. Ziehl-Neelsen stain.

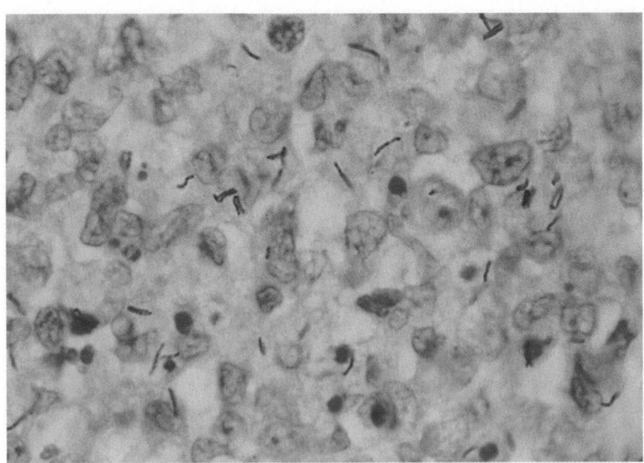

FIGURE 24.12. *Mycobacterium avium–intracellulare* lymphadenitis. Foamy histiocytes with numerous acid-fast bacilli. Ziehl-Neelsen stain.

HISTOCHEMISTRY

The Ziehl-Neelsen (Figs. 24.11 and 24.12), Kinyoun, Fite-Faraco, and Grocott methenamine silver (Fig. 24.13) stains easily show numerous MAI bacilli within polygonal or spindle-shaped histiocytes.

IMMUNOHISTOCHEMISTRY

The histiocytes stain with antibodies against CD68 and lysozyme, in contrast to the cells of Kaposi sarcoma, which stain with antibodies for CD31 and CD34 markers (18). It has been reported that the lymphocytes accompanying the aggregates of histiocytes in mycobacteriosis do not include B cells or natural killer T cells, as they do in the better-formed granulomas of other infections (22,23). The ratio of CD4+ to CD8+ cells is greater than 2 in the former case and less than 1 in the latter according to the same studies.

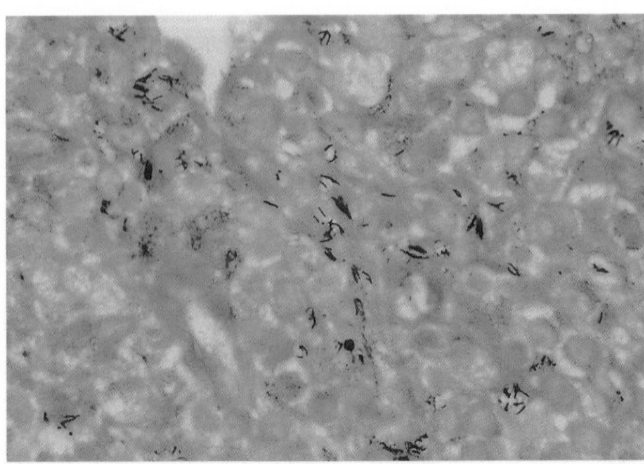

FIGURE 24.13. *Mycobacterium avium–intracellulare* lymphadenitis. Foamy histiocytes with numerous silver-stained bacilli. Gomori methenamine silver stain.

Checklist

MYCOBACTERIUM AVIUM–INTRACELLULARE LYMPHADENITIS

HIV-positive persons
Low CD4+ T-cell count
Multiple enlarged lymph nodes
Effaced architecture
Lymphocyte depletion
Sheets of large, pale, striated histiocytes
Abundant intracellular acid-fast bacilli also positive for S-100 protein and Grocott methenamine silver
Rare granulomas and giant cells
Lack of necrosis, calcification, fibrosis
Spindle-cell (histoid) form possibly staining for actin and desmin

Immunostaining of the mycobacteria within the histiocytes for protein S-100 provides an additional means of differentiating among these lesions (18,24) (Fig. 24.14). Specific antibodies for desmin, actin, and tubulin also stain intracellular MAI organisms, although this finding has not been confirmed by all reported studies (16,17).

The polymerase chain reaction has been successfully used to identify various mycobacteria in pathologic materials. The presence of *M. tuberculosis* and MAI organisms could be also ascertained with polymerase chain reaction in paraffin sections; however, the sensitivity of the technique was not significantly greater than that of the acid-fast stains (25).

DIFFERENTIAL DIAGNOSIS

- *M. tuberculosis* lymphadenitis shows more necrosis in the exudative phase and more granulomas, giant cells, and fibrosis in the proliferative phase. Few acid-fast bacilli are generally found, in contrast to the large number present in MAI lymphadenitis.
- *Histoplasma* lymphadenitis: Sheets of large epithelioid cells containing yeasts that stain with Grocott methenamine silver; absence of acid-fast bacilli.
- *Cryptococcus* lymphadenitis: Sheets of large epithelioid cells containing yeasts that stain with mucicarmine; absence of acid-fast bacilli.
- Sarcoidosis lymphadenopathy: Well-organized granulomas with giant cells, plasma cells, and peripheral fibrocollagen; absence of acid-fast bacilli.
- Spindle cell tumors (leiomyosarcoma, fibrosarcoma) and pseudotumors of lymph nodes: Absence of acid-fast bacilli.
- Kaposi sarcoma: Erythrocyte-containing slitlike spaces, cells positive for CD31 and CD34 markers; absence of acid-fast bacilli.

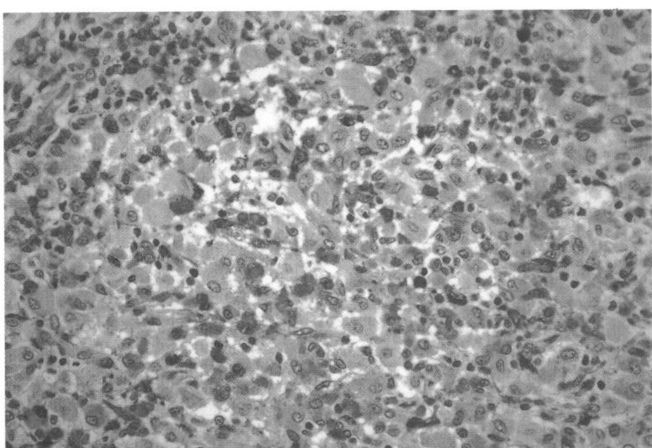

FIGURE 24.14. *Mycobacterium avium–intracellulare* lymphadenitis. Foamy histiocytes with large amounts of S-100-positive bacilli. S-100/alkaline phosphatase stain.

REFERENCES

1. Sinnott JT, Emmanuel PJ. Mycobacterial infections in the transplant patient. Semin Respir Infect 1990;5:65–73.
2. Zakowski P, Fliegel S, Berlin GW, et al. Disseminated *Mycobacterium avium–intracellulare* infection in homosexual men dying of acquired immunodeficiency. JAMA 1982;248:2980–2982.
3. Greene JB, Sidju GS, Lewin S, et al. *Mycobacterium avium–intracellulare*: a cause of disseminated life-threatening infection in homosexuals and drug abusers. Ann Intern Med 1982;97:539–546.
4. Pitchenik AE, Cole C, Russell BW, et al. Tuberculosis, atypical mycobacteriosis, and the acquired immunodeficiency syndrome among Haitian and non-Haitian patients in South Florida. Ann Intern Med 1984;101: 641–645.
5. Edelman AS, Zolla-Pazner S. AIDS: a syndrome of immune dysregulation, dysfunction, and deficiency. FASEB J 1989;3:22–30.
6. Ioachim HL. Immunopathogenesis of human immunodeficiency virus infection. Cancer Res 1990;50:5612s–5617s.

7. Klatt EC, Jensen DF, Meyer PR. Pathology of *Mycobacterium avium–intracellulare* infection in acquired immunodeficiency syndrome. Hum Pathol 1987;18:709–714.
8. Ioachim HL. Pathology of AIDS. Textbook and color atlas. Philadelphia: JB Lippincott Co, 1989.
9. Ioachim HL. Biopsy diagnosis in human immunodeficiency virus infection and acquired immunodeficiency syndrome. Arch Pathol Lab Med 1990;114:284–295.
10. Mufarrij AA, Greco MA, Antopol SC, et al. The histopathology of cervical lymphadenitis caused by *Mycobacterium avium–Mycobacterium intracellulare* complex in an immunocompromised host. Hum Pathol 1982;13:78–81.
11. Farhi DC, Mason UG, Horsburgh CR. Pathologic findings in disseminated *Mycobacterium avium–intracellulare* infection: a report of 11 cases. Am J Clin Pathol 1986;85:67–73.
12. Wade HW. The histoid variety of lepromatous leprosy. Int J Lepr 1963;31:129–142.
13. Sekosan M, Cleto M, Senseng C, et al. Spindle cell pseudotumors in the lungs due to *Mycobacterium tuberculosis* in a transplant patient. Am J Surg Pathol 1994;18:1065–1068.
14. Wood C, Nickoloff BJ, Todes-Taylor NR. Pseudotumor resulting from atypical mycobacterial infection: a "histoid" variety of *Mycobacterium avium–intracellulare* complex infection. Am J Clin Pathol 1985;83:524–527.
15. Brandwein M, Choi HH, Strauchen J, et al. Spindle cell reaction to nontuberculous mycobacteriosis in AIDS mimicking a spindle cell neoplasm: evidence for dual histiocytic and fibroblast-like characteristics of spindle cells. Virchows Arch A Pathol Anat Histopathol 1990;416:218–221.
16. Umlas J, Federman M, Crawford C, et al. Spindle cell pseudotumor due to *Mycobacterium avium–intracellulare* in patients with acquired immunodeficiency syndrome (AIDS). Positive staining of mycobacteria for cytoskeleton filaments. Am J Surg Pathol 1991;15:1181–1187.
17. Chen KTK. Mycobacterial spindle cell pseudotumor of lymph nodes. Am J Surg Pathol 1992;16:276–281.
18. Logani S, Lucas DR, Cheng JD, et al. Spindle cell tumors associated with mycobacteria in lymph nodes of HIV-positive patients. Kaposi sarcoma with mycobacteria and mycobacterial pseudotumor. Am J Surg Pathol 1990;23:656–661.
19. Wolf DA, Wu CD, Medeiros U. Mycobacterial pseudotumors of lymph node. A report of two cases diagnosed at the time of intraoperative consultation using touch imprint preparations. Arch Pathol Lab Med 1995;119:811–814.
20. Berk RS, Moon M, Highbee R, et al. Actin-like material in *Pseudomonas aeruginosa.* Infect Immun 1985;50:483–487.
21. Gobel U. Supramolecular structures in mycoplasmas. Yale J Biol Med 1983;56:695–700.
22. Van Den Oord JJ, De Wolf-Peters C, Facchetti F, et al. Cellular composition of hypersensitivity-type granulomas. Hum Pathol 1984;15:559–565.
23. Brincker H, Pedersen NT. Immunological marker patterns in granulomatous lymph node lesions. Histopathology 1989;15: 495–503.
24. Taskin M, Hoda R, Santagada E, et al. S100 may identify granulomas of *Mycobacterium avium–intracellulare.* Mod Pathol 1996;9:132A.
25. Perosio PM, Frank TS. Detection and species identification of mycobacteria in paraffin sections of lung biopsy specimens by the polymerase chain reaction. Am J Clin Pathol 1993;100:643–647.

25

MYCOBACTERIUM LEPRAE LYMPHADENITIS

DEFINITION

Lymphadenitis caused by infection with *Mycobacterium leprae.*

ETIOLOGY

Morphologically, *M. leprae* is almost indistinguishable from *Mycobacterium tuberculosis* but is slightly less acid-resistant in its staining properties (1). The human leprosy bacillus is an obligate intracellular parasite that is notable for its limited host range and its failure to grow *in vitro,* which has prevented progress in research and the development of vaccines. A leprosy-like disease was reproduced in armadillos, and the leprosy bacillus was grown in the mouse footpad (2). In humans, the transmission of leprosy is by direct contact through skin abrasions or mucous membranes of the mouth or nose. Infectivity is not high, even among close family contacts (3).

EPIDEMIOLOGY

About 13 million people are estimated to have leprosy around the world; 60% of the cases occur in Asia (3,4), and 3.5 million of these are in India (2). The prevalence is not high—1% to 5%, even in endemic areas. In the United States, the number of cases has increased, and leprosy is reported among immigrants from countries where the disease is endemic (3,4).

PATHOGENESIS

The clinicopathologic manifestations of leprosy directly reflect the relationship between infectious agent and host. The host response is determined by the host immune status, which appears to be affected in leprosy by a diminished number of circulating T cells (5). The disease takes two principal forms, lepromatous and tuberculoid, which represent opposite extremes of the immune response; a spectrum of intermediate lesions and manifestations is seen (6). Studies in which HLA typing is used indicate that individual receptivity for leprosy is genetically determined and that the tuberculoid form is related to an HLA-linked recessive gene (7).

CLINICAL SYNDROME

Persons of any age may become infected; however, in areas of high endemicity, the disease is usually diagnosed in the first three decades of life (1). In lepromatous leprosy, cellular resistance against *M. leprae* is minimal, and patients may present with erythematous or hypopigmented skin macules, papules, nodules, plaques, or diffuse infiltrations. The lepromatous lesions are poorly defined and tend to become confluent. In this, the progressive phase of the disease, the lesions contain numerous lepra cells and large numbers of acid-fast bacilli. There is a deficiency of helper T cells specific for *M. leprae* antigens, and of suppressor T cells specific for *M. leprae* (8). The lepromin test result is generally negative. In tuberculoid leprosy, specific cellular immunity is pronounced, and skin lesions are sharply defined and localized. They include few lepra cells and rare bacilli; a proliferation of fibrous tissues is seen, and the lepromin test result is positive.

A distinctive feature of leprosy is involvement of nerves, which may occur in any phase of the disease. *M. leprae* is the only mycobacterium that regularly invades nerves (1). *M. leprae* multiplies in the skin histiocytes and the Schwann cells of nerves. Thus, the most characteristic clinical feature of leprosy is the association of skin and nerve lesions. Another distinctive feature of leprosy is the distribution of lesions in cooler parts of the body, particularly the skin, mucous membranes of the upper respiratory tract (turbinates, nasal septum, larynx), anterior part of the eye, testes, nerve trunks that are close to the skin surface, and lymph nodes that drain dermal lesions (9). When tests for syphilis are performed on

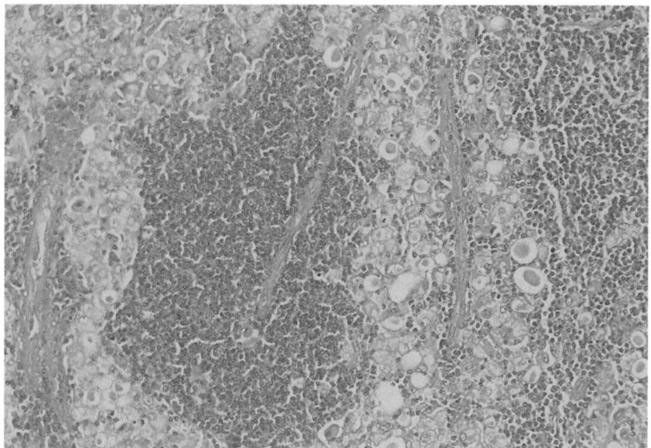

FIGURE 25.1. Lepromatous lymphadenitis. Large aggregates of foamy macrophages and globi (*right*) replace the lymphoid cells in parafollicular and medullary areas. Hematoxylin and eosin stain. (Courtesy of Dr. Wayne M. Meyers, Armed Forces Institute of Pathology, Washington, DC.)

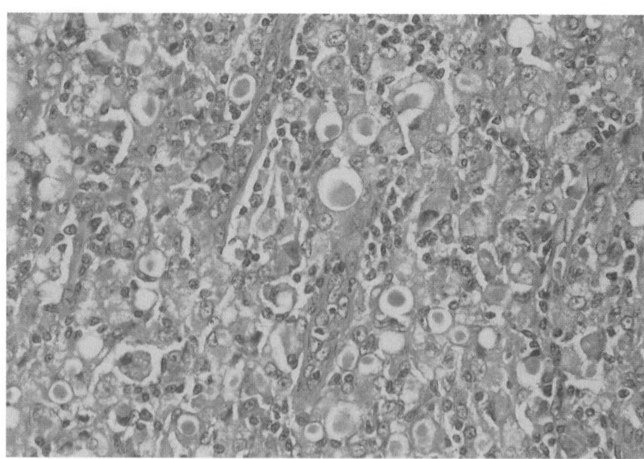

FIGURE 25.3. Lepra cells and globi in lepromatous leprosy replacing nodal lymphoid tissues. Hematoxylin and eosin stain. (Courtesy of Dr. Wayne M. Meyers, Armed Forces Institute of Pathology, Washington, DC.)

the sera of patients with moderately or advanced lepromatous leprosy, the results are frequently false-positive (1).

HISTOPATHOLOGY

Like those of other organs, lymph node lesions show a spectrum of changes that extends from lepromatous to tuberculoid leprosy. In a study of 77 lymph nodes from 62 patients with leprosy, representing the entire disease spectrum, Turk and Waters (10) documented the correlation of histologic lesions with clinical stage and lepromin test result.

In lepromatous leprosy lymphadenitis, the lymph nodes may be considerably enlarged. The paracortical areas are largely depleted of lymphocytes, which are replaced by sheets of histiocytes, including frequent lepra cells that contain large numbers of mycobacteria (Figs. 25.1 and 25.2). In early lesions, only one or a few bacilli are present in the cytoplasm of histiocytes. In advanced cases, typical foamy histiocytes or lepra cells containing masses of acid-fast bacilli (globi) are commonly seen (Figs. 25.2 and 25.3). Cells situated in the subcapsular region of the lymph nodes appear to be more heavily parasitized with bacilli than do those in deeper areas (10). The numbers of bacilli in histiocytes vary between microglobi and large globi, but after the containing cells degenerate, the bacilli are released free in the tissues (Fig. 25.4). The germinal centers are prominent, and large aggregates of plasma cells are present at the corticomedullary junction and in the medullary cords.

In tuberculoid leprosy lymphadenitis, the lymph nodes are generally smaller and the germinal centers inconspicuous. Non-necrotizing granulomas, similar to those of sarcoidosis, are scattered throughout the nodal parenchyma (Figs. 25.5 and 25.6). The histiocytes have the typical appearance of

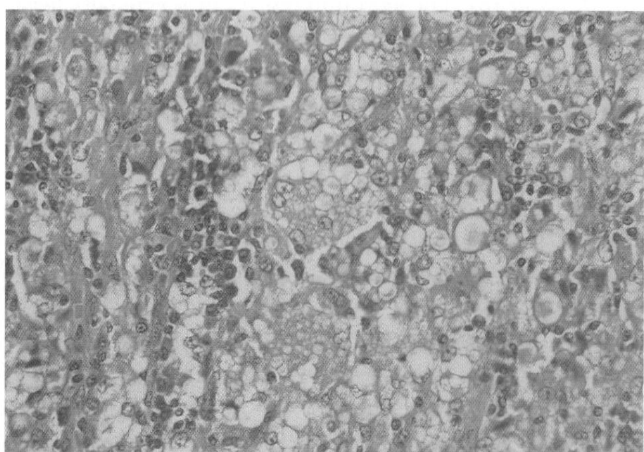

FIGURE 25.2. Foamy macrophages, or lepra cells, containing large amounts of bacilli replacing lymphoid tissues. Hematoxylin and eosin stain. (Courtesy of Dr. Wayne M. Meyers, Armed Forces Institute of Pathology, Washington, DC.)

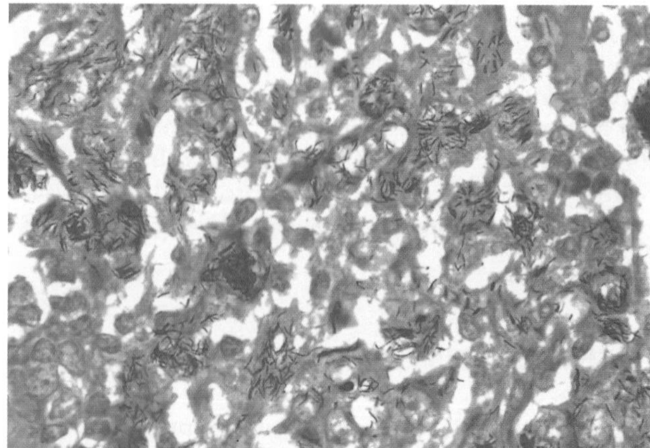

FIGURE 25.4. Lymph node section stained with Fite-Faraco stain shows large numbers of acid-fast bacilli in lepra cells and large globi. Fite-Faraco stain. (Courtesy of Dr. Wayne M. Meyers, Armed Forces Institute of Pathology, Washington, DC.)

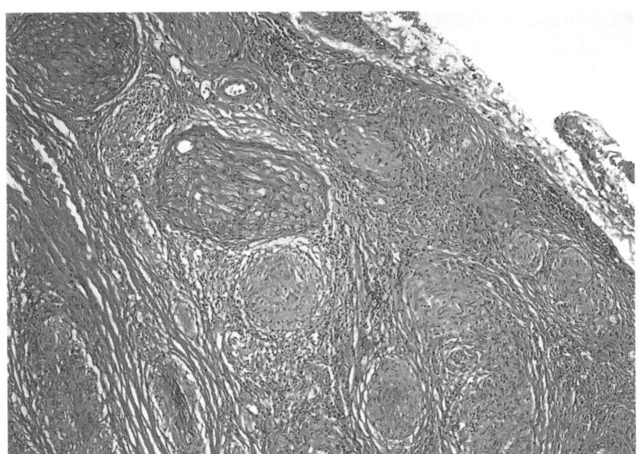

FIGURE 25.5. Inguinal lymph node with tuberculoid leprosy. Multiple granulomas in the perinodal tissues adjacent to nerves with degenerative lesions. Hematoxylin, phloxine, and saffron stain.

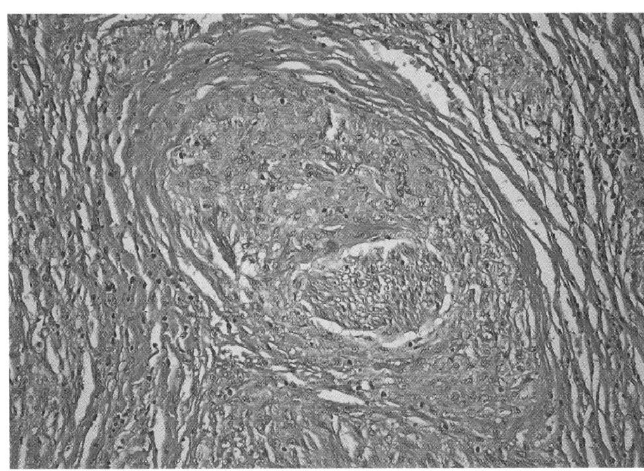

FIGURE 25.6. Same section as in Fig. 25.5. Degenerated nerve surrounded by epithelioid giant cell granuloma. Hematoxylin, phloxine, and saffron stain.

epithelioid cells and are arranged concentrically. Multinucleated giant cells of the Langhans type are present in the center of granulomas. The periphery is occupied by thick cuffs of lymphocytes that separate the granulomas, although these may occasionally coalesce. Nerves in the adjacent tissues degenerate and may be surrounded by granulomas (Fig. 25.6). Lepra cells are not seen, and acid-fast bacilli are very rare if they are present at all. In borderline leprosy, intermediate histologic patterns develop, whereas in patients treated for long periods, the lepromatous infiltrates are broken up by broad bands of lymphocytes that progressively repopulate the paracortical areas (10). The histoid leprosy described by Wade (11) is characterized by spindle-shaped histiocytes containing phagocytosed bacilli oriented parallel to the long axis of the cell. This form of leprosy appears to develop after prolonged medical treatment.

Checklist

MYCOBACTERIUM LEPRAE LYMPHADENITIS

- Cutaneous lesions
- Nerve involvement
- Enlarged lymph nodes
- Lepromatous leprosy
  - Paracortical areas depleted of lymphocytes
  - Aggregates of plasma cells
  - Sheets of histiocytes
  - Lepra cells with globi present
  - Acid-fast bacilli present
  - Lepromin test negative
  - Low level of specific immunity
- Tuberculoid leprosy
  - Non-necrotizing granulomas
  - Epithelioid cells, lymphocytes
  - Lepra cells absent
  - Acid-fast bacilli absent
  - Lepromin test positive
- Histoid leprosy
  - Spindle-shaped histiocytes
  - Abundant acid-fast bacilli

LABORATORY TESTS

Bacteriologic diagnosis is accomplished by staining acid-fast bacilli in lymph node smears, imprints, or sections with the Fite-Faraco, Ziehl-Neelsen, or Kinyoun stain (Fig. 25.4). The lepromin test is performed by intradermal injection of heat-killed *M. leprae* organisms. Patients with lepromatous leprosy show no reaction, whereas patients with tuberculoid leprosy have a papulonodular reaction that is maximal at 3 to 4 weeks. Histologically, the lesion consists of non-necrotizing epithelioid granulomas.

DIFFERENTIAL DIAGNOSIS

- All granulomatous lymphadenitides (tuberculosis, sarcoidosis, syphilis, brucellosis, lymphogranuloma venereum, fungal infections) must be considered in the differential diagnosis of leprosy lymphadenitis. As emphasized by Binford and Meyers (1), this is a difficult differential diagnosis, and because of the very serious consequences of a positive diagnosis, the formula "consistent with" or "compatible with" should not be used in this case. A positive diagnosis must take into account cutaneous lesions, involvement of nerves, the presence of acid-fast bacilli, and the result of a lepromin test.
- *Mycobacterium avium–intracellulare* lymphadenitis, with its sheets of histiocytes filled with acid-fast bacilli, closely resembles lepromatous lymphadenitis, and the distinction relies on epidemiologic, clinical, and serologic features.
- Spindle-shaped histiocytes stuffed with acid-fast *M. avium–intracellulare* bacilli may be indistinguishable from the spindle-shaped histiocytes of histoid leprosy.
- Fibroma, fibrosarcoma, and dermatofibrosarcoma resemble histoid leprosy; however, acid-fast bacilli are not present.

REFERENCES

1. Binford CH, Meyers WM. Leprosy. In: Binford CH, Connor DH, eds. Pathology of tropical and extraordinary diseases, vol 1. Washington, DC: Armed Forces Institute of Pathology, 1976: 205–225.
2. Storrs EE, Binford CH. Experimental lepromatous leprosy in nine-banded armadillos (*Dasypus novemcinctus Linn*). Am J Pathol 1978;92:813–816.
3. Shepard CC. Leprosy today. N Engl J Med 1982;307:1640–1641.
4. Bloom BR. Learning from leprosy: a perspective on immunology and the third world. J Immunol 1986;137:1–10.
5. Van Voorhis WC, Kaplan G, Sarno EN, et al. The cutaneous infiltrates of leprosy: cellular characteristics and the predominant T-cell phenotypes. N Engl J Med 1982;307:1593–1597.
6. Ridley DS, Jopling WH. Classification of leprosy according to immunity: a five-group system. Int J Lepr 1966;34:255.
7. De Vries RRP, van Eden W, van Rood JJ. HLA-linked control of the course of *M. leprae* infections. Lepr Rev 1981;52[Suppl 1]: 109–119.
8. Slack MPE. Mycobacterial infections. In: McGee, ed. Oxford textbook of pathology, vol 1. Oxford: Oxford University Press, 1992:481–484.
9. Binford CH. Pathology—the doorway to the understanding of leprosy. Am J Clin Pathol 1969;51:681–698.
10. Turk JL, Waters MFR. Immunological significance of changes in lymph nodes across the leprosy spectrum. Clin Exp Immunol 1971;8:363–376.
11. Wade HW. The histoid variety of lepromatous leprosy. Int J Lepr 1963:129–142.

PART III

SECTION FOUR

FUNGAL LYMPHADENITIDES

In the population at large, mycotic infections are generally restricted to the skin; however, in persons debilitated by chronic disease, treated for long periods with broad-spectrum antibiotics, or immunosuppressed by radiation and chemotherapy, deep-seated organs may be involved. Most fungi are regular saprophytes that may become pathogenic under such conditions. The AIDS epidemic has been accompanied by a substantial increase in visceral and disseminated mycoses and in other opportunistic infections. Some of these, such as histoplasmosis and coccidioidomycosis, are particularly prominent in the regions where they are normally endemic, becoming in such areas the most frequent complications of AIDS. In the present chapter, only the fungal infections that may affect lymph nodes are discussed.

26

CRYPTOCOCCUS LYMPHADENITIS

DEFINITION

Lymphadenitis caused by infection with *Cryptococcus neoformans.*

ETIOLOGY

C. neoformans is a saprophytic, monomorphic fungus that forms yeasts but not hyphae. The yeasts are round, about 10 μm in diameter, refractile, and surrounded by a thick mucopolysaccharide capsule. Budding is more common in *Cryptococcus* organisms than in any other yeasts. Single or double buds with narrow bases form that detach easily, reproducing the mother cell. Rapidly growing organisms may form chains of budding cells resembling hyphae (1,2). They are easily isolated from clinical specimens, forming moist, mucoid white colonies on Sabouraud agar. The cell walls stain with Grocott methenamine silver (GMS) and characteristically with mucicarmine and periodic acid–Schiff (PAS) stains.

PATHOGENESIS

C. neoformans is present worldwide, particularly in soil contaminated by pigeon excreta or the debris of pigeon roosts (2). *C. neoformans* is not highly pathogenic. The virulence factors are related to the capsule and include proteases, phospholipases, melanin, mannitol, and others, which interfere with phagocytosis and destruction of the organism (3). The infection is acquired by inhaling yeasts. In the lung, these generate a primary focus; lymphangitis and involvement of a regional lymph node follow, resulting in what is called a *primary pulmonary lymph node complex of cryptococcosis* (4). In normal, immunocompetent persons, this remains clinically occult and eventually undergoes fibrosis. Immunodeficient persons may acquire a new aerogenous infection, or an old, occult lesion may be reactivated.

According to the data of the Centers for Disease Control and Prevention, cryptococcosis occurs in about 7% of AIDS patients, although its incidence is probably higher in large urban locations (5).

CLINICAL SYNDROME

Cryptococcosis is one of the few fungal infections that affects both immunocompetent and immunodeficient persons (6). It generally starts as a primary pulmonary lymph node complex, which in immunocompetent persons becomes fibrosed and occult. In people susceptible to the infection because of neutropenia, diabetes, renal insufficiency, or corticosteroid therapy, cryptococcosis may become disseminated, with predominant organ localization, and involve the meninges and central nervous system (4,7,8). In AIDS, cryptococcosis may be the presenting manifestation or appear together with other opportunistic infections. The lymph nodes may be affected in relation to an occult focus of cryptococcosis or as part of the disseminated form (9). Involved lymph nodes show multiple nodular, confluent lesions that may be visible on radiologic examination (7).

HISTOPATHOLOGY

In lymph nodes, the lesions consist of scattered or confluent noncaseous granulomas. They are composed of lymphocytes, epithelioid cells, and numerous multinucleated giant cells containing large numbers of phagocytosed organisms. These are in the form of yeasts that may be barely visible as unstained circular forms with hematoxylin and eosin stain (Fig. 26.1) but are stained a brilliant red with PAS or mucicarmine stain (Fig. 26.2). The selective staining can be attributed to the 3- to 5-μm-thick mucopolysaccharide capsules of *C. neoformans* yeasts that appear as clear, concentric spaces on the regular stains (10,11). Large numbers of degenerating yeasts release abundant gelatinous fluid that accumulates and forms cystic spaces surrounded by collagenous tissue (10) (Figs. 26.3 and 26.4).

The diagnosis requires identification of *C. neoformans* organisms by serologic testing, culture, or histopathologic staining. The yeasts stain well with hematoxylin and eosin,

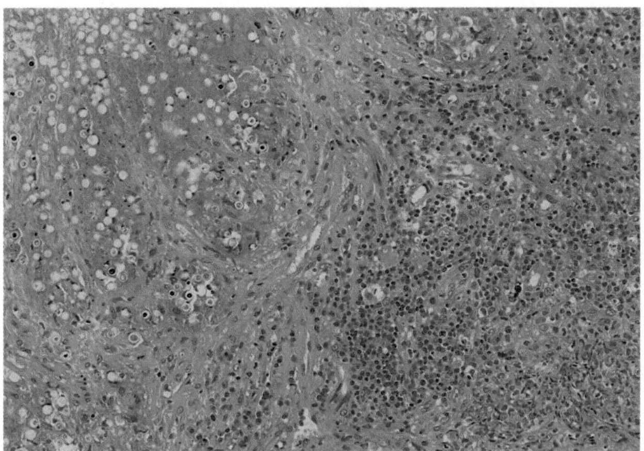

FIGURE 26.1. *Cryptococcus* lymphadenitis showing replacement of lymphoid tissues by histiocytes with engulfed yeasts and gelatinous substance. Hematoxylin, phloxine, and saffron stain.

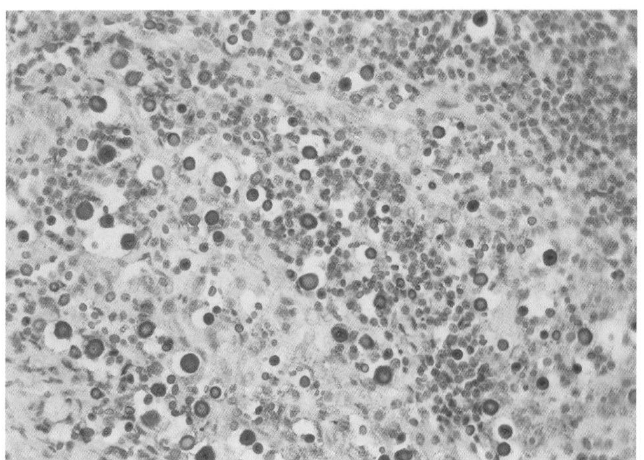

FIGURE 26.2. *Cryptococcus* yeasts in lymph node stained brilliant red. Mucicarmine stain.

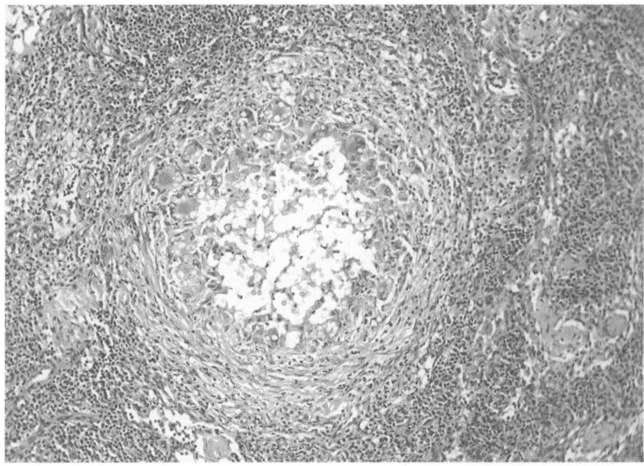

FIGURE 26.3. Cryptococcal cyst filled with yeasts and gelatinous substance surrounded by fibrous pseudocapsule. Hematoxylin, phloxine, and saffron stain.

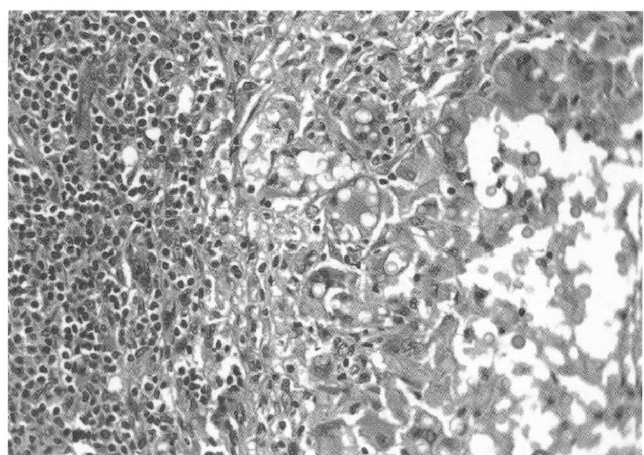

FIGURE 26.4. Wall of cryptococcal cyst lined by histiocytes and giant cells containing multiple yeasts. Hematoxylin, phloxine, and saffron stain.

PAS, and the GMS stain (Fig. 26.5). India ink can detect them in smears of sputum or cerebrospinal fluid or in touch preparations. Typically, however, the diagnosis relies on the unique property of the capsules to stain bright red with mucicarmine (10).

DIFFERENTIAL DIAGNOSIS

- *Histoplasma* lymphadenitis: The yeasts are slightly smaller, although they show similar budding. Granulomas and yeast-containing giant cells are also present; however, the yeasts have no capsules and do not stain with mucicarmine.
- *Pneumocystis* lymphadenitis: The organisms have different shapes and do not stain with mucicarmine.
- *Mycobacterium* lymphadenitis: The granulomas and epithelioid and giant cells may be similar, but the organisms are acid-fast bacilli and do not stain with mucicarmine.

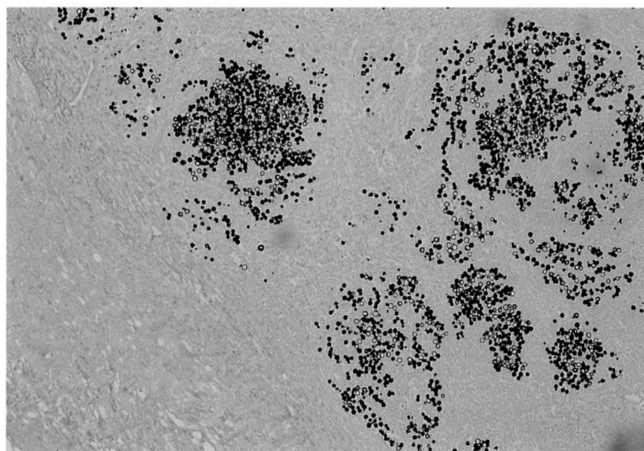

FIGURE 26.5. *Cryptococcus* yeasts in lymph node—single, budding, and in clusters. Grocott methenamine silver stain.

Checklist

CRYPTOCOCCUS LYMPHADENITIS

Immunodeficiency background
Frequent in AIDS patients
Monomorphic fungus
Single, narrow-based budding yeasts
Thick mucopolysaccharide capsule
Strong staining with mucicarmine and PAS stains
Non-necrotizing granulomas
Epithelioid cells and yeast-filled giant cells
Cystic areas with gelatinous content

REFERENCES

1. Binford CH, Dooley JR. Cryptococcosis. In: Binford CH, Connor DH, eds. Pathology of tropical and extraordinary diseases, vol 2. Washington, DC: Armed Forces Institute of Pathology, 1976:572–574.
2. Chandler FW, Watts JC. Cryptococcosis. In: Connor DH, Chandler FW, Schwartz DA, et al., eds. Pathology of infectious diseases, vol 2, Appleton & Lange, 1997.
3. Buchanan KL, Murphy JW. What makes *Cryptoccoccosis neoformans* a pathogen? Emerging Infect Dis 1998;4:71–83.
4. Baker RD. The primary pulmonary lymph node complex of cryptococcosis. Am J Clin Pathol 1976;65:83–92.
5. Centers for Disease Control. Update: acquired immunodeficiency syndrome—United States. MMWR Morb Mortal Wkly Rep 1986;35:542.
6. Myerowitz RL. Local and disseminated cryptococcosis. In: Myerowitz RL, ed. The pathology of opportunistic infections. New York: Raven Press, 1983:145–160.
7. Kerkering TM, Duma RJ, Shadomy S. The evolution of pulmonary cryptococcosis. Ann Intern Med 1981;94:611–616.
8. Lai KK, Rosenberg AE. A 55-year-old man with a destructive bone lesion 17 months after liver transplantation. N Engl J Med 1999;340:1981–1988.
9. Kovacs JA, Kovacs AA, Polis M, et al. Cryptococcosis in the acquired immunodeficiency syndrome. Ann Intern Med 1985;103:533.
10. Ioachim HL. Pathology of AIDS. Textbook and color atlas. Philadelphia: JB Lippincott Co, 1989:50–52.
11. Ioachim HL. Biopsy diagnosis in human immunodeficiency virus infection and acquired immunodeficiency syndrome. Arch Pathol Lab Med 1990;114:284–294.

27

HISTOPLASMA LYMPHADENITIS

DEFINITION

Lymphadenitis caused by infection with *Histoplasma capsulatum.*

ETIOLOGY

H. capsulatum is a thermally dimorphic fungus. Its natural habitat is the soil, particularly when contaminated by excreta of chickens, birds, and bats (1). There, the organism exists in the mycelial phase at ambient temperature. Infection occurs when spores or hyphae are inhaled into the lungs. At the higher temperature of the body, *H. capsulatum* converts to its intracellular yeast form, which has little potential for infection (1,2). Plated on Sabouraud dextrose agar, it forms large, cottony mycelial colonies with prominent, cross-walled hyphae. The yeasts have rigid cell walls and average 3 μm in diameter. Tissue fixatives cause the protoplasm to retract from the rigid walls and leave a clear space, which gives the erroneous impression of an unstained capsule (1).

EPIDEMIOLOGY

Histoplasmosis is endemic in Central America and in the eastern and central United States. In areas of high endemicity, such as the central valleys of the Mississippi and Ohio rivers, more than 80% of the population is sensitized (3). It has been estimated on the basis of histoplasmin skin tests that occult infection with *H. capsulatum* is three to four times more frequent in the U.S. population than occult infection with *Mycobacterium tuberculosis* (4). Because of the high infectivity rate, disseminated histoplasmosis may occur in as many as 5% of AIDS patients in Ohio and Mississippi and 6.7% of those in Guatemala (5,6).

PATHOGENESIS

In the normal population, infections with *Histoplasma* organisms remain occult, although occasionally, in special circumstances of heavy infection, outbreaks of histoplasmosis do occur (7). During an outbreak in Indiana, disseminated histoplasmosis developed in 4.2% of immunocompetent persons and 55.2% of patients who were immunosuppressed (8). Widely disseminated histoplasmosis may occur in patients with Hodgkin lymphoma and acute leukemias treated with corticosteroids and cytotoxic drugs (9). AIDS patients in endemic areas are at high risk for acquiring histoplasmosis, and virulent forms of disease with dissemination are frequent (8,10,11). In normal, immunocompetent persons, infection with airborne spores of *Histoplasma* usually results in the formation of a minute (5-mm), subpleural, caseated, calcified nodule in the lower lobe of lung and a calcified area in the regional hilar lymph node; these form a primary complex entirely similar to the one commonly seen in tuberculosis (12,13). In contrast, extensive lesions involving most organs develop in immunodeficient persons, particularly patients with AIDS. The lymph nodes and other components of the mononuclear phagocyte system (bone marrow, spleen, and liver) are the usual locations. The number of CD4+ T cells is greatly decreased in disseminated histoplasmosis, usually to below 75/mL (5). In their absence, macrophages become engorged with yeasts, which remain intact and are transported to various organs to disseminate the disease (11).

CLINICAL SYNDROME

The clinical presentation of disseminated histoplasmosis is nonspecific; sometimes, fever and weight loss are the only symptoms. Because the fungi are transported by histiocytes, the reticuloendothelial system is primarily affected, and therefore the bone marrow, lymph nodes, spleen, and liver are most likely to be involved (11). In a summary of reported series of cases of disseminated histoplasmosis in AIDS patients, bone marrow cultures were positive for organisms in 83% of cases, and bone marrow histologic sections were positive in 40% of cases in the form of discrete granulomas or lymphohistiocytic aggregates (14). The adrenal gland is also frequently involved, 80% in one series of cases, with necrosis and Addison disease in 10% (9–11). Any organ can be affected. Whereas pulmonary histoplas-

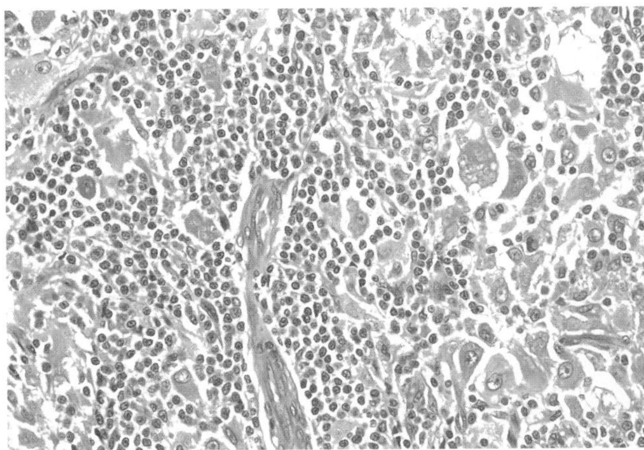

FIGURE 27.1. *Histoplasma* lymphadenitis. Large, pale histiocytes and giant cells scattered or clustered in the nodal cortex. Hematoxylin, phloxine, and saffron stain.

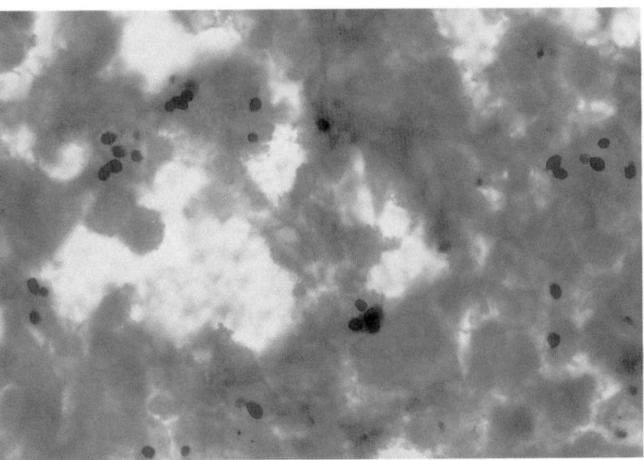

FIGURE 27.3. Histiocyte yeasts, single and in clusters, with budding forms in tissue imprint. Grocott methenamine silver stain.

mosis in immunocompetent people is generally benign, in immunodeficient persons, severe and often fatal disease results from extension to the lungs, heart, and brain (11).

HISTOPATHOLOGY

The lymph node cortex and medulla are replaced initially by granulomas composed of epithelioid and giant cells; these coalesce and form vast sheets of histiocytes containing large numbers of yeasts (15,16) (Fig. 27.1). The latter appear as small, round, unstained, empty-looking intracytoplasmic vacuoles after hematoxylin and eosin (H&E) staining (Fig. 27.2). The yeasts of *H. capsulatum* are round or oval, have a diameter of 2 to 4 μm, and multiply by narrow-based buds. Like other fungi, they stain selectively with the Grocott methenamine silver stain (Fig. 27.3). The macrophages engulf the yeasts but are unable to destroy them, so that abundant replication of the organisms takes place inside the cells and continuous proliferation of the phagocytic histiocytes (Fig. 27.2). The yeast-laden macrophages replace normal tissues and often undergo central necrosis; the yeasts are then released to infect newly attracted histiocytes (1,2). The histologic appearance resembles that of lepromatous leprosy and mycobacteriosis because the pathogenic mechanisms are similar (i.e., proliferation of nonreactive macrophages) (2). Old lesions in the lungs or lymph nodes, with a central area of caseous necrosis and calcium deposits and a capsule of fibrous tissue, may be indistinguishable radiologically and even histologically from those of tuberculosis (14) (Fig. 27.4).

LABORATORY TESTS

Histopathologic examination is the most reliable and commonly used method of diagnosing histoplasmosis. Serologic tests, such as complement fixation and immunodiffusion, and blood culture techniques are also available. However,

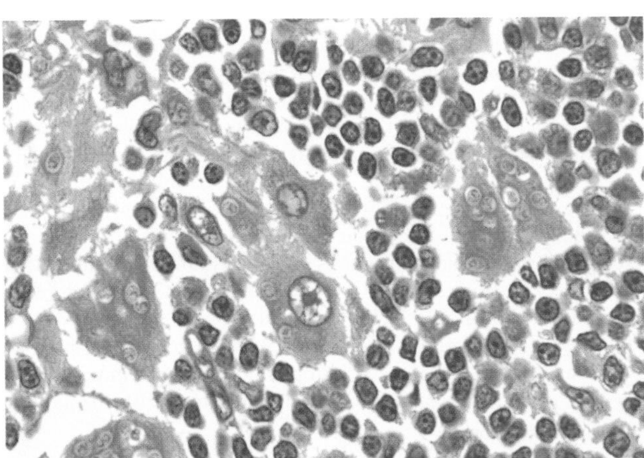

FIGURE 27.2. Same section. Histiocytes and giant cells containing numerous yeasts are seen as unstained, empty-looking vacuoles. Hematoxylin, phloxine, and saffron stain.

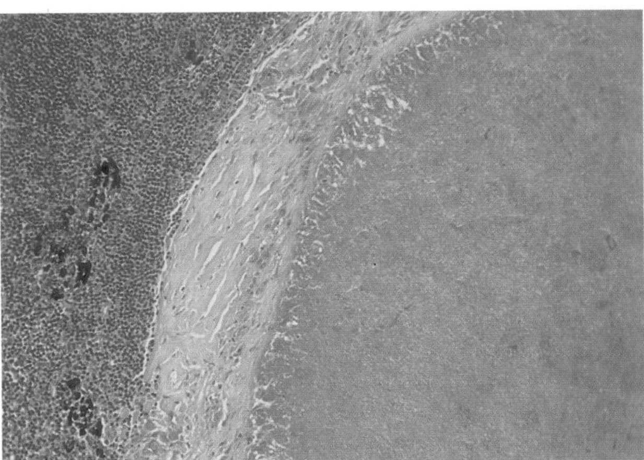

FIGURE 27.4. Large area of caseous necrosis with thick fibrous capsule in hilar anthracotic lymph node. *Histoplasma* pneumonitis and lymphadenitis. Grocott methenamine silver stain.

Checklist

HISTOPLASMA LYMPHADENITIS

Persons from endemic areas (central United States)
Immunodeficiency background
High incidence in AIDS patients in endemic areas
Dimorphic fungus
Mycelia in nature, yeasts in mammalian body
Narrow-based, budding yeasts
Epithelioid and giant cell granulomas
Yeast-filled histiocytes and giant cells
Necrotic, partially fibrosed areas of primary foci of infection
Stain with Grocott methenamine silver
Do not stain with mucicarmine, periodic acid–Schiff, H&E

serologic tests may yield false-positive and false-negative results, particularly in immunosuppressed patients (17).

DIFFERENTIAL DIAGNOSIS

- *Cryptococcus* lymphadenitis is similar histologically. The yeasts are similar in size and budding forms. With H&E staining, they also appear as empty, round spaces within the cytoplasm of macrophages, and they also stain with Grocott methenamine silver.
- Mucicarmine and periodic acid–Schiff clearly stain the capsule of *Cryptococcus* organisms; *Histoplasma* organisms remain unstained, so that differentiation is easy.
- *Leishmania* organisms resemble those of *Histoplasma* but do not stain with silver.
- *Toxoplasma* organisms are much smaller and not intracellular.
- *Blastomyces* organisms are larger and have broad-based buds.
- *Pneumocystis* organisms are distinguished by the absence of budding and the presence of pink proteinaceous material.
- *Mycobacterium* lymphadenitis is similar histologically; however, the organisms are not fungi but acid-fast bacilli.

REFERENCES

1. Binford CH, Dooley JR. Histoplasmosis. In: Binford CH, Connor DH, eds. Pathology of tropical and extraordinary diseases, vol 2. Washington, DC: Armed Forces Institute of Pathology, 1976:578–581.
2. Goodwin RA, Shapiro JL, Thurman GH, et al. Disseminated histoplasmosis: clinical and pathologic correlations. Medicine 1980;59:1–33.
3. Nardell EA, Mark EJ. Fibrosing mediastinitis due to histoplasmosis. N Engl J Med 1989;320:380–389.
4. Edwards LB, Acquaviva FA, Livesay VT, et al. An atlas of sensitivity to tuberculin, PPD-B and histoplasmin in the United States. Am Rev Respir Dis 1969;99[Suppl]:1–132.
5. Hajjeh RA. Disseminated histoplasmosis in persons infected with human immunodeficiency virus. Clin Infect Dis 1995;21[Suppl I]:S108–S110.
6. Segura L, Rojas M, Pelaez N, et al. Disseminated histoplasmosis in human immunodeficiency virus type I infection: risk factors in Guatemala. Clin Infect Dis 1997;25:343–344.
7. Wheat LJ, Slama TG, Eitzen HE, et al. Large urban outbreak of histoplasmosis: clinical features. Ann Intern Med 1981;94:331–337.
8. Wheat LJ, Slama TG, Zeckel ML. Histoplasmosis in the acquired immune deficiency syndrome. Am J Med 1985;78:203–210.
9. Kauffman CA, Israel KS, Smith JW, et al. Histoplasmosis in immunosuppressed patients. Am J Med 1978;65:923–932.
10. Bonner JR, Alexander WJ, Dismukes WE, et al. Disseminated histoplasmosis in patients with the acquired immune deficiency syndrome. Arch Intern Med 1984;144:2178–2181.
11. Levitz SM, Mark EJ. Histoplasmosis. N Engl J Med 1998;339: 1835–1843.
12. Vanek J, Schwarz J. The gamut of histoplasmosis. Am J Med 1971;50:89–104.
13. Reynolds RJ, Penn RL, Grafton WE, et al. Tissue morphology of *Histoplasma capsulatum* in acute histoplasmosis. Am Rev Respir Dis 1984;130:317–320.
14. Kurtin PJ, McKinsey DS, Gupta MR, et al. Histoplasmosis in patients with acquired immunodeficiency syndrome. Am J Clin Pathol 1990;93:367–372.
15. Ioachim HL. Pathology of AIDS. Textbook and color atlas. Philadelphia: JB Lippincott Co, 1989:56–58.
16. Ioachim HL. Biopsy diagnosis in human immunodeficiency virus infection and acquired immunodeficiency syndrome. Arch Pathol Lab Med 1990;114:284–294.
17. Paya CV, Roberts GD, Cockerill FR. Laboratory methods for the diagnosis of disseminated histoplasmosis: clinical importance of the lysis-centrifugation blood culture technique. Mayo Clin Proc 1987;62:480–485.

28

COCCIDIOIDOMYCOSIS LYMPHADENITIS

DEFINITION

Lymphadenitis caused by infection with *Coccidioides immitis.*

EPIDEMIOLOGY

Coccidioidomycosis is endemic in the southwestern United States, particularly southern California, Arizona, New Mexico, and western Texas, in Mexico, and in parts of Central and South America (1,2). In these endemic areas, the incidence of coccidioidomycosis increased during the 1990s (3–5). The mycelial form of the fungus inhabits the soil of desert regions with only brief, intense rainy season, conditions best met in the Sonoran Life Zone, where coccidioidomycosis is prevalent (1). In the United States, 100,000 infections occur annually, and of these, 1 in 200 becomes disseminated life-threatening disease (2). In New York, an average of 30 hospital discharges per year with the diagnosis of coccidioidomycosis have been recorded in the past few years (6). The incidence of coccidioidomycosis is high in AIDS patients who live in endemic areas; in a study of 27 AIDS patients in Tucson, 7 (26%) had the disease (7).

ETIOLOGY

Winds can carry the fungus *C. immitis* for long distances along with contaminated soil, so that epidemics of coccidioidomycosis develop in both animals and humans (8). The dimorphic fungus can grow as a mold in mycelial form in the natural environment and in the laboratory at 25° to 30°C, or as a yeast in spherule form in the tissues or when incubated at 37°C (3). The mycelial form of *C. immitis* consists of septate hyphae, 2 to 4 μm in width, that produce alternating, barrel-shaped arthroconidia. The forms seen in infected tissues are yeasts; the branching, septate hyphae are rarely found in tissues, mostly in necrotic and cavitated areas (9,10). The yeasts, called *sporangia,* appear as fairly large spherules, 20 to 60 μm in diameter, with a thick, brown, double-contoured capsule containing multiple small (2 to 5 μm), round endospores. Tissue sections usually exhibit a mixture of small, immature and large, mature sporangia, in addition to degenerated forms with broken capsules and partially released endospores. The endospores give rise to long, thin, branching, and septate hyphae. The arthrospores, which are the component parts of the hyphae, break into small, lightweight microorganisms that are easily airborne and highly infectious. Coccidioidomycosis is one of the infections for which laboratory workers are at highest risk (11). For this reason, when *C. immitis* infection is suspected, the specimens sent to the laboratory must be clearly labeled and strict precautions taken at autopsy to avoid spreading the infection.

PATHOGENESIS

In normal persons, the primary lesion is pulmonary and develops after spores are inhaled. The lesion shows a predilection for the right lung and upper lobes; it is usually subpleural and involves satellite lymph nodes, as in tuberculosis and histoplasmosis (10). In patients with AIDS, most cases of coccidioidomycosis, like those of histoplasmosis, represent reactivation of an earlier latent infection, sometimes years after a visit to an endemic area (2). Patients on long-term dialysis, renal transplant recipients, and patients on immunosuppressive therapy in endemic areas are particularly at risk. Thus, *C. immitis* is the most common single agent of infection in the transplant population in Arizona, causing severe disease with high rates of dissemination and mortality (12). A study of *C. immitis* isolates from patients in New York City, a nonendemic area, revealed genotypes similar to those in Arizona, an indication of travel-related acquisition of the disease (6).

CLINICAL SYNDROME

Primary coccidioidomycosis is usually pulmonary, developing after highly infectious aerosolized arthroconidia are inhaled. In about 40% of people, a mild, flulike respiratory syndrome, sometimes referred to as *San Joaquin Valley fever,* appears and then resolves spontaneously (13). Most infections in the endemic areas are asymptomatic and are recognized retrospectively by a positive reaction on a skin test (l). In about 1% of cases, chronic, progressive coccidioidal pneumonia develops, with cavitation resembling that of tuberculosis. Also, mainly in AIDS patients, severe forms of extrathoracic disseminated infection may develop, involving most organs and leading to death (14). Immunocompromised persons and infants are at highest risk for coccidioidomycosis (2). In most studies, more than 75% of patients were older than 55 years and had cancer or AIDS (6).

HISTOPATHOLOGY

In the lung, the primary lesion appears radiographically as a coin lesion; this is surgically removed and examined to rule out a possible tumor (10). It usually consists of a central area of caseous necrosis surrounded by lymphocytes and fibrosis (Fig. 28.1). Non-necrotic tissues are infiltrated by epithelioid and giant cells containing fungi in the form of sporangia (10,11,14) (Fig. 28.2). In the involved lymph nodes, granulomas, single or coalescent with areas of necrosis, similar to the lesions of tuberculosis and histoplasmosis, are seen. They are composed of epithelioid cells, giant cells of the Langhans or foreign body type, lymphocytes, and some plasma cells (14,15). Scattered throughout are thick-walled, immature sporangia, 10 to 40 μm in diameter, and mature sporangia, up to 60 μm in diameter, containing a dozen or more endospores. Other organisms are degenerated, with incomplete capsules, partially releasing their spores (Fig. 28.3). The latter are small, round spherules seen within giant cells or free in areas of fibrosis (11,15). The endospores may give rise to long, thin, branching, septate hyphae in a few areas of the lymph nodes (11). The clusters of endospores may be surrounded by a radiating, eosinophilic corona of Splendore-Hoepli material, which indicates an immunologic host reaction to fungal antigens (1). The optimal stains for the fungal organisms are period acid–Schiff and specifically Grocott methenamine silver (Fig. 28.4).

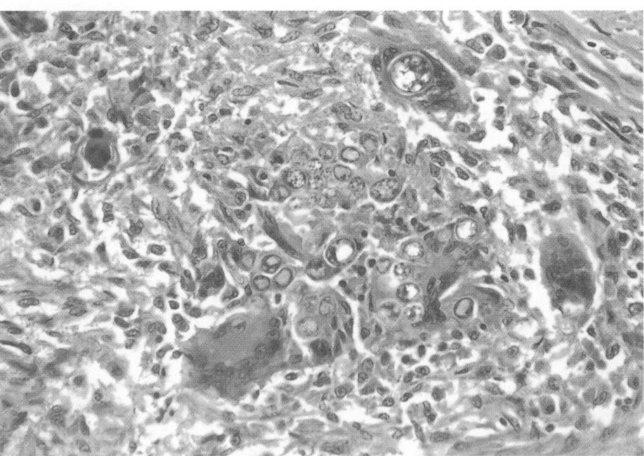

FIGURE 28.2. Granulomatous infiltrates composed of lymphocytes, plasma cells, histiocytes, and giant cells containing viable and degenerated sporangia. Hematoxylin, phloxine, and saffron stain.

LABORATORY TESTS

The diagnosis should be confirmed by the following:

- Culture on Sabouraud dextrose agar
- Serology
- Immunofluorescence
- Delayed-type hypersensitivity reaction on skin testing

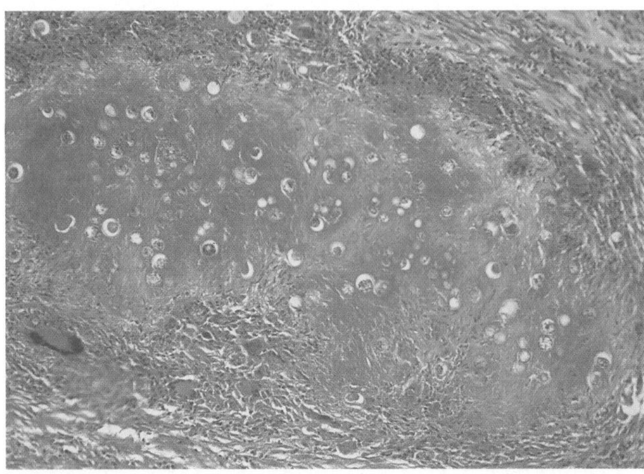

FIGURE 28.1. Peritoneal lymph node with area of caseous necrosis, including degenerated empty cysts, surrounded by histiocytes and giant cells. Hematoxylin, phloxine, and saffron stain.

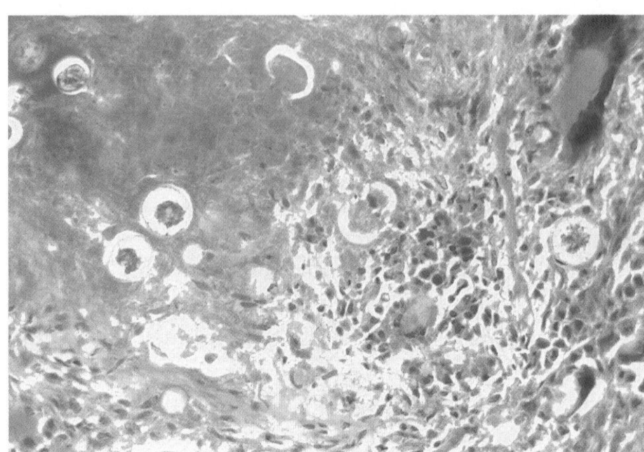

FIGURE 28.3. Degenerated empty cysts in area of necrosis and sporangia engulfed by giant cells. Hematoxylin, phloxine, and saffron stain.

Checklist

COCCIDIOIDOMYCOSIS LYMPHADENITIS

Persons from endemic areas (southwestern United States)
Immunodeficiency background
High incidence in AIDS patients from endemic areas
Dimorphic fungus with yeast and hyphae forms
Sporangium with multiple endospores and thick, double capsule
Cysts and spores that stain with methenamine silver
Necrotizing granulomas
Giant cells containing sporangia

DIFFERENTIAL DIAGNOSIS

- Histoplasmosis lymphadenitis: The yeasts are smaller, without sporangia and endospores. Necrosis is less common.
- *Cryptococcus* lymphadenitis: The yeasts are smaller and have a capsule that stains strongly with mucicarmine stain.
- *Mycobacterium* lymphadenitis: Acid-fast bacilli are present instead of yeasts.

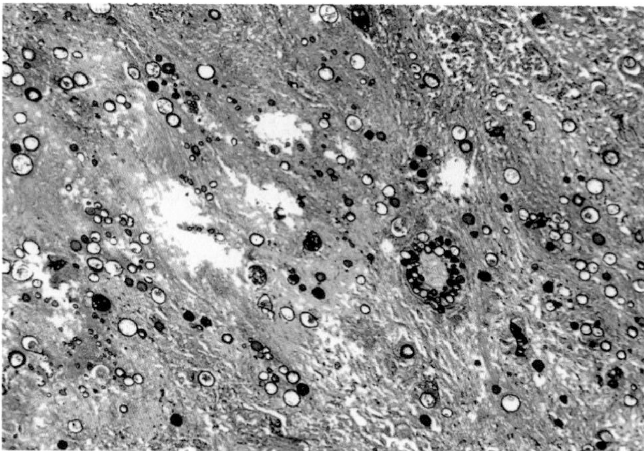

FIGURE 28.4. Sporangia, free spores, and degenerated cysts of coccidioidomycosis. Grocott methenamine silver stain.

REFERENCES

1. Chandler FW, Watts JC. Pathologic diagnosis of fungal infections. Chicago: American Society of Clinical Pathologists Press, 1988:13–23.
2. Stevens DA. Current concepts: coccidioidomycosis. N Engl J Med 1995;332:1077–1182.
3. Centers for Disease Control and Prevention. Coccidioidomycosis—United States, 1991–1992. MMWR Morb Mortal Wkly Rep 1993;42:21–24.
4. Pappagianis D. Marked increase in cases of coccidioidomycosis in California: 1991, 1992 and 1993. Clin Infect Dis 1994;19[Suppl 1]:S14–S18.
5. Kirkland TM, Fierer J. Coccidioidomycosis: a reemerging infectious disease. Emerging Infect Dis 1996;2:192–199.
6. Chaturvedi V, Ramani R, Gromadzki S, et al. Coccidioidomycosis in New York State. Emerging Infect Dis 2000;6:25–29.
7. Bronnimann DA, Adam RD, Galgiani JN, et al. Coccidioidomycosis in the acquired immunodeficiency syndrome. Ann Intern Med 1987;106:372–379.
8. Larone DH, Mitchell TG, Walsh TJ. *Histoplasma, Blastomyces, Coccidioides* and other dimorphic fungi causing systemic mycoses. In: Murray PR, et al., eds. Manual of clinical microbiology. Washington, DC: American Society for Microbiology Press, 1999:1259–1274.
9. Flynn NM, Hoeprich PD, Kawachi MM, et al. An unusual outbreak of wind-borne coccidioidomycosis. N Engl J Med 1979;301:358–361.
10. Deppich LM, Donowho EM. Pulmonary coccidioidomycosis. Am J Clin Pathol 1972;58:489–500.
11. Medeiros AA, Mark EJ. A 51-year-old woman with chest pain and a coin lesion. Case Records 1980;302:2218–2223.
12. Cohen IM, Galgiani JN, Potter D, et al. Coccidioidomycosis in renal replacement therapy. Arch Intern Med 1982;142:489–494.
13. Drutz DJ, Cantanzaro A. A state of the art coccidioidomycosis. Am Rev Respir Dis 1978;117:727–771.
14. Ioachim HL. Pathology of AIDS. Textbook and color atlas. Philadelphia: JB Lippincott Co, 1989:60–62.
15. Ioachim HL. Biopsy diagnosis in human immunodeficiency virus infection and acquired immunodeficiency syndrome. Arch Pathol Lab Med 1990;114:284–294.

29

PNEUMOCYSTIS LYMPHADENITIS

DEFINITION

Lymphadenitis caused by infection with *Pneumocystis carinii.*

SYNONYM

P. carinii infection of lymph nodes.

ETIOLOGY

P. carinii, the agent of pneumocystosis, was previously considered to be a protozoan because of the presence of filopodia on its trophozoites. Subsequent studies, however, have shown that its ribosomal RNA has sequences of the fungus type and consequently that *P. carinii* represents a species of fungus (1).

EPIDEMIOLOGY

Although *P. carinii* organisms are ubiquitous in nature, normal persons of the general population become immune in early childhood, and infections in immunocompetent persons are not known to occur. By the middle of the twentieth century, *P. carinii* pneumonia (PCP) had not yet been recognized in North America (2). Cases of *Pneumocystis* infection were recorded in malnourished children in underdeveloped countries and in persons with congenital immunodeficiencies. The disease became more common with the increased use of immunosuppressive therapies in organ transplant recipients and cancer patients (3,4). Since 1981, pneumocystosis has been recognized as the most common opportunistic infection associated with AIDS. At the peak of the epidemic of HIV infection, PCP developed in 60% to 85% of AIDS patients and was the most common cause of death (5–8).

PATHOGENESIS

P. carinii organisms affect most mammalian species and can be found in hosts with no clinical or histologic evidence of disease. They may remain for long intervals in latent or inactive states. Activation and replication are stimulated and permitted by immunodeficiency. Pneumonia developed in 100% of experimental rats without *P. carinii* inoculation after 2 to 4 months of corticosteroid administration (2). In humans, *P. carinii* organisms are normally controlled and kept in latent cyst form by cellular immunity. When the number of CD4+ T cells is severely decreased, as in AIDS, sporozoites are released from the cysts, become trophozoites, increase in size, and mature into new cysts (2). Patients with CD4+ T-cell counts of less than 200/mm^3 are at highest risk for PCP (9).

CLINICAL SYNDROME

In AIDS patients, *Pneumocystis* infection is with few exceptions limited to the lungs; it results in severe, acute, bilateral pneumonia, which is fatal if not treated (6–8). Sometimes, the presentation is insidious, and the symptoms, which are nonspecific, develop slowly. In either case, the lesion is a foamy, granular, eosinophilic, intraalveolar fibrinous exudate containing numerous *P. carinii* organisms (10). With the introduction of anti-*Pneumocystis* drugs, particularly pentamidine, survival has increased; however, occasional cases of disseminated pneumocystosis have been reported (11–17). Although administering pentamidine as an aerosol rather than intravenously cleared the lungs of *Pneumocystis* organisms, it failed to prevent dissemination of the infection because the serum levels generated were insufficient to eradicate the organisms (18–21). In its rare disseminated form, pneumocystosis may involve bone marrow, lymph nodes, liver, spleen, heart, kidney, thyroid, adrenals, and other organs (10–23). Clinical symptoms and signs reflect the organs affected, and autopsies have confirmed widespread dissemination of the disease.

HISTOPATHOLOGY

The lymph nodes, more commonly the mediastinal and retroperitoneal nodes, are markedly enlarged and show irregularly shaped, creamy yellowish, necrotic areas on section (19,21). Microscopically, such areas consist of

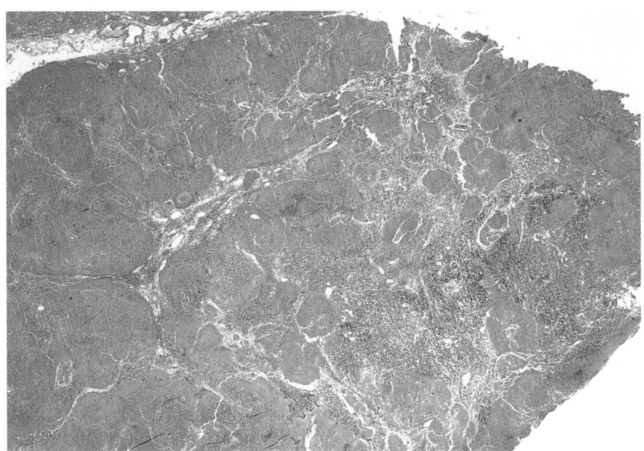

FIGURE 29.1. *Pneumocystis* lymphadenitis. Mediastinal lymph node with innumerable granulomas replacing almost the entire lymphoid parenchyma. Hematoxylin, phloxine, and saffron stain.

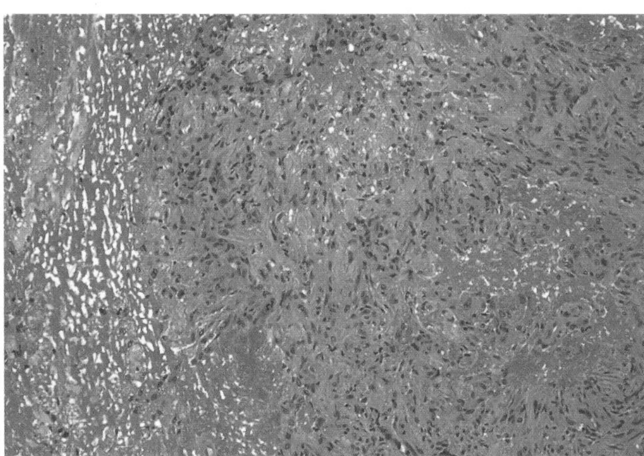

FIGURE 29.3. Necrotic tissues and fibrinous exudates admixed with reactive lymphocytes, histiocytes, and giant cells. Hematoxylin, phloxine, and saffron stain.

necrotic tissues admixed with the characteristic, strongly eosinophilic, periodic acid–Schiff-positive, fibrinous foamy exudate of the *Pneumocystis* infection (Figs. 29.1 and 29.2). Reactive inflammatory cells are usually not present. Occasionally, epithelioid cells and multinucleated giant cells may be present in some organs at the periphery of necrotic areas (24) (Fig. 29.3). Staining with Grocott methenamine silver (GMS) reveals numerous round or helmet-shaped collapsed *P. carinii* cysts within the fibrinous exudate (Fig. 29.4). Monoclonal antibodies specific for antigens expressed by *Pneumocystis* are available and can be used in addition to the GMS stain for identification (25). Polymerase chain reaction is more sensitive than other techniques and applicable to induced sputum and bronchoalveolar lavage specimens; however, it may produce false-positive results (26).

DIFFERENTIAL DIAGNOSIS

- Tuberculous lymphadenitis: Necrotizing tuberculosis may affect lymph nodes, particularly mediastinal and retroperitoneal nodes. The gross appearance and the microscopic necrotic areas, sometimes with epithelioid and giant cells, may be similar, but special stains reveal the presence of acid-fast bacilli in one case and GMS-positive cysts in the other.
- *Histoplasma* lymphadenitis may also result in extensive necrosis with epithelioid and giant cells. GMS stains both organisms and reveals their morphologic differences.
- *Cryptococcus* lymphadenitis: The yeasts are mucicarmine-positive.
- Necrotizing lymphadenitis: No microorganisms are identified by special stains.

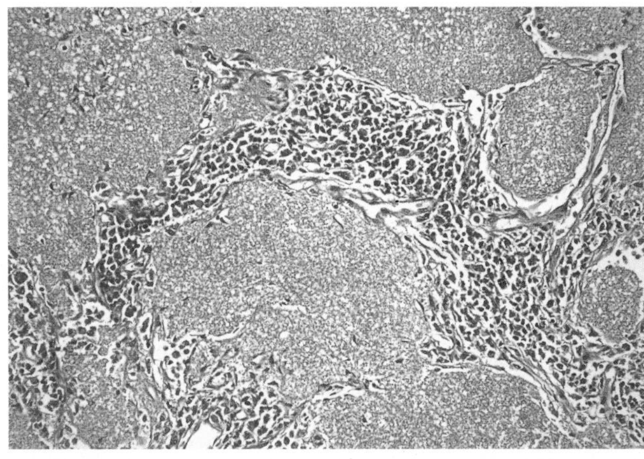

FIGURE 29.2. Necrotic tissues with characteristic foamy eosinophilic appearance surrounded by histiocytes, lymphocytes, and rare giant cells. Hematoxylin, phloxine, and saffron stain.

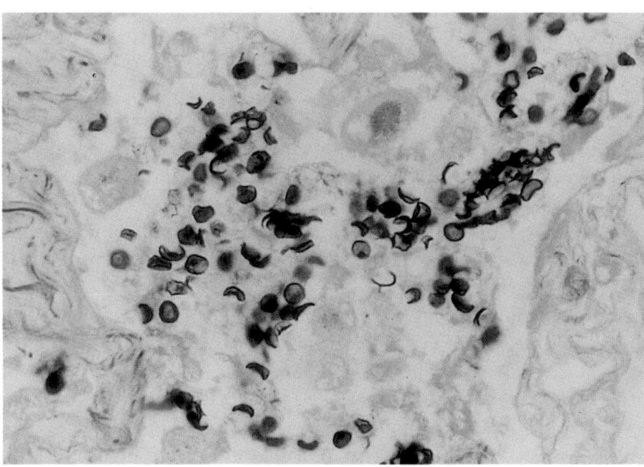

FIGURE 29.4. Silver-staining round or helmet-shaped collapsed *P. carinii* cysts in necrotic mediastinal lymph node. Grocott methenamine silver stain.

Checklist

PNEUMOCYSTIS LYMPHADENITIS

Patient infected with HIV
CD4+ T cells markedly decreased in number
Bilateral *P. carinii* pneumonia or disseminated pneumocystosis
Enlarged mediastinal or retroperitoneal lymph nodes
Coalescent necrotic areas
Fibrinous, foamy exudate that stains with periodic acid–Schiff
Lack of inflammatory response
Round or helmet-shaped *P. carinii* cysts that stain with GMS

- Kikuchi lymphadenitis: Necrotic areas are accompanied by an inflammatory response. The result of GMS staining is negative.
- Metastatic carcinomas in lymph nodes: Tumor cells can usually be recognized at the periphery of necrotic areas.

REFERENCES

1. Edman JC, Kovacs JA, Masur H, et al. Ribosomal RNA sequence shows *Pneumocystis carinii* to be a member of fungi. Nature 1988;334:519.
2. Hughes WT. *Pneumocystis carinii* pneumonia. N Engl J Med 1977;297:1381–1383.
3. Dutz W. *Pneumocystis carinii* pneumonia. Pathol Annu 1970;5: 309–341.
4. Price RA, Hughes WT. Histopathology of *Pneumocystis carinii* infestation and infection in malignant disease in childhood. Hum Pathol 1974;5:737–752.
5. Gottlieb MS, Schroff R, Schanker HM, et al. *Pneumocystis carinii* pneumonia and mucosal candidiasis in previously healthy homosexual men. N Engl J Med 1981;305:1425–1431.
6. Masur H, Michelis MA, Greene JB, et al. An outbreak of community-acquired *Pneumocystis carinii* pneumonia: initial manifestation of cellular immune dysfunction. N Engl J Med 1981;305: 1431–1438.
7. Murray JF, Garay SM, Hopewell PC, et al. Pulmonary complications of the acquired immunodeficiency syndrome: an update. Report of the second National Heart, Lung, and Blood Institute workshop. Am Rev Respir Dis 1987;135:504–509.
8. Gal AA, Koss MN, Strigle S, et al. *Pneumocystis carinii* infection in the acquired immune deficiency syndrome. Semin Diagn Pathol 1989;6:287–299.
9. Leoung GS, Feigal DW, Montgomery AB, et al. Aerosolized pentamidine for prophylaxis against *Pneumocystis carinii* pneumonia. N Engl J Med 1990;323:769–775.
10. Ioachim HL. Pathology of AIDS. Textbook and color atlas. Philadelphia: JB Lippincott Co, 1989:68–70, 159–160.
11. Heyman MR, Rasmussen P. *Pneumocystis carinii* involvement of the bone marrow in acquired immune deficiency syndrome. Am J Clin Pathol 1987;87:780–783.
12. Macher AM, Bardenstein DS, Zimmerman LE, et al. *Pneumocystis carinii* choroiditis in a male homosexual with AIDS and disseminated pulmonary and extrapulmonary *P. carinii* infection [Letter]. N Engl J Med 1987;316:1092.
13. Radin DR, Baker EL, Klatt EC. Visceral and nodal calcification in *Pneumocystis carinii* infection. AJR Am J Roentgenol 1990; 154:27–31.
14. Cote RJ, Rosenblum M, Telzak E, et al. Disseminated *Pneumocystis carinii* infection causing extrapulmonary organ failure: clinical, pathologic and immunohistochemical analysis. Mod Pathol 1990;3:25–30.
15. Ravalli S, Garcia RL, Vincent RA. Disseminated *Pneumocystis carinii* infection in the acquired immune deficiency syndrome. N Y State J Med 1990:155–157.
16. Grimes MM, LaPook JD, Bar MH, et al. Disseminated *Pneumocystis carinii* infection in a patient with acquired immune deficiency syndrome. Hum Pathol 1987;18:307–308.
17. Unger PA, Rosenblum M, Krown SE. Disseminated *Pneumocystis* in a patient with AIDS. Hum Pathol 1988;19:113–116.
18. Raviglione MC, Garner GR, Mullen MP. *Pneumocystis carinii* in bone marrow [Letter]. Ann Intern Med 1988:253.
19. De Roux S, Adsay V, Ioachim HL. Disseminated Pneumocystosis without pulmonary involvement in AIDS patient on prophylactic aerosolized pentamidine treatment. Arch Pathol Lab Med 1991;115:1137–1140.
20. Telzak EE, Cote RJ, Gold JWM, et al. Extrapulmonary *Pneumocystis carinii* infections. Rev Infect Dis 1990;12:380–386.
21. Ellison E, Yuen SY, Lawson L, et al. Fine-needle aspiration diagnosis of extrapulmonary *Pneumocystis carinii* lymphadenitis in a human immunodeficiency virus positive patient. Diagn Cytopathol 1995;12:251–253.
22. Barnett RN, Hull JG, Vortel V, et al. *Pneumocystis carinii* in lymph nodes and spleen. Arch Pathol 1969;88:175.
23. Afessa B, Green WR, Williams WA, et al. *Pneumocystis carinii* pneumonia complicated by lymphadenopathy and pneumothorax. Arch Intern Med 1988;148:2651–2654.
24. Bleiweiss IJ, Jagirdar JS, Klein MJ, et al. Granulomatous *Pneumocystis carinii* pneumonia in three patients with the acquired immune deficiency syndrome. Chest 1988;94:580–583.
25. Kovacs JA, Gill V, Swan JC, et al. Prospective evaluation of a monoclonal antibody in diagnosis of *Pneumocystis carinii* pneumonia. Lancet 1986;2:1.
26. Sun T. Current topics in protozoal diseases. Am J Clin Pathol 1994;102:16–29.

PART III

SECTION FIVE

PROTOZOAL LYMPHADENITIDES

Parasitic protozoa are major causes of disease, particularly in developing countries. They do not secrete exotoxins but are able, according to species, to colonize the gastrointestinal tract, invade the circulating blood, or develop within cells. Among the important parasites of humans are the many types of plasmodia, amebae, cryptosporidia, trypanosomatids, and others. Only some are etiologic agents of lymphadenitides. *Toxoplasma, Leishmania,* and *Filaria* are common in various parts of the world and may cause specific lymphadenitides.

30

TOXOPLASMA LYMPHADENITIS

DEFINITION

Lymphadenitis caused by infection with the protozoan *Toxoplasma gondii.*

SYNONYM

Piringer-Kuchinka lymphadenopathy.

EPIDEMIOLOGY

Toxoplasmosis is a common parasitic disease worldwide. The infection, which is mostly asymptomatic, is prevalent in warm and humid climates, where almost all people have antibodies to *Toxoplasma,* and is infrequent in cold and dry areas (1,2). In the United States, toxoplasmosis is the most common parasitic infection. It is estimated that 50% of Americans have antibodies, indicative of chronic asymptomatic infection, and every year about 3,000 children are infected at birth (3). In France, 70% to 90% of persons older than 20 years have positive serologic findings (4). *T. gondii* organisms infect a wide variety of mammals and birds, but the definitive host is the cat (3). Rodents may also serve as intermediate hosts, as in a reported case of *Toxoplasma* lymphadenitis transmitted to a patient by his pet rabbit (5).

ETIOLOGY

The parasite has a complex life cycle. The cat is the definitive host for the sexual stage of reproduction, during which trophozoites multiply in the intestinal epithelium and produce oocysts that are eliminated in the stool. Human beings and other mammals, the intermediate hosts, are infected through the ingestion of oocysts from contaminated soil or infected, undercooked meat (2,3). More unusual modes of infection are transplacental transfer of *T. gondii* from mother to fetus and transmission of *Toxoplasma* organisms with a transplanted kidney to a susceptible immunodeficient recipient (6). In intermediate hosts, the ingested oocysts are disrupted by digestive enzymes and the trophozoites are released into the intestine, where they spread through lymphatics and blood vessels and are carried by macrophages into the internal organs (7). Within macrophages, particularly in immunodeficient hosts, the trophozoites multiply rapidly, forming large clusters of small (2 to 6 μm diameter), crescent-shaped entities called *tachyzoites.* In immunocompetent hosts, as immunity is established, the parasites are segregated in cysts partially synthesized by the host. Protected by the cyst walls, bradyzoites multiply slowly, as their name implies, and may persist for long periods of time. Thus, in humans, *Toxoplasma* organisms exist in two forms, trophozoites in the circulation and bradyzoites within intracellular cysts; the third form, the oocyst, is found only in cats.

CLINICAL FEATURES

Toxoplasmosis may occur as one of three major clinical syndromes: *Toxoplasma* lymphadenitis in the general population, systemic toxoplasmosis in immune-deficient patients, and fetal toxoplasmosis transmitted by transplacental infection.

In immunologically compromised hosts, such as patients who have leukemia, lymphoma, or AIDS or are receiving immunosuppressive therapy, *T. gondii* infection becomes acutely disseminated, usually progressing to involve the central nervous system (8–14). In a study of brain biopsy specimens in patients with AIDS, toxoplasmic encephalitis was the diagnosis in 71% of cases (13). When associated with severe immune deficiency, toxoplasmosis often results in death from myocarditis, pneumonitis, chorioretinitis, or encephalitis (15,16). Similar infections may occur in an immunosuppressed host when *Toxoplasma* organisms are inadvertently transmitted with a transplanted kidney (6). Fetal toxoplasmosis, the result of congenital infection, occurs in 1 of every 1,000 live births in the United States. The chance of transmitting the infection transplacentally is greater during the last trimester; however, the damage to the fetus is greater when transmission occurs in early pregnancy (7). It is generally a serious systemic illness that produces symptomatic cerebral and ocular lesions. In affected children, the brain lesions are usually periventricular with characteristic focal calcifications.

In normal adults, the most common manifestation is a localized lymphadenopathy. It may be entirely asymptomatic or accompanied by mild, nonspecific symptoms such as fever and myalgia. *Toxoplasma* is considered to be the etiologic agent of 15% to 20% of all unexplained lymphadenopathies, particularly those involving cervical lymph nodes (3,17).

The posterior cervical lymph nodes are most commonly and characteristically involved (18). However, other cervical, supraclavicular, and occipital lymph nodes may be affected, and occasionally generalized lymphadenopathy, sometimes accompanied by moderate hepatosplenomegaly, may occur (3,17). The lymph nodes may be tender or painless on palpation, and the enlargement may last from a few days to more than a year, usually resolving spontaneously in a matter of weeks. At palpation, the lymph node is firm but not rock hard, 0.5 to 3 cm in diameter, and not ulcerated (16).

HISTOPATHOLOGY

The histologic criteria originally described by Piringer-Kuchinka and colleagues (19) and Saxen and colleagues (20) have been repeatedly confirmed (21,22), and it is generally accepted that *Toxoplasma* lymphadenitis can be diagnosed histologically and confirmed by serologic assays (21–24).

The lymph node architecture is altered by the lymphoid follicles, which are markedly hyperplastic, comprising reactive germinal centers; by numerous, widely scattered epithelioid cells; and by aggregates of monocytoid cells. The reactive follicles, clusters of epithelioid cells, and patches of monocytoid cells constitute a triad characteristic of *Toxoplasma* lymphadenitis (Fig.30.1). The follicles are enlarged mainly by the intensely reactive germinal centers. These include increased numbers of centroblasts, many in mitosis, and macrophages containing nuclear debris (tingible bodies) (Fig. 30.2).

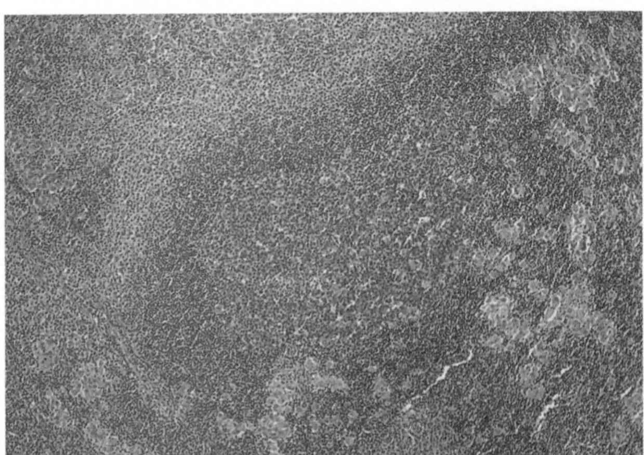

FIGURE 30.1. Characteristic triad of *Toxoplasma* lymphadenitis: enlarged follicle with reactive germinal center, area of monocytoid cells (*top* and *left*) outside the mantle zone, and clusters of epithelioid cells (*right* and *bottom*) encroaching on lymphoid follicle.

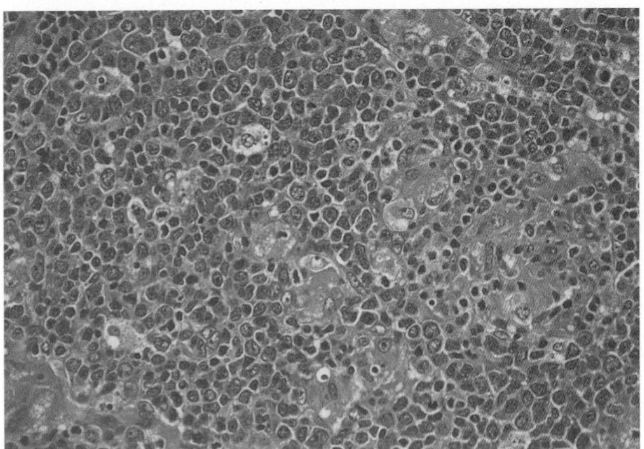

FIGURE 30.2. Reactive germinal center with tingible-body macrophages and epithelioid cells penetrating from the right.

The monocytoid cells are assembled in islands and sheets around and within the nodal sinuses, sometimes adjacent to blood vessels (Fig. 30.3). They are large, flat cells with sharp, visible cell borders, clear cytoplasm, and relatively small, darkly stained nuclei (Fig. 30.4). Nucleoli are inconspicuous and mitoses are absent (Fig. 30.5). These cells, described as monocytoid because of a morphologic resemblance, are in fact B cells expressing surface immunoglobulins and cytoplasmic B-cell markers (24,25) (Figs. 30.6 and 30.7). Although common in toxoplasmosis, they are not specific and can be seen in other lymphadenitides, notably in the acute stage of HIV infection (26).

The epithelioid cells, singly and in clusters, are scattered throughout the cortex and paracortex (Fig. 30.8). Charac-

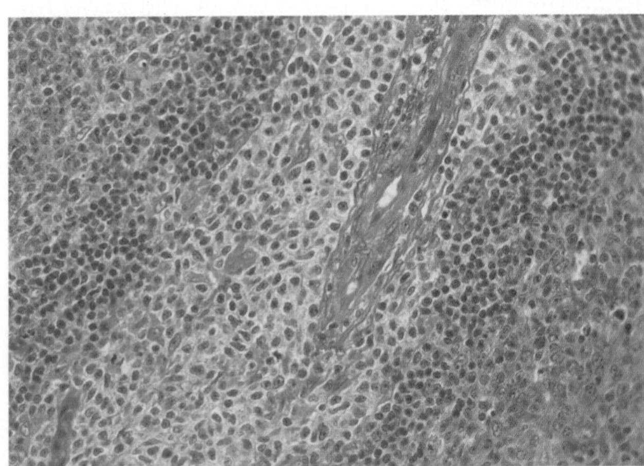

FIGURE 30.3. Area of monocytoid cells surrounding blood vessel.

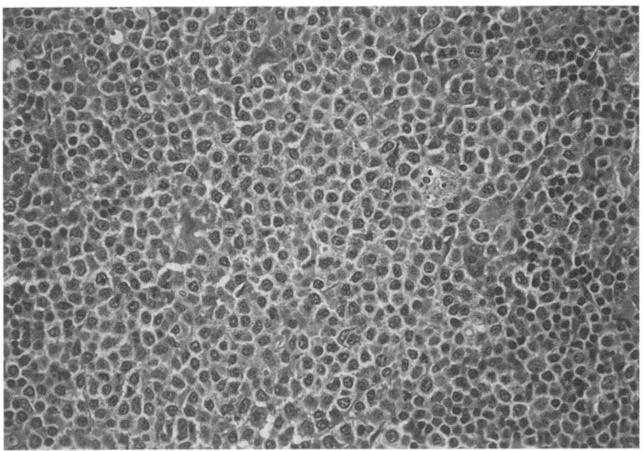

FIGURE 30.4. Monocytoid cells are monomorphic, with abundant clear cytoplasm and round, dark, centrally located nuclei.

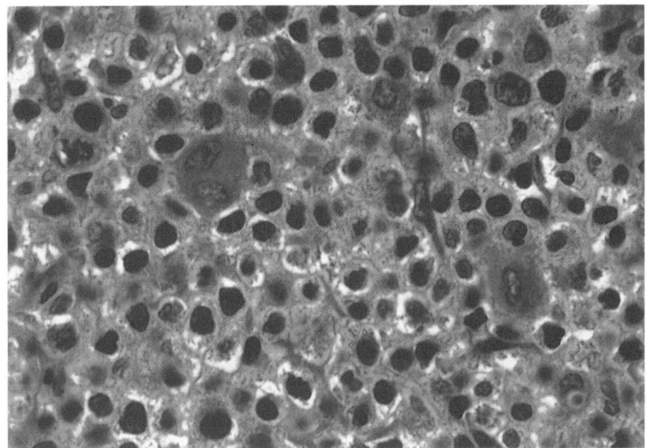

FIGURE 30.5. Monocytoid cells with hyperchromatic, structureless nuclei and pale-staining cytoplasm. Inconspicuous nucleoli and mitoses.

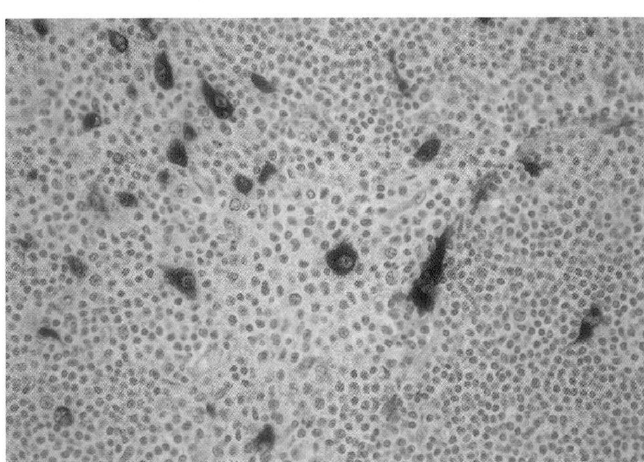

FIGURE 30.6. Area of monocytoid cells immunostained for CD68 antigen shows staining of incidental histiocytes but not of monocytoid cells.

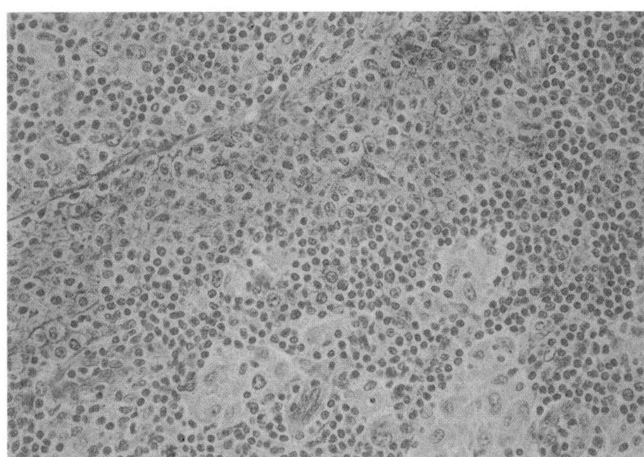

FIGURE 30.7. Area of monocytoid cells immunostained for CD20 antigen shows staining of monocytoid cells, indicating their B-cell origin.

teristic of toxoplasmosis is encroachment by epithelioid cells on follicles and germinal centers, so that their contours are blurred. Although the numbers of epithelioid cells are sometimes considerable, they do not form round, organized granulomas, as they do in sarcoidosis (Fig. 30.9). They also do not induce necrosis and are not accompanied by fibrosis. Multinucleated giant cells are not part of the toxoplasmic epithelioid cell proliferation.

The lymph node sinuses are distended and lined by hyperplastic endothelial cells. Plasma cells are usually present, but neutrophils and eosinophils are not. Activated lymphocytes are frequent. Vascular proliferation and deposition of fibrocollagen are minimal.

Toxoplasma organisms, appearing as clusters of trophozoites free or within macrophages, are rarely seen [in 1% of cases in a series of the Armed Forces Institute of Pathology (2) and in no cases in another series (22)]. In contrast, in immunodeficient patients, particularly in patients with AIDS,

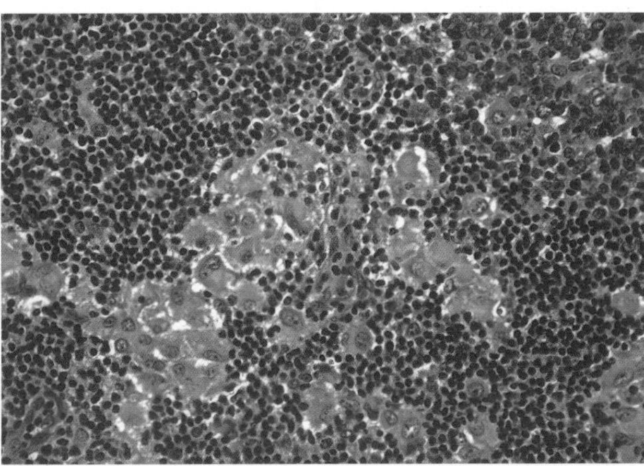

FIGURE 30.8. Clusters of epithelioid cells without formation of granulomas in paracortex.

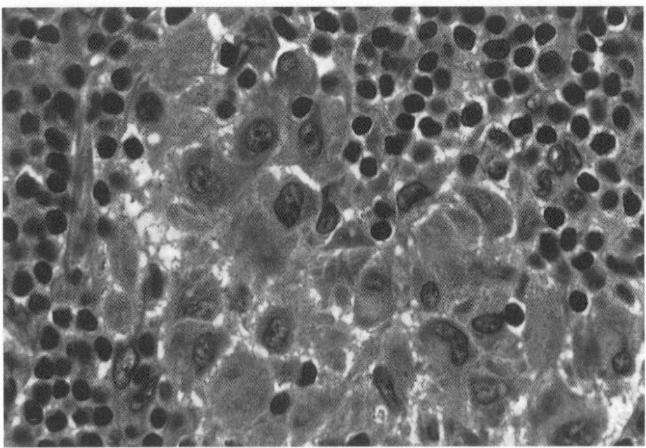

FIGURE 30.9. Epithelioid cells have abundant, pale-staining cytoplasm and ovoid nuclei with one or two conspicuous nucleoli and no visible mitoses.

free *Toxoplasma* trophozoites may be noted in the tissues (27). Trophozoites represent the invasive form and are responsible for the manifestations of the acute infection. They are best recognized by their crescent shapes in Giemsa-stained tissue imprints and smears (7). *Toxoplasma* cysts are even less common and are found in only a few cases in involved lymph nodes (28) (Fig. 30.10). Their presence indicates chronic, but not necessarily acute, infection. Both trophozoites and cysts can be also identified immunohistochemically with anti-*Toxoplasma* antibodies in tissue sections (29).

The question of whether *Toxoplasma* lymphadenitis can be diagnosed histologically has been raised and tested repeatedly. Piringer-Kuchinka et al. (19), who originally described the histologic picture of *Toxoplasma* lymphadenitis, subjected their cases to serologic testing and obtained high titers with the Sabin-Feldman dye test and the complement fixation test in 46 of 49 patients. More recently, in a study of 667 cases originally suspected of having *Toxoplasma* lymphadenitis, high titers of specific antibodies were obtained in 80% of cases; conversely, 85% to 95% of cases with high antibody titers exhibited the characteristic histology (24). Thus, it can be concluded that *Toxoplasma* lymphadenitis can be diagnosed histologically with a fairly high degree of accuracy when the elements of the characteristic triad (i.e., reactive germinal centers, perifollicular clusters of epithelioid cells, and aggregates of monocytoid cells) coexist. The diagnosis of *Toxoplasma* lymphadenitis is clinically significant for its differentiation from lymphoma, the potential risk to pregnancy, and the indication to investigate the possible involvement of other organs (16).

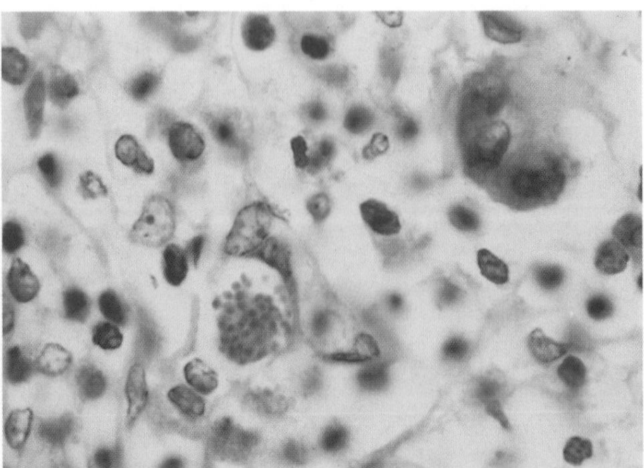

FIGURE 30.10. Rare observation of *Toxoplasma* organisms in lymph node. Numerous trophozoites engulfed by macrophage (*center*) in paracortical area, which also contains epithelioid cells and a multinucleated giant cell (*upper right*).

CYTODIAGNOSIS

Fine needle aspiration of enlarged lymph nodes is increasingly used as a first-line, less invasive, less costly diagnostic procedure. In *Toxoplasma* lymphadenitis, an aspirate stained with Giemsa or Diff-Quick stain shows a polymorphous population of small inactive or large activated lymphocytes, epithelioid cells, plasma cells, and tingible-body macrophages. No evidence of giant cells, granulomas, or suppurative or caseating necrosis is noted. These findings suggestive of toxoplasmosis must then be confirmed by serologic testing (30).

ELECTRON MICROSCOPY

Characteristic ultrastructural features of *T. gondii* are paired organelles, dense bodies, conoid nuclei at the rounded posterior end, and double-layered pellicles (29).

IMMUNOHISTOCHEMISTRY/MOLECULAR PATHOLOGY

T. gondii can be identified *in situ* with the use of commercially available anti-*Toxoplasma* antibodies, fluorescein-labeled for frozen sections or peroxidase-labeled for paraffin-embedded tissues. This method permits faster and easier recognition of trophozoites and cysts on tissue sections and smears than does hematoxylin and eosin or Giemsa stain (7,29). *Toxoplasma* genomes can be identified in fresh or paraffin-embedded tissues with a sensitive and specific polymerase chain reaction technique (31). With this method, *Toxoplasma* DNA was reliably detected in *Toxoplasma* encephalitis and myocarditis in AIDS patients, but not in *Toxoplasma* lymphadenitis in immunocompetent patients, in whom only one of nine cases produced positive results (31).

LABORATORY TESTS

A tentative histologic diagnosis of *Toxoplasma* lymphadenitis must be confirmed by serologic tests.

- The classic Sabin-Feldman dye test, which is highly sensitive and specific, is based on the observation that *Toxoplasma* organisms do not stain with alkaline methylene blue if they have been exposed to antibody-containing serum. Because of the occurrence of *Toxoplasma* antibodies in a large segment of the general population, a test result is considered diagnostic only if a change from a negative to a positive result or from a low titer to rapidly climbing titers occurs (from 0 to 1:256 or higher is considered significant) (17), or if a strikingly high stable titer of 1:64,000 or higher is seen (1). The long-used test requires live *Toxoplasma* organisms and therefore has been replaced by the indirect immunofluorescence test.
- In the indirect immunofluorescence test, purified air-dried smears of a *Toxoplasma* suspension, stored at −20°C, are used to measure immunoglobulin M (IgM) and IgG antibodies to cell wall antigens. The IgM antibodies are first detected a few days after infection; they rise to a peak and decrease during a few weeks or months. A titer of 1:80 or higher is indicative of recent infection (3,7). The IgG antibodies reach a peak titer of 1:1,000 or higher 6 to 8 weeks after infection; this titer persists for months or years (3,7).
- Complement-fixing antibodies appear much later, are considered positive when they rise from 0 to 1:8 or higher (17), and may prove useful in patients who already have a high titer in the dye test.
- Indirect hemagglutination tests also produce peak values at 4 to 6 months (7).
- Intraperitoneal inoculation: Suspected material is inoculated into mice. *Toxoplasma* tachyzoites are present in the exudate that develops after 4 to 6 days. This is a highly reliable means of diagnosis (2).

DIFFERENTIAL DIAGNOSIS

- Sarcoidosis lymphadenopathy has well-formed granulomas with multinucleated giant cells, in contrast to toxoplasmosis, in which the proliferation of epithelioid cells is diffuse and giant cells are absent.
- Dermatopathic lymphadenopathy includes melanin pigment and lipids, in addition to a large collection of histiocytes.
- Infectious mononucleosis lymphadenitis shows reactive germinal centers and a massive proliferation of immunoblasts without the clusters of epithelioid cells characteristic of toxoplasmosis, cat-scratch disease, and brucellosis. Lupus erythematosus lymphadenopathies have distinct areas of necrosis.
- Leishmaniasis lymphadenitis may manifest only as lymph node involvement. The histology may be entirely similar to that of toxoplasmosis, in which case the distinction can be made by electron microscopy (32).

Checklist

TOXOPLASMA LYMPHADENITIS

Worldwide distribution
Most common parasitic infection in the United States
Cat definitive host and source of contamination
T. gondii in humans: trophozoites as rapidly multiplying form or cysts as latent form
Clinical forms of toxoplasmosis
- Toxoplasmosis lymphadenitis in immunocompetent hosts
- Systemic toxoplasmosis in immunodeficient hosts
- Fetal toxoplasmosis acquired by transplacental infection

Posterior cervical lymph nodes most commonly affected
Characteristic histologic triad
- Reactive germinal centers
- Perifollicular and intrafollicular clusters of epithelioid cells
- Patches of monocytoid cells

Absence of necrosis, fibrosis, granulomas, neutrophils, eosinophils
In situ identification of *T. gondii* with labeled antibodies
Reliable serologic tests available to confirm histologic diagnosis

- HIV lymphadenitis, pattern A, shows aggregates of monocytoid cells and reactive follicles but no clusters of epithelioid cells. Immune stainings for HIV p24 can resolve a difficult differential diagnosis.
- Non-Hodgkin lymphomas may include clusters of epithelioid cells indistinguishable from those of toxoplasmosis; however, the general structure is destroyed and the cellularity is more uniform. In contrast, in *Toxoplasma* lymphadenitis, the follicular architecture is preserved and the cell populations are diverse (15).
- Tumor-reactive lymphadenopathy is characterized by marked hyperplasia of histiocytes, generally confined to the sinuses.
- Lennert lymphoma is characterized by large numbers of epithelioid cells; however, recent reports indicate that it does not represent a well-defined entity and that epithelioid cells may be seen in a variety of lymphomas that must be diagnosed by their characteristic features (15).
- Hodgkin lymphoma, lymphocytic and histiocytic type, shows effacement of follicles and the presence of lymphocyte and histiocyte cells (popcorn cells).
- Malignant histiocytosis: Obliteration of nodal architecture, cells with highly atypical nuclei and numerous atypical mitoses.

Determining the identity of the microorganisms involves distinguishing *T. gondii* from *Histoplasma capsulatum,* a fungus, which also is characterized by the presence of multiple organisms within a cell. However, *Histoplasma* organisms are present only in histiocytes, whereas *Toxoplasma* organisms invade any parenchymal cell; in addition, the cell wall of *Histoplasma* organisms stains strongly with periodic acid–Schiff stain (6). *Leishmania* organisms are differentiated from *T. gondii* organisms by the characteristic presence of a kinetoplast. *Pneumocystis carinii* organisms are differentiated by their failure to stain with hematoxylin and eosin.

REFERENCES

1. Remington JS, Jacobs L, Kaufman HE. Toxoplasmosis in the adult. N Engl J Med 1960;262:180–186, 237–241.
2. Frenkel JK. Toxoplasmosis. In: Binford CH, Connor DH, eds. Pathology of tropical and extraordinary diseases, vol 1. Washington, DC: Armed Forces Institute of Pathology, 1976:284–301.
3. Krick JA, Remington JS. Current concepts in parasitology—toxoplasmosis in the adult: an overview. N Engl J Med 1978;298: 550–553.
4. Garin Y, Audouin J, Diebold J. La lymphadénite toxoplasmique: aspects histopathologiques et étude en immunofluorescence. Arch Anat Cytol Pathol 1977;25:221–226.
5. Ishikawa T, Nishino H, Ohara M, et al. The identification of a rabbit-transmitted cervical toxoplasmosis mimicking malignant lymphoma. Am J Clin Pathol 1990;94:107–110.
6. Myerowitz RL. Toxoplasmosis. In: Myerowitz RL, ed. The pathology of opportunistic infections. New York: Raven Press, 1983:225–235.
7. Sun T. Toxoplasmosis. In: Sun T, ed. Sexually related infectious diseases. New York: Field, Rich, 1986:227–237.
8. Hakes TB, Armstrong D. Toxoplasmosis: problems in diagnosis and treatment. Cancer 1983;52:1535–1540.
9. Gleason TH, Hamlin WB. Disseminated toxoplasmosis in the compromised host. Arch Intern Med 1974;134:1059–1062.
10. Ruskin J, Remington JS. Toxoplasmosis in the compromised host. Ann Intern Med 1976;84:193–199.
11. Petito CK, Cho E-S, Lemann W, et al. Neuropathology of acquired immunodeficiency syndrome (AIDS): an autopsy review. J Neuropathol Exp Neurol 1986;45:635–646.
12. Moskowitz LB, Hensley GT, Chan JC, et al. Brain biopsies in patients with acquired immune deficiency syndrome. Arch Pathol Lab Med 1984;108:368–371.
13. Levy RM, Bredesen DE, Rosenblum ML. Neurological manifestations of the acquired immunodeficiency syndrome (AIDS): experience at UCSF and review of the literature. J Neurosurg 1985; 62:475–495.
14. Moskowitz LB, Hensley GT, Chan JC, et al. The neuropathology of acquired immune deficiency syndrome. Arch Pathol Lab Med 1984;108:867–872.
15. Miettinen M, Fransilla K. Malignant lymphoma simulating lymph node toxoplasmosis. Histopathology 1982;6:129–140.
16. McCabe RE, Brooks RG, Dorfman RF, et al. Clinical spectrum in 107 cases of toxoplasmic lymphadenopathy. Rev Infect Dis 1987;9:754–774.
17. Jones TC, Kean BH, Kimball AC. Toxoplasmic lymphadenitis. JAMA 1965;192:87–91.
18. Gray GF Jr, Kimball AC, Kean BH. The posterior cervical lymph node in toxoplasmosis. Am J Pathol 1972;69:349–358.
19. Piringer-Kuchinka A, Martin I, Thalhammer O. Uber die vorzuglich cervico-nuchale Lymphadenitis mit kleinherdiger Epithelioid zellwucherung. Virchows Arch A Pathol Anat Histopathol 1958;331:522–535.
20. Saxen E, Saxen L, Gronroos P. Glandular toxoplasmosis: a report on 23 histologically diagnosed cases. Acta Pathol Microbiol Scand 1958;44:319–328.
21. Stansfeld AG. The histological diagnosis of toxoplasmic lymphadenitis. J Clin Pathol A 1961;14:565–573.
22. Dorfman RF, Remington JS. Value of lymph node biopsy in the diagnosis of acute acquired toxoplasmosis. N Engl J Med 1973;289:878–881.
23. Putschar WGJ. Can toxoplasmic lymphadenitis be diagnosed histologically? [Editorial]. N Engl J Med 1973;289:913–914.
24. Miettinen M. Histologic differential diagnosis between lymph node toxoplasmosis and other benign lymph node hyperplasias. Histopathology 1981;5:205–216.
25. Sheibani K, Fritz RM, Winberg CD, et al. "Monocytoid" cells in reactive follicular hyperplasia with and without multifocal histiocytic reactions: an immunohistochemical study of 21 cases including suspected cases of toxoplasmic lymphadenitis. Am J Clin Pathol 1984;81:453–458.
26. Ioachim HL, Cronin W, Roy M, et al. Persistent lymphadenopathies in individuals at high risk for HIV infection. Clinicopathologic correlations and long-term follow-up in 79 cases. Am J Clin Pathol 1990;93:208–218.
27. Ioachim HL. Toxoplasmosis. In: Pathology of AIDS. Philadelphia: JB Lippincott Co, 1989:71–73.
28. Cohen C, Trapuckd S. *Toxoplasma* cyst with toxoplasmic lymphadenitis. Hum Pathol 1984;15:396–397.
29. Andres TL, Dorman SA, Winn WC Jr, et al. Immunohistochemical demonstration of *Toxoplasma gondii.* Am J Clin Pathol 1981;75:431–434.
30. Gupta RK. Fine needle aspiration cytodiagnosis of toxoplasmic lymphadenitis. Acta Cytol 1997;41:1031–1034.
31. Weiss LM, Chen Y-Y, Berry GJ, et al. Infrequent detection of *Toxoplasma gondii* genome in toxoplasmic lymphadenitis. Hum Pathol 1992;23:154–158.
32. Daneshbod K. Localizing lymphadenitis due to *Leishmania* simulating toxoplasmosis. Value of electron microscopy for differentiation. Am J Clin Pathol 1978;69:462–467.

31

LEISHMANIA LYMPHADENITIS

ETIOLOGY

Leishmania donovani, a protozoan, is transmitted by sandflies (*Phlebotomus* species). In human tissues, the leishmanias, or amastigotes, appear as small, ovoid or round organisms, 1.5 to 3 μm in diameter (1). They have a thin cell membrane, a large nucleus, and a rod-shaped kinetoplast. The parasites multiply by binary fission within histiocytes; these eventually burst and release the amastigotes, which then infect new histocytes (1). The natural reservoirs of *Leishmania* organisms are various animals, including dogs and cats.

EPIDEMIOLOGY

Leishmaniasis is endemic in Asia, South America, Africa, and the Mediterranean regions. Travelers from other parts of the world may acquire the disease (2,3).

CLINICAL SYNDROME

The various clinical forms of leishmaniasis depend on the protozoan species and the geographic site (2). Visceral leishmaniasis, or kala-azar, the most severe and extensive form of the disease, prevails in areas where the climate favors the propagation of sandflies, such as the Indian subcontinent (1). Cutaneous leishmaniasis, manifesting as ulcers of the skin with scarring at the site of sandfly bites, is more common in South America. Both the visceral and cutaneous forms of leishmaniasis are accompanied by regional lymphadenitis. In Iran, visceral leishmaniasis is common in children and associated with palpable lymph nodes in 5% of cases (4). In addition, leishmaniasis may be solely localized to the lymph nodes, without any evidence of visceral or cutaneous involvement (2–5). *Leishmania* lymphadenitis was reported in American service personnel overseas and in patients in other countries under the name of *localized lymph node leishmaniasis without any other clinical manifestations* (2,4).

HISTOPATHOLOGY

In one study of 19 cases of localized *Leishmania* lymphadenitis, peripheral lymph nodes in all areas, from submandibular to inguinal, were involved (4). The lymph nodes are moderately enlarged, firm, and adherent to the surrounding tissues. The lymphoid follicles are hyperplastic with reactive germinal centers. Multiple small collections of histiocytes and epithelioid cells are scattered in the cortex and medulla, creating a "starry sky" pattern (Fig. 31.1) and often involving the lymphoid follicles; the pattern is similar to the distribution of epithelioid cells in toxoplasmic lymphadenitis. Larger collections of histiocytes may accumulate under and even within the lymph node capsule. Some granuloma-like aggregates of epithelioid cells (Fig. 31.2) also include a few multinucleated giant cells (Fig. 31.3). Areas of necrosis may be present in the center of granulomas with bodies that stain with hematoxylin, some of which are dead organisms (4) (Fig. 31.2). A few histiocytes in the cortex contain abundant intracytoplasmic, small (1 to 2 μm), basophilic organisms, the amastigotes or Leishman-Donovan bodies, which stain strongly with hematoxylin (Fig.31.4). Plasma cells are inconspicuous. As the immunity develops, the granulomatous reaction predominates and the leishmanias are hard to find (1). Granulomas with giant cells are usually devoid of parasites (2). In some patients, an anergic response is characterized by numerous large histiocytes (Fig. 31.4) and giant cells (Figs. 31.5 and 31.6); these contain multiple intracellular amastigotes (Fig. 31.7) and produce a starry sky pattern (4). In others, necrosis is present, possibly the result of a strong antigen–antibody interaction (4–6).

ELECTRON MICROSCOPY

The Leishman-Donovan amastigotes are round to oval bodies within vacuoles within histiocytic macrophages. They have a round nucleus with a peripheral chromatic central nucleolus, a rod-shaped kinetoplast, and a target-shaped basal body. A double-layered membrane is present that may adhere to a nearby organism (2,4).

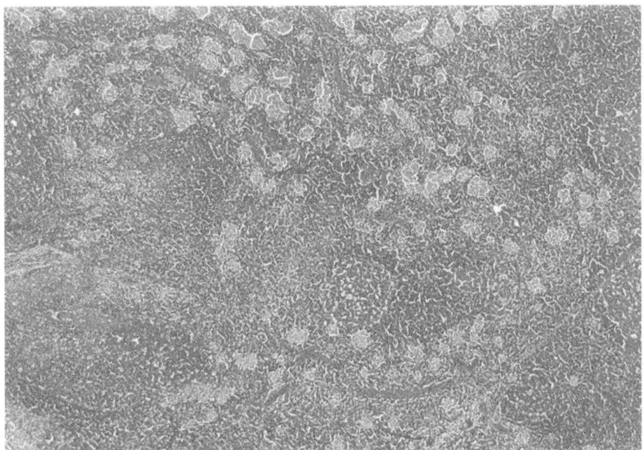

FIGURE 31.1. *Leishmania* lymphadenitis. Numerous small granulomas in the cortex producing a starry sky pattern. Hematoxylin and eosin stain. (From Azadeh B, Sells PG, Ejeckam GC, et al. Localized *Leishmania* lymphadenitis. Immunohistochemical studies. Am J Clin Pathol 1994;102:11–15, with permission. Slide courtesy of Dr. B. Azadeh.)

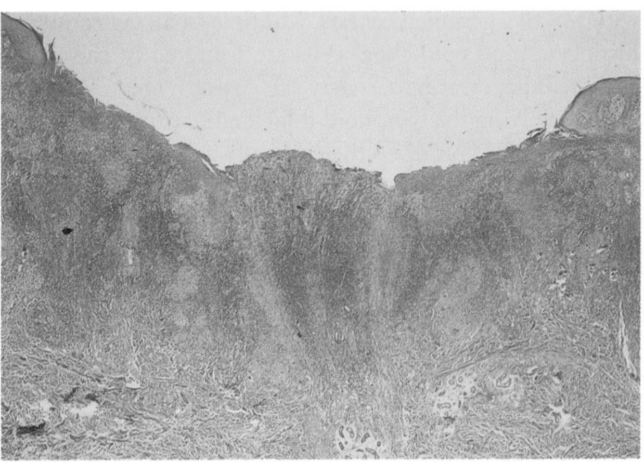

FIGURE 31.2. *Leishmania* lymphadenitis with multiple granulomas, some with areas of necrosis (*bottom*). Hematoxylin, phloxine, and saffron stain.

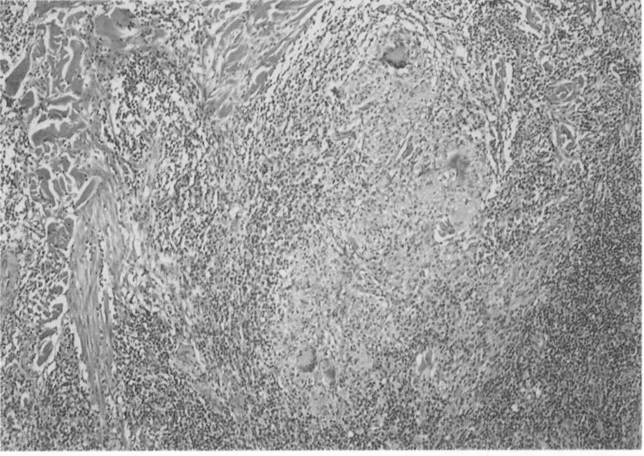

FIGURE 31.3. Same lymph node as in Fig. 31.2. Large confluent granulomas with multinucleated giant cells. Hematoxylin, phloxine, and saffron stain.

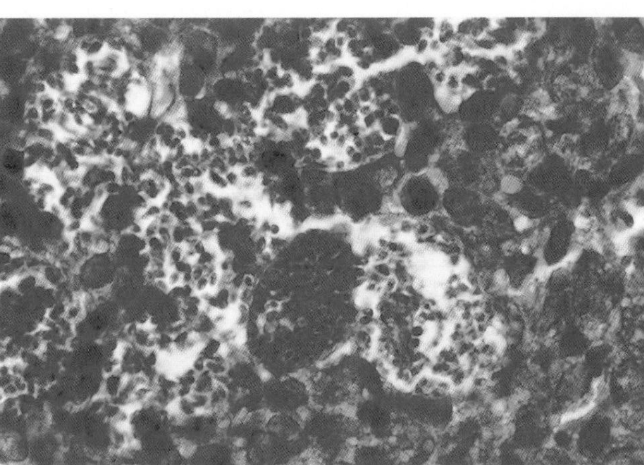

FIGURE 31.4. *Leishmania* lymphadenitis. Numerous *Leishmania* amastigotes within a histiocyte and free in the tissues. Hematoxylin and eosin stain. (From Azadeh B, Sells PG, Ejeckam GC, et al. Localized *Leishmania* lymphadenitis. Immunohistochemical studies. Am J Clin Pathol 1994;102:11–15, with permission. Slide courtesy of Dr. B. Azadeh.)

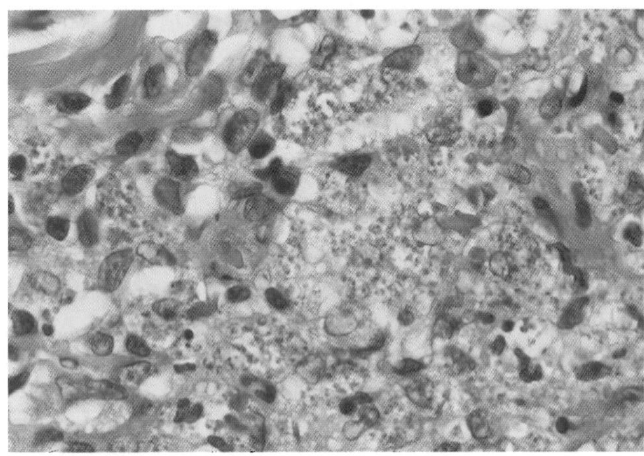

FIGURE 31.5. *Leishmania* lymphadenitis in HIV-infected immunodeficient patient; a large number of amastigotes are free in the tissues. Hematoxylin, phloxine, and saffron stain.

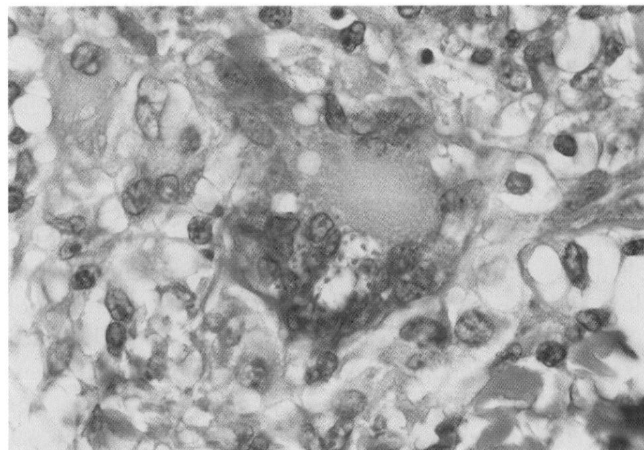

FIGURE 31.6. Same lymph node as in Fig. 31.5. Engulfed amastigotes within multinucleated giant cell. Hematoxylin, phloxine, and saffron stain.

Checklist

LEISHMANIA LYMPHADENITIS

Microscopic protozoa transmitted by sandflies
Cutaneous and localized or visceral and systemic
Lymphadenitis and perilymphadenitis
Granulomas forming starry sky pattern
Necrosis more common in immunodeficient patients
Histiocytes and giant cells with intracellular amastigotes
Round organisms that stain strongly with hematoxylin
Double-layered membrane, kinetoplast

IMMUNOHISTOCHEMISTRY

Antiserum raised in rabbits against live amastigotes was used in lymph node sections in a peroxidase–antiperoxidase staining (6). Positive staining of *Leishmania* organisms and diffuse staining of granulomas containing the amastigote antigens was obtained. The plasma cells in the inflammatory infiltrates were predominantly of the immunoglobulin G (IgG) and IgE classes.

DIFFERENTIAL DIAGNOSIS

- *Toxoplasma* lymphadenitis: Necrosis and fibrosis, present in *Leishmania* lymphadenitis, are not features of *Toxoplasma* lymphadenitis. The size and shape of the two organisms are identical; however, the rod-shaped kinetoplast and target-shaped basal body seen under the electron microscope are unique to *Leishmania* organisms. Serologic tests specific for *Toxoplasma* are available.
- *Histoplasma* lymphadenitis: The yeasts resemble the *Leishmania* organisms; however, the former are not stained by hematoxylin and are stained by Grocott methenamine silver stain, whereas the opposite is true for the latter.
- Cat-scratch lymphadenitis: Tissue necrosis surrounded by epithelioid cells is present; however, the organisms are clusters of bacilli stained by Warthin-Starry silver stain.
- Mycobacterial lymphadenitis: Tissue necrosis surrounded by epithelioid cells is present; however, the organisms are acid-fast bacilli.
- Sarcoidosis lymphadenitis: Necrosis is rare and limited, and microorganisms are not present.

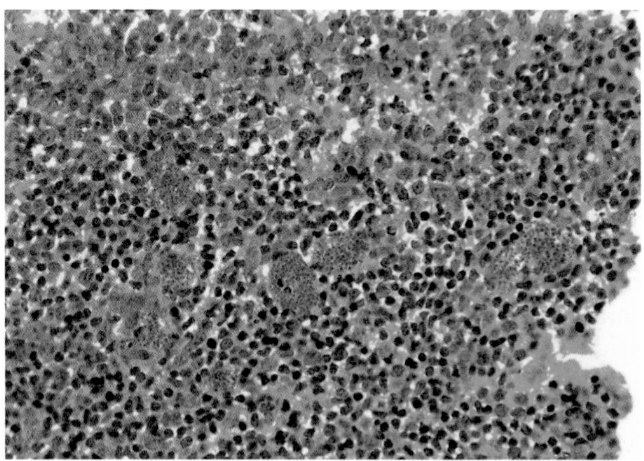

FIGURE 31.7. *Leishmania* lymphadenitis. Immunostaining for *Leishmania* antigen shows numerous amastigotes within macrophages. Rabbit anti-L tropica antiserum/peroxidase stain. (From Azadeh B, Sells PG, Ejeckam GC, et al. Localized *Leishmania* lymphadenitis. Immunohistochemical studies. Am J Clin Pathol 1994;102:11–15, with permission. Slide courtesy of Dr. B. Azadeh.)

REFERENCES

1. Connor DH, Neafie RC. Cutaneous leishmaniasis. In: Binford CH, Connor DH, eds. Pathology of tropical and extraordinary diseases, vol 1. Washington, DC: Armed Forces Institute of Pathology, 1976:258–272.
2. Daneshbod K. Localized lymphadenitis due to *Leishmania* simulating toxoplasmosis. Am J Clin Pathol 1978;69:462–467.
3. Kern F, Pedersen JK. Leishmaniasis in the United States. A report of ten cases in military personnel. JAMA 1973;226:872–874.
4. Azadeh B. "Localized" leishmania lymphadenitis: a light and electron microscopic study. Am J Trop Med Hyg 1985;34:447–455.
5. Bell DW, Carmichael JAG, Williams RS, et al. Localized leishmaniasis of lymph nodes. Report of four cases. Br Med J 1958;1:740–743.
6. Azadeh B, Sells PG, Ejeckam GC, et al. Localized leishmania lymphadenitis. Immunohistochemical studies. Am J Clin Pathol 1994;102:11–15.

32

FILARIA LYMPHADENITIS

DEFINITION

Lymphadenitis caused by infection with filarial parasites.

ETIOLOGY

Filaria organisms are nematode worms of various species with a distinct geographic distribution. *Wuchereria bancrofti* is prevalent in Africa and Central and South America. *Brugia malayi* and *Brugia timor* are more common in Asia and South America (1,2). In North America, cases of *Brugia* filariasis acquired from animals, *B. beaveri* from raccoons and *B. lepori* from rabbits, have been reported (3,4). Most cases have been from the northeastern United States; occasional cases have occurred in the South, Midwest, and even New York City (5). According to the World Health Organization, lymphatic filariasis affects more than 90 million people throughout the world (6).

PATHOGENESIS

In humans, adult *Filaria* worms colonize lymphatic vessels and lymph nodes, where they can live for years. The female worms discharge microfilariae into the blood, which is ingested by various species of mosquitoes. In the mosquitoes, which act as intermediate hosts and vectors, the microfilariae metamorphose into infective larvae, which through the insect bite penetrate the skin, enter the circulation, and migrate to a suitable location, where they develop into adult worms (1).

CLINICAL SYNDROME

Bancroftian filariae may be as long as 100 mm and up to 200 μm wide, whereas *Brugia* filariae are slender and threadlike, with a diameter of 40 to 75 μm. In men, they are most commonly found in the lymphatics of the epididymis and testis, and in women in the lymphatics of the breast (6). They also invade the lymphatics of the legs and the inguinal and pelvic lymph nodes. The lymphatics become occluded and inflamed. Dead and degenerated parasites in particular elicit intense inflammatory reactions, which have been misinterpreted in some cases as testicular torsion and mammary fibroadenoma or carcinoma (6). Cervical, axillary, and inguinal lymph nodes may be enlarged and tender (3). In the acute phase, fever, headache, muscle pains, and nausea may be present (1). Blockage of the lymphatics in the lower limbs may cause elephantiasis of the legs, more often in elderly persons (7). Primary immune deficiency or secondary immune suppression allows the development of filariae and dissemination of the infection (7). *Brugia* filariasis with severe lymphedema was reported in a 7-month-old American child with congenital immune deficiency (7).

HISTOPATHOLOGY

The lymphatic spaces containing filariae in the lymph nodes, male genitalia, breasts, and legs are dilated and lined by thickened endothelium. They are surrounded by a chronic inflammatory infiltrate consisting of lymphocytes, plasma cells, eosinophils, and histiocytes. In time, a granulomatous reaction of epithelioid and giant cells develops. Viable microfilariae in lymphatics usually do not cause lesions, whereas degenerating parasites provoke an intense inflammatory reaction in which microabscesses and granulomas form around a central area of necrosis and coagulated lymph containing the parasite (Figs. 32.1 and 32.2). The worms are 30 to 75 μm wide and have a thin cuticle with fine transverse striations (3). Eventually, the dead worms become calcified and surrounded by a dense fibrous capsule (Fig. 32.3). Microfilariae can be identified in the peripheral blood, particularly at night. Surgical removal of the involved lymphatics or lymph node may be curative; otherwise, antifilarial drugs are administered.

LABORATORY TESTS

Elevated titers of immunoglobulin G to *Brugia* antigens can be assessed. An enzyme-linked immunosorbent assay that measures antifilarial antibody levels is available (4).

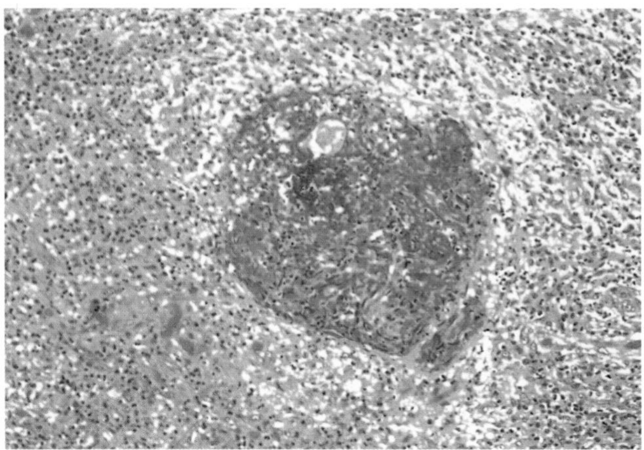

FIGURE 32.1. Central area of necrosis and coagulated lymph, including filarial cyst and giant cells, surrounded by abundant inflammatory infiltrate in inguinal lymph node. Hematoxylin, phloxine, and saffron stain.

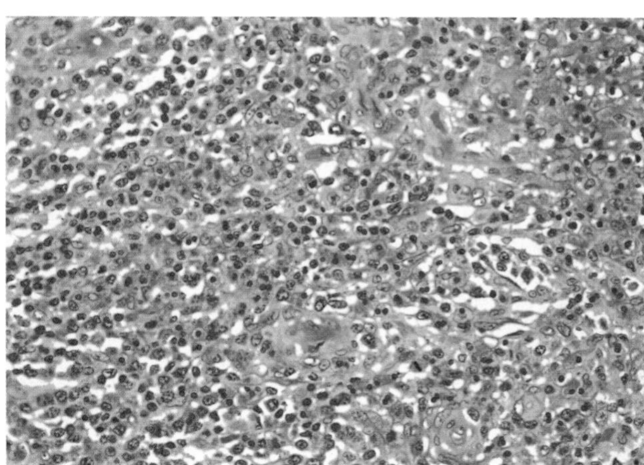

FIGURE 32.2. Necrotic area (*upper right*) with abundant inflammatory infiltrate comprising lymphocytes, plasma cells, histiocytes, and numerous eosinophils. Hematoxylin, phloxine, and saffron stain.

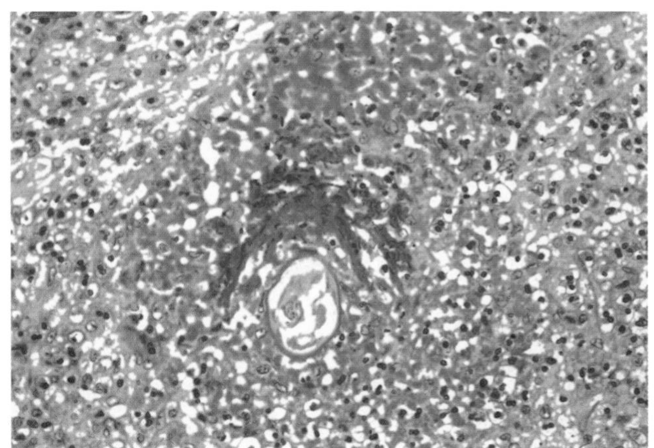

FIGURE 32.3. Dead, calcified filarial organism within fibrosed cyst, tissue necrosis, foreign body giant cells, and inflammatory infiltrate. Hematoxylin, phloxine, and saffron stain.

DIFFERENTIAL DIAGNOSIS

- Cat-scratch lymphadenitis similarly shows a central necrotic zone surrounded by microabscess and granuloma. The presence of microfilariae or organisms that stain with Warthin-Starry stain can make the diagnosis.
- *Toxoplasma* lymphadenitis: Epithelioid granulomas are present, but not necrosis and microabscesses.
- Hodgkin lymphoma: The presence of necrosis, eosinophilia, and epithelioid cells may be common. A search for microfilariae or Reed-Sternberg cells is required.

REFERENCES

1. Meyers WM, Neafie RC, Connor DH. Bancroftian and Malayan filariasis. In: Binford CH, Connor DH, eds. Pathology of tropical

Checklist

FILARIA LYMPHADENITIS

Endemic in tropical countries
Transmitted by mosquitoes
Lymphatics of epididymis, testis, breast, legs
Inguinal, axillary, cervical lymph nodes
Viable worms with little or no reaction
Degenerating worms with marked inflammatory reaction
Necrotic center, microabscesses, eosinophilia, granulomas
Blocked lymphatics, elephantiasis

and extraordinary diseases. Washington, DC: Armed Forces Institute of Pathology, 1976:340–352.
2. Orihel TC, Beaver PC. Zoonotic *Brugia* infections in North and South America. Am J Trop Med Hyg 1989;40:638–647.
3. Baird JK, Alpert LI, Friedman R, et al. North American brugian filariasis: report of nine infections of humans. Am J Trop Med Hyg 1986;35:1205–1209.
4. Eberhard ML, DeMeester LJ, Martin BW, et al. Zoonotic *Brugia* infection in Western Michigan. Am J Surg Pathol 1993;17:1058–1061.
5. Rosenblatt R, Baver PC, Orihel TC. A filarial infection apparently acquired in New York City. Am J Trop Med Hyg 1962;11:641–645.
6. Jungmann P, Figueredo-Silva J, Dreyer G. Bancroftian lymphangitis in northeastern Brazil: a histopathological study of 17 cases. J Trop Med Hyg 1992;95:114–118.
7. Simmons CF, Winter HS, Berde C, et al. Zoonotic filariasis with lymphedema in an immunodeficient infant. N Engl J Med 1984; 310:1243–1245.

PART IV

LYMPHADENOPATHIES

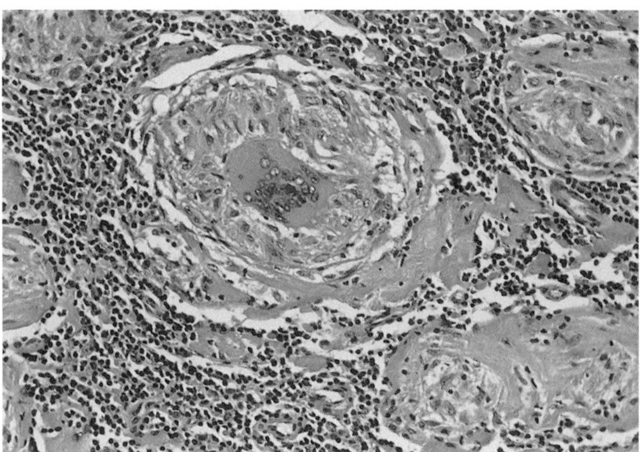

Lymphadenopathies are reactive processes of lymph nodes in response to a variety of exogenous and endogenous stimulants. The etiology and pathogenesis of many lymphadenopathies are still unknown; thus, the category remains heterogeneous and poorly defined. Possible causes of lymphadenopathies include microorganisms not yet identified, autoimmune diseases, immune deficiency and dysregulation, foreign bodies, medical procedures, and tumors. Lymphadenopathies are non-neoplastic processes, so their recognition and differential diagnosis are of great importance.

Classifying entities of unknown etiologies and overlapping histologic patterns is a tentative and imperfect process. We have chosen the term *lymphadenopathies* for lymph node lesions in which no infectious agent has been identified, in contrast to *lymphadenitides* (described in Part III), which are causally related to microorganisms. We have further subclassified lymphadenopathies into reactive lymphadenopathies (Section One), lymphadenopathies associated with clinical syndromes (Section Two), iatrogenic lymphadenopathies (Section Three), vascular lymphadenopathies (Section Four), foreign body lymphadenopathies (Section Five), and lymph node inclusions (Section Six).

PART IV

SECTION ONE

REACTIVE LYMPHADENOPATHIES

33

REACTIVE LYMPHOID HYPERPLASIA

DEFINITION

Enlargement of lymph nodes or other lymphoid organs as a consequence of hyperplasia of some or all of the cellular components, reflecting stimulation of the lymphoid cells by a variety of antigens and representing a benign, reversible process.

ETIOLOGY

The causes of reactive lymphoid hyperplasia (RLH) would make a long list of bacteria, viruses, chemicals, environmental pollutants, drugs, altered tissue components, and numerous other substances acting as antigens or allergens. The hyperplastic lymph node reaction to some of these noxious agents includes characteristic morphologic features, the recognition of which is helpful in determining cause. The various lymphadenitides and lymphadenopathies described in the following chapters belong to this category.

In some cases, specific microorganisms can be detected on regular sections and identified by special stains, *in situ* hybridization, or other procedures, so that an etiologic diagnosis is possible. In others, characteristic morphologic patterns may suggest an etiologic diagnosis without proving it directly; such a situation must be clearly indicated in the final diagnosis. Still, the cases of RLH in which an etiologic agent is identified represent only a fraction, probably fewer than 10%, of all hyperplastic lymph nodes. Most enlarged lymph nodes involved by RLH or atypical lymphoid hyperplasia do not exhibit morphologic patterns indicative of specific agents, and therefore the cause of RLH is listed as unknown. Of practical importance is the need for biopsy and expert histopathologic examination to rule out neoplasia, particularly lymphoma, which RLH may simulate.

PATHOGENESIS

An essential function of lymph nodes is to filter the lymph that is drained from their tributary regions. Thus, a large variety of substances are carried to the lymph nodes. Some of these are amorphous foreign bodies, which are simply phagocytosed and degraded; others are antigenic and therefore able to trigger an immune reaction. The reactions of lymph nodes to foreign substances are diverse and difficult to separate into specific patterns. Stansfeld (1) distinguishes predominantly inflammatory reactions, caused mainly by bacteria and fungi, and predominantly immune reactions, which are more often the effects of viruses or drugs. The immune responses may be predominantly of B-cell type, characterized morphologically by either follicular hyperplasia or plasmacytosis, or predominantly of T-cell type, with a characteristic pattern of T-cell hyperplasia (1). Specific morphologic features of non-neoplastic lesions of lymph nodes permit them to be distinguished from malignant lesions (2). Lymphadenitides and lymphadenopathies tend to exhibit one of four characteristic histologic patterns: follicular, sinus, diffuse, or mixed (3). These represent expansions of the normal follicular, paracortical, medullary, and sinusoidal lymph node compartments (4). The histologic pattern seen on a tissue section captures only one point in time during the life of a lesion, reaction, or reparatory process. The patterns vary with the particular etiologic agent and the age, history, and immune competence of the host. Therefore, combined, overlapping architectural features are a more common finding than clearly defined histologic patterns on biopsy specimens of non-neoplastic lymph nodes.

CLINICAL SYNDROME

Enlarged lymph nodes may be the expression of a local lesion or systemic disease, and the clinical symptoms will reflect the underlying disorder accordingly. In children, enlarged lymph nodes are not uncommon. Non-neoplastic diagnoses were made in 68% of peripheral lymph node biopsy specimens from 85 children, and almost half were "benign reactive hyperplasia" (5). In a child up to 12 years of age, a palpable lymph node not exceeding 10 mm in diameter can be considered a normal finding, whereas lymph nodes larger than 3 mm in diameter in newborns or children past the age of 12 years are potentially abnormal and must be explored further (6). Axillary, epitrochlear, and inguinal lymph nodes in children are frequently enlarged as a result of trauma and infections that result from play habits or exposure to animals (7). Cervical nodes may be enlarged because of upper respiratory infection, and enlarged cervical nodes are less cause for alarm than enlarged nodes in the supraclavicular area or lower neck, which may indicate mediastinal disease (7). In children between 1 and 6 years old, only 28% of cervical lymph nodes infected with atypical mycobacteria were detected with Ziehl-Neelsen or auramine O stain (5). Lymph nodes that are firm to hard, sometimes adherent to deep tissues, suggest malignancy, whereas soft or fluctuant nodes indicate inflammation (7). Fever, weight loss, pallor, and malaise are important symptoms that must be taken into consideration in the evaluation of lymph node disease in both children and adults (8).

In the elderly, RLH of lymph nodes is uncommon; because their humoral immune response is subdued (9) the proliferation and expansion of germinal centers is far less apparent than in younger persons (10). In a United States study of 58 lymph node biopsy specimens from patients age 60 years or older, reactive follicular hyperplasia was associated with an inflammatory cause (rheumatoid arthritis, thrombophlebitis, or skin infection) in only 12 cases (20%), whereas lymphoma was present concurrently or subsequently in 18 cases (31%) (10). Reactive lymphadenopathies in older patients may have an occult neoplastic cause, so that careful study is required to rule out lymphoma (10). In a study of Japanese patients age 60 years or older, florid reactive follicular hyperplasia was accompanied by immunologic abnormalities (most often resulting from rheumatoid arthritis or multicentric Castleman disease) in 16 of 23 cases (70%), and malignant lymphoma developed in none (11).

Negative or nondiagnostic lymph node biopsy results showing only a general reactive pattern that does not indicate a specific diagnosis constitute a frequent problem for pathologists and clinicians. In review studies of lymph node biopsies, 37% to 59% of them were nondiagnostic, but during follow-up of the same patients, a disease related to the initial indication for lymph node biopsy, usually lymphoma, developed in 25% within 8 months and in 50% within 5 years (12,13). These results suggest that clinicians should not hesitate to recommend a repeated biopsy when systemic symptoms and nonlocalized adenopathies persist (13). In children, nondiagnostic biopsies, most often with a follicular pattern, are frequent. In one study, they accounted for 37% of 100 cases, and 74% of the patients were alive and well 5 to 20 years after the biopsy (14).

HISTOPATHOLOGY

A pathologic entity as heterogeneous and loosely defined as RLH may, not unexpectedly, exhibit a variety of morphologic patterns. This is because each of the major lymph node tissue components may be involved in the reactive process, resulting in effacement of the original architecture and the formation of new histologic structures. Although clearly defined patterns are not usually observed, several attempts have been made to classify the variants of RLH. According to the predominance of various lymph node components, four major histologic patterns have been described in the reactive process (3).

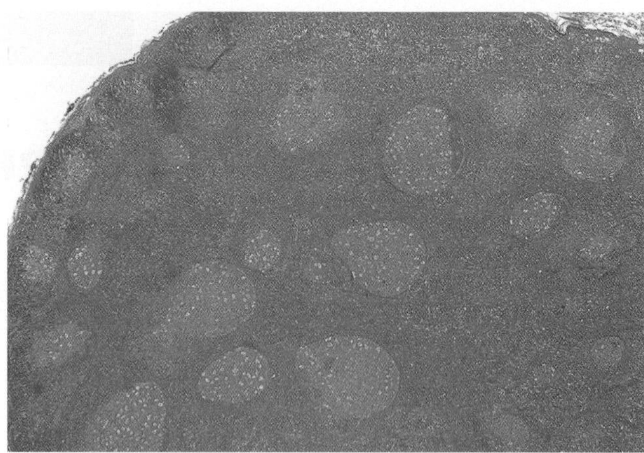

FIGURE 33.1. Reactive lymphoid hyperplasia, follicular pattern. Numerous enlarged lymphoid follicles with prominent germinal centers in cortex and corticomedullary junction area. Hematoxylin and eosin stain.

Follicular Pattern

The lymph node follicles are numerous and enlarged (Fig. 33.1), located not only in one row in the cortex but in two and three rows in the paracortex, corticomedullary junction, and even medulla (15). They vary considerably in size and shape, occasionally coalesce, and display dumbbell (Fig. 33.2) or other bizarre configurations. The mantle zone and germinal center are sharply demarcated in a reactive follicle

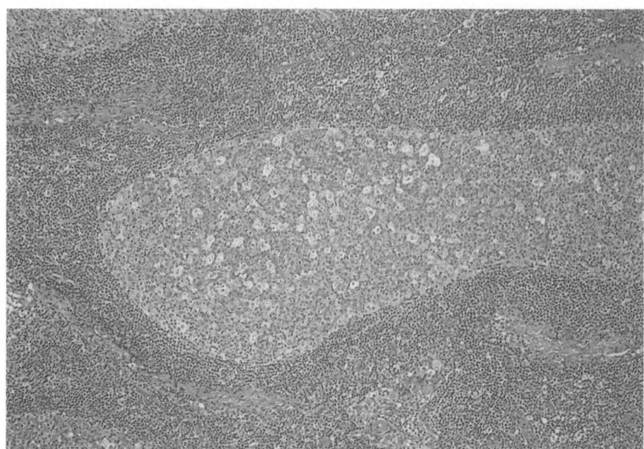

FIGURE 33.2. Reactive lymphoid hyperplasia with dumbbell-shaped follicle.

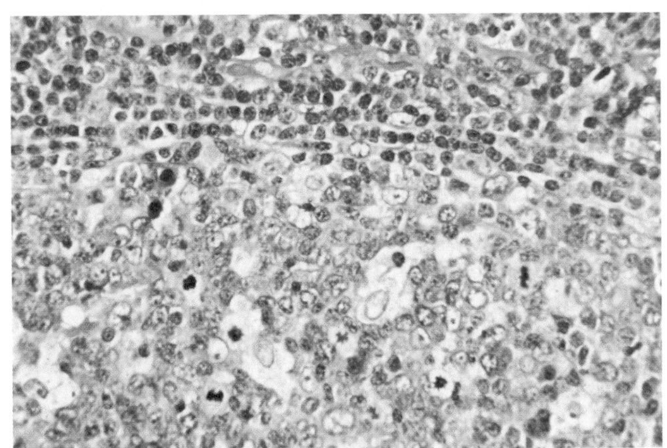

FIGURE 33.3. Sharply demarcated mantle zone (*top*) and germinal center (*bottom*) in reactive follicle.

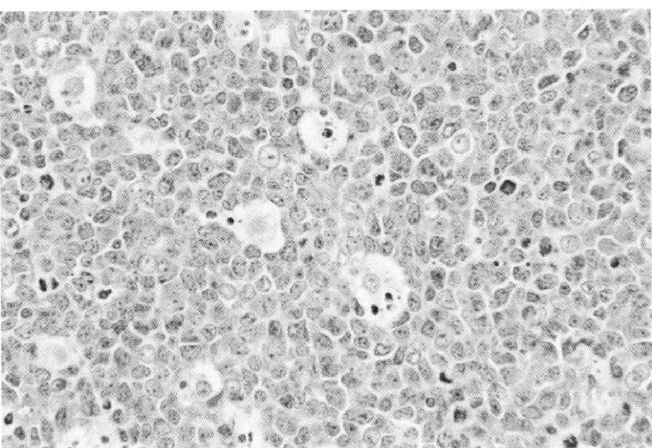

FIGURE 33.4. Reactive lymphoid hyperplasia of cervical lymph node. Germinal center with cleaved and noncleaved follicle center cells and tingible-body macrophages containing engulfed nuclear debris. Hematoxylin and eosin stain.

(Fig. 33.3). The germinal centers are prominent and hyperplastic (Figs. 33.1 and 33.2) and comprise a mixture of small and large lymphoid cells with both cleaved and noncleaved nuclei that include frequent mitoses. They also exhibit cellular destruction in the form of scattered nuclear debris and tingible-body macrophages (Fig. 33.4). A thick, peripheral layer of small, mature lymphocytes encircles the germinal center, clearly separating the follicle from the surrounding nodal parenchyma (Figs. 33.1–33.3). Silver staining reveals a slightly compressed reticulin network around the expanding reactive lymphoid follicles, but not as much compression as is seen in follicular lymphoma (FL). Large numbers of lymphocytes may infiltrate the capsule and perinodal fat or surround the lymphatics and blood vessels (Fig. 33.5); sometimes the appearance resembles the invasion of extranodal tissues seen in lymphomas and leukemias.

The follicular pattern is characteristic of a humoral immune reaction, involving the predominant stimulation and proliferation of B cells. In children and adolescents with RLH, the follicles often reach huge proportions (16). In adults, clinical suspicion of a salivary gland tumor frequently leads to biopsy of parotid or submandibular lymph

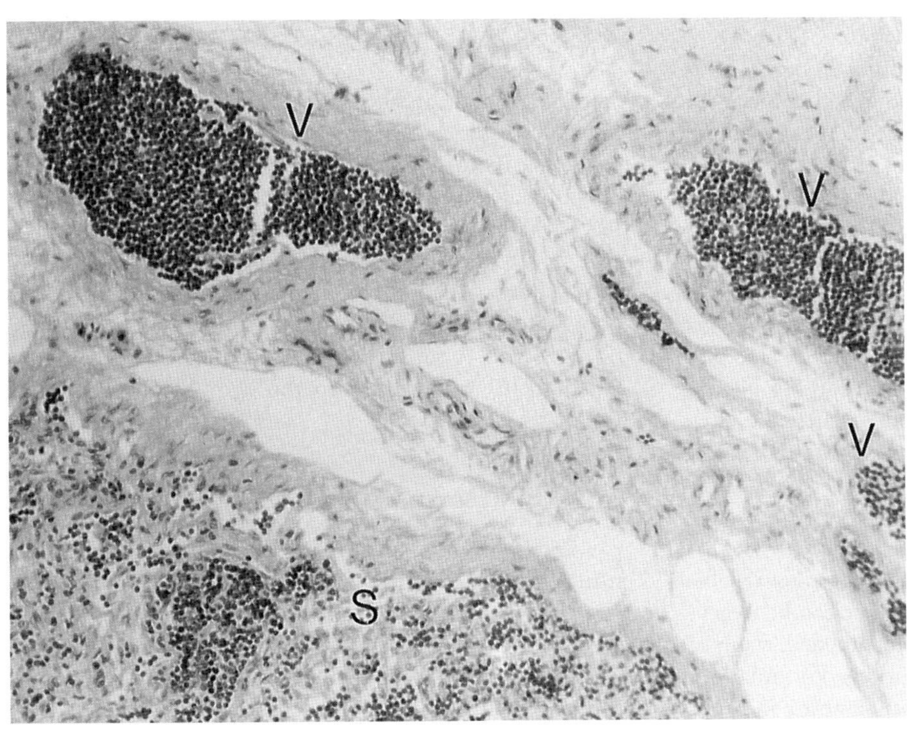

FIGURE 33.5. Reactive lymphoid hyperplasia in cervical lymph node of a 9-year-old boy. Subcapsular sinus (*S*) with marked histiocytosis. Perinodal blood vessels (*V*) and lymphatics packed with lymphocytes resembling leukemia. Hematoxylin, phloxine, and saffron stain.

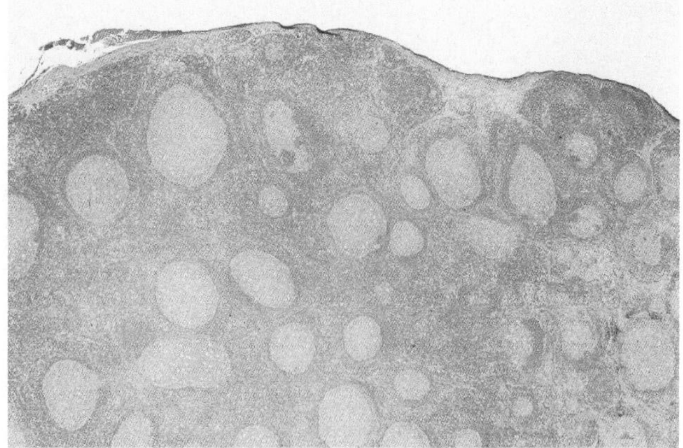

FIGURE 33.6. Enlarged cervical lymph node from a child with sore throat, fever, and spontaneous regression. Hyperplastic follicles with reactive germinal centers and thick mantle zones. Hematoxylin and eosin stain.

nodes enlarged by reactive giant follicles (16) (Fig. 33.6). A follicular pattern is characteristically present in syphilitic lymphadenitis (see Chapter 21), HIV lymphadenitis (see Chapter 15), rheumatoid lymphadenopathy (see Chapter 41), and angiofollicular lymph node hyperplasia (Castleman disease; see Chapter 43). The reaction may vary from one that involves just one or a few germinal centers to an extensive reaction that includes large numbers of follicles with enlarged germinal centers obliterating the paracortex and encroaching on the medulla, sinuses, and sometimes even the perinodal fat. Unlike the nodules of FL, however, the reactive follicles do not infiltrate the surrounding adipose tissues to a large extent, even when highly stimulated (1). In cases of prolonged antigenic stimulation, the reactive germinal centers may grow to giant size and coalescing irregular shapes, resembling the pieces of a jigsaw puzzle (1).

The presence of numerous follicles throughout the cortical and medullary zones of the lymph node biopsy specimen make the morphologic distinction between exaggerated RLH and FL a difficult one. Nathwani et al. (17) exhaustively investigated the reliability of multiple histologic and cytologic criteria. The follicles in RLH, compared with those in FL, are less numerous, less evenly distributed, and more irregularly shaped (17). The number of follicles per unit area is greater in FL than in RLH (17), although the distributions of the follicular diameters overlap (18). FL forms evenly distributed, back-to-back follicles throughout the lymph node with decreased interfollicular tissue (17). Densely compacted reticulin fibers between neoplastic follicles can be visualized with a silver stain. In contrast, the lymph node stroma in RLH is looser.

Although monomorphism (cellular monotony) favors FL, cytologic features, such as nuclear shape, are less reliable than histologic pattern (17). Cytology alone can be treacherous; for example, malignant lymphoma, follicular, mixed small cleaved and large cell type (Working Formulation) and reactive follicular hyperplasia contain a nearly indistinguishable variety of both small and large follicle center cells (centrocytes and centroblasts). However, mitotic figures are significantly more numerous in RLH than in FL (17). Additional features of RLH include the persistence, at least in part, of a lymphocytic mantle around the germinal centers, and tingible-body macrophages within the germinal centers create a characteristic "starry sky" pattern (1).

Sinus Pattern

All lymph node sinuses are markedly enlarged, compressing the nodal parenchyma (Fig. 33.7). They appear prominent even on low-power microscopic observation, dilated by abundant fluid and an excessive proliferation of histiocytes that partially obliterate their lumina (Fig. 33.8). The medulla is enlarged by a proliferation of histiocytes and of plasma cells, each forming, on occasion, solid cords and sheets. The sinus pattern is particularly noticeable in sinus histiocytosis with massive lymphadenopathy (Rosai-Dorfman disease; see Chapter 37) and in lymph nodes draining malignant tumors (see Chapter 44).

Monocytoid B lymphocytes resembling monocytes/histiocytes with abundant pale cytoplasm, round to slightly indented nuclei, open chromatin, and inconspicuous nucleoli distend the subcapsular and medullary lymph node sinuses in toxoplasmosis (see Chapter 30) (19), AIDS-related lymphadenopathy (20) (see Chapter 15), and other infectious and reactive conditions (21). Monocytoid B lymphocytes are found adjacent to hyperplastic, but not atrophic, follicles (20,21). They must be distinguished from monocytoid B-cell lymphoma or marginal zone B-cell lymphoma (22) (see Chapter 63).

Diffuse Pattern

The lymph node architecture is effaced, and the lymphoid follicles, germinal centers, and nodal sinuses are inconspicuous. The entire lymph node parenchyma consists of sheets of lymphocytes admixed with immunoblasts and occasional macrophages; a typically mottled appearance is the result (Fig. 33.9). Postcapillary venules may be prominent.

A diffuse pattern of lymphoid hyperplasia is common in lymphadenitides of viral origin (see Chapter 10), lymphadenopathy associated with anticonvulsant therapy (see Chapter 46), and dermatopathic lymphadenopathy (see Chapter 42).

Mixed Pattern

Combinations of follicular, diffuse, and sinus patterns constitute the mixed pattern. Thus, enlarged lymphoid follicles with prominent germinal centers may coexist with a marked interfollicular proliferation of immunoblasts and occasionally with distended sinuses and a proliferation of histiocytes.

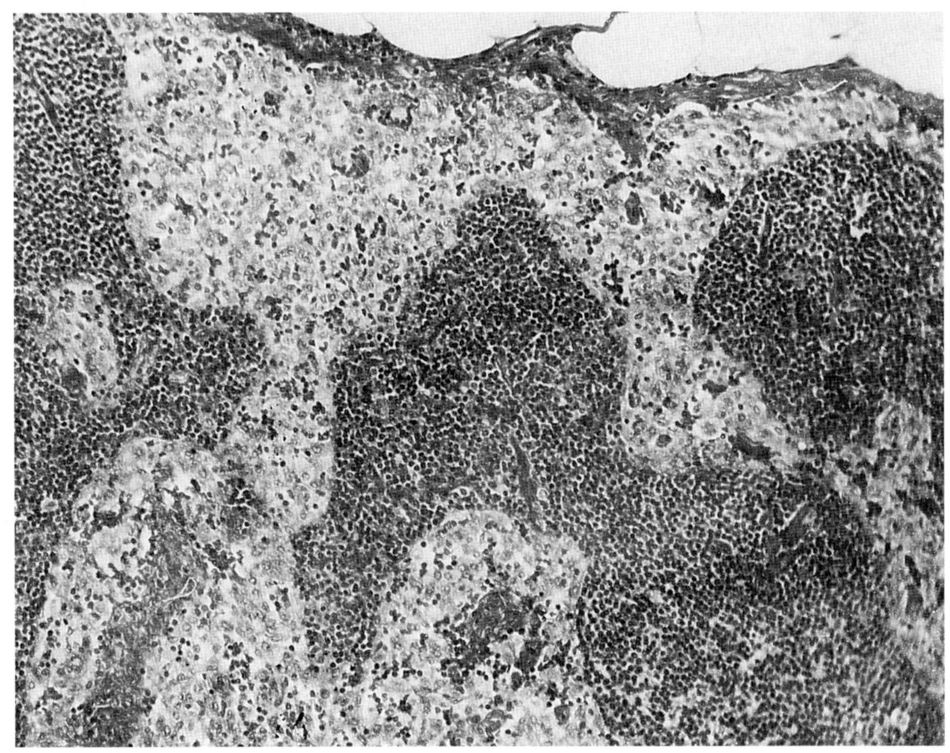

FIGURE 33.7. Reactive lymphoid hyperplasia with sinus pattern. Distended sinuses with abundant histiocytic proliferation in tumor-reactive lymph node. Hematoxylin and eosin stain.

Mixed hyperplastic patterns can be seen in infectious mononucleosis (see Chapter 9) and *Toxoplasma* lymphadenitis (see Chapter 30).

IMMUNOHISTOCHEMISTRY

A predominantly B-cell response is characterized by hyperplasia of germinal centers and therefore by a follicular pattern. Monoclonal antibodies directed against B lymphocytes, such as L26 (CD20), Leu-14 (CD22), and B4 (CD19), and particularly against centrocytes and centroblasts, such as LN-1 and LN-2, can be used to demonstrate the B cells. Because the population of follicles is heterogeneous, T cells and various kinds of histiocytes are also present. To differentiate between RLH and FL, the monoclonality of the latter must be demonstrated. This is achieved by the detection of membrane monoclonal light chain immunoglobulins. Unfortunately, this crucial differential test requires unfixed cells, fresh in suspension for flow cytometry or frozen for cryostat sections.

Immunohistochemical staining detects the expression of

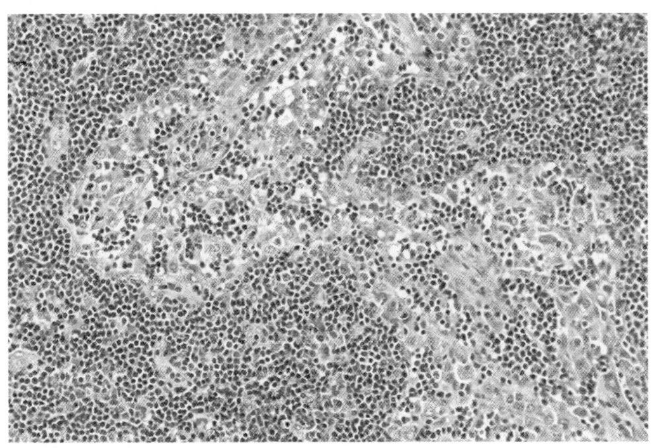

FIGURE 33.8. Numerous histiocytes in distended cortical sinus. Hematoxylin, phloxine, and saffron stain; ×200.

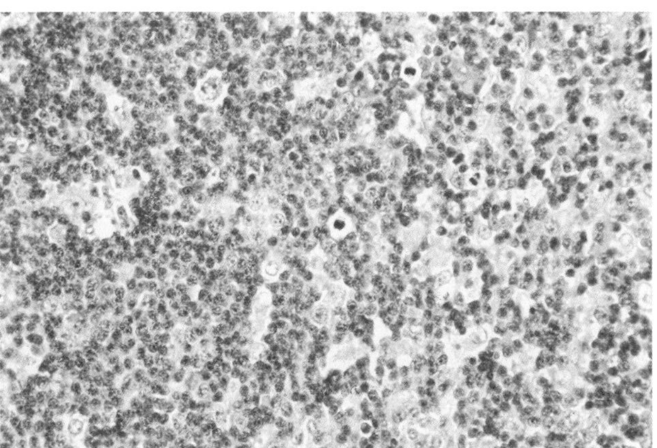

FIGURE 33.9. Reactive lymphoid hyperplasia with diffuse pattern; lymph node architecture effaced, follicles and sinuses inconspicuous. Admixture of small and activated lymphocytes, histiocytes, and interdigitating dendritic cells resulting in mottled appearance. Hematoxylin and eosin stain.

bcl-2 protein in fixed lymph node tissue. In RLH, bcl-2 protein is strongly expressed in mantle zone B-cells and moderately expressed in paracortical T cells; the germinal centers are negative for bcl-2 protein (23,24) (Fig. 33.10). In FL, neoplastic follicles overproduce bcl-2 protein and exhibit intense staining (23,24) except in a minority of cases (25) (see Chapter 64). Another useful antibody in differentiating RLH from FL on formalin-fixed paraffin sections is MT-2, which normally marks mantle B-zone cells but not the cells of germinal centers and aberrantly marks the cells of FL (26). Therefore, the germinal centers of RLH are negative and the nodules of FL are positive for MT-2 staining on paraffin sections.

A predominantly T-cell response is suspected when the follicles are small or absent and the interfollicular areas representing the T-cell zones or paracortex are widened and contain numerous postcapillary venules and activated lymphocytes or immunoblasts (1). Monoclonal antibodies can reveal the T-cell zones: pan-T-cell markers such as CD2, CD3, CD5, and CD7 or the T cell-associated marker UCHL-1 (CD45RO). Clonality cannot be determined by immunophenotype in the case of T-cell reactive proliferations, although neoplasia may be suspected if loss of one or more of the pan-T-cell antigens is noted.

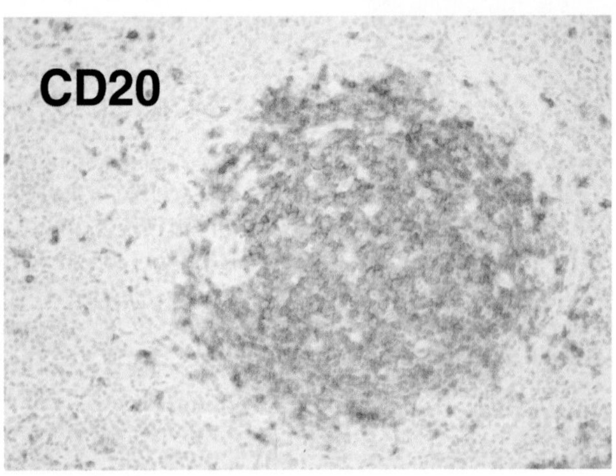

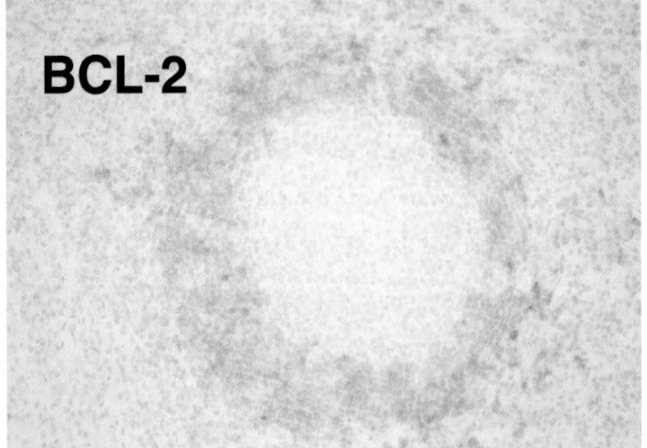

FIGURE 33.10. Top: Reactive follicle expresses CD20 (B-cell marker) in both mantle zone and germinal center. **Bottom:** Reactive follicle expresses bcl-2 protein only in mantle zone. Germinal center lacks bcl-2 protein. Immunoperoxidase stain.

GENE REARRANGEMENT ANALYSIS

Despite all efforts, in some cases, usually because of unavailable fresh or frozen tissues, the distinction between RLH and FL cannot be made reliably by histologic or immunohistochemical means. In such cases, gene rearrangement analysis is indicated for the detection of neoplastic monoclonality (27). The translocation of immunoglobulin heavy chain and bcl-2 can be detected in follicular lymphomas by the polymerase chain reaction. This breakpoint is not detectable in RLH when standard assay conditions are used (28).

DIFFERENTIAL DIAGNOSIS

As previously mentioned, the diagnosis of RLH includes two essential components: the elimination of malignant disease and the determination of cause. Although ruling out neoplasia is by far the more important, identifying the cause of lymphoid hyperplasia strongly supports a nonmalignant diagnosis and provides an indication for treatment. The entities discussed below most closely resemble the histologic patterns of RLH.

- Atypical lymphoid hyperplasia may also show enlarged lymph nodes with nodular and diffuse proliferative patterns. The cellular atypia is far greater, however, and the appearance of the lesions is highly suggestive of malignancy. In contrast, RLH, although its pattern is abnormal, does not give the impression of a malignant condition (29).
- Follicular (nodular) lymphoma: Lymph node architecture is obliterated. Nodules are of similar sizes and shapes. The cells are more closely packed. Component cells are more uniform, although their nuclei appear markedly indented and atypical. Mitoses are less frequent, and tingible-body macrophages are absent. Nodules have no peripheral rims of mature lymphocytes, and therefore their borders appear poorly demarcated. Substantial invasion of capsule and perinodal fibroadipose tissues is present (30). Cell surface markers are monoclonal light chain immunoglobulins.
- Diffuse lymphomas of small and large cell types: Cell population is more uniform than in RLH and generally does not include plasma cells and macrophages. Nuclei are atypical and nucleoli prominent. Significant invasion of capsule and perinodal tissues. Cell surface markers are monoclonal light chain immunoglobulins.
- Hodgkin lymphoma, lymphocyte predominance type and mixed cellularity type, may resemble RLH of diffuse or mixed pattern by architectural effacement and mixed cell population. Must be differentiated by demonstrating the presence of Reed-Sternberg cells, Hodgkin cells, and fibrosis.

Checklist

REACTIVE LYMPHOID HYPERPLASIA

Follicular Pattern
Numerous, enlarged, oddly shaped follicles
Prominent germinal centers
Peripheral rim of mature lymphocytes
Nonhomogeneous lymphocyte population
Frequent mitoses
Many apoptotic cells in germinal center
Tingible-body macrophages
Polyclonal surface immunoglobulins
Germinal centers negative for bcl-2

Sinus Pattern
Prominent sinuses
Histiocyte hyperplasia
Proliferation of plasma cells
Polyclonal surface immunoglobulins

Diffuse Pattern
Effacement of architecture
Proliferation of immunoblasts
Mottled appearance
Mixed cell population
Plasma cells, macrophages
Polyclonal surface immunoglobulins

Mixed Pattern
Effacement of architecture
Combinations of follicular, sinus, and diffuse patterns
Mixed cell populations
Plasma cells, macrophages
Polyclonal surface immunoglobulins

REFERENCES

1. Stansfeld AG. Inflammatory and reactive disorders. In: Stansfeld AG, ed. Lymph node biopsy interpretation. New York: Churchill Livingstone, 1985:85–141.
2. Butler JJ. Non-neoplastic lesions of lymph nodes of man to be differentiated from lymphomas. NCI Monogr 1969;32:233–255.
3. Dorfman RF, Warnke R. Lymphadenopathy simulating the malignant lymphomas. Hum Pathol 1974;5:519–550.
4. van der Valk P, Meijer CJ. The histology of reactive lymph nodes. Am J Surg Pathol 1987;11:866–882.
5. Benjamin DR. Granulomatous lymphadenitis in children. Arch Pathol Lab Med 1987;111:750–753.
6. Barnes LA. Manual of pediatric diagnosis. Chicago: Year Book, 1972:46–47.
7. Carpentieri U, Smith LR, Daeschner CW. Approach to a child with enlarged lymph nodes. Tex Med 1983;79:58–60.
8. Greenfield S, Jordan MC. The clinical investigation of lymphadenopathy in primary care practice. JAMA 1978;240:1388–1393.
9. Johnson JT, Myers EN. Evaluation of cervical masses in the elderly. Geriatrics 1983;38:99–106.
10. Osborne BM, Butler JJ. Clinical implications of nodal reactive follicular hyperplasia in the elderly patient with enlarged lymph nodes. Mod Pathol 1991;4:24–30.
11. Kojima M, Nakamura S, Shimizu K, et al. Florid reactive follicular hyperplasia in elderly patients. A clinicopathological study of 23 cases. Pathol Res Pract 1998;194:391–397.
12. Saltzstein SL. The fate of patients with nondiagnostic lymph node biopsies. Surgery 1965:58;659–662.
13. Sinclair S, Beckman E, Ellman L. Biopsy of enlarged, superficial lymph nodes. JAMA 1974;228:602–603.
14. Kissane JM, Gephardt GN. Lymphadenopathy in childhood: long-term follow-up in patients with nondiagnostic lymph node biopsies. Hum Pathol 1974;5:431–439.
15. Cottier H, Turk J, Sobin L. A proposal for a standardized system of reporting human lymph node morphology in relation to immunological function. Bull World Health Organ 1972;47:375– 408.
16. Osborne BM, Butler JJ, Variakojis D, et al. Reactive lymph node hyperplasia with giant follicles. Am J Clin Pathol 1982;78:493–499.
17. Nathwani BN, Winberg CD, Diamond LW, et al. Morphologic criteria for the differentiation of follicular lymphoma from florid reactive follicular hyperplasia: a study of 80 cases. Cancer 1981;48:1794–1806.

18. Ratech H, Sheibani K, Nathwani BN, et al. Immunoarchitecture of the "pseudofollicles" of well-differentiated (small) lymphocytic lymphoma: a comparison with true follicles [published erratum appears in Hum Pathol 1988;19:495]. Hum Pathol 1988;19:89–94.
19. Sheibani K, Fritz RM, Winberg CD, et al. "Monocytoid" cells in reactive follicular hyperplasia with and without multifocal histiocytic reactions: an immunohistochemical study of 21 cases including suspected cases of toxoplasmic lymphadenitis. Am J Clin Pathol 1984;81:453–458.
20. Sohn CC, Sheibani K, Winberg CD, et al. Monocytoid B lymphocytes: their relation to the patterns of the acquired immunodeficiency syndrome (AIDS) and AIDS-related lymphadenopathy. Hum Pathol 1985;16:979–985.
21. Plank L, Hansmann ML, Fischer R. The cytological spectrum of the monocytoid B-cell reaction: recognition of its large cell type. Histopathology 1993;23:425–431.
22. Kojima M, Nakamura S, Itoh H, et al. Occurrence of monocytoid B-cells in reactive lymph node lesions. Pathol Res Pract 1998;194:559–565.
23. Zutter M, Hockenbery D, Silverman GA, et al. Immunolocalization of the Bcl-2 protein within hematopoietic neoplasms. Blood 1991;78:1062–1068.
24. Kondo E, Nakamura S, Onoue H, et al. Detection of bcl-2 protein and bcl-2 messenger RNA in normal and neoplastic lymphoid tissues by immunohistochemistry and *in situ* hybridization. Blood 1992;80:2044–2051.
25. Ratech H. Molecular pathology of low-grade malignant lymphomas. Med Oncol 1995;12:167–176.
26. Browne G, Tobin B, Carney DN, et al. Aberrant MT2 positivity distinguishes follicular lymphoma from reactive follicular hyperplasia in B5- and formalin-fixed paraffin sections. Am J Clin Pathol 1991;96:90–94.
27. Williams ME, Lee JT, Innes DJ, et al. Immunoglobulin gene rearrangement in abnormal lymph node hyperplasia. Am J Clin Pathol 1991;96:746–754.
28. Segal GH, Scott M, Jorgensen T, et al. Standard polymerase chain reaction analysis does not detect t(14;18) in reactive lymphoid hyperplasia. Arch Pathol Lab Med 1994;118:791–794.
29. Schroer KR, Franssila KO. Atypical hyperplasia of lymph nodes: a follow-up study. Cancer 1979;44:1155–1163.
30. Rappaport H. Tumors of the hematopoietic system. Washington, DC: Armed Forces Institute of Pathology, 1966:426–442.

34

ATYPICAL LYMPHOID HYPERPLASIA

DEFINITION

Hyperplasia with atypical histologic or cytologic features of lymph nodes (or of other lymphoid organs), suggestive but not diagnostic of lymphoma.

PATHOGENESIS

Atypical lymphoid hyperplasia (ALH) is neither a clinical nor a pathologic entity, but rather a diagnostic category comprising borderline cases in which a definite determination of benign or malignant lesion cannot be made by microscopic examination (1). Some of these cases may represent early lymphomas, and others, abnormal lymph node reactions to various antigenic stimulants.

In persons with primary immunodeficiency diseases, such as ataxia telangiectasia or Wiskott-Aldrich syndrome, the incidence of lymphomas is increased (2), and these patients also show atypical lymph node reactions that cannot be classified. In a series of 35 lymphoreticular disorders that developed in patients with primary immunodeficiency, three (8.5%) were unclassifiable and considered to represent reactive phenomena in immunologically abnormal hosts (3).

In several retrospective studies of lymph node biopsies, patient follow-up was used to assess the subsequent course of nondiagnostic lesions and lesions diagnosed as atypical hyperplasia. In one review of 379 biopsies of peripheral lymph nodes, 158 were nondiagnostic and 12 were diagnosed as atypical hyperplasia. Lymphomas developed in seven of these patients (4). Sinclair and associates (1) reviewed 135 biopsies of enlarged superficial lymph nodes. Fifty (27%) of these were nondiagnostic, and lymphomas occurred in nine. In the series of Saltzstein (5), 105 of 177 patients undergoing lymph node biopsy had no specific pathologic diagnosis; however, 56 (53%) in the next 6 months showed a disease related to the initial indication for biopsy. In a survey of 600 cases referred for a second histologic opinion after an initial biopsy of Hodgkin disease, Symmers (6) found the diagnosis to be incorrect in 283 cases (47%). In 14 cases, he considered the lesion to be unclassifiable, and seven of these patients died with lymphomas and seven recovered completely. Finally, when Schroer and Franssila (7) reviewed 70 cases in which a diagnosis of atypical hyperplasia of lymph nodes had been made, they found that a malignant lymphoproliferative disease had developed in 37% of the patients during the following 2 to 13 years. The atypical hyperplasia represented 3.1% of all lymph node biopsies performed during the same period (7).

Some clinicopathologic entities, such as progressive transformation of germinal centers (see Chapter 35), iatrogenic lymphadenopathies (see Chapters 45 and 46), Kikuchi lymphadenopathy (see Chapter 38), rheumatoid lymphadenopathy (see Chapter 41), HIV lymphadenitis (see Chapter 15), angioimmunoblastic lymphadenopathy/lymphoma (see Chapter 74), and others, exhibit features of ALH and possibly were included in this category before they were described as separate entities.

Lymphoproliferative disorders are hyperplastic reactions of lymphoid tissues that develop in recipients of organ transplants (8,9) (see Chapter 80). They may also develop in persons with primary or acquired immunodeficiency (10) (see Chapters 79 and 81). Lymphoproliferative disorders may encompass a whole spectrum of lymphoid proliferations, from benign reactive lymphoid hyperplasia (RLH) to non-Hodgkin lymphoma (NHL) of high-grade large cell type. Whereas a diagnosis at either of the two extremes of this spectrum is not particularly difficult, in a significant number of cases, a histologic determination of benign or malignant cannot readily be made, and such lesions are therefore referred to as *lymphoproliferative lesions.* The term is noncommittal and reflects the difficulty of reaching a firm histologic diagnosis. The microscopic appearance is essentially that of ALH, showing various types of histologic or cytologic atypia. The observations of spontaneous regression of lymphomas after discontinuance of immunosuppressive treatment raise further questions about the accuracy of histologic diagnosis in some cases of atypical lymphadenopathies.

Artifactual changes in cytology and histology are commonly produced by faulty techniques in the processing of lymph nodes. Uneven fixation, incomplete dehydration, and poor staining can cause tissue alterations that are often misinterpreted as atypical or even malignant changes. Although it has been frequently stated (11–13), it cannot be overemphasized that the correct reading and interpretation of lymph node sections requires nearly perfect processing techniques. It is reasonable to assume that the diagnosis of ALH will be made less frequently in the future, as the processing of lymph nodes improves and the interpretation of changes is facilitated by a better characterization of old and new entities. Nevertheless, if a clear conclusion cannot be reached and if the diagnosis of ALH is a matter of concern, the clinician should not hesitate to suggest a repeated lymph node biopsy.

CLINICAL SYNDROME

Systemic symptoms such as fever, night sweats, anorexia, and fatigue appear to be more common in patients in whom lymphomas ultimately develop than in those in whom they do not (1). It also seems that lymph node enlargement limited to one area correlates with a more favorable prognosis than does generalized enlargement. Abnormal peripheral blood counts and morphology are generally unfavorable prognostic features. Although the clinical information is contributory and should be considered in every case, most authors agree that the final pathologic diagnosis must be based exclusively on histologic findings (7,11).

HISTOPATHOLOGY

Atypical lymphoid hyperplasia has no characteristic histologic pattern. In some cases, the architecture is nodular, and in others, it is diffuse (7). Both patterns are similar to those described in RLH (see Chapter 33).

In the nodular type of ALH, the number of lymph node follicles is increased, and their size and shape vary greatly. Elongated, angulated, and dumbbell-shaped nodules, frequently coalescing, are common (14). The germinal centers are large and include various types of cells and frequent mitoses. In children, RLH may be particularly exuberant, resulting in enlarged lymph nodes with numerous follicles and hyperreactive germinal centers that may not exhibit the usual starry sky pattern with numerous tingible-body macrophages (Fig. 34.1).

In general, the nodular type is easier to distinguish from its malignant counterpart, and its clinical course is more often benign (7). In children, in whom the nodular (follicular) type of reactive hyperplasia is common, the age of the patient is an essential feature in the differential diagnosis with follicular lymphoma because the latter is almost never encountered in children.

The diffuse type of ALH is more difficult to classify and differentiate from the various forms of Hodgkin lymphoma (HL) and NHL. About 50% of the cases classified as ALH, diffuse type, in the series of Schroer and Franssila (7) eventually evolved into lymphomas. The effacement of follicles and sinuses suggests lymphoma (Fig. 34.2); however, in both types, nodular and diffuse, the atypia is mainly cytologic (Fig. 34.3). Either numerous large cells with fairly abundant cytoplasm containing vesicular nuclei with multiple nucleoli or large cells with large nuclei, thick nuclear membranes, and prominent nucleoli resembling immunoblasts are seen (Fig. 34.4). Both cell types exhibit numerous mitoses. These atypical cells are present in clusters or singly, admixed with other cell types, as in iatrogenic (see Chapters 45 and 46) or angioimmunoblastic (see Chapter 74) lymphadenopathies (Fig. 34.4). Eosinophils, sometimes in increased numbers (Fig. 34.5), plasma cells, histiocytes, and even Hodgkin-like and Reed-Sternberg-like cells may occasionally be present, making the differential diagnosis with HL difficult. In other types of ALH, less cellular variation is seen, the cellular proliferation consisting basically of

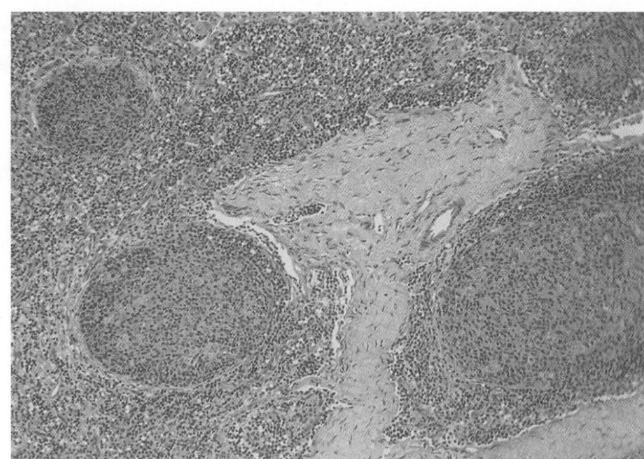

FIGURE 34.1. Atypical lymphoid follicular hyperplasia in submaxillary lymph node of a 6-year-old boy. The hyperplastic follicles are large, without evident tingible-body macrophages or mantle zones. Hematoxylin, phloxine, and saffron stain.

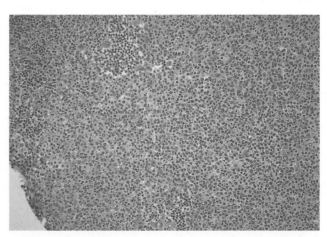

FIGURE 34.2. Lymph node with complete effacement of follicles and sinuses in HIV-positive patient. Hematoxylin, phloxine, and saffron stain.

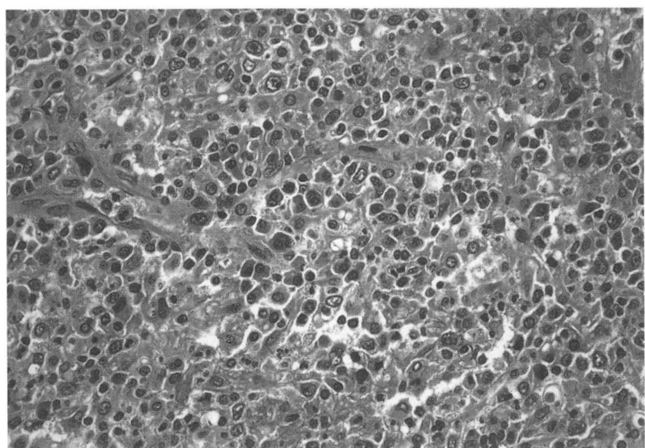

FIGURE 34.3. Atypical lymphoid hyperplasia marked by a mixture of small and large lymphoid cells, often with atypical hyperchromatic nuclei. Hematoxylin, phloxine, and saffron stain.

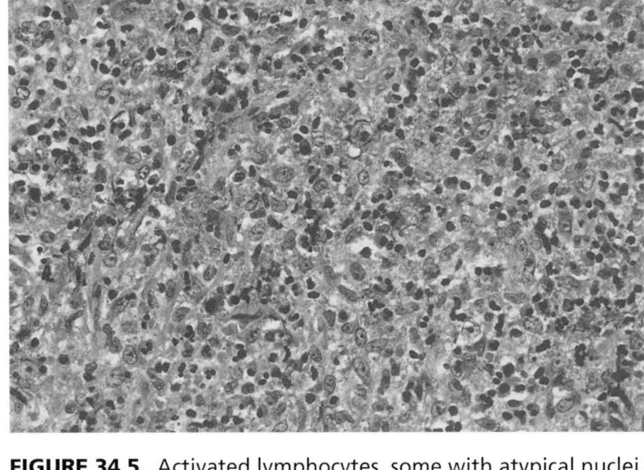

FIGURE 34.5. Activated lymphocytes, some with atypical nuclei, admixed with eosinophils and lymphocytes. Hematoxylin, phloxine, and saffron stain.

one type, such as the immunoblasts that predominate in infectious mononucleosis (Fig. 34.6), cells with clear cytoplasm and atypical nuclei (Fig. 34.7), or of a mixture of two cell populations—small, mature lymphocytes and large, atypical lymphoid cells, as described above, forming patterns that mimic the mixed types of lymphocytic lymphomas. The lymphoproliferative disorders that develop in immunodeficient patients are characterized by diffuse proliferations of atypical lymphocytes and immunoblasts; these result in the effacement of nodal architecture (8–10) (Fig. 34.2).

In considering the changes of ALH, it is important to remember that solid aggregates of uniform, atypical lymphoid cells forming islands or cords are not consistent with ALH because they constitute one of the hallmarks of malignant lymphomas. Generally, in cases classified as ALH, the extent and degree of cellular atypia correlate positively with the frequency of future malignant development (15).

IMMUNOHISTOCHEMISTRY

In cases of ALH in which a diagnosis of NHL is suspected, the uncertainty can usually be resolved with an immunophenotypic study. With the use of frozen sections or flow cytometry on cell suspensions, the monoclonality or polyclonality of light chain immunoglobulins (Igs) on the membranes of B cells can be determined (Fig. 34.8). In differentiating nodular aggregates of atypical lymphoid cells from follicular lymphoma, immunostaining for bcl-2 (Fig. 34.9) or MT-2 (Figs. 34.10 and 34.11) is helpful; staining is positive in the latter case and negative in the former.

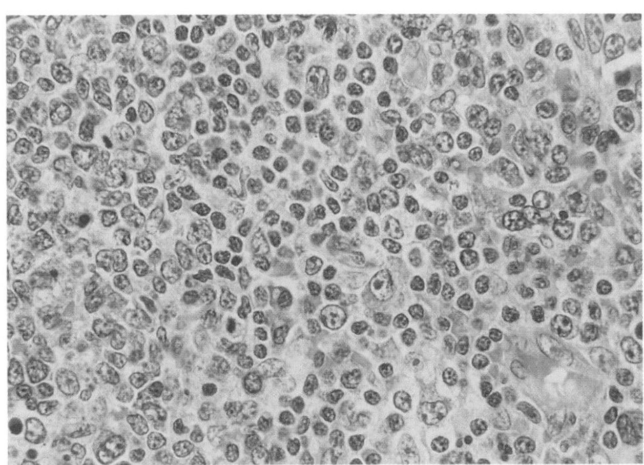

FIGURE 34.4. Atypical lymphoid hyperplasia, including numerous lymphoid cells with large, irregular vesicular nuclei and prominent nucleoli, in angioimmunoblastic lymphadenopathy. Hematoxylin, phloxine, and saffron stain.

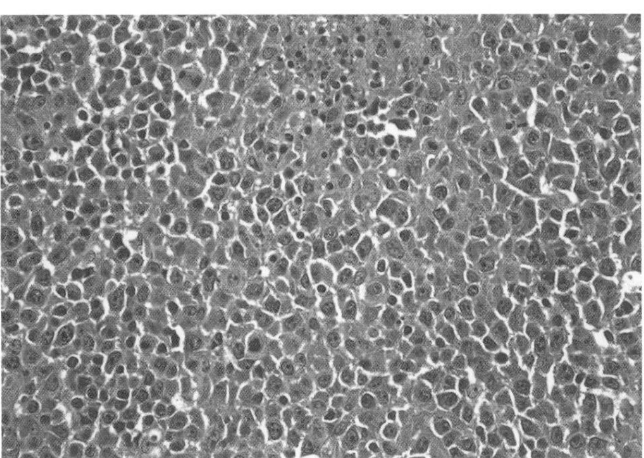

FIGURE 34.6. Sheets of immunoblasts with focal areas of necrosis (*top*) in infectious mononucleosis lymphadenitis. Hematoxylin, phloxine, and saffron stain.

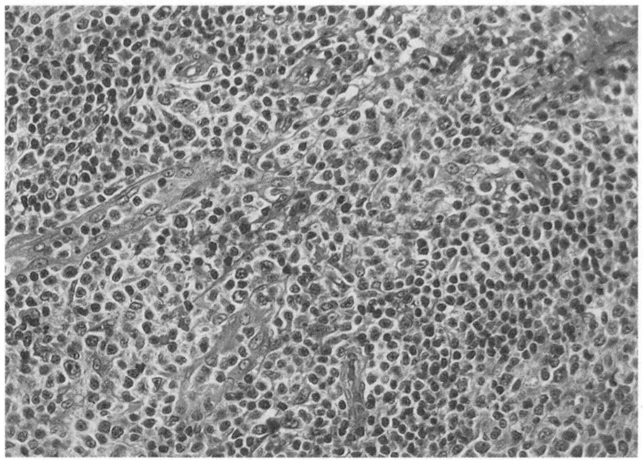

FIGURE 34.7. Aggregates of lymphoid cells with clear cytoplasm and occasional atypical nuclei. Hematoxylin, phloxine, and saffron stain.

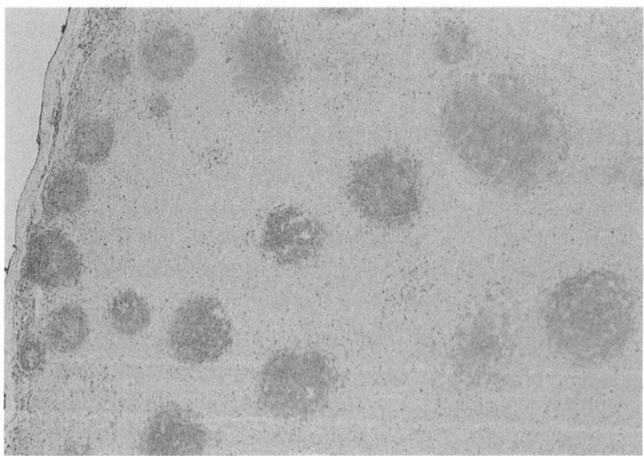

FIGURE 34.8. Reactive lymph node with numerous hyperplastic lymphoid follicles. L26/peroxidase stain.

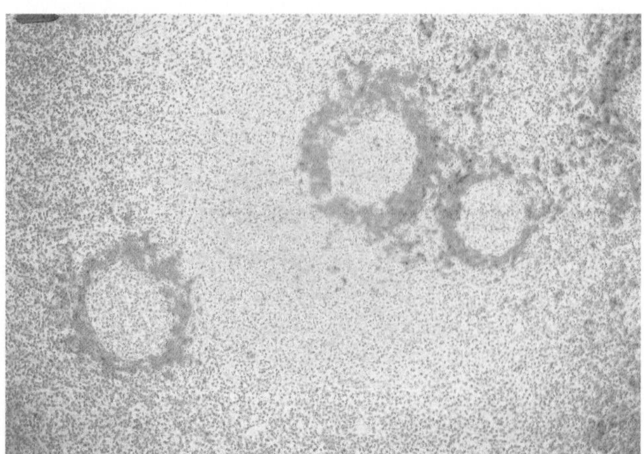

FIGURE 34.9. Same lymph node. Immunostaining for bcl-2 shows lack of germinal center staining; in contrast, positive staining of mantle zone indicates a non-neoplastic process. bcl-2/peroxidase stain.

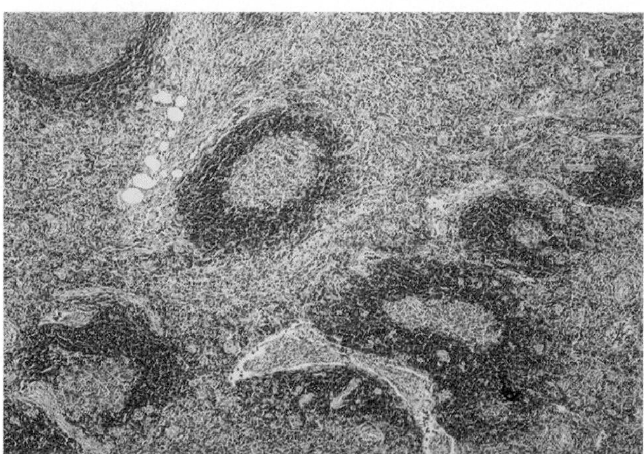

FIGURE 34.10. Reactive lymphoid follicles immunostained with MT-2 antibodies showing non-neoplastic pattern, similar to that obtained with bcl-2 in Fig. 34.9.

GENE REARRANGEMENT ANALYSIS

Even with the use of immunohistochemistry, the question of malignancy may still not be resolved in a good number of cases with histologic features of ALH—for example, proliferations of T lymphocytes in which monoclonality is not demonstrable by immunophenotyping, some B-cell lymphomas that do not express membrane Igs, and T cell-rich B-cell lymphomas (so-called because the large number of reactive T cells overshadows the smaller number of malignant B lymphocytes) (16,17). In such cases, the study of gene rearrangements can provide the answer. Southern blot analysis of extracted DNA can demonstrate clonal Ig or T-cell receptor gene rearrangements and therefore the presence of a malignant cell population (18). In a study of 11 patients in whom lymph node biopsy showed abnormal hyperplasia with histopathologic findings suggestive but not diagnostic of lymphoma and in whom immunophenotyping was in-

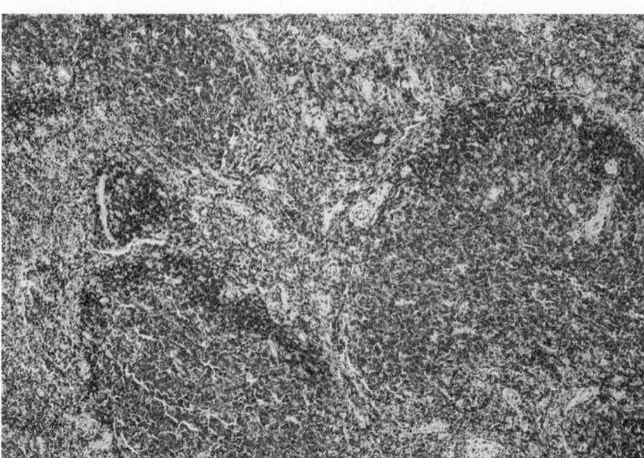

FIGURE 34.11. MT-2 antibody staining of follicular lymphoma produces a pattern that is the reverse of the non-neoplastic proliferation in Fig. 34.10. MT-2/peroxidase stain.

Checklist

ATYPICAL LYMPHOID HYPERPLASIA

Lymphadenopathy, isolated or regional
Nodular or diffuse pattern with effaced architecture
Cell population mixed
Capsule minimally involved
Nuclear atypia
Nucleolar prominence
Mitoses variable
Cell surface markers polyclonal
Clonal gene rearrangements absent

conclusive, gene rearrangement study was undertaken (19). Six of these patients had an Ig gene rearrangement and were found to have NHL of B-cell type on repeated biopsy after 8 days to 46 months. Three patients without a detectable gene rearrangement showed no evidence of NHL at follow-up reevaluation after 36 to 60 months. However, in two patients with negative results on Southern blot analysis, lymphomas developed at 2.5 and 45 months, respectively. These two false-negative results can be explained if the lymph nodes that were examined were uninvolved by NHL at the time of exploration or contained fewer than 2% to 5% of malignant clone cells, which is about the threshold proportion for Southern blot detection (19).

Many cases of clonal rearrangements detected in atypical lymphoid lesions that did not progress to lymphoma for very long periods of time have been reported. Others even regressed when the effects of promoting factors such as *Helicobacter pylori* infection in MALT (mucosa-associated lymphoid tissue) lymphomas and immunosuppression in transplant recipients ended (20,21). With the genotype methods of molecular pathology, Southern blot, and particularly the sensitive technique of polymerase chain reaction, cellular clones can be detected in many lymphoid populations that are chronically stimulated (22); however, not all of them progress to lymphoma. It is therefore reasonable to agree with the concept put forward by R. Collins that clonality is not equivalent to malignancy and that Ig gene rearrangement is not necessarily diagnostic of malignant lymphoma (23). Thus, clonal small lymphocytic lesions should be assumed to be malignant if they are multifocal and produce solid mass lesions. In other cases, ALH lesions composed of small lymphocytes and limited in extent, even when Ig gene rearrangements are present, may be designated as *clonal disorders of uncertain malignant potential* (23).

DIFFERENTIAL DIAGNOSIS

- RLH may show similar histologic patterns (see Chapter 33) without the cellular atypia characteristic of ALH. A diagnosis of RLH, in contrast to one of ALH, does not imply suspicion of malignancy.
- Follicular (nodular) lymphoma shows nodules that vary only slightly in size and shape and are evenly distributed throughout the cortex and medulla of the lymph node (11). The nodules have no peripheral rim of small lymphocytes and appear poorly demarcated. The stroma between the expanding nodules appears compressed; the compression is well demonstrated by reticulin staining. The cells inside and outside the nodules are similar. Mitoses are fewer in number, and macrophages are absent. Cell surface markers are monoclonal Igs.
- Diffuse lymphomas of small and large cell types: The cell population is more uniform than in ALH and does not include plasma cells, eosinophils, or macrophages. Extensive invasion of the capsule and pericapsular tissues is seen. The reticulin pattern is altered. The nuclei are more atypical. Mitoses may be frequent. Cell surface markers are monoclonal.
- HL, lymphocyte predominance type, contains lymphocytic and histiocytic (L & H) (popcorn) cells.
- HL, classic type, contains Hodgkin cells and Reed-Sternberg cells that are CD15+, CD30+, and CD20−, the opposite of the atypical cells in ALH.
- Malignant histiocytosis: High grade of cellular atypia, prominent nucleoli, numerous mitoses, areas of necrosis.

REFERENCES

1. Sinclair S, Beckman E, Ellman L. Biopsy of enlarged superficial lymph nodes. JAMA 1974;228:602–603.
2. Gatti RA, Good RA. Occurrence of malignancy in immunodeficiency disease: a literature review. Cancer 1971;28:89–98.
3. Frizzera G, Rosai J, Dehner PL, et al. Lymphoreticular disorders in primary immunodeficiencies. New findings based on an up-to-date histologic classification of 35 cases. Cancer 1980;46:692– 699.
4. Moore RD, Weisberger AS, Bowerfind ES. An evaluation of lymphadenopathy in systemic disease. Arch Intern Med 1957;99: 751–759.
5. Saltzstein SL. The fate of patients with nondiagnostic lymph node biopsies. Surgery 1965;58:659–662.

6. Symmers W St C Sr. Survey of the eventual diagnosis in 600 cases referred for a second histological opinion after an initial biopsy diagnosis of Hodgkin's disease. Am J Clin Pathol 1968;21:650–653.
7. Schroer KP, Franssila KO. Atypical hyperplasia of lymph nodes: a follow-up study. Cancer 1979;44:1155–1163.
8. Cleary ML, Sklar J. Lymphoproliferative disorder in cardiac transplant recipients are multiclonal lymphomas. Lancet 1984; 12:489–493.
9. Frizzera G, Hanto DW, Gajl-Peczalska J, et al. Polymorphic diffuse B-cell hyperplasias and lymphomas in renal transplant recipients. Cancer Res 1981;41:4262–4279.
10. Canioni D, MacKelvie P, Debure A, et al. Lymphadenopathy in renal transplant patients treated with immunosuppressive antibodies (OKT3 and antithymocyte globulin). A report of nine cases. Am J Surg Pathol 1989;13:87–96.
11. Butler JJ. Non-neoplastic lesions of lymph nodes of man to be differentiated from lymphomas. NCI Monogr 1969;323:233–255.
12. Dorfman RF, Warnke R. Lymphadenopathy simulating the malignant lymphomas. Hum Pathol 1974;5:519–550.
13. Banks PM. Technical aspects of specimen preparation and special studies. In: Jaffe ES, ed. Surgical pathology of lymph nodes and related organs. Philadelphia: WB Saunders, 1985:1–22.
14. Rappaport H. Tumors of the hematopoietic system. In: Atlas of tumor pathology, Section III, Fascicle 8. Washington, DC: Armed Forces Institute of Pathology, 1966:426–442.
15. Brubaker DB, Shiteside TL. Differentiation between benign and malignant human lymph nodes by means of immunologic markers. Cancer 1979;43:1165–1176.
16. Osborne BM, Butler JJ, Pugh WC. The value of immunophenotyping on paraffin sections in the identification of T cell-rich B-cell large cell lymphomas: lineage confirmed by JH rearrangements. Am J Surg Pathol 1990;14:933–938.
17. Macon WR, Williams ME, Greer JP, et al. T cell-rich B-cell lymphomas: a clinicopathologic study of 17 cases. Am J Surg Pathol 1992;16:351–364.
18. Williams ME, Innes DJ, Borowitz MJ, et al. Immunoglobulin and T-cell receptor gene rearrangements in human lymphoma and leukemia. Blood 1987;69:79–87.
19. Williams ME, Lee JT, Innes DJ, et al. Immunoglobulin gene rearrangement in abnormal lymph node hyperplasia. Am J Clin Pathol 1991;96:746–775.
20. Wotherspoon AC, Doglioni C, et al. Regression of primary low-grade B-cell gastric lymphoma of mucosa-associated lymphoid tissue type after eradication of *Helicobacter pylori.* Lancet 1993; 342:575–577.
21. Starzl TE, Nalesnik MA, Porter KA, et al. Reversibility of lymphomas and lymphoproliferative lesions developing under cyclosporine-steroid therapy. Lancet 1984;1:584–587.
22. Torlakovic E, Cherwitz DL, Jessurun J, et al. B-cell gene rearrangement in benign and malignant lymphoid proliferations of mucosa-associated lymphoid tissue and lymph nodes. Hum Pathol 1997;28:166–173.
23. Collins RD. Is clonality equivalent to malignancy: specifically, is immunoglobulin gene rearrangement diagnostic of malignant lymphoma? [Editorial]. Hum Pathol 1997;28:757–759.

35

PROGRESSIVE TRANSFORMATION OF GERMINAL CENTERS

DEFINITION

Progressive transformation of germinal centers (PTGC) is a benign lymphadenopathy. Large nodules containing small lymphocytes of the mantle zone type, in a background of reactive follicular hyperplasia (RFH), partially replace the normal lymph node architecture. A minority of patients have both PTGC and nodular lymphocyte predominance Hodgkin lymphoma (NLPHL).

SYNONYMS

Progressively transformed germinal centers, progressively transformed follicular centers.

EPIDEMIOLOGY

The frequency of PTGC in enlarged lymph nodes with RFH may be as high as 10% (1), but this is difficult to determine because most studies rely on referral material. Data from the Kiel Lymph Node Registry identified PTGC in 30 of 820 (3.5%) cases of nonspecific lymphadenitis (2). It has long been recognized that PTGC develops in a minority of patients with NLPHL either in different lymph nodes [5 of 206 (2%)] (3) or in the same lymph node [31 of 171 (18%)] (4). A review of 50 patients with PTGC includes 5 with concurrent NLPHL (10%), 15 with previous Hodgkin lymphoma (HL) of all types (30%), and 31 without prior or subsequent HL (62%) (5). Therefore, new lymphadenopathy in a patient in whom NLPHL was previously diagnosed should not be judged *a priori* as recurrent disease without a confirmatory lymph node biopsy. In the majority of patients, PTGC is unassociated with either prior or subsequent HL (1,2).

PATHOGENESIS

The etiology and pathogenesis of PTGC are unknown. PTGC was originally described in association with NLPHL (3,4,6) but can be seen in a variety of reactive lymphadenopathies (6). Because mitoses are scarce, an increase of small lymphocytes in PTGC probably depends on migration, not proliferation (3). Various hypotheses have been proposed to explain the origin of PTGC: a preneoplastic stage of NLPHL (3,7,8); one of the possible destinies of the follicular center (9); follicle centers inappropriately overrun with mantle zone cells (10); and premature arrest at an early transition stage between primary and secondary follicles because of incomplete blastic transformation of B cells (11).

CLINICAL SYNDROME

Progressive transformation of germinal centers characteristically presents as a single, asymptomatic, enlarged lymph node in young men in the second decade of life (2,5). It is most often seen in the neck (1,2), then in the inguinal and axillary regions (2). Recurrent PTGC may involve the same or different lymph node groups (1,2,5). In the overwhelming majority of patients, PTGC does not predict the development of HL, nor does PTGC have any relationship to HL (1,2,5). In some cases, PTGC occurs during, preceding, or following HL, mostly of the lymphocyte predominance type, but in a few cases of the nodular sclerosis or mixed cellularity type (2,5). An interval as long as 13 years may separate the diagnoses of PTGC and NLPHL (8,12). Approximately 20% (23 of 110) of patients with PTGC are 16 years old or younger (1). Although the initial clinical presentation in children and adults is similar, PTGC tends to recur at a higher rate, and multiple times, in children (1). Occasionally, generalized lymphadenopathy unassociated with NLPHL develops in children with PTGC (2).

HISTOPATHOLOGY

In half of cases one to three PTGC (2), and in a few cases up to 15 PTGC, can be identified in a single tissue section (1).

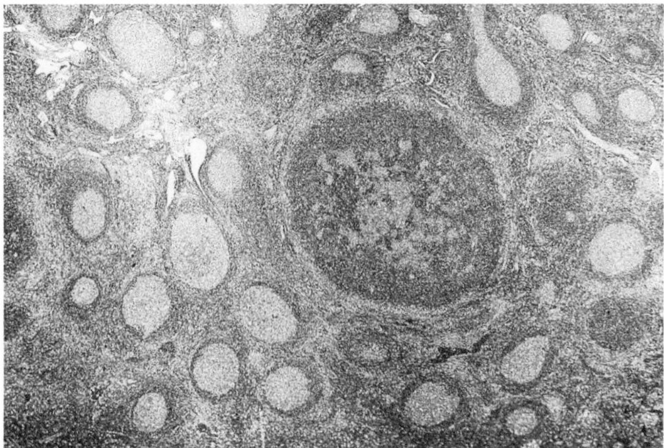

FIGURE 35.1. Progressive transformation of germinal centers. Partial replacement of lymph node architecture by nodule three to five times the diameter of surrounding reactive follicles. Hematoxylin and eosin stain.

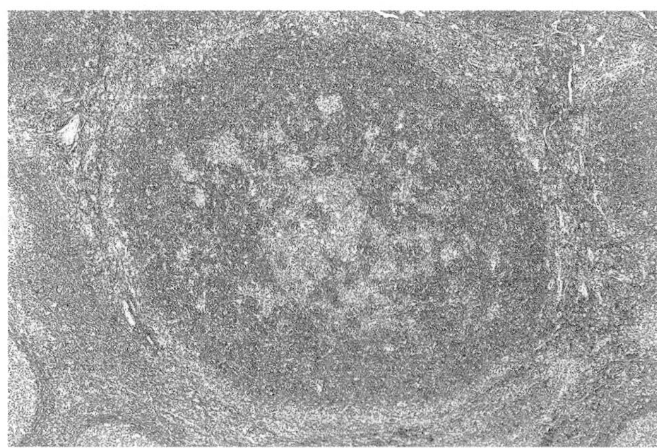

FIGURE 35.2. Progressive transformation of germinal centers. Same lymph node as in Fig. 35.1 at higher magnification. Small lymphocytes replace germinal center cells and blur mantle zone boundary. Hematoxylin and eosin stain.

However, no more than two or three PTGC cluster together (1). Small lymphocytes progressively infiltrate and expand the germinal centers, producing nodules two to four times the diameter of background reactive follicles. The large nodules partially replace the normal lymph node (1,3,4,6) (Fig. 35.1). As the large nodules continue to accumulate small lymphocytes in aggregates of various sizes and shapes, the boundary between the germinal center and mantle zone blurs, leaving behind only a few residual germinal center cells (Fig. 35.2). Sometimes, small lymphocytes organize concentrically in the poorly demarcated periphery (11). Nonetheless, the interfollicular area is not involved (3). PTGC do not polarize, although transitional forms between RFH and PTGC can be found (3,7) (Fig. 35.3). No lymphocytic and histiocytic (L&H) variants, so-called popcorn cells (see Chapter 58), or classic, diagnostic Reed-Sternberg

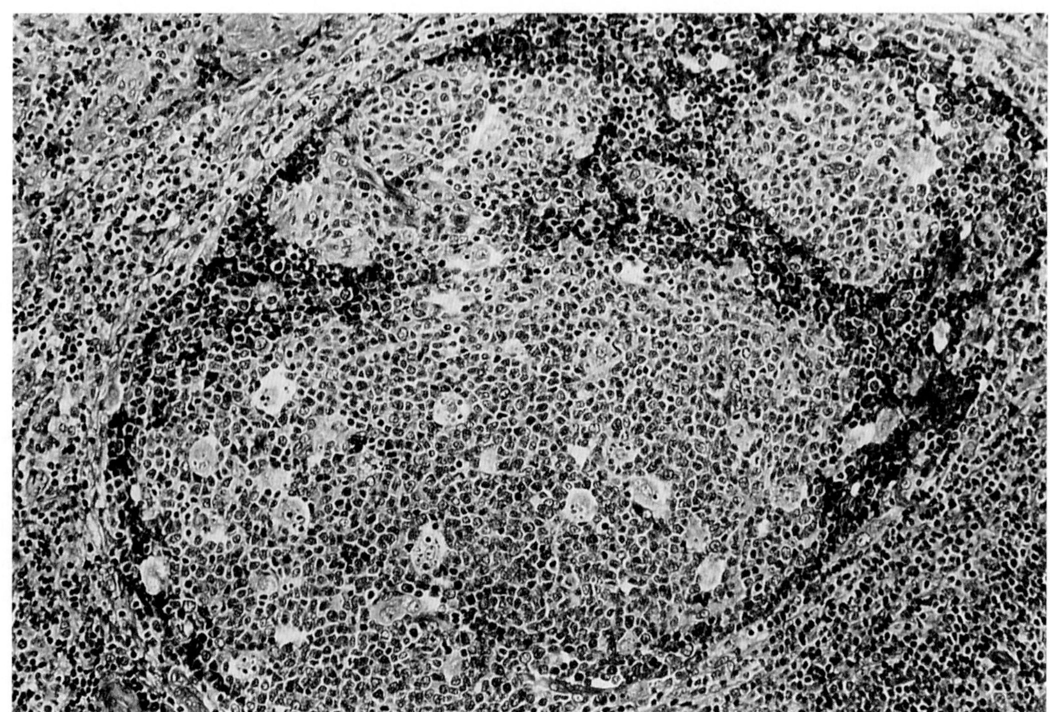

FIGURE 35.3. Progressive transformation of germinal centers. Transitional form retaining some recognizable reactive follicular hyperplasia. Growth of small, mature, darkly staining lymphocytes into reactive germinal center with numerous tingible-body macrophages. Hematoxylin, phloxine, and saffron stain.

Checklist

PROGRESSIVE TRANSFORMATION OF GERMINAL CENTERS

Young male patients
Single, asymptomatic enlarged lymph node
Partial lymph node involvement
Large lymphocytic nodule in a background of RFH
Small lymphocytes interspersed with residual germinal center cells
Polyclonal mantle zone B-cell phenotype
No Reed-Sternberg cells or L&H variants

cells (see Chapter 57) are seen. Tingible-body macrophages, plasma cells, and eosinophils are rare to absent. Epithelioid cells are uncommon and seldom form groups around a PTGC (3,5), but when present, they mainly affect lymph nodes from children rather than adults (1). PTGC and NLPHL occur in the same lymph node simultaneously in the presence of abundant RFH (4). However, no reliable morphologic features predict which cases of PTGC will be associated with HL (1). Exceptionally florid PTGC, with up to 123 (mean, 67) PTGC per lymph node, tends to involve multiple anatomic sites, persist, and recur (13). Lymph nodes showing florid RFH in AIDS do not contain PTGC (5,14).

IMMUNOHISTOCHEMISTRY

The major lymphocytic population in PTGC is phenotypically equivalent to polyclonal mantle zone B cells expressing CD20, CD24, CD45RA, surface membrane immunoglobulin M (sIgM), sIgD, and HLA-DR (11,12). The B cells occur in well-circumscribed, confluent nodules (12). CD4+ helper/inducer T cells predominate over CD8+ suppressor/cytotoxic T cells (11). T cells and CD57+ cells are randomly distributed (11,12), only rarely forming T-cell rosettes (12). Although some CD38+ terminally differentiated B cells can be found in reactive secondary follicles (15), they are generally absent in PTGC (11). The follicular dendritic meshwork in PTGC is controversial. Some investigators find that it is abnormally sparse, vague, and broken up, lacking sharply circumscribed foci, and lacking a concentric pattern at the periphery of the nodule because of a reduced number of dendritic processes (8,11). Others report a well-circumscribed, tightly concentric arrangement of follicular dendritic cells (12). Because anti-Ig staining does not reveal the typical RFH "lacelike" pattern, it is not likely that antigen–antibody complexes coat the follicular dendritic reticulum cells in PTGC (11). Without fixed antigen–antibody complexes, an initiator for the development of an immune response in secondary follicles is lacking.

DIFFERENTIAL DIAGNOSIS

- NLPHL: Nodules replace the entire lymph node; presence of Reed-Sternberg variants (L&H, or "popcorn," cells); irregularly distributed B cells in a "moth-eaten" pattern; aggregates of T cells and many T-cell rosettes around large B cells (12,16).
- Follicular lymphoma: Nodules in a back-to-back arrangement; infiltration of the perinodal fat; uniform population of small cleaved, mixed, or large cells; no reactive germinal centers (17).

REFERENCES

1. Osborne BM, Butler JJ, Gresik MV. Progressive transformation of germinal centers: comparison of 23 pediatric patients to the adult population. Mod Pathol 1992;5:135–140.
2. Hansmann ML, Fellbaum C, Hui PK, et al. Progressive transformation of germinal centers with and without association to Hodgkin's disease. Am J Clin Pathol 1990;93:219–226.
3. Poppema S, Kaiserling E, Lennert K. Hodgkin's disease with lymphocytic predominance, nodular type (nodular paragranuloma) and progressively transformed germinal centres—a cytohistological study. Histopathology 1979;3:295–308.
4. Burns BF, Colby TV, Dorfman RF. Differential diagnostic features of nodular L & H Hodgkin's disease, including progressive transformation of germinal centers. Am J Surg Pathol 1984;8:253–261.
5. Osborne BM, Butler JJ. Clinical implications of progressive transformation of germinal centers. Am J Surg Pathol 1984;8:725–733.
6. Muller-Hermelink H-K, Lennert K. Phases of germinal center development. In: Lennert K, Stein H, Mohri N, et al., eds. Malignant lymphomas other than Hodgkin's disease. Berlin: Springer-Verlag, 1978:38.
7. Poppema S, Kaiserling E, Lennert K. Nodular paragranuloma and progressively transformed germinal centers. Ultrastructural

and immunohistologic findings. Virchows Arch B Cell Pathol Mol Pathol 1979;31:211–225.

8. Crossley B, Heryet A, Gatter KC. Does nodular lymphocyte predominant Hodgkin's disease arise from progressively transformed germinal centres? A case report with an unusually prolonged history. Histopathology 1987;11:621–630.
9. Lennert K, Stein H. The germinal center: morphology, histochemistry, and immunohistology. In: Christophers E, Goos M, eds. Lymphoproliferative disease of the skin. New York: Springer-Verlag, 1982:3–15.
10. Stein H, Gerdes J, Mason DY. The normal and malignant germinal centre. Clin Haematol 1982;11:531–559.
11. van den Oord JJ, de Wolf-Peeters C, Desmet VJ. Immunohistochemical analysis of progressively transformed follicular centers. Am J Clin Pathol 1985;83:560–564.
12. Nguyen PL, Ferry JA, Harris NL. Progressive transformation of germinal centers and nodular lymphocyte predominance Hodgkin's disease: a comparative immunohistochemical study. Am J Surg Pathol 1999;23:27–33.
13. Ferry JA, Zukerberg LR, Harris NL. Florid progressive transformation of germinal centers. A syndrome affecting young men, without early progression to nodular lymphocyte predominance Hodgkin's disease. Am J Surg Pathol 1992;16:252–258.
14. Srigley JR, Barlogie B, Butler JJ, et al. Lymphadenopathy and malignant lymphoma in homosexual males: acridine orange DNA-RNA flow cytometric observations. Lab Invest 1984;50:44A.
15. Bhan AK, Nadler LM, Stashenko P, et al. Stages of B-cell differentiation in human lymphoid tissue. J Exp Med 1981;154:737–749.
16. Kamel OW, Gelb AB, Shibuya RB, et al. Leu 7 (CD57) reactivity distinguishes nodular lymphocyte predominance Hodgkin's disease from nodular sclerosing Hodgkin's disease, T cell-rich B-cell lymphoma and follicular lymphoma. Am J Pathol 1993;142:541–546.
17. Osborne BM, Butler JJ. Follicular lymphoma mimicking progressive transformation of germinal centers. Am J Clin Pathol 1987;88:264–269.

PART IV

SECTION TWO

LYMPHADENOPATHIES ASSOCIATED WITH CLINICAL SYNDROMES

36

KIMURA LYMPHADENOPATHY

DEFINITION

Kimura lymphadenopathy is a chronic inflammatory disorder prevalent in Asians. It involves subcutaneous tissues and lymph nodes and is characterized by angiolymphoid proliferation and eosinophilia.

SYNONYM

Kimura disease

ETIOLOGY

Endemic in Asia and sporadic in other geographic regions, Kimura disease is suggestive of an infectious origin, but no pathogen has been demonstrated.

CLINICAL FEATURES

The disease, described in 1948 by Kimura and co-workers (1) and earlier reported in a Chinese medical journal (2), is endemic in Asia, occurring primarily in China, Japan, and Indonesia (3). In the West, Kimura disease is sporadic and was for a time considered to be the late stage of a condition called *angiolymphoid hyperplasia with eosinophilia* (ALHE), described by Wells and Whimster in 1969 (4). Subsequent studies made the distinction between the two entities, as delineated in the differential diagnosis (5–7). Essentially, Kimura disease is located deep in the subcutaneous tissues and in almost all cases involves the regional lymph nodes; in contrast, ALHE is largely restricted to the dermis (3,8,9). It occurs predominantly in young adults; the age range is 27 to 40 years, and the male-to-female ratio of 3:1 indicates a male predominance. The onset is insidious, and the manifestations are enlarging nodular masses in the head and neck areas, most frequently infraauricular or retroauricular. The lesions are single in 60% of cases and multiple, occasionally symmetric, in the rest (7). On occasion, the salivary glands (particularly the parotid), oral cavity, axilla, groin, and limbs are involved (10). Cases of eosinophilic infiltrates in skeletal muscles, prostate, and kidney have also been reported, the latter resulting in a nephrotic syndrome (3,10). Peripheral blood eosinophilia (10% to 50%) and elevated serum levels of immunoglobulin E (IgE) are constant features of Kimura disease (3,7). The skin and lymph node lesions do not ulcerate, and although recurrences are common, the disease has a benign course (2,10). The best clinical results are obtained with radiation therapy; both surgical excision and steroid treatments are associated with high rates of recurrence (11,12).

HISTOPATHOLOGY

Lymphoid infiltrates with the formation of follicles and germinal centers, accompanied by plasma cells, mast cells, and particularly large numbers of eosinophils, are present in the subcutis. Thin-walled capillaries are also present. The lymph nodes, enlarged to a diameter of 1 to 4 cm and frequently adherent to one another, show markedly hyperplastic follicles with reactive germinal centers and a well-defined peripheral mantle (9) (Fig. 36.1). Diffuse eosinophilia, eosinophilic microabscesses, and infiltration of germinal centers, sometimes resulting in folliculolysis, are part of the process (Figs. 36.2 and 36.3). Polykaryocytes of the Warthin-Finkeldey type, characterized by an overlapping, grapelike arrangement of nuclei, are common, often located within the germinal centers (Fig. 36.4). In areas of eosinophilia, crystalline structures are sometimes seen in the cytoplasm of histiocytes or extruded in the stroma as Charcot-Leyden crystals (3). Vascular hyperplasia is present, mostly of postcapillary venules, and is more pronounced in the mantle zone of the germinal centers (10) (Fig.36.5). Sclerosis develops in older lesions, accompanied by vascular atrophy and sinus obliteration, while the eosinophils still persist (10).

IMMUNOHISTOCHEMISTRY

Deposits of IgE in the germinal centers can be demonstrated with anti-IgE antibodies in immunofluorescence or by immunoperoxidase staining. Variable amounts of IgA and

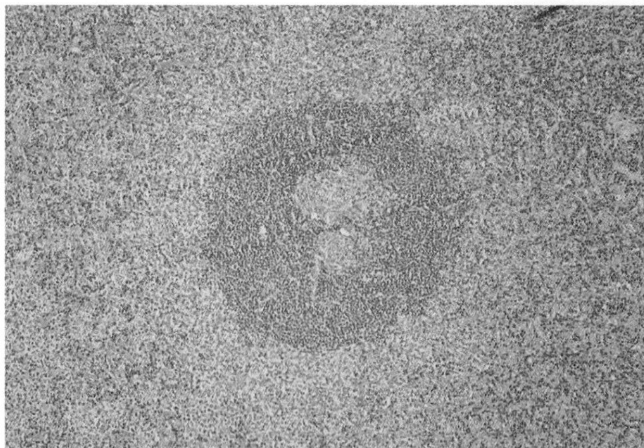

FIGURE 36.1. Kimura lymphadenopathy. Involuted follicle with hyperplasia of mantle zone and abundant eosinophilia in the surrounding cortical area. Hematoxylin, phloxine, and saffron stain.

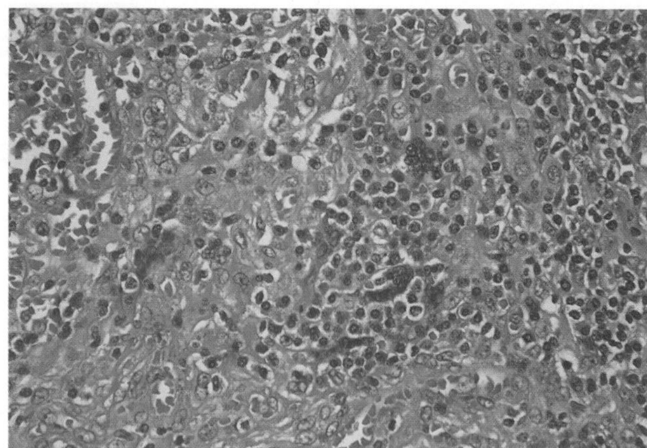

FIGURE 36.4. Kimura lymphadenopathy. Warthin-Finkeldey polykaryocytes and eosinophils, and proliferation of capillaries in cervical lymph node. Hematoxylin, phloxine, and saffron stain.

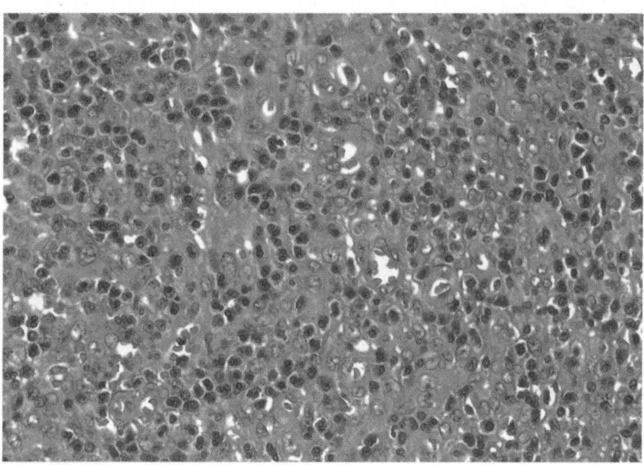

FIGURE 36.2. Kimura lymphadenopathy. Abundant diffuse eosinophilia in paracortex. Hematoxylin, phloxine, and saffron stain.

complement components C1g and C3 may also be deposited in the germinal centers (3). The vascular endothelial cells stain strongly with factor VIII and with *Ulex europaeus* agglutinin (UEA-1) (7). The polykaryocytes are of the Warthin-Finkeldey type and therefore probably of helper T-cell origin (13).

CYTOPATHOLOGY

Fine needle aspiration attempted in three cases of parotid and submandibular lymph node masses produced smears composed of dissociated and clustered endothelial cells, eosinophils, lymphocytes, and Warthin-Finkeldey giant cells. In two cases, the diagnosis of Kimura lymphadenopathy was suggested; however, in the third case, prominent nucleoli in some cells led to an erroneous diagnosis of Hodgkin lymphoma. Excision biopsy and histologic diagnosis are therefore recommended for confirmation in such cases (14).

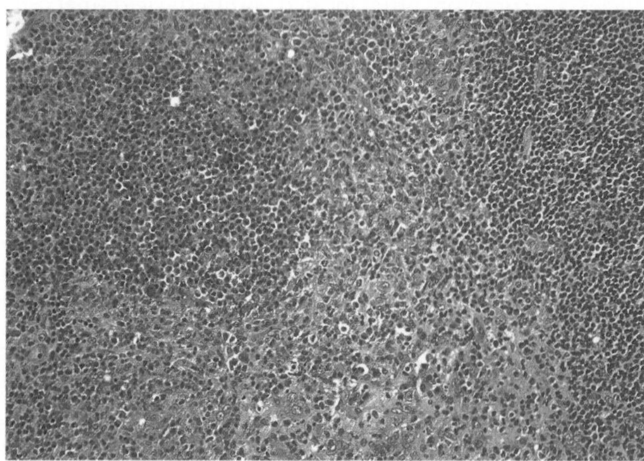

FIGURE 36.3. Kimura lymphadenopathy. Eosinophilic microabscess in cervical lymph node. Hematoxylin, phloxine, and saffron stain.

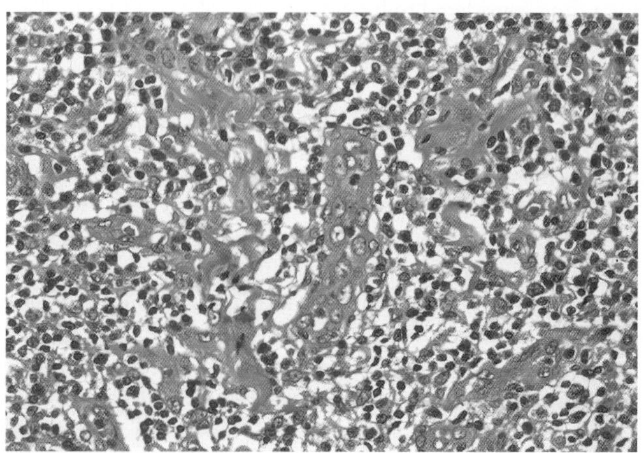

FIGURE 36.5. Kimura lymphadenopathy. Vascular proliferation with hyperplasia of endothelial cells. Hematoxylin, phloxine, and saffron stain.

Checklist

KIMURA LYMPHADENOPATHY

More common in Asians
Predominance in young men
Predilection for neck and periauricular areas
Deep-seated subcutaneous nodules
Concomitant or exclusive involvement of regional lymph nodes
Occasional involvement of salivary glands and kidneys
Hyperplastic lymphoid follicles with prominent germinal centers
Hyperplasia and endothelial cells in postcapillary venules
Abundant eosinophil infiltration, often involving germinal centers
Polykaryocytes of Warthin-Finkeldey type
Deposition of IgE in germinal centers
Peripheral blood eosinophilia and elevated levels of IgE

DIFFERENTIAL DIAGNOSIS

- ALHE, because of some histologic similarities, has occasionally been confused with or mistaken for an early stage of Kimura disease. In contrast with Kimura disease, which is common in Asians and seated deep in the subcutaneous tissues, ALHE occurs in Caucasians, involves the superficial skin, forming clusters of papules, and is characterized by hypertrophic endothelial cells that protrude into or occlude the lumina. More importantly, lymphadenopathy is an essential part of Kimura disease and is not present in ALHE.
- Hodgkin disease, mixed cellularity type, has in common with Kimura disease eosinophils, plasma cells, and sclerosis but lacks hyperplastic germinal centers and deposits of IgE. The presence of Reed-Sternberg cells confirms the diagnosis.
- Castleman disease includes vascular hyperplasia but lacks eosinophilia, and the germinal centers are involuted and hyalinized rather than hyperplastic.
- Dermatopathic lymphadenopathy may be associated with follicular hyperplasia and sclerosis and is distinguished by deposits of hemosiderin, melanin, and lipids.
- Lymphadenopathy of drug reaction may show eosinophilia but usually is not restricted to one group of lymph nodes.
- Parasitic lymphadenitis is marked by eosinophilia but also by the formation of granulomas and by remnants of parasites.

REFERENCES

1. Kimura T, Yoshimura S, Ishikawa E. On the unusual granulation combined with hyperplastic changes of lymphatic tissue. Trans Soc Pathol Jpn 1948;37:179–180.
2. Kung ITM, Gibson JB, Bannatyne PM. Kimura's disease: a clinico-pathological study of 21 cases and its distinction from angiolymphoid hyperplasia with eosinophilia. Pathology 1984;16:39–44.
3. Kuo T-T, Shih L-Y, Chan H-L. Kimura's disease. Involvement of regional lymph nodes and distinction from angiolymphoid hyperplasia with eosinophilia. Am J Surg Pathol 1988;12:843–854.
4. Wells GC, Whimster IW. Subcutaneous angiolymphoid hyperplasia with eosinophilia. Br J Dermatol 1969;81:1–15.
5. Rosai J, Gold J, Landy R. The histiocytoid hemangiomas. A unifying concept embracing several previously described entities of skin, soft tissue, large vessels, bone and heart. Hum Pathol 1979;10:707–730.
6. Googe PB, Harris NL, Mihm MC Jr. Kimura's disease and angiolymphoid hyperplasia with eosinophilia: two distinct histopathological entities. J Cutan Pathol 1987;14:263–271.
7. Urabe A, Tsuneyoshi M, Enjoji M. Epithelioid hemangioma versus Kimura's disease: a comparative clinicopathologic study. Am J Surg Pathol 1987;11:758–766.
8. Reed RJ, Terazakis N. Subcutaneous angioblastic lymphoid hyperplasia with eosinophilia (Kimura's disease). Cancer 1972;29:489–497.
9. Helander SD, Peters MS, Kuo T-T, et al. Kimura's disease and angiolymphoid hyperplasia with eosinophilia: new observations from immunohistochemical studies of lymphocytes markers, endothelial antigens, and granulocyte proteins. J Cutan Pathol 1995;22:319–326.
10. Hui PK, Chan JKC, Ng CS, et al. Lymphadenopathy of Kimura's disease. Am J Surg Pathol 1989;13:177–186.
11. Kim GE, Kim WC, Yang WI, et al. Radiation treatment in patients with recurrent Kimura's disease. Int J Radiat Oncol Biol Phys 1997;38:607–612.
12. Hareyama M, Oouchi A, Nagakura H, et al. Radiotherapy for Kimura's disease: the optimum dosage. Int J Radiat Oncol Biol Phys 1998;40:647–651.
13. Kamel OW, LeBrun DP, Berry GJ, et al. Warthin-Finkeldey polykaryocytes demonstrate a T-cell immunophenotype. Am J Clin Pathol 1992;97:179–183.
14. Jayaram G, Peh KB. Fine-needle aspiration cytology in Kimura's disease. Diagn Cytopathol 1995;13:295–299.

37

SINUS HISTIOCYTOSIS WITH MASSIVE LYMPHADENOPATHY

DEFINITION

A rare type of benign histiocytosis characterized histologically by intracellular engulfment of lymphocytes.

SYNONYMS

Rosai-Dorfman disease

Histiocytose lipidique ganglionnaire pseudotumorale de Destombes

Lymphadenitis with massive hemophagocytic sinus histiocytosis of Lennert

ETIOLOGY

The etiology of sinus histiocytosis with massive lymphadenopathy (SHML) remains unknown. Although the clinical manifestations and histologic appearance are suggestive of an infectious process, no microorganism has yet been identified.

CLINICAL FEATURES

Initial reports by Destombes (1) and Rosai and Dorfman (2,3) described this disorder as a massive, bilateral, mostly cervical lymphadenopathy of young black children. A review of 423 cases published or recorded by 1990 in a registry of cases maintained at the Yale University School of Medicine revealed a much broader spectrum of the disease (4). The age of patients ranged from newborn to 74 years (mean, 20.6 years) (4). The distribution was worldwide, all races were affected, and males outnumbered females almost 6 to 4 (4). In addition to affecting lymph nodes, still the principal site, SHML in the form of pseudotumors was reported to occur in about one-third of cases in the orbit (5), ear (6), upper respiratory tract (7), gastrointestinal tract (8), meninges (4,9), and other extranodal sites (10,11). Some patients experience a short, nonspecific febrile episode, occasionally with pharyngitis and night sweats, before the lymph nodes become enlarged. In most cases, however, localized lymphadenopathy is the only manifestation at onset and during the full course of the disease. With the exception of patients in whom a few aggressive forms of the disease involve vital organs and occasionally cause death, most remain generally healthy; however, large, sometimes deforming, but painless lymph nodes may persist for several years. In most cases, the disease is self-limited and eventually recedes. Rare fatal outcomes tend to occur in patients with generalized lymphadenopathy and immune dysfunction, manifested by hematologic auto-antibodies, inflammatory joint disease, glomerulonephritis, or Wiskott-Aldrich syndrome (12). The cause of death may be a consequence of the immunologic abnormality (13). In more aggressive forms, combinations of corticosteroids and alkylating agents have been used, but no effective treatment has yet been devised (14). SHML is infrequently associated with non-Hodgkin (4,15,16) or Hodgkin lymphomas (17,18).

IMMUNOLOGY

Some patients have one or more immune disorders, such as polyarthralgia, asthma, or hemolytic anemia, preceding or associated with the onset of SHML (4). Abnormalities in serum protein levels are detected in a majority of patients, who usually show moderate polyclonal hypergammaglobulinemia. In the patients tested, a reversal in the ratio of CD4 to CD8 circulating lymphocytes was recorded (4).

HISTOPATHOLOGY

Large, matted lymph nodes exhibit fibrosis of the capsule and pericapsular fibrofatty tissues. The architecture is altered by marked dilatation of the sinuses (Fig. 37.1) and effacement of the follicles and germinal centers (Fig. 37.2). The sinuses are distended and obstructed by static lymph

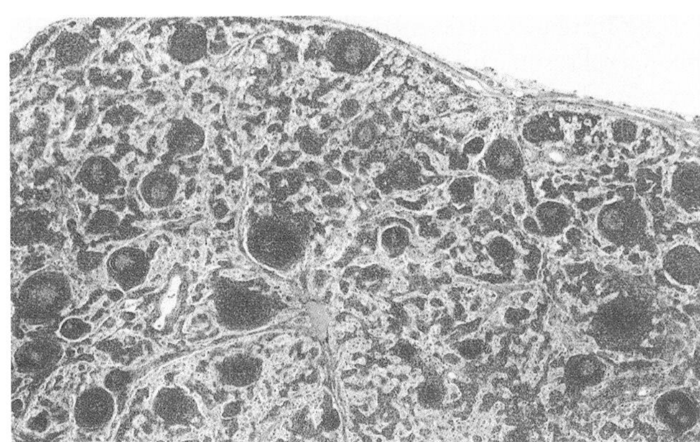

FIGURE 37.1. Sinus histiocytosis with massive lymphadenopathy. Markedly widened sinuses alter normal lymph node architecture. Hematoxylin and eosin stain.

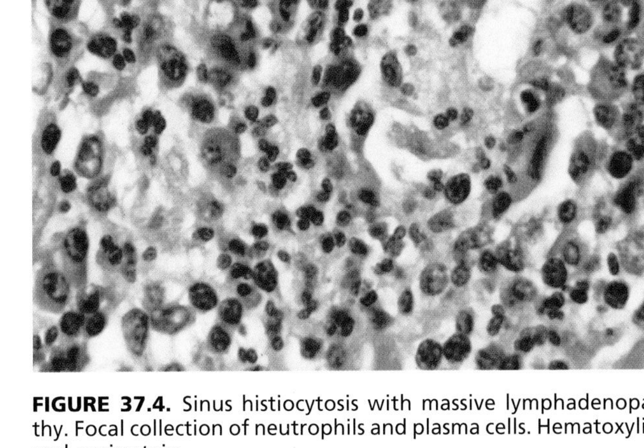

FIGURE 37.4. Sinus histiocytosis with massive lymphadenopathy. Focal collection of neutrophils and plasma cells. Hematoxylin and eosin stain.

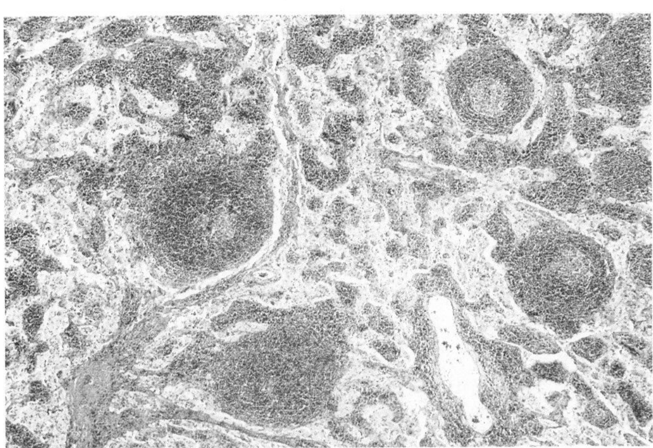

FIGURE 37.2. Sinus histiocytosis with massive lymphadenopathy. Sinuses excessively dilated by lymph and macrophages compress follicles, causing a loss of germinal centers, and replace lymphoid parenchyma. Hematoxylin and eosin stain.

(Fig. 37.3) and a mixed population of cells, including polymorphonuclear leukocytes (Fig. 37.4). The predominant cells in the sinuses and medulla are histiocytes, which exhibit much morphologic variation and marked phagocytic properties (Fig. 37.5). These characteristic SHML cells are generally large and irregularly shaped, with abundant, acidophilic, sometimes vacuolated cytoplasm and one or several markedly indented nuclei, prominent nucleoli, and rare mitoses (Fig. 37.6). The intracytoplasmic vacuoles contain engulfed lymphocytes, erythrocytes, or neutrophils (Fig. 37.7). The cells engulfed by histiocytes are usually contained in an intracytoplasmic vacuole, protected from cytolytic enzymes (Figs. 37.5–37.7). Some cells, particularly lymphocytes in the vacuoles, are viable, reproducing the phenomenon of *emperipolesis* (Fig. 37.8); others are degraded, often forming nuclear fragments (19). Some vacuoles include only nuclear debris or lipids that stain with Sudan black, and as many as 20 engulfed cells may be present

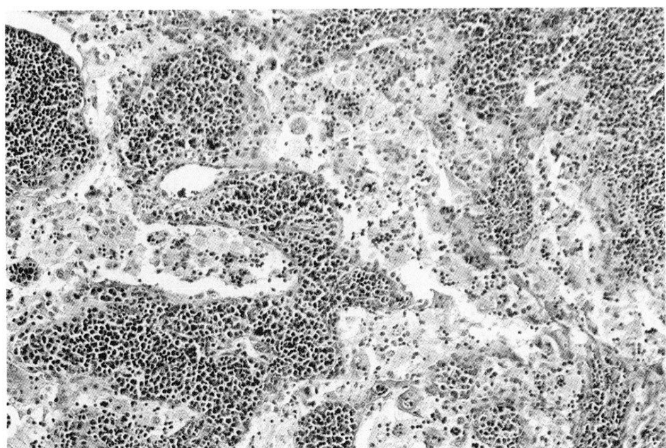

FIGURE 37.3. Sinus histiocytosis with massive lymphadenopathy. Markedly distended sinus with hyperplasia of sinus histiocytes, proliferation of plasma cells and macrophages, and deposits of proteinaceous material. Hematoxylin and eosin stain.

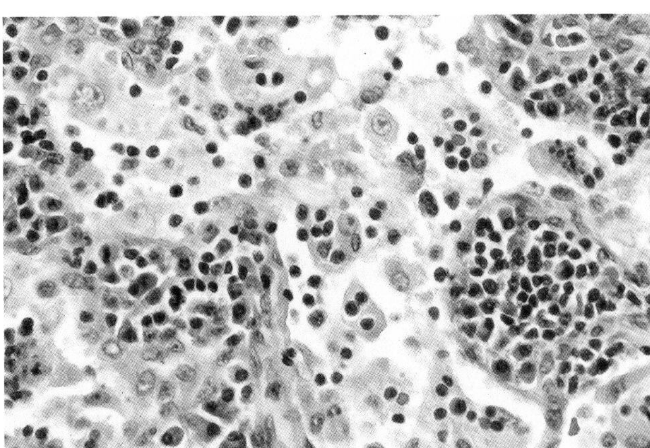

FIGURE 37.5. Sinus histiocytosis with massive lymphadenopathy. Cell debris, proteinaceous deposits, histiocytes, and large macrophages containing multiple lymphocytes within intracytoplasmic vacuoles (emperipolesis). Hematoxylin and eosin stain.

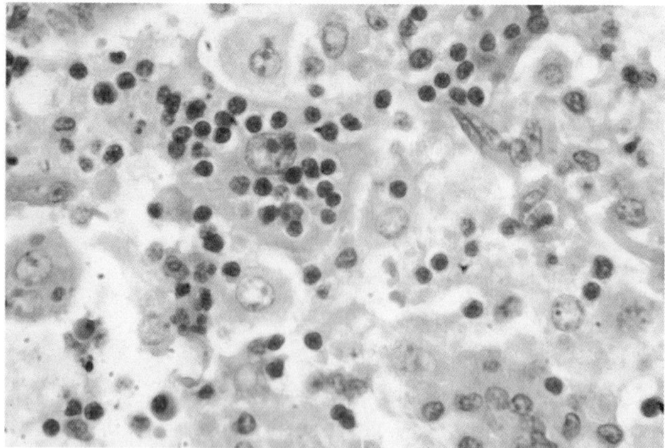

FIGURE 37.6. Sinus histiocytosis with massive lymphadenopathy. Large phagocytic histiocytes with abundant cytoplasm and vesicular nuclei containing numerous lymphocytes within intracytoplasmic vacuoles. Hematoxylin and eosin stain.

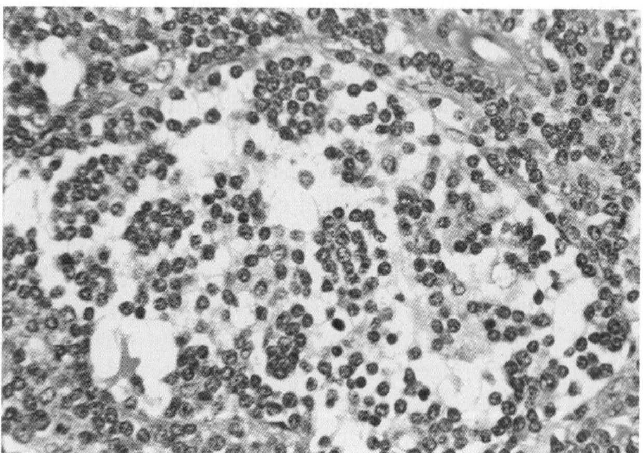

FIGURE 37.7. Sinus histiocytosis with massive lymphadenopathy. Numerous engulfed lymphocytes in extremely active emperipolesis obscure histiocyte nuclei. Hematoxylin and eosin stain.

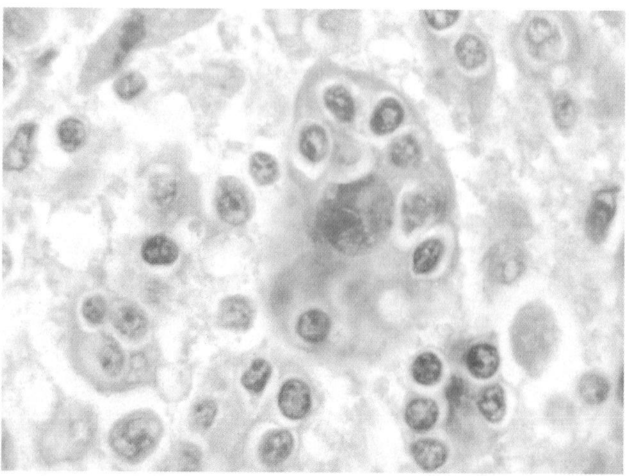

FIGURE 37.8. Sinus histiocytosis with massive lymphadenopathy. Large phagocytic histiocyte with centrally located nucleus and multiple intracytoplasmic vacuoles containing viable lymphocytes (emperipolesis). Hematoxylin and eosin stain.

in one histiocyte. The medullary pulp includes numerous plasma cells, some binucleated, mature lymphocytes, and on occasion large, compact aggregates of lipid-laden histiocytes. Eosinophils are rare. Necrosis is not present. The lymphocytes are of both T- and B-cell types. Both lymphocytes and plasma cells have different classes of immunoglobulins, in accordance with the polyclonality of hypergammaglobulinemia. The histopathologic (3,19–21) and electron microscopic (19,22–25) features of SHML have been amply described and illustrated in earlier articles (Fig. 37.9). Based on ultrastructural features, three different types of histiocyte have been identified: cells with smooth cytoplasmic borders and moderate amounts of cytoplasmic lipid (type 1), cells with numerous interdigitating filiform processes (type 2), and large cells with abundant lipid and myelin figures (type 3) (24,25). The latter more frequently exhibit lymphocyte-containing vacuoles. Inside the vacuoles, the lymphocytes are in various states of preservation (25). The phenomenon of emperipolesis ("wandering in and around") of lymphocytes can be demonstrated in tissue culture (22,26).

CYTOLOGY

Fine needle aspiration (FNA) smears are typically highly cellular, with many histiocytes, phagocytosed lymphocytes, and a reactive lymphoid background (27,28). Most histiocytes have a bland nucleus and abundant, pale, sometimes vacuolated cytoplasm. Atypical histiocytes contain hyperchromatic nucleoli with prominent nucleoli, and some histiocytes are huge (28). In FNA preparations, phagocytosed lymphocytes do not appear surrounded by a "halo," as they often do in tissue sections because of a fixation artifact (3). This can lead to difficulty in distinguishing emperipolesis from overlapping lymphocytes. In FNA smears of early SHML lesions, prominent germinal centers yield many lymphocytes and occasional immunoblasts (28). In later stages, numerous plasma cells and Russell bodies predominate (29–31).

IMMUNOHISTOCHEMISTRY

The SHML cells stain strongly with antibodies directed toward pan-macrophage antigens such as CD14 (Leu-M3; Becton, Dickinson), EBM11 (Dako), and HAM56 (Enzo) (25,32,33). In most cases, they also stain with antibodies to α_1-antichymotrypsin and α_1-antitrypsin, which suggests lysosomal activity (25), although lysozyme may be variable or undetectable (32,34). These results indicate that the SHML cells belong to the macrophage–histiocyte family. It is not yet clear, however, which particular member of the family they represent because almost all cases of SHML express S100 protein (25,32,33,35) (Fig 37.10), a characteristic marker for interdigitating dendritic cells in lymph nodes

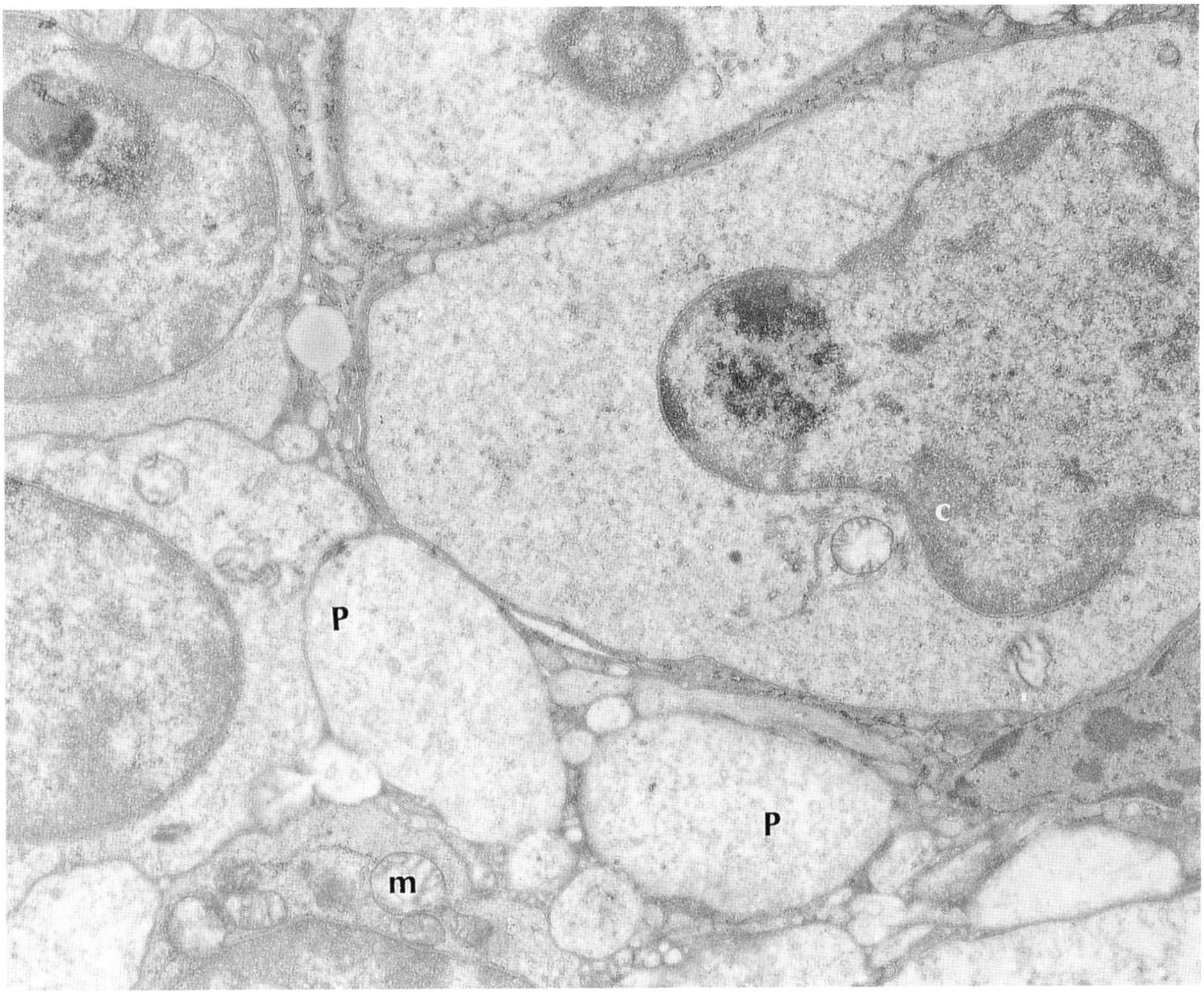

FIGURE 37.9. Sinus histiocytosis with massive lymphadenopathy. Large histiocyte with multiple interlocked cell processes (*P*), abundant cytoplasm, few mitochondria (*m*), and irregularly shaped nucleus with finely dispersed chromatin (*c*). ×12,600.

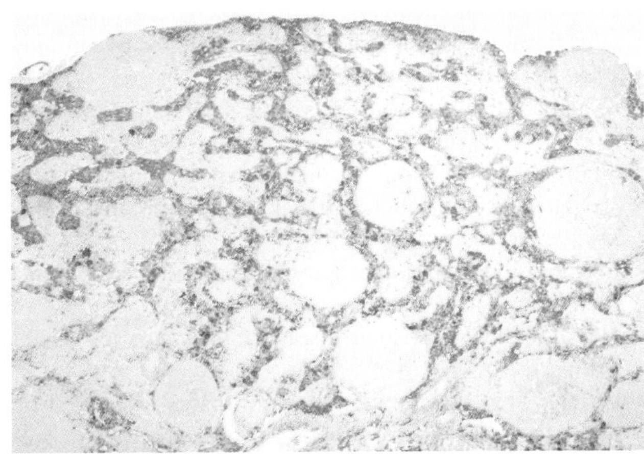

FIGURE 37.10. Sinus histiocytosis with massive lymphadenopathy. Histiocytes expressing S100 protein outline distended sinuses. Immunoperoxidase stain.

and Langerhans cells in skin; however, SHML cells and Langerhans cells differ morphologically. Both SHML cells and Langerhans cells express aspartic proteinases: cathepsin D (found in antigen-presenting cells) and cathepsin E (marking the macrophage lineage). SHML cells express a pattern of adhesion molecules characteristic of circulating monocytes: CD11b+, CD11c+, CD18+, CD62L+, and CD103+ (36). Although CD1a is usually not detected in SHML cells, conflicting results have been reported (32,37,38). For example, normal interdigitating reticulum cells, Langerhans cells, and SHML cells, but not macrophages, stain positively with the anti-CD1a monoclonal antibody 010 in paraffin sections (39). On the other hand, some investigators find rare CD1a+ cells in a particular case or only few CD1a+ cases of SHML (34,40,41). The LN-3 antibody reveals that Langerhans cells, but not SHML cells, express HLA-DR (major histocompatability class II antigen) (38). A majority of SHML cells are intensely positive for CD14 (Leu-M3), CD11c (Leu-M5),

Checklist

SINUS HISTIOCYTOSIS WITH MASSIVE LYMPHADENOPATHY

Children and adolescents
Febrile episode
Polyclonal hypergammaglobulinemia
Massive lymphadenopathy
Cervical site
Long duration
Good general condition
Spontaneous regression
Effacement of follicles
Dilatation of sinuses
Proliferation of sinus histiocytes
Lipid-laden macrophages
Absence of necrosis
Lack of mitoses
SHML cells with engulfed lymphocytes (emperipolesis)
SHML cells positive for macrophage markers
SHML cells positive for S100 protein
SHML cells positive for lysosomal activity

CD68 (KP1), S100 protein, and DRC-1 (which identifies dendritic reticulum cell meshworks in B-cell follicles and veiled cells); a minority of SHML cells are positive for CD4 (Leu-3A) and CD30 (Ki-1) (42). Because normal macrophages express CD4 and activated macrophages can express CD30 (43), these results suggest that SHML cells represent macrophages recently derived from circulating monocytes, possibly activated by T cells (33). Inside the SHML cells, the engulfed lymphocytes are of both B- and T-cell types (33).

CYTOGENETICS

Only two SHML cases have been studied; one showed a normal karyotype, and the other had a minor hypodiploid clone lacking chromosome 20 (42).

MOLECULAR DIAGNOSIS

T-cell and B-cell antigen receptor genes were in a germline configuration in one SHML case (32). In two female patients with SHML, polymerase chain reaction analysis of X-linked polymorphic regions of the human androgen receptor (HUMARA) locus revealed a polyclonal proliferation (44). Serologic findings of Epstein-Barr virus infection were present in more than half of SHML cases (4), but the results of *in situ* hybridization studies for latent or lytic Epstein-Barr virus infection were negative in paraffin sections (45). Although *in situ* hybridization studies detect human herpesvirus 6 in SHML tissues, it remains unclear exactly which cells are infected (46).

DIFFERENTIAL DIAGNOSIS

- Sinus histiocytosis: Nonspecific reaction of lymph nodes to infections and neoplasia. Lymphophagocytosis not present. Results of staining for S100 protein positive in only a few isolated cells.
- Malignant histiocytosis: Cells aggregated in clusters or islands; marked nuclear atypia, frequent mitoses.
- Granulomatous lesions: Epithelioid cells arranged in typical patterns, multinucleated giant cells, occasional necrosis.
- Eosinophilic granuloma: Large numbers of eosinophils present.
- Hand-Schüller-Christian disease: Characteristic skeletal lesions.
- Letterer-Siwe disease: Common in infants, characteristic skin lesions.
- Hodgkin disease: Absence of sinus distention, presence of Reed-Sternberg cells.

REFERENCES

1. Destombes P. Adenitis with lipid excess, in children or young adults, seen in the Antilles and in Mali (4 cases) [in French]. Bull Soc Pathol Exot Filiales 1965;58:1169–1175.
2. Rosai J, Dorfman RF. Sinus histiocytosis with massive lymphadenopathy. A newly recognized benign clinicopathological entity. Arch Pathol 1969;87:63–70.
3. Rosai J, Dorfman RF. Sinus histiocytosis with massive lymphadenopathy: a pseudolymphomatous benign disorder. Analysis of 34 cases. Cancer 1972;30:1174–1188.
4. Foucar E, Rosai J, Dorfman R. Sinus histiocytosis with massive lymphadenopathy (Rosai-Dorfman disease): review of the entity. Semin Diagn Pathol 1990;7:19–73.
5. Foucar E, Rosai J, Dorfman RF. The ophthalmologic manifestations of sinus histiocytosis with massive lymphadenopathy. Am J Ophthalmol 1979;87:354–367.
6. Foucar E, Rosai J, Dorfman RF. Sinus histiocytosis with massive lymphadenopathy. Arch Otolaryngol 1978;104:687–693.
7. Biller HF, Pilch BZ. Case records of the Massachusetts General Hospital. Weekly clinicopathological exercises. Case 52-1981. A 51-year-old man with upper-airway obstruction and lymphadenopathy. N Engl J Med 1981;305:1572–1580.
8. Osborne BM, Hagemeister FB, Butler JJ. Extranodal gastrointestinal sinus histiocytosis with massive lymphadenopathy. Clinically presenting as a malignant tumor. Am J Surg Pathol 1981;5: 603–611.
9. Kessler E, Srulijes C, Toledo E, et al. Sinus histiocytosis with massive lymphadenopathy and spinal epidural involvement: a case report and review of the literature. Cancer 1976;38:1614–1618.
10. Buchino JJ, Byrd RP, Kmetz DR. Disseminated sinus histiocytosis with massive lymphadenopathy: its pathologic aspects. Arch Pathol Lab Med 1982;106:13–16.
11. Mir R, Aftalion B, Kahn LB. Sinus histiocytosis with massive lymphadenopathy and unusual extranodal manifestations. Arch Pathol Lab Med 1985;109:867–870.
12. Foucar E, Rosai J, Dorfman RF. Sinus histiocytosis with massive lymphadenopathy. An analysis of 14 deaths occurring in a patient registry. Cancer 1984;54:1834–1840.
13. Foucar E, Rosai J, Dorfman RF, et al. Immunologic abnormalities and their significance in sinus histiocytosis with massive lymphadenopathy. Am J Clin Pathol 1984;82:515–525.
14. Komp DM. The treatment of sinus histiocytosis with massive lymphadenopathy (Rosai-Dorfman disease). Semin Diagn Pathol 1990;7:83–86.
15. Rangwala AF, Zinterhofer LJ, Nyi KM, et al. Sinus histiocytosis with massive lymphadenopathy and malignant lymphoma. An unreported association. Cancer 1990;65:999–1002.
16. Koduru PR, Susin M, Kolitz JE, et al. Morphological, ultrastructural, and genetic characterization of an unusual T-cell lymphoma in a patient with sinus histiocytosis with massive lymphadenopathy. Am J Hematol 1995;48:192–200.
17. Falk S, Stutte HJ, Frizzera G. Hodgkin's disease and sinus histiocytosis with massive lymphadenopathy-like changes. Histopathology 1991;19:221–224.
18. Maia DM, Dorfman RF. Focal changes of sinus histiocytosis with massive lymphadenopathy (Rosai-Dorfman disease) associated with nodular lymphocyte predominant Hodgkin's disease. Hum Pathol 1995;26:1378–1382.
19. Lennert K, Niedorf HR, Blumcke S, et al. Lymphadenitis with massive hemophagocytic sinus histiocytosis. Virchows Arch B Cell Pathol 1972;10:14–29.
20. Diebold J, Tixier P, Baufine-Ducrocq H, et al. Lymphadenopathy caused by hemophagocytic sinus histiocytosis (Destombes-Rosai-Dorfman syndrome). Immunologic and histopathologic study of a new case [in French]. Ann Anat Pathol (Paris) 1976;21: 347–356.
21. Lampert F, Lennert K. Sinus histiocytosis with massive lymphadenopathy: fifteen new cases. Cancer 1976;37:783–789.
22. Karpas A, Arno J, Cawley J. Sinus histiocytosis with massive lymphadenopathy—properties of cultured histiocytes. Eur J Cancer 1973;9:729–732.
23. Ioachim HL. Lymph nodes and spleen. In: Johannessen JV, ed. Electron microscopy in medicine, vol 5. New York: McGraw-Hill, 1981:431–436.
24. Sanchez R, Sibley RK, Rosai J, et al. The electron microscopic features of sinus histiocytosis with massive lymphadenopathy: a study of 11 cases. Ultrastruct Pathol 1981;2:101–119.
25. Lopez P, Estes ML. Immunohistochemical characterization of the histiocytes in sinus histiocytosis with massive lymphadenopathy: analysis of an extranodal case. Hum Pathol 1989;20: 711–715.
26. Ioachim HL. Emperipolesis of lymphoid cells in mixed cultures. Lab Invest 1965;14:1784–1794.
27. Patel KD, Rege JD, Naik LP. Fine-needle aspiration cytology of sinus histiocytosis with massive lymphadenopathy: a case report. Diagn Cytopathol 1996;15:221–223.
28. Stastny JF, Wilkerson ML, Hamati HF, et al. Cytologic features of sinus histiocytosis with massive lymphadenopathy. A report of three cases. Acta Cytol 1997;41:871–876.
29. Layfield LJ. Fine needle aspiration cytologic findings in a case of sinus histiocytosis with massive lymphadenopathy (Rosai-Dorfman syndrome). Acta Cytol 1990;34:767–770.
30. Pettinato G, Manivel JC, d'Amore ES, et al. Fine needle aspiration cytology and immunocytochemical characterization of the histiocytes in sinus histiocytosis with massive lymphadenopathy (Rosai-Dorfman syndrome). Acta Cytol 1990;34:771–777.
31. Trautman BC, Stanley MW, Goding GS, et al. Sinus histiocytosis with massive lymphadenopathy (Rosai-Dorfman disease): diagnosis by fine-needle aspiration. Diagn Cytopathol 1991;7:513–516.
32. Bonetti F, Chilosi M, Menestrina F, et al. Immunohistological analysis of Rosai-Dorfman histiocytosis. A disease of S-100 + CD1-histiocytes. Virchows Arch A Pathol Anat Histopathol 1987;411:129–135.
33. Eisen RN, Buckley PJ, Rosai J. Immunophenotypic characterization of sinus histiocytosis with massive lymphadenopathy (Rosai-Dorfman disease). Semin Diagn Pathol 1990;7:74–82.
34. Paulli M, Rosso R, Kindl S, et al. Immunophenotypic characterization of the cell infiltrate in five cases of sinus histiocytosis with massive lymphadenopathy (Rosai-Dorfman disease). Hum Pathol 1992;23:647–654.
35. Miettinen M, Paljakka P, Haveri P, et al. Sinus histiocytosis with massive lymphadenopathy. A nodal and extranodal proliferation of S-100 protein positive histiocytes? Am J Clin Pathol 1987;88: 270–277.
36. Quaglino P, Tomasini C, Novelli M, et al. Immunohistologic findings and adhesion molecule pattern in primary pure cutaneous Rosai-Dorfman disease with xanthomatous features. Am J Dermatopathol 1998;20:393–398.
37. Sacchi S, Artusi T, Torelli U, et al. Sinus histiocytosis with massive lymphadenopathy. Leuk Lymphoma 1992;7:189–194.
38. Paulli M, Feller AC, Boveri E, et al. Cathepsin D and E co-expression in sinus histiocytosis with massive lymphadenopathy (Rosai-Dorfman disease) and Langerhans' cell histiocytosis: further evidences of a phenotypic overlap between these histiocytic disorders. Virchows Arch 1994;424:601–606.

39. Krenacs L, Tiszalvicz L, Krenacs T, et al. Immunohistochemical detection of CD1A antigen in formalin-fixed and paraffin-embedded tissue sections with monoclonal antibody 010. J Pathol 1993;171:99–104.
40. Maennle DL, Grierson HL, Gnarra DG, et al. Sinus histiocytosis with massive lymphadenopathy: a spectrum of disease associated with immune dysfunction. Pediatr Pathol 1991;11:399–412.
41. Perrin C, Michiels JF, Lacour JP, et al. Sinus histiocytosis (Rosai-Dorfman disease) clinically limited to the skin. An immunohistochemical and ultrastructural study. J Cutan Pathol 1993;20:368–374.
42. Sacchi S, Artusi T, Selleri L, et al. Sinus histiocytosis with massive lymphadenopathy: immunological, cytogenetic and molecular studies. Blut 1990;60:339–344.
43. Andreesen R, Brugger W, Lohr GW, et al. Human macrophages can express the Hodgkin's cell-associated antigen Ki-1 (CD30). Am J Pathol 1989;134:187–192.
44. Paulli M, Bergamaschi G, Tonon L, et al. Evidence for a polyclonal nature of the cell infiltrate in sinus histiocytosis with massive lymphadenopathy (Rosai-Dorfman disease). Br J Haematol 1995;91:415–418.
45. Tsang WY, Yip TT, Chan JK. The Rosai-Dorfman disease histiocytes are not infected by Epstein-Barr virus. Histopathology 1994;25:88–90.
46. Levine PH, Jahan N, Murari P, et al. Detection of human herpesvirus 6 in tissues involved by sinus histiocytosis with massive lymphadenopathy (Rosai-Dorfman disease). J Infect Dis 1992;166:291–295.

38

KIKUCHI-FUJIMOTO LYMPHADENOPATHY

DEFINITION

Subacute necrotizing lymphadenopathy associated with mild fever, more common in Asia, predominantly in young women.

SYNONYM

Histiocytic necrotizing lymphadenopathy

ETIOLOGY

The etiology of necrotizing lymphadenitis is unknown. Although a viral infection is suggested by the clinical and histologic features, no infectious agent has been identified so far. The results of an investigation for the presence of Epstein-Barr virus (EBV) and human herpesvirus type 6 (HHV-6) were negative (1). In a recent study of cervical lymphadenopathies in Korean patients, HHV-8 was detected by polymerase chain reaction and Southern blot analysis in 8 of 26 cases of Kikuchi-Fujimoto lymphadenopathy and in none of 40 cases of various unrelated lymphadenopathies (2). In an earlier work in a different population, HHV-8 was not found in any of seven cases of Kikuchi-Fujimoto lymphadenopathy (3).

CLINICAL FEATURES

Described independently in 1972 by Kikuchi (4) and Fujimoto et al. (5), this subacute necrotizing lymphadenitis has been recognized frequently in Asia and sporadically in Western countries. The patients are predominantly women, and although the age range is wide, the average age is less than 30 years (6–10). The cervical lymph nodes are involved in almost all cases; involvement is more often unilateral but sometimes bilateral at multiple locations or systemic (8–11). The lymphadenopathy, which is painless, is either unaccompanied by symptoms or associated with moderate fever, chills, myalgia, sore throat, and skin rashes. The course is benign, with spontaneous resolution of the adenopathy in a few weeks or months and rare recurrences (6–11). Involvement of extranodal sites is unusual but well documented, particularly in Asia, where Kikuchi disease is relatively common (12). In a report of five cases, the patients presented with cutaneous involvement in addition to the typical necrotizing lymphadenopathy. Cutaneous eruptions on the upper body in some cases resembled those of systemic lupus (12). In one reported fatal case, of a 38-year old Chinese man, fever and systemic necrotizing lymphadenitis were associated with necrotizing myocarditis (13). The liver and spleen were moderately enlarged in only a few of the reported cases. Leukopenia with mild lymphocytosis and occasional atypical lymphocytes may occur in some cases (10). Bone marrow biopsy, when performed, revealed no abnormalities (6).

HISTOPATHOLOGY

The lymph node architecture is partially maintained, and residual follicles have reactive germinal centers. Patchy areas of necrosis, irregularly shaped and occasionally confluent, are randomly distributed, often appearing as wedge-shaped regions in the cortex (Fig. 38.1). The necrosis consists of brightly eosinophilic fibrinoid deposits including nuclear fragments surrounded by large accumulations of pale-staining histiocytes (Fig. 38.2). Sometimes, the tissue necrosis is represented only by isolated apoptotic cells scattered throughout large aggregates of histiocytes admixed with cellular debris and nuclear dust (Fig. 38.3). Some authors consider histiocytic proliferation rather than necrosis to be the characteristic feature of Kikuchi-Fujimoto lymphadenopathy, and they even include in this entity cases that lack overt necrosis, showing only scattered cells with pyknosis or karyorrhexis (1,9) (Fig. 38.4). The cellular debris is actively phagocytosed by numerous histiocytes, cells with abundant cytoplasm and peripheral, compressed, crescentic nuclei re-

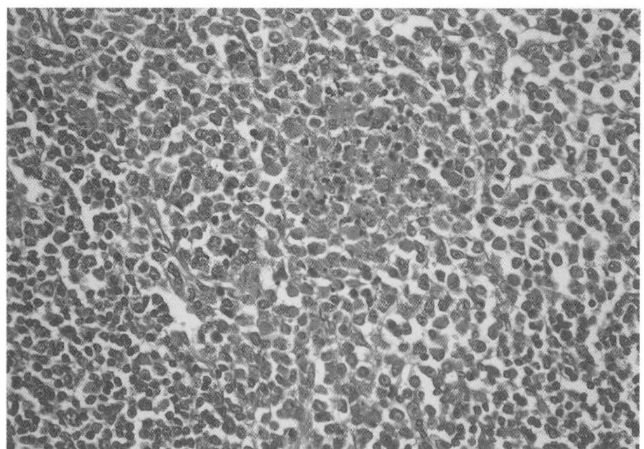

FIGURE 38.1. Kikuchi lymphadenopathy of a cervical lymph node. Area of tissue necrosis with extensive apoptosis, mostly of histiocytes. Hematoxylin, phloxine, and saffron stain.

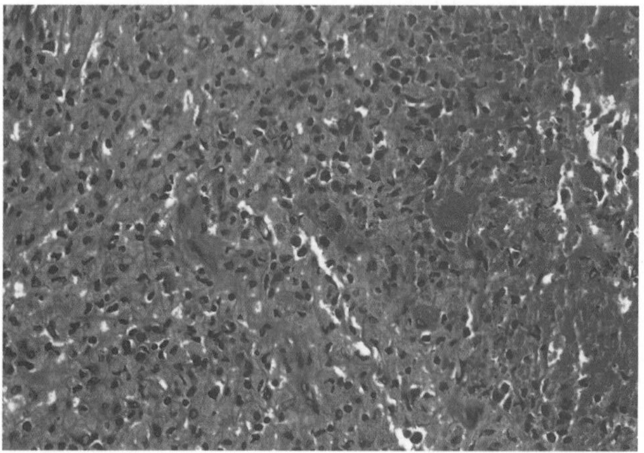

FIGURE 38.2. Fibrinoid necrosis with abundant nuclear fragments in cortical area. Hematoxylin, phloxine, and saffron stain.

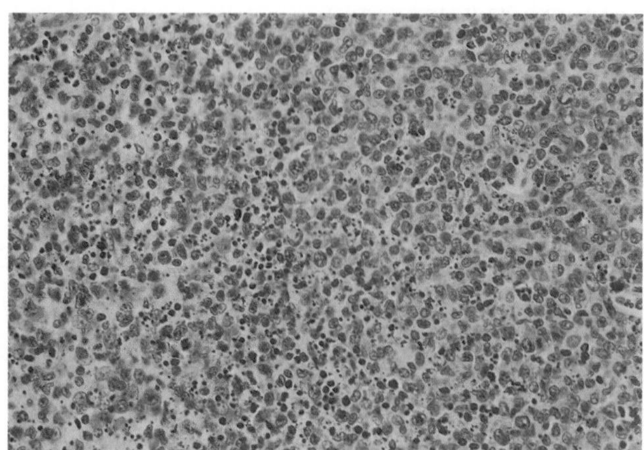

FIGURE 38.3. Extensive apoptosis in area of histiocytic proliferation. Abundant nuclear debris but no leukocytic infiltration. Hematoxylin, phloxine, and saffron stain.

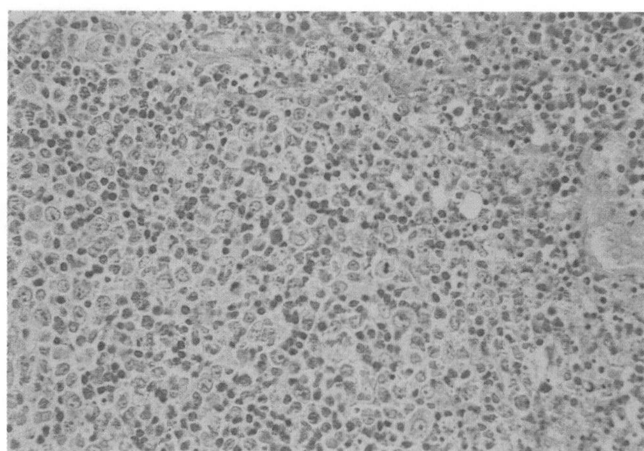

FIGURE 38.4. Sheets of proliferating histiocytes in Kikuchi lymphadenopathy. Hematoxylin, phloxine, and saffron stain.

sembling signet ring cells (11). The areas of histiocytosis also include small lymphocytes, activated T lymphocytes, and a moderate number of plasma cells. A consistent absence of neutrophils and eosinophils is a distinctive feature of this lesion (14) (Fig. 38.5). At the periphery of necrotic areas are nests of plasmacytoid monocytes and immunoblasts. Usually, a degree of perilymphadenitis is present, with lymphocytes, often apoptotic, and histiocytes infiltrating the perinodal adipose tissues (11). According to the predominant histologic features, four subtypes can be distinguished: (a) lymphohistiocytic, characterized by cellular proliferation; (b) phagocytic, with numerous histiocytes and single-cell necrosis; (c) necrotic, with distinct foci of necrosis; and (d) foamy cell type, in which vacuolated histiocytes aggregate around necrotic foci (10).

Early lesions may show minimal necrosis and phagocytosis, being formed by aggregates of immunoblasts (transformed lymphocytes) and plasmacytoid monocytes, so that

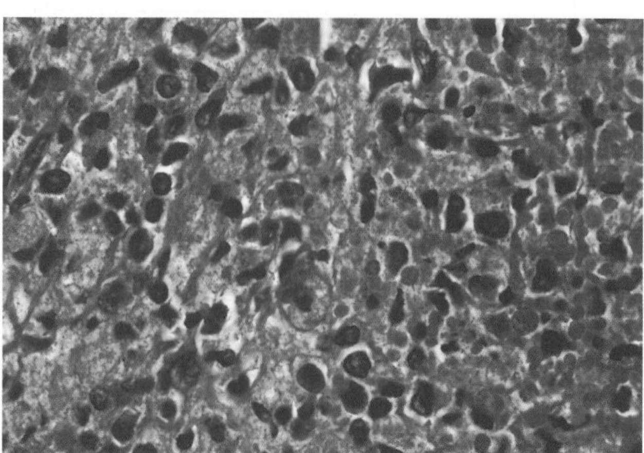

FIGURE 38.5. Area of necrosis with apoptotic cells but no inflammatory cells. Hematoxylin, phloxine, and saffron stain.

lymphoma may be suspected (15). In a second stage, individual cell apoptosis and confluent necrosis prevail, whereas resorption of necrosis and repopulation with normal cells are seen in the resolution phase of the process (15). In cases with skin involvement, necrotic keratinocytes and vacuolar interface changes are seen, with superficial dense dermal lymphohistiocytic and deep perivascular infiltrates, abundant karyorrhectic debris, and the characteristic absence of polynuclear leukocytes (12).

ULTRASTRUCTURE

Under the electron microscope, the histiocytes appear as large cells with phagolysosomes containing phagocytosed nuclear debris and myelin-like inclusions (16). The plasmacytoid monocytes comprise a well-developed endoplasmic reticulum with numerous parallel cisternae, a feature that contrasts with their lack of immunoglobulins or any other secretory products (17). Tubuloreticular structures, described as intertwined, membrane-bound tubules, seen in viral lymphadenitides such as those caused by HIV (18) and in autoimmune diseases such as systemic lupus (19), have also been found in 14 of 15 cases of Kikuchi-Fujimoto lymphadenopathy within histiocytes, immunoblasts, and endothelial cells (16). Interferon-α, a frequent component of antiviral defense reactions, is related to the presence of tubuloreticular structures and has been identified with the use of a polyclonal antibody in many histiocytes of this lymphadenopathy (20).

IMMUNOHISTOCHEMISTRY

Staining of the histiocytes, which represent the majority of the infiltrating cells, for lysozyme and with antibodies against CD68, Mac 387, and KiMiP1 confirms their histiocytic nature (10) (Fig. 38.6). The lymphocytes in the involved zones are predominantly T cells, with CD8+ (cytotoxic/suppressor) cells far more numerous than CD4+ (helper) cells. The plasmacytoid monocytes are stained by antibody LN-2 for the marker CD74 (10). The origin of these cells is still controversial, with more recent studies demonstrating that they represent activated monocytes rather than T cells, as originally postulated (17,21).

DIFFERENTIAL DIAGNOSIS

Kikuchi-Fujimoto lymphadenopathy is a rare disease in Western countries; however, it is important that it be included in the differential diagnosis of necrotizing lymphadenopathies, such as tuberculosis, lupus erythematosus, and lymphoma, because its course and treatment are entirely different.

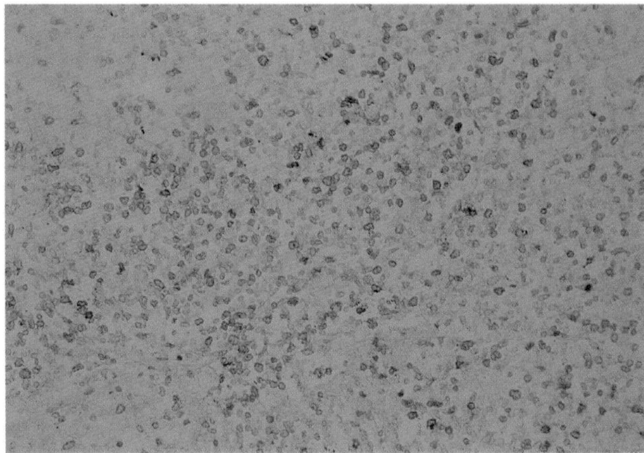

FIGURE 38.6. Histiocytic proliferation in Kikuchi cervical lymphadenopathy. CD68 antibody/peroxidase stain.

- Lymph node infarction: Ischemic necrosis without nuclear debris involving the entire lymph node and sparing only a narrow subcapsular rim.
- Systemic lupus lymphadenitis: The foci of fibrinoid necrosis with nuclear debris may be similar; however, hematoxylin bodies and lesions of vasculitis are also present.
- Necrotizing granulomatous lesions of *tuberculosis, histoplasmosis, leprosy,* and *cat-scratch disease* display characteristic proliferations of epithelioid cells and giant cells and granuloma formation. Etiologic agents can be identified by special stainings.
- Necrotizing lymphadenitis in *syphilis* is usually accompanied by perivascular plasma cell infiltrates, in *Yersinia* infection by eosinophils, and in *bacterial* infection by accumulations of neutrophils.
- Necrotizing lymphadenitis in acute *EBV* infection is accompanied by lymphocyte depletion and occasional hemophagocytosis by histiocytes (22). Results of tests for antibodies to EBV-specific antigens are positive.
- Necrotic foci in *allergic reactions* are surrounded by eosinophils and plasma cells.
- Necrosis in *lymphomas,* although occasionally very extensive, shows lymphoma cells in the peripheral areas.
- Non-Hodgkin lymphoma: Because of sinus obliteration and a proliferation of plasmacytoid monocytes, Kikuchi-Fujimoto lymphadenopathy may be misdiagnosed as lymphoma. However, the reactive follicles and the mixture of lymphocytes and histiocytes exhibit nonmalignant morphologic features.

Checklist

KIKUCHI-FUJIMOTO LYMPHADENOPATHY

Predominance in young women and Asian populations
Cervical lymph nodes
Occasional mild fever, sore throat, myalgia
Benign course, spontaneous remission
Lymph node slightly enlarged
Architecture partially preserved
Patchy areas of necrosis
Marked apoptosis
Nuclear debris
Aggregates of histiocytes, nonphagocytic and phagocytic, with crescentic nuclei
Activated T lymphocytes (immunoblasts)
Plasmacytoid monocytes
Absence of neutrophils and eosinophils
Histiocytes C68+; T cells CD8+ (predominant)
Intracytoplasmic tubuloreticular structures

REFERENCES

1. Kikuchi M. Histiocytic necrotizing lymphadenitis (Kikuchi-Fujimoto disease) in Japan. Am J Surg Pathol 1991;15:l97.
2. Huh J, Kang GH, Gong G, et al. Kaposi's sarcoma-associated herpesvirus in Kikuchi's disease. Hum Pathol 1998;29:1091–1096.
3. Chadburn A, Cesarman E, Nador RG, et al. Kaposi's sarcoma-associated herpesvirus sequences in benign lymphoid proliferation not associated with human immunodeficiency virus. Cancer 1997;80:788–797.
4. Kikuchi M. Lymphadenitis showing focal reticulum cell hyperplasia with nuclear debris and phagocytosis [in Japanese]. Nippon Ketsueki Gakkai Zasshi 1972;35:379–380.
5. Fujimoto Y, Kozima Y, Yamaguchi K. Cervical subacute necrotizing lymphadenitis. A new clinicopathological entity [in Japanese]. Naika 1972;20:920–927.
6. Turner RR, Martin J, Dorfman RF. Necrotizing lymphadenitis. A study of 30 cases. Am J Surg Pathol 1983;7:115–123.
7. Unger PD, Rappaport KM, Strauchen JA. Necrotizing lymphadenitis (Kikuchi's disease). Report of four cases of an unusual pseudolymphomatous lesion and immunologic marker studies. Arch Pathol Lab Med 1987;111:1031–1034.
8. Dorfman RF. Histiocytic necrotizing lymphadenitis of Kikuchi and Fujimoto. Arch Pathol Lab Med 1987;111:1026–1029.
9. Chamulak GA, Brynes RK, Nathwani BN. Kikuchi-Fujimoto disease mimicking malignant lymphoma. Am J Surg Pathol 1990; 14:514–523.
10. Kuo TT. Kikuchi's disease (histiocytic necrotizing lymphadenitis). A clinicopathologic study of 79 cases with an analysis of histologic subtypes, immunohistology and DNA ploidy. Am J Surg Pathol 1995;19:798–809.
11. Tsang WY, Chan JK, Ng CS. Kikuchi's lymphadenitis. A morphologic analysis of 75 cases with special reference to unusual features. Am J Surg Pathol 1994;18:219–231.
12. Spies J, Foucar K, Thompson CT, et al. The histopathology of cutaneous lesions of Kikuchi's disease (necrotizing lymphadenitis). A report of five cases. Am J Surg Pathol 1999;23:1040–1047.
13. Chan JKC, Wong K-C, Ng C-S. A fatal case of multicentric Kikuchi's histiocytic necrotizing lymphadenitis. Cancer 1989;63: 1856–1862.
14. Pileri S, Kikuchi M, Helbron D, et al. Histiocytic necrotizing lymphadenitis without granulocytic infiltration. Virchows Arch A Pathol Anat Histopathol 1982;395:257–271.
15. Nathwani BN. Kikuchi-Fujimoto disease. Am J Surg Pathol 1991;15:196–197.
16. Imamura M, Ueno H, Matsuura A, et al. An ultrastructural study of subacute necrotizing lymphadenitis. Am J Pathol 1982;107: 292–299.
17. De Vos R, De Wolf-Peeters C, Facchetti F, et al. Plasmacytoid monocytes in epithelioid cell granulomas: ultrastructural and immunoelectron microscopic study. Ultrastructural Pathol 1990; 14:291–302.
18. Sidhu GS, Stahl RE, El Sadr W, et al. The acquired immunodeficiency syndrome: an ultrastructural study. Hum Pathol 1985; 16:377–386.
19. Grimley PM, Barry DW, Schaff Z, et al. Lupus-type tubular structures in human lymphoid cell cultures. Arthritis Rheum 1973;16:550.
20. Sumiyoshi Y, Kikuchi M, Takeshita M, et al. Alpha-interferon in Kikuchi's disease. Virchows Arch B Cell Pathol Mol Pathol 1991; 61:201–207.
21. Feller AC, Lennert K, Stein H, et al. Immunohistology and etiology of histiocytic necrotizing lymphadenitis: report of three instructive cases. Histopathology 1983;7:825–839.
22. Reisman RP, Greco MA. Virus-associated hemophagocytic syndrome due to Epstein-Barr virus. Hum Pathol 1984;15:290–293.

39

SARCOIDOSIS LYMPHADENOPATHY

DEFINITION

Sarcoidosis is a systemic granulomatous disease of worldwide distribution and unknown cause.

EPIDEMIOLOGY

Sarcoidosis occurs worldwide, affecting persons of all races and ages. A seasonal clustering is observed, with more cases occurring in winter and early spring (1). Adults between 20 and 40 years of age are usually affected. Sarcoidosis occurs twice as frequently in women as in men, 10 times more frequently in blacks than in whites, and only very rarely in children (2–4). In the United States, the incidence is approximately 5 cases per 100,000 in the white population and 40 cases per 100,000 in the black population (5). A worldwide survey comparing 3,676 patients in nine different countries showed similar pathologic lesions and clinical presentations (3,4). However, a number of studies indicate that sarcoidosis affects blacks more acutely and more severely than people of other races (6–8).

ETIOLOGY

Because its clinical manifestations overlap those of other diseases, and because specific diagnostic tests are not available, the cause of sarcoidosis is still unknown (9). Community outbreaks and clusters of cases, suggestive of an infectious origin, have often been reported. Supporting this hypothesis are cases in which sarcoidosis was inadvertently transmitted by cardiac and bone marrow transplantation (10,11). Of a variety of infectious agents, mycobacteria have been considered most likely to be involved in the etiology of sarcoidosis. Since its original description a century ago, sarcoidosis has been considered to be related to tuberculosis based on clinical and pathologic similarities (12). Indeed, the granulomatous lesions characteristic of sarcoidosis resemble to a great extent those produced by *Mycobacterium tuberculosis* and *Mycobacterium leprae* organisms. The theory that a mycobacterium causes sarcoidosis was substantiated by the detection of mycobacterial DNA and ribosomal RNA in affected tissues by means of the polymerase chain reaction (13,14). The mycobacteria involved in the origin of sarcoidosis may be nontuberculous forms, cell wall-deficient forms, or L-forms, which may explain the repeated failures to stain, culture, or otherwise identify the pathogenic agent of sarcoidosis (12,15). Granulomas induced by beryllium and other dusts or particulate substances also closely resemble those of sarcoidosis, an observation that has given rise to the hypothesis that noninfectious environmental agents, triggering exaggerated immune responses during repeated exposures, may cause the disease (12). However, although the granulomatous lesions may be indistinguishable, berylliosis induces only localized lesions, whereas sarcoidosis is a systemic disease that affects multiple organs.

PATHOGENESIS

Genetic factors have a part in the pathogenesis of sarcoidosis, although a single gene does not seem to be responsible (9). A predisposition to respond to particular antigens with exaggerated cellular reactions appears to be genetic. Serologic studies have identified primary associations with major histocompatibility loci, such as class I HLA-A1 and HLA-B8, similar to those found in some autoimmune disorders (5,16).

Essentially all organs may be involved by sarcoidosis, and more than one organ is involved at a given time. The most common sites, in decreasing order of frequency, are the pulmonary hilar lymph nodes, lungs, peripheral lymph nodes, liver, eyes, skin, bones, salivary glands, and other organs (17). Although the thoracic lymphadenopathies overshadow the pulmonary lesions, which sometimes are inapparent, recent studies have shown that in most cases sarcoidosis begins with an initial focus of alveolitis (5). Subsequently, the process evolves with the development of characteristic granulomas followed by fibrosis. Cardiac sarcoidosis is the most common cause of death in sarcoidosis as a consequence of the fibrosis produced (18). Underlying these lesions are severe alterations of immune mechanisms manifested both at the site of involvement and systemically. In fact, the disorder is not a state of generalized anergy and is not associated with an increased incidence of cancer, as was previously believed, but it is associated with greatly increased cellular activity in the organs involved (6). The number of CD4+ T cells is decreased in the peripheral blood of patients with sarcoidosis, whereas in the tissues involved, an increased ratio of CD4+ to CD8+ T cells indicates a state of cell-mediated hyperreactivity (19,20). In addition to the accumulations of T cells and monocytes, numerous B cells and plasma cells are present, indicating the production of immunoglobulins at the sites of granuloma formation (21,22). Hypergammaglobulinemia as a result of uncontrolled B-cell activation and circulating immune complexes is also a common finding in sarcoidosis (3). Circulating monocytes are attracted to the areas of granuloma formation, where they are transformed into epithelioid and giant cells (23–25). The epithelioid cells synthesize angiotensin-converting enzyme, a glycoprotein component of the renin–angiotensin system, and lysozyme; both are present in increased amounts in serum and tissues involved by granulomas (26). Hypercalcemia and hypercalciuria, which may be prominent features of sarcoidosis, are related to increased plasma levels of 1,25-dihydroxyvitamin D, or calcitriol, which is also produced by the epithelioid cells of sarcoid granulomas (27). Thus, a chronic cascade of inflammatory processes occurs in which unknown antigens drive a hyperactive cellular immune response, with T cells producing interferon-γ and interleukin 2, and the epithelioid cells releasing a variety of cytokines, chemoattractants, and other proinflammatory mediators (5,9,28).

CLINICAL SYNDROME

Sarcoidosis may present with an acute onset of symptoms, such as fever, weight loss, and erythema nodosum, which is associated with a good prognosis, or with a chronic course, including pulmonary, pericardial, or myocardial involvement, which indicates an unfavorable course (5). Cardiac sarcoidosis, which is more common than previously thought and difficult to diagnose clinically, may be the cause of arrhythmias and sudden death (18). The disease is more severe and more persistent in blacks and in the elderly. In most cases, however, sarcoidosis remits spontaneously, with complete cure. Because sarcoidosis is a multisystem disease, the patterns of presentation may vary; however, the most common lesions are respiratory, ocular, and dermatologic (4). In the United States, more than half of patients present with chronic respiratory symptoms and few general signs (9).

Lymphadenopathies are frequently present in cases of sarcoidosis, and the pulmonary hilar lymph nodes are most commonly affected (77% of cases) (29). Bilateral and symmetric involvement of peribronchial lymph nodes in the absence of peripheral or mediastinal lymphadenopathy and with few or no pulmonary infiltrates is almost pathognomonic for sarcoidosis (30). Iritis, uveitis, sinusitis, erythema nodosum, and bone and joint lesions may also appear as manifestations of sarcoidosis, either singly or in association with the pulmonary and lymph node lesions. Frequent accompanying findings are an elevated erythrocyte sedimentation rate, elevated levels of angiotensin-converting enzyme, reversal of the albumin–globulin ratio, hypergammaglobulinemia, hypercalcemia, hypercalciuria, and abnormal serum liver chemistries (31). Biopsy specimens of the gums, nose, lungs, or lymph nodes demonstrating the characteristic sarcoid granulomas and a positive Kveim test result are the findings that positively identify sarcoidosis.

HISTOPATHOLOGY

The characteristic histologic feature of sarcoidosis in all tissues is the noncaseating granuloma. In the involved lymph nodes, the architecture is partially or totally replaced by numerous, closely packed, well-demarcated granulomas (32) (Figs. 39.1 and 39.2). Sometimes, the granulomas are less well demarcated (Fig. 39.3) and may even coalesce (Fig. 39.4). They are composed predominantly of epithelioid cells (Fig. 39.5) with scattered multinucleated giant cells (Fig.39.6), lymphocytes, plasma cells, and fibroblasts. CD4+ and CD8+ T lymphocytes and to a lesser extent B lymphocytes form a concentric rim around the epithelioid granuloma (Figs. 39.5 and 39.6). The epithelioid cells are arranged in concentric rows, forming "perimeters of defense" against antigens presumed to be in the central areas of the granulomas (23–25) (Fig. 39.5). The granulomas in sarcoidosis are of the high-turnover type, and cells are actively replaced (23).

The epithelioid cells are transformed bone marrow monocytes and thus are members of the mononuclear phagocyte system (33). In contrast to the macrophages (also derived from monocytes), the epithelioid cells exhibit

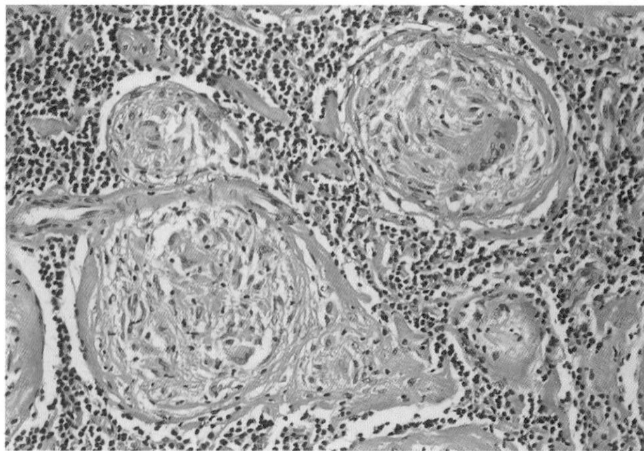

FIGURE 39.1. Sarcoidosis of hilar lymph node. Numerous, closely packed, nodular granulomas evenly placed in lymphoid parenchyma. Hematoxylin, phloxine, and saffron stain.

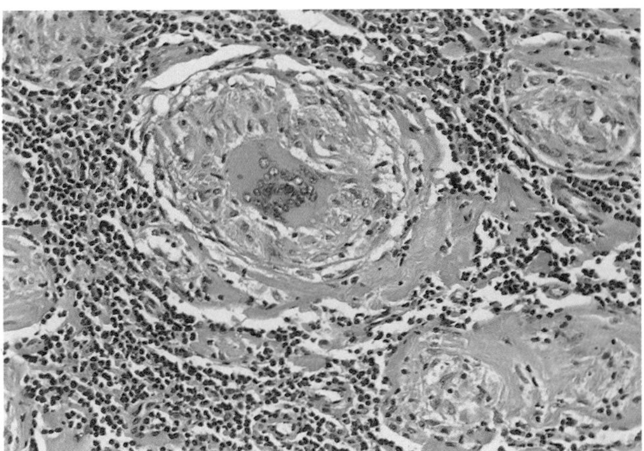

FIGURE 39.2. Same section as in Fig. 39.1. Granuloma of epithelioid cells with central multinucleated giant cell, peripheral lymphocytes, and collagen. Hematoxylin, phloxine, and saffron stain.

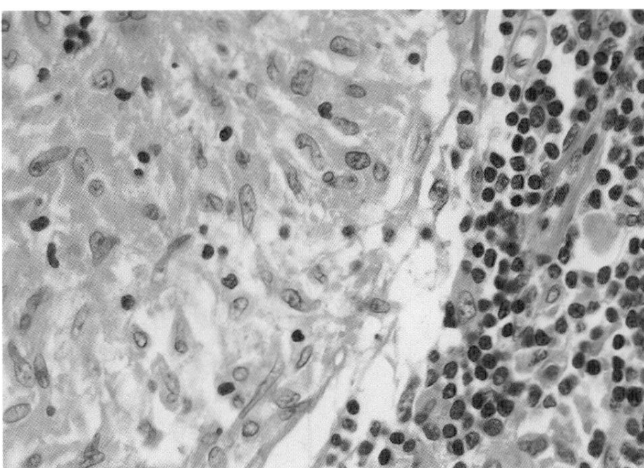

FIGURE 39.5. Epithelioid cells directed toward center of granuloma (*upper left corner*) form a "perimeter of defense." Peripheral rim of lymphocytes (*right*). Hematoxylin, phloxine, and saffron stain.

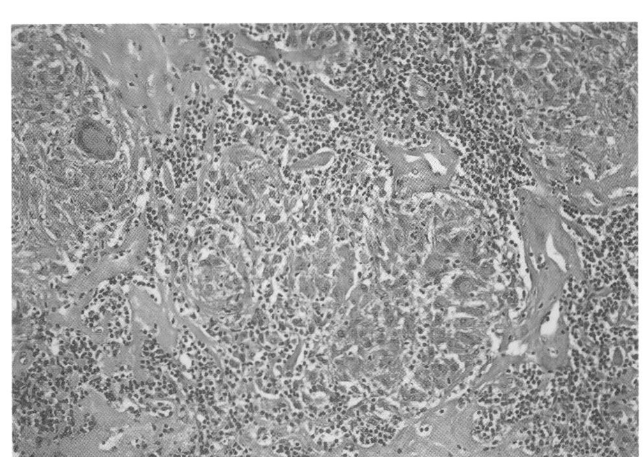

FIGURE 39.3. Non-necrotizing, less well-formed granulomas with giant cells and deposits of collagen. Hematoxylin, phloxine, and saffron stain.

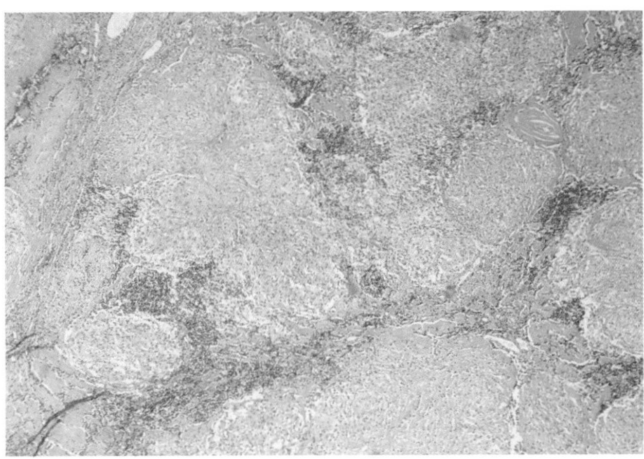

FIGURE 39.4. Coalescing granulomas in sarcoidosis with small focus of central necrosis (*upper left*). Hematoxylin, phloxine, and saffron stain.

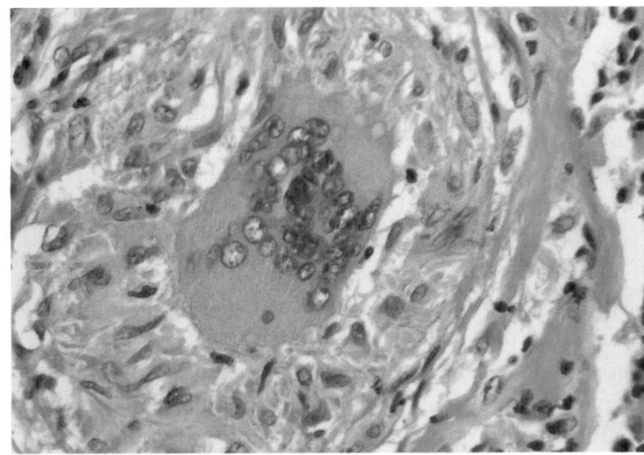

FIGURE 39.6. Multinucleated giant cell, palisading epithelioid cells, and collagen fibers (*right*). Hematoxylin, phloxine, and saffron stain.

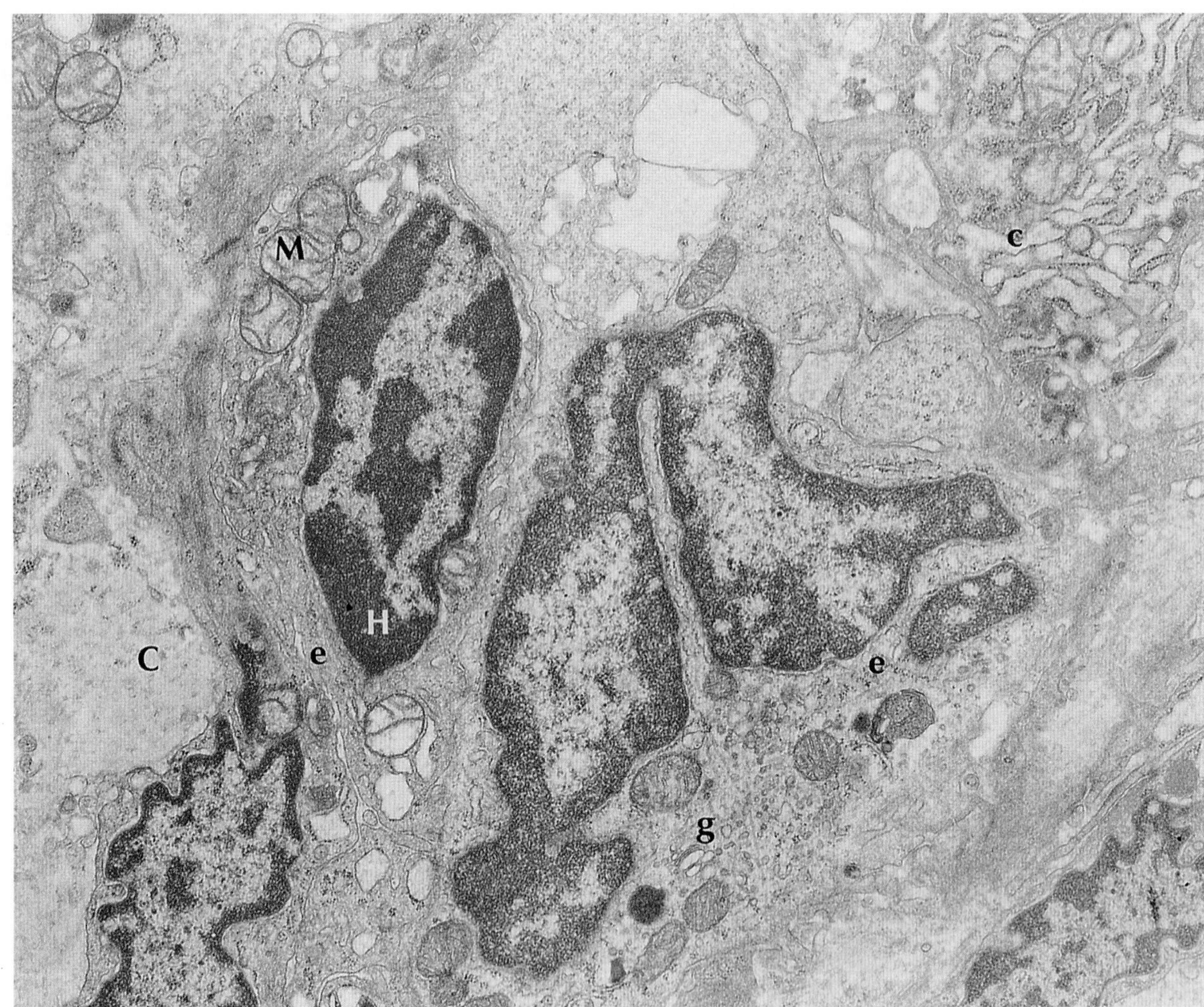

FIGURE 39.7. Sarcoid granuloma in hilar lymph node with epithelioid cells of secretory type containing well-developed, rough endoplasmic reticulum (*e*) with distended cisternae (*C*), Golgi body (*g*), numerous mitochondria (*M*), and indented nuclei with abundant heterochromatin (*H*). Marked deposits of collagen (*left*). ×12,400.

marked secretory activity. Currently, they are known to secrete more than 40 different moieties into the extracellular tissues (34). Among the enzymes secreted by the epithelioid cells are angiotensin-converting enzyme, lysozyme, glucuronidase, collagenase, and calcitriol (4). The ultrastructure of epithelioid cells reflects their secretory activity, showing prominent Golgi bodies, mucoprotein-containing secretory vesicles, and abundant endoplasmic reticulum (4,35) (Fig. 39.7). The multinucleated giant cells are of the Langhans type and are produced by the fusion of epithelioid cells under the stimulation of a particular lymphokine (25). As a result, they exhibit similar nuclear and cytoplasmic features (Fig. 39.8). The presence of angiotensin-converting enzyme in the cytoplasm of synthesizing epithelioid cells can be shown with specific antibodies and immunofluorescence or immunoperoxidase staining (26) (Fig. 39.9). Although necrosis is uncommon, small foci of central fibrinoid necrosis may be seen occasionally (Fig. 39.4), and the presence of focal necrosis should not exclude the diagnosis of sarcoidosis. Extensive, confluent necrosis is not seen in sarcoidosis.

The central areas also comprise deposits of immunoglobulins and various inclusion bodies, such as asteroid, Schaumann, or Hamazaki-Wesenberg bodies. All are formed in epithelioid or giant cells and may be extruded into the extracellular space. The asteroid bodies present in 2% to 9% of cases (26) are organic protein structures, mostly complex lipoproteins (2), and appear as 10- to 25-μm, reddish pink, spider-like, spiculated, stellate inclusions (Figs. 39.10 and 39.11). Schaumann bodies are concentrically laminated, dark blue, oval structures composed of a protein matrix impregnated with calcium phosphate or carbonate and iron (2). They are strongly basophilic and when fully formed look like a raspberry (4). Their presence was noted in 48% to 88% of cases in various studies (26). Hamazaki-Wesenberg bodies, noted in 11% to 68% of lymph nodes affected by sarcoidosis, are giant lysosomes (Fig. 39.12) that are usu-

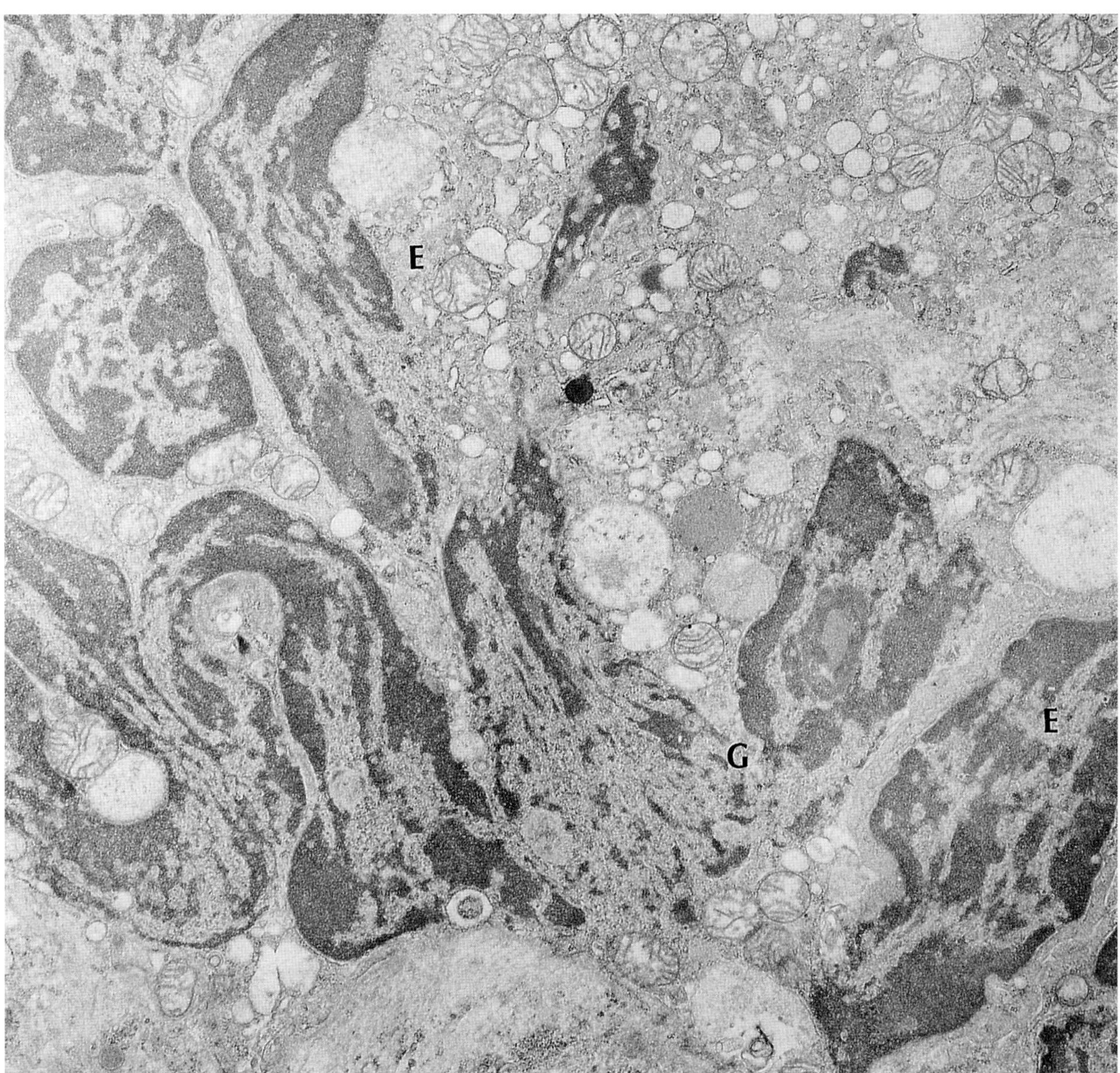

FIGURE 39.8. Epithelioid cells of secretory type (*E*) and multinucleated giant cell (*G*). ×16,200.

ally present extracellularly at or near the peripheral sinus of involved lymph nodes and almost always outside the granulomas (26). Stained with Gomori silver stain, they appear as clusters of budding, yeastlike organisms (Fig. 39.13) that can easily be mistaken for fungi (26). All the inclusion bodies probably represent the end result of autophagic activity and are thus a form of residual body (4). None is considered to contain any causative agent. The results of stainings for acid-fast bacilli and fungi are negative. Calcification is not observed in the granulomas of sarcoidosis. At a later stage, fibroblasts, mast cells, collagen fibers, and proteoglycans accumulate at the periphery of granulomas, forming dense bands of fibrosis. The fibrosis generated by sarcoidosis may be abundant in various organs, often interfering with cardiac and pulmonary function (5,20,24,28). Sarcoid-like granulomas have been reported to occur during the course of various neoplasias, particularly lymphomas, and in other unrelated diseases (36); coexistence in the same lymph node of active sarcoidosis and metastatic carcinoma is also possible.

HISTOCHEMISTRY

Epithelioid granulomas, even when unaccompanied by necrosis, must be investigated for microorganisms by staining for acid fast bacilli (Ziehl-Neelsen, Kinyoun) and fungi (Gomori methenamine silver). Negative results on staining do not entirely exclude an infectious origin. In a study of 92 patients with epithelioid granulomas in which the spe-

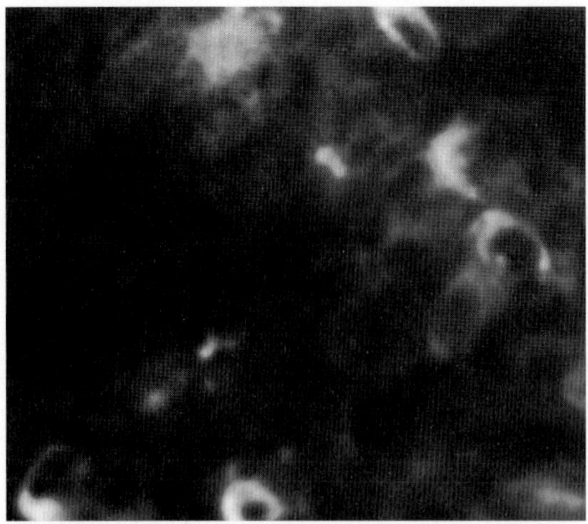

FIGURE 39.9. Cytoplasmic fluorescence in epithelioid cells of sarcoid granuloma in lymph node after incubation with rabbit anti-angiotensin II and fluorescein isothiocyanate-labeled goat antirabbit immunoglobulin. ×500. (From Rosen Y, Vuletin JC, Pertschuk LP, et al. Sarcoidosis, from the pathologist's vantage point. Pathol Annu 1979;14:405–439, with permission.)

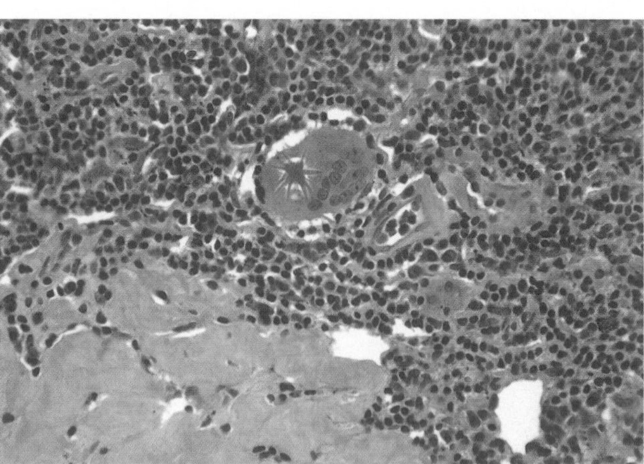

FIGURE 39.10. Asteroid body in the form of a spider-like, brilliant red cytoplasmic inclusion within multinucleated giant cell of sarcoid granuloma. Hematoxylin, phloxine, and saffron stain.

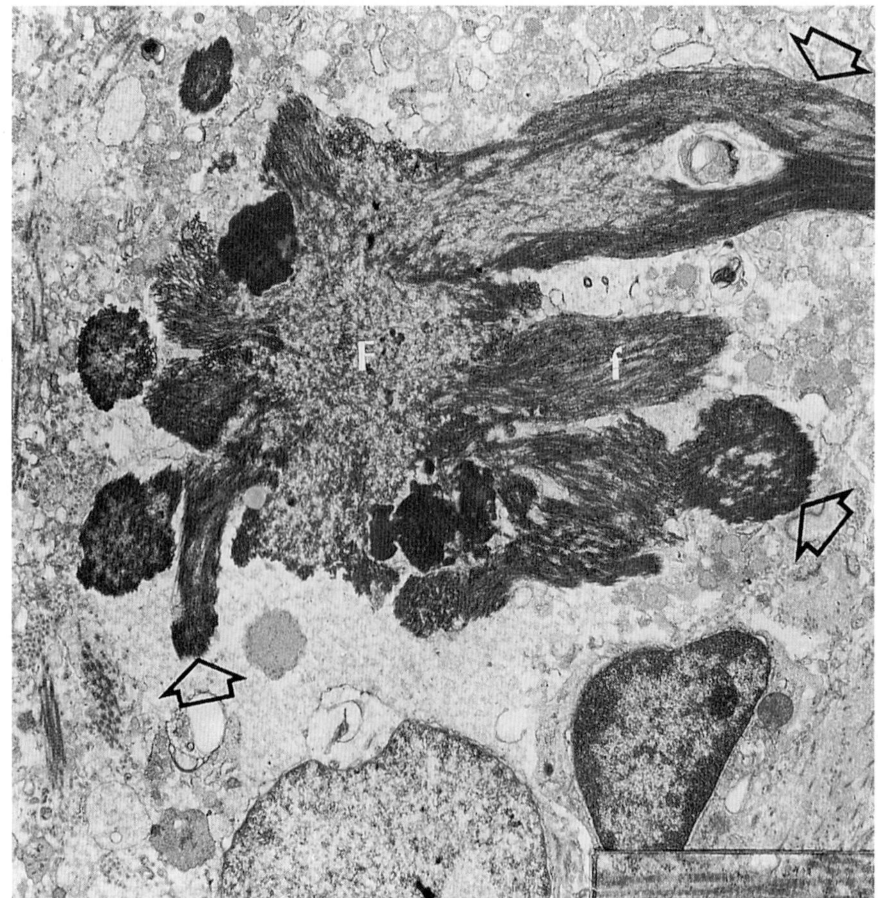

FIGURE 39.11. Asteroid body within the cytoplasm of a multinucleated giant cell. Flocculent central area has fibrillar peripheral arm. ×7,750. **Inset:** Characteristic periodic banding of collagen in peripheral arm. (From Rosen Y, Vuletin JC, Pertschuk LP, et al. Sarcoidosis, from the pathologist's vantage point. Pathol Annu 1979;14:405–439, with permission.)

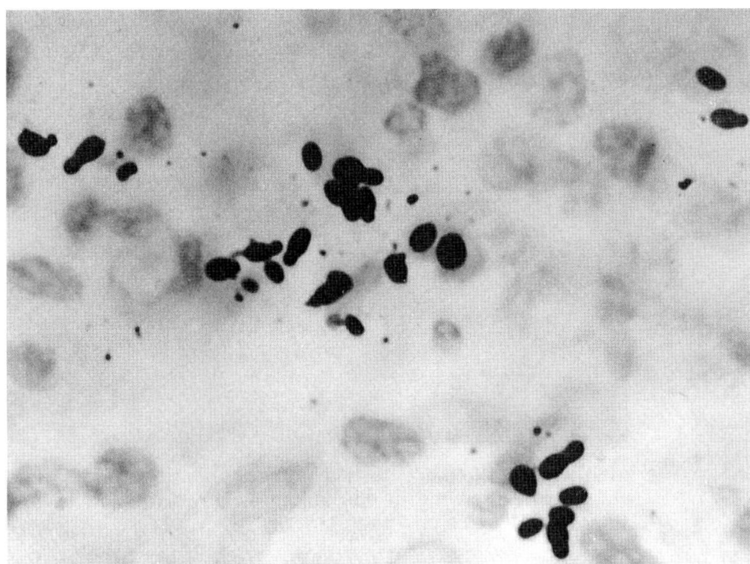

FIGURE 39.12. Hamazaki-Wesenberg bodies with fungus-like budding in the peripheral sinus of lymph node with sarcoidosis. Grocott methenamine silver stain. (From Rosen Y, Vuletin JC, Pertschuk LP, et al. Sarcoidosis, from the pathologist's vantage point. Pathol Annu 1979;14:405–439, with permission.)

cific histologic stainings did not detect any microorganisms, microbiologic cultures were positive in 10 patients (10.9%) for mycobacteria or fungi, whereas the remaining 82 patients had sarcoidosis (37). Further etiologic investigations may be pursued with the use of polymerase chain reaction technology.

IMMUNOHISTOCHEMISTRY

The lymphocytes associated with the granulomas in the active phase of the lesion are predominantly CD4+ (helper) T cells that stain with CD3, CD4, and CD45RO (UCHL-1) antibodies (Fig. 39.14). As the lesions become less active, the

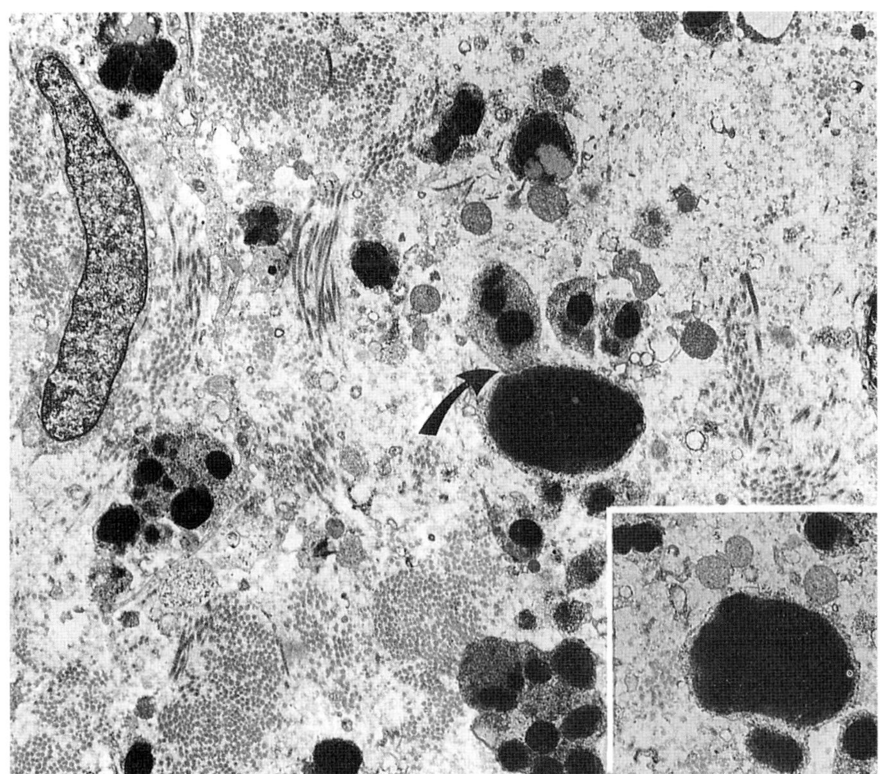

FIGURE 39.13. Same lesion as in Fig. 39.12. Hamazaki-Wesenberg bodies show heterogeneous inner structure and occasional budding. **Inset:** Hamazaki-Wesenberg body with morphologic appearance of giant lysosome. (From Rosen Y, Vuletin JC, Pertschuk LP, et al. Sarcoidosis, from the pathologist's vantage point. Pathol Annu 1979;14:405–439, with permission.)

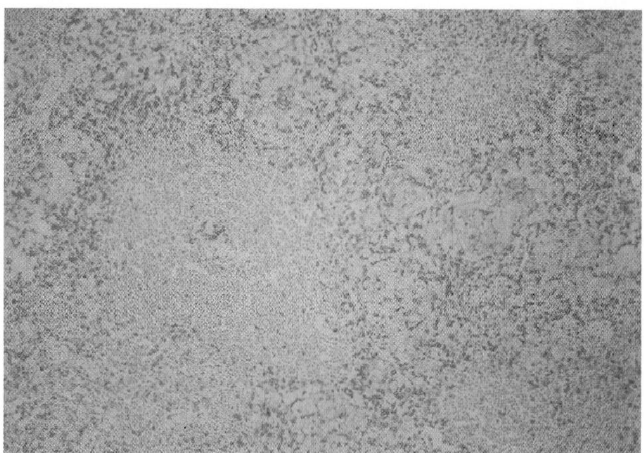

FIGURE 39.14. Sarcoidosis lymphadenopathy. T lymphocytes at the periphery of granulomas. UCHL-1/peroxidase stain.

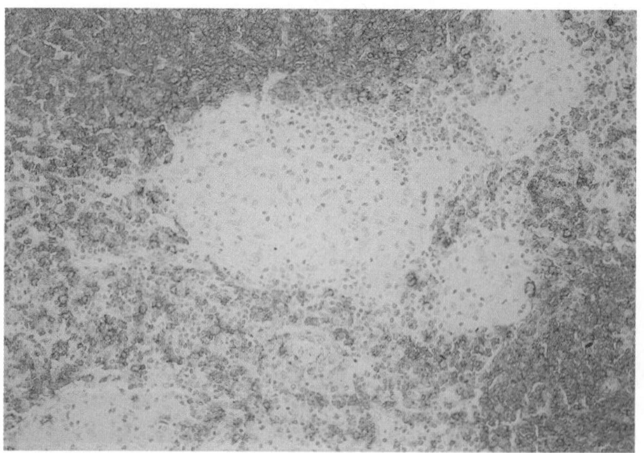

FIGURE 39.15. Sarcoidosis lymphadenopathy. B lymphocytes in large numbers between granulomas. L26/peroxidase stain.

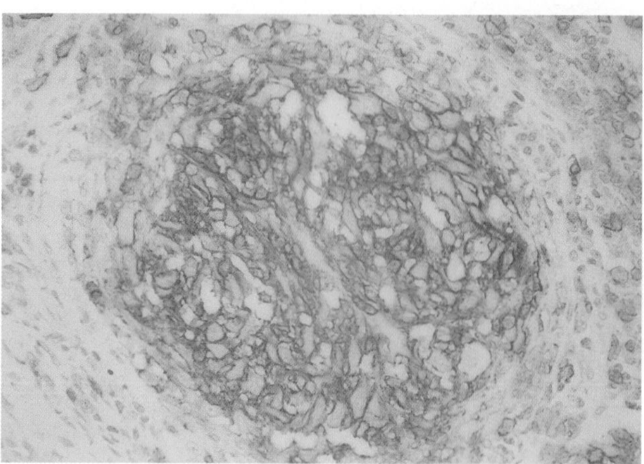

FIGURE 39.16. Sarcoidosis lymphadenopathy. Sialophorin secreted by epithelioid cells in granuloma. Anti-CD43/peroxidase stain.

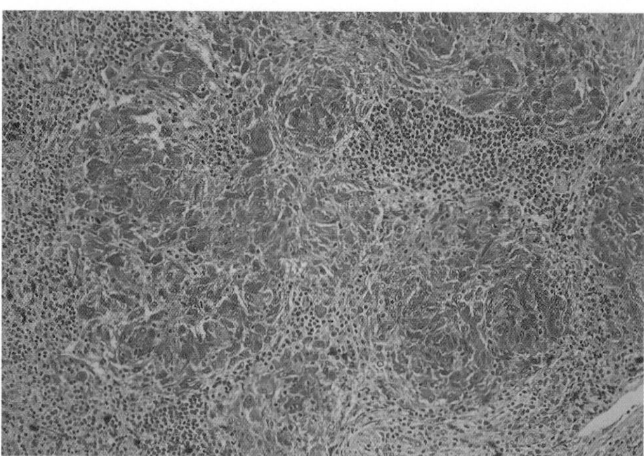

FIGURE 39.17. Sarcoidosis lymphadenopathy. Cytoplasmic staining of lysozyme in epithelioid cells of granulomas. Antilysozyme/alkaline phosphatase stain.

number of CD4+ T cells decreases, and the ones still present are mostly CD8+ (suppressor) T cells (5,27). Although most of the lymphocytes in granulomas are T cells, numerous B cells and frequent plasma cells are also seen, indicating the production of immunoglobulins (Fig. 39.15). Fibroblasts increase in number as the granuloma's age, and early fibrosis is recognized by deposition of intracellular reticulin, which is then gradually replaced by dense bands of collagen. The epithelioid and giant cells in sarcoid granulomas show strong staining for sialophorin (Fig. 39.16) and lysozyme (Figs. 39.17 and 39.18), but not for HAM56 and Leu-M1, which, however, stain the occasional macrophages (Fig. 39.19).

DIFFERENTIAL DIAGNOSIS

The granulomas of sarcoidosis can usually be distinguished from other granulomas by their characteristically sharp de-

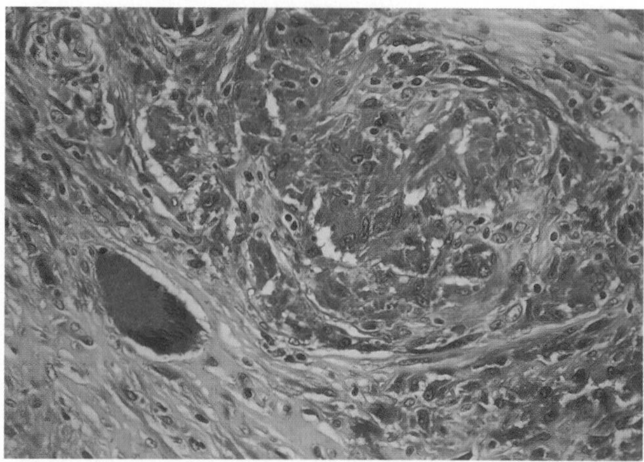

FIGURE 39.18. Same lesion as in Fig. 39.17. Abundant intracytoplasmic red staining of lysozyme in giant cell (*left*) and epithelioid cells. Antilysozyme/alkaline phosphatase stain.

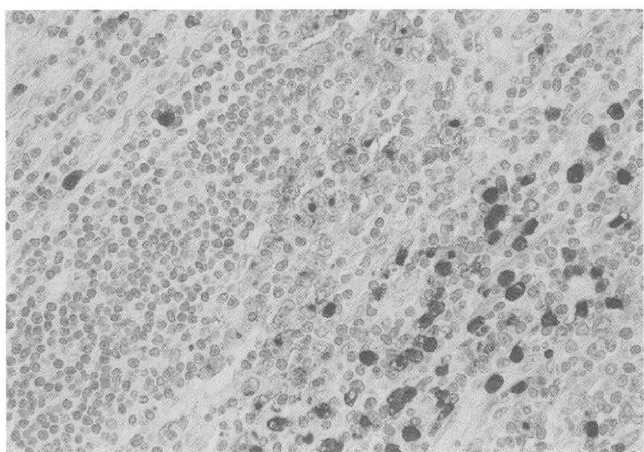

FIGURE 39.19. Sarcoidosis granuloma in cervical lymph node. Results of staining with Leu-M1 antibody are positive for macrophages scattered throughout the lymph node but negative for the epithelioid cells of the sarcoid granuloma. Leu-M1/alkaline phosphatase stain.

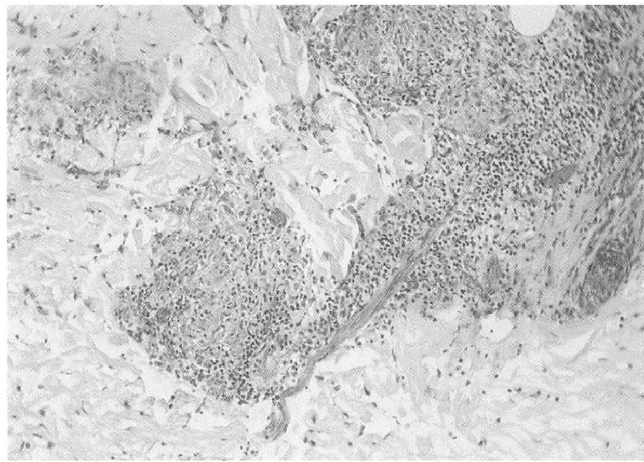

FIGURE 39.20. Positive Kveim-Siltzbach skin test result. Sarcoid granulomas in skin of forearm 4 weeks after injection of antigen.

marcation, close proximity to each other, and lack of necrosis. Nevertheless, acid-fast and methenamine silver staining, to rule out mycobacteria and fungi, must always be part of the differential diagnosis of granulomas.

- Tuberculous granulomas are not as well organized; they frequently coalesce and exhibit variable degrees of caseous necrosis. Acid-fast staining shows rare rod-shaped, brilliantly stained organisms. Cultures for organisms are positive. The absence of necrosis or acid-fast bacilli does not rule out tuberculosis; however, in tuberculosis, the pulmonary lesions are obvious, and the hilar lymphadenopathy, contrary to that in sarcoidosis, is bilateral in fewer than 10% of cases.
- Nontuberculous *Mycobacterium* granulomas, usually *M. avium–intracellulare*: Ill-defined granulomas or simply sheets of epithelioid cells, lack of necrosis and fibrosis; large numbers of intracellular acid-fast bacilli.
- *Histoplasma* granulomas: Focal or confluent caseous necrosis, positive staining of yeasts with methenamine silver, positive cultures. Bilateral involvement of hilar lymph nodes is uncommon.
- *Cryptococcus* granulomas: Well-formed granulomas, minimal fibrosis, positive staining with methenamine silver, periodic acid–Schiff, and mucicarmine.
- Beryllium and a few other metal dusts and organic antigens may cause disease that clinically and histologically is indistinguishable from sarcoidosis (38–39).
- Lymphoma: Mediastinal lymph nodes are more commonly involved in lymphoma, peribronchial lymph nodes in sarcoidosis. All other signs and symptoms of sarcoidosis are absent.

CONFIRMATORY TESTS AND SYMPTOMS

No diagnostic blood, skin, or radiologic imaging tests are specific for sarcoidosis (9). Kveim-Siltzbach skin test results were positive in 78% of cases of sarcoidosis in comparative studies conducted in nine countries (3). A saline suspension of human sarcoid tissue is prepared and 0.15 mL is injected intradermally and very superficially into the flexor surface of the forearm (3). Any palpable nodule developing at the site during the next 6 weeks is sampled and examined histologically for the presence of typical sarcoid granulomas (40) (Fig. 39.20).

Other findings are the following:

Hypergammaglobulinemia in up to 80% of cases (>3.5 g/100 mL).

Hypercalciuria with or without hypercalcemia in 11% of cases (>11.5 mg/100 mL) (3).

Pulmonary infiltrates, skin granulomas (erythema nodosum), eye lesions (iritis, uveitis), fleeting arthralgia involving large joints.

Stainings and cultures negative for mycobacteria and fungi.

Depression of delayed hypersensitivity (mumps, tuberculin, dinitrochlorobenzene).

Depression of lymphoblastic transformation of lymphocytes in contact with lectins.

Elevated levels of angiotensin-converting enzyme and lysozyme in involved lymph nodes and serum.

Demonstration of angiotensin-converting enzyme within epithelioid cells by specific antibody and immunofluorescence or peroxidase staining.

Family involvement (frequency of sarcoidosis of 1.5% among first-degree relatives vs. 0.07% in the general population) (19).

Response to corticosteroid therapy.

Results of biopsy of minor salivary glands positive in 58% of patients with sarcoidosis (41); skin biopsy and transbronchial lung biopsy used as less invasive procedures than biopsy of mediastinal lymph nodes or liver (9).

Checklist

SARCOIDOSIS LYMPHADENOPATHY

Adults 20 to 40 years old
Increased prevalence in blacks (10-fold greater) and women (twofold greater)
Multisystemic (lungs, lymph nodes, skin, eyes, joints)
Pulmonary hilar lymphadenopathy, bilateral
Round, single, closely apposed granulomas
Necrosis absent or focal
Noncaseating granulomas
Epithelioid cells positive for lysozyme, negative for HAM56 and Leu-M1
Langhans-type giant cells
Asteroid bodies, Schaumann bodies
Hamazaki-Wesenberg bodies
CD4+ T cells, CD8+ T cells, B cells, plasma cells
Fibroblasts, collagen fibers
Calcification absent
Acid-fast bacilli absent
Methenamine silver staining negative
Kveim test result positive
Hypergammaglobulinemia
Hypercalciuria
Angiotensin-converting enzyme level elevated
Lysozyme level elevated
Depressed cell-mediated immune response
Response to corticosteroid therapy

REFERENCES

1. Bardinas F, Morera J, Fite E, et al. Seasonal clustering of sarcoidosis. Lancet 1989;2:455–456.
2. Cunningham JA. Sarcoidosis. Pathol Annu 1967;2:31–47.
3. James DG, Neville E. Pathobiology of sarcoidosis. Pathobiol Annu 1977;7:31–63.
4. James DG, Williams WJ. Sarcoidosis and other granulomatous disorders. Philadelphia: WB Saunders, 1985.
5. Thomas PD, Hunninghake GW. Current concepts of the pathogenesis of sarcoidosis. Am Rev Respir Dis 1987;135:747–760.
6. Siltzbach LE, James DG, Neville E, et al. Course and prognosis of sarcoidosis around the world. Am J Med 1974;57:847–852.
7. Edmundstone WM, Wilson AG. Sarcoidosis in Caucasians, blacks and Asians in London. Br J Dis Chest 1985;79:27–36.
8. Rybicki BA, Major M, Popovich J Jr, et al. Racial differences in sarcoidosis incidence: a 5-year study in a health maintenance organization. Am J Epidemiol 1997;145:234–241.
9. Newman LS, Rose CS, Maier LA. Sarcoidosis. N Engl J Med 1997;336:1224–1234.
10. Burke WMJ, Keogh A, Maloney PL, et al. Transmission of sarcoidosis via cardiac transplantation. Lancet 1990;336: 1579.
11. Heyll A, Meckenstock G, Aul C, et al. Possible transmission of sarcoidosis via allogeneic bone marrow transplantation. Bone Marrow Transplant 1994;14:61–64.
12. Moller DR. Etiology of sarcoidosis. Clin Chest Med 1997;18: 695–706.
13. Bocart D, Lecossier D, DeLassence A, et al. A search for mycobacterial DNA in granulomatous tissues from patients with sarcoidosis using the polymerase chain reaction. Am Rev Respir Dis 1992;145:1142.
14. Popper HH, Klemen H, Hoefler G, et al. Presence of mycobacterial DNA in sarcoidosis. Hum Pathol 1997;28:796–800.
15. Muscovic EA. Sarcoidosis and mycobacterial L-forms. Pathol Annu 1987;13:69–164.
16. Lenhart K, Kolck V, Bartova A. HLA antigens associated with sarcoidosis. Dis Markers 1990;8:23–29.
17. Siltzbach LE. Sarcoidosis: clinical features and management. Med Clin North Am 1967;51:483–502.
18. Perry A, Vuitch F. Causes of death in patients with sarcoidosis. Arch Pathol Lab Med 1995;119:167–172.
19. Hunninghake GW, Crystal RG. Pulmonary sarcoidosis: a disorder mediated by excess helper T-lymphocyte activity at sites of disease activity. N Engl J Med 1981;305:429–434.
20. Viale G, Codecasa L, Bulgheroni P, et al. T-cell subsets in sarcoidosis: an immunocytochemical investigation of blood, bronchoalveolar lavage fluid, and prescalenic lymph nodes from eight patients. Hum Pathol 1986;17:476–481.
21. Hunninghake GW, Fulmer JD, Young RC, et al. Localization of the immune response in sarcoidosis. Am Rev Respir Dis 1979; 120:49–57.

22. Semenzato G, Zezzutto A, Pizzolo G, et al. Immunohistological study in sarcoidosis: evaluation at different sites of disease activity. Clin Immunol Immunopathol 1984;30:29–40.
23. Spector WG. The macrophage: its origins and role in pathology. Pathobiol Annu 1974;4:33–65.
24. Adams DO. The granulomatous inflammatory response. Am J Pathol 1976;84:164–191.
25. Epstein WL. Granuloma formation in man. Pathobiol Annu 1977;7:1–31.
26. Rosen Y, Vuletin JC, Pertschuk LP, et al. Sarcoidosis, from the pathologist's vantage point. Pathol Annu 1979;14:405–439.
27. Papapoulos SE, Clemens TL, Fraher LJ, et al. 1,25-Dihydroxycholecalciferol in the pathogenesis of the hypercalcemia of sarcoidosis. Lancet 1979;1:627–630.
28. Inoue Y, King TE Jr, Tinkle SS, et al. Human mast cell basic fibroblast growth factor in pulmonary fibrotic disorder. Am J Pathol 1996;149:2037–2054.
29. Winterbauer RH, Belic N, Moores KD, et al. A clinical interpretation of bilateral hilar adenopathy. Ann Intern Med 1973;78: 65–71.
30. Hodgson CH, Olson AM, Good CA. Bilateral hilar adenopathy: its significance and management. Ann Intern Med 1955;43:83–99.
31. Salman SD, Graeme-Cook F. A 63-year-old woman with bilateral maxillary sinus opacification and mediastinal lymphadenopathy. N Engl J Med 1990;322:116–123.
32. Ioachim HL. Granulomatous lesions of lymph nodes. In: Ioachim HL, ed. Pathology of granulomas. New York: Raven Press, 1983:151–187.
33. Van Furth R, Cohn ZA, Hirsch JG, et al. The mononuclear phagocyte system: a new classification of macrophages, monocytes and their precursor cells. Bull World Health Organ 1972; 46:845–852.
34. Davies P, Bouney RJ. Secretory products of mononuclear phagocytes—a brief review. J Reticuloendothelial Soc 1979;36:37–48.
35. Ioachim HL. Lymph nodes and spleen. In: Johannessen JV, ed. Electron microscopy in human medicine, vol 5. New York: McGraw-Hill, 1981:385–464.
36. Atwood WG, Miller RC, Nelson CT. Sarcoidosis and the malignant lymphoreticular diseases. Arch Dermatol 1966;94:144–150.
37. Hsu RM, Connors AF, Tomashefski JF. Histologic, microbiologic, and clinical correlates of the diagnosis of sarcoidosis by transbronchial biopsy. Arch Pathol Lab Med 1996;120:364–368.
38. Newman LS. Beryllium disease and sarcoidosis: clinical and laboratory links. Sarcoidosis 1995;12:7–19.
39. De Vuyst P, Dumortier P, Schandene L, et al. Sarcoid-like lung granulomatosis induced by aluminum dusts. Am Rev Respir Dis 1987;135:493–497.
40. Munro CS, Mitchell DN. The Kveim response: still useful, still a puzzle. Thorax 1987;42:321–331.
41. Nessan VJ, Jacoway JR. Biopsy of minor salivary glands in the diagnosis of sarcoidosis. N Engl J Med 1979;301:922–924.

40

SYSTEMIC LUPUS LYMPHADENOPATHY

DEFINITION

Lymphadenopathy associated with active systemic lupus erythematosus (SLE).

SYNONYM

Lupus lymphadenopathy

CLINICAL FEATURES

Systemic lupus erythematosus is prevalent in white adults between the ages of 11 and 40 years and 3.5 times more common in women than in men (1). The lymph nodes are commonly involved in SLE, and moderate or marked enlargement of lymph nodes, localized or generalized, was recorded in 66.7% of 210 cases reviewed (1). In a more recent study of 90 cases of SLE, lymphadenopathy was present in 23 of the patients (26%) (2). The higher incidence of lymphadenopathy in earlier studies may be related to the inclusion of a considerable number of autopsy cases, whereas the lower incidence in the recent studies may be a consequence of the effect of steroid treatments (2). Cervical lymph nodes were most often involved (43%), followed by mesenteric (21%), axillary (18%), inguinal (17%), and retroperitoneal nodes (1). Pulmonary hilar and mediastinal lymphadenopathy in SLE has also been reported (3). In 12% of cases, the lymphadenopathy was generalized (1). Patients with lymphadenopathy tend to be younger (mean age, 36 years) than those without it (mean age, 45 years), and the prevalence of lymph node involvement is higher in children than in adults (2,4,5). The incidence of lymphoma is significantly increased in persons with immunodeficiency diseases, and lymphoma has also been reported in patients with SLE (6,7). In one report, lymphomas occurred in four women 2 months to 12 years after the onset of SLE (7). Previously, 14 cases with this association, all in women, had been reported in the literature. In four, the diagnoses had been made simultaneously, and in two, lymphoma preceded SLE. Of 12 patients, four had Hodgkin disease and eight had non-Hodgkin lymphoma (7).

CLINICAL SYNDROME

The clinical features of SLE are pleomorphic, affecting multiple organ systems. Constitutional symptoms include fever, fatigue, weight loss, and mucocutaneous lesions (e.g., skin rashes, oral ulcers, vasculitis, alopecia). Arthritis, glomerulonephritis, pleural effusions or polyserositis, retinitis, and myocarditis may also be present (2,4). Lymphadenopathies appear to be associated with more active forms of disease causing relatively severe symptoms, often hepatosplenomegaly, and higher levels of antinuclear antibodies (2). Because the diagnosis of SLE rests on well-defined clinical and serologic criteria, biopsy of enlarged lymph nodes is now rarely performed in SLE.

HISTOPATHOLOGY

The lymph nodes are soft and only slightly enlarged, seldom exceeding 3 cm in diameter (8). On section, foci of necrosis or hemorrhage may be recognized (Fig. 40.1). Occasionally, the necrosis is so extensive that the lymph node is fragmented during removal (8). Before the introduction of steroid treatment, necrosis was present in about 25% of lymph nodes at biopsy, and more often at autopsy (9). Steroid treatment has changed the course of SLE and has probably decreased the prevalence of necrosis (8).

The nodal architecture is effaced, and the lymphoid follicles are inconspicuous because of massive edema and sinus dilation. Random foci of necrosis, sometimes confluent, include a mixture of live and dead cells and are characterized by a peripheral area that ends abruptly, without inflammatory cells or granulation tissue (Fig. 40.1). Cells in apoptosis and scattered nuclear debris are commonly present. Characteristic of SLE lymphadenopathy are the "hematoxylin bodies," which are extracellular clumps, 5 to 12 μm in diameter, of amorphous, necrotic material (Figs. 40.2 and 40.3). They resemble those commonly seen in crushed areas of small cell carcinoma of the lung and stain heavily with hematoxylin, periodic acid–Schiff (PAS), and Feulgen stains. They are composed of aggregates of nuclear DNA (a result of extensive karyorrhexis and karyopyknosis), polysac-

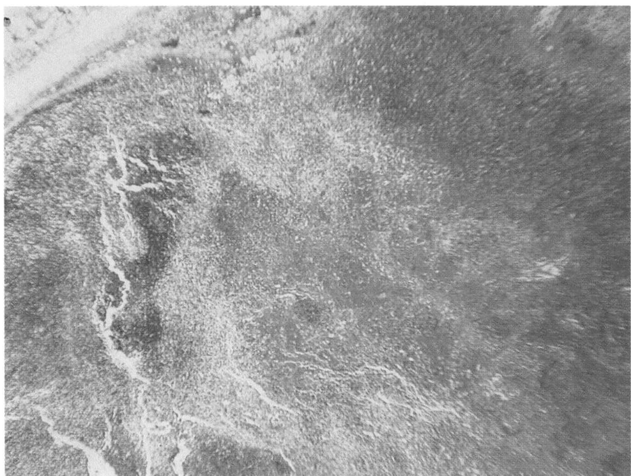

FIGURE 40.1. Axillary lymph node in systemic lupus erythematosus. Multiple confluent foci of fibrinoid necrosis and effacement of architecture. Hematoxylin, phloxine, and saffron stain.

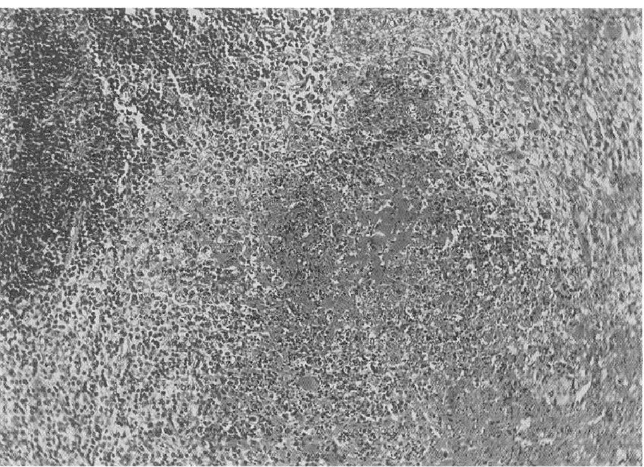

FIGURE 40.2. Same section as in Fig. 40.1. Focus of fibrinoid necrosis surrounded by apoptotic cells, abundant hematoxylin bodies, nuclear debris, macrophages, lymphocytes, and plasma cells. Hematoxylin, phloxine, and saffron stain.

charides, and immunoglobulins (10,11). The cell population includes immunoblasts, plasma cells, lymphocytes, and macrophages containing nuclear debris (Fig. 40.3). The immunoblasts have large, vesicular nuclei with prominent nucleoli. Some may have multilobate nuclei, resembling megakaryocytes (1), but they should not be confused with Reed-Sternberg cells. The plasma cells often contain PAS-positive bodies. Polymorphonuclear leukocytes, both neutrophils and eosinophils, are very rare, a feature that helps to differentiate SLE lymphadenopathy from other forms of

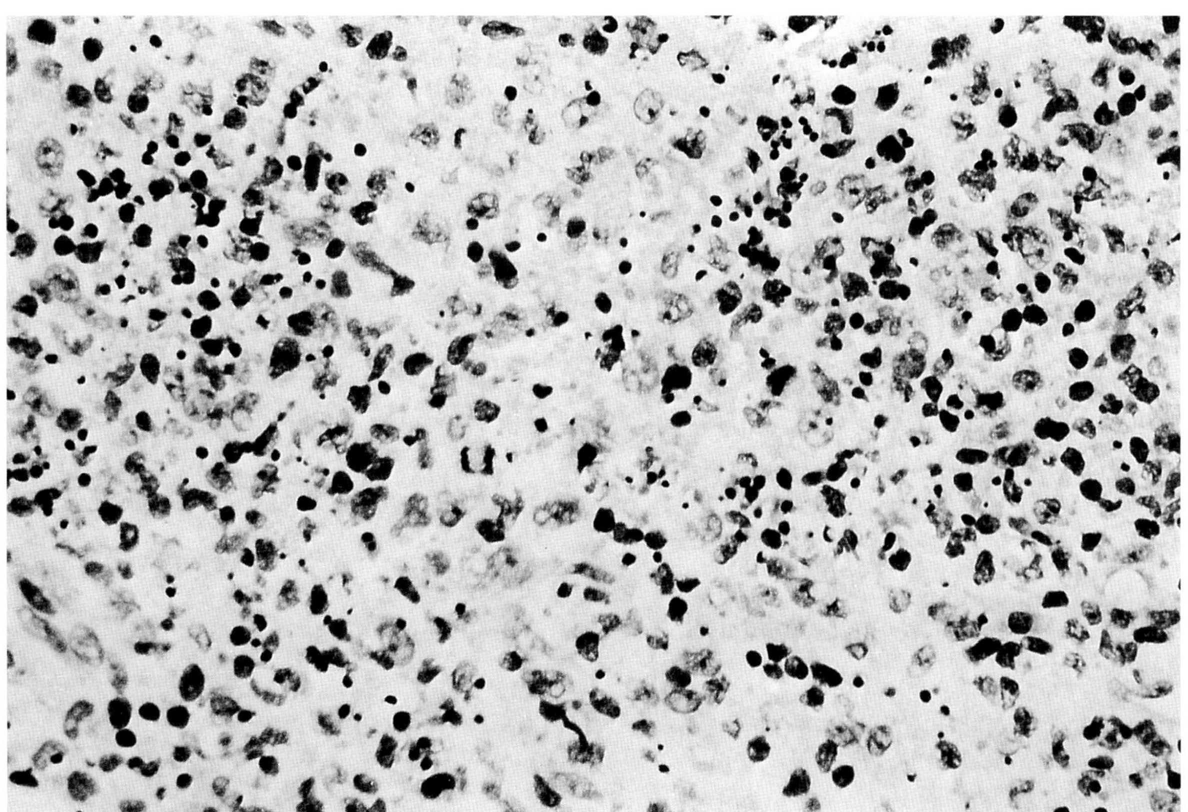

FIGURE 40.3. Cervical lymph node in systemic lupus erythematosus. Foci of necrosis with extensive cellular apoptosis, nuclear debris, numerous scattered hematoxylin bodies, and immunoblasts with occasional mitoses. Hematoxylin, phloxine, and saffron stain.

necrotizing lymphadenitis (12). The blood vessels are lined by hyperplastic endothelial cells. They may show the Azzopardi phenomenon—that is, deposits of hematoxylin-staining nuclear material resulting from fibrinoid necrosis of vessel walls (1). Surrounding the larger vessels, degenerated collagen and deposited gammaglobulins may form perivascular "onion skin" cuffs. Granulomas are not noted, and fibrosis is absent.

The SLE cell phenomenon—phagocytosis of lymphocytic nuclear debris by neutrophils that can be observed in pleural fluid—is also characteristic of this disease.

A positive result of the lupus band test on a punch biopsy specimen of skin consists of a continuous line of immunoreactive deposits along the epidermal–dermal junction; a positive result is obtained in 50% to 60% of patients with SLE (4).

IMMUNOHISTOCHEMISTRY

When a battery of monoclonal antibodies was used to stain frozen sections of an enlarged axillary lymph node in a patient with SLE, two predominant cell populations were seen around the necrotic areas: Leu-M1+ histiocytes and OKT8+ (CD8+) (cytotoxic/suppressor) T cells. The uninvolved areas of the lymph node showed the usual cell populations (13). The finding of increased numbers of suppressor T cells is in accordance with pathogenetic concepts of SLE in which the dysfunction of CD8+ suppressor T cells is considered to be a major contributing factor in the dysregulation of B cells, the production of auto-antibodies, and even potentially neoplastic proliferations.

LABORATORY TESTS

The diagnosis is based on the demonstration of specific auto-antibodies directed against native (double-stranded) and denatured (single-stranded) DNA (14). Elevated antinuclear antibody titers are also associated with infections and tumors; however, a titer of 1:320 or higher on an immunofluorescence assay has a specificity of almost 97% in the diagnosis of SLE (15).

DIFFERENTIAL DIAGNOSIS

- Necrotizing lymphadenopathy of Kikuchi and Fujimoto lacks hematoxylin bodies and vascular fibrinoid necrosis. Immunohistochemical staining is not contributory (13).
- Infectious mononucleosis lymphadenopathy shows hyperplastic follicles with reactive germinal centers, including marked phagocytosis of nuclear debris that results in a starry sky pattern and mottled paracortical areas. Results of EBER *in situ* hybridization for Epstein-Barr virus are positive.
- Cat-scratch lymphadenitis includes neutrophils, granulomas, microabscesses, and bacilli that stain with Warthin-Starry stain.
- Luetic lymphadenitis: Necrosis lacks hematoxylin bodies. Epithelioid and giant cells are present. Spirochetes that stain with the Warthin-Starry stain may be demonstrated. Confirmation is made by serologic tests.
- Mycobacterial lymphadenitis: Necrosis is accompanied by epithelioid and multinucleated giant cells. Acid-fast bacilli are present.
- Tularemia lymphadenitis: Contact with wild animals or tick bites. Necrotic areas with abundant inflammatory cells, mainly neutrophils.

Checklist

SYSTEMIC LUPUS LYMPHADENOPATHY

Architecture effaced
Follicles inconspicuous
Necrosis focal or confluent
Nuclear debris and hematoxylin bodies
Immunoblasts
Neutrophils and eosinophils absent
Granulomas absent
Vasculitis with fibrinoid necrosis
Vascular encrustation with hematoxylin-positive nuclear material
Sinuses distended
Fibrosis absent
Predominance of CD8+ (suppressor) T cells

REFERENCES

1. Fox RA, Rosahn PD. The lymph nodes in disseminated lupus erythematosus. Am J Pathol 1943;19:74–99.
2. Shapira Y, Weinberger AA, Wysenbeck AJ. Lymphadenopathy in systemic lupus erythematosus. Prevalence and relation to disease manifestations. Clin Rheumatol 1996;15:335–338.
3. Kassan S, Moss ML, Reddick RL. Progressive hilar and mediastinal lymphadenopathy in systemic lupus erythematosus on corticosteroid therapy. N Engl J Med 1976;294:1382–1383.
4. Bloom BJ, Zukerberg LR. A nine-year old girl with fever and cervical lymphadenopathy. N Engl J Med 1999;340:1491–1497.
5. King KK, Kornreich HK, Bernstein BH, et al. The clinical spectrum of systemic lupus erythematosus in childhood. Arthritis Rheum 1977;20:287.
6. Smith CK, Cassidy JT, Bole GG. Type I dysgamma-globulinemia, systemic lupus erythematosus and lymphoma. Am J Med 1970;48:1134–1119.
7. Green JA, Dawson AA, Walker W. Systemic lupus erythematosus and lymphoma. Lancet 1978;2:753–755.
8. Paradinas F. Lymphadenopathy in autoimmune disorders—systemic lupus erythematosus. In: Stansfeld AG, ed. Lymph node biopsy interpretation. New York: Churchill Livingstone, 1985: 165–168.
9. Klemperer P, Pollack AD, Baehr C. Pathology of disseminated lupus erythematosus. Arch Pathol Lab Med 1941;32:569–631.
10. Moore RD, Weisberger AS, Bowerfind ES. Histochemical studies of lymph nodes in disseminated lupus erythematosus. Arch Pathol Lab Med 1956;62:472–478.
11. Godman GD, Deitch AD, Klemperer P. The composition of the LE and hematoxylin bodies of systemic lupus erythematosus. Am J Pathol 1958;34:1–23.
12. Robinson DR, Long JC. A 19-year-old woman with fever and lymphadenopathy. N Engl J Med 1979;301:881–887.
13. Medeiros LJ, Kaynor B, Harris NL. Lupus lymphadenitis: report of a case with immunohistologic studies on frozen sections. Hum Pathol 1989;20:295–299.
14. Fudenberg HH, Stites DP, Caldwell JL, et al. Basic and clinical immunology. Los Altos, CA: Lange Medical, 1976:363–365.
15. Tan EM, Feltkamp TEW, Smolen JS, et al. Range of antinuclear antibodies in "healthy" individuals. Arthritis Rheum 1997;40: 1601–1611.

41

RHEUMATOID LYMPHADENOPATHY

DEFINITION

Generalized lymphadenopathy accompanying rheumatoid arthritis (RA).

PATHOGENESIS

Systemic lymphadenopathy may occur in 50% to 75% of patients with RA (1,2). Ranging from mild to severe, the lymphadenopathy is not restricted to the lymph nodes draining the affected joints; rather, it represents the involvement of lymphoid tissues in RA, which is conceived of as a generalized disease. Reactive follicles with prominent germinal centers are seen in both lymph nodes and synovium, and a lacy network of early complement components (C1q, C4, C3c, C3d) and immunoglobulin M (IgM) rheumatoid factor decorates the follicular dendritic cells (3). The production of interleukin 6 may contribute to lymphadenopathy in RA (4).

Lymphadenopathies, some with similar histologic changes, may occur in other, related conditions, such as juvenile RA, or Still disease (5), Felty syndrome (in 40% to 50% of cases) (6), and adult-onset Still disease (7). Sjögren syndrome (5,8), Hashimoto thyroiditis (5), dermatomyositis (9), polyarteritis nodosa (9), scleroderma (9), and other autoimmune and collagen diseases may also be accompanied by regional or generalized lymphadenopathy. More specific clinical and histologic features are associated with systemic lupus lymphadenopathy (see Chapter 40).

CLINICAL SYNDROME

The axillary, cervical, and supraclavicular lymph nodes are most often involved, but enlarged inguinal, epitrochlear, and preauricular nodes and enlarged nodes in the forearm, thigh, and other unusual places have been found (1,10,11). The lymph nodes are palpable, mobile, and nontender. The spleen is moderately enlarged (5% to 20% of cases), particularly in Still disease (juvenile RA associated with splenomegaly and lymphadenopathy) and Felty syndrome (RA in adults accompanied by splenomegaly, lymphadenopathy, and leukopenia). Episodes of fever, anemia, and weight loss are often associated with rheumatoid lymphadenopathy. In RA and other autoimmune diseases, hyperglobulinemia and cryoglobulinemia are common (5). Patients with adult-onset Still disease exhibit spiking fever, cutaneous eruptions that are sometimes pruritic, and generalized lymphadenopathy (7). In all these syndromes, lymph node enlargement may precede the arthritis and raise a clinical suspicion of lymphoma. A B-cell lymphoproliferative disorder or Hodgkin disease may develop in patients with RA who are receiving long-term methotrexate (12).

HISTOPATHOLOGY

Marked follicular hyperplasia is noted in both the cortex and the medulla (13,14) (Fig 41.1). The follicular pattern is characteristic (11) and may constitute a problem in the differential diagnosis with nodular (follicular) lymphoma (11,15). The follicles vary in size and shape and often coalesce to form bizarre, sometimes dumbbell-shaped structures (14). Lymphoid infiltration of the capsule and perinodal fibrofatty tissues with occasional formation of extranodal follicles occurs often (1,11). The germinal centers are prominent (Fig. 41.1) and include frequent cells in mitosis, macrophages containing nuclear debris, and deposits of amorphous, hyaline-like material that stains with periodic acid–Schiff but not Congo red (11,16). Similar hyaline material can be found in systemic sclerosis (16). A minority of lymph nodes in patients with RA contain sarcoid-like granulomas (16). Cracking artifacts, caused by pressure from enlarged follicles, may be present in the perifollicular areas (1). The deep cortex and the medulla include large numbers of plasma cells that may form clusters or solid sheets (Figs. 41.2 and 41.3). Occasionally, plasma cells are found in the germinal centers (11). Binucleated plasma cells and Russell bodies are common. Neutrophils are also present and may form aggregates with foci of cellular necrosis (11). The sinuses and capillaries are distended and lined by hyperplastic endothelial cells. The lumina contain polymorphonuclear leukocytes and lymphocytes. The reactive lymph nodes in RA have features similar to those of the lymphoid cells in the affected

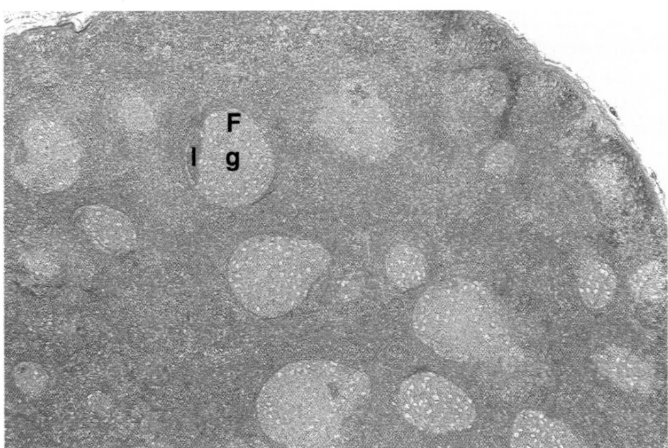

FIGURE 41.1. Axillary lymph node of a 32-year-old woman with rheumatoid arthritis. Lymphoid follicles (*F*) are enlarged and irregularly shaped, with prominent germinal centers (*g*) and peripheral layers of small, mature lymphocytes (*l*). Hematoxylin and eosin stain.

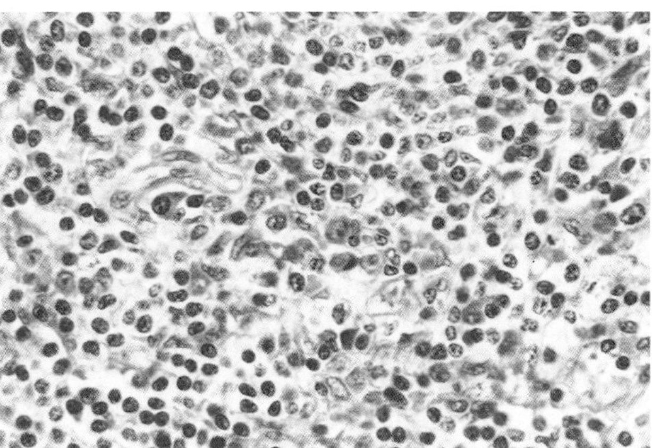

FIGURE 41.2. Rheumatoid lymphadenopathy. Large medullary aggregates of plasma cells. Hematoxylin and eosin stain.

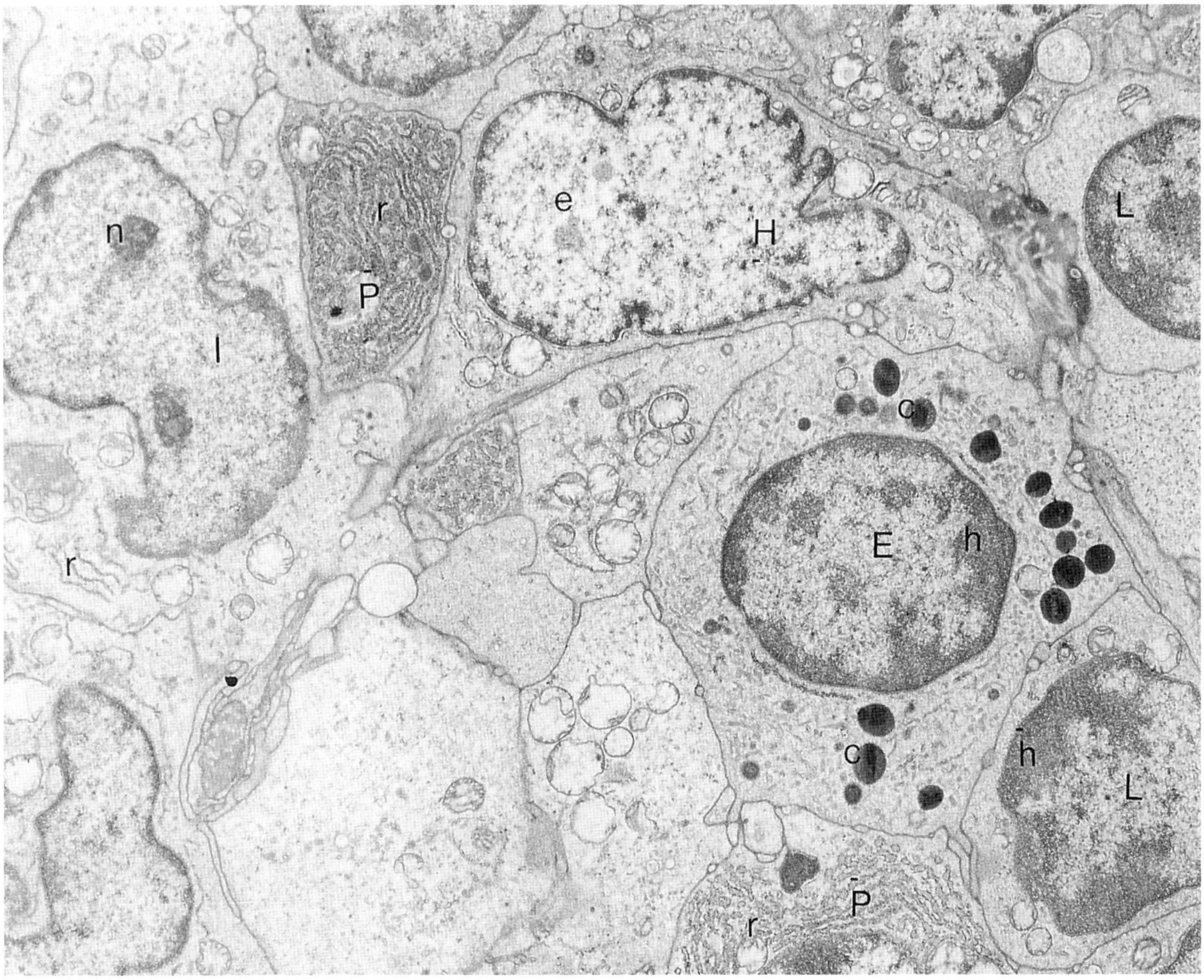

FIGURE 41.3. Rheumatoid lymphadenopathy. Plasma cells (*P*) with abundant, granular endoplasmic reticulum (*r*); eosinophil (*E*) with cytoplasmic granules containing crystalline bars (*c*) and nucleus with heterochromatin (*h*); lymphocytes (*L*) with scarce cytoplasm, few mitochondria, and nucleus with heterochromatin; immunoblast (*I*) with abundant cytoplasm, few profiles of endoplasmic reticulum, and nucleus with prominent nucleoli (*n*); and histiocyte (*H*) with lysosome and nucleus with euchromatin (*e*). ×9,600.

Checklist

RHEUMATOID LYMPHADENOPATHY

Follicular hyperplasia involving cortex and medulla
Irregularly shaped, coalescing follicles
Prominent germinal centers
Infiltration of capsule and pericapsular tissues
Marked plasmacytosis
Clusters of neutrophils with focal necrosis
Distended sinuses
Endothelial hyperplasia
Rheumatoid factor test results positive

synovia, which proliferate abundantly, forming follicles with germinal centers (1). After corticosteroid therapy, follicular hyperplasia and prominence of germinal centers resolve and become inapparent. In a study of eight cases of adult-onset Still disease (7), the lymph node histology was different from that of rheumatoid lymphadenopathy. Instead of follicular hyperplasia, effacement of the nodal architecture was noted, but a marked paracortical hyperplasia with numerous atypical immunoblasts was present, sometimes simulating malignant lymphoma (7).

LABORATORY TESTS

The laboratory tests for rheumatoid factors are:

- Antibodies to altered gamma globulin, the so-called rheumatoid factors detected by agglutination tests (latex fixation test). These tests are very sensitive, yielding positive results in about 70% of cases, but they are not very specific because the results may be also positive in the presence of granulomatous disease, chronic liver disease, and subacute bacterial endocarditis.
- Tube dilution tests, in which human IgG is adsorbed on particulate carriers such as latex or bentonite, are more sensitive and can provide titers.
- The sensitized sheep red cell test (Rose-Waaler test) depends on the binding of specific antibodies and thus is highly specific.
- Radioimmunoassay for IgM rheumatoid factor.

DIFFERENTIAL DIAGNOSIS

- Follicular lymphoma: Lymph node architecture not preserved. Nodules round and more homogeneous. Germinal centers not as apparent. Plasma cells absent.
- Syphilitic lymphadenitis: Follicular hyperplasia, vasculitis, and perivasculitis particularly noted in the pericapsular tissues. Giant cells and occasional formation of granulomas. Spirochetes present.

REFERENCES

1. Motulsky AG, Weinberg S, Saphir O, et al. Lymph nodes in rheumatoid arthritis. Arch Intern Med 1952;90:660–676.
2. Robertson MD, Hart FD, White WF, et al. Rheumatoid lymphadenopathy. Ann Rheum Dis 1968;27:253–260.
3. Imai Y, Sato T, Yamakawa M, et al. A morphological and immunohistochemical study of lymphoid germinal centers in synovial and lymph node tissues from rheumatoid arthritis patients with special reference to complement components and their receptors. Acta Pathol Jpn 1989;39:127–134.
4. Numata Y, Matsuura Y, Onishi S, et al. Interleukin-6 positive follicular hyperplasia in the lymph node of a patient with rheumatoid arthritis. Am J Hematol 1991;36:282–284.
5. Paradinas F. Rheumatoid arthritis and related conditions. In: Stansfeld AG, ed. Lymph node biopsy interpretation. New York: Churchill Livingstone, 1985:168–169.
6. Pruzanski W. Lymphadenopathy associated with dysgammaglobulinemia. Semin Hematol 1980;17:44–62.
7. Valente RM, Banks PM, Conn DL. Characterization of lymph node histology in adult onset Still's disease. J Rheumatol 1989; 16:349–354.
8. McCurley TL, Collins RD, Ball E. Nodal and extranodal lymphoproliferative disorders in Sjögren's syndrome: a clinical and immunopathologic study. Hum Pathol 1990;21:482–492.
9. Symmers WSC. Lymphadenitis associated with connective tissue diseases. In: Symmers WSC, ed. Systemic pathology. New York: Churchill Livingstone, 1978:690–693.
10. Cruickshank B. Lesions of lymph nodes in rheumatoid arthritis and disseminated lupus erythematosus. Scottish Med J 1958;3: 110–117.
11. Nosanchuk JS, Schnitzer B. Follicular hyperplasia in lymph nodes from patients with rheumatoid arthritis. A clinicopathologic study. Cancer 1969;24:243–254.
12. Chevrel G, Berger F, Miossec P, et al. Hodgkin's disease and B cell lymphoproliferation in rheumatoid arthritis patients treated with methotrexate: a kinetic study of lymph node changes. Arthritis Rheum 1999;42:1773–1776.
13. Butler JJ. Non-neoplastic lesions of lymph nodes of man to be differentiated from lymphomas. NCI Monogr 1969;32: 233–255.
14. Dorfman RF, Warnke R. Lymphadenopathy simulating the malignant lymphomas. Hum Pathol 1974;5:519–550.
15. Hartsock RJ. Reactive lesions in lymph nodes. In: Rebuck JW, Berard CW, Abell MR, eds. The reticuloendothelial system. International Academy of Pathology Monograph No. 16. Baltimore: Williams & Wilkins, 1975:153–184.
16. McCluggage WG, Bharucha H. Lymph node hyalinisation in rheumatoid arthritis and systemic sclerosis. J Clin Pathol 1994; 47:138– 42.

42

DERMATOPATHIC LYMPHADENOPATHY

DEFINITION

Reactive paracortical lymph node hyperplasia associated with chronic dermatoses and characterized by an increased number of interdigitating reticulum cells (IRCs), Langerhans cells (LCs), and histiocytes with lipid and melanin deposits.

SYNONYM

Lipomelanotic reticulosis

PATHOGENESIS

Lymphadenopathy associated with chronic dermatologic lesions represents the lymph node reaction to the drainage of melanin and various skin antigens. In a series of 906 consecutive lymph node biopsies, dermatopathic lymphadenopathy (DL) occurred in 40 cases (4.8%), twice as often in male as in female patients (1). Associated skin lesions are commonly exfoliative or eczematoid: pemphigus, psoriasis, neurodermatitis, eczema, and atrophia senilis (2–4). The skin disorder may be present 6 months to 6 years before a lymph node biopsy is performed (2). In one study, 12% of the patients had no clinical skin disease (1). Reflecting the drainage of the skin lesions, 70% of patients with cutaneous T-cell lymphoma (CTCL) or Sézary syndrome had palpable lymph nodes at the time of diagnosis (5). Distinguishing between DL and CTCL is important because lymph node involvement in the course of CTCL or Sézary syndrome is a significant indicator of a poor prognosis (6,7). Several studies have attempted to define the histologic or immunophenotypic signs of lymph node involvement by CTCL or Sézary syndrome because, in the early stages, the regional lymph nodes show only the changes of DL (8–11). Most authors have concluded that minimal histologic changes in regional lymph nodes draining CTCL are not characteristic and are not a basis for a confident distinction between DL and CTCL infiltrating lymph nodes (12–14). Approximately one-sixth of more than 1,000 axillary lymph nodes from 50 consecutive radical mastectomies contained mild to moderate dermatopathic changes, but only one patient had active skin disease—that is, contact dermatitis (15). DL does not always correlate with contemporary skin irritation; sometimes, it may reflect healed dermatitis (15).

CLINICAL SYNDROME

Axillary and inguinal lymph nodes are most commonly involved, although generalized superficial lymphadenopathy may also occur. In two cases, external mammary lymph nodes involved by DL presented clinically as lateral breast masses (2,16). The lymph nodes are moderately enlarged, firm, movable, and nontender. On cut section, the surface is tan with occasional brown, pigmented foci. Peripheral blood eosinophilia is frequently present; sometimes the percentage is as high as 35% (2). Pruritus occurs in almost all cases. DL is often associated with CTCL or nodal lymphoma (1).

HISTOPATHOLOGY

The architecture is generally maintained with a paracortical T-zone expansion (Fig. 42.1). The lymphoid follicles and germinal centers are present; they are usually hyperplastic in early stages (13) (Fig. 42.2) but compressed and atrophic in later stages. The lesions consist of irregularly shaped, pale-staining patches of IRCs, LCs, and histiocytes (Fig. 42.3), generally located in the cortex toward the periphery of the node (1). Some histiocytes contain lipids and appear foamy (Fig 42.4); others are heavily laden with pigments (Fig. 42.5) such as melanin and, less frequently, hemosiderin (17). Appropriate staining with Sudan black B for lipid, Fontana silver for melanin (Fig. 42.6), and Prussian blue for iron (Fig. 42.7) is needed to identify the phagocytosed materials. Intermingled with the histiocytes are variable numbers of plasma cells, eosinophils, and occasionally neutrophils. The lymph node medulla contains pronounced infiltrates of plasma cells, and the medullary sinuses are distended and filled with histiocytes, plasma

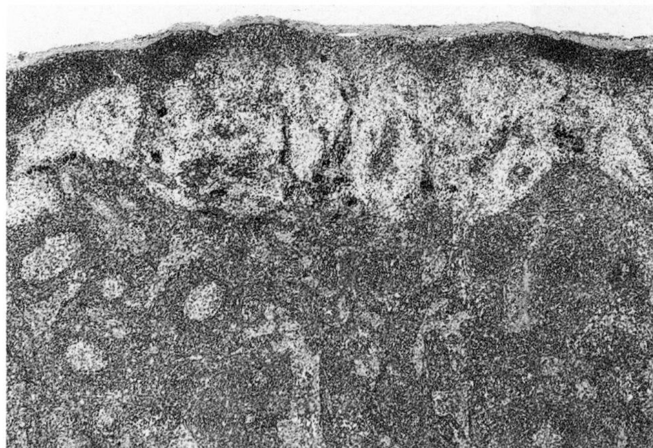

FIGURE 42.1. Dermatopathic lymphadenopathy of axillary lymph node. Large, confluent, palely stained areas of histiocytic aggregates in the cortex. Hematoxylin and eosin stain.

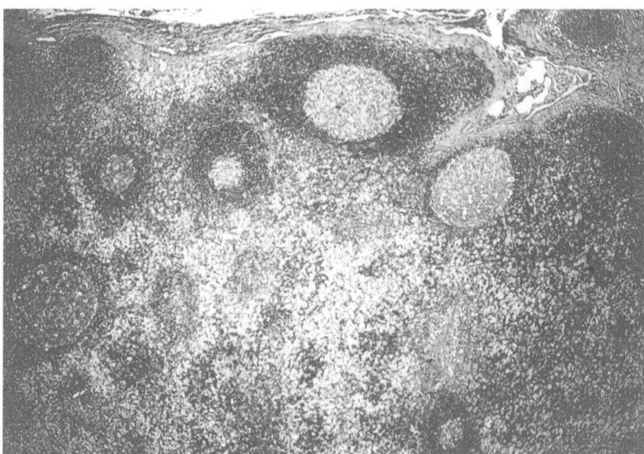

FIGURE 42.2. Dermatopathic lymphadenopathy with hyperplastic follicles and paracortical T zone slightly expanded by pale histiocytes and interdigitating reticulum cells. Hematoxylin and eosin stain.

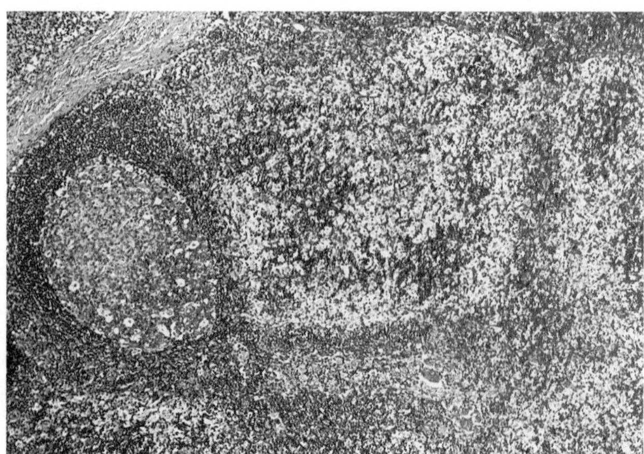

FIGURE 42.3. Dermatopathic lymphadenopathy. **Left:** Reactive follicle with prominent germinal center. **Right:** Variegated color ("mottling") in expanded paracortical T zone caused by numerous histiocytes, interdigitating reticulum cells, and pigment. Hematoxylin and eosin stain.

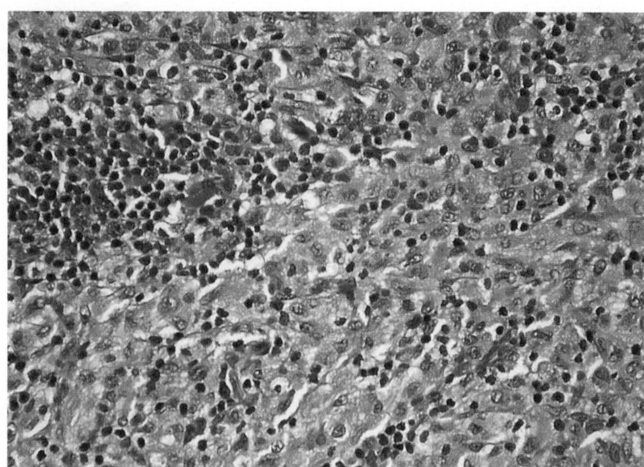

FIGURE 42.4. Dermatopathic lymphadenopathy. Aggregates of histiocytes with large, flat, sometimes foamy cytoplasm and small, central nuclei with interspersed plasma cells and lymphocytes. Hematoxylin, phloxine, and saffron stain.

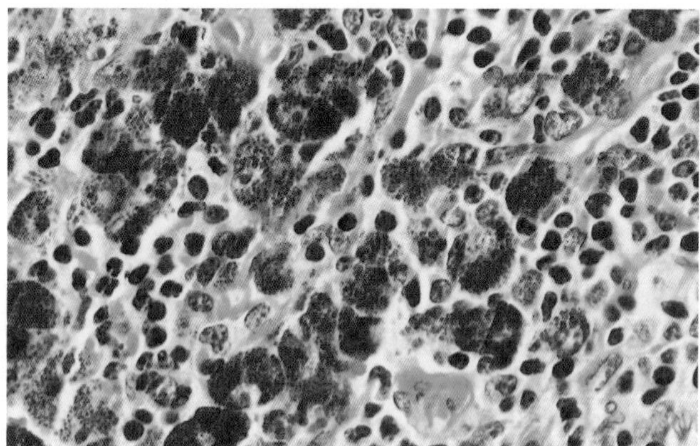

FIGURE 42.5. Dermatopathic lymphadenopathy. Numerous pigment-containing histiocytes. Hematoxylin and eosin stain.

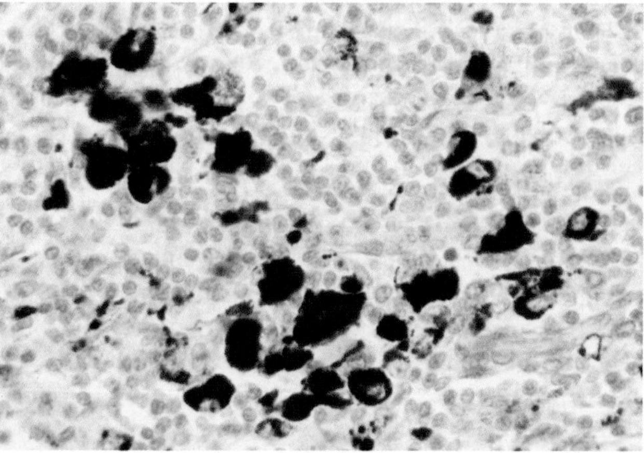

FIGURE 42.6. Melanin-laden histiocytes in dermatopathic lymphadenopathy. Cytoplasm of histiocytes is filled with melanin, so that the nuclei are barely visible. Fontana stain.

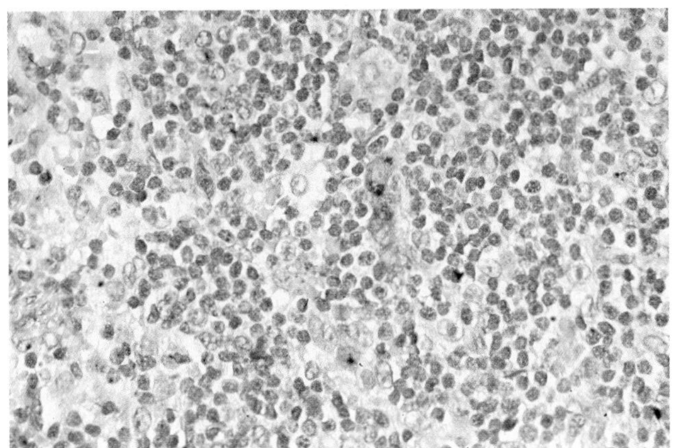

FIGURE 42.7. Hemosiderin-laden histiocytes in dermatopathic lymphadenopathy. Prussian blue stain.

cells, and eosinophils. Capillary hyperplasia is moderate. In persons with hyperpigmented skin, mild changes of histiocytic proliferation and phagocytosis of lipids and melanin pigment occur frequently; however, the diagnosis of DL should be applied only when the lymph nodes are definitely enlarged (18). The histiocytes proliferating in the pale-staining paracortical areas of DL are of various kinds. They include phagocytic histiocytes (macrophages) containing melanin, lipids, or hemosiderin, IRCs, and LCs migrating from the dermis (13,19). The nuclei of these specialized cells have complex, delicately folded membranes and contrast with the round or ovoid nuclei of the histiocytes in the lymph node sinuses (15). They derive from the bone marrow and are involved in antigen presentation to T lymphocytes. A few atypical, cerebriform, small lymphocytes can be seen in DL in patients with or without CTCL (13,20).

CYTOCHEMISTRY

Fontana silver staining (Fig. 42.6) can prove the presence of melanin in enlarged lymph nodes. Prussian blue staining for hemosiderin pigment (Fig. 42.7) does not exclude the simultaneous presence of melanin. Therefore, both stainings should be performed.

ELECTRON MICROSCOPY

In DL, IRCs are more frequent than LCs (19,21). Both IRCs and LCs have complex, indented, delicate nuclear contours and irregular, finger-like, cytoplasmic extensions (20–25). IRCs, in comparison with LCs, may contain more abundant hyperplastic smooth endoplasmic reticulum, lipid droplets, and fibrogranular bodies (21), and also more prominent tubulovesicular complexes and melanin granules (23). However, the Birbeck granule, found in LCs but not in IRCs, is the most reliable ultrastructural feature for separating the two cell types (19–25).

IMMUNOHISTOCHEMISTRY

Both IRCs and LCs stain positively for the following markers: CD1a, HLA-DR, S100 protein, and membrane adenosine triphosphatase (15,19,22,23). Lysozyme is present in histiocytes, which are usually located within sinuses, but not in IRCs or LCs (14). The histiocytes are well stained with HAM56 or CD68. Stained for the S100 protein, IRCs and LCs appear similar, with spider-like processes, and can be distinguished only by observation under the electron microscope of Birbeck granules within the LCs (19). The T cells are predominantly of the CD4+ (helper) type. The subsets of T cells and histiocytes are no different in lymph nodes involved with DL than in lymph nodes involved with DL and early CTCL (11,14). Based on the lack of expression of proliferating cell nuclear antigen, neither IRCs nor LCs divide in the lymph node (25). This suggests that IRCs and LCs either migrate from the skin as fully developed antigen-presenting cells or transform locally in the lymph node in response to antigenic influx (25). One can diagnose CTCL in lymph nodes if pan-T-cell marker expression is drastically reduced (26). However, a false-negative result may be obtained in cases of DL only minimally infiltrated by CTCL cells (14,26).

MOLECULAR DIAGNOSIS

Demonstrating a clonal T-cell antigen receptor gene rearrangement is more accurate than histologic studies for diagnosing early CTCL in lymph nodes that simulate DL (27) and is also superior for predicting clinical behavior (28).

DIFFERENTIAL DIAGNOSIS

- Advanced CTCL infiltrating lymph nodes partially or totally obliterates the nodal architecture (29). Isolated or small aggregates of atypical lymphocytes with deeply indented, cerebriform nuclei may occasionally be seen in DL, but they do not occur in large sheets. Molecular studies are required to diagnose early CTCL in lymph nodes.
- Hodgkin lymphoma may show similar pale-staining patches of histiocytes; however, typical Reed-Sternberg cells and mononuclear variants are also present.

Checklist

DERMATOPATHIC LYMPHADENOPATHY

Chronic, exfoliative skin condition
Pruritus, eosinophilia
Axillary, inguinal lymphadenopathy
Architecture preserved
Follicular hyperplasia
Paracortical, palely stained, confluent areas
CD1a+ and S100 protein+ IRCs and LCs
Melanin-, hemosiderin-, lipid-laden macrophages
Plasma cells, eosinophils
Potential association with CTCL and presence of CTCL cells

REFERENCES

1. Cooper RA, Dawson PJ, Rambo ON. Dermatopathic lymphadenopathy: a clinicopathologic analysis of lymph node biopsy over a fifteen-year period. Calif Med 1967;106:170–175.
2. Hurwit E. Dermatopathic lymphadenitis: focal granulomatous lymphadenitis associated with chronic generalized skin disorders. J Invest Dermatol 1942;5:197–204.
3. Laipply TC. Lipomelanotic reticular hyperplasia of lymph nodes. Report of 6 cases. Arch Intern Med 1948;81:19–36.
4. Lennert K, Elschner H. Zur kenntnis der lipomelanotischen reticulo(cyto)se. Frankfurt Z Pathol 1954;65:559–577.
5. Bunn PA Jr, Huberman MS, Whang-Peng J, et al. Prospective staging evaluation of patients with cutaneous T-cell lymphomas. Demonstration of a high frequency of extracutaneous dissemination. Ann Intern Med 1980;93:223–230.
6. Epstein EH Jr, Levin DL, Croft JD Jr, et al. Mycosis fungoides. Survival, prognostic features, response to therapy, and autopsy findings. Medicine (Baltimore) 1972;51:61–72.
7. Fuks ZY, Bagshaw MA, Farber EM. Prognostic signs and the management of the mycosis fungoides. Cancer 1973;32:1385–1395.
8. Matthews MJ. Surgical pathology of mycosis fungoides and Sézary syndrome. In: Jaffe ES, ed. Surgical pathology of the lymph nodes and related organs. Philadelphia: WB Saunders, 1985:329–357.
9. Sausville EA, Worsham GF, Matthews MJ, et al. Histologic assessment of lymph nodes in mycosis fungoides/Sézary syndrome (cutaneous T-cell lymphoma): clinical correlations and prognostic import of a new classification system. Hum Pathol 1985; 16:1098–1109.
10. Wechsler J, Diebold J, Gerard-Marchant R. Lymph node histopathologic aspects in cutaneous lymphomas of the mycosis fungoides or Sézary syndrome type. Retrospective study of 98 biopsies. Ann Pathol 1987;7:122–129.
11. Willemze R, Scheffer E, Meijer CJ. Immunohistochemical studies using monoclonal antibodies on lymph nodes from patients with mycosis fungoides and Sézary's syndrome. Am J Pathol 1985;120:46–54.
12. Colby TV, Burke JS, Hoppe RT. Lymph node biopsy in mycosis fungoides. Cancer 1981;47:351–359.
13. Burke JS, Colby TV. Dermatopathic lymphadenopathy. Comparison of cases associated and unassociated with mycosis fungoides. Am J Surg Pathol 1981;5:343–352.
14. Burke JS, Sheibani K, Rappaport H. Dermatopathic lymphadenopathy. An immunophenotypic comparison of cases associated and unassociated with mycosis fungoides. Am J Pathol 1986;123:256–263.
15. Gould E, Porto R, Albores-Saavedra J, et al. Dermatopathic lymphadenitis. The spectrum and significance of its morphologic features. Arch Pathol Lab Med 1988;112:1145–1150.
16. Heymann AD, Rotterdam HZ. Dermatopathic lymphadenitis presenting as lateral breast mass. JAMA 1978;240:1622–1623.
17. Dorfman RF, Warnke R. Lymphadenopathy simulating the malignant lymphomas. Hum Pathol 1974;5:519–550.
18. Butler JJ. Non-neoplastic lesions of lymph nodes of man to be differentiated from lymphomas. NCI Monogr 1969;32: 233–255.
19. Rausch E, Kaiserling E, Goos M. Langerhans cells and interdigitating reticulum cells in the thymus-dependent region in human dermatopathic lymphadenitis. Virchows Arch B Cell Pathol 1977;25:327–343.
20. Herrera GA. Light microscopic, S-100 immunostaining, and ultrastructural analysis of dermatopathic lymphadenopathy, with and without associated mycosis fungoides. Am J Clin Pathol 1987;87:187–195.
21. Poblete MT, Figueroa CD, Caorsi I. Ultrastructural characteristics of the interdigitating dendritic cell in dermatopathic lymphadenopathy of mycosis fungoides patients. J Pathol 1987; 151:263–269.
22. van der Oord JJ, de Wolf-Peeters C, de Vos R, et al. The paracortical area in dermatopathic lymphadenitis and other reactive conditions of the lymph node. Virchows Arch B Cell Pathol Mol Pathol 1984;45:289–299.
23. Asano S, Muramatsu T, Kanno H, et al. Dermatopathic lymphadenopathy. Electron microscopic, enzyme-histochemical and immunohistochemical study. Acta Pathol Jpn 1987;37: 887–900.
24. Shamoto M, Osada A, Shinzato M, et al. A comparative study on Langerhans cells in lymph nodes with dermatopathic lymphadenopathy and histiocytosis X cells. Adv Exp Med Biol 1995;378:139–141.
25. Shamoto M, Osada A, Shinzato M, et al. Do epidermal Langerhans cells, migrating from skin lesions, induce the paracortical hyperplasia of dermatopathic lymphadenopathy? Pathol Int 1996;46:348–354.
26. Weiss LM, Wood GS, Warnke RA. Immunophenotypic differences between dermatopathic lymphadenopathy and lymph node

involvement in mycosis fungoides. Am J Pathol 1985;120: 179–185.
27. Weiss LM, Hu E, Wood GS, et al. Clonal rearrangements of T-cell receptor genes in mycosis fungoides and dermatopathic lymphadenopathy. N Engl J Med 1985;313:539–544.
28. Lynch JW Jr, Linoilla I, Sausville EA, et al. Prognostic implications of evaluation for lymph node involvement by T-cell antigen receptor gene rearrangement in mycosis fungoides. Blood 1992;79:3293–3299.
29. Vonderheid EC, Diamond LW, van Vloten WA, et al. Lymph node classification systems in cutaneous T-cell lymphoma. Evidence for the utility of the Working Formulation of Non-Hodgkin's Lymphomas for Clinical Usage. Cancer 1994;73: 207–218.

43

CASTLEMAN LYMPHADENOPATHY

DEFINITION

In the original report by Castleman and co-workers (1), the lesion was described as a large, benign, asymptomatic mass of mediastinal lymph nodes that resembled thymoma both clinically and histologically. In subsequent observations, the definition was broadened to include extramediastinal lymph nodes and the spleen (2–4). The entity was further expanded by the description of two histologic variants (2) and the inclusion of multicentric cases (5–9), and it eventually came to be considered a benign, systemic lymphoproliferative disorder (10–12).

SYNONYMS

Castleman disease
Angiofollicular lymph node hyperplasia
Giant lymph node hyperplasia
Angiomatous lymphoid hamartoma

VARIANTS

- Localized
  - Hyaline-vascular type
  - Plasma cell type
- Multicentric

PATHOGENESIS

Since the initial description by Castleman and co-workers in 1956, many articles on the subject of Castleman lymphadenopathy have reported new cases and redefined the syndrome. In line with the original definition (1), earlier papers reported tumor-like masses of lymphoid tissues in the mediastinum or pericardium, and these were considered to be hamartomatous (13–15). Castleman and collaborators later redefined the syndrome to include, in addition to the initially described lymphoid vascular type, a variant characterized by the presence of large numbers of plasma cells, and they allowed that it may occur not only in the mediastinum but also in lymph nodes in other locations (2). Subsequently, multicentric cases were included, and now, in its current version, Castleman lymphadenopathy is considered to be a systemic disease with general manifestations that involves multiple organs. The cause is still unknown, and therefore the only unifying features of the numerous cases reported remain two largely nonspecific histologic patterns. One pattern is characterized by reactive follicles with hyperplastic or involuted and hyalinized germinal centers and marked interfollicular vascular proliferation. This pattern, nonspecific and relatively common, is often seen in association with various disorders of immune regulation. Thus, Castleman-like changes have been described in autoimmune disease (11,12), primary immune deficiencies (11,12), Kaposi sarcoma (15–18), and the late phase (pattern C) of HIV lymphadenitis (19,20). The second pattern, characterized by large accumulations of plasma cells, is equally nonspecific and common to a variety of lymphadenopathies associated with rheumatoid arthritis (11), lues (10), angioimmunoblastic lymphadenopathy (10–11), and the POEMS syndrome (*p*eripheral neuropathy, *o*rganomegaly, *e*ndocrinopathy, *m*onoclonal M protein, *s*kin lesions) (21–24). The latter, a multisystem syndrome, may be related to high levels of interleukin 6 (IL-6) or other cytokines found in the serum and cerebrospinal fluid of some patients with the POEMS syndrome and possibly produced by the lymphoid cells of Castleman lymphadenopathy (22–24).

The lymphoid hyaline-vascular lesions tend to be localized; they are less likely to be associated with clinical manifestations or systemic disease and are more often amenable to surgical cure. In contrast, the plasma cell proliferative lesions are more likely to be part of a systemic disease and are associated with a higher risk for chronic infections and progression to lymphoma (8–11). Mixed or transitional forms, described by the original proponents of the two variants, and progression from the plasma cell to the hyaline or vascular form (2,9,25) generally have not been confirmed, and the two forms usually do not coexist or occur successively (10). Reports of lymphomas that developed months or years after a diagnosis of Castleman lymphadenopathy raised the question of a relationship between the two entities (8,9). The idea that the lymphoid changes in Castleman lymphadenopathy represent precursor stages of lymphomas seemed to be confirmed by immunohistologic and genotypic studies detecting the presence of monoclonal populations of B cells in Castleman lymphadenopathy (26,27). However, cases of lymphoma in Castleman lymphadenopathy remain rare exceptions, and the significance of small populations of monoclonal lymphoid cells is unknown. Whether they represent the beginning of lymphomas or simply the expansion of cellular clones that under conditions of immune dysregulation result in various autoimmune disorders is still uncertain (28). With so much dissimilarity among the clinical, morphologic, and therapeutic features of its variant types, Castleman disease, as presently defined, appears to be a highly heterogeneous entity defined by characteristic (albeit nonspecific) histologic patterns that are probably related to conditions of immune deregulation.

In a search for a putative etiologic agent, sequences of human herpesvirus type 8 (HHV-8), known to be associated with Kaposi sarcoma, were found in 100% of HIV-positive and 50% of HIV-negative cases of multicentric Castleman disease with and without associated Kaposi sarcoma (29,30). A monoclonal antibody against latent nuclear antigen 1 (LNA-1) of HHV-8 was used to demonstrate nuclear staining of B cells in the mantle zone (30). Whether HHV-8 represents an etiologic or a passenger agent is unclear. Recently, an unusual cluster of cases of rapidly progressing multicentric Castleman disease was reported (31). The plasma cell type of Castleman disease developed in the lymph nodes, liver, and bone marrow of four patients with AIDS. All were positive for HHV-8 and Kaposi sarcoma, and died shortly thereafter while undergoing active anti-HIV treatment.

CLINICAL SYNDROME

The symptoms recorded by the numerous reports in the literature differ for the two histologic variants.

Hyaline-Vascular Type

In earlier publications, the hyaline-vascular type was reported to be far more common than the plasma cell type and to affect much younger patients (2). As more cases of multicentric Castleman disease were recognized, the differences in incidence and age range between the two forms appeared to decrease (9,10). No sex difference is noted between the types of Castleman lymphadenopathy. However, the locations and clinical symptoms differ. The hyaline-vascular lesions are usually localized, often in the mediastinum, and not infrequently they are asymptomatic and discovered on routine radiographic examination of the chest. In a few cases, symptoms of tracheobronchial compression have occurred. Because of the localized nature of these benign tumors, their surgical removal, when complete, has been curative in all patients.

Plasma Cell Type

The plasma cell type usually is not restricted to the mediastinum and most often is accompanied by systemic manifestations (32). Older patients, more often with mesenteric or retroperitoneal tumors, are included in this group. The symptoms include fever, sweats, weight loss, and fatigue. The most frequently found laboratory abnormalities are anemia, an elevated erythrocyte sedimentation rate, hypergammaglobulinemia, hypoalbuminemia, hypoferremia, and hypotransferrinemia. The hypergammaglobulinemias associated with this syndrome are polyclonal, indicating their nonmalignant nature (2,4,25).

Refractory hypochromic anemia, often recorded in cases of angiofollicular lymph node hyperplasia of the plasma cell variant, has been shown to be associated with a circulating anti-erythropoietin factor (3,21). Splenomegaly was present in 11 patients and hepatomegaly in 8 of 16 cases with multicentric angiofollicular lymph node hyperplasia (9). Severe peripheral neuropathies (3,4), growth retardation in an 11-year-old girl (corrected with the removal of the tumor) (3), and delayed puberty in an adolescent girl (3,33) have also been reported in association with these lymphoid neoplasms.

The course of Castleman disease is variable, ranging from stable and persistent to more aggressive and relapsing; occasionally, the disease progresses to malignant lymphoma (9). Because of the small number of cases that have been followed in each category, the prognosis cannot be based on clinical or histologic criteria. It is generally agreed that the unicentric lymphoid or vascular types of lesions have a more favorable course than the multicentric plasma cell types. The localized type may be curable by surgical or radiation treatment, whereas the multifocal type exhibits a more aggressive course that requires systemic therapy with steroids or cytostatic drugs.

HISTOPATHOLOGY

Two distinct histologic variants have been described in Castleman lymphadenopathy (2,25). At present, it is not clear whether the variants represent two stages of one syndrome, two different host reactions to the same etiologic agent, or two unrelated clinicopathologic entities. In both cases, the involved lymph nodes are enlarged, occasionally as much as 3 to 7 cm in their greatest dimension (12). The masses are well circumscribed, solitary, or multinodular (Fig. 43.1).

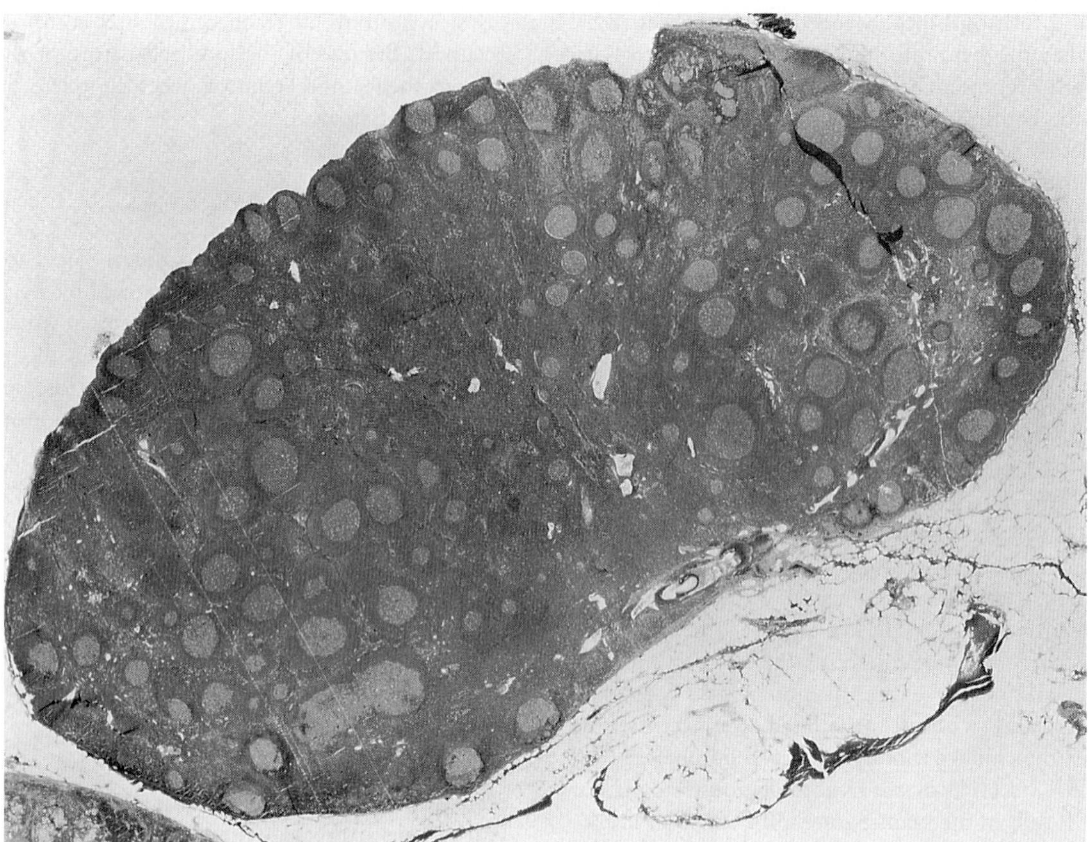

FIGURE 43.1. Castleman lymphadenopathy, hyaline-vascular type, of supraclavicular lymph node (3 × 5 cm). Lymphoid follicles in greatly increased numbers are present throughout the nodal parenchyma. Germinal centers of variable sizes are surrounded by concentric cuffs of lymphocytes. Hematoxylin and eosin stain.

Hyaline-Vascular Type

This more commonly observed histologic pattern may represent an advanced stage of the disease. The nodal architecture is altered by an increased number of lymphoid follicles, which are not restricted to the cortical area but evenly distributed throughout the entire parenchyma (Figs. 43.1 and 43.2). The follicles, however, may be unusually small and their germinal centers transfixed by radially penetrating capillaries, so that a characteristic "lollipop" structure often forms (Figs. 43.3 and 43.4). Many of the capillaries are ensheathed with collagen or surrounded by wide cuffs of hyaline substance. The germinal centers are involuted, poorly cellular, and partly or totally replaced by deposits of hyaline (Figs. 43.4 and 43.5) that are clearly revealed with periodic acid–Schiff stain. Surrounding the small germinal centers are multiple concentric layers of lymphocytes (Fig. 43.2). The regular layering of lymphocytes in onionskin fashion results in another characteristic feature of this pattern, the "target" appearance of the lymphoid follicles (Fig. 43.6). Markedly hyperplastic follicular dendritic cells may form concentric rings with lymphocytes trapped between them—hence the onionskin pattern (34). The lymphocytes are small and uniform (Fig. 43.3). Mitoses are not noted. Between the follicles are numerous blood vessels, mostly postcapillary venules, lined by hyperplastic endothelial cells and surrounded by fibrocollagen (Fig. 43.7). The lymph node sinuses are not distended, becoming sometimes quite inapparent (35). A morphometric study found no significant

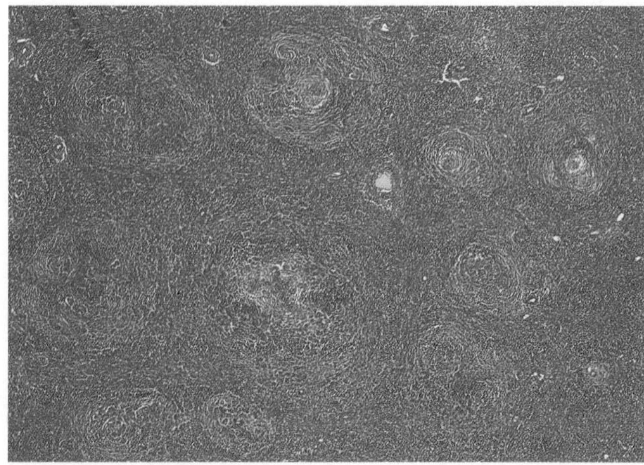

FIGURE 43.2. Lymphoid follicles in large numbers with small, involuted, and partly collagenized germinal centers. Hematoxylin, phloxine, and saffron stain.

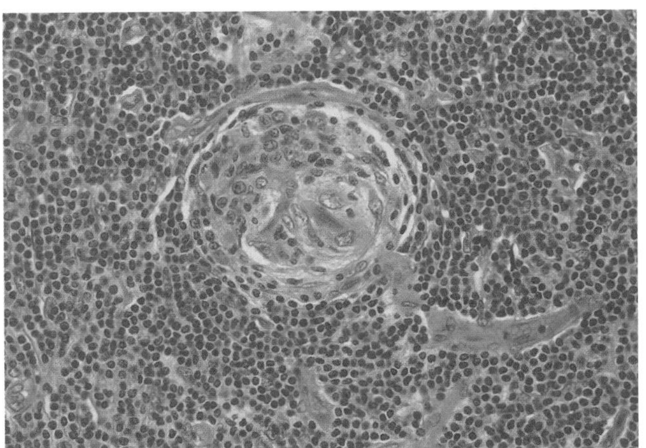

FIGURE 43.3. Lymphoid follicle with partially involuted germinal center transfixed by penetrating arteriole and surrounded by mantle of small lymphocytes. Hematoxylin, phloxine, and saffron stain.

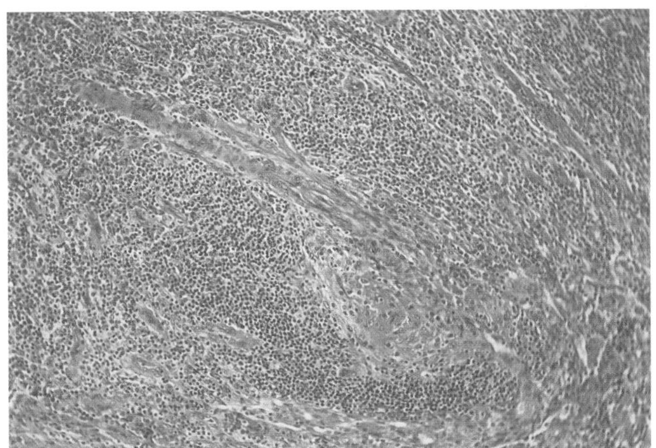

FIGURE 43.4. Lymphoid follicle with involuted, collagenized germinal center and penetrating arteriole ("lollipop" follicle). Hematoxylin, phloxine, and saffron stain.

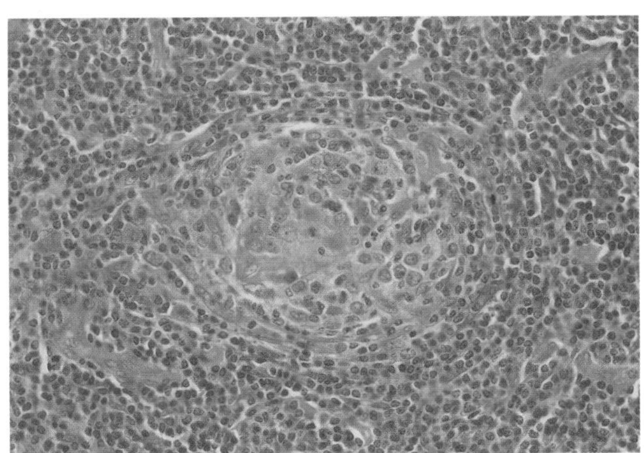

FIGURE 43.5. Involuted hyalinized follicle with indistinct lymphocytic mantle. Hematoxylin, phloxine, and saffron stain.

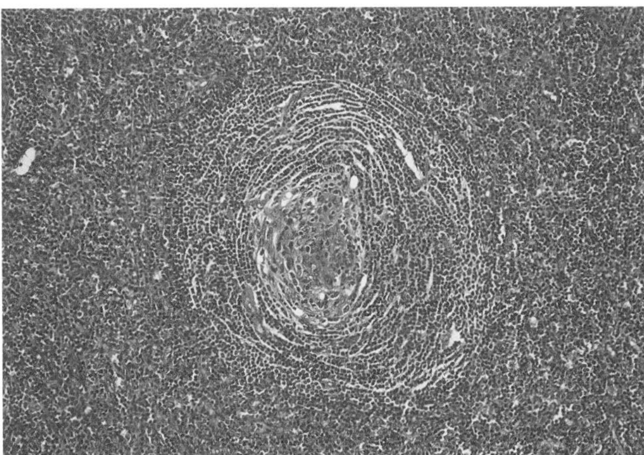

FIGURE 43.6. Target follicle with partly hyalinized germinal center and concentric layers of small, uniform lymphocytes. Hematoxylin, phloxine, and saffron stain.

differences in follicle size, numbers of mitotic figures, or amount of hyaline change between the two types of Castleman lymphadenopathy (35).

Plasma Cell Type

The plasma cell type is more commonly multicentric and may represent an earlier stage of the disease. Follicular hyperplasia may be predominant, with large germinal centers surrounded by narrow peripheral cuffs of mature lymphocytes (Figs. 43.8 and 43.9). These germinal centers are active, with frequent cells in mitosis and macrophages containing nuclear debris. Coexistent with the hyperplastic follicles or replacing them entirely are the involuted, atrophic, or hyalinized follicles and hyperplastic blood vessels with collagenized walls (Fig. 43.10) described in the preceding section. The interfollicular areas and medulla, regardless of the follicle type, are occupied by large sheets of plasma cells,

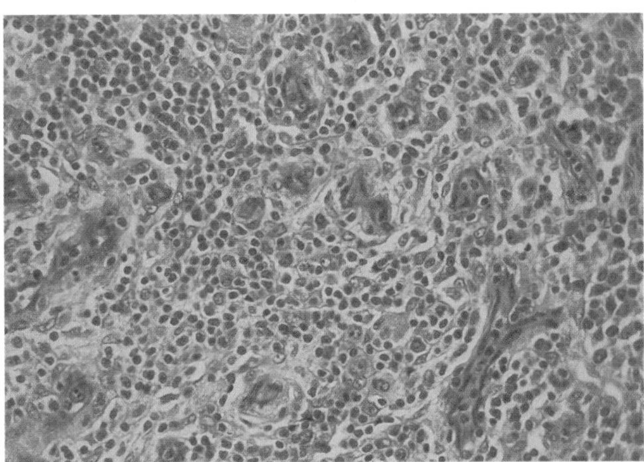

FIGURE 43.7. Numerous blood vessels with hyperplastic endothelial cells surrounded by cuffs of collagen. Hematoxylin, phloxine, and saffron stain.

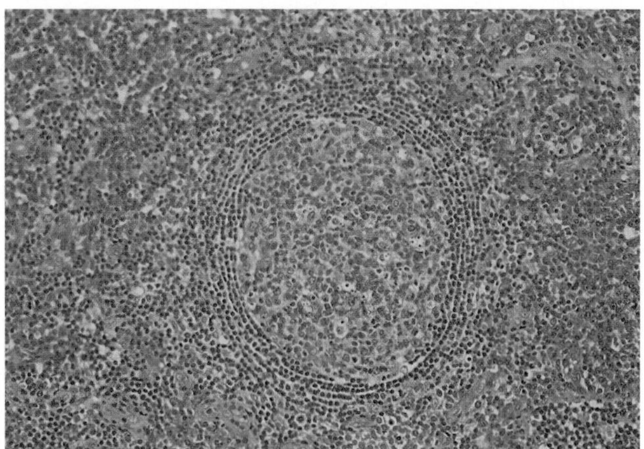

FIGURE 43.8. Hyperplastic follicle with reactive germinal center and mantle of concentric small lymphocytes. Hematoxylin, phloxine, and saffron stain.

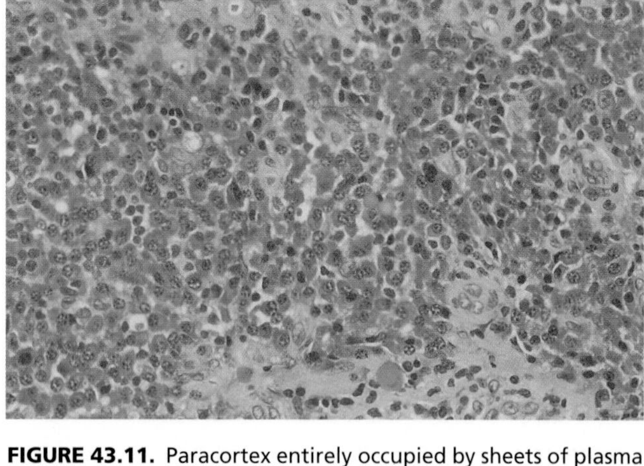

FIGURE 43.11. Paracortex entirely occupied by sheets of plasma cells, some binucleated, some with Dutcher bodies and Russell bodies. Hematoxylin, phloxine, and saffron stain.

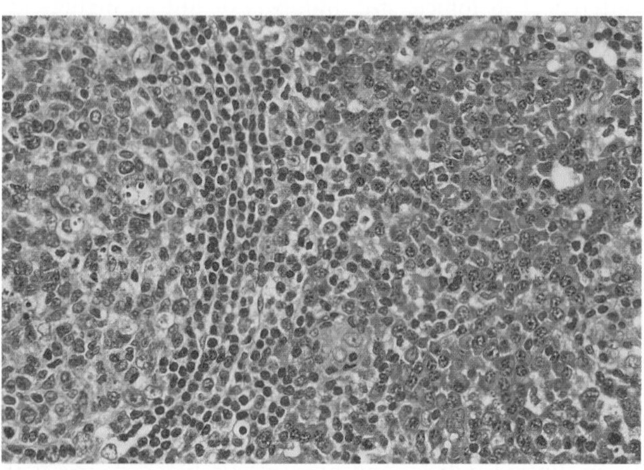

FIGURE 43.9. Reactive germinal center (*left*), concentric layers of lymphocytes, and perifollicular plasma cells. Hematoxylin, phloxine, and saffron stain.

some mature and some immature, with occasional binucleated and atypical forms (Figs. 43.9 and 43.11). Russell bodies may be also present (Fig. 43.12). Intermingled with the plasma cells are immunoblasts, plasmacytoid monocytes, lymphocytes, and occasional histiocytes.

Sequential lymph node biopsies in two studies of patients with Castleman disease showed persistence of the same histologic pattern in 8 of 14 and in 5 of 7 patients; conversions from one type to another were uncommon (9,10). Lymph nodes from different locations showed similar histologic patterns. In the case of systemic lymphoproliferative disorders with morphologic features of Castleman disease (Fig. 43.13), lymphoid infiltrates (nodular or diffuse) were also seen in the spleen, lungs, and bone marrow (10). Unusual locations (e.g., intrapericardial and epidural) have also been reported (14,36). In cases in which Kaposi sarcoma coexisted in the same lymph node, the two lesions could be adjacent or intermingled (7,18).

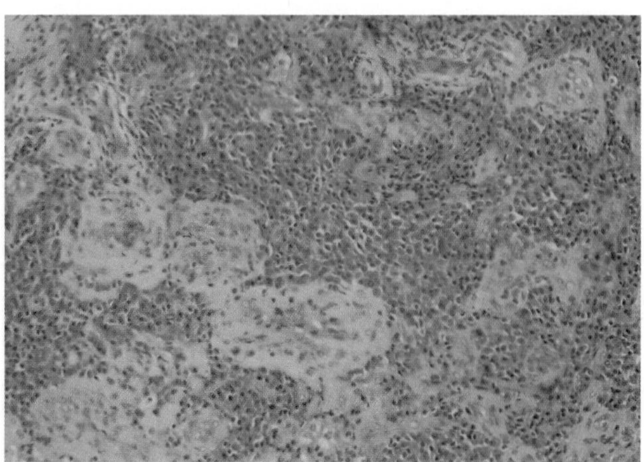

FIGURE 43.10. Blood vessels ensheathed by thick layers of collagen in paracortex filled with plasma cells. Hematoxylin, phloxine, and saffron stain.

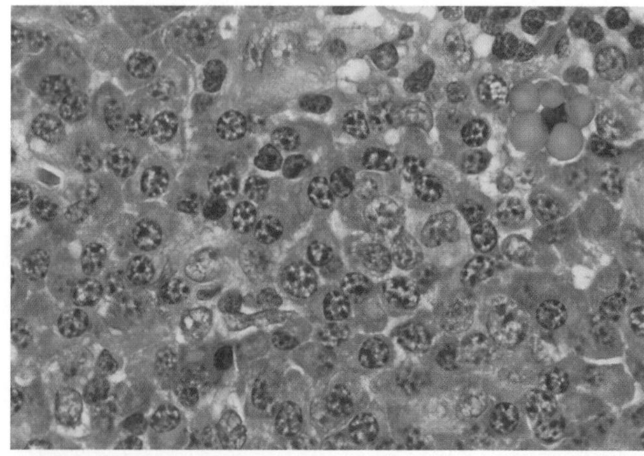

FIGURE 43.12. Sheets of plasma cells in paracortex with prominent paranuclear hof and Russell bodies (*upper right*). Hematoxylin, phloxine, and saffron stain.

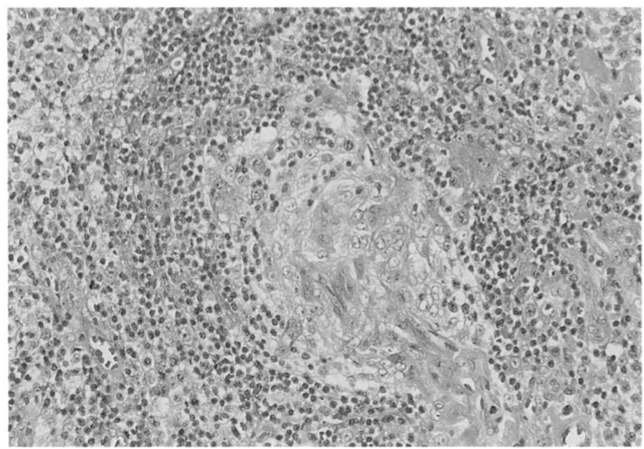

FIGURE 43.13. Multicentric Castleman disease showing fibrosing lymph node follicle surrounded by lymphocytes, plasma cells, and immunoblasts. Hematoxylin and eosin stain.

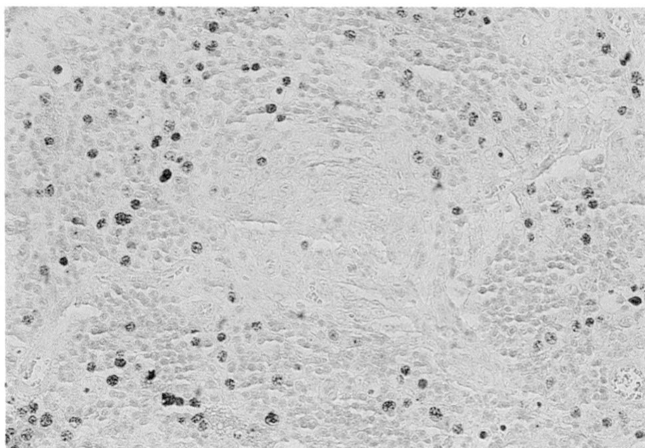

FIGURE 43.14. Same section as in Fig. 43.13, immunostained with monoclonal antibody LN-53 shows nuclear staining for latent nuclear antigen 1 in lymphocytes and immunoblasts. LN-53/peroxidase stain. (Courtesy of P. K. Bhattacharya, M.D.)

Castleman disease, whether localized or multicentric, remains a poorly understood entity, and difficult problems are encountered in the diagnosis and clinical management. More recently published series agree that although the unicentric form can be cured by surgical removal, the multicentric forms of either histologic type may benefit only from steroid or chemotherapy given in an early phase (37–39). It is likely that the localized and systemic forms of Castleman disease are in fact different clinical disorders with similar histologic features.

IMMUNOHISTOCHEMISTRY

In Castleman disease, B lymphocytes and plasma cells produce polyclonal immunoglobulins (Igs), which explains the frequently observed hypergammaglobulinemia associated with the plasma cell type (6,8,40). Immunoperoxidase stainings reveal that the plasma cells contain intracytoplasmic IgG, IgA, and IgM and both κ and λ chains in the normal ratio, and that the IgM+ cells are more commonly perifollicular, whereas the IgG+ and IgA+ cells are mainly in the interfollicular areas (6). In the plasma cell form, abundant production of IL-6 by B cells in the germinal centers and by many immunoblasts in the mantle zone and interfollicular areas results in high serum levels of IL-6 and marked proliferation of plasma cells (22–24). IL-6, a soluble protein secreted by lymphoid cells, stimulates the proliferation of B cells and maturation into plasma cells (39). In the hyaline-vascular form, no significant expression of IL-6 is detected. The lymphocyte-depleted follicles show a greatly increased population of follicular dendritic cells, whereas the interfollicular areas show marked vascular proliferation and frequent T-zone plasmacytoid cells (23). The follicular dendritic cells are stained with S100 antibody, specifically with DRC-1 (on frozen section) and CNA-42 (on paraffin sections). The expression of IL-6 by lymphoid cells and histiocytes is demonstrated with rabbit antihuman IL-6 antibody. The presence of HHV-8 in the form of LNA-1 in immunoblasts located in the mantle follicular zone is demonstrated by immunostaining with monoclonal antibody LN-53 (30) (Fig. 43.14).

DIFFERENTIAL DIAGNOSIS

Hyaline-Vascular Type

- Thymomas include nests of epithelial cells with squamous differentiation, which can be identified by immunostaining for cytokeratins. Vascular hyperplasia is not a feature of thymomas.
- Follicular hyperplasia of reactive lymphadenopathies: Whatever the cause, such follicles are large and contain tingible-body macrophages. The target/onionskin pattern is not seen in acute reactive lymphadenopathies.
- *Toxoplasma* lymphadenitis: The reactive follicles are infiltrated by epithelioid cells.
- HIV lymphadenitis, pattern C (burnout phase) has in common involuted follicles with hyalinized germinal centers and interfollicular vascular proliferation. HIV serum antibody testing is necessary for a definitive diagnosis.
- Kaposi sarcoma lymphadenopathy may exhibit involuted, hyalinized follicles; however, it is distinguished by cleft-like vascular spaces lined by spindle-shaped cells.
- Follicular lymphoma has a pattern of evenly distributed nodules of similar size and shape. They are composed of closely packed cells with atypical nuclei.

Plasma Cell Type

- Angioimmunoblastic lymphadenopathy: The nodal architecture is effaced and the sinuses are markedly

Checklist

CASTLEMAN LYMPHADENOPATHY

Localized

Hyaline-vascular type
More common
Younger patients
Isolated lymph node mass
Often mediastinal
Frequently asymptomatic
Numerous, small lymphoid follicles
Transfixing, collagen-ensheathed arterioles ("lollipop" follicle)
Hyaline deposits in germinal centers
Concentric layering of lymphocytes (target follicles)
Inapparent sinuses
Interfollicular vascular hyperplasia
Small, inactive lymphocytes
Absence of mitoses

Plasma cell type
Older patients
Systemic symptoms
Possible associations
- Anemia
- Hypergammaglobulinia
- Peripheral neuropathies
- Kaposi sarcoma
- POEMS syndrome

Hyperplastic lymphoid follicles
Active germinal centers
Interfollicular sheets of plasma cells
Plasmacytoid monocytes
Polyclonal immunoglobulins

Multicentric
Atypical lymphoproliferative disorder
Plasma cell type more common
Older patients
Severe systemic symptoms
Multiple lymphoid organs involved
High levels of IL-6 in lymph nodes and serum
Kaposi sarcoma/HHV-8 often present
HIV infection often associated

dilated. It lacks the follicular pattern of Castleman lymphadenopathy.

- Sinus histiocytosis with massive lymphadenopathy has inconspicuous follicles and grossly distended sinuses with emperipolesis.
- Plasmacytoma: Sheets of typical and atypical plasma cells without preservation of lymphoid follicles. The rich vascularity of angiofollicular lymphoid hyperplasia is not present. The plasma cells are monoclonal.

REFERENCES

1. Castleman B, Iverson L, Mendez V. Localized mediastinal lymph node hyperplasia resembling thymoma. Cancer 1956;9:822–830.

2. Keller AR, Hochholzer L, Castleman B. Hyaline-vascular and plasma-cell types of giant lymph node hyperplasia of the mediastinum and other locations. Cancer 1972;29:670–683.
3. Burgert EO Jr, Gilchrist GS, Fairbanks VF, et al. Intraabdominal angiofollicular lymph node hyperplasia (plasma cell variant) with an antierythropoietic factor. Mayo Clin Proc 1975;50:542–546.
4. Gaba AR, Stein RS, Sweet DL, et al. Multicentric giant lymph node hyperplasia. Am J Clin Pathol 1978;69:86–90.
5. Marti S, Pahissa A, Guardia J, et al. Multicentric giant follicular lymph node hyperplasia. Favorable response to radiotherapy. Cancer 1983;51:808–810.
6. Tanda F, Massarelli G, Costanzi G. Multicentric giant lymph node hyperplasia. Hum Pathol 1983;14:1053–1058.
7. Chen KTK. Multicentric Castleman's disease and Kaposi's sarcoma. Am J Surg Pathol 1984;8:287–293.
8. Kessler E. Multicentric giant lymph node hyperplasia. A report of seven cases. Cancer 1985;56:2446–2451.
9. Weisenburger DD, Nathwani BN, Winberg CD, et al. Multicentric angiofollicular lymph node hyperplasia: a clinicopathologic study of 16 cases. Hum Pathol 1985;16:162–172.
10. Frizzera G, Massarelli G, Banks PM, et al. A systemic lymphoproliferative disorder with morphologic features of Castleman's disease. Pathological findings in 15 patients. Am J Surg Pathol 1983;7:211–231.
11. Frizzera G. Castleman's disease: more questions than answers. Hum Pathol 1985;16:202–205.
12. Frizzera G. Systemic Castleman's disease. Am J Surg Pathol 1991;15:192.
13. Lattes R, Pachter MR. Benign masses of probable hamartomatous nature: analysis of 12 cases. Cancer 1962;15:197–214.
14. Fisher ER, Sieracki JC, Goldenberg DM. Identity and nature of isolated lymphoid tumors (so-called nodal hyperplasia, hamartoma, and angiomatous hamartoma). Cancer 1970;25: 1286–1300.
15. Virmani R, McAllister HA, Bewtra C, et al. Intrapericardial giant lymph node hyperplasia. Am J Surg Pathol 1982;6:475–481.
16. Perlow LS, Taff ML, Orsini JM, et al. Kaposi's sarcoma in a young homosexual man. Association with angiofollicular lymphoid hyperplasia and a malignant lymphoproliferative disorder. Arch Pathol Lab Med 1983;107:510–513.
17. Dickson D, Ben-Ezra JM, Reed J, et al. Multicentric giant lymph node hyperplasia, Kaposi's sarcoma, and lymphoma. Arch Pathol Lab Med 1985;109:1013–1018.
18. Xerri L, Guigou V, Lepidi H, et al. Lymphadenopathic tumor exhibiting intermingled features of Kaposi's sarcoma, malignant lymphoma, and angiofollicular hyperplasia. Arch Pathol Lab Med 1991;115:1162–1166.
19. Ioachim HL. Pathology of AIDS. Textbook and color atlas. Philadelphia: JB Lippincott Co, 1989.
20. Ioachim HL, Cronin W, Roy M, et al. Persistent lymphadenopathies in individuals at high risk for HIV infection. Clinicopathologic correlations and long-term follow-up in 79 cases. Am J Clin Pathol 1990;93:208–218.
21. Chan JKC, Fletcher CDM, Hicklin GA, et al. Glomeruloid hemangioma. A distinctive cutaneous lesion of multicentric Castleman's disease associated with POEMS syndrome. Am J Surg Pathol 1990;14:1036–1046.
22. Mandler RN, Kerrigan DP, Smart J, et al. Castleman's disease in POEMS syndrome with elevated interleukin-6. Cancer 1992;69: 2697–2703.
23. Hsu S-M, Xie S-S, Waldron JA, et al. Expression of interleukin-6 in Castleman's disease. Hum Pathol 1993;24:833–839.
24. Soubrier MJ, Dubost J-J, Sauvezie BJM, et al. POEMS syndrome: a study of 25 cases and a review of the literature. Am J Med 1994;97:543–553.
25. Flendrig JA, Schillings PHM. Benign giant lymphoma: the clinical signs and symptoms. Folia Med Neerl 1969;12:119.
26. Hall PA, Donaghy M, Cotter FE, et al. An immunohistological and genotypic study of the plasma cell form of Castleman's disease. Histopathology 1989;14:333–346.
27. Radaskiewizs TR, Hansmann M-L, Lennert K. Monoclonality and polyclonality of plasma cells in Castleman's disease of the plasma cell variant. Histopathology 1989;14:11–24.
28. Isaacson PG. Castleman's disease. Commentary. Histopathology 1989;14:429–432.
29. Soulier J, Grollet L, Oksenhendler E, et al. Kaposi's sarcoma-associated herpesvirus-like DNA sequences in multicentric Castleman's disease. Blood 1995;86:1276–1280.
30. Dupin N, Fisher C, Kellam P, et al. Distribution of human herpesvirus-8 latently infected cells in Kaposi's sarcoma, multicentric Castleman's disease and primary effusion lymphoma. Proc Natl Acad Sci U S A 1999;96:4546–4551.
31. Zietz C, Bogner JR, Goebel F-D, et al. An unusual cluster of cases of Castleman's disease during highly active antiretroviral therapy for AIDS. N Engl J Med 1999;340:1923–1924.
32. Yu GMS, Carson JW. Giant lymph-node hyperplasia, plasma-cell type, of the mediastinum, with peripheral neuropathy. Am J Clin Pathol 1976;66:46–53.
33. Massey GV, Kornstein MJ, Wahl D, et al. Angiofollicular lymph node hyperplasia (Castleman's disease) in an adolescent female. Clinical and immunologic findings. Cancer 1991;68:1 365–1372.
34. Diebold J, Bientz M, Daussy M, et al. Hyperplasie lymphoide angiofolliculaire de localisation mediastinale. Étude en immunofluorescence directe. Rev Fr Mal Respir 1976;4: 373–378.
35. Menke DM, Camoriano JK, Banks PM. Angiofollicular lymph node hyperplasia. A comparison of unicentric, multicentric, hyaline vascular, and plasma cell types of disease by morphometric and clinical analysis. Mod Pathol 1992;5:525–530.
36. Alper G, Crumrine PK, Hamilton RL, et al. Unusual case of inflammatory spinal epidural mass (Castleman syndrome). Pediatr Neurol 1996;15:60–62.
37. Herrada J, Cabanillas F, Rice L, et al. The clinical behavior of localized and multicentric Castleman disease. Ann Intern Med 1998;128:657–662.
38. Bowne WB, Lewis JL, Filippa DA, et al. The management of unicentric and multicentric Castleman's disease. A report of 16 cases and a review of the literature. Cancer 1999;85:706–717.
39. Shahidi H, Myers JL, Kvale PA. Castleman's disease. Mayo Clin Proc 1995;70:969–977.
40. Diamond LW, Braylan RC. Immunological markers and DNA content in a case of giant lymph node hyperplasia (Castleman's disease). Cancer 1980;46:730–735.

44

TUMOR-REACTIVE LYMPHADENOPATHY

DEFINITION

Reactive, usually enlarged, regional lymph nodes draining tumor areas.

PATHOGENESIS

Regional lymph nodes tributary to tumor-bearing organs are considered anatomic barriers to tumor spread. They are also the site where specific immune interactions between tumor antigens and responding lymphoid cells takes place. According to these concepts, the primary antitumor function of lymph nodes is not merely filtration but also immunologic tumor surveillance (1). Consequently, the regional lymph nodes are commonly enlarged as a result of reactive lymphadenopathy, tumor metastasis, or both. In response to tumor-associated antigens, the various cell populations of regional lymph nodes react in different ways, giving rise to a multitude of morphologic patterns. Numerous studies have been devoted to the analysis of such reactions, in an effort to understand the mechanisms of lymph node metastases. Some studies have correlated various histologic patterns of reactive lymph nodes with the dissemination of tumors (2–11), whereas others have investigated the capacity of their lymphocytes to transform *in vitro* when in contact with antigens (12,13). Tumor-associated antigens, shed by tumor cells or released by cell death, in addition to viable tumor cells, are carried by lymph to the draining lymph nodes, providing constant nonspecific and specific stimulation. Thus, various defense reactions may be triggered, including phagocytosis, production of antibodies, and sensitization of lymphocytes (14). Such reactions were investigated in various studies by determining the amounts and types of immunoglobulins in pericancerous human lymph nodes (14) and by immunohistochemically detecting epitopes of tumor-associated glycoproteins in the draining lymph nodes. Thus, uninvolved regional lymph nodes in resected colon carcinomas were investigated immunohistochemically to detect tumor-associated antigens (15). Sinus macrophages, lymphatic endothelial cells, and especially follicular dendritic cells in the unaffected lymph nodes showed immune reactions with monoclonal antibodies against epitopes of some tumor- or colon-associated glycoproteins that were similar to their reaction to the carcinoma cells of the colonic tumor. Although the morphologic changes of lymph nodes draining tumor-bearing organs provide evidence for antitumor immune reactivity, not many studies have been devoted to the investigation of this important segment of tumor metastasis. Most studies were performed in the 1970s, and very few studies taking advantage of newer technologies have been reported to date.

CLINICAL SYNDROME

Understanding the process of lymph node metastasis is of major theoretic importance and also of practical value. Recognition of the histologic patterns of lymph node reactivity to the presence of tumors is a common objective of the study of biopsy and surgical specimens. Not infrequently, markedly enlarged and firm lymph nodes removed as part of radical tumor excision reveal no tumor metastasis on microscopic examination. In a study of 163 patients with renal cell carcinoma, 43 patients had enlarged lymph nodes with a diameter of 1 to 2.2 cm on computed tomography (16). Of these, 18 patients (42%) had metastases of renal cell carcinoma, but 25 patients (58%) had only follicular hyperplasia or inflammatory changes, often associated with involvement of the renal vein or necrosis. The study concluded that radiologic and even gross examination findings of enlarged lymph nodes should not be interpreted as metastatic unless they are so proven by cytologic (fine needle aspiration) or histologic (biopsy) examination. The presence of lymph node metastasis constitutes an essential factor in the tumor–node–metastasis (TNM) prognostic system. Moreover, a number of studies have investigated possible correlations between patterns of lymph node reactivity and prognosis, so far without firm, conclusive results (2,4,5,7,8,10,17).

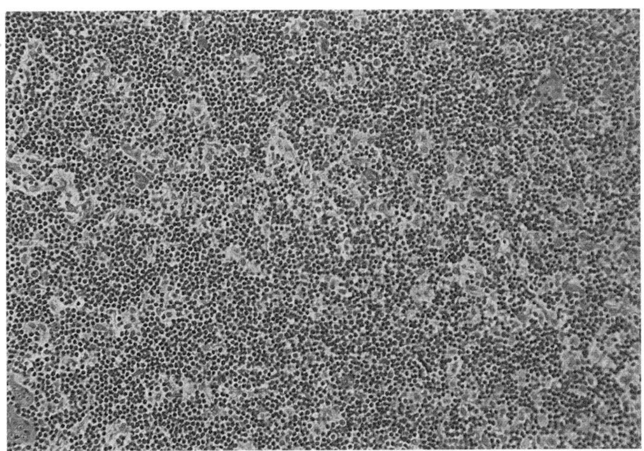

FIGURE 44.1. Lymphocyte predominance pattern of uninvolved axillary lymph node in breast cancer. Enlarged paracortical T-cell area includes numerous histiocytes. Hematoxylin, phloxine, and saffron stain.

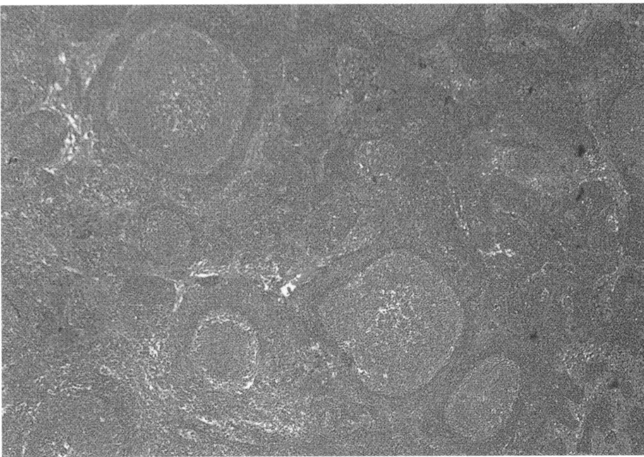

FIGURE 44.3. Germinal center predominance pattern of uninvolved axillary lymph node in breast cancer with enlarged follicles and reactive germinal centers. Hematoxylin, phloxine, and saffron stain.

HISTOPATHOLOGY

A proposal for a standardized system of reporting human lymph node morphology in relation to immune reaction was published in 1973 by the World Health Organization (18). The authors recommended a topographic examination of the lymph node sections with separate descriptions of the functional areas: cortex with follicles and germinal centers, paracortex, sinuses, and medullary cords. Studies of regional lymph nodes in tumors of various organs have attempted to identify histologic patterns of reactions, possibly with prognostic implications (6–10). One of four major histologic patterns is usually seen, and often combinations thereof.

Lymphocyte Predominance

Lymph nodes are enlarged particularly because of the increased number of lymphocytes in the paracortical areas (T-cell zone) (Figs. 44.1 and 44.2). The lymphoid follicles are effaced and the germinal centers mostly inapparent, whereas the paracortex is markedly thickened. Such lymphoid hyperplasia may or may not be associated with sinus histiocytosis. The pattern is thought to reflect changes related to cellular immunity and to be associated with an earlier diagnosis, a better prognosis, and longer survival (7–11).

Germinal Center Predominance

The lymph nodes are similarly enlarged, but the increase in volume is caused by hyperplasia of follicles, particularly the germinal centers (B-cell zone) (Figs. 44.3 and 44.4). The germinal centers are prominent and composed mostly of large, primitive cells with numerous mitoses. The medullary cords are also enlarged and contain increased numbers of plasma cells. Sinus histiocytosis may coexist with these changes, which are considered to be associated with humoral immunity and a less favorable prognosis (7–9).

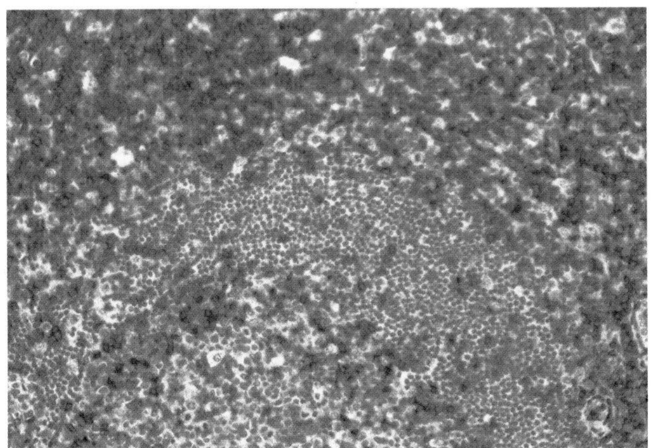

FIGURE 44.2. Lymphocyte predominance pattern in same uninvolved reactive lymph node as in Fig. 44.1 showing CD43+ T cells. Anti-CD43/peroxidase stain.

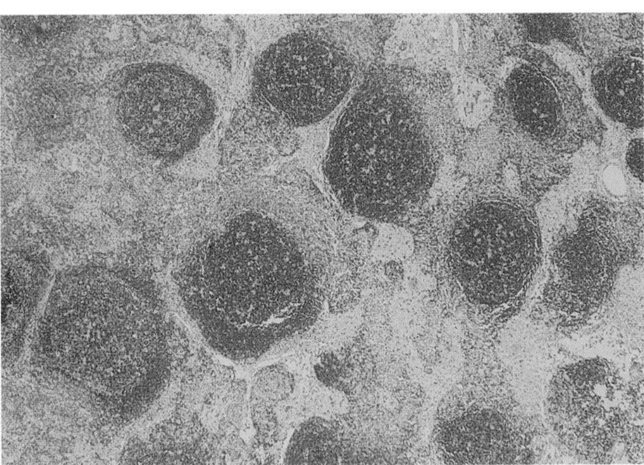

FIGURE 44.4. Germinal center predominance pattern in same uninvolved reactive lymph node as in Fig. 44.3 showing CD20+ B cells. L26 (anti-CD20)/peroxidase stain.

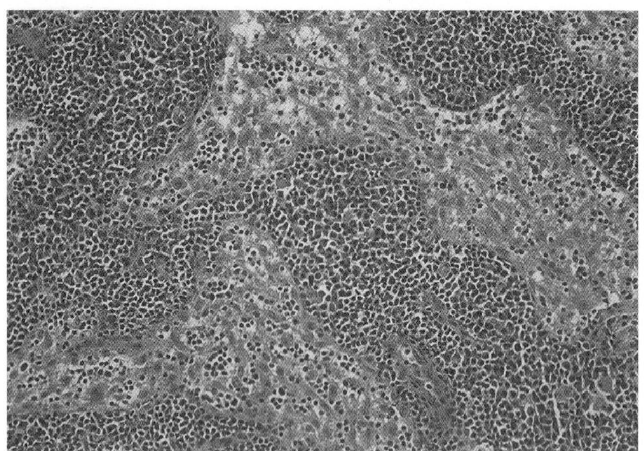

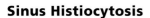

FIGURE 44.5. Sinus histiocytosis pattern of enlarged (2.8-cm diameter) axillary lymph node in breast cancer. Largely distended sinuses are filled with histiocytes and macrophages. Hematoxylin, phloxine, and saffron stain.

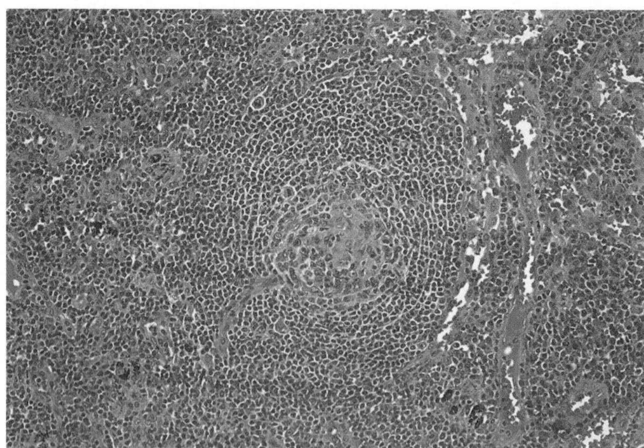

FIGURE 44.7. Lymphocyte depletion pattern with involuted, partly hyalinized germinal center and reactive, dilated sinuses. Hematoxylin, phloxine, and saffron stain.

Sinus Histiocytosis

A predominance of sinuses characterizes this morphologic pattern, which can occur in isolation or together with one of the preceding patterns. The lymph node is enlarged by markedly distended sinuses and hyperplasia of the sinus histiocytes (Figs. 44.5 and 44.6). The pale staining of histiocytes and endothelial cells that line the branching lumina contrasts strongly with the dark staining of lymphocytic areas and produces the characteristic appearance of sinus histiocytosis. This reactive pattern has been generally associated with a more favorable prognosis (2,3).

Lymphocyte Depletion

The lymph node is of normal or diminished size, and the lymphocytic population is depleted. The loosely packed lymphocytes are separated by deposits of amorphous substance and areas of fibrocollagen (Fig. 44.7). The vessels have thick walls with hyaline deposits. Diffuse fibrosis and patchy deposition of hyaline involve both the cortex and medulla. These changes are considered to reflect an exhausted ("burnt out") lymph node and to be associated with metastases and a poor prognosis (7,8,11).

The patterns described according to the World Health Organization proposals are not mutually exclusive. They usually represent a predominant pattern and are often combined. The prognostic value of the histologic patterns has been contested by some authors (10).

IMMUNOHISTOCHEMISTRY

The presence of metastases in reactive lymph nodes is sometimes difficult to establish. Sinus histiocytosis may be difficult to distinguish from some types of metastatic carcinoma, such as lobular carcinoma of the breast (Fig. 44.8) (see Chapter 94). Immunohistochemical stainings with cytokeratin anti-

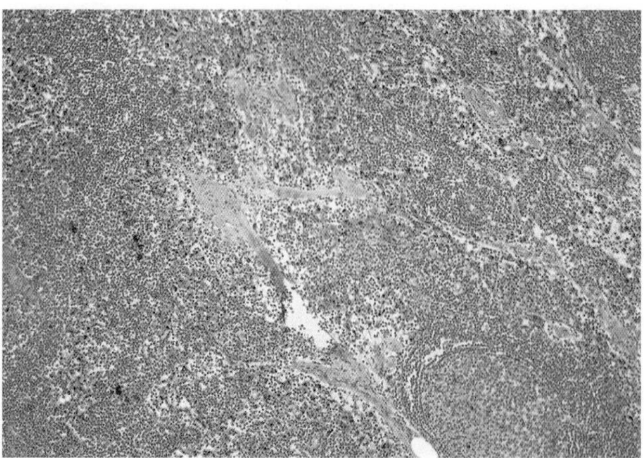

FIGURE 44.6. Sinus histiocytosis pattern of same lymph node as in Fig. 44.5, with CD68+ histiocytes and macrophages filling the distended sinus. Anti-CD68/peroxidase stain.

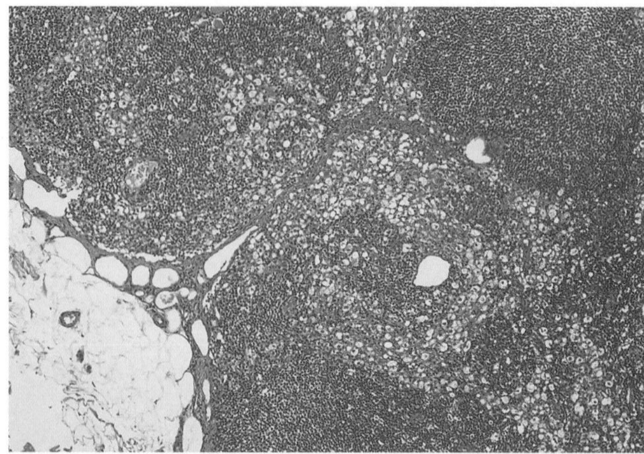

FIGURE 44.8. Metastatic lobular breast carcinoma resembling lymph node with reactive sinus histiocytosis. Hematoxylin, phloxine, and saffron stain.

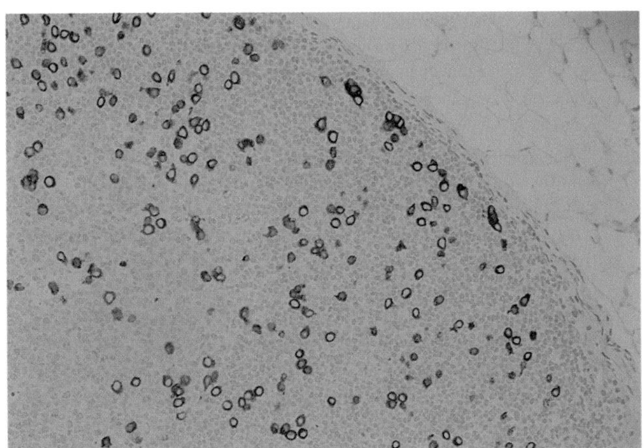

FIGURE 44.9. Metastatic lobular breast carcinoma in lymph node. Immunostaining with cytokeratin (*CK*) reveals the epithelial nature of the cells. Anti-CK/peroxidase stain.

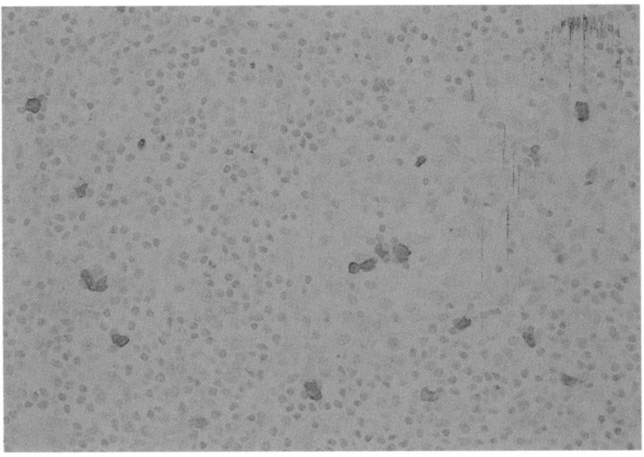

FIGURE 44.10. Axillary lymph node uninvolved by tumor with cytokeratin-positive histiocytes. Anti-CD68/peroxidase stain.

bodies are very useful, not only in the detection of micrometastases but also in differential diagnosis (Fig. 44.9). However, the clinician should be aware that not all cytokeratin-positive cells in lymph nodes are carcinoma cells; dendritic cells and endothelial cells are also stained (Fig. 44.10). Equally difficult may be the distinction between markedly reactive sinus histiocytosis and various types of large cell ymphomas. The use of a panel of B- and T-cell marker antibodies to identify the lymphoid cells and the use of histiocyte/monocyte marker antibodies to highlight the histiocytes is indicated for this particular problem. Immunostaining for carcinoembryonic antigen or other tumor-associated antigens is indicated to detect them in tumor-draining lymph nodes.

DIFFERENTIAL DIAGNOSIS

- Metastatic carcinoma: The presence of excessive sinus histocytosis must not divert the clinician from the search for small foci of carcinoma cells, which sometimes coexist. Occasional findings of necrotic debris, fragments of keratin, or psammoma bodies indicate metastatic carcinoma. Particularly difficult to distinguish are metastases of poorly differentiated carcinomas, such as nasopharyngeal carcinoma, in which the anaplastic cells are accompanied by large numbers of lymphocytes. Serial sections, mucicarmine staining, and particularly cytokeratin antibodies CK7 and CK20 in addition to carcinoembryonic antigen in immunohistochemical staining must be used to detect and identify suspected carcinomas.
- Malignant histiocytosis and histiocytic lymphoma grow in sheets without the characteristic sinus pattern of sinus histocytosis. The nuclei are pleomorphic, and mitoses are frequent.
- Sinus histiocytosis with massive lymphadenopathy (Rosai-Dorfman) exhibits a sinus pattern but also shows lymphocytes within cytoplasmic vacuoles of histiocytes (emperipolesis).
- Anaplastic large cell lymphoma exhibits a sinus pattern, but the cells have hyperchromatic, pleomorphic nuclei and frequent mitoses. Immunohistochemical staining is positive for CD30 and anaplastic lymphoma kinase antibodies.

Checklist

TUMOR-REACTIVE LYMPHADENOPATHY

History of regional tumor
Enlarged lymph nodes
Absence of metastatic tumor cells confirmed by immunohistochemical cytokeratin staining
Absence of desmoplastic reaction
Paracortical hyperplasia (T-cell response)
Germinal center hyperplasia (B-cell response)
Distended sinuses with histiocytosis
Lymphocyte depletion

REFERENCES

1. Santin AD. Lymph node metastases: the importance of the microenvironment. Cancer. 2000;88:175–179.
2. Black MM, Speer FD. Sinus histiocytosis of lymph nodes in cancer. Surg Gynecol Obstet 1958;106:163.
3. Black MM. Reactivity of the lymphoreticuloendothelial system in human cancer. Prog Clin Cancer 1965;1:26.
4. Mattheiem W. La réaction d'hyperplasie histiocytaire des ganglions pelviens dans l'epithélioma du col utérin: valeur pronostique comparée aux critères classiques. Bull Cancer (Paris) 1962; 49:421.
5. Silverberg SG, Chitale AR, Hind AD, et al. Sinus histiocytosis and mammary carcinoma: study of 363 radical mastectomies and a historical review. Cancer 1970;26:1177–1184.
6. Fisher ER, Saffer EA, Fisher B. Studies concerning the regional lymph node in cancer. VI. Correlation of lymphocyte transformation of regional node cells and some histopathologic discriminants. Cancer 1973;32:104–111.
7. Tsakraklides V, Anastassiades OT, Kersey JH. Prognostic significance of regional lymph node histology in uterine cervical cancer. Cancer 1973;31:860–868.
8. Tsakraklides V, Olson P, Kersey JH, et al. Prognostic significance of the regional lymph node histology in cancer of the breast. Cancer 1974;34:1259–1267.
9. Pratt DJ, Brynes RK, Vardiman JW, et al. Mesocolic lymph node histology is an important prognostic indicator for patients with carcinoma of the sigmoid colon: an immunomorphologic study. Cancer 1975;35:1388–1397.
10. Fisher ER, Gregorio R, Redmond C, et al. Pathologic findings from the National Surgical Adjuvant Breast Project (Protocol No. 4). II. The significance of regional node histology other than sinus histiocytosis in invasive mammary cancer. Am J Clin Pathol 1976;65:21–30.
11. Kaufman M, Wirth K, Scheurer J, et al. Immunomorphological lymph node changes in patients with operable bronchogenic squamous cell carcinoma. Cancer 1977;39:2271–2377.
12. Fisher B, Saffer EA, Fisher ER. Studies concerning the regional lymph node in cancer. III. Response of regional lymph node cells from breast and colon cancer patients to PHA stimulation. Cancer 1972;30:1202–1215.
13. Fisher B, Saffer EA, Fisher ER. Studies concerning the regional lymph node in cancer. VII. Thymidine uptake by cells from nodes of breast cancer patients relative to axillary location and histopathologic discriminants. Cancer 1974;33:271–279.
14. Burtin P, Loisillier F, Buffe D, et al. Immunoglobulin-producing cells in human pericancerous lymph nodes. Cancer 1969;23: 80–87.
15. Mariani-Costantini R, Muraro R, Ficari F, et al. Immunohistochemical evidence of immune responses to tumor-associated antigens in lymph nodes of colon carcinoma patients. Cancer 1991;67:2880–2886.
16. Studer UE, Scherz S, Scheidegger J, et al. Enlargement of regional lymph nodes in renal cell carcinoma is often not due to metastases. J Urol 1990;144: 243–245.
17. Tsakraklides V, Wanebo HJ, Sternberg SS, et al. Prognostic evaluation of regional lymph node morphology in colorectal cancer. Am J Surg 1975;129:174.
18. Cottier H, Turk J, Sobin L. A proposal for a standardized system of reporting human lymph node morphology in relation to immunological function. Am J Clin Pathol 1973;26:317–331.

PART IV

SECTION THREE

IATROGENIC LYMPHADENOPATHIES

Lymphadenopathies may occur in patients treated with a variety of immunomodulatory drugs. Drugs such as prednisone, azathioprine, methotrexate, cyclosporine, and others are used to diminish the symptoms of hyperimmune reactions in recipients of organ transplants and in patients with autoimmune diseases. However, treatments intended to modulate immune reactions, particularly when extended for long periods of time, have the inadvertent effect of inducing a variety of lymphoproliferative disorders (1–10). These range from benign reactive lymphadenopathies to atypical lymphoproliferative lesions to Hodgkin and non-Hodgkin lymphomas. A particular feature of such lymphoproliferations is that they may regress on cessation of treatment. In some cases, even lymphomas with demonstrated monoclonality have regressed after the discontinuation of immunomodulatory drugs.

The development of lymphadenopathy after immunomodulatory treatments, particularly methotrexate, is described in Chapter 45; the development after anticonvulsant therapy is described in Chapter 46, and after immunosuppressive treatments in the context of organ transplantation in Chapter 80.

REFERENCES

1. Nalesnik MA, Makowka L, Starzt LE. The diagnosis and treatment of posttransplant lymphoproliferative disorders. Curr Probl Surg 1988;25:376–472.
2. Ellman MH, Hurwitz H, Thomas C, et al. Lymphoma developing in a patient with rheumatoid arthritis taking low dose weekly methotrexate. J Rheumatol 1991;18:1741–1743.
3. Shiroky JB, Frost A, Skelton JE, et al. Complications of immunosuppression associated with weekly low dose methotrexate. J Rheumatol 1991;18:1172–1175.
4. Kingsmore SF, Hall BD, Allen NB, et al. Association of methotrexate, rheumatoid arthritis and lymphoma. Report of 2 cases and literature review. J Rheumatol 1992;19:1462–1465.
5. Taillan B, Garnier G, Castanet J, et al. Lymphoma developing in a patient with rheumatoid arthritis taking methotrexate. Clin Rheumatol 1993;12:93–94.
6. Kamel OW, van de Rijn M, LeBrun DP, et al. Lymphoid neoplasms in patients with rheumatoid arthritis and dermatomyositis: frequency of Epstein-Barr virus and other features associated with immunosuppression. Hum Pathol 1994;25:638–643.
7. Thomason RW, Craig FE, Banks PM, et al. Epstein-Barr virus and lymphoproliferation in methotrexate treated rheumatoid arthritis. Mod Pathol 1996;9:261–266.
8. Kamel OW, Weiss LM, van de Rijn M, et al. Hodgkin's disease and lymphoproliferations resembling Hodgkin's disease in patients receiving long-term low-dose methotrexate therapy. Am J Surg Pathol 1996;20:1279–1287.
9. Georgescu L, Quinn GC, Schwartzman S, et al. Lymphoma in patients with rheumatoid arthritis: association with the disease state or methotrexate treatment. Semin Arthritis Rheum 1997;26:794–804.
10. Kamel OW. Iatrogenic lymphoproliferative disorders in nontransplantation settings. Semin Diagn Pathol 1997;14:27–34.

45

DRUG-INDUCED LYMPHADENOPATHY

METHOTREXATE

DEFINITION

Lymphadenopathy associated with methotrexate (MTX) therapy.

PATHOGENESIS

Methotrexate, formerly known as *amethopterin,* is an antimetabolite used in the treatment of adult rheumatoid arthritis (RA), severe psoriasis, post-transplantation reactions, and certain neoplastic diseases. The drug may be highly toxic to the bone marrow, liver, and kidneys, and meticulous care is required when it is administered. However, rheumatologists use MTX in small doses for extended treatments in place of gold and azathioprine because it is faster-acting and more effective (1–3). It has been estimated that the number of annual prescriptions reaches 1.25 million; 50% to 60% of these are for patients with RA (4). The enlarged lymph nodes that develop in some patients on long-term MTX therapy may look like atypical reactive lymphadenopathy, resemble Hodgkin lymphoma or large cell immunoblastic lymphoma, or indeed be a type of lymphoma, as demonstrated by clonal immunoglobulin gene rearrangement (5,6). Virtually all these pseudolymphomas and lymphomas are of B-cell type and positive for Epstein-Barr virus (EBV), like the lymphoproliferative lesions associated with immunosuppressive treatments (6–8). Also like such lesions, the Hodgkin and non-Hodgkin lymphomas related to MTX treatment may regress spontaneously when the drug is withheld (4–6). However, immunosuppression may not be the sole cause of MTX-related lymphomas; the effect of MTX on the lymphoid system is probably complex, and RA itself is associated with lymphoproliferative lesions (see Chapter 41).

CLINICAL FEATURES

Single or multiple lymphadenopathies, usually indolent, may develop. Enlargement of cervical, axillary, inguinal, and deep-seated retroperitoneal or pelvic lymph nodes has been reported. In many cases, the enlargement regressed after MTX was discontinued, even when prednisone was not (5).

HISTOPATHOLOGY

In a recent case, effacement of the follicles and extension of the paracortical areas comprised an atypical lymphoid proliferation (Fig. 45.1). This consisted of a mixed cell population, including small and transformed lymphocytes, plasmacytoid lymphocytes, cells with large and small cleaved nuclei, and cells with large vesicular nuclei and prominent nucleoli that resembled Hodgkin cells or Reed-Sternberg cells (Fig. 45.2). In other cases, the histology more closely resembles that of Hodgkin lymphoma, particularly of the lymphocyte predominance type (Figs. 45.2 and 45.3), and in still others, the lesions cannot be distinguished from those of large cell lymphomas. In such cases, the definitive diagnosis depends on immunophenotyping and gene rearrangement analysis.

IMMUNOHISTOCHEMISTRY

In general, the Hodgkin-like and Reed-Sternberg-like cells are CD20+ (Figs. 45.4 and 45.5) and CD30+ but CD15−. In some cases, however, the Reed-Sternberg cells are CD15+, and such cases are more likely to progress and behave like Hodgkin lymphoma (5).

MOLECULAR PATHOLOGY

Southern blot analysis or polymerase chain reaction has shown some cases to be monoclonal with respect to immunoglobulin genes, thus confirming the histologic appearance of large cell lymphoma. In *situ* hybridization studies have revealed expression of EBV-encoded RNA transcripts, and immunohistochemical staining has demonstrated the pres-

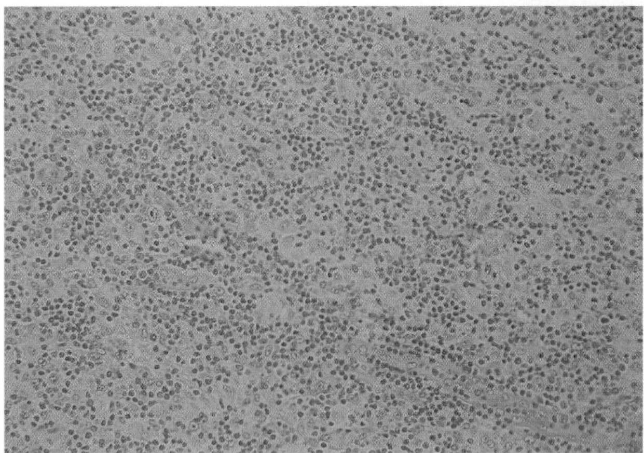

FIGURE 45.1. Systemic lymphadenopathies that developed in a 75-year-old woman after treatment for 14 years with methotrexate for rheumatoid arthritis. Altered nodal architecture with effaced follicles and expanded paracortex. Hematoxylin and eosin stain.

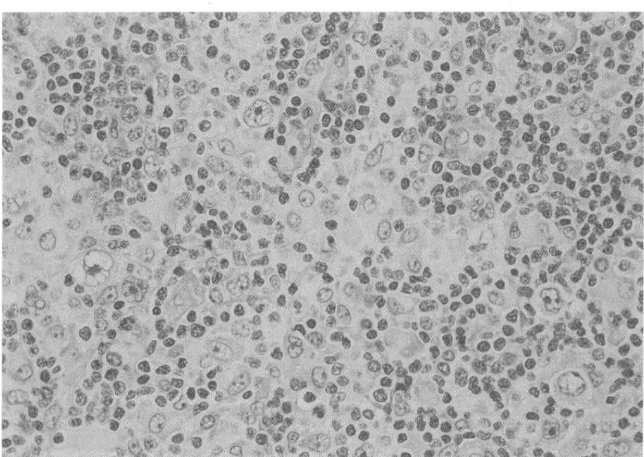

FIGURE 45.2. Same lymph node section as in Fig. 45.1. Small lymphocytes and transformed lymphocytes (immunoblasts), some with lobate vesicular nuclei and prominent nucleoli, resembling lymphocytic and histiocytic ("popcorn") cells, Hodgkin cells, and Reed-Sternberg cells. Hematoxylin and eosin stain.

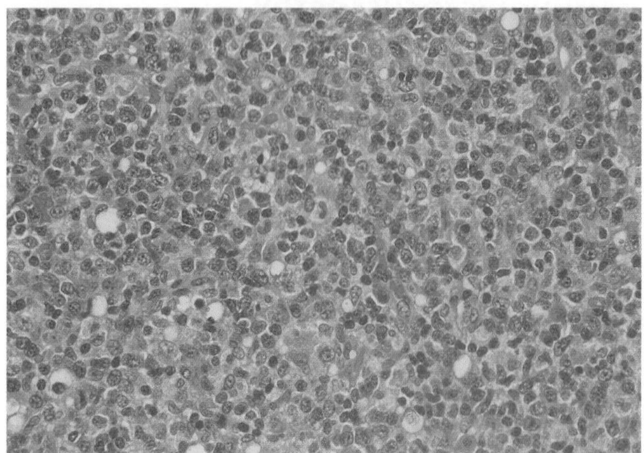

FIGURE 45.3. Methotrexate lymphadenopathy with effaced architecture and mixed cell populations comprising lymphocytes, plasmacytoid lymphocytes, and immunoblasts, some with large nuclei and prominent nucleoli, resembling Hodgkin cells. Hematoxylin, phloxine, and saffron stain.

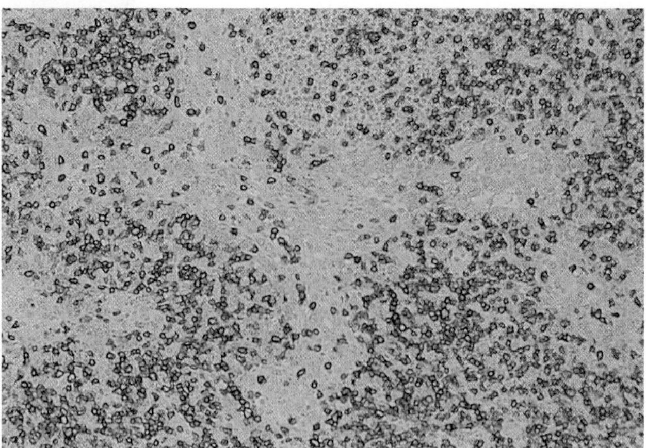

FIGURE 45.4. Small lymphocytes, but not the large, transformed lymphocytes, are immunostained for T-cell marker. Anti-CD3/peroxidase stain.

ence of latent membrane protein, usually in the Reed-Sternberg and Hodgkin cells (4–9). Thus, 33% to 41% of cases in different series have been positive for EBV (4,7). The EBV genome in the MTX-related lymphadenopathies is clonal, as in the transplantation-related lymphoproliferative disorders (9). The lymphadenopathies that regress after the cessation of MTX treatment have been mainly EBV-positive (9).

DIFFERENTIAL DIAGNOSIS

The two ends of the spectrum of lymphoproliferative lesions (i.e., benign reactive hyperplasias and lymphomas) can be identified by their usual histologic features. However, the lesions of atypical hyperplasias resembling lymphomas, often with Reed-Sternberg-like cells, may be indistinguishable without the help of immunohistochemistry and molecular analysis. In such cases, discontinuation of MTX therapy is recommended.

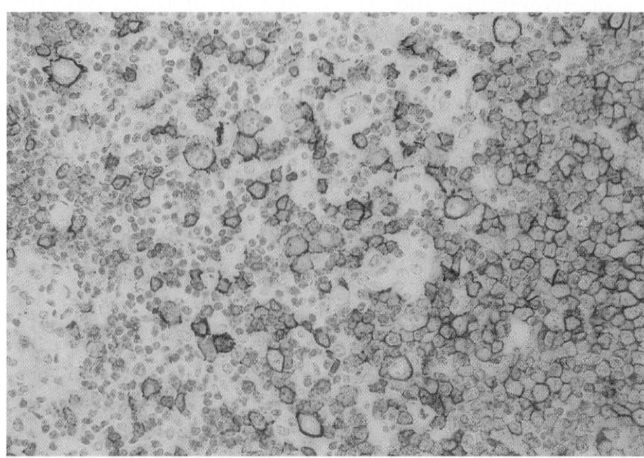

FIGURE 45.5. Large, transformed lymphocytes, including Hodgkin-like cells, are immunostained for B-cell marker CD20. L26/peroxidase stain.

Checklist

DRUG-INDUCED LYMPHADENOPATHY: METHOTREXATE

History of RA or autoimmune disease
MTX therapy
Lymphadenopathy, regional or generalized
Effacement of follicles
Mixed lymphoid population, including immunoblasts and plasmacytoid lymphocytes
Hodgkin-like, Reed-Sternberg-like cells
CD15−, CD30+, CD20+
EBV+
Regression after cessation of treatment

REFERENCES

1. Weinstein A, Marlowe S, Korn J, et al. Low-dose methotrexate treatment of rheumatoid arthritis: long-term observations. Am J Med 1985;79:331–337.
2. Weinblatt ME, Weissman BN, Holdswort DE, et al. Long-term prospective study of methotrexate in the treatment of rheumatoid arthritis: 84-month update. Arthritis Rheum 1992;35:129–137.
3. Kremer IM, Phelps CT. Long-term prospective study of the use of methotrexate in the treatment of rheumatoid arthritis: update after a mean of 90 months. Arthritis Rheum 1992;35:138–145.
4. Georgescu L, Quinn GC, Schwartzman S, et al. Lymphoma in patients with rheumatoid arthritis: association with the disease state or methotrexate treatment. Semin Arthritis Rheum 1997;26:794–804.
5. Kamel OW, Weiss LM, van de Rijn M, et al. Hodgkin's disease and lymphoproliferations resembling Hodgkin's disease in patients receiving long-term low-dose methotrexate therapy. Am J Surg Pathol 1996;20:1279–1287.
6. Thomason WR, Craig FE, Banks PM, et al. Epstein-Barr virus and lymphoproliferation in methotrexate-treated rheumatoid arthritis. Mod Pathol 1996;9:261–266.
7. Kamel OW, van de Rijn M, LeBrun DP, et al. Lymphoid neoplasms in patients with rheumatoid arthritis and dermatomyositis: frequency of Epstein-Barr virus and other features associated with immunosuppression. Hum Pathol 1994;25:638–643.
8. Ferraccioli GF, Casatta L, Bartoli E, et al. Epstein-Barr virus-associated Hodgkin's lymphoma in a rheumatoid arthritis patient treated with methotrexate and cyclosporin A [Letter]. Arthritis Rheum 1995;6:867–868.
9. Kamel OW. Iatrogenic lymphoproliferative disorders in nontransplantation settings. Semin Diagn Pathol 1997;14:27–34.

46

DRUG-INDUCED LYMPHADENOPATHY

ANTICONVULSANTS

DEFINITION

Lymphadenopathy associated with a systemic hypersensitivity reaction to arene oxide-producing anticonvulsant drugs: phenytoin (Dilantin), carbamazepine (Tegretol), and phenobarbital (1).

SYNONYMS

Anticonvulsant hypersensitivity syndrome
Carbamazepine lymphadenopathy
Dilantin lymphadenopathy
Phenytoin lymphadenopathy

PATHOGENESIS

The triad of fever, rash, and lymphadenopathy is a feature of the anticonvulsant hypersensitivity syndrome (AHS) (1). Dilantin, the commercial name of phenytoin (diphenylhydantoin), is the anticonvulsant drug most often associated with this syndrome (2), but carbamazepine (Tegretol) (3) and phenobarbital also cause AHS (1). Lymph node abnormalities usually appear early, within weeks to months, after the initiation of anticonvulsant drug therapy; these include lymphoid hyperplasia (4), a particular type of angioimmunoblastic lymphadenopathy (AILD) (5,6), immunoblastic proliferation (7), and rarely infarction (8). Dermatopathic lymphadenitis (9) is probably secondary to skin rash, and not a direct effect of the drug. In numerous "pseudolymphomas," the lymph node histology simulates malignancy, but the lymphadenopathy regresses spontaneously after the drug is withdrawn (10–12). Hodgkin lymphoma or non-Hodgkin lymphoma develops after long-term anticonvulsant therapy in rare patients (7,10,11,13). Some lymphomas appear during drug administration (13), immediately following reactive lymphadenopathy (11), or after disappearance of lymphadenopathy and a prolonged asymptomatic period (7,10). In one patient, lymphoblastic lymphoma developed after phenytoin exposure *in utero* (14). It remains controversial whether anticonvulsant exposure truly increases the risk for malignancy (7,12,15).

Siblings of patients affected with AHS are at increased risk for the development of AHS, which suggests a genetic basis (16). An allergic hypersensitivity mechanism may explain why AHS does not depend on anticonvulsant dosage or serum levels (17), and in one patient, rechallenge with a small amount of drug was fatal (18). Alternatively, toxic metabolites may be pathogenic; cytochrome P-450 metabolizes phenytoin, carbamazepine, and phenobarbital to arene oxide derivatives, which must be detoxified by epoxide hydrolase. The genetic absence or mutation of this enzyme could cause an accumulation of toxic compounds (18).

CLINICAL SYNDROME

Fever, rash, and lymphadenopathy are typical clinical features of AHS (1). Hepatitis is present to some degree in most patients, and although it is rare, liver failure is the most frequent cause of death (1). Gingival hyperplasia develops in some patients treated with long-term phenytoin; it regresses on drug withdrawal (19). Fever, skin rashes of various kinds, eosinophilia, gum hyperplasia, and lymphadenopathy usually appear weeks to months after the initiation of anticonvulsant therapy (10,20). Rashes, fever, hepatosplenomegaly, facial edema, and nausea may also accompany carbamazepine-associated lymphadenopathy (1,3,12,20). AHS laboratory findings may include hypogammaglobulinemia or hypergammaglobulinemia, eosinophilia, leukopenia, and atypical lymphocytosis (1,20). Symptoms, including lymphadenopathy, regress after anticonvulsants are discontinued, but they may reappear if the same drug is resumed. Skin lesions may mimic those of cutaneous T-cell lymphoma (21,22). A number of cases of Hodgkin lymphoma and non-Hodgkin lymphoma have developed after prolonged anticonvulsant therapy. Most authors, however, believe that the risk is very small. A much greater hazard is misclassifying a benign lymphadenopathy as a malignant lymphoma (7,19).

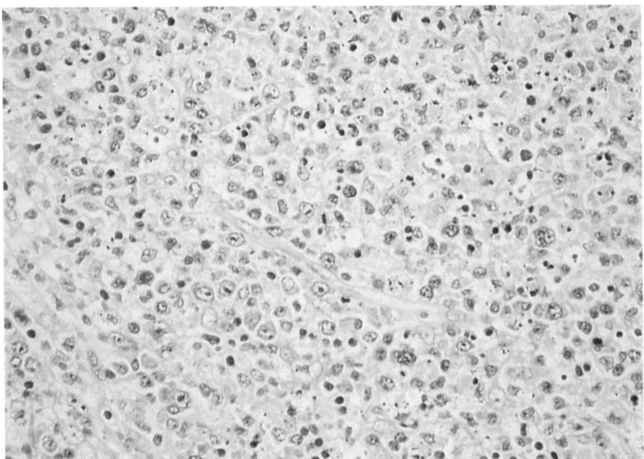

FIGURE 46.1. Phenytoin lymphadenopathy in a 29-year-old man after 11 years of treatment. Diffuse infiltrate of lymphocytes and immunoblasts, including Reed-Sternberg-like cells. Hematoxylin, phloxine, and saffron stain.

The misdiagnosis of anticonvulsant therapy-associated lymphadenopathies as AILD is also disadvantageous; despite their atypical appearance, such lymphadenopathies usually regress after treatment is discontinued, whereas non–drug-related AILD is fatal in about 75% of cases because of infectious or lymphomatous complications (23).

HISTOPATHOLOGY

The lymph nodes are markedly enlarged and show varying degrees of architectural effacement. This is caused by a diffuse, mixed cellular proliferation and scattered small foci of necrosis. The cellular infiltrates include numerous large immunoblasts with occasional nuclear atypia and frequent mitoses (Figs. 46.1 and 46.2). Eosinophils, plasma cells, and neutrophils are also present. Reed-Sternberg cells are not present; however, atypical large transformed lymphocytes with Reed-Sternberg-like nuclei may be seen. Fibrosis is minimal. Patterns of reactive follicular hyperplasia (Fig. 46.3), AILD-like changes (Fig. 46.4), and immunoblastic proliferation (Fig. 46.2) have been described (7). The lymphadenopathies associated with anticonvulsant drugs usually affect the parafollicular areas in the form of a pleomorphic hyperplasia with a predominance of activated, immunoblastic lymphocytes (19).

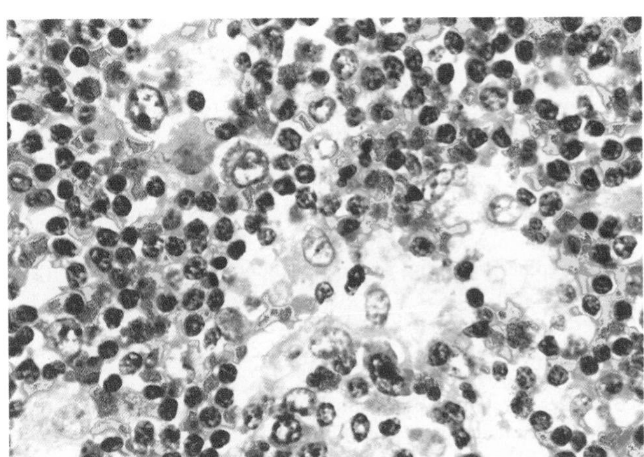

FIGURE 46.2. Phenytoin lymphadenopathy. Atypical immunoblasts with vesicular nuclei and large nucleoli. Hematoxylin and eosin stain.

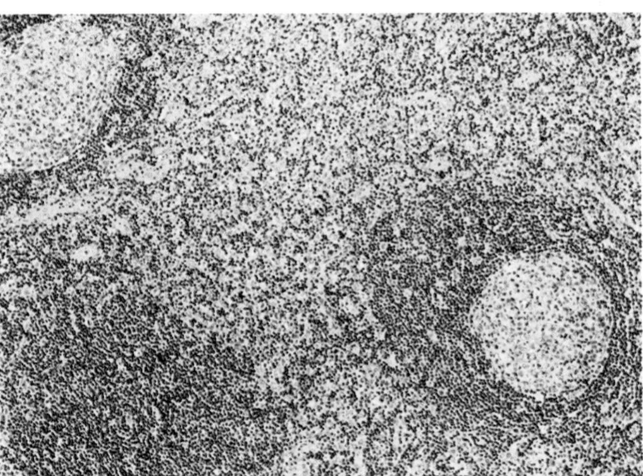

FIGURE 46.3. Phenobarbital lymphadenopathy in a 3-year-old boy treated for seizures. Reactive follicles are widely separated by an expanded paracortical T zone. Hematoxylin and eosin stain.

IMMUNOHISTOCHEMISTRY

The lymphadenopathies in which immunohistochemical studies have been performed were polyclonal. A few re-

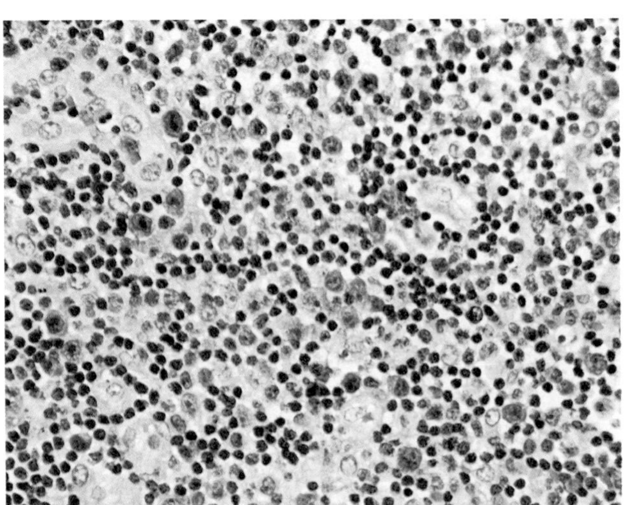

FIGURE 46.4. Same lymph node as in Fig. 46.3. Increased vascularity and scattered immunoblasts in the paracortex simulate angioimmunoblastic lymphadenopathy. Hematoxylin and eosin stain.

Checklist

LYMPHADENOPATHY ASSOCIATED WITH ANTICONVULSANT THERAPY

History of convulsive disorder and anticonvulsant treatment
Fever, skin rashes, eosinophilia
Hyperplastic gingivitis
Generalized lymphadenopathy
Effacement of follicles
Diffuse, mixed cellular infiltrates
Proliferation of immunoblasts
Eosinophils, plasma cells
Focal necrosis
Regression after cessation of treatment

ported monoclonal cases were of B-cell type, and in one case, the immunoblasts expressed T-cell markers plus activation marker CD30 (12) (Fig. 46.5). Most cases of phenytoin lymphadenopathy do not express CD30 (7), but this criterion is not completely reliable. The immunoblasts in infectious mononucleosis are usually CD30+ (24,25).

MOLECULAR DIAGNOSIS

Antigen receptor gene rearrangement studies indicate the absence of a monoclonal B-cell (26) or T-cell (27) population.

CONFIRMATORY TESTS

Regression of symptoms after cessation of anticonvulsant therapy confirms the diagnosis.

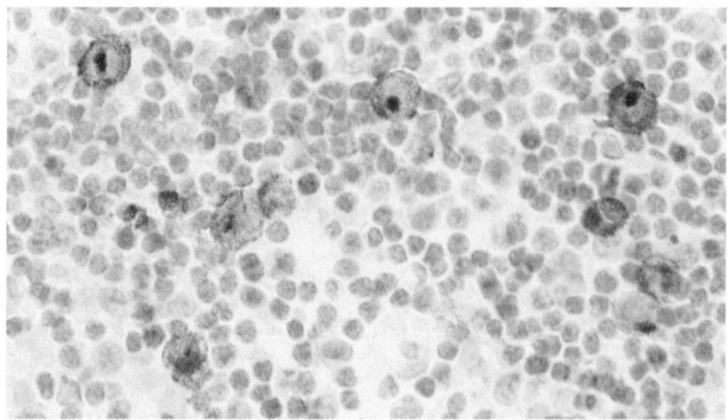

FIGURE 46.5. Same lymph node as in Figs. 46.3 and 46.4. Scattered immunoblasts express CD30 (Ki-1) in a dotlike and membrane distribution. Immunoperoxidase stain.

DIFFERENTIAL DIAGNOSIS

- Viral lymphadenitides, such as infectious mononucleosis, have a starry sky pattern with marked activity of germinal centers and no eosinophils. Occasionally, the two lesions may be indistinguishable. CD30 expression is usually present in infectious mononucleosis but absent in phenytoin lymphadenopathy.
- AILD may be indistinguishable because its pathogenesis is not clearly defined and it can also be drug-induced.
- Hodgkin lymphoma may appear similar, in which case the diagnosis must be confirmed by using strict criteria for the identification of Reed-Sternberg cells.
- Ki-1 anaplastic large cell lymphoma exhibits aggregates of highly atypical immunoblasts, often in a sinusoidal distribution.

REFERENCES

1. Vittorio CC, Muglia JJ. Anticonvulsant hypersensitivity syndrome. Arch Intern Med 1995;155:2285–2290.
2. Powers NG, Carson SH. Idiosyncratic reactions to phenytoin. Clin Pediatr (Phila) 1987;26:120–124.
3. De Vriese AS, Philippe J, Van Renterghem DM, et al. Carbamazepine hypersensitivity syndrome: report of 4 cases and review of the literature. Medicine (Baltimore) 1995;74:144–151.
4. Yates P, Stockdill G, McIntyre M. Hypersensitivity to carbamazepine presenting as pseudolymphoma. J Clin Pathol 1986; 39:1224–1228.
5. Frizzera G, Moran EM, Rappaport H. Angio-immunoblastic lymphadenopathy. Diagnosis and clinical course. Am J Med 1975;59:803–818.
6. Lukes RJ, Tindle BH. Immunoblastic lymphadenopathy. A hyperimmune entity resembling Hodgkin's disease. N Engl J Med 1975;292:1–8.
7. Abbondazo SL, Irey NS, Frizzera G. Dilantin-associated lymphadenopathy. Spectrum of histopathologic patterns. Am J Surg Pathol 1995;19:675–686.

8. Harris NL, Widder DJ. Phenytoin and generalized lymphadenopathy [Letter]. Arch Pathol Lab Med 1983;107: 663–664.
9. Severson GS, Harrington DS, Burnett DA, et al. Dermatopathic lymphadenopathy associated with carbamazepine: a case mimicking a lymphoid malignancy [Letter]. Am J Med 1987;83: 597–599.
10. Saltzstein SL, Ackerman LV. Lymphadenopathy induced by anticonvulsant drugs mimicking clinically and pathologically malignant lymphomas. Cancer 1959;12:164–182.
11. Gams RA, Neal JA, Conrad FG. Hydantoin-induced pseudopseudolymphoma. Ann Intern Med 1968;69:557–568.
12. Katzin WE, Julius CJ, Tubbs RR, et al. Lymphoproliferative disorders associated with carbamazepine. Arch Pathol Lab Med 1990;114:1244–1248.
13. Hyman GA, Sommers SC. The development of Hodgkin's disease and lymphoma during anticonvulsant therapy. Blood 1966;28:416–427.
14. Murray JC, Hill RM, Hegemier S, et al. Lymphoblastic lymphoma following prenatal exposure to phenytoin. J Pediatr Hematol Oncol 1996;18:241–243.
15. Li FP, Willard DR, Goodman R, et al. Malignant lymphoma after diphenylhydantoin (Dilantin) therapy. Cancer 1975;36: 1359–1362.
16. Gennis MA, Vemuri R, Burns EA, et al. Familial occurrence of hypersensitivity to phenytoin. Am J Med 1991;91:631–634.
17. Silverman AK, Fairley J, Wong RC. Cutaneous and immunologic reactions to phenytoin. J Am Acad Dermatol 1988;18:721–741.
18. Schmidt D, Kluge W. Fatal toxic epidermal necrolysis following reexposure to phenytoin: a case report. Epilepsia 1983;24: 440–443.
19. Symmers WS. Bribery. Pathol Annu 1984;19:347–358.
20. Segal GH, Clough JD, Tubbs RR. Autoimmune and iatrogenic causes of lymphadenopathy. Semin Oncol 1993;20:611–626.
21. Rijlaarsdam U, Scheffer E, Meijer CJ, et al. Mycosis fungoides-like lesions associated with phenytoin and carbamazepine therapy. J Am Acad Dermatol 1991;24:216–220.
22. Sakai C, Takagi T, Oguro M, et al. Erythroderma and marked atypical lymphocytosis mimicking cutaneous T-cell lymphoma probably caused by phenobarbital. Intern Med 1993;32: 182–184.
23. Steinberg AD, Seldin MF, Jaffe ES, et al. NIH conference. Angioimmunoblastic lymphadenopathy with dysproteinemia. Ann Intern Med 1988;108:575–584.
24. Abbondanzo SL, Sato N, Straus SE, et al. Acute infectious mononucleosis. CD30 (Ki-1) antigen expression and histologic correlations [see Comments]. Am J Clin Pathol 1990;93: 698–702.
25. Segal GH, Kjeldsberg CR, Smith GP, et al. CD30 antigen expression in florid immunoblastic proliferations. A clinicopathologic study of 14 cases. Am J Clin Pathol 1994;102:292–298.
26. Jeng YM, Tien HF, Su IJ. Phenytoin-induced pseudolymphoma: reevaluation using modern molecular biology techniques. Epilepsia 1996;37:104–107.
27. Braddock SW, Harrington D, Vose J. Generalized nodular cutaneous pseudolymphoma associated with phenytoin therapy. Use of T-cell receptor gene rearrangement in diagnosis and clinical review of cutaneous reactions to phenytoin. J Am Acad Dermatol 1992;27:337–340.

PART IV

SECTION FOUR

VASCULAR LYMPHADENOPATHIES

A variety of vascular disorders may affect the lymph nodes, resulting in ischemic infarction, benign vascular proliferations, or malignant vascular neoplasms.

Lymph nodes are well vascularized, and therefore ischemic infarction is uncommon. Occasional obstruction of blood flow may occur in the case of compression by tumor, vascular embolization and thrombosis, or surgical intervention in the region (see Chapter 47).

Non-neoplastic angiomatosis in lymph nodes arising in the high endothelial venules of the paracortex is a characteristic feature of angioimmunoblastic lymphadenopathy (see Chapter 74), Castleman lymphadenopathy (see Chapter 43), Kimura lymphadenopathy (see Chapter 36), HIV lymphadenitis, type C (see Chapter 15), and others. Bacillary angiomatosis, a tumor-like proliferation of capillaries and arterioles, is caused by a microorganism named *Bartonella henselae* (see Chapter 19). A peculiar process of lymph node angiomatosis is the vascular transformation of sinuses in which the vasoproliferative process selectively involves the nodal sinuses, expanding through subcapsular, intermediate, and medullary sinuses without involvement of the lymphoid parenchyma or the lymph node capsule (see Chapter 48). Some of these conditions may be related to the release of angiogenesis factors by activated lymphoid cells. The importance of vascular lymphadenopathies is that they can be confused with the vascular neoplasms of lymph nodes (see Chapters 84 and 85).

47

LYMPH NODE INFARCTION

DEFINITION

Massive necrosis of coagulative type involving most of the nodal parenchyma and sparing only a narrow subcapsular rim.

PATHOGENESIS

Because of their abundant vascularity and well-developed anastomoses, lymph nodes are rarely infarcted (1). Only a limited number of cases are recorded in the literature (2,3). In most of these, occlusive vascular thrombosis affected hilar or intranodal veins. Both superficial and deep-seated lymph nodes may be involved (4,5). The five patients reported in one study (1) were middle-aged; two had a history of vascular disease, and three had undergone recent surgery in the area drained by the infarcted lymph nodes. In all cases, thrombosis of intranodal and hilar veins was noted. Thrombophlebitis and vascular surgery in the region of the affected nodes has occasionally been mentioned, as has local trauma caused by fine needle aspiration biopsy of lymph nodes (6,7). Cases have also been reported in which lymph node infarction was accompanied by acute febrile disease of unknown origin. The patients were young, and the appearance was that of an acute viral infection with spontaneous recovery (4). However, such cases may represent necrotizing lymphadenopathy or Kikuchi disease (see Chapter 38) rather than lymph node infarction (8). The most common cause of massive lymph node infarction is involvement by tumor, either primary lymphoma or metastatic carcinoma. In a series of cases reported from the M.D. Anderson Cancer Center (6,9), malignant tumor was present at the site or elsewhere in about 30% of cases in one series and in as many as 81% of cases (13 of 16) when the patients underwent biopsy from 2 days to 6 months later. Thus, a massively infarcted lymph node should always raise the suspicion of underlying lymphoma.

In the largest published study of lymph node infarction, 51 cases were collected from medical centers in Europe and America during a 30-year period (10). Of these, 20 were associated with lymphoma at the time of infarction or during the following 2 years. After the interval of 2 years, the outcome was excellent, which perhaps indicates that lymphoma was present although not yet diagnosed at the time of infarction (10). Lymphomas and metastatic tumors probably cause infarction by vascular thrombosis or tumor expansion with impairment of vascular flow in small arteries and veins. The remaining 31 cases were not associated with lymphoma, and the cause of infarction was not always apparent. The type of coagulative necrosis indicates the ischemic nature of necrosis. Among the causes other than lymphoma suggested by various studies are viral infections, drug reactions, systemic lupus, local mechanical pressure, and particularly vascular thrombosis. In superficial lymph nodes, the major arteries and veins enter the node through the hilar region. This vascular distribution may explain the sparing of the subcapsular lymphoid tissues in lymph node infarction (1,10). In contrast, in deep lymph nodes, which lack a hilum, necrosis is more extensive (5,10).

CLINICAL SYNDROME

Clinically, it is very difficult to distinguish between lymph node infarction and lymphoma (10). Persons of either sex and a wide range of ages may be affected in both conditions, and fever and local pain may accompany both. Because lymphoma may be associated with the infarction of an entire lymph node as well as other lymph nodes, additional lymph nodes must be obtained to rule out the possibility of simultaneous malignancy (10). Furthermore, because lymphoma is so often diagnosed subsequently, follow-up of patients with lymph node infarction for the first 2 years is advisable (10).

HISTOPATHOLOGY

The involved lymph nodes show massive ischemic infarction; usually, only a narrow peripheral rim of cortical tissue is spared (Fig. 47.1). Almost the entire nodal parenchyma is necrotic and strongly eosinophilic, and ghosts of lymphocytes, often lymphoma cells (Fig. 47.2), and of other tissue components are seen. However, the reticulin network is pre-

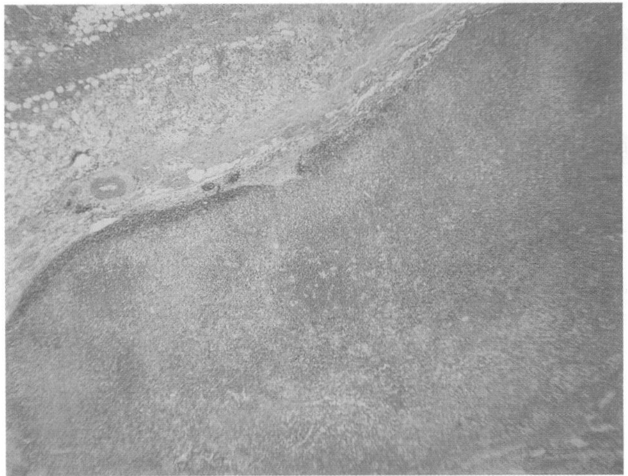

FIGURE 47.1. Infarcted lymph node with narrow rim of subcapsular preserved lymphocytes surrounding massive necrosis of nodal parenchyma. Hematoxylin, phloxine, and saffron stain.

served, as shown by silver staining. In general, the subtotal type of necrosis occurs in superficial lymph nodes (axillary, inguinal), whereas extensive necrosis more often occurs in deep lymph nodes (mesenteric) (10) (Fig. 47.3). In a region marginal to the necrotic nodal tissues, in the perinodal fibroadipose tissues, an abundant inflammatory exudate composed of fibrin and polymorphonuclear leukocytes is usually seen. This early, acute inflammatory reaction gradually changes to a chronic inflammatory infiltrate in which lymphocytes are the predominant cell type. By the third week, a zone of granulation tissue containing numerous newly formed capillaries is closely apposed to the necrotic tissues (Fig. 47.4). Thus, the sequence of inflammatory events is remarkably similar in both morphology and timing to that in myocardial infarction (1).

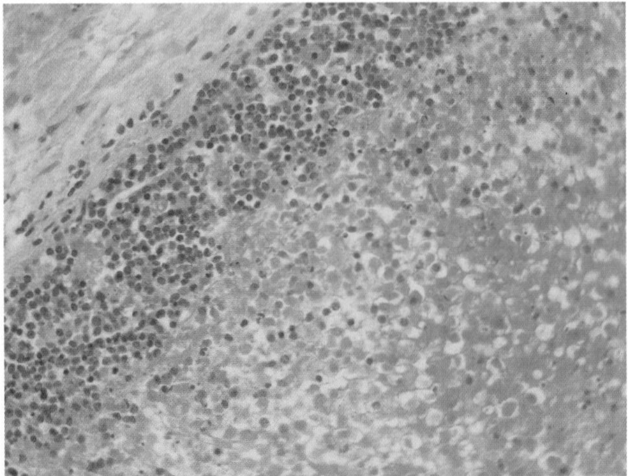

FIGURE 47.2. Same lymph node as in Fig. 47.1. Capsule (*upper left*), preserved lymphocytes in subcapsular area, and tissue necrosis with ghost cells (*right*). Hematoxylin, phloxine, and saffron stain.

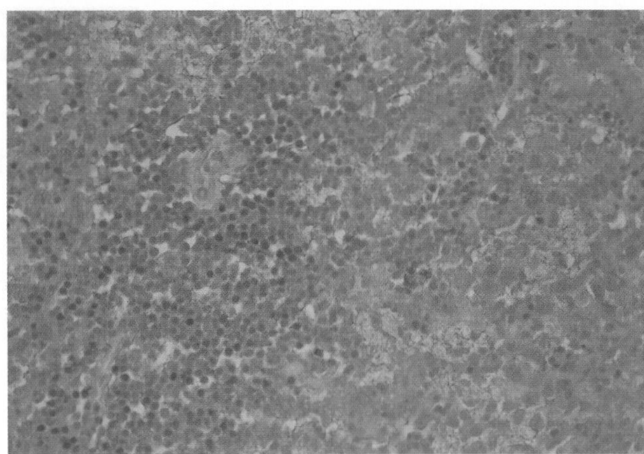

FIGURE 47.3. Infarcted mesenteric lymph node with small B-cell lymphoma. Ghost cells and few remaining viable cells. Hematoxylin, phloxine, and saffron stain.

Months after infarction, regeneration may take place, probably as a consequence of the initial preservation of the reticulin network and the rich nodal vascularization. The recolonization of the infarcted lymph node derives from the peripheral rim of lymphoid cells that remains unaffected because of the abundant anastomotic vasculature of the lymph node capsule. Thrombi, fresh or in various stages of organization and recanalization, are present in veins of the lymph node hilus, capsule, or parenchyma. The arteries are usually patent, and the nerves may show wallerian degeneration.

IMMUNOHISTOCHEMISTRY

Immunostaining of both necrotic tissues and viable tissues of the infarcted lymph nodes yields similar results. When a panel of T cell- and B cell-associated antibodies was used on

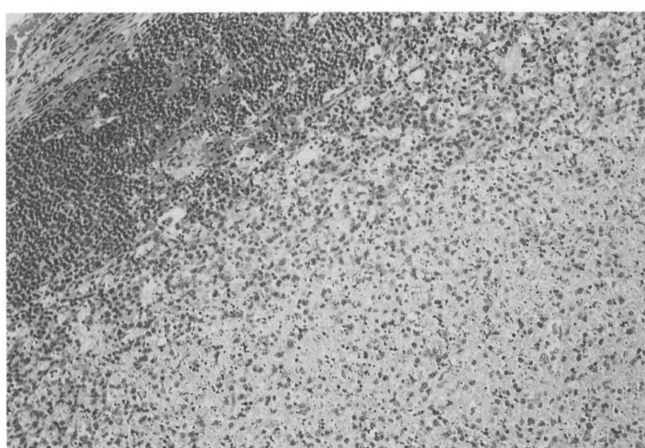

FIGURE 47.4. Axillary lymph node infarction of unknown cause. Newly formed vessels in the peripheral rim of preserved lymphocytes (*upper left*). Hematoxylin, phloxine, and saffron stain.

Checklist

LYMPH NODE INFARCTION

Massive ischemic necrosis, subtotal in superficial lymph nodes, more extensive in deep lymph nodes
Peripheral rim of spared lymphoid tissue
Ghostlike necrotic lymphocytes or lymphoma cells
Preservation of reticulin network
Marginal inflammatory infiltrates
Thrombosis of hilar or intranodal vessels
Necrotizing tissues reactive in immunohistochemical and molecular analysis

paraffin-embedded sections, the necrotic tissues were specifically stained, indicating the feasibility of immunohistochemical studies of infarcted tissues for diagnostic purposes (11). Thus, acid-fast and silver stainings may be applied to detect bacteria, and monoclonal antibodies for the immunohistochemical identification of lymphoma.

GENE REARRANGEMENTS

DNA extracted from necrotic infarcted tissues was used to demonstrate clonal immunoglobulin gene rearrangements by Southern blot hybridization in a case in which extensive tissue necrosis made morphologic diagnosis very difficult (12). Both immunohistochemistry and DNA hybridization can be used as auxiliary techniques when a diagnosis of lymphoma is suspected in an infarcted lymph node.

DIFFERENTIAL DIAGNOSIS

- Necrotizing lymphadenitis of Kikuchi and Fujimoto is characterized by patchy necrosis, partially preserved architecture, and an absence of granulocytes. It is more common in Asians and young women.
- Necrotizing granulomatous lesions of tuberculosis, leprosy, lymphogranuloma venereum, and cat-scratch disease can be distinguished by the presence of epithelioid cells surrounding the foci of necrosis and the identification of specific microorganisms by special stainings.
- Necrotic areas of syphilis are accompanied by a proliferation of epithelioid cells and by lesions of vasculitis with perivascular cuffs of plasma cells.
- Necrotic foci in hypersensitivity reactions are surrounded by cellular infiltrates that include eosinophils and plasma cells.
- Malignant Hodgkin and non-Hodgkin lymphomas can be diagnosed in infarction-free areas. When the tumor necrosis is extensive and complete, the diagnosis is difficult and relies on the size and disposition of the residual ghostlike cells. Examining additional sections and levels, in addition to reticulin staining, may be helpful in such cases (6).

REFERENCES

1. Davies JD, Stansfeld AG. Spontaneous infarction of superficial lymph nodes. J Clin Pathol 1972;25:689–696.
2. Elie H, Joubert B, Mandard JC. Infarctus ischémique spontané massif d'un ganglion lymphatique cervical. Ann Pathol 1982; 2:240–242.
3. Kiesler J, Dirschmid K. Der Lymphknoteninfarkt. Pathologe 1984;5:33–36.
4. Benisch BM, Howard RG. Lymph node infarction in two young men. Am J Clin Pathol 1975;63:818–823.
5. Watts IC, Sebek BA, McHenry MC, et al. Idiopathic infarction of intraabdominal lymph nodes. Am J Clin Pathol 1980;74: 687–690.
6. Davies JD. Lymph node infarction. In: Stansfeld AG, ed. Lymph node biopsy interpretation. New York: Churchill Livingstone, 1985:144–147.
7. Davies JD, Webb AJ. Segmental lymph-node infarction following fine-needle aspiration. J Clin Pathol 1982;35:855–857.
8. Turner RR, Martin J, Dorfman FR. Necrotizing lymphadenitis. Am J Sur Pathol 1983;7:115–123.
9. Cleary KR, Osborne BM, Butler JJ. Lymph node infarction foreshadowing malignant lymphoma. Am J Surg Pathol 1982;6: 435–442.
10. Maurer R, Schmid U, Davies JD, et al. Lymph-node infarction and malignant lymphoma: a multicentre survey of European, English and American cases. Histopathology 1986;10:571–588.
11. Norton AJ, Ramsay AD, Isaacson PG. Antigen preservation in infarcted lymphoid tissue. A novel approach to the infarcted lymph node using monoclonal antibodies effective in routinely processed tissues. Am J Surg Pathol 1988;12:759–767.
12. Laszewski MJ, Belding PJ, Feddersen RM, et al. Clonal immunoglobulin gene rearrangement in the infarcted lymph node syndrome. Am J Clin Pathol 1991;96:116–120.

48

VASCULAR TRANSFORMATION OF SINUSES

DEFINITION

Benign vascular proliferation of lymph nodes with characteristic sinus distribution.

PATHOGENESIS

Vascular transformation of sinuses (VTS) is a rare condition in which the vasoproliferative process is restricted to the lymph node sinuses and does not involve the parenchyma, capsule, or perinodal fibroadipose tissues (1–5). In the original description, the cause of VTS was believed to be thrombosis of the perinodal veins, which had been identified in all three cases (1). In experiments in rabbits, VTS was reproduced by occluding efferent lymphatics and veins (6). Lymphatic or venous obstructions, sometimes at more distal sites, caused by a variety of conditions—tumors, congestive heart failure, thrombosis of major vessels, surgical procedures, and radiotherapy—were identified in other reports and in a survey of 76 cases (4,5,7). Despite this frequent association, vascular obstruction alone may not explain the exuberant proliferation of vessels within the lymph node sinuses, which occurred in some cases in lymph nodes draining cancer or hemangioma without vascular occlusion (8). It has been suggested that angiogenesis factors released by activated lymphoid cells under conditions not fully understood may induce the proliferation of blood vessels in the lymph node sinuses (5,8). Other types of benign vascular proliferation in lymph nodes have been described under the names of *nodal angiomatosis* (9,10) and *hemangiomatoid lesion* (11), and in association with infectious processes such as toxoplasmosis (12), HIV infection (13,14), and bacillary angiomatosis (15). Some of these entities are poorly defined, and differentiating between them and Kaposi sarcoma (KS) remains difficult because of overlapping histologic patterns and poorly understood mechanisms of vascular proliferation.

CLINICAL SYNDROME

In most cases, VTS, like other vascular proliferations of lymph nodes, is an incidental finding in lymph nodes excised during tumor surgery. Occasionally, such lymph nodes are moderately enlarged, and so biopsy specimens are obtained for microscopic diagnosis. The age and sex of patients were about evenly distributed in a review of a large series of cases (5). Lymph nodes at any location may be affected (8). By itself, the vascular transformation of lymph nodes causes no ill effect; however, differentiating it from malignant vascular tumors of lymph nodes, such as KS and angiosarcoma, is of great importance.

HISTOPATHOLOGY

The subcapsular, intermediate, and medullary sinuses are distended and filled with proliferating blood vessels that form an anastomosing network of small vascular channels lined by hyperplastic endothelial cells (1) (Figs. 48.1–48.3). The changes occur in the marginal sinuses or in all the sinuses, sometimes even affecting the afferent and efferent lymphatics (8). Although the lymphoid follicles and paracortex are not directly involved, the expanding sinuses compress and diminish the parenchyma, markedly altering the lymph node architecture (Figs. 48.4 and 48.5). An important feature is the lack of capsular involvement (Fig. 48.3), which helps to differentiate VTS from KS (5). The authors of a study of 76 cases of VTS described four histologic patterns: (a) cleftlike spaces lined by flat endothelial cells; (b) rounded vascular spaces engorged with blood and lined by plump endothelial cells; (c) solid, composed of spindle and plump cells; and (d) plexiform, with intercommunicating vascular channels (5). All are associated with varying numbers of extravasated erythrocytes, deposits of hemosiderin, partial thrombosis, and fibrosis. Nodal angiomatosis, an entity described earlier (9) and considered by some authors to be no different from VTS (5), was indeed presented in similar terms, including endothelium-lined channels and slitlike and round vascular lumina. The sparing of lymphoid follicles was also noted, but the selective sinus involvement of VTS was not mentioned (9).

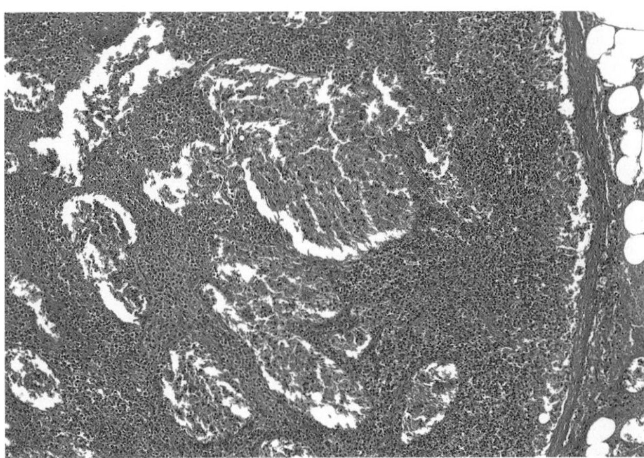

FIGURE 48.1. Vascular transformation of sinuses in cervical lymph node of patient with carcinoma of parotid gland. Marginal, cortical, and medullary sinuses are greatly distended and filled with blood. No metastatic tumor in the lymph node. Hematoxylin, phloxine, and saffron stain.

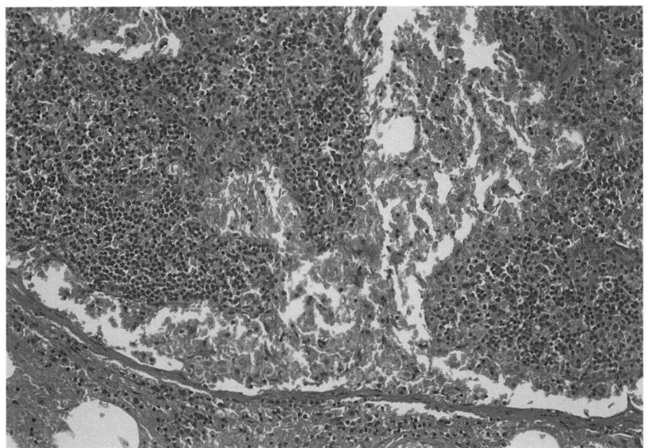

FIGURE 48.2. Same lymph node as in Fig. 48.1. Marginal and cortical sinuses show vascular transformation and congestion. Hematoxylin, phloxine, and saffron stain.

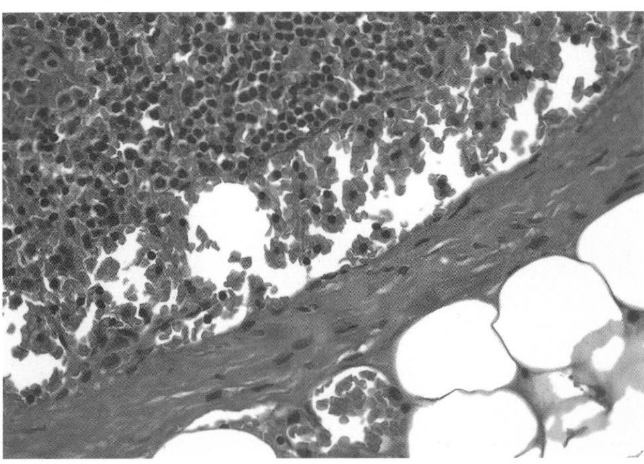

FIGURE 48.3. Small, endothelium-lined vascular spaces have formed within the distended marginal sinus. The capsule is not involved. Hematoxylin, phloxine, and saffron stain.

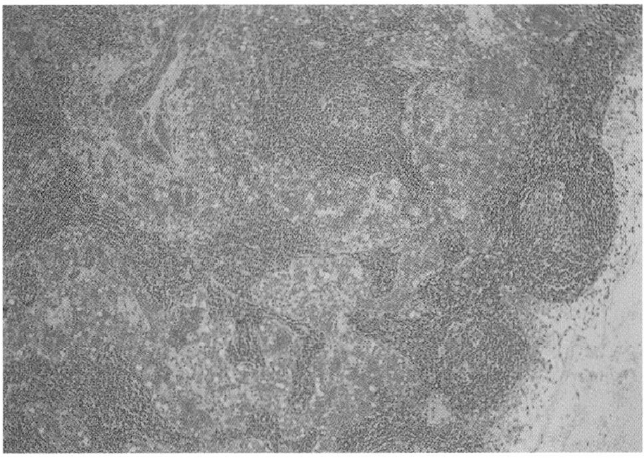

FIGURE 48.4. Vascular transformation of sinuses in axillary lymph nodes. Sinuses greatly distended and filled with blood; lymphoid follicles with reactive germinal centers not affected. Hematoxylin, phloxine, and saffron stain.

DIFFERENTIAL DIAGNOSIS

- KS, the most important entity to separate from the various benign vascular proliferations in lymph nodes, has many histologic features in common, so the distinction is particularly difficult. The morphologic characteristics of malignancy, such as nuclear atypia, an increased number of mitoses, and the predominance of spindle cells over vascular structures proposed by some authors (3,4,10), are not particularly useful because they are frequently lacking in KS. More reliable differential features seem to be a random distribution and capsular involvement in KS, which are not seen in VTS. Hyaline globules that stain with periodic acid–Schiff are common in KS but do not occur in VTS (8).

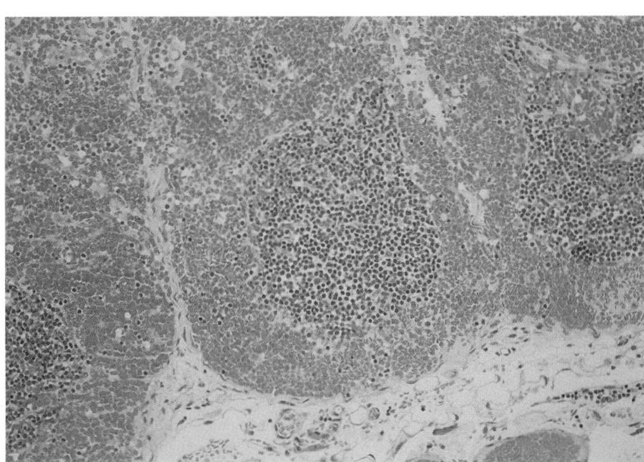

FIGURE 48.5. Same lymph node as in Fig. 48.4. Lymphoid parenchyma atrophied by compression. No hemorrhages are seen, blood being contained in the distended sinuses. Hematoxylin, phloxine, and saffron stain.

Checklist

VASCULAR TRANSFORMATION OF SINUSES

Vascular proliferation within lymph node sinuses
Association with vascular obstruction
Cleftlike, rounded, solid, and plexiform patterns
Erythrocyte extravasation
Fibrosis
No nuclear atypia
No frequent mitoses
No capsular involvement

- Bacillary angiomatosis has capillary nodules that are randomly distributed and lacks fibrosis. Warthin-Starry stain shows bacillary organisms.
- Hemangioma and hemangioendothelioma have aggregates of vessels of various types in well-circumscribed nodules that replace the nodal parenchyma. No sinus pattern is seen. Medullary or hilar sites are more likely.
- Angiosarcoma is invasive, replacing the lymph node parenchyma, and the cells exhibit nuclear atypia and frequent mitoses.

REFERENCES

1. Haferkamp O, Rosenau W, Lennert K, et al. Vascular transformation of lymph node sinuses due to venous obstruction. Arch Pathol 1971;92:81–83.
2. Maurer R, Schmid U, Davies ID, et al. Lymph node infarction and malignant lymphoma: a multicenter survey of European, English and American cases. Histopathology 1986;10:571–588.
3. Michal M, Koza V. Vascular transformation of lymph node sinuses—a diagnostic pitfall: histopathologic and immunohistochemical study. Pathol Res Pract 1989;185:441–444.
4. Ostrowski ML, Siddiqui T, Barnes RE, et al. Vascular transformation of lymph node sinuses, a process displaying a spectrum of histologic features. Arch Pathol Lab Med 1990;114:656–660.
5. Chan JKC, Warnke RA, Dorfman RF. Vascular transformation of sinuses in lymph nodes. A study of its morphological spectrum and distinction from Kaposi's sarcoma. Am J Surg Pathol 1991; 15:732–743.
6. Steinman G, Foldi E, Foldi M, et al. Morphologic findings in lymph nodes after occlusion of their efferent lymphatic vessels and veins. Lab Invest 1982;47:43.
7. Scherrer C, Maurer R. La transformation vasculaire sinusienne du ganglion lymphatique: analyse morphologique et immunohistochimique de six cas. Ann Pathol (Paris) 1985;5:231–238.
8. Tsang WYW, Chang JKC, Dorfman RF, et al. Vasoproliferative lesions of the lymph node. Pathol Annu 1994;29:63–133.
9. Fayemi AO, Toker C. Nodal angiomatosis. Arch Pathol 1975;99: 170–172.
10. Bedrosian SA, Goldman RL. Nodal angiomatosis: relationship to vascular transformation of lymph nodes [Letter]. Arch Pathol Lab Med 1984;108:864–865.
11. Lott MF, Davies JD. Lymph node hypervascularity: hemangiomatoid lesions and pan-nodal vasodilatation. J Pathol 1983; 140:209–219.
12. Rousselet M-C, Saint-André J-P, Beaufils J-M, et al. Benign vascular proliferation in a lymph node following acute toxoplasmosis. A differential diagnosis from Kaposi's sarcoma. Arch Pathol Lab Med 1988;112:1264–1266.
13. Tenner-Racz K, Kruse R, Schmidt H, et al. Vascular sinus transformation in AIDS: a pathologic condition of lymph nodes resembling Kaposi's sarcoma. Ann Pathol 1988;58:92A.
14. Ioachim HL, Cronin W, Roy M, et al. Persistent lymphadenitis in individuals at high risk for HIV infection: clinicopathologic correlations and long-term follow-up in 79 cases. Am J Clin Pathol 1990;93:208–218.
15. Chan JKC, Lewin KJ, Lombard CM, et al. Histopathology of bacillary angiomatosis of lymph node. Am J Surg Pathol 1991;15: 430–437.

PART IV

SECTION FIVE

FOREIGN BODY LYMPHADENOPATHIES

A variety of substances of endogenous and exogenous origin, when carried to the regional lymph nodes, trigger cellular reactions. The histiocytes, cells endowed with phagocytic ability, are the main reactants against such foreign bodies. They transform into macrophages, epithelioid cells, and multinucleated giant cells in an effort to segregate, phagocytose, digest, and dissolve the foreign materials. Because these arrive through the lymph node sinuses, the foreign body lymphadenopathies generally display a histologic sinus pattern, particularly involving the subcapsular sinus. The foreign substances drained by the lymph nodes may be of endogenous origin (e.g., proteins and lipids) or exogenous origin (frequently iatrogenic, a result of specific treatment modalities). The more common foreign body lymphadenopathies are further described.

49

PROTEINACEOUS LYMPHADENOPATHY

DEFINITION

Enlarged lymph node with partial or total replacement of normal architecture by deposits of acellular amorphous material with the characteristic features of amyloid or of other proteinaceous substances.

SYNONYM

Amyloid lymphadenopathy

PATHOGENESIS

The prevalence of lymph node involvement in primary or secondary amyloidosis is estimated at 17% to 37% of cases (1,2); however, very rarely is amyloid lymphadenopathy the major or only organ presentation (2–5). Among 40,000 lymph node biopsies recorded in the Lymph Node Registry in Kiel, amyloid lymphadenopathy was the presenting feature in only 10 (6).

Amyloid appears to be deposited in lymph nodes independently of its distribution in other tissues; conversely, lymph nodes draining organs heavily affected by amyloidosis may be entirely unaffected (7). More often than amyloid, other proteinaceous substances, representing different by-products of abnormal immune reactions, may be deposited in the lymph nodes during the course of various diseases (5,8), including immunoblastic lymphadenopathy (9), nodular (follicular) lymphoma (8,10), and Hodgkin disease (11). Such substances may be related to amyloid, but they differ from it histologically and ultrastructurally (5). The morphologic alterations of the involved lymph nodes are similar, regardless of the nature of the deposited substance, which cannot be ascertained under the light microscope without special stainings. Almost all cases reported have immunoglobulin (Ig) abnormalities, generally hypergammaglobulinemia with elevated levels of IgM or IgA (5,8). Amyloid appears fibrillar on electron microscopy and exhibits a β-pleated sheet structure on roentgenographic diffraction, which determines its characteristic staining and optical features (12,13). Thus, amyloid binds Congo red and shows green birefringence under polarized light when stained with Congo red (14). Among the proteins that form β-pleated sheets, those derived from Ig light chains are designated *AL*. The two isotypes of AL, λ and κ, are designated *Aλ* and *Aκ*, respectively (13). Within the AL groups, light chains of the λ class are more often associated with amyloid than light chains of the κ class (15). A second group is characterized by amyloid fibril protein AA and is associated with reactive or secondary amyloidosis (16).

CLINICAL SYNDROME

In 90% of cases of primary amyloidosis, a monoclonal M protein is present in serum, urine, or cerebrospinal fluid (17). In 20% of patients with AL amyloidosis, an association with multiple myeloma is noted (17). The identification of AL protein in the amyloid of a lymph node indicates the presence of plasma cell dyscrasia with amyloidosis, idiopathic amyloidosis, or a lymphoproliferative neoplasm. For such patients, further investigation would include bone marrow examination, investigation of light chains in the urine, and serum protein studies (16). The identification of AA protein in a proteinaceous lymphadenopathy suggests reactive systemic amyloidosis, which may be associated with various conditions, including rheumatoid arthritis, ankylosing spondylitis, Crohn disease, tuberculosis, osteomyelitis, leprosy, and neoplasia (16). In 22% (10 of 44) of uremic patients with lymphadenopathy, lymph node amyloid deposits, usually type AA, were found in vascular, follicular, or diffuse patterns (18). AL amyloid can cause abrupt hemorrhagic lymph node swelling that is followed by incomplete waning (19).

HISTOPATHOLOGY

The involved lymph nodes are moderately enlarged. The architecture is regionally obliterated, with occasional well-preserved areas. Masses of acellular, amorphous, and eosinophilic material replace most of the nodal tissues (Figs. 49.1 and

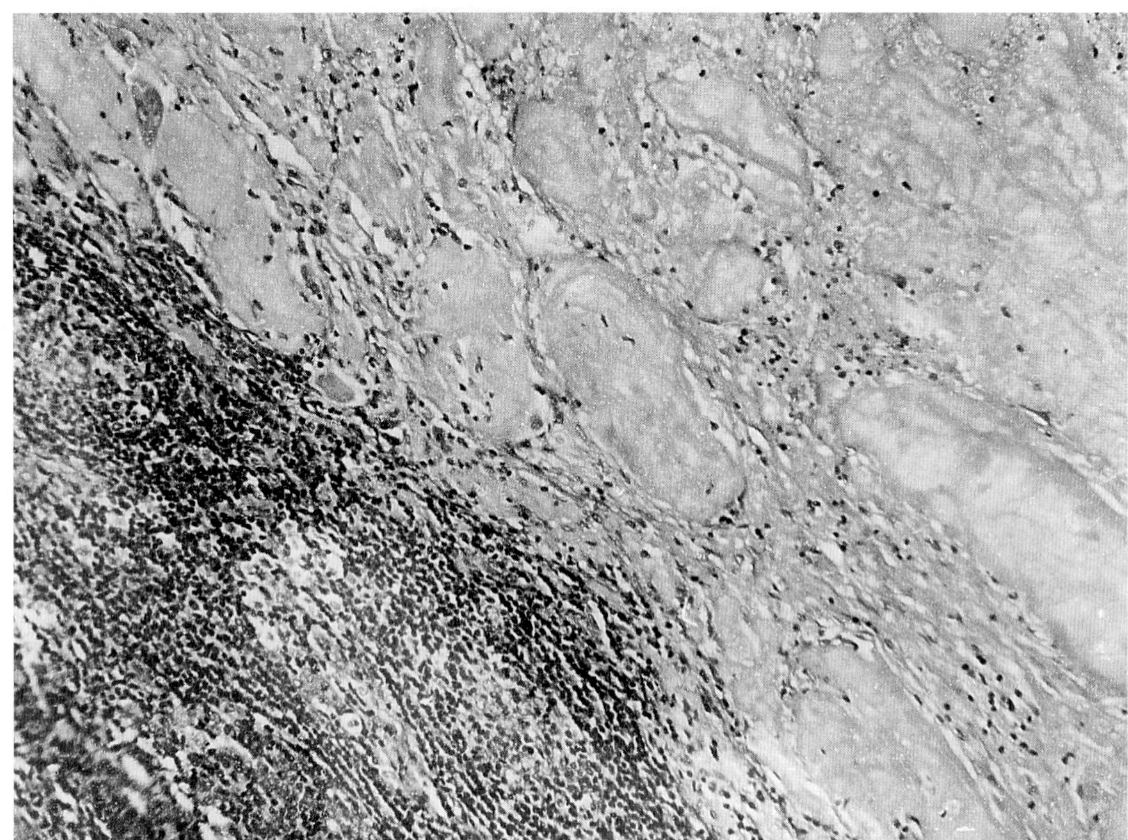

FIGURE 49.1. Amyloid lymphadenopathy with large nodules of amorphous deposits replacing nodal parenchyma. Hematoxylin and eosin stain.

49.2). A few residual atrophic follicles may be present within the amorphous deposits. The deposited substance is sometimes arranged concentrically around blood vessels (5), and at other times in large, coalescing nodules or patches (8) (Figs. 49.3 and 49.4). Lymphoid cells, mostly mature lymphocytes and plasma cells, persist at the periphery or are sprinkled throughout the amorphous deposits (Figs. 49.3 and 49.4). Occasional multinucleated giant cells, some containing intracytoplasmic amyloid, may be seen (15). Bands of collagen fibers and areas of hyalinization are also present. With the metachromatic dyes crystal violet and toluidine blue, amyloid stains rose pink; with Congo red, it stains orange (Fig. 49.4) and then intensely apple green under polarized light. By contrast, strongly positive diastase-resistant, periodic acid–Schiff (PAS) staining of an amorphous substance, with negative results of amyloid staining, indicates a glycoprotein (possibly paraamyloid) (8) (Fig 49.2). The latter, commonly referred to as a *proteinaceous precipitate,* has been reported in isolation and in association with nodular lymphoma (8,10), Waldenström macroglobulinemia (5), carcinoma (5), and immunoblastic lymphadenopathy (9). Lymphoplasmacytic lymphoma can be associated with localized amyloid (20). Extracellular deposits of non-amyloid Ig, of either monoclonal (21) or polyclonal origin (22), can also enlarge lymph nodes.

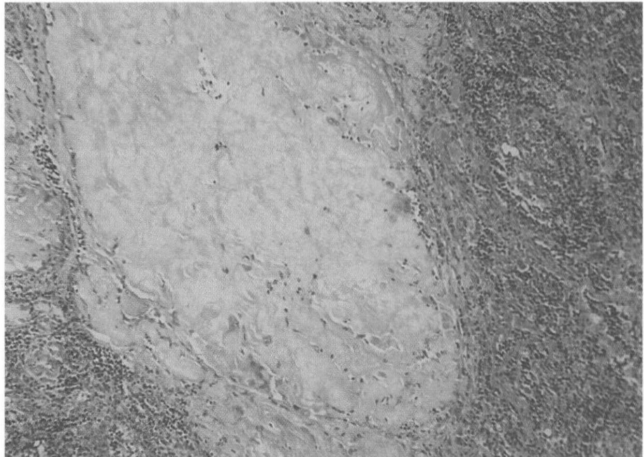

FIGURE 49.2. Proteinaceous lymphadenopathy. Masses of acellular, amorphous, periodic acid–Schiff (PAS)-positive proteinaceous material obliterate normal lymph node structure. PAS stain.

Four patterns of lymph node amyloid deposition were described in one study of 12 cases: vessel involvement only, follicular, diffuse, and a combination of follicular and diffuse (16). However, the small number of cases in each group does not allow for significant morphologic–clinical correlations.

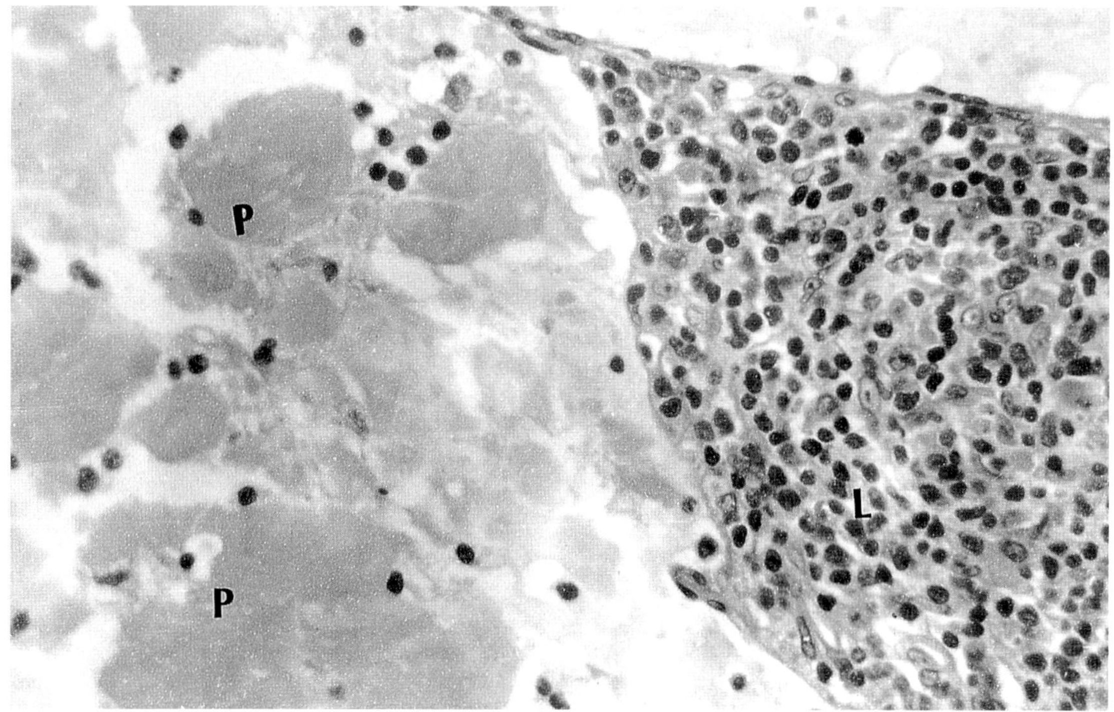

FIGURE 49.3. Paraaortic lymph node with nodular masses of periodic acid–Schiff-positive proteinaceous material (*P*). Residual lymphoid cells (*L*) appear unaffected. Hematoxylin, phloxine, and saffron stain.

ELECTRON MICROSCOPY

Under the electron microscope (Fig. 49.5), amyloid deposits are recognized by a characteristic meshwork of randomly distributed, nonbranching, fine (7.5 nm in diameter) fibrils that crisscross into and out of the plane of section (12). In contrast, non-amyloid proteinaceous material appears as deposits of a tightly packed substance of great electron density. Occasionally, proteinaceous material in lymph nodes appears as concentric lamellae separated by collagen fibrils (5).

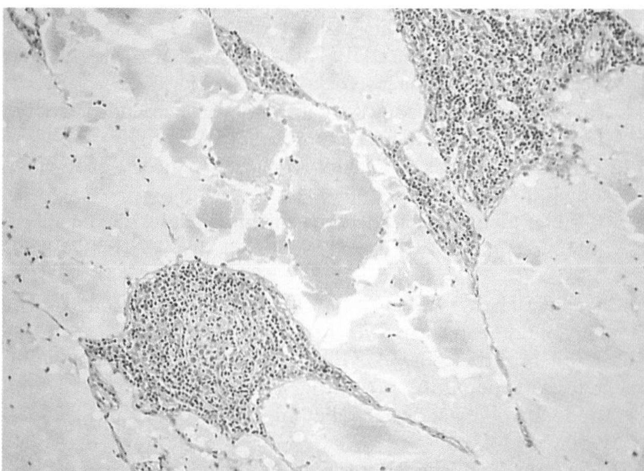

FIGURE 49.4. Extensive replacement of lymph node parenchyma by proteinaceous Congo red-positive substance with well-preserved lymphoid tissue. Congo red stain.

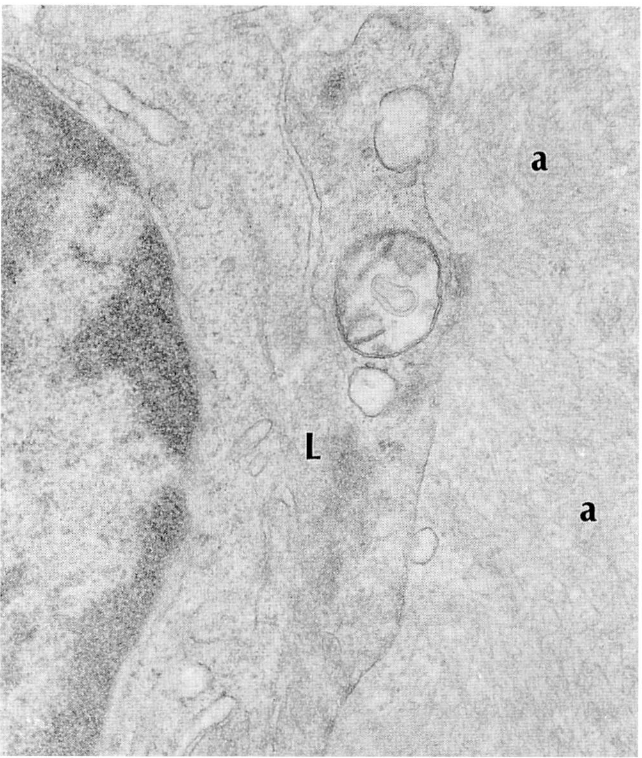

FIGURE 49.5. Amyloid lymphadenopathy showing longitudinal and transverse sections of randomly distributed amyloid fibrils (*a*) next to a lymphoid cell (*L*). ×32,000.

Checklist

PROTEINACEOUS LYMPHADENOPATHY

Primary or secondary amyloidosis
Ig abnormalities
Partial or total nodal replacement
Acellular, amorphous, eosinophilic masses
Concentric perivascular, follicular, or diffuse deposits
Amyloid or proteinaceous (non-amyloid) deposits
Positive amyloid stainings, or positive D-PAS and negative amyloid stainings
Characteristic amyloid fibrillar structure by electron microscopy

IMMUNOHISTOCHEMISTRY

Immunofluorescence staining with antibodies directed against κ or λ light chains can be used to identify amyloid deposits under the fluorescence microscope. In cases of secondary amyloidosis, the findings are of mixed Ig light chains, or more likely entirely negative. Anti-amyloid A protein antibody and the avidin–biotin peroxidase technique can also be used to identify amyloid deposits.

LABORATORY TESTS

- Congo red with examination under polarized light, methyl violet, crystal violet, and thioflavine-T staining to identify amyloid.
- Masson trichrome, van Gieson trichrome stainings to identify collagen.
- PAS staining before and after diastase (D-PAS) to identify glycoprotein.
- Electron microscopic examination to identify amyloid and collagen fibrils in amorphous deposits.
- Electrophoresis and immunoelectrophoresis to investigate possible Ig abnormalities.
- Lymphangiography to show enlarged lymph nodes of various sizes with irregular margins and filling defects, without lymphatic obstruction (2).

DIFFERENTIAL DIAGNOSIS

- Hodgkin disease, nodular sclerosis type, has broad bands of acellular collagen that is characteristically birefringent; however, the cellular infiltrates show features of Hodgkin lymphoma.
- Follicular lymphoma with proteinaceous precipitates is diagnosed by the morphology of the cellular areas.
- Diffuse histiocytic lymphoma with bands of sclerosis is similarly differentiated on the basis of cell morphology (5).

REFERENCES

1. MacKenzie DH. Amyloidosis presenting as lymphadenopathy. Br Med J 1963;2:1449–1450.
2. Ko HS, Davidson JW, Pruzanski W. Amyloid lymphadenopathy. Ann Intern Med 1976;85:763–764.
3. Brandt K, Carthcart ES, Cohen AS. A clinical analysis of the course and prognosis of 42 patients with amyloidosis. Am J Med 1968;44:955–969.
4. Scheurlen PG, Haun W, Mausle E, et al. Generalized tumorous lymph node amyloidosis with polyneuropathy and macroglobulinaemia [in German; author's translation]. Dtsch Med Wochenschr 1973;98:1947–1951.
5. Osborne BM, Butler JI, Mackay B. Proteinaceous lymphadenopathy with hypergammaglobulinemia. Am J Surg Pathol 1979;3:137–145.
6. Newland JR, Linke RP, Kleinsasser O, et al. Lymph node enlargement due to amyloid. Virchows Arch A Pathol Anat Histopathol 1983;399:233–236.
7. Symmers WSC Sr. Primary amyloidosis: a review. J Clin Pathol 1956;9:187–211.
8. Rosas-Uribe A, Variakojis D, Rappaport H. Proteinaceous precipitate in nodular (follicular) lymphomas. Cancer 1973;31:532–542.
9. Palutke M, Khilanani P, Weise R. Immunologic and electron microscopic characteristics of a case of immunoblastic lymphadenopathy. Am J Clin Pathol 1976;65:929–941.
10. Talerman A, Platenburg HP. Follicular lymphoma with deposits of amorphous hyaline material. J Pathol 1974;112:27–31.
11. Massarelli G, Bosincu L, Costanzi G. Proteinaceous material in Hodgkin's disease [Letter]. Hum Pathol 1975;6:638–639.
12. Franklin EC, Zucker-Franklin D. Current concepts of amyloid. Adv Immunol 1972;15:249–304.
13. Glenner GG. Amyloid deposits and amyloidosis: the betafibrilloses [second of two parts]. N Engl J Med 1980;302:1333–1343.
14. Puchtler H, Sweat F, Levine M. On the binding of Congo red by amyloid. J Histochem Cytochem 1962;10:355–364.
15. Kahn H, Strauchen JA, Gilbert HS, et al. Immunoglobulin-related amyloidosis presenting as recurrent isolated lymph node involvement. Arch Pathol Lab Med 1991;115:948–950.
16. Newland JR, Linke RP, Lennert K. Amyloid deposits in lymph nodes: a morphologic and immunohistochemical study. Hum Pathol 1986;17:1245–1249.

17. Castano EM, Frangione B. Human amyloidosis, Alzheimer disease and related disorders. Lab Invest 1988;58:122–132.
18. Guz G, Ozdemir BH, Sezer S, et al. High frequency of amyloid lymphadenopathy in uremic patients. Ren Fail 2000;22:613–621.
19. Hanley JP, MacLean FR, Evans JL, et al. Hemorrhagic lymphadenopathy as a presenting feature of primary AL amyloidosis. Pathology 2000;32:21–23.
20. Simmonds PD, Cottrell BJ, Mead GM, et al. Lymphadenopathy due to amyloid deposition in non-Hodgkin's lymphoma. Ann Oncol 1997;8:267–270.
21. Banerjee D, Mills DM, Hearn SA, et al. Proteinaceous lymphadenopathy due to monoclonal nonamyloid immunoglobulin deposit disease. Arch Pathol Lab Med 1990;114: 34–39.
22. Michaeli J, Niesvizky R, Siegel D, et al. Proteinaceous (angiocentric sclerosing) lymphadenopathy: a polyclonal systemic, nonamyloid deposition disorder. Blood 1995;86:1159–1162.

50

LIPID LYMPHADENOPATHY

DEFINITION

Lymphadenopathy with foreign body reaction to lipids of endogenous or exogenous origins.

PATHOGENESIS

Foreign body reactions to lipids, in the form of lipogranulomas or lipogranulomatosis, may involve lymph nodes and sometimes other components of the reticuloendothelial system (bone marrow, liver, spleen). They are a relatively common finding in patients who are elderly or obese, and in those with diabetes mellitus or hyperlipidemia (1,2). Long-term total parenteral nutrition can lead to massive splenomegaly, hepatomegaly, and lymphadenopathy as the lipid component accumulates in macrophages (3). Lipogranulomatosis may develop in lymph nodes draining the biliary system, notably the cholecystic lymph nodes, in patients with cholelithiasis (4). Other endogenous sources of lipids are hematomas, cholesterol deposits, xanthomatous lesions, tumors, fat emboli, and necrotic fat (4). Exogenous lipids may be inhaled and cause lipoid pneumonia; other sources of exogenous lipids are contrast media used in lymphangiography or bronchography, lipid-based substances injected into hemorrhoids, and oils used as depot vehicles to allow the slow release of injected drugs (2).

HISTOPATHOLOGY

The lipids that drain with lymph into the lymph nodes are seen more frequently in the subcapsular and medullary sinuses. Lipid granulomas are formed by the accumulation of histiocytes and multinucleated giant cells around the globules of fat, which may be confluent, forming microcysts or small, empty-looking vacuoles (Fig. 50.1). Phagocytosed inside the macrophages, the lipid vacuoles are always smaller than the single vacuole of normal fat cells (4). In frozen sections, the fatty globules can be revealed by Sudan black or scarlet red stainings. In paraffin sections, the fat has been dissolved by the xylene treatment and appears as empty spaces. Such spaces, microcysts, and vacuoles are lined by fine cytoplasmic films of giant cells that stretch to encircle the foreign body (Fig. 50.2). Epithelioid cells are part of the reaction, but they do not form well-defined granulomas. The multinucleated giant cells are of foreign body type (Fig. 50.3). Lymphocytes, plasma cells, and sometimes eosinophils may accompany the cellular proliferation. Eventually, sometimes in days or weeks but at other times in months or years, the exogenous fat is removed (2). In hyperlipidemia, the lipid granulomas consist of foamy cells and Touton-type giant cells. Foamy cells are also part of the process in some infectious diseases (e.g., Whipple disease, leishmaniasis), storage diseases (e.g., Niemann-Pick, Gaucher, or Fabry disease), and diseases of un-

Checklist

LIPID LYMPHADENOPATHY

History of infection, inhalation
History of cholelithiasis, diabetes, obesity
Sinus histiocytosis
Lipid microcysts, droplets
Foreign body giant cells with intracytoplasmic vacuoles
Histiocytes, macrophages, epithelioid cells
Atrophy and fatty metamorphosis

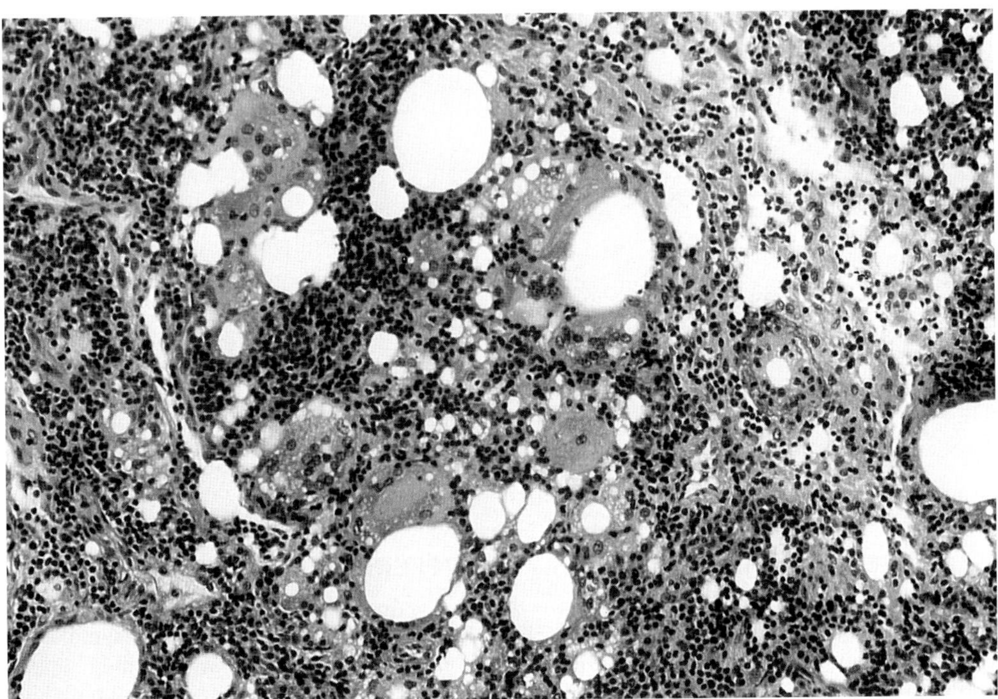

FIGURE 50.1. Lipid lymphadenopathy of peribiliary lymph node in patient with pancreatic carcinoma. Microcysts and globules of fat of various sizes, histiocytes, and giant cells replace nodal parenchyma. Hematoxylin, phloxine, and saffron stain.

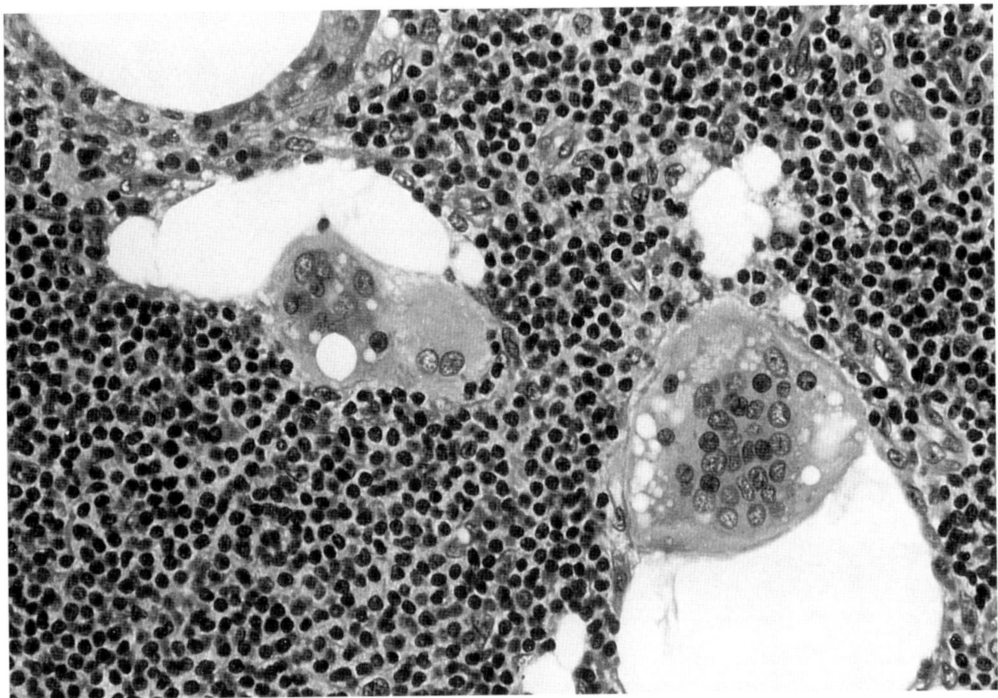

FIGURE 50.2. Same lymph node as in Fig. 50.1. Microcysts with lipid droplets within multinucleated giant cells. Hematoxylin, phloxine, and saffron stain.

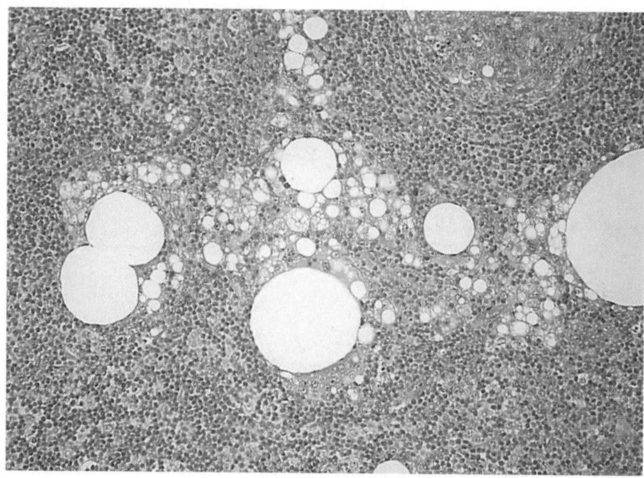

FIGURE 50.3. Lipid lymphadenopathy of peribiliary lymph node in patient with cholelithiasis. Lipid droplets, coarse to very fine, surrounded by cytoplasmic film of foreign body giant cells. Hematoxylin, phloxine, and saffron stain.

known cause (e.g., histiocytosis X, Hand-Schüller-Christian disease).

Lymph nodes may undergo atrophy and fatty replacement as a result of obesity, physiologic regression in the elderly, or radiation treatment of tumors (5). In such cases, partial or total fatty metamorphosis takes place, and only a few clusters or a narrow peripheral rim of lymphocytes remains by which the lymph nodes can be recognized (Figs. 50.4 and 50.5).

DIFFERENTIAL DIAGNOSIS

- Whipple disease: The macrophages contain characteristic inclusions that stain with periodic acid–Schiff, and foreign body giant cells are not present.
- Silicone lymphadenopathy: The material in the vacuoles, although mostly washed away during processing, still stains palely with eosin or shows a few fine, flakelike fragments.

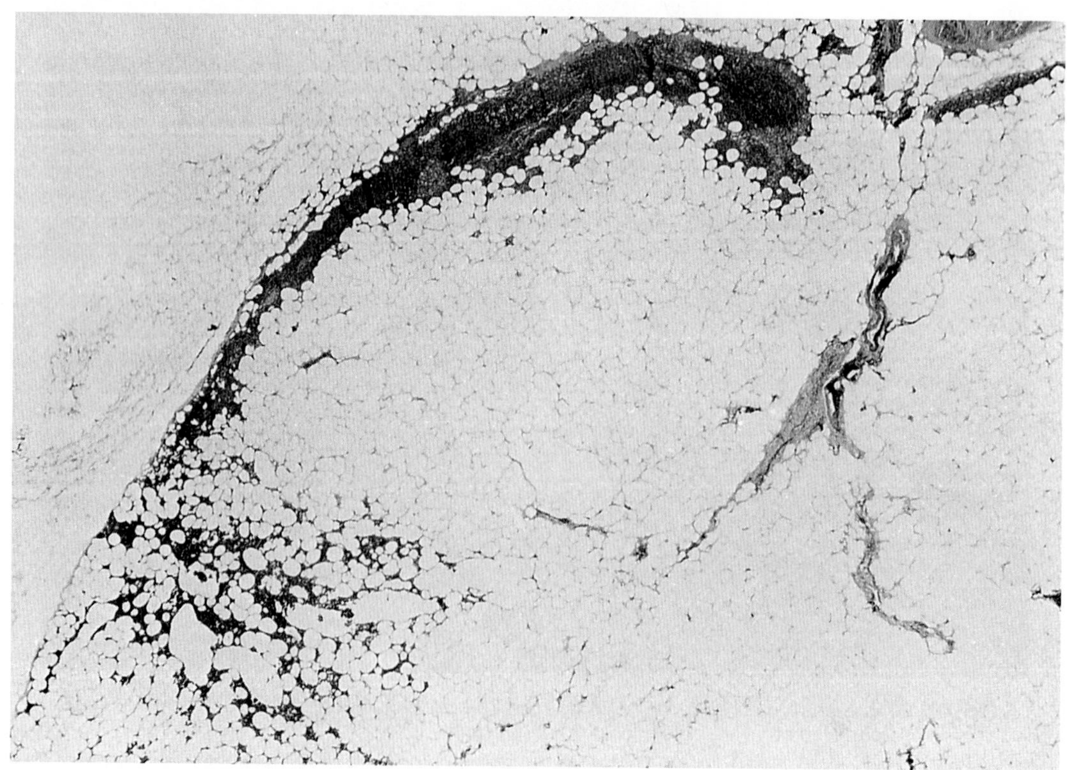

FIGURE 50.4. Pelvic lymph node after radiation treatment. Fatty metamorphosis of lymph node parenchyma with residual peripheral rim of lymphocytes. Hematoxylin and eosin stain.

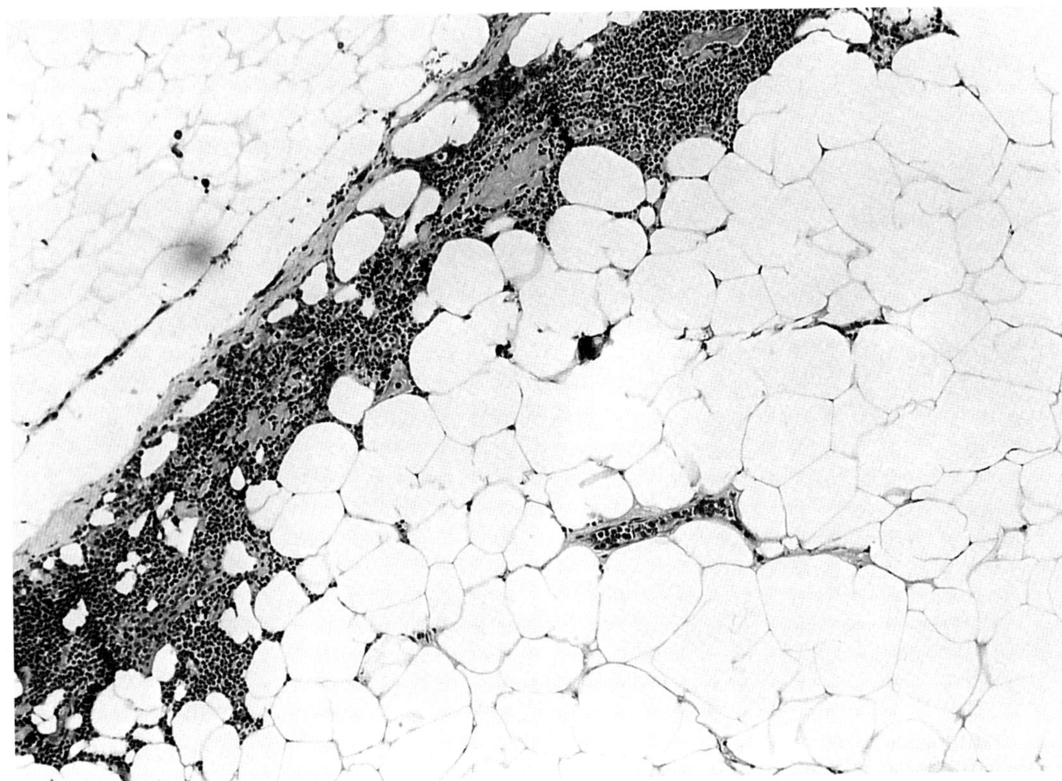

FIGURE 50.5. Same lymph node as in Fig. 50.4. Only subcapsular narrow rim of lymphocytes remains; entire nodal parenchyma has been replaced by mature adipose tissue. Hematoxylin and eosin stain.

LYMPHANGIOGRAPHY-ASSOCIATED LYMPHADENOPATHY

DEFINITION

Lymphadenopathy developing in the regional lymph nodes as a result of lymphangiography.

PATHOGENESIS

When lymphangiography was introduced in 1952, enabling radiologic visualization of the lymphatics, a water-soluble contrast medium was initially used; this was subsequently replaced by low-viscosity iodized oil contrast media such as lipiodol, Ethiodol, and others (6). Angiographic media usually contain organic iodine and an oil base such as the one derived from ethyl esters of poppyseed oil that is a component of Ethiodol, a substance more fluid than lipiodol (7). Ordinarily, 4 to 15 mL of contrast medium may be injected into an adult, depending on the site under investigation. A total of 15 mL is sufficient to show the lymphatics of both legs and fill the sinuses of inguinal, iliac, and periaortic lymph nodes (6). The medium is retained in the lymph nodes for a period of a few weeks to several months, and traces have been found as much as 4 years later (6). The cellular reaction in draining lymph nodes is essentially directed against the oily vehicle, and in this sense lymphangiography-associated lymphadenopathy is in fact a lipid lymphadenopathy (see earlier in this chapter). Lymphangiography was formerly used to a large extent in the staging of Hodgkin lymphoma, a practice that has been gradually abandoned as radiation and chemotherapy have become more effective.

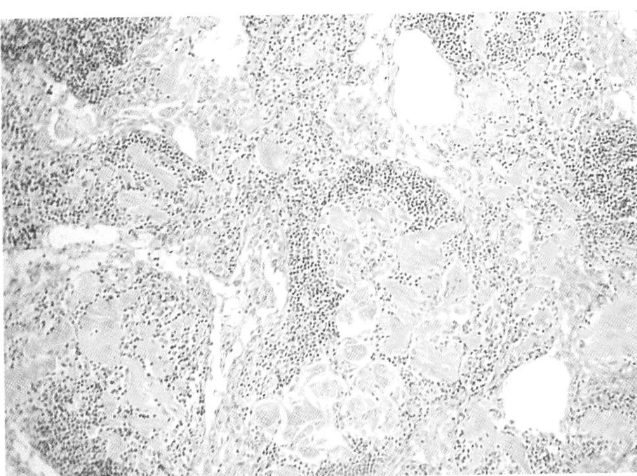

FIGURE 50.6. Lymph node architecture disrupted by oil droplets and accumulations of epithelioid and giant cells. Hematoxylin, phloxine, and saffron stain.

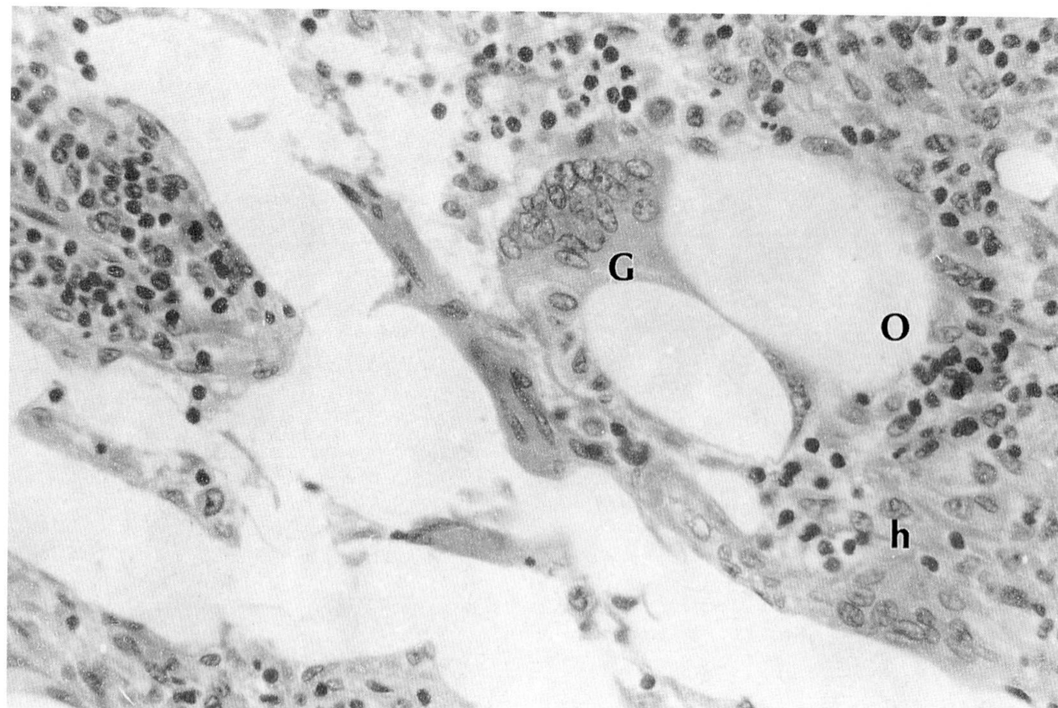

FIGURE 50.7. Oil droplets (*O*) encircled by multinucleated giant cells (*G*) and histocytes (*h*). Hematoxylin, phloxine, and saffron stain.

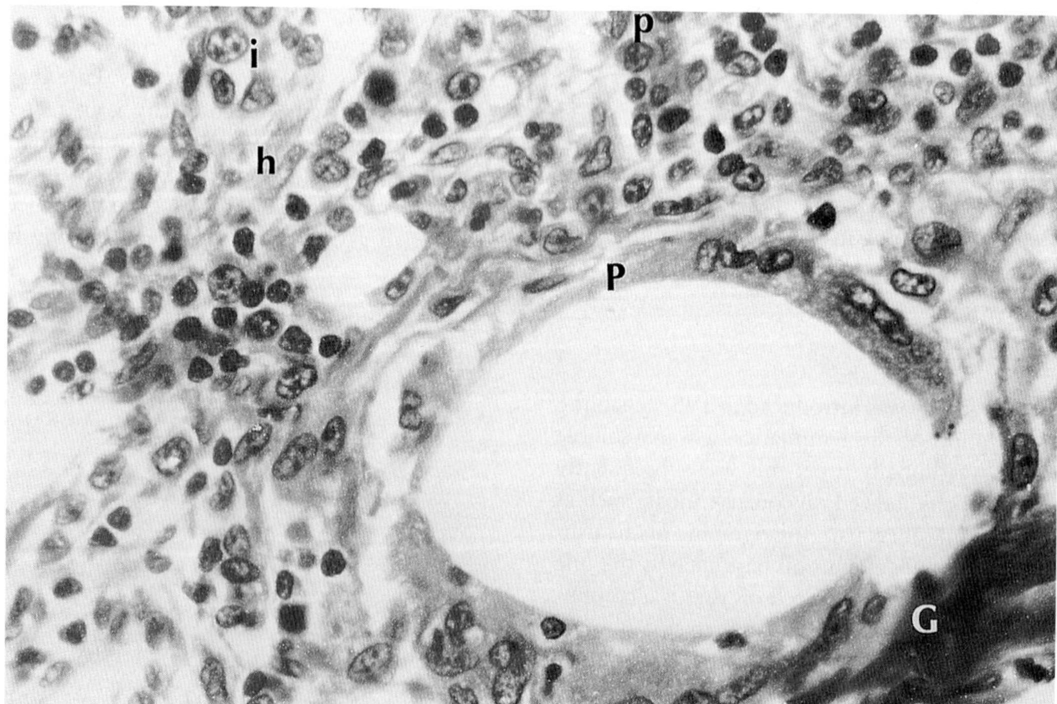

FIGURE 50.8. Foreign body multinucleated giant cell (*G*) surrounding oil droplet with fine film of cytoplasm (*P*). Histiocytes (*h*), plasma cells (*p*), and immunoblasts (*i*) accompany the giant cells. Hematoxylin, phloxine, and saffron stain.

Checklist

LYMPHANGIOGRAPHY-ASSOCIATED LYMPHADENOPATHY

History of lymphangiography
Sinus histiocytosis, notably of subcapsular sinus
Compressed follicles
Droplets appearing as empty spaces encircled by multinucleated giant cells
Histocytes, eosinophils, plasma cells

HISTOPATHOLOGY

The lymphoid follicles are diminished, the germinal centers are hypoplastic, and sinus histiocytosis is predominant. Oil droplets that appear as empty spaces, varying from the size of a few lymphocytes to that of a follicle, are scattered throughout the nodal parenchyma (Fig. 50.6). Each is surrounded by histiocytes and multinucleated giant cells of foreign body type (Fig. 50.7). The giant cells usually include oval, uniform nuclei grouped in the central area and rarely show the peripheral nuclear distribution of Langhans cells (7). Frequently, only fine cytoplasmic processes of these cells are inserted between the oil and the lymphoid tissues (Fig. 50.8). In the first few days, neutrophils and occasional eosinophils and plasma cells may be noted near the lipid deposits. The giant cell reaction appears later and persists as long as unresorbed oil is present. Some lipid droplets have wavy or scalloped margins that suggest resorption of oil (7). However, the process is slow, and the morphologic changes may still be present months or years after lymphangiography. The giant cells disappear gradually; fibrosis and scarring do not usually occur. In lymph nodes involved by malignant processes, the lipid vacuoles are small because of increased tissue pressure, and the giant cells are less frequent. In patients who have undergone two or more lymphangiograms, lymph node hyperplasia may occur as a reaction to the contrast media (8). The enlarged follicles remain unopacified and produce an image of granularity or foaminess on the lymphangiogram that can be misinterpreted as relapsing lymphoma (8,9). Because magnetic resonance imaging carried out after lymphangiography cannot discriminate opacified pelvic lymph nodes from subcutaneous or retroperitoneal adipose tissue, it is recommended that magnetic resonance studies be done first (10).

DIFFERENTIAL DIAGNOSIS

- Fungal infections may show macrophages and multinucleated giant cells with empty-looking intracytoplasmic vacuoles. Gomori methenamine silver staining visualizes the yeasts.
- *Mycobacterium avium–intracellulare* and tuberculous lymphadenitides: Acid-fast stainings show the presence of engulfed bacilli.
- Sarcoidosis forms well-defined granulomas without intracellular or extracellular vacuoles.
- Silicone lymphadenopathy: The foreign material may appear as lightly stained fluid or flakes. It can be visualized by polarized light.

REFERENCES

1. Rywlin AM, Ortega R. Lipid granulomas of the bone marrow. Am J Clin Pathol 1972;57:457–462.
2. Symmers WS. The lymphoreticular system. In: Symmers WS, ed. Systemic pathology, vol. 2. New York: Churchill Livingstone, 1978:558–559.
3. Perez-Jaffe LA, Furth EE, Minda JM, et al. Massive macrophage lipid accumulation presenting as hepatosplenomegaly and lymphadenopathy associated with long-term total parenteral nutrition therapy for short bowel syndrome. Hum Pathol 1998;29: 651–655.
4. Carr I, Murari PJ, Pettigrew NM. Lymph nodes and spleen. In: Silverberg SG, ed. Principles and practice of surgical pathology. New York: Churchill Livingstone, 1990:394.
5. Smith T. Fatty replacement of lymph nodes mimicking lymphoma relapse. Cancer 1986;58:2686–2688.
6. Symmers WS. The lymphoreticular system. In: Symmers WS, ed. Systemic pathology, vol 2. New York: Churchill Livingstone, 1978:558–559.
7. Ravel R. Histopathology of lymph nodes after lymphangiography. Am J Clin Pathol 1966;46:335–340.
8. Castellino PA. Observations on "reactive (follicular) hyperplasia" as encountered in repeat lymphography in the lymphomas. Cancer 1974;34:2042–2050.
9. Butler JJ. Non-neoplastic lesions of lymph nodes of man to be differentiated from lymphomas. NCI Monogr 1969;32:233–255.
10. Buckwalter KA, Ellis JH, Baker DE, et al. Pitfall in MR imaging of lymphadenopathy after lymphangiography. Radiology 1986; 161:831–832.

51

SILICONE LYMPHADENOPATHY

DEFINITION

Lymphadenopathy of regional lymph nodes caused by the presence of silicone carried from tributary organs.

PATHOGENESIS

Silicone consists of polymers of dimethylsiloxane. When repeating units are polymerized, a whole range of synthetic substances with chains of varying length is created; short chains produce liquid silicone, longer chains form gels, and cross-linking of chains results in silicone rubber or elastomer (1). Because silicone is not biodegradable and elicits little or no reaction from human tissues, it is widely utilized in the manufacture of implants for reconstructive, cosmetic, and orthopedic surgery (2,3). The most frequent applications of silicone are in mammoplasty and joint prostheses. Originally, in cosmetic breast augmentation and breast reconstruction after mastectomy, liquid silicone (dimethicone) was injected directly into the breast. This technique was abandoned because the silicone tended to migrate as a result of gravity and absorption, so that disfiguring complications developed (4). In experiments performed in mice, low-molecular-weight silicones from breast implants that were injected subcutaneously disseminated to virtually all tissues and organs (5). The regional lymph nodes in particular receive silicone carried from tributary organs (3,6–8). To prevent this from happening, silicone was mixed with various fatty acids, with the intention of inducing fibrosis around the injected fluid. However, fatty substances induce foreign body giant cell reactions and scarring. Another substance used in the past to coat breast implants was polyurethane foam, which is deposited as triangular solid particles among reacting foreign body giant cells (9,10). Best tolerated are the presently used silicone bags containing silicone gels or saline solutions. However, even these may occasionally rupture, leak, or simply release microscopic particles through "bleeding" from the surface of the implant (11). Such particles, when carried to regional lymph nodes, may induce silicone lymphadenopathy (3,7,8).

CLINICAL SYMPTOMS

Enlarged axillary lymph nodes may be clinically indistinguishable from metastatic breast cancer. On occasion, even internal mammary lymph nodes, which are relatively inaccessible to biopsy, may be affected by silicone migration (12). Therefore, the axilla of a patient with a silicone gel implant must be monitored routinely, particularly after a mammary tumor has been excised, and lymph node biopsy performed when necessary (13). Evidently, the presence of a silicone or another foreign body lymphadenopathy does not preclude the coexistence of neoplasia in the same lymph nodes. Lymphoma in axillary nodes with silicone lymphadenopathy has been reported, as has metastatic prostatic adenocarcinoma in pelvic lymph nodes with foreign body histiocytosis as a reaction to total joint arthroplasty (8,14,15). When corrective silicone prostheses are placed in the small joints of fingers, hands, and feet deformed by rheumatoid arthritis, silicone is ultimately carried to the regional lymph nodes (16). The incidence of silicone lymphadenopathy in patients with joint prostheses has been estimated to be as low as 1.8% (17) and as high as 13% (18). In general, unilateral lymphadenopathies in persons with mammary or joint prostheses, even when they develop years after implantation of the device, must be evaluated (16,19). Silicone may enter the general circulation and be found in various organs, as has been observed in patients on hemodialysis or with valve prostheses (1). It has been claimed that silicone may cause a variety of systemic symptoms and diseases, including autoimmune, neurologic, and neoplastic conditions. This subject remains highly controversial and is the basis of unending medical debates and liability suits.

HISTOPATHOLOGY

The tissue reaction to silicone depends mainly on particle size. When silicone lymphadenopathy is caused by particles of elastomer, a typical non-necrotizing granulomatous reaction with epithelioid cells and giant cells of foreign body type surrounding the silicone particles is observed (1,16). In

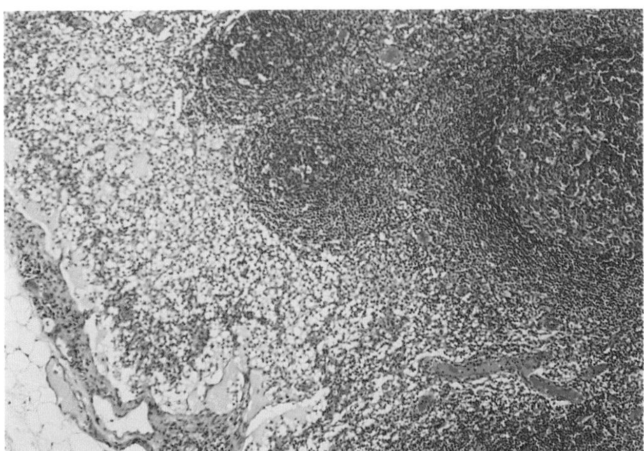

FIGURE 51.1. Axillary lymph node of silicone-implanted breast. Large areas of lymph node cortex parenchyma replaced by sheets of clear cells. Reactive germinal center in adjacent follicles. Hematoxylin, phloxine, and saffron stain.

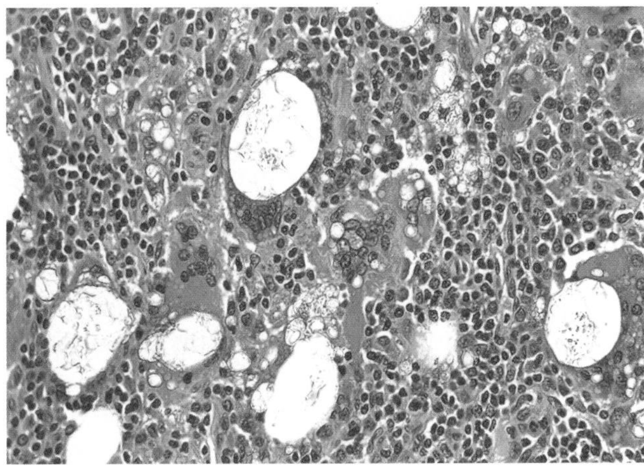

FIGURE 51.3. Histiocytes surrounded by foreign body giant cells contain vacuoles with fine strands of refractile material. Hematoxylin, phloxine, and saffron stain.

contrast, when droplets of liquid silicone arrive in the sinuses of the draining lymph nodes, no noticeable cellular reaction occurs. The silicone appears in the form of round vacuoles of various sizes within the sinuses or lymphoid parenchyma. Their numbers may be negligible, or aggregated clusters may occupy as much as 60% of the section (3) (Fig. 51.1). The vacuoles may be entirely empty if silicone has been washed away during processing, or they may contain a thin, peripheral layer of lightly staining fluid. In addition to extracellular silicone, which at low magnification appears as a lacy pattern, fine vacuoles within histiocytes may result in a bubbly or foamy aspect with peripheralized nuclei (Fig. 51.2). Sometimes, a fine strand of refractile unstained material can be seen (Fig. 51.3). Silicone lymphadenopathy does not comprise atypical nuclei, mitoses, necrosis, or fibrosis. When numerous foreign body giant cells containing fragments, crystals, or polarizable foreign bodies are present, these are caused not by silicone but by other materials used in the prostheses (1,9,10) (Fig. 51.3).

HISTOCHEMISTRY

Silicone is not stained by hematoxylin and eosin, periodic acid–Schiff (PAS), trichrome, mucin, or oil red-O stains and is not birefringent in polarized light (3). The silicone-containing histiocytes are identified by staining with anti-

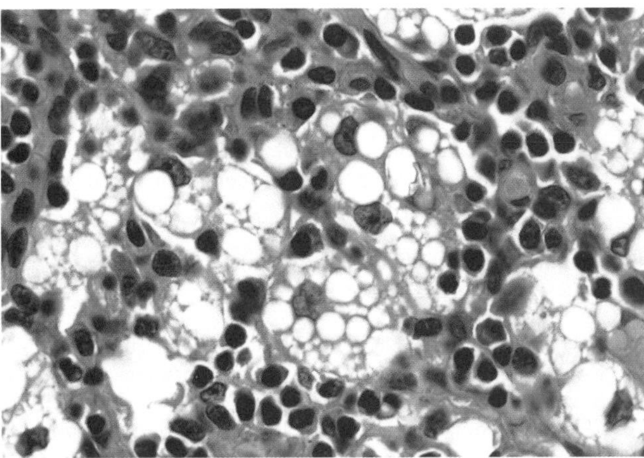

FIGURE 51.2. Histiocytes with clear, empty-looking cytoplasm and peripheral nuclei or multiple intracytoplasmic droplets, which create a bubbly or foamy appearance. Hematoxylin, phloxine, and saffron stain.

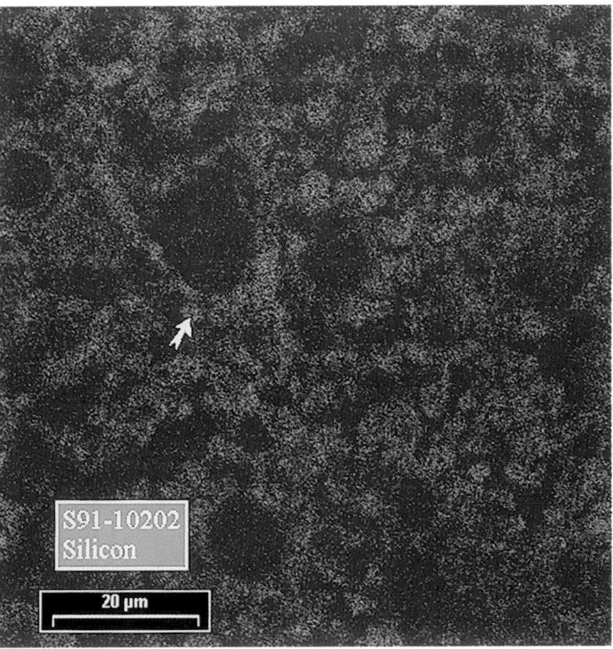

FIGURE 51.4. Electron micrograph of lymph node with electron-opaque flakes of silicone.

Checklist

SILICONE LYMPHADENOPATHY

History of cosmetic, reconstructive, or orthopedic surgery
Enlarged regional lymph nodes (axillary, inguinal)
Partial lymph node involvement
Extracellular empty-looking vacuoles of various sizes
Histiocytes with intracellular foamy vacuoles
Intracellular clear substance unstained by hematoxylin and eosin, oil red-O, PAS, mucicarmine
Foreign body multinucleated giant cells, occasionally
EDXEA silicone peak

bodies against the CD68 histiocyte marker. The foreign body giant cells stain for CD68 and CD44 cellular activation marker (20).

ELECTRON MICROSCOPY

Glutaraldehyde preserves the silicone well, which appears as electron-opaque fragmented spicules or flakes (Fig. 51.4). With the technique of energy-dispersive x-ray elemental analysis (EDXEA), an elemental silicone peak is obtained and confirms the diagnosis (3) (Fig. 51.5).

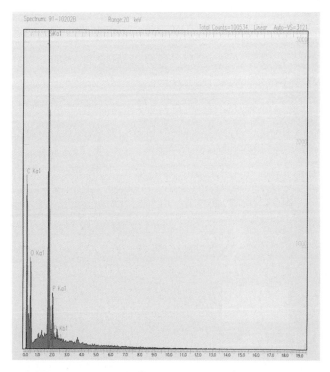

FIGURE 51.5. Energy dispersive x-ray elemental analysis (EDXEA) of lymph node showing elemental silicone peak.

DIFFERENTIAL DIAGNOSIS

- Lipogranuloma: The vacuoles of fat are coarse, in contrast to the fine, foamy vacuoles of silicone.
- Fat necrosis is accompanied by frequent foreign body giant cells.
- Metastatic lobular carcinoma of the breast is an essential and often difficult differential diagnosis; staining with PAS and mucicarmine makes the distinction.
- Metastatic signet ring cell carcinoma: Sometimes very similar histologically. Positive staining with PAS and mucicarmine.
- Metastatic renal clear cell carcinoma: Cytokeratin- and vimentin-positive.
- Non-Hodgkin lymphoma, signet ring cell type: CD45 (LCA)+, CD20 (L26)+.

REFERENCES

1. Travis WD, Balogh K, Abraham JL. Silicone granulomas: report of three cases and review of the literature. Hum Pathol 1985;16: 19–27.
2. Demergian V. Experiences with the newer subcutaneous implants material. Surg Clin North Am 1963;43:1313–1321.
3. Truong LD, Cartwright J Jr, Goodman MD, et al. Silicone lymphadenopathy associated with augmentation mammaplasty. Morphologic features of nine cases. Am J Surg Pathol 1988; 12:484–491.
4. Symmers W St C. Silicone mastitis in "topless" waitresses and some other varieties of foreign body mastitis. Br Med J 1968;3: 19–22.
5. Kala SV, Lykissa ED, Neely MW, et al. Low molecular weight silicones are widely distributed after a single subcutaneous injection in mice. Am J Pathol 1998;152:645–649.
6. Wintsch W. Smahel J. Clodius L. Local and regional lymph node response to ruptured gel-filled mammary prostheses. Br J Plast Surg 1978;31:349–352.
7. Hausner RJ, Schoen FJ, Mendez-Fernandez HA, et al. Migration of silicone gel to axillary lymph nodes after prosthetic mammaplasty. Arch Pathol Lab Med 1981;105:371–372.

8. Benjamin E, Ahmed A, Rashid ATMF, et al. Silicone lymphadenopathy: a report of two cases, one with concomitant malignant lymphoma. Diagn Histopathol 1982;5:133–141.
9. Fitzgibbons PL. Breast prosthesis reaction [Letter to the Editor]. Am J Surg Pathol 1996;20:505.
10. Bleiweiss IJ, Copeland M. Breast prosthesis reaction [Letter to the Editor]. Am J Surg Pathol 1996;20:505–506.
11. Noone RB. A review of the possible health implications of silicone breast implants. Cancer 1997;79:1747–1756.
12. Kao CC, Rand RP, Holt CA, et al. Internal mammary silicone lymphadenopathy mimicking recurrent breast cancer. Plast Reconstr Surg 1997;99:225–229.
13. Kulber DA, Mackenzie D, Steiner JH, et al. Monitoring the axilla in patients with silicone gel implants. Ann Plast Surg 1995;35:580–584.
14. Cook PD, Osborne BM, Connor RL, et al. Follicular lymphoma adjacent to foreign body granulomatous inflammation and fibrosis surrounding silicone breast prosthesis. Am J Surg Pathol 1995;19:712–717.
15. Peoch M, Ducros V, Barnoud R, et al. Foreign body histiocytosis reaction after hip replacement with concomitant metastatic adenocarcinoma in the same lymph node. Hum Pathol 1998;29:95–98.
16. Rogers LA, Longtine JA, Garnick MC, et al. Silicone lymphadenopathy in a long distance runner: complication of a silastic prosthesis. Hum Pathol 1988;19:1237–1239.
17. Jassim KA, Weerasinghe BD. Silicone lymphadenopathy, synovitis, and osteitis complicating big toe silastic prostheses. J R Coll Surg Edinb 1986;32:29–33.
18. Lazaro MA, Garcia MD, deBenyacar MA, et al. Lymphadenopathy secondary to silicone hand joint prostheses. Clin Exp Rheumatol 1990;8:17–22.
19. Roux SP, Bertucci GM, Ibarra JA, et al. Unilateral axillary adenopathy secondary to a silicone wrist implant: report of a case detected at screening mammography. Radiology 1996;198:345–346.
20. Abbondanzo SL, Young UL, Wei MQ, et al. Silicone gel-filled breast and testicular implant capsules: a histologic and immunophenotypic study. Mod Pathol 1999;12:706–713.

52

LYMPHADENOPATHY OF METAL DEBRIS ASSOCIATED WITH JOINT PROSTHESES

DEFINITION

Lymphadenopathy caused by abraded metal debris drained from sites of joint prostheses.

PATHOGENESIS

The use of metal prostheses to replace large joints has become a common practice during the past decade. As a consequence, cases have been reported of the presence of metal wear debris in local and distant lymph nodes and in bone marrow, liver, and spleen (1–5). Stainless steel, cobalt, chromium, titanium, zirconium, nickel, barium, and ceramic are used to construct hip and knee prostheses; cementing materials, particularly polyethylene, are also used. Most modern joint prostheses are made of stainless steel or cobalt–chrome alloy. Polyethylene or ceramic is used to fashion the articulating surface and polymethylacrylate to cement the prosthesis in place (1,4). The amount of metal carried to distant organs is highest in patients with loose and worn prostheses, and the superficial coating is the main source of debris (2). However, levels of metal may also be raised in patients whose prostheses show no visible wear, and, to a lesser extent, in those who have hip screws; such increases indicate the potential for widespread dissemination of foreign materials (2). The largest number of particles carried to the regional lymph nodes are of polyethylene, which is easily abraded and causes most of the reactive histiocytic proliferation. Titanium dioxide, deposited as black pigment in the cells, may cause intense damage in the form of necrosis and fibrosis in the lungs and lymph nodes of workers inhaling titanium in paint factories (6).

CLINICAL SYNDROME

Depending on the nature of the materials used in the manufacture of joint prostheses, wear debris is released in the periarticular tissues. Tissue macrophages clear the debris by draining particulate material to the regional lymph nodes. When wear is excessive, the removal system is overloaded, and a local intense foreign body giant cell reaction ensues that contributes to further wear of the prosthesis (1). An important consequence of this process is the reactive enlargement of the pelvic lymph nodes; these drain the lymphatics of the hip and also collect the lymphatics of the pelvic area. Therefore, enlarged pelvic lymph nodes in a person with a hip prosthesis may become a source of concern and possible misdiagnosis when coexisting cancers of the prostate or uterine cervix are present (1).

HISTOPATHOLOGY

The cut surface of the enlarged lymph nodes appears dark brown or black (3). The sinuses are markedly distended, and a marked proliferation of large, foamy histiocytes that stain with periodic acid–Schiff may replace part of the lymphoid tissues, forming coalescing nests and sheets (Fig. 52.1). The vacuolated, foamy, or totally clear histiocytes contain polyethylene or silicone (Fig. 52.2). In addition, the cells contain metal particles in the shape of needles or flakes (Figs. 52.2 and 52.3). These are 0.5 to 5 μm in largest dimension, irregularly shaped, and black on hematoxylin and eosin staining. Some particles may be as large as 100 μm and are usually contained in large, multinucleated giant cells (1) (Fig. 52.3). The metal particles are strongly birefringent under polarized light. In cases with extensive wear damage to the prosthesis, necrosis in the lymph nodes has been recorded (2).

ELECTRON MICROSCOPY

Energy dispersive x-ray elemental analysis (EDXEA) shows characteristic peaks for cobalt–chromium and titanium in the involved lymph nodes (3,6). Usually, about 90% of the

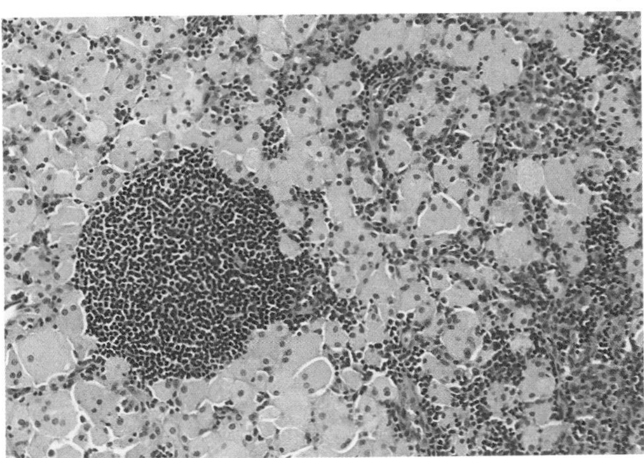

FIGURE 52.1. Lymph node in which lymphoid tissues are largely replaced by nests and sheets of large, foamy, polyethylene-containing histiocytes. Hematoxylin, phloxine, and saffron stain.

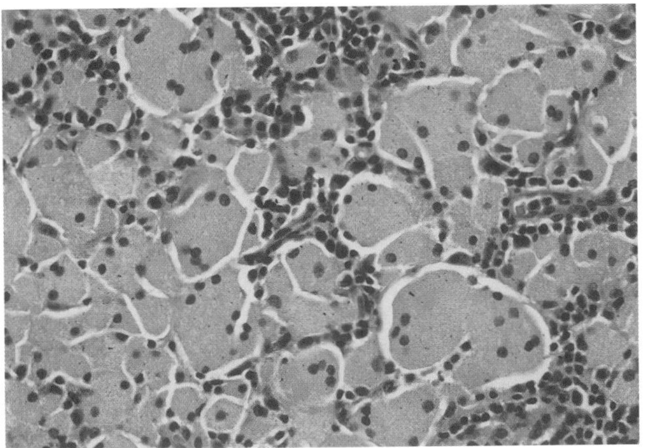

FIGURE 52.2. Foamy histiocytes containing polyethylene and black metal needles. Hematoxylin, phloxine, and saffron stain. (Courtesy of Dr. J. Albores- Saavedra.)

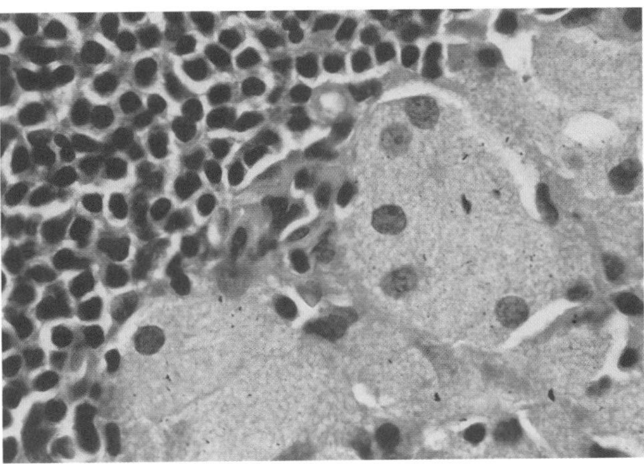

FIGURE 52.3. Foamy histiocytes, some forming multinucleated foreign body giant cells, with black cobalt–chromium needles and flakes. Hematoxylin, phloxine, and saffron stain. (Courtesy of Dr. J. Albores- Saavedra.)

particles are cobalt–chromium and 10% are titanium (3). The histiocytes are immunoreactive for lysozyme, α_1-antitrypsin, α_1-antichymotrypsin, and cathepsin D. They are negative for cytokeratin, PSA, PSAP, and S100 protein (3).

DIFFERENTIAL DIAGNOSIS

- Sinus histiocytosis and nests of histiocytes/epithelioid cells are part of many reactive lymphadenopathies, including mycobacteriosis, toxoplasmosis, Whipple disease, Gaucher disease, and Rosai-Dorfman lymphadenopathy. The distinction is made by observing the metal particles after regular staining or in polarized light.
- *Mycobacterium tuberculosis, Mycobacterium avium,* and *Mycobacterium leprae* may produce similar lesions. Therefore, staining for acid-fast bacilli should be routinely performed for any lesions comprising epithelioid cells, giant cells, granulomas, and necrosis.

Checklist

LYMPHADENOPATHY OF METAL DEBRIS ASSOCIATED WITH JOINT PROSTHESES

Persons with large joint prostheses
Enlarged lymph nodes
Dark brown or black cut surface
Sinus histiocytosis
Nests and sheets of histiocytes, epithelioid cells, and foreign body giant cells
Needle-like flakes of black foreign material
Often associated with clear histiocytes containing silicone
Identification by EDXMA

- Fungal infections also should be ruled out by routinely staining suspect lesions with Grocott methenamine silver (GMS). In a reported case, iron, phosphorus, and calcium deposited in a lymph node formed structures resembling hyphae and elicited a histiocytic reaction. The differential diagnosis of the "pseudofungi" was made by GMS staining and EDXEA (7).
- The presence of metastatic carcinoma of prostate, bladder, or uterine cervical origin in the enlarged pelvic lymph nodes can be ascertained by cytokeratin immunostaining.

REFERENCES

1. Gray MH, Talbert ML, Talbert WM, et al. Changes seen in lymph nodes draining the sites of large joint prostheses. Am J Surg Pathol 1989;13:1050–1056.
2. Case CP, Langkamer VG, James C, et al. Widespread dissemination of metal debris from implants. J Bone Joint Surg Br 1994;76: 701–712.
3. Albores-Saavedra J, Vuitch F, Delgado R, et al. Sinus histiocytosis of pelvic lymph nodes after hip replacement. A histiocytic proliferation induced by cobalt–chromium and titanium. Am J Surg Pathol 1994;18:83–90.
4. Basle MF, Bertrand G, Guyetant S, et al. Migration of metal and polyethylene particles from articular prostheses may generate lymphadenopathy with histiocytosis. J Biomed Mater Res 1996;30: 157–163.
5. Benz EB, Sherburne B, Hayek JE, et al. Lymphadenopathy associated with total joint prostheses. A report of two cases and a review of the literature. J Bone Joint Surg Am 1996;78:588–593.
6. Moran CA, Mullick FG, Ishak KG, et al. Identification of titanium in human tissues: probable role in pathologic processes. Hum Pathol 1991;22:450–454.
7. Connelly J, Ro JY, Cartwright J. Pseudofungi in a lymph node. A case report with energy dispersive x-ray elemental analysis. Arch Pathol Lab Med 1991;115:1166–1168.

53

GOLD LYMPHADENOPATHY

DEFINITION

Lymphadenopathy caused by intramuscular injections of gold and deposits in lymph nodes.

PATHOGENESIS

In chrysotherapy for rheumatoid arthritis, gold sodium thiomalate is injected intramuscularly for long periods of time (1,2). In one reported case, of a woman with a 33-year history of severe progressive rheumatoid arthritis and marked deformities of her hands and feet, intramuscular solid sodium thiomalate had been administered every 2 weeks for 10 years (2). Following intramuscular administration, 90% of the gold compound is bound to protein, and approximately 40% of each dose is eliminated in urine and feces (3). Gold toxicity is manifested by a number of complications, including dermatitis, thrombocytopenic purpura, nephritis, and vasculitis. Some 25% to 50% of patients must discontinue therapy because of toxicity (1,2). Lymph node complications may present as nodal infarction (4), but more commonly gold lymphadenopathy develops when gold particles are transported to the lymph nodes, where they are dispersed throughout the nodal sinuses and parenchyma. The lymph node reaction is that of foreign body lymphadenopathy.

HISTOPATHOLOGY

The lymph node follicles are enlarged, sometimes irregularly shaped and coalescing. The germinal centers are reactive and contain tingible-body macrophages (2). The sinuses are dilated and filled with histiocytes. Foreign material, in the form of black or colorless, round or rectangular, platelike crystalline structures, is dispersed throughout the sinuses and nodal parenchyma, more often within the cytoplasm of multinucleated giant cells and histiocytes (1,2). The foreign material does not polarize (1) (Fig. 53.1).

ELECTRON MICROSCOPY

Radiographic microanalysis performed with a transmission electron microscope and the energy-dispersive x-ray elemental analysis (EDXEA) device shows characteristic gold peaks (1,2) (Fig. 53.2). Ultrastructurally, gold particles appear as electron-dense granules and filaments, or as rods (1).

DIFFERENTIAL DIAGNOSIS

- Microcalcifications in intramammary or axillary lymph nodes detected during scanning mammography: Findings must be correlated with the history and histologic findings (4).

Checklist

GOLD LYMPHADENOPATHY

History of rheumatoid arthritis and chrysotherapy
Hyperplastic follicles with reactive germinal centers
Extracellular and intracellular dense granular or platelike structures
Multinucleated giant cells
Histiocytes with phagocytosed foreign bodies
EDXEA gold peak

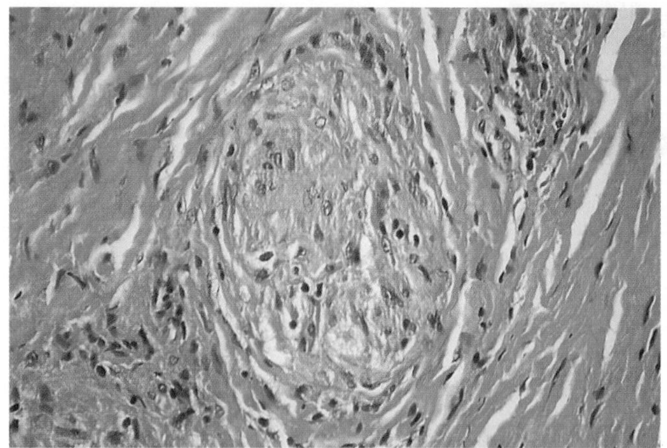

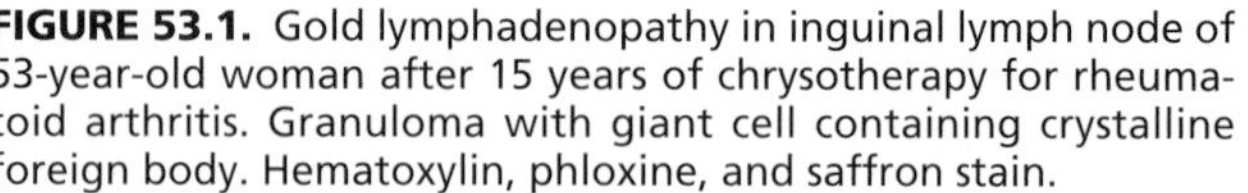

FIGURE 53.1. Gold lymphadenopathy in inguinal lymph node of 53-year-old woman after 15 years of chrysotherapy for rheumatoid arthritis. Granuloma with giant cell containing crystalline foreign body. Hematoxylin, phloxine, and saffron stain.

- Silicone lymphadenopathy: Morphology may be similar. The distinction must be made by the history and eventually by EDXEA (5,6).

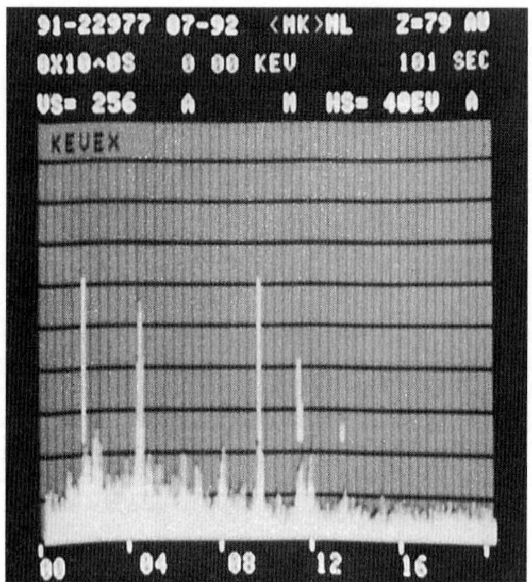

FIGURE 53.2. Energy-dispersive x-ray elemental analysis (EDXEA) of lymph node with foreign body showing characteristic gold peaks (Mα Lα Lβ). (Courtesy of J. A. Terzakis, M.D.)

REFERENCES

1. Carter TR. Intramammary lymph node gold deposits simulating microcalcifications on mammogram. Hum Pathol 1988;19:992–994.
2. Rollins SD, Craig JP. Gold-associated lymphadenopathy in a patient with rheumatoid arthritis. Histologic and scanning electron microscopic features [see Comments]. Arch Pathol Lab Med 1991; 115:175–177.
3. Gottlieb NL, Page WF, Appelrouth DJ, et al. Antecedent tonsillectomy and appendectomy in rheumatoid arthritis. J Rheumatol 1979;6:316–323.
4. Spark RP. Gold-associated lymphadenopathy in a patient with rheumatoid arthritis [Letter; Comment]. Arch Pathol Lab Med 1991;115:861–862.
5. Travis WD, Balogh K, Abraham JL. Silicone granulomas: report of three cases and review of the literature. Hum Pathol 1985;16:19–27.
6. Abraham JL. Silicone in gold-associated lymphadenopathy [Letter; Comment]. Arch Pathol Lab Med 1991;115:862.

PART IV

SECTION SIX

LYMPH NODE INCLUSIONS

Metastases of malignant tumors frequently lodge in the regional lymph nodes, indicating by their presence the capacity of a particular neoplasm to disseminate and form new colonies at distant sites. The finding of carcinoma or melanoma cells in a lymph node significantly worsens the prognosis of malignant disease.

As a consequence of developmental heterotopia, nonneoplastic squamous cells, glandular formations, or nests of nevus cells may be also present in lymph nodes. Although far less common than tumor metastases, such benign inclusions must be carefully considered to avoid confusion with their malignant counterparts.

54

EPITHELIAL CELL INCLUSIONS IN LYMPH NODES

DEFINITION

Clusters of benign, well-differentiated epithelial cells in lymph nodes.

PATHOGENESIS

The presence of epithelial cells in lymph nodes is usually the result of metastasis from a regional carcinoma. Their detection is of great clinical importance because it determines the staging, and consequently the treatment, of malignant tumors. Far less often, benign epithelial cells unrelated to the existence of a malignant tumor may also be present in various lymph nodes. Their origin is not well understood, although several theories have been proposed, including transportation of detached epithelial cells as a kind of benign metastasis (1–3), developmental heterotopia (4–7), and metaplasia of local multipotential cells (8–10). Because lymph node epithelial inclusions raise different problems of pathogenesis and differential diagnosis, depending on their location and histologic appearance, the various types are discussed separately.

Upper Cervical Lymph Nodes

Salivary gland acini and ducts may be found randomly distributed within the upper cervical lymph nodes. They are considered to represent aberrant or heterotopic parotid gland tissue in lymph nodes (4). Ectopic parotid glands or portions thereof are often detected within parotid gland lymph nodes at biopsies performed in the course of inflammatory or neoplastic lymphadenopathies (11) (Fig. 54.1) (see Chapter 16).

Lower Cervical Lymph Nodes

Incidental findings of colloid-containing thyroid follicles at radical dissection of the neck for various squamous carcinomas or melanomas of the head and neck have been reported occasionally (12–15) (Figs. 54.2 and 54.3). None of these was detected grossly, and the incidence was only about 1 in 100 neck dissections (13). When the thyroid glands were later examined histologically, no primary carcinomas were found.

However, Butler and colleagues (14) showed the presence of an occult primary carcinoma of the thyroid in 16 of 22 patients who had thyroid follicles incidentally found in regional cervical lymph nodes. The authors believe that the benign histologic appearance and lack of a papillary component in the thyroid follicles present in cervical lymph nodes do not preclude their being metastatic. Although clinically occult, the primary thyroid carcinoma in the studied cases was found after careful sectioning of the gland, and it usually contained papillary in addition to follicular areas.

Whether thyroid follicles within cervical lymph nodes represent metastases of occult thyroid carcinomas or embryonic malformations has not been resolved, and definitive diagnosis may not be always possible.

Axillary Lymph Nodes

Nodules composed of mammary ducts, cysts, and myoepithelial cells have been observed in axillary lymph nodes (1,16,17) (Fig. 54.4). The breast was the site of fibrocystic disease but not of carcinoma, and the axillary lymph node inclusions were explained by embryonic malformation or by lymphatic transport of nonmalignant cells (benign metastasis) (1). Only one report of a cystic squamous epithelial axillary lymph node inclusion occurring in a patient with breast carcinoma has been published (18).

Mediastinal Lymph Nodes

Glandlike structures lined by columnar epithelial cells were seen in mediastinal lymph nodes (3,10) and were considered to be of mesothelial origin. Some of these patients had pleuritis with pleural effusions, and the lymph node inclusions were interpreted as pleural cells that had entered lymphatic spaces and been transported to the mediastinal lymph nodes (3).

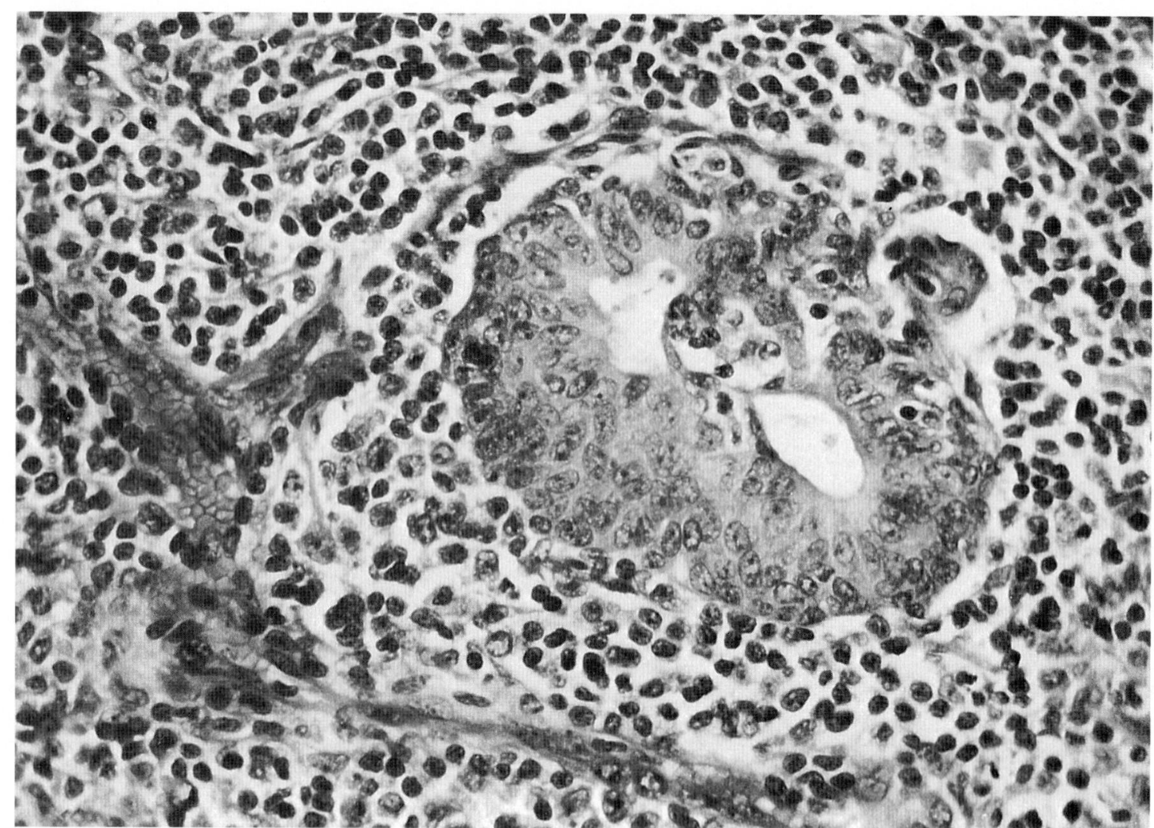

FIGURE 54.1. Salivary gland inclusion in parotid lymph node. Salivary gland duct with hyperplastic lining epithelium lies within the nodal lymphoid tissue. Hematoxylin, phloxine, and saffron stain.

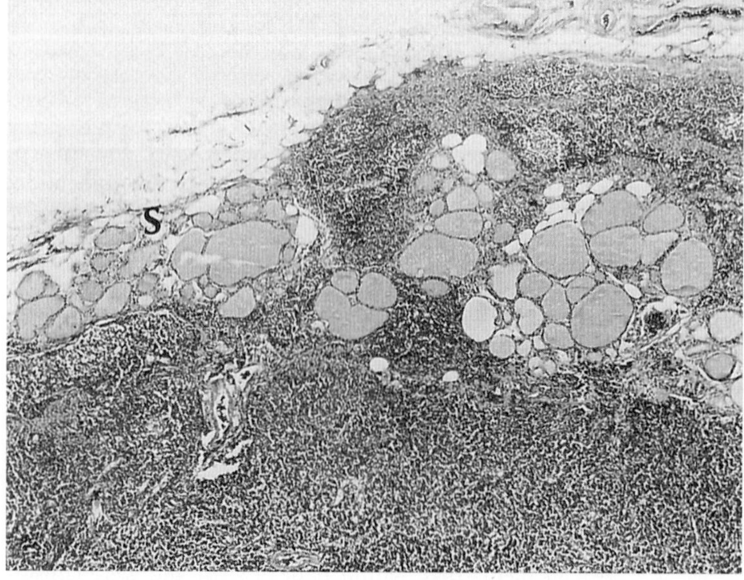

FIGURE 54.2. Thyroid inclusions in cervical lymph node; several clusters of colloid-filled follicles in the peripheral sinus (*S*). (From Nicastri AD, Foote FW Jr, Frazell EL. Benign thyroid inclusions in cervical lymph nodes. JAMA 1965;194:113–116, with permission.)

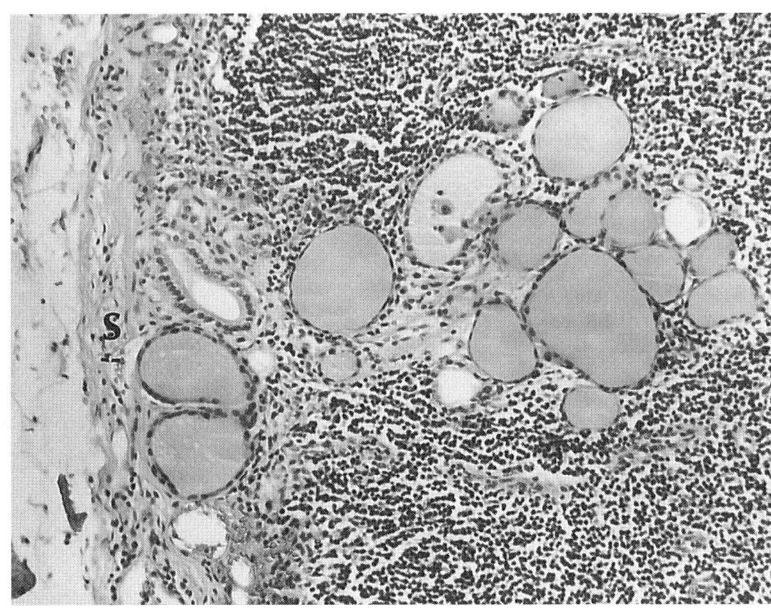

FIGURE 54.3. Same lymph node as in Fig. 54.2. Nonpapillary, colloid-containing follicles lined by flattened cuboidal epithelium in peripheral sinus (*S*). ×540.

Mesenteric Lymph Nodes

Colonic glands of benign histologic appearance were observed in the mesenteric lymph nodes (19,20) of patients undergoing colectomy for colonic carcinoma (19). The colonic carcinoma was only focal in a villous adenoma, and the glands in the mesenteric lymph nodes appeared benign and were thought to represent embolization caused by the surgical procedure (19).

Renal Lymph Nodes

Renal tubular inclusions associated with proteinaceous material identified as Tamm-Horsfall protein were seen in regional lymph nodes excised with Wilms tumors in children (21). The epithelial cells may have been derived from nephrons damaged by tumor obstruction or in other cases from squamous metaplasia of calyceal urothelium (21). Remnants of wolffian ducts were another proposed origin (6).

Peritoneal Lymph Nodes

Benign glandular inclusions were first and most often observed in pelvic and paraaortic lymph nodes removed from women during laparotomy or radical surgery (2,5–9,22–24) (Figs. 54.5–54.8). Their prevalence was reported to be 12% in a study of 50 female patients operated on for various gy-

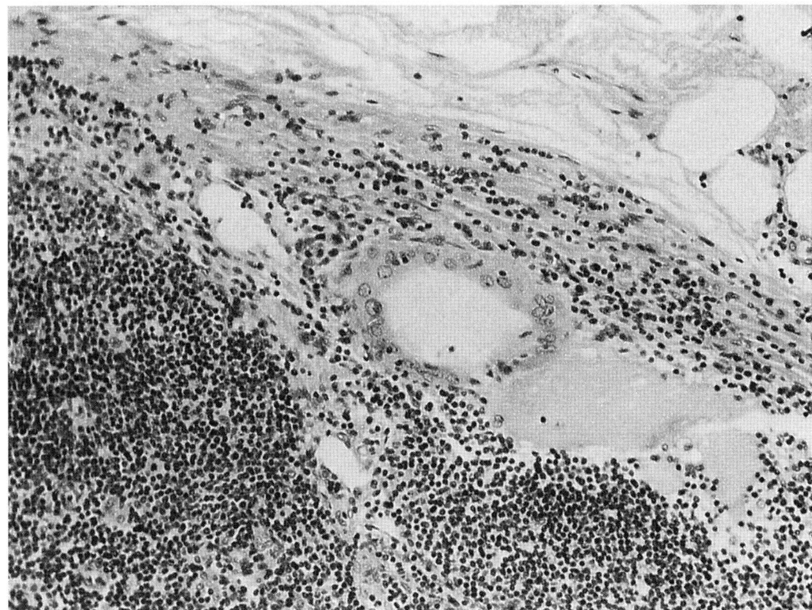

FIGURE 54.4. Mammary gland inclusion in axillary lymph node. Isolated glandlike structure lined by epithelium of normal appearance in subcapsular area. Hematoxylin and eosin stain.

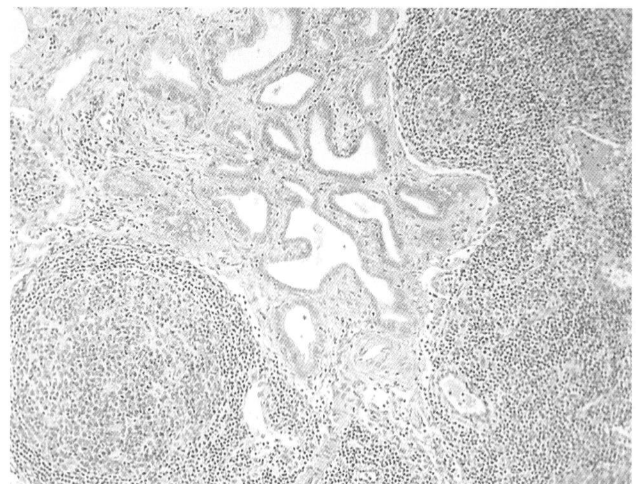

FIGURE 54.5. Glandular inclusions in peritoneal lymph node of 42-year-old woman with no neoplastic disease. The glands have bizarre shapes, are lined by low columnar epithelium, and are surrounded by fibrocollagen. Hematoxylin, phloxine, and saffron stain.

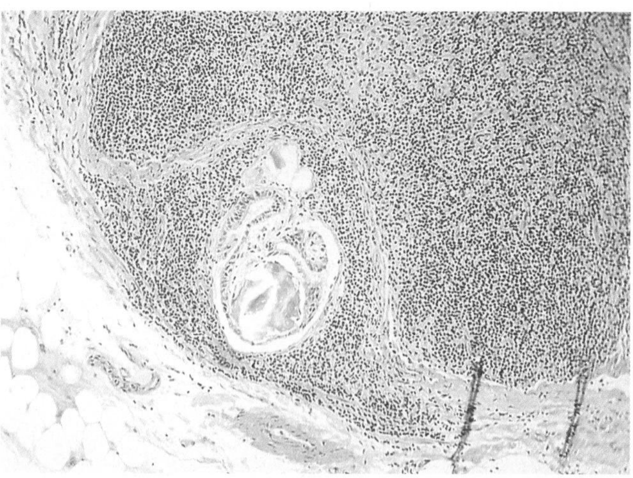

FIGURE 54.6. Same lymph node as in Fig. 44.5. Cluster of glands of nonmalignant appearance lying within lymphoid tissue in the absence of endometrial stroma. Hematoxylin, phloxine, and saffron stain.

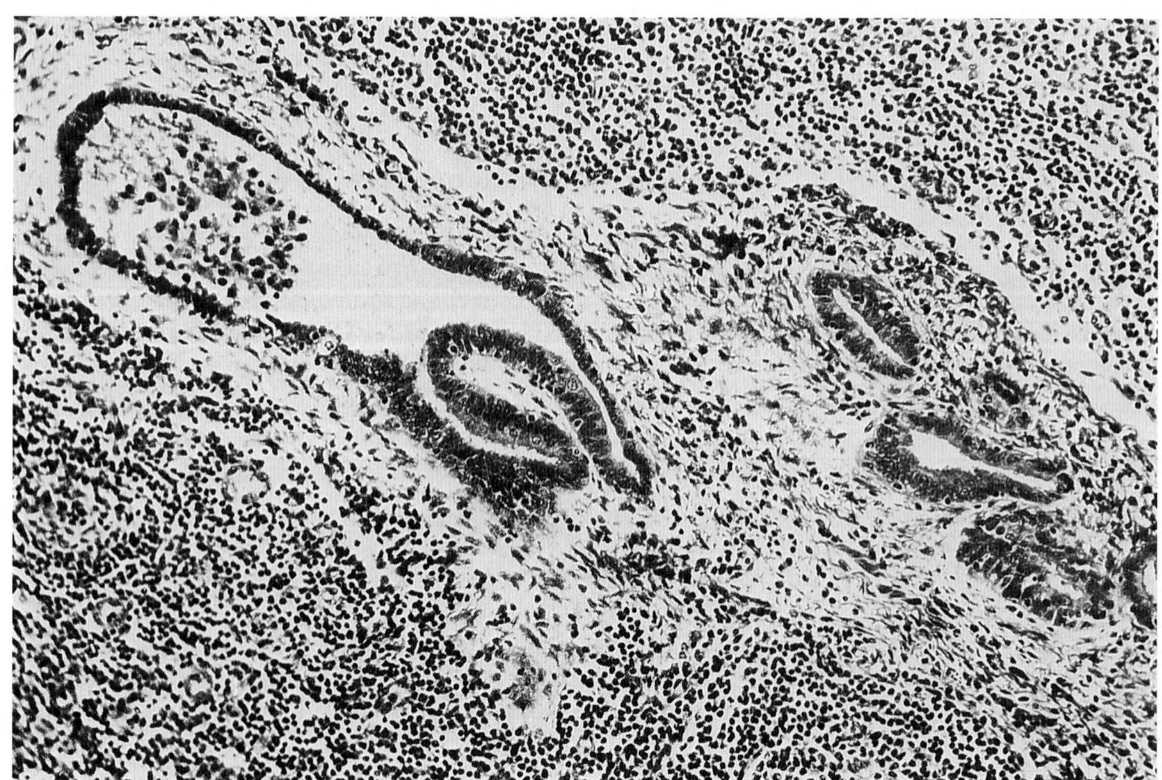

FIGURE 54.7. Glandular inclusions in the pelvic lymph nodes of a 45-year-old woman with squamous cell carcinoma of uterine cervix. (Courtesy of Dr. K. R. Zinsser.)

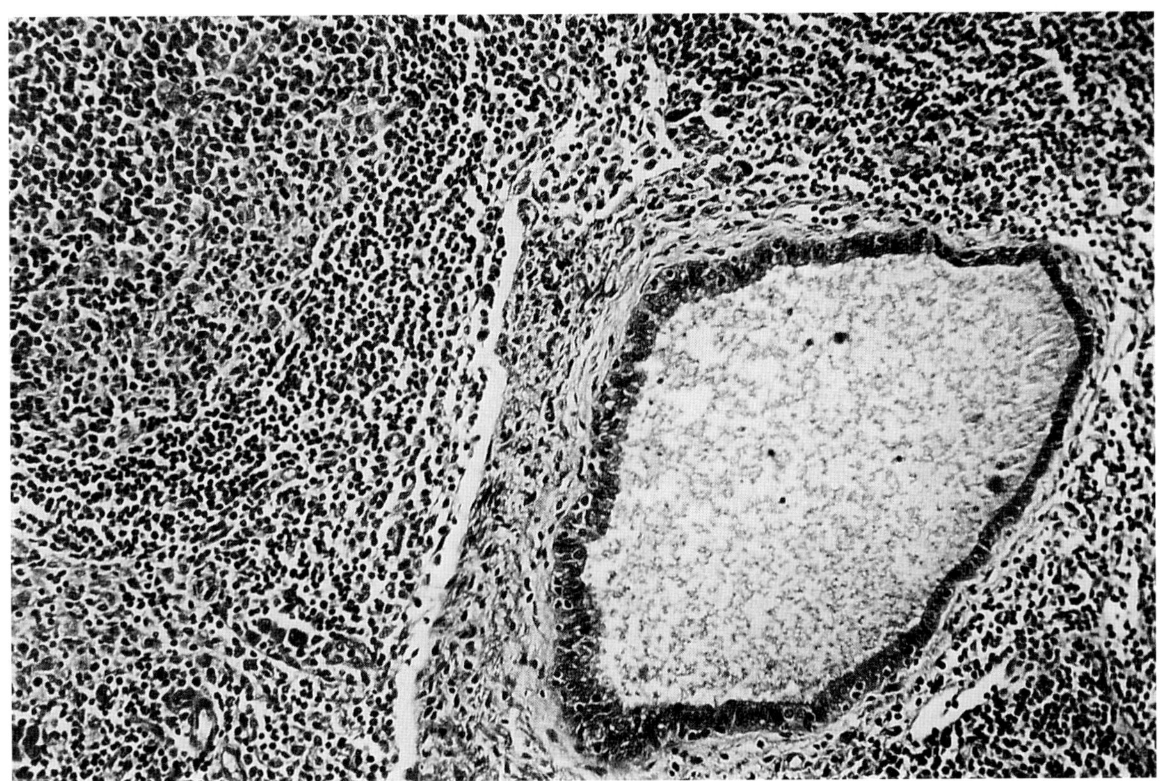

FIGURE 54.8. Glandular inclusions in paraaortic lymph node of 22-year-old woman with clear cell adenocarcinoma of vagina. Isolated, distended gland lined by well-differentiated epithelium. (Courtesy of Dr. K. R. Zinsser.)

necologic conditions (5), 14.8% in a survey of 128 cases (2), and as high as 40.8% in an earlier meticulous study of radical resections for cervical carcinoma (22). Epithelial inclusions were found in 14% of abdominal lymph nodes from 50 random autopsies of female patients and in none of those from 50 autopsies of male patients (8). Glandular inclusions in women may be found not only in abdominal lymph nodes but also in the ovaries, parametria, and pelvic peritoneum. In some of these cases, the glands are surrounded by endometrial stroma and therefore qualify as endometriosis. Other glands, however, may have ciliated epithelium, papillae, sometimes even psammoma bodies, and no stroma (7). Such glands resemble not endometrial but tubal or ovarian germinal epithelium and are devoid of accompanying stroma. The presence of ectopic epithelium resembling that of fallopian tube, a condition termed *endosalpingiosis,* may be congenital or acquired (23). Some authors have found endosalpingiosis in patients with chronic salpingitis, particularly salpingitis isthmica nodosa, who also tended to have ectopic pregnancies and spontaneous abortions (7). Such endothelium was thought to be transferred by ruptured inflammatory adhesions between the tube and other pelvic sites (2,5). Others consider glandular inclusions with a tubal or ovarian epithelial lining to be the result of müllerian differentiation, occurring in nests of totipotential cells of the coelomic epithelium. Although all the series of cases published indicate an absence of pelvic lymph node glandular inclusions in men (2,5,6,8), two such cases have been reported in the literature (25,26). The presence of benign glandular inclusions in the abdominal lymph nodes of men supports the theory of metaplasia of peritoneal mesothelium, as both wolffian ducts in males and müllerian ducts in females originate from the embryonal coelomic epithelium (25).

CLINICAL SYNDROME

The benign epithelial inclusions of lymph nodes are incidental findings and therefore unaccompanied by any symptoms. However, their clinical importance may be considerable because when they are misdiagnosed as metastatic carcinoma, extensive, costly, and sometimes damaging investigative and therapeutic procedures may follow.

HISTOPATHOLOGY

Cervical lymph nodes with inclusions of salivary glands (Fig. 54.1) may show enlarged reactive follicles with germinal centers containing tingible-body macrophages, patches of monocytoid cells, immunoblasts, plasma cells, and vascular proliferations, all caused by viral infections and typically seen in HIV lymphadenitis (11). In addition, scattered throughout the reactive lymph nodes are salivary acini and ducts, some lined by metaplastic squamous epithelium and others forming keratin cysts or solid epithelial islands. They represent inclusions of salivary glands within reactive cervical lymph nodes, not salivary glands infiltrated and destroyed by lymphocytes such as those in Sjögren or Mikulicz syndrome (11).

Cervical lymph nodes with inclusions of thyroid tissue (Figs. 54.2 and 54.3) show clusters of colloid follicles lined by low cuboidal epithelium. The nuclei are not atypical. Papillary structures and psammoma bodies are not present. Characteristically, the follicles lie within the peripheral sinus or near it (13).

Axillary lymph nodes containing heterotopic mammary epithelium show an aggregate of small mammary ducts, usually located in the subcapsular area (1) (Fig. 54.4). The ducts are composed of epithelial and myoepithelial cells. Morphologic variation is frequent, with cystic spaces lined by apocrine epithelium or by squamous cells that may form keratin. However, the epithelial cells do not show cytologic features of malignancy, such as hyperchromatism, nuclear pleomorphism, and mitoses. No inflammatory or desmoplastic reaction is present.

Mediastinal lymph nodes may contain cystic structures in the subcapsular area lined by a single layer of tall columnar epithelium on a well-defined basement membrane. In a reported case, no ciliated or goblet cells were present that suggested respiratory tract epithelium (10). In other cases, spaces between cells in small clusters within the nodal sinuses, so-called mesothelial windows, suggested an origin in the mesothelial cells of the pleurae, an origin confirmed by immunohistochemical study (3). The cells had bland nuclei, a low nuclear-to-cytoplasmic ratio, and no mitoses, features indicating their benign nature.

Mesenteric lymph nodes in an adenocarcinomatous colectomy specimen contained several simple tubular colonic glands in nodal sinuses (19). The glands had a benign appearance, were confined to the lumina, and were not accompanied by an inflammatory or fibrotic reaction.

Renal lymph nodes of pediatric Wilms tumors had dense proteinaceous material and cells in the sinuses in 29 of 45 cases (21). The hyaline material reacted positively with antisera against Tamm-Horsfall protein, whereas the cells were usually arranged in small alveolar or tubular configurations. Cytologically, they appeared benign.

Pelvic and abdominal lymph nodes with epithelial inclusions are slightly enlarged and show multiple glandular units located more often in the lymph node capsule and cortex (Figs. 54.5–54.8), sometimes also the medulla, but not in the sinuses or germinal centers (8). The glands form focal aggregates and vary in size and shape. The lining cells are cuboidal or tall, columnar, sharply demarcated, sometimes pseudostratified, and often ciliated.

Occasional infoldings of the epithelium with formation of papillae can be seen (5,7). Intraluminal mucin may be present that is stainable with Alcian blue (5). Nuclear pleomorphism, prominent nucleoli, and mitoses are not present (Fig. 54.8). Occasionally, microcalcification and psammoma bodies are noted. The histologic appearance is well differentiated and clearly benign, resembling ovarian germinal inclusion cysts or normal tubal epithelium. In contradistinction with endometriosis, periglandular endometrial stroma and hemorrhages are absent.

IMMUNOHISTOCHEMISTRY

Positive staining of intranodal cells with anticytokeratin monoclonal antibodies such as AE1/3 or CAM5.2 may be used to confirm their epithelial origin. A staining pattern positive for cytokeratins but negative for epithelial membrane antigen, Leu-M1, and carcinoembryonic antigen is indicative of mesothelial cells (3). In addition, mesothelial cells express calretinin (27).

Checklist

EPITHELIAL CELL INCLUSIONS IN LYMPH NODES

- Aggregates of epithelial structures in capsular or cortical sites
- Salivary glands in upper cervical lymph nodes
- Thyroid follicles devoid of papillae in lower cervical lymph nodes
- Mammary ducts and cysts in axillary lymph nodes
- Cell clusters with mesothelial windows in mediastinal lymph nodes
- Glands lined by salpingeal or ovarian epithelium in pelvic lymph nodes of women
- Benign histologic appearance of all epithelial structures
- Lack of nuclear pleomorphism and mitoses
- Lack of vascular, lymphatic, and sinus invasion

DIFFERENTIAL DIAGNOSIS

- Metastatic carcinoma: Early metastases are usually located in the marginal sinus. Blood vessels, lymphatics, and medullary sinuses may also be involved. The carcinoma cells generally exhibit neoplastic features, particularly pleomorphic nuclei and mitoses. In later stages, nodal metastases are surrounded by fibrous tissue; however, particularly on frozen sections, epithelial inclusions may be difficult to distinguish from the well-differentiated corresponding carcinomas. In the case of thyroid inclusions, multiple sections must be examined for the presence of papillary structures, which clearly make the diagnosis of thyroid carcinoma.
- Endometriosis in abdominal lymph nodes includes periglandular endometrial stroma and accumulations of hemosiderin-laden macrophages.

REFERENCES

1. Edlow DW, Carter D. Heterotopic epithelium in axillary lymph nodes: report of a case and review of the literature. Am J Clin Pathol 1973;59:666–673.
2. Zinsser KR, Wheeler JE. Endosalpingiosis in the omentum: a study of autopsy and surgical material. Am J Surg Pathol 1982;6: 109–117.
3. Brooks JS, LiVolsi VA, Pietra GG. Mesothelial cell inclusions in mediastinal lymph nodes mimicking metastatic carcinoma. Am J Clin Pathol 1990;93:741–748.
4. Brown RB, Gaillard RA, Turner JA. The significance of aberrant or heterotopic parotid gland tissue in lymph nodes. Ann Surg 1953;138:850–856.
5. Kheir SM, Mann WJ, Wilkerson JA. Glandular inclusions in lymph nodes. The problem of extensive involvement and relationship to salpingitis. Am J Surg Pathol 1981;5:353–359.
6. Farhi DC, Silverberg SG. Pseudometastases in female genital cancer. Pathol Annu 1982;17:47–76.
7. Shen SC, Bansal M, Purrazzella R, et al. Benign glandular inclusions in lymph nodes, endosalpingiosis, and salpingitis isthmica nodosa in a young girl with clear cell adenocarcinoma of the cervix. Am J Surg Pathol 1983;7:293–300.
8. Karp LA, Czernobilsky B. Glandular inclusions in pelvic and abdominal para-aortic lymph nodes. A study of autopsy and surgical material in males and females. Am J Clin Pathol 1969;52:212–218.
9. Kempson RL. Consultation case: benign glandular inclusions in iliac lymph nodes. Am J Surg Pathol 1978;2:321–325.
10. Longo S. Benign lymph node inclusions. Hum Pathol 1976;7: 349–354.
11. Ioachim HL, Ryan JR, Blaugrund SM. Salivary gland lymph nodes. The site of lymphadenopathies and lymphomas associated with human immunodeficiency virus infection. Arch Pathol Lab Med 1988;112:1224–1228.
12. Gerard-Marchant R. Thyroid follicle inclusions in cervical lymph nodes. Arch Pathol 1964;77:633.
13. Nicastri AD, Foote FW, Frazell EL. Benign thyroid inclusions in cervical lymph nodes. JAMA 1965;194:1–4.
14. Butler JJ, Tulinius H, Ibanez ML, et al. Significance of thyroid tissue in lymph nodes associated with carcinoma of the head, neck or lung. Cancer 1967;20:103–112.
15. Meyer JS, Steinberg LS. Microscopically benign thyroid follicles in cervical lymph nodes. Serial section study of lymph node inclusions and entire thyroid gland in 5 cases. Cancer 1969;24: 302–311.
16. Garrett R, Ada AEV. Epithelial inclusion cysts of axillary lymph node: report of a case simulating adenocarcinoma. Cancer 1957; 10:173.
17. Silton RM. More glandular inclusions. Am J Surg Pathol 1979;3: 285–286.
18. Fraggetta F, Vasquez E. Epithelial inclusion in axillary lymph node associated with a breast carcinoma: report of a case with a review of the literature. Pathol Res Pract 1999;195:263–266.
19. Perrone T. Embolization of benign colonic glands to mesenteric lymph nodes. Am J Surg Pathol 1985;9:538–541.
20. Gritsman AY, Schwartz AM. Benign glandular inclusions. Arch Pathol Lab Med 1985;109:389–390.
21. Weeks DA, Beckwith JB, Mierau GW. Benign nodal lesions mimicking metastases from pediatric renal neoplasms: a report of the National Wilms' Tumor Study Pathology Center. Hum Pathol 1990;21:1239–1244.
22. Huhn FO. Drüseneinschlüsse in Beckenlymphknoten der Frau. Virchow's Arch 1962;335:84–100.
23. Burmeister RE, Fechner RE, Franklin RR. Endosalpingiosis of the peritoneum. Obstet Gynecol 1969;34:310–318.
24. Ehrmann RL, Federschneider JM, Knapp RC. Distinguishing lymph node metastases from benign glandular inclusions in low-grade ovarian carcinoma. Am J Obstet Gynecol 1980;136:737–746.
25. Huntrakoon M. Benign glandular inclusions in the abdominal lymph nodes of a man. Hum Pathol 1985;16:644–646.
26. Tazelaar HD, Vareska G. Benign glandular inclusions. Hum Pathol 1986;17:100–101.
27. Barberis MC, Faleri M, Veronese S, et al. Calretinin. A selective marker of normal and neoplastic mesothelial cells in serous effusions. Acta Cytol 1997;41:1757–1761.

55

NEVUS CELL INCLUSIONS IN LYMPH NODES

DEFINITION

Aggregates of nevus cells in the lymph node hilus, capsule, or trabeculae.

PATHOGENESIS

Aggregates of nevus cells within peripheral lymph nodes have been reported occasionally (1–8). Two explanations have been considered; however, neither has been generally accepted for lack of satisfactory documentation. According to one opinion, nevus cells in the lymph nodes may represent arrested aberrant embryonal migration from the neural crest. Johnson and Helwig (1), discussing this possibility, indicated that reports of blue nevi in unusual locations, such as the prostate, uterine cervix, and vagina, provide similar examples of abnormal embryonal migration. According to another opinion, the nevus cells migrate to the lymph nodes in adult life and therefore represent "benign metastases" from a cutaneous site (2,4,8). The mechanism of this cell transfer, possibly through lymph or blood vessels, is not clear. Bell and co-workers (4), studying serial sections of 124 nevi, found frequent subendothelial hillocks of nevus cells protruding into the lumina of lymphatic vessels and occasional free clusters of cells in the vascular spaces. The breaching of the lymphatic endothelial lining shown in this study provides support for the idea that benign nevus cells can embolize, lodge, and grow in the regional lymph nodes without evidence of further malignant invasion.

Another peculiar aspect of aberrant nevus cells is their exclusive location in superficial skin-draining lymph nodes (2,8). All 46 cases of lymph node nevus inclusions reported as of 1977 were located in peripheral lymph nodes; no inclusions in visceral lymph nodes were reported (3,4). Among all the cases, the axillary lymph nodes were by far the most frequently involved group. Whether this is because of special local conditions or because the axillary lymph nodes are more often examined is not known. In a study of lymph nodes removed for various visceral and cutaneous lesions, nevus cells were found in 6.2% of all axillary lymph nodes examined (2). However, in the extensive study by Ridolfi and associates (3), nevus cell aggregates were present in only 3 of 17,504 lymph nodes (0.017%) obtained from 909 mastectomies (0.33% of cases), and in 3 of 2,607 lymph nodes (0.12%) obtained from 100 dissections for malignant melanoma (3% of cases).

In most cases of nevus cell inclusions, the lymph nodes were removed as part of cancer diagnostic or therapeutic procedures. The primary tumors were carcinomas or, in a few instances, malignant melanomas; however, no morphologic resemblance to the nevus cell inclusions was noted. In the cases in which malignant melanoma was not the primary tumor, the follow-up histories revealed no metastases or deaths from melanoma, support for the benign nature of the aberrant nevus cells.

HISTOPATHOLOGY

Nevus cell inclusions in lymph nodes are an incidental finding because they do not cause clinical symptoms or physical enlargement and their only importance is possible confusion with metastatic melanoma. In most reported cases, clusters of nevus cells were located in the connective tissues of the lymph node capsule (Fig. 55.1), hilus, or trabeculae. Nevus cells have never been reported to occur in the marginal sinus, the usual site of metastatic tumors, and in only three cases were they noted within the lymph node parenchyma (3,9). The nevus cells (Figs. 55.2 and 55.3) form cords, nests, or linear strands and include occasional slitlike spaces, similar to those often seen in dermal nevi (4). Rarely does blue nevus involve the lymph node capsule (5,6). If melanocytes are found in the lymph node marginal sinus synchronously with a pigmented skin lesion, the possibility of a metastatic malignancy should be seriously considered (10–12).

In a few reported cases, nevus cells of benign morphologic appearance were noted within the walls and lumina of afferent lymphatics (2,8). The cells are monomorphic, with indistinct borders and fine, pink cytoplasm containing brown,

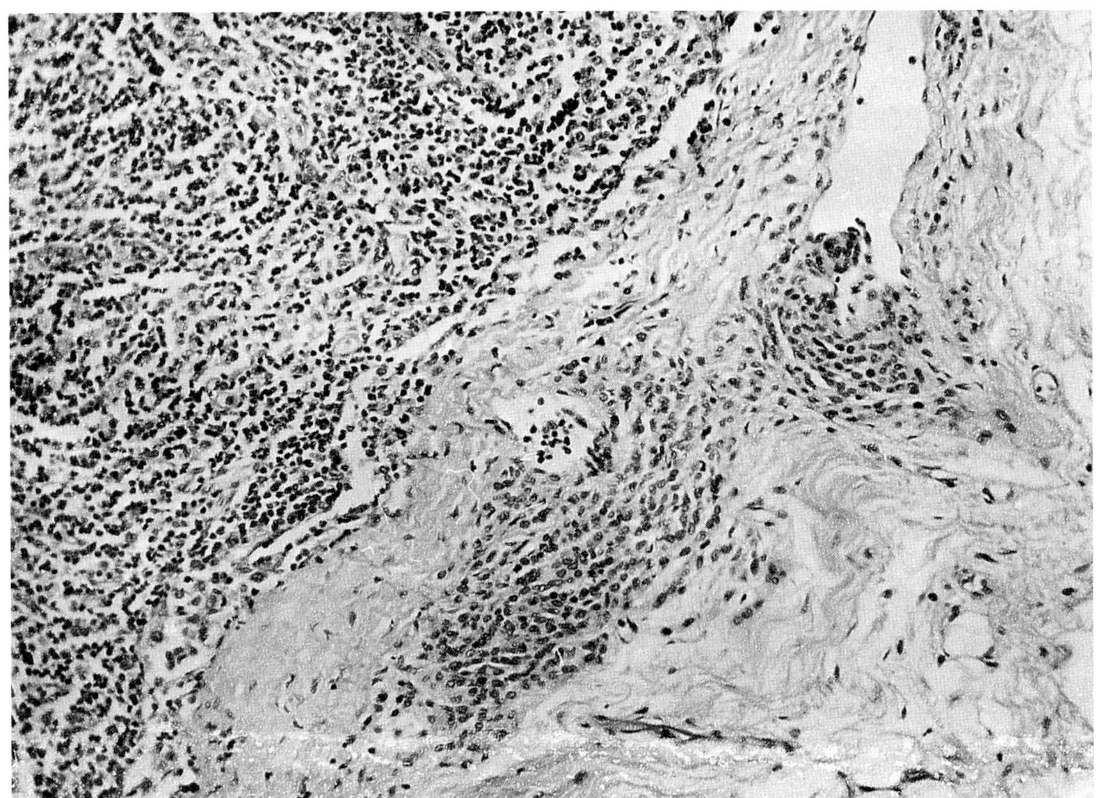

FIGURE 55.1. Axillary lymph node with two capsular aggregates of nevus cells. Lymph node cortex (*left*), capsular aggregate of nevus cells (*center*), and subendothelial hillock of nevus cells protruding into the lumen of a capsular lymphatic vessel (*right*). Hematoxylin, phloxine, and saffron stain.

granular melanin pigment. The nuclei are round or oval and the nucleoli inconspicuous, and mitoses are not noted. In morphologic appearance, clustering patterns, the presence of melanin pigment, the lack of prominent nucleoli, and the absence of mitoses, these cells resemble those of common intradermal nevi and suggest the benign nature of this lesion.

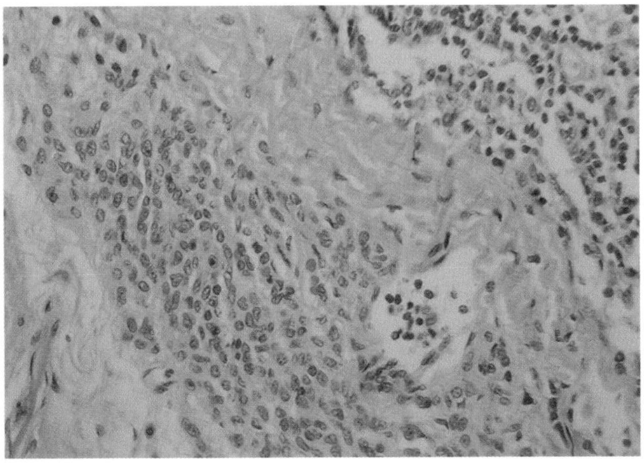

FIGURE 55.2. Inclusion of nevus cells in lymph node capsule. Hematoxylin, phloxine, and saffron stain.

ELECTRON MICROSCOPY

Examination under the electron microscope of a nevus cell aggregate in the axillary lymph node of a patient with breast cancer showed uniform, round nevus cells with indented nuclei, dispersed chromatin, randomly oriented cy-

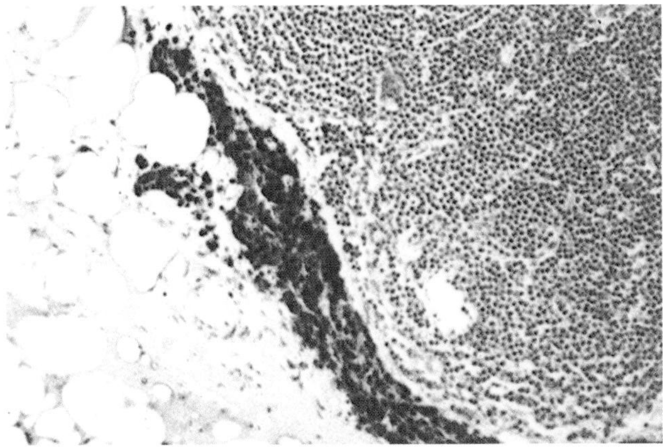

FIGURE 55.3. Lymph node cortex (*right*) and S100 protein+ nevus cells in lymph node capsule (*center*). Immunoperoxidase stain.

Checklist

NEVUS CELL INCLUSIONS IN LYMPH NODES

Aggregates of nevus cells in the lymph node capsule, hilum, or trabeculae
Marginal sinus not involved; parenchyma very rarely involved
Monomorphic cell population
Lack of nuclear pleomorphism and nucleolar prominence
Absence of mitoses

toplasmic fibrils, and a few mature melanosomes (7). The appearance was indistinguishable from that of an intradermal nevus.

DIFFERENTIAL DIAGNOSIS

- Malignant melanoma metastatic to lymph nodes, particularly in cases with a known melanoma primary, is the main diagnostic concern. In contrast to the benign nevus inclusions, metastatic melanoma cells are always located in the marginal sinus or nodal parenchyma. Cell size, nuclear atypia, nucleolar prominence, and frequency of mitoses are the characteristic features.

REFERENCES

1. Johnson WT, Helwig EB. Benign nevus cells in the capsule of lymph nodes. Cancer 1969;23:747–753.
2. McCarthy SW, Palmer AA, Bale PM, et al. Naevus cells in lymph nodes. Pathology 1974;6:351–358.
3. Ridolfi RL, Rosen PP, Thaler H. Nevus cell aggregates associated with lymph nodes: estimated frequency and clinical significance. Cancer 1977;39:164–171.
4. Bell ME, Hill DP, Bhargava MK. Lymphatic invasion in pigmented nevi. Am J Clin Pathol 1979;72:97–100.
5. Lamovec J. Blue nevus of the lymph node capsule. Report of a new case with review of the literature. Am J Clin Pathol 1984;81:367–372.
6. Mancini L, Gubinelli M, Fortunato C, et al. Blue nevus of the lymph node capsule. Report of a case. Pathologica 1992;84:547–550.
7. Erlandson RA, Rosen PP. Electron microscopy of a nevus cell aggregate associated with an axillary lymph node. Cancer 1982;49:269–272.
8. Subramony C, Lewin JR. Nevus cells within lymph nodes. Possible metastases from a benign intradermal nevus. Am J Clin Pathol 1985;84:220–223.
9. Hruban RH, Eckert F, Baricevic B. Melanocytes of a melanocytic nevus in a lymph node from a patient with a primary cutaneous melanoma associated with a small congenital nevus. Am J Dermatopathol 1990;12:402–407.
10. Shih L, Hawkins DB. Recurrent postauricular blue nevus with lymph node involvement. Otolaryngol Head Neck Surg 1987;97:491–494.
11. Gonzalez-Campora R, Diaz-Cano S, Vazquez-Ramirez F, et al. Cellular blue nevus with massive regional lymph node metastases. Dermatol Surg 1996;22:83–87.
12. Smith NM, Evans MJ, Pearce A, et al. Cytogenetics of an atypical Spitz nevus metastatic to a single lymph node. Pediatr Pathol Lab Med 1998;18:115–122.

PART

V

LYMPHOMAS

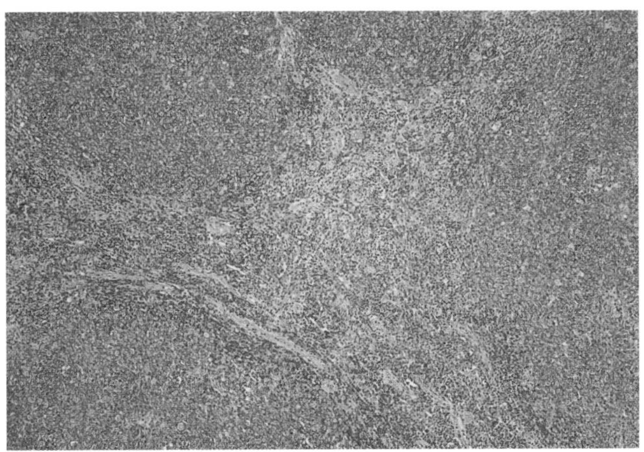

For the hematopathologist involved in scientific research, lymphomas and leukemias present the most challenging field of medical investigation, one in which immunity and neoplasia interface and in which new concepts and tech-niques are constantly tested. For the practicing pathologist, the important task of correctly diagnosing and classifying leukemias and lymphomas arises frequently and can be difficult. To establish the treatment and determine the prognosis, Hodgkin and non-Hodgkin lymphomas must be identified and phenotyped. Non-Hodgkin lymphomas must be differentiated from Hodgkin lymphomas, and both must be separated from the various types of non-neoplastic lymphadenopathies. Once identified, they must be charac-terized morphologically, immunologically, and genotypi-cally. An array of diagnostic methods and a wide variety of reagents and techniques, unmatched by those in any other area of diagnostic pathology, are available. It is incumbent on the practicing pathologist to set up standards and select methods that are most likely to facilitate the proper diag-nosis at a reasonable cost.

In 2001, the American Cancer Society estimated 63,600 new cases of lymphoma: 7,400 of Hodgkin lymphoma and 56,200 of non-Hodgkin lymphoma, 35,000 cases in men and 28,600 in women. These statistics indicate that lymphoma is the fifth most common malignant neoplasm in persons of both sexes in the United States. In children, leukemias and lymphomas are among the most common forms of neoplasia; however, the survival rates have considerably improved during the past decade. The epidemiology of lymphomas is varied, with considerable geographic differences observed in the age of populations affected and in the predominant forms of disease. In the Western hemisphere and in higher socioeconomic groups, B-cell lymphomas, less aggressive types, and cases in older persons are more frequent. In the Orient, T-cell lymphomas are more frequent, and in underdeveloped countries, highly aggressive lymphomas affecting younger persons are more common.

The clinical management of lymphomas depends on

correct diagnosis and classification. Through the years, the definition, typing, and classification of lymphomas have continuously evolved. In the last two decades, our unders-tanding of the immune system has increased rapidly, and the methods by which it is studied have improved. These achievements have had to be integrated into the nomen-clature and classification of lymphomas. At the same time, efforts have been made to devise categories and types of lymphomas to allow better reproducibility. In the next chapter, the nomenclature and classification of lymphomas are considered in relation to their clinical significance.

PART V

SECTION ONE

NOMENCLATURE AND CLASSIFICATION OF LYMPHOMAS

56

NOMENCLATURE AND CLASSIFICATION OF LYMPHOMAS

Traditionally, tumors of various organs have been named and classified according to their histogenesis. This concept is based on the assumption that tumors originate in the cells and tissues that they resemble morphologically and, further, that the degree of resemblance indicates the stage of tumor cell differentiation (reflected in the qualifiers *well differentiated* and *poorly differentiated*).

In the past two decades, rapid progress in immunology and molecular biology has led to important discoveries related to the origin and function of lymphocytes. These in turn are reflected in conceptual changes in the nomenclature and classification of lymphomas. The earlier observation that small, mature-looking circulating lymphocytes, when stimulated by lectins or antigens (2), can transform into large, immature-looking blast cells involved in DNA synthesis and mitotic activity (Fig. 56.1) brought into question the appropriateness of estimating cellular differentiation on the basis of morphology alone (3). Activated lymphocytes or immunoblasts that in the past, according to their size and structure, were considered to represent reticulum cells, histiocytes, or primitive stem cells are in fact transformed lymphocytes engaged in protein production and immune activity. Similarly deceiving is the structure of small lymphocytes, which appear as "mature, well-differentiated, end-of-the-line cells" yet can change both their structure and function to the level of primitive blast cells.

The heterogeneity of lymphocytes is another major discovery that has had a lasting impact on our understanding of lymphomas (4,5). With the aid of newly developed methods, the T- and B-cell types of lymphocytes can be identified, and subpopulations of these groups can be recognized by their surface markers and secretory products. Again, the microscopic appearance of cells is deceiving because distinct populations of lymphocytes may be morphologically indistinguishable.

In the 1970s, numerous investigators, applying modern immunologic methods to the study of lymphoma, made important contributions to the recognition of new types of neoplasms (3,6–16). Before then, the classification of Rappaport (16) (Table 56.1), published in 1966, had been used internationally, having received broad acceptance for its high reproducibility and good clinicopathologic correlations. Lukes and Collins (3,17) and Lennert and associates (6,18) were the first to develop classifications based on evidence of lymphocyte transformation and the existence of T- and B-cell systems. Additional classifications that were subsequently proposed considerably increased the terminology used in this field (19–22). The large number of publications on lymphomas has added to the inherent complexity of the subject, making the understanding of this group of neoplasms particularly difficult. The classic Rappaport classification was modified to include newly described entities and to correct terms such as *nodular lymphoma* and *histiocytic lymphoma,* which were no longer in agreement with the new conceptual changes (22). Lukes and collaborators, in multiparameter studies of large numbers of cases correlating morphologic features with immunophenotypes, showed that most non-Hodgkin lymphomas (NHLs) in the Western world, between 75% and 81% in their series, are of B-cell origin, a conclusion confirmed by all subsequent studies (23–25). The Kiel classification, based on the concepts introduced by Lennert, was updated to incorporate new data on histogenesis, morphology, and immunologic cell function (26). The Kiel classification was widely used in Europe but remained largely unfamiliar in the United States. The classification published by the World Health Organization (WHO) was criticized for reintroducing previously abandoned histogenetic terms (21). The British classification proposed by Bennett et al. (19) and classifications by Dorfman (20) and Mann et al. (27) replaced many of the discredited histogenetic names with new terms and definitions; however, they were not widely accepted.

The profusion of nomenclature and classification systems has contributed to a forbidding image of lymphomas that not infrequently discourages their study. The lack of agreement and the use of different classifications in textbooks, laboratory investigations, and clinical trials still prevents effective communication between workers in the field, particularly between pathologists and clinicians. Yet, as Nathwani (28) points out in a critical analysis of this sub-

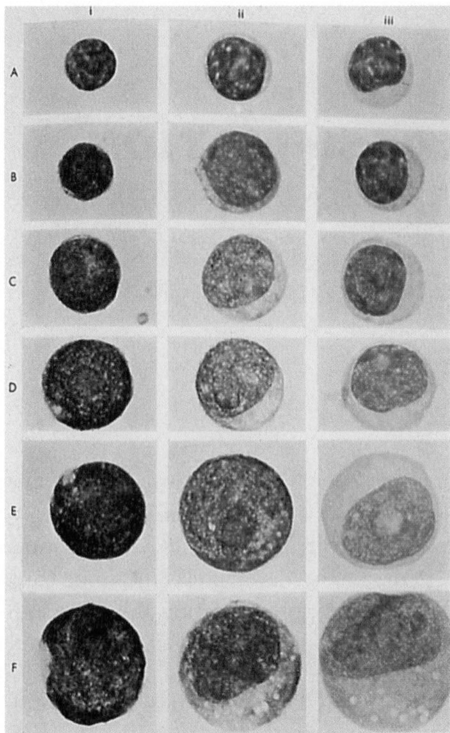

FIGURE 56.1. Transformation of normal human lymphocytes in culture induced by phytohemagglutinin: *row A,* at zero hours; *row B,* at 24 hours; *rows C–F,* at 48 hours. (From Yoffey JM, et al. Morphological studies in the culture of human leucocytes with phytohaemagglutinin. Br J Haematol 1965;11:488, with permission.)

ject, the fact that the similarities between the various classification systems in use are far more numerous than the differences indicates the possibility of achieving a consensus on one classification system. A major effort in this sense was the elaborate study of 1,175 NHLs by a panel of international experts that resulted in a new classification, the Working Formulation for Clinical Usage (29) (Table 56.2). The NHLs were categorized according to the classifications most commonly used at the time. A large part of the nomenclature in the Working Formulation was derived from the concepts of Lukes and Collins (17). As Lennert et al. (6) had previously attempted to do, it added an important clinical feature by dividing the lymphomas into low-,

TABLE 56.1. CLASSIFICATION OF NON-HODGKIN LYMPHOMAS

Nodular	Diffuse
Lymphocytic, well-differentiated	
Lymphocytic, poorly differentiated	
Mixed cell (lymphocytic and histiocytic)	
Histiocytic	
Undifferentiated	

From Rappaport H. Tumors of the hematopoietic system. In: Atlas of Tumor Pathology, Section III, Fasc. 8. Washington, DC: Armed Forces Institute of Pathology, 1966, with permission.

TABLE 56.2. A WORKING FORMULATION OF NON-HODGKIN LYMPHOMAS FOR CLINICAL USAGE: RECOMMENDATIONS OF AN EXPERT INTERNATIONAL PANEL

Low-grade
- Malignant lymphoma
  - Small lymphocytic
    - Consistent with chronic lymphocitic leukemia; plasmacytoid
- Malignant lymphoma, follicular
  - Predominantly small cleaved
    - Diffuse areas; sclerosis
- Malignant lymphoma, follicular
  - Mixed, small cleaved and large cell
    - Diffuse areas; sclerosis

Intermediate-grade
- Malignant lymphoma, follicular
  - Predominantly large cell
    - Diffuse areas; sclerosis
- Malignant lymphoma, diffuse
  - Small cleaved
    - Sclerosis
- Malignant lymphoma, diffuse
  - Mixed, small and large cell
    - Sclerosis; epithelioid cell component
- Malignant lymphoma, diffuse
- Large cell
    - Cleaved; noncleaved; sclerosis

High-grade
- Malignant lymphoma
  - Large cell, immunoblastic
    - Plasmacytoid; clear cell; polymorphic; epithelioid cell component
- Malignant lymphoma
  - Lymphoblastic
    - Convoluted; nonconvoluted
- Malignant lymphoma
  - Small noncleaved
    - Burkitt; follicular areas

Miscellaneous
- Composite
- Mycosis fungoides
- Histiocytic
- Extramedullary plasmacytoma
- Unclassifiable
- Other

From the National Cancer Institute-sponsored study of classifications of non-Hodgkin's lymphomas. Summary and description of a working formulation for clinical usage. Cancer 1982;49:2112–2135, with permission.

intermediate-, and high-grade categories, with prognostic implications. The stated goal at the time of publication was that the Working Formulation was not intended to be a new classification system but rather a means of "translating" among the various systems in existence to facilitate clinical comparisons of case reports and therapeutic trials (29). In the years since 1982, mainly because of its clinical correlations, the Working Formulation has become the NHL classification system generally used in the United States and many other countries.

In the past two decades, unprecedented technologic progress made possible detailed analyses of cellular biochemistry, immunology, and genetics. Materials and methods for probing nuclear DNA, determining immunophenotypic profiles, and detecting chromosome translocations became available and led to expanded knowledge and improved diagnosis. In the field of lymphomas, the existence of new populations of lymphoid cells was recognized, and new types of neoplasms were described. Among these were mantle cell lymphoma, marginal zone and monocytoid lymphomas as new types of B-cell neoplasms, and peripheral T-cell lymphoma, adult T-cell lymphoma, and anaplastic large cell lymphoma as new types of T-cell neoplasms.

Including the newly described forms of lymphomas in the existing classifications proved difficult, and awkward terms and ambiguous categories, noted by various authors, often resulted (30,31). To incorporate the new knowledge (31,32), an updated Kiel classification, in which the NHLs were divided into B- and T-cell types, was published in 1988 (26) (Table 56.3). However, the diagnostic reproducibility and clinical relevance of the group of T-cell lymphomas in the updated Kiel classification were criticized (30). Changes in the Working Formulation, originally a purely morphologic classification, were also advocated to account for new entities and reflect the immunophenotypes of lymphomas. Here again, the B-cell lymphomas proved easier to include because the Working Formulation, when it was created, was defined in accordance with the already known categories of B-cell lymphomas. In the case of the T-cell lymphomas, described later, the maturation scheme of normal T-cell counterparts on which the classification rests was far less clearly defined.

TABLE 56.3. UPDATED KIEL CLASSIFICATION OF NON-HODGKIN LYMPHOMAS

B-cell	T-cell
Low-grade	**Low grade**
*Lymphocytic—chronic lymphocytic and pro lymphocytic leukemia; hairy cell leukemia	Lymphocytic—chronic lymphocytic and pro lymphocytic leukemia
	Small, cerebriform cell-mycosis fungoides, Sézary syndrome
Lymphoplasmacytic/cytoid (LP immunocytoma)	Lymphoepithelioid (Lennert lymphoma)
Plasmacytic	Angioimmunoblastic (AILD, LgX)
*Centroblastic/centrocytic	
—follicular ± diffuse	T zone
—diffuse	Pleomorphic, small cell (HTLV-T±)
High-grade	**High-grade**
Centroblastic	Pleomorphic, medium and large cell (HTLV-T±)
*Immunoblastic	Immunoblastic (HTLV-T±)
*Large cell anaplastic (Ki-l+)	Large cell anaplastic (Ki-l+)
Burkitt lymphoma	
*Lymphoblastic	Lymphoblastic
Rare types	**Rare types**

AILD, angioimmunoblastic T-cell lymphoma; LgX, lymphogranulomatosis X; HTLV; human T-cell lymphotropic virus.
* Indicates some degree of correspondence, either in morphology or in functional expression, between categories in the two columns.
From Stansfield AG, Diebold J, Noel H, et al. Updated Kiel classification for lymphomas. Lancet 1998;1:292–293, with permission.

In 1994, an international group of hematopathologists with particular interest and expertise in lymphomas published a proposal for a new classification of lymphomas with the following title: "A Revised European-American Classification of Lymphoid Neoplasms: a Proposal from the International Lymphoma Study Group" (32) (Table 56.4). Generally known by its acronym, REAL, the new classification has been widely publicized and generally accepted on both sides of the Atlantic. As stated in its introduction, the REAL classification is not based on the histogenesis of lymphoma cells. Although this would be a desirable mode for a scientific classification, it is recognized that it is not entirely possible at the present time. Not all types of lymphomas can be traced to specific stages in the differentiation of normal lymphoid cells, and not infrequently, some well-defined lymphomas cannot be matched to any normal cell counterpart. Instead, the REAL classification takes the practical approach of categorizing lymphomas not by their presumed cell of origin but by their morphologic, immunologic, and genetic features. In this way, the REAL classification becomes a "list" of well-defined clinicopathologic entities (32). Some categories are provisional, depending on further progress in defining them, and others that do not fit into the categories of the list "are best left unclassified reflecting the fact that we do not yet understand everything about lymphomas or the immune system" (32). In the future, newly recognized entities can be readily added to the list.

The REAL proposal raised some concerns among clinicians, who argued that a classification based on the separation of lymphomas according to their B- or T-cell origin is not clinically useful (33,34). They also were concerned that some entities have no good clinical correlation, and that in many cases the identification of various entities relies on specialized techniques, such as molecular biology and cytogenetics, that are not largely available (33,34). Some pathologists expressed concerns about inconsistencies in the nomenclature, the absence of tumor grading, and the equal listing of both frequent and rare types of lymphomas (35). However, the REAL classification offered important advantages, among them the inclusion of newly described types of lymphomas, the definition of generally recognized clinicopathologic entities, and the unification of American and European classifications. Although generally based on the updated Kiel classification, the REAL proposal also included features of the Lukes-Collins classification, which gave it an international character. To evaluate the reproducibility and clinical relevance of the

TABLE 56.4. LIST OF LYMPHOID NEOPLASMS RECOGNIZED BY THE INTERNATIONAL LYMPHOMA STUDY GROUP

B-cell neoplasms
- I. Precursor B-cell neoplasm: precursor B-lymphoblastic leukemia/lymphoma
- II. Peripheral B-cell neoplasms
  1. B-cell chronic lymphocytic leukemia/prolymphocytic leukemia/small lymphocytic lymphoma
  2. Lymphoplasmacytoid lymphoma/immunocytoma
  3. Mantle cell lymphoma
  4. Follicle center lymphoma, follicular
     Provisional cytologic grades: I (small cell), II (mixed small and large cell), III (large cell)
     Provisional subtype: diffuse, predominantly small cell type
  5. Marginal zone B-cell lymphoma
     Extranodal (MALT type ± monocytoid B cells)
     Provisional subtype: nodal (± monocytoid B cells)
  6. Provisional entity: splenic marginal zone lymphoma (± villous lymphocytes)
  7. Hairy cell leukemia
  8. Plasmacytoma/plasma cell myeloma
  9. Diffuse large B-cell lymphoma*
     Subtype: primary mediastinal (thymic) B-cell lymphoma
  10. Burkitt lymphoma
  11. Provisional entity: high-grade B-cell lymphoma, Burkitt-like*

T-cell and putative NK-cell neoplasms
- I. Precursor T-cell neoplasm: precursor T-lymphoblastic lymphoma/leukemia
- II. Peripheral T-cell and NK-cell neoplasms
  1. T-cell chronic lymphocytic leukemia/prolymphocytic leukemia
  2. Large granular lymphocyte leukemia (LGL)
     T-cell type
     NK-cell type
  3. Mycosis fungoides/Sézary syndrome
  4. Peripheral T-cell lymphomas, unspecified*
     Provisional cytologic categories: medium-sized cell, mixed medium and large cell, large cell, lymphoepithelioid cell
     Provisional subtype: hepatosplenic $\gamma\delta$ T-cell lymphoma
     Provisional subtype: subcutaneous panniculitic T-cell lymphoma
  5. Angioimmunoblastic T-cell lymphoma (AILD)
  6. Angiocentric lymphoma
  7. Intestinal T-cell lymphoma (± enteropathy-associated)
  8. Adult T-cell lymphoma/leukemia (ATL/L)
  9. Anaplastic large cell lymphoma (ALCL), CD30−, T- and null-cell types
  10. Provisional entity: anaplastic large-cell lymphoma, Hodgkin-like

Hodgkin disease (HD)
- I. Lymphocyte predominance
- II. Nondular sclerosis
- III. Mixed cellularity
- IV. Lymphocyte depletion
- VI. Provisional entity: lymphocyte-rich classic HD

* These categories are thought likely to include more than one disease entity.
MALT, mucosa-associated lymphoid tissue; NK, natural killer.
From the Non-Hodgkins Lymphoma Classification Project. A clinical evaluation of the International Lymphoma Study Group. Classification of non-Hodgkin lymphoma. Blood 1997;89;3909–3918, with permission.

REAL proposal, a study of 1,403 cases of NHL at nine locations around the world was organized and classified by five expert hematopathologists (36). With use of the new classification, a diagnostic accuracy of 85% and a diagnostic reproducibility of 85% were achieved for the major lymphoma types. Immunophenotyping improved the diagnostic accuracy by 10% to 45% (36). These results were considered satisfactory for the practical use of the proposed classification. Subsequently, the REAL classification, with modifications suggested by the clinical study, was adopted as the new WHO classification of lymphomas (37) (Table 56.5).

No classification can be expected to be ideal or immutable, and the imperfections and inconsistencies of those currently in use reflect our present level of understanding. As progress in hematopathology and related fields continues, new nomenclatures and classifications will be forthcoming. Meanwhile, for daily practice and scientific communication, we must strive to provide a correct and usable language.

In the following chapters, the Hodgkin lymphomas (HLs) and NHLs are described according to the new WHO classification.

B-CELL LYMPHOMAS

The normal differentiation of the B-lymphocyte lineage from stem cells to plasma cells occurs successively in the fetal liver, bone marrow, and lymph nodes. The characteristic marker of B lymphocytes is the presence of immunoglobulins, which act as the cell surface antigen receptor. The genes that code for antibody are rearranged in the course of differentiation from stem cell to pre-B cell (38). Understanding the stages of B-lymphocyte maturation has facilitated the recognition of the relationships between the various types of B-cell lymphomas and leukemias.

In North America and Europe, B-cell lymphomas represent all follicular lymphomas and 80% to 90% of diffuse lymphomas, whereas T-cell lymphomas are more common in Asia (39). They are distinguished by cell type and patterns of growth. The cell types have been defined according to cell size (small, intermediate, large) and nuclear shape (cleaved, noncleaved). The cell size is determined by comparing lymphoma cells with coexisting histiocytes or endothelial cells and indicating whether their nuclei are smaller or larger. The nuclear shape indicates whether the lymphoma cells are in a dividing (centroblast/noncleaved) or nondividing (centrocyte/cleaved) phase of the cell cycle. The growth pattern may be nodular or diffuse. The aggregation of lymphoma cells into nodules indicates a follicular origin and a tendency to re-form the original structures. Both cell type and growth pattern relate to the rate of cell multiplication and invasiveness and therefore are important prognostic indicators. As tumor cells mutate and select, lymphomas progress to more aggressive, more malignant forms. Thus, the progression of lymphomas is from small cells to large cells, from cleaved

TABLE 56.5. WORLD HEALTH ORGANIZATION CLASSIFICATION OF LYMPHOID NEOPLASMS

B-cell neoplasms
- Precursor B-cell neoplasm
  - *Precursor B-lymphoblastic leukemia/lymphoma (precursor B-cell acute lymphoblastic leukemia)*
- **Mature (peripheral) B-cell neoplasms****
  - *B-cell chronic lymphocytic leukemia/small lymphocytic lymphoma*
  - B-cell prolymphocytic leukemia
  - Lymphoplasmacytic lymphoma
  - Splenic marginal zone B-cell lymphoma (± villous lymphocytes)
  - Hairy cell leukemia
  - *Plasma cell myeloma*/plasmacytoma
  - *Extranodal marginal zone B-cell lymphoma of MALT type*
  - Nodal marginal zone B-cell lymphoma (± monocytoid B cells)
  - *Follicular lymphoma*
  - *Mantle cell lymphoma*
  - *Diffuse large B-cell lymphoma*
    - Mediastinal large B-cell lymphoma
    - Primary effusion lymphoma
  - *Burkitt lymphoma/Burkitt cell leukemia*

T- and NK-cell neoplasms
- **Precursor T-cell neoplasm**
  - *Precursor T-lymphoblastic lymphoma/leukemia (precursor T-cell acute lymphoblastic leukemia)*
- **Mature (peripheral) T-cell neoplasms****
  - T-cell prolymphocytic leukemia
  - T-cell granular lymphocytic leukemia
  - Aggressive NK-cell leukemia
  - Adult T-cell lymphoma/leukemia (HTLV-*T*+)
  - Extranodal NK/T-cell lymphoma, nasa type
  - Enteropathy-type T-cell lymphoma
  - Hepatosplenic γδ T-cell lymphoma
  - Subcutaneous panniculitis-like T-cell lymphoma
  - *Mycosis fungoides*/Sézary syndrome
  - Anaplastic large cell lymphoma. T/null-cell, primary cutaneous type
  - *Peripheral T-cell lymphoma, not otherwise characterized*
  - *Angioimmunoblastic T-cell lymphoma*
  - *Anaplastic large cell lymphoma, T/null-cell, primary systemic type*

Hodgkin lymphoma (Hodgkin disease)
- Nodular lymphocyte predominance Hodgkin lymphoma
- Classic Hodgkin lymphoma
  - *Nodular sclerosis Hodgkin lymphoma (grades 1 and 2)*
  - Lymphocyte-rich classic Hodgkin lymphoma
  - *Mixed cellularity Hodgkin lymphoma*
  - Lymphocyte depletion Hodgkin lymphoma

MALT, mucosa-associated lymphoid tissue; NK, natural killer; HTLV, human
T-cell lymphotropic virus.
From Harris NL, Jaffe ES, Diebold J, et al. The World Health Organization classification of hematological malignancies: report of the clinical advisory meeting, Airlie House, VA, November 1997. Mod Pathol 2000;13:193–207, with permission.

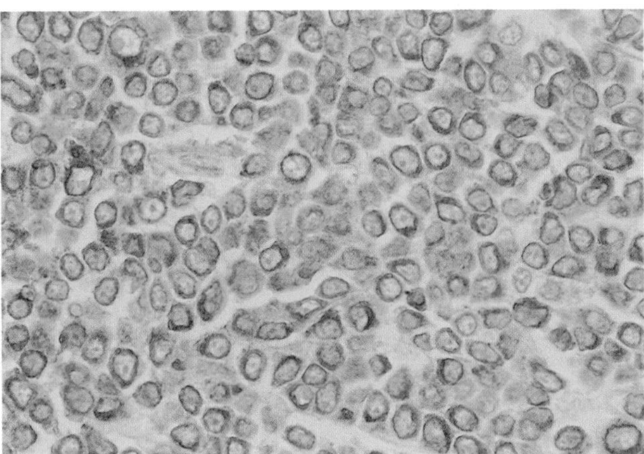

FIGURE 56.2. Diffuse large B-cell lymphoma with strong membrane staining for CD74, a pan-B-cell marker. CD74/peroxidase stain.

nuclei to noncleaved nuclei, and from nodular to diffuse patterns. In terms of lymphoma behavior, cell size and shape are more important than pattern of growth. Most B-cell lymphomas arise in the germinal centers of the lymph node follicles. The normal cell population of germinal centers includes small and large, cleaved and noncleaved cells. From these normal precursors, a variety of lymphomas may emerge, ranging from low-grade to high-grade. In contrast to the normal heteroclonal lymphoid population of follicles, the lymphoma cells are monoclonal and therefore similar morphologically, and they express the same immunoglobulin light chain. The B-cell origin of lymphomas can be identified by immunostaining with monoclonal antibodies (MAbs) specific for B-cell markers, such as CD19 or CD20 (Fig. 56.2). Further dissection of the B-cell lymphoma class into the component individual types is achieved by multiparameter analysis, in which definition of immunophenotype is of utmost importance. The five types of B-cell small cell lymphomas can be distinguished by determining their constellation of antigenic markers, which are identified by the appropriate MAbs (Table 56.6). Determining the type of B-cell lymphomas is essential for establishing the prognosis and treatment of such tumors. The neoplastic nature of B-cell lymphomas can be revealed by the demonstration of

TABLE 56.6. PHENOTYPE OF SMALL B-CELL LYMPHOMAS

	B-CLL/SLL	LPL	MCL	FL	MZL
CD5	+	∓	+	−	−
CD10	−	−	−	±	−
CD23	+	−	−	∓	∓
CD43	+	∓	+	−	∓
sIg	+	+	+	+	+
cytoIg	∓	+	−	−	±
bcl-1	∓	−	+	−	−
bcl-6	−	−	−	+	−

B-CLL/SLL, B-cell chronic lymphocytic leukemia/small lymphocytic lymphoma; LPL, lymphoplasmacytic lymphoma; MCL, mantle cell lymphoma; FL, follicular lymphoma; MZL, nodal marginal zone B-cell lymphoma; +, almost always positive; ±, positive more often than negative; ∓, negative more often than positive; −, almost always negative; sIg, surface immunoglobulin; cytoIg, cytoplasmic immunoglobulin.

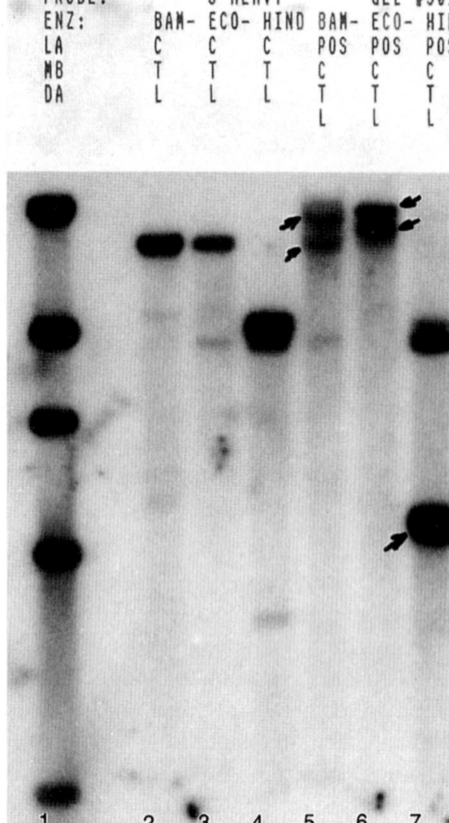

FIGURE 56.3. Autoradiograph of genomic DNA extracted from an axillary lymph node hybridized with a probe that recognizes the joining region of immunoglobulin heavy chain gene. *Lane 1* indicates molecular weights. *Lanes 2–7* show *Bam*HI, *Eco*RI, and *Hind*III digests of placental DNA (control, *lanes 2–4*) and lymphoma DNA (*lanes 5–7*). A comparison of lanes 2–4 with lanes 5–7, respectively, shows extra bands (*arrows*), indicating clonal rearrangements of immunoglobulin heavy chain genes. (Courtesy of Dennis M. Todd, Ph.D., Gencare Biomedical Research Corp.)

monoclonal light chain immunoglobulin restriction and by the presence of clonal gene rearrangements (Fig. 56.3).

Admixed with the homogeneous lymphoma cells are other normal components of the lymphoid follicles, such as helper T cells and dendritic reticular cells. In the normal follicle, the T-cells are predominantly CD4+ helper cells, which cooperate in the immune response by secreting cytokines and activating the B cells (38). In the B-cell lymphomas, the T cells are still present, sometimes in very large numbers, in the T cell-rich B-cell lymphomas (Fig. 56.4) (see Chapter 67). Occasionally, reactive T cells may obscure underlying lymphoma B cells, potentially causing a misinterpretation of immunophenotypes.

The REAL/WHO classification distinguishes within both B- and T-cell lymphomas two major categories: *precursor* and *mature.* The precursor B- and T-cell lymphomas comprise the lymphoblastic lymphomas and leu-kemias, which derive from progenitor cells that have not yet been activated by antigen and are still in an undifferentiated stage. All other lymphomas representing different stages of differentiation are included in the mature category. The names of the various mature lymphomas are related to their presumed cell of origin (mantle cell lymphoma), presumed function in the immune system [mucosa-associated lymphoid tissue (MALT) lymphoma], or location (mediastinal large B-cell lymphoma), or the traditional clinicopathologic name may be used (Burkitt lymphoma, mycosis fungoides).

Lymphomas originating in the cells of the germinal centers are follicular center cell lymphomas, and their growth pattern can be nodular or diffuse. Frequently, confusion is caused by the terms *follicular lymphoma* and *follicular center cell lymphoma,* which are not synonymous but are often used interchangeably. *Follicular lymphoma* is a B-cell lymphoma, composed of cleaved or noncleaved cells, growing in a nodular pattern. *Follicular center cell lymphoma* refers to cell type; the cells are of follicular origin—that is, cleaved or noncleaved B cells with a nodular or a diffuse pattern.

B-cell lymphomas constitute a broad spectrum extending from small cell to large cell types with, by implication, low-grade to high-grade clinical behavior. The term *grade* is defined by size and shape of cells and nuclei, density of chromatin, and number of mitoses (proliferation fraction), which may indicate tumor aggressiveness and clinical behavior. Lymphomas composed of cells that resemble small, nonactivated, mature-appearing lymphocytes in size and shape are the most common in the Western hemisphere. They are also the types of lymphomas most frequently seen in older persons. Some B-cell lymphomas are recognized by their characteristic histologic patterns, which in some cases (e.g., follicular lymphoma) are by definition of B-cell type. Other histologic types of lymphoma, although almost always of B-cell type, still include a small minority (1% to 3% in the case of small lymphocytic lymphomas) of T-cell

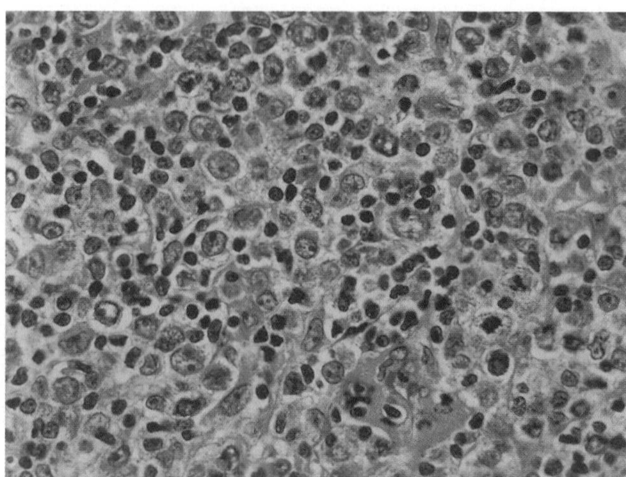

FIGURE 56.4. T cell-rich B-cell lymphoma. Numerous reactive small T lymphocytes partially obscure the large lymphoma B cells in the background. Hematoxylin, phloxine, and saffron stain.

types. Lymphomas related to certain pathogenetic conditions, such as immune deficiencies, are of B-cell type with only very rare exceptions (40). The degree of involvement of bone marrow and peripheral blood, which results in the clinical picture of lymphoma/leukemia, varies with cell type and stage of disease. The individual types of B-cell lymphomas are described in Chapters 60 through 70.

T-CELL LYMPHOMAS

The differentiation of T cells occurs predominantly in the thymus, where the pre-T cells migrate from the bone marrow. The early thymocytes enter the thymic cortex, at which time the rearrangement of T-cell antigen receptor genes takes place (41). The thymocytes at this time express CD7, a pan-T-cell antigen that persists on mature T lymphocytes, and also CD5 and CD2, the sheep erythrocyte receptor. As differentiation proceeds and the thymocytes move from the thymic cortex to the thymic medulla, at an intermediate level of maturation, CD4 and CD8 are both expressed on the same cell; later, they separate into CD4+ and CD8+ mature T cells.

As in the B-cell lineage, lymphomas and leukemias may originate at various levels of the T-cell pathway. In the Western hemisphere, neoplasms of T-cell origin are less common than those of B-cell origin, representing 15% to 20% of acute lymphocytic leukemias and 10% to 20% of NHLs (39). They were characterized later, after the main NHL classifications had been devised. As a result, knowledge of T-cell lymphomas has lagged behind, and the Working Formulation classification generally used is not applicable to T-cell neoplasms.

A convenient way to classify T-cell neoplasms is to separate them into thymic (precursor) and post-thymic (mature, peripheral) categories, depending on the stage of differentiation of the presumed cells of origin (Table 56.5). The thymic T-cell neoplasms constitute 15% to 30% of acute lymphoblastic leukemias and 80% to 90% of lymphoblastic lymphomas of T-cell type (42).

The phenotypes of the *precursor T-cell lymphomas* seem to correspond roughly with the multiple stages of normal thymocyte maturation (see Chapter 59). These neoplasms exhibit a phenotype of cellular immaturity characterized by fine and delicate chromatin, inconspicuous nucleoli, and the presence of intranuclear terminal deoxynucleotidyl transferase (TdT). However, regardless of the antigens expressed, all precursor T-cell lymphomas behave in a biologically aggressive fashion.

The *mature (post-thymic) lymphomas* are a heterogeneous category that includes such dissimilar clinicopathologic entities as the following, among others: virus-induced adult T-cell lymphomas, endemic in southern Japan; mycosis fungoides and its leukemic form, Sézary syndrome; T-cell leukemia with cells bearing natural killer cell surface markers; anaplastic large cell lymphomas. Mycosis fungoides (cutaneous T-cell lymphoma), a skin-based lymphoproliferative disease involving lymph nodes secondarily (see Chapter 72), must be distinguished from reactive mimickers (see Chapter 42). The human T-cell leukemia virus (HTLV-1) is etiologically linked to adult T-cell lymphoma/leukemia (see Chapter 71). Anaplastic large cell lymphoma is pathogenetically related to the t(2;5) translocation, which is a 2p23 chromosomal structural alteration causing deregulated expression of ALK, an oncogene with tyrosine kinase enzymatic activity (see Chapters 8 and 75).

The largest group, the *peripheral T-cell lymphomas, not otherwise specified,* are characterized by a diffuse pattern of growth, frequently a mixed population of large and small cells, an inflammatory background that often includes eosinophils or epithelioid cells, and a mature T-cell immunophenotype (43). They have been divided into many categories based on morphologic heterogeneity, clinical diversity, and, when known, unique pathogenesis. Although the morphologic spectrum of this category is broad, the histologic subtypes have not been shown to have prognostic relevance. The immunophenotypes of the peripheral T-cell lymphomas comprise some, but not all, of the pan-T-cell markers (Fig. 56.5) in addition to CD4 or CD8, the former far more common than the latter (43,44). It is usual for T-cell lymphomas to lose pan-T-cell antigens and express anomalous T-cell antigen profiles (39).

The rearrangement of the T-cell receptor (TCR) chain gene is a consistent clonal marker of most T-cell lymphomas (45) (Fig. 56.6).

Just as the majority of normal, mature T cells express the $\alpha\beta$ TCR, the majority of peripheral T-cell neoplasms in lymph nodes also express the $\alpha\beta$ TCR. A minority of T-cell malignancies expressing the $\gamma\delta$ TCR tend to develop in subcutaneous tissue, liver, or spleen.

All the T-cell neoplasms have clonally rearranged TCR genes; they are divided into precursor and mature (periph-

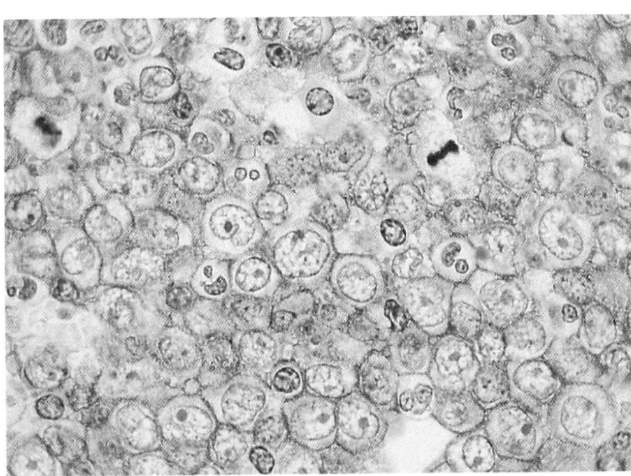

FIGURE 56.5. Peripheral T-cell lymphoma with large cells, pleomorphic nuclei, prominent nucleoli, and frequent mitoses showing membrane staining for CD43. CD43/peroxidase stain.

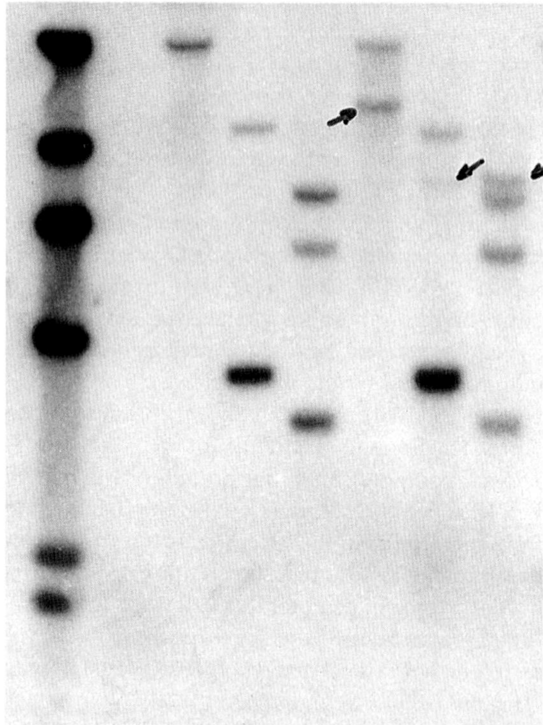

FIGURE 56.6. Autoradiograph of genomic DNA extracted from a mediastinal lymph node mass hybridized with a probe recognizing T-cell receptor β chain gene. *Lane 1* indicates molecular weights. *Lanes 2–7* show *Bam*HI, *Eco*RI, and *Hind*III digests of placental DNA (control, *lanes 2–4*) and lymphoma DNA (*lanes 5–7*). A comparison of lanes 2–4 with lanes 5–7, respectively, shows extra bands (*arrows*), indicating clonal rearrangements of T-cell receptor β chain gene, diagnostic of T-cell lymphoma. (Courtesy of Dennis M. Todd, Ph.D., Gencare Biomedical Research Corp.)

eral) types. The precursor T-cell neoplasms originate from bone marrow, thymus, and lymph nodes. The peripheral T-cell neoplasms often develop in lymph nodes, but also extranodally. Natural killer cell lymphomas retain germline TCR genes, usually involving extranodal anatomic sites but rarely occurring primarily in lymph nodes.

HODGKIN LYMPHOMA

The disease that bears the name of Thomas Hodgkin, who in 1832 reported the first seven cases of this neoplasm, has been the subject of intensive research; however, the etiology and pathogenesis remain largely unknown (Fig. 56.7). The cause of the disease is still obscure, the histogenesis of the characteristic cells is unclear, and the relationship with other kinds of lymphomas is controversial.

Fortunately, major advances have been made in the diagnosis and treatment of Hodgkin disease. As a result, a malignant neoplasm that was uniformly fatal at the turn of the twentieth century presently has a cure rate of more than 90%. Although Hodgkin disease is a neoplasm of the lymphoid organs, the name *Hodgkin disease* was used because of its uncertain origin, and it was distinguished from all other lymphomas (the NHLs) to emphasize the unique features of this clinicopathologic entity. Because the treatment of HL is so effective, it is extremely important to differentiate it from both benign lymphoid reactions and NHLs.

Recently, substantial progress has been made in understanding the histogenesis of the characteristic Hodgkin/Reed-Sternberg cells. In polymerase chain reaction analysis of single cells isolated by micromanipulation, immunoglobulin gene rearrangements in the Reed-Sternberg cells indicate a clonal origin in the cells of the follicular germinal center. The lymphocytic and histiocytic cells of lymphocyte predominance Hodgkin disease express B-cell markers

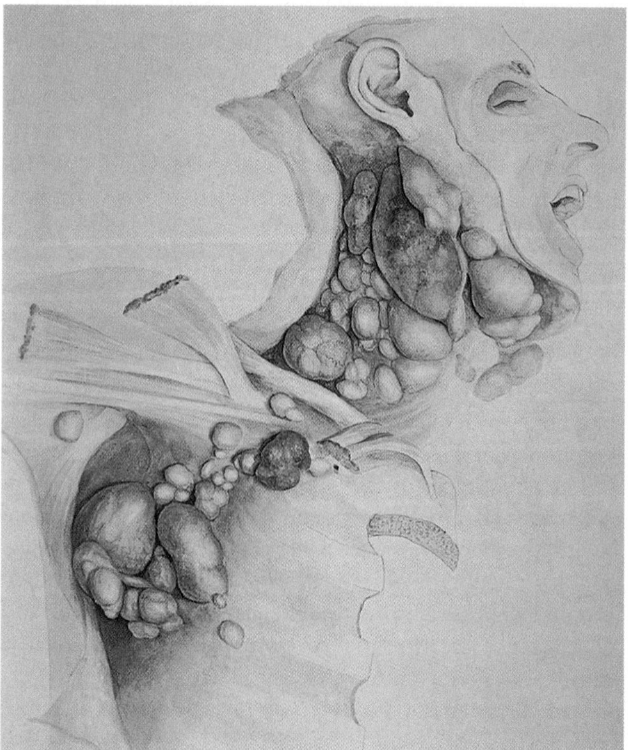

FIGURE 56.7. Enlarged lymph nodes in the neck and axilla of a patient with Hodgkin lymphoma. Original paintings of Sir Robert Carswell from his *Cases and Descriptions,* Manuscript 1, 1828:145–149. London, University College Library. (From Dawson PJ. The original illustrations of Hodgkin's disease. Ann Diagn Pathol 1999;3:386–393, with permission of University College, London, and the American Medical Association.)

and similarly seem to represent aberrant forms of B-cell lymphomas.

The REAL/WHO system, which in fact notes that Hodgkin disease is a particular type of B-cell lymphoma, has decided at least temporarily to classify it separately. The name of this particular neoplasm is HL with two major types: nodular lymphocyte predominance and classic. The latter is further subtyped, as shown in the new WHO classification (Table 56.5). All types and subtypes of HL are described in Chapters 57 and 58.

REFERENCES

1. Greenlee RT, Hill-Harmon MB, Murray T, et al. Cancer statistics 2001. CA Cancer J Clin 2001;51:15–36.
2. Nowell PC. Phytohemagglutinin: an initiation of mitosis in cultures of normal human leukocytes. Cancer Res 1960;20:462–466.
3. Lukes RJ, Collins RD. Immunologic characterization of human malignant lymphomas. Cancer 1974;34:1488–1503.
4. Jondal M, Holm G, Wigzell H. Surface markers on human T and B lymphocytes. J Exp Med 1972;136:207–215.
5. Bhan AK, Nadler LM, Stashenko P, et al. Stages of B-cell differentiation in human tissue. J Exp Med 1981;154:737–749.
6. Lennert K, Mohri N, Stein N, et al. The histopathology of malignant lymphoma. Br J Haematol 1975;31[Suppl]:193–203.
7. Aisenberg AC, Long JC. Lymphocyte surface characteristics in malignant lymphoma. Am J Med 1975;58:300–306.
8. Leech JH, Glick AD, Waldron JA, et al. Malignant lymphomas of follicular center cell origin in man. I. Immunologic studies. J Natl Cancer Inst 1975;54:11–21.
9. Jaffe ES, Shevach EM, Sussman EH, et al. Membrane receptor sites for the identification of lymphoreticular cells in benign and malignant conditions. Br J Cancer 1975;31[Suppl 2]:107–120.
10. Gajl-Peczalska KJ, Bloomfield CD, Coccia PF, et al. B- and T-cell lymphomas: analysis of blood and lymph nodes in 87 patients. Am J Med 1975;59:674–685.
11. Seligman M, Brouet JC, Preud'Homme JL. Immunologic classification of non-Hodgkin's lymphomas: current status. Cancer Treat Rep 1977;61:1179–1185.
12. Whiteside TL, Rowlands DT Jr. T-cell and B-cell identification in the diagnosis of lymphoproliferative disease. Am J Pathol 1977;88:754–792.
13. Berard CW, Jaffe ES, Braylan RC, et al. Immunologic aspects and pathology of malignant lymphomas. Cancer 1978;42:911–921.
14. Johansson B, Klein E, Haglund S. Correlation between the presence of surface localized immunoglobulin (Ig) and the histological type of human malignant lymphomas. Clin Immunol Immunopathol 1976;5:119–132.
15. Siegal FP, Filippa DA, Koziner B. Surface markers in leukemias and lymphomas. Am J Pathol 1978;90:451–460.
16. Rappaport H. Tumors of the hematopoietic system. In: Atlas of tumor pathology. Washington, DC: Armed Forces Institute of Pathology, 1966: section III, fascicle 8.
17. Lukes RJ, Collins RD. New approaches to the classification of the lymphomata. Br J Cancer 1975;31[Suppl 2]:1–28.
18. Lennert K, Mohri N. Histopathology and diagnosis of non-Hodgkin's lymphomas. In: Malignant lymphomas other than Hodgkin's disease. New York: Springer-Verlag, 1978.
19. Bennett MH, Farrer-Brown G, Henry K, et al. Classification of non-Hodgkin's lymphomas. Lancet 1974;2:405–406.
20. Dorfman RF. The non-Hodgkin's lymphomas. In: Rebuck JW, Berard CW, Abell MR, eds. The reticulo-endothelial system. Baltimore: Williams & Wilkins, 1975:262–281 (International Academy of Pathology Monograph No. 16).
21. Mathé G, Rappaport H, O'Connor GT, et al. Histological and cytological typing of neoplastic diseases of hematopoietic and lymphoid tissues. In: World Health Organization international histological classification of tumors, No. 14. Geneva: World Health Organization, 1976.
22. Rappaport H, Braylan RC. Changing concepts in the classification of malignant neoplasms of the hematopoietic system. In: Rebuck JW, Berard CW, Abell MR, eds. The reticulo-endothelial system. Baltimore: Williams & Wilkins, 1975: 1–19 (International Academy of Pathology Monograph No. 16).
23. Lukes RJ, Parker JW, Taylor CR, et al. Immunologic approach to non-Hodgkin's lymphomas and related leukemias: analysis of the result of multiparameter studies of 425 cases. Semin Hematol 1978;15:322–352.
24. Lukes RJ. The immunologic approach to the pathology of malignant lymphomas. Am J Clin Pathol 1979;72:657–669.
25. Lukes RJ, Collins RD. B-cell neoplasms. In: Tumors of the hematopoietic system. Washington, DC: Armed Forces Institute of Pathology, 1992:93–97 (series II, fascicle 28).
26. Stansfeld AG, Diebold J, Noel H, et al. Updated Kiel classification for lymphomas. Lancet 1988;1:292–293.
27. Mann RB, Jaffe ES, Berard CW. Malignant lymphomas: a conceptual understanding of morphologic diversity. Am J Pathol 1979;94:103–192.
28. Nathwani BN. A critical analysis of the classifications of non-Hodgkin's lymphomas. Cancer 1979;44:347–384.
29. National Cancer Institute-sponsored study of classifications of Non-Hodgkin's lymphomas. Summary and description of a working formulation for clinical usage. Cancer 1982;49:2112–2135.
30. Wright DH. Updated Kiel classification for lymphomas [Editorial]. J Pathol 1989;157:283–284.
31. Burke JS. The histopathologic classification of non-Hodgkin's lymphomas: ambiguities in the working formulation and two newly reported categories. Semin Oncol 1990;17:3–10.
32. Harris NL, Jaffe ES, Stein H, et al. A revised European-American Classification of lymphoma neoplasms: a proposal from the International Lymphoma Study Group. Blood 1994;84:1361–1392.
33. Rosenberg SA. Classification of lymphoid neoplasms. Blood 1994;84:1359–1360.
34. Longo DL. The real classification of lymphoid neoplasms: one clinician's view. Principles and practice of oncology 1995;9:1–12.
35. Ioachim HL. The revised European-American classification of lymphoid neoplasms. Cancer 1996;78:1–9.
36. The Non-Hodgkin's Lymphoma Classification Project. A clinical evaluation of the International Lymphoma Study Group. Classification of non-Hodgkin lymphoma. Blood 1997;89:3909–3918.
37. Harris NL, Jaffe ES, Diebold J, et al. The World Health Organization classification of hematological malignancies: report of the clinical advisory committee meeting, Airlie House, Virginia, November 1997. Mod Pathol 2000;13:193–207.
38. Roitt I. The recognition of antigen. In: Essential immunology. Oxford: Blackwell Science, 1997:43–63.
39. Warnke RA, Weiss LM, Chan JKC, et al. Tumors of the lymph nodes and spleen. Washington, DC: Armed Forces Institute of Pathology, 1995: series III, fascicle 14.

40. Ioachim HL. The opportunistic tumors of immune deficiency. Adv Cancer Res 1990;54:301–317.
41. Magrath I. Lymphocyte ontogeny: a conceptual basis for understanding neoplasia of the immune system. In: Magrath I, ed. The Non-Hodgkin's lymphomas. Baltimore: Williams & Wilkins, 1990:29–48.
42. Cossman J. T-cell neoplasms and Hodgkin's disease. In: Berard CW, Dorfman RF, Kaufman N, eds. Malignant lymphoma. Baltimore: Williams & Wilkins, 1987:104–123 (International Academy of Pathology Monograph No. 29).
43. Jaffe ES. An approach to the classification of post-thymic T-cell malignancies. In: Hanaoka M, et al., eds. Lymphoid malignancy. Field & Wood, 1990:91–95.
44. Weiss LM, Crabtree GS, Rouse RV, et al. Morphologic and immunologic characterization of 50 peripheral T-cell lymphomas. Am J Pathol 1985;118:316–324.
45. Flug F, Pellici PG, Bonetti F, et al. T-cell receptor gene rearrangements as markers of lineage and clonality in T-cell neoplasms. Proc Natl Acad Sci U S A 1985;82:3460–3464.

PART V

SECTION TWO

HODGKIN LYMPHOMA

57

HODGKIN LYMPHOMA

CLASSIC

HODGKIN LYMPHOMA

DEFINITION

Lymphoma characterized by a heterogeneous cellularity comprising a minority of specific neoplastic cells and a majority of reactive non-neoplastic cells.

SYNONYM

Hodgkin disease

EPIDEMIOLOGY

The wide geographic variation in the incidence of Hodgkin lymphoma (HL) supports the belief that the disease is caused by an environmental, probably infectious, agent (1). In the United States and western Europe, HL is a common form of cancer in young adults (2), with 3.5 to 5 cases occurring per 100,000 population per year in persons between the ages of 15 and 35 years (3). In Japan, the incidence is almost three times lower (4). Statistics of the American Cancer Society estimate 7,400 new cases of HL, 3,900 in men and 3,500 in women, for the year 2001 in the United States (5). In economically developed countries with a high standard of living, HL is rare in children and more frequent in young adults, displaying the histologic types that are associated with a favorable prognosis. In underdeveloped countries and populations with poor socioeconomic conditions, the incidence is highest in children, and the histologic types associated with a poor prognosis predominate (6).

In relation to age, the distribution curve is bimodal, with the first peak between 15 and 34 years and the second peak after 54 years (7). Nodular sclerosis and lymphocyte predominance, the histologic types with a favorable prognosis, are significantly more common in younger persons and in women (8–11), an observation interpreted by some as an indication that HL is not a single etiologic entity but may comprise at least two distinct diseases, possibly induced by different agents (12).

Hodgkin lymphoma occurs slightly more often in men than in women. The overall ratio is 1.34:1.00; it is approximately equal in younger patients, and a male predominance was noted in a series of older patients (13). In AIDS patients and transplant recipients, HLs are far less common than non-Hodgkin lymphomas (NHLs) (14,15). Still, their incidence is significantly increased, and AIDS patients carry a risk for HL 10 times greater than that of persons without AIDS (16).

ETIOLOGY

Extensive investigations directed at a variety of etiologic factors have failed so far to reveal the cause of HL. Clusters of HL cases have been reported in families and in social groups of unrelated persons, observations that focus attention on genetic and other host factors and, alternatively, on various environmental agents (13,17). The potential role of Epstein-Barr virus (EBV) has been a favorite subject of study because of its strong association with other types of lymphomas. Furthermore, epidemiologic studies indicate a relationship between EVB and infectious mononucleosis, which is associated with a fourfold increased risk for the subsequent development of HL (18). When Southern blot hybridization with a DNA probe was used to examine 16 HL biopsy specimens, monoclonal EBV DNA was detected in 20% of them (19). *In situ* hybridization applied to the same cases showed the EBV nucleic acid to be localized to the Reed-Sternberg (R-S) cells. These findings were confirmed by a large study of 198 HL, 151 NHL, and 34 nonmalignant lymph nodes; by the polymerase chain reaction (PCR), EBV-specific DNA sequences were detected in 58% of HL cases (20).

The EBV-positive cells were monoclonal, suggesting that the EBV infection had occurred before the clonal cell proliferation (19). EBV-positive R-S cells are found in 40% to 50% of cases by *in situ* hybridization with EBER probe (21) (Fig. 57.1).

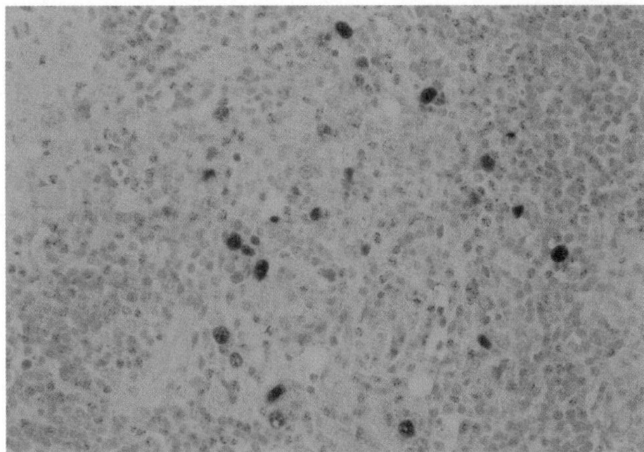

FIGURE 57.1. Cervical lymph node with Hodgkin lymphoma, mixed cellularity, showing multiple large cells with positive nuclear staining for Epstein-Barr virus. *In situ* hybridization with EBER probe.

Hodgkin lymphoma is more likely to be EBV-positive in very young and very old patients (22), and in HIV-infected patients, up to 100% of cases are EBV-positive (23). However, EBV alone may not provide the answer to the cause of HL because in numerous typical cases, the same techniques were unable to demonstrate the presence of EBV, and in at least one study, the number of EBV-positive cases of HL was not higher than the number of EBV-positive cases of benign hyperplastic lymphadenopathies (24).

CLASSIFICATION

In contrast to malignant neoplasms in general and lymphomas in particular, which are characteristically composed of clonal monomorphic populations of cells, HL presents as a mixture of different cells assembled in a variety of histologic patterns. Also unlike any other neoplasm, HL comprises of a minority of neoplastic cells, the R-S cells and their variants, and a majority of reactive inflammatory cells, which form the bulk of the tumor. These include lymphocytes of various kinds, plasma cells, polynuclear neutrophils and eosinophils, histiocytes, and fibroblasts. Attempts were made at various times to identify recognizable histologic patterns among the admixture of cells that constitute HL. An early classification by Jackson and Parker in 1944 (25) divided HL into three subtypes—paragranuloma, granuloma, and sarcoma—a nomenclature suggesting that HL begins as a benign inflammatory condition and eventually evolves into a malignant tumor (Table 57.l). Because the vast majority of cases belonged to the granuloma category, this classification was of limited practical use. In 1966, Lukes and Butler (26) introduced a new classification comprising six subtypes; shortly afterward, at the Rye conference, this was simplified to four subtypes (Table 57.1). This classification was widely accepted by pathologists and clinicians because it correlated well with survival (Fig. 57.2), and it remained the dominant classification for the next 30 years. With the introduction of immunophenotyping, it became apparent that the type of HL designated lymphocyte predominance is different from the classically described forms and may even represent a different clinicopathologic entity. This belief was expressed at an international conference held in 1994 on the subject (27) and subsequently defined in the revised European-American classification of lymphoid neoplasms (REAL) (28). With further modifications, included in the presently accepted World Health Organization (WHO) classification of lymphomas (29), HL is divided into two major entities, *lymphocyte predominance* and *classic,* with the latter further subtyped (Table 57.1). Although under the general heading of HL, we are discussing the two entities in separate chapters to emphasize the multiple differential features.

TABLE 57.1. CLASSIFICATIONS OF HODGKIN LYMPHOMA

Jackson-Parker (1944)
Paragranuloma
Granuloma
Sarcoma
Lukes-Butler (1966)
Lymphocyte predominance
Nodular
Diffuse
Nodular sclerosis
Mixed cellularity
Lymphocyte depletion
Diffuse fibrosis
Reticular
Rye conference (1966)
Lymphocyte predominance
Nodular sclerosis
Mixed cellularity
Lymphocyte depletion
REAL (1994)
Lymphocyte predominance, nodular
Classic
Nodular sclerosis
Lymphocyte-rich
Mixed cellularity
Lymphocyte depletion

REAL, revised European-American lymphoma (classification).

CLASSIC HODGKIN LYMPHOMA

DEFINITION

Histologic types of HL characterized by the presence of R-S cells and their variants.

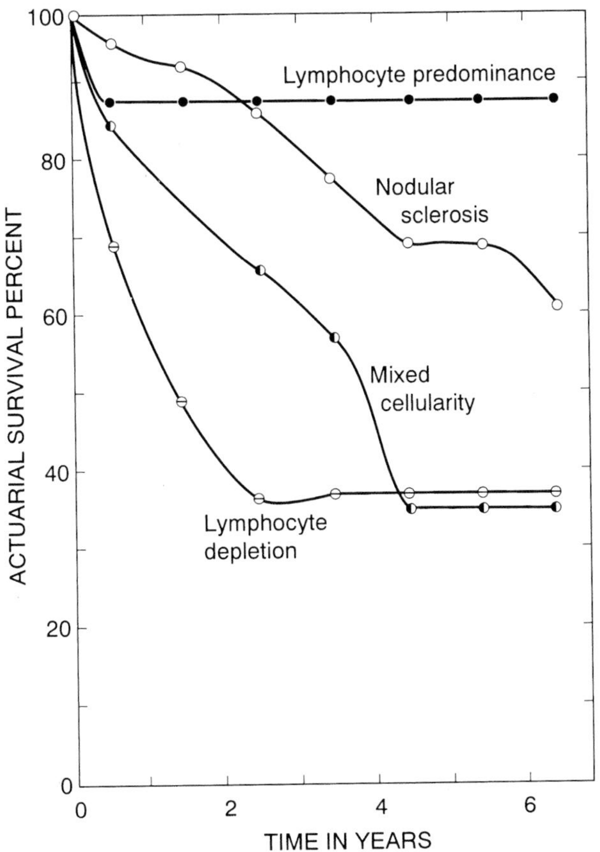

FIGURE 57.2. Hodgkin disease: survival versus histologic type (all stages). Actuarial survival in 176 cases of Hodgkin lymphoma shows good correlation with the histologic types. (From Keller AR, Kaplan HS, Lukes RJ, et al. Correlation of histopathology with other prognostic indicators in Hodgkin's disease. Cancer 1968;22: 487–499, with permission.)

SYNONYMS

Hodgkin lymphoma: nodular sclerosis (NS), mixed cellularity (MC), and lymphocyte depletion (LP)

Hodgkin lymphoma: granuloma and sarcoma

PATHOGENESIS

The localization and spread of HL were long considered to be random and therefore unpredictable. Lymphomas, including HLs, were considered to arise multifocally within the reticuloendothelial system, so that the term *metastasis* was rarely used in the context of these tumors, as it is for carcinomas and sarcomas (30). This concept derived mainly from observations of advanced disease in which multiple organs were involved; more recently, with the benefit of early diagnosis and the help of modern staging procedures, it has been recognized that HL may start unifocally and at first involve a single lymph node or a single group of lymph nodes. The involved lymph nodes are enlarged and often firm, particularly in NS, in which bands of fibrosis delineate vague nodular areas (Fig. 57.3).

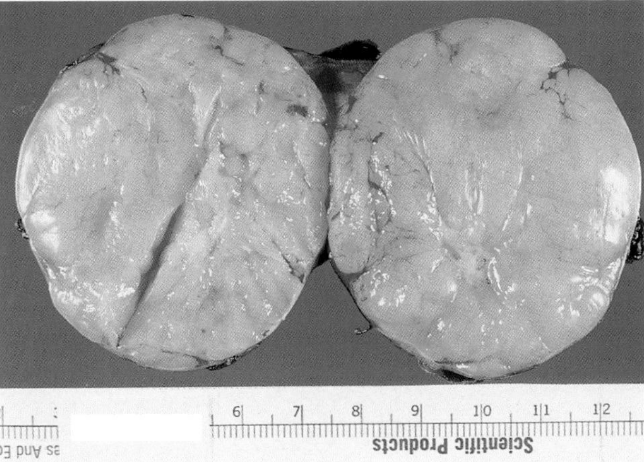

FIGURE 57.3. Axillary lymph node with nodular sclerosis Hodgkin lymphoma shows vague nodularity and whitish areas of fibrosis.

Even within a lymph node, the involvement may be focal, and diseased areas may contrast with uninvolved areas of normal parenchyma (17,31,32) (Fig. 57.4). To avoid missing foci of HL, particularly in lymph nodes that are not grossly enlarged, the whole lymph node should be processed and multiple, preferably semiserial sections examined. The initial foci of HL are usually situated in the interfollicular areas of the cortex (the T-cell zone) without apparent relation to sinuses or capillaries.

Hodgkin lymphoma spreads mostly by contiguity, from one chain of lymph nodes to another, as demonstrated by the mapping studies of Kaplan (33).

The cervical and supraclavicular lymph nodes are most frequently involved, particularly in cases with limited disease (stages I and II) (Fig. 57.5). Abdominal lymph nodes

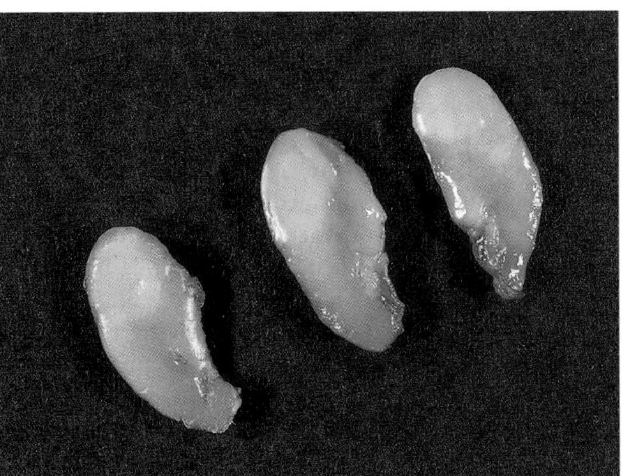

FIGURE 57.4. Cervical lymph node partially involved by Hodgkin lymphoma. Microscopically, the lesion is restricted to the upper pole, which grossly shows enlargement and discoloration.

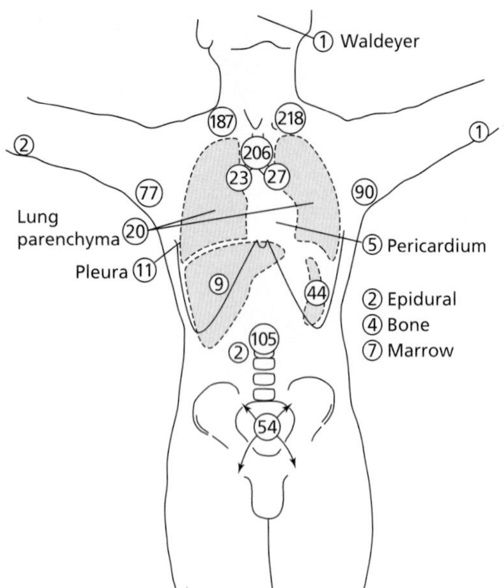

FIGURE 57.5. Frequency of involvement of various lymph node sites in a series of 340 untreated patients with Hodgkin lymphoma according to the mapping of H. Kaplan. (From Kaplan HS. Hodgkin's disease. Cambridge, MA: Harvard University Press, 1972, with permission.)

usually are not affected if the cervical or mediastinal lymph nodes are not involved (32,33). From the axillary lymph nodes, HL spreads to infraclavicular, supraclavicular, and low cervical lymph nodes of the same side and not to the opposite side.

Correlations between anatomic location and histologic type have been noted. Of all the histologic types, NS is most likely to spread by contiguity, whereas noncontiguous dissemination, when it occurs, is more than twice as frequent in MC and LD types (10). HL in the mediastinal lymph nodes is usually of the NS type, which in stage I is 15 times more common in the mediastinum than all other histologic types combined according to the original study by Lukes and Butler (26) and confirmed by others (9,10). MC and LD types are seldom restricted to a single site or region (33) and are more likely to involve extralymphatic organs and tissues (11). Involvement of the left supraclavicular nodes is often followed by abdominal paraaortic node involvement, whereas involvement of the right supraclavicular nodes tends to be associated with mediastinal adenopathy. Paraaortic lymph node involvement usually precedes involvement of the spleen, which in turn is followed by liver or bone marrow involvement, or both (Fig. 57.6). Of all the histologic types, NS shows the greatest propensity to spread by contiguity, whereas noncontiguous dissemination, when it occurs, is more than twice as frequent in the MC and LD types (11).

In about 10% of cases, the pattern of contiguous lymphatic spread is not evident (33). The involvement of noncontiguous lymph nodes and the dissemination of HL to bone marrow, spleen, and liver suggest blood vessel invasion, which is estimated to occur in more than 20% of cases (34) (Fig. 57.7). Rappaport and colleagues (34) demonstrated invasion of veins in 6% to 14% of diagnostic lymph node biopsy specimens. Silver staining of elastic fibers may reveal the presence of vascular invasion, an aggravating factor that indicates extensive disease and the need for systemic rather than regional therapy (35,36). Although not restricted to the LD type, the invasion of blood vessels is more frequently associated with this histologic form (36).

The consistency of histologic types in the presence of multiple localizations and between nonsynchronous lesions has been debated. It is generally believed that simultaneous lesions tend to be of similar histologic type (10,37), whereas during the natural course of the disease, a transition from less malignant to more malignant histologic types commonly occurs (37,38).

The clinical stages of Hodgkin disease are currently evaluated according to the Ann Arbor classification as modified by the Cotswolds Conference in 1989 (39,40) (Table 57.2). The staging procedure as originally formulated required exhaustive surgical and radiologic investigations, including laparotomy, lymph node biopsies, splenectomy, liver and bone marrow biopsies, computed tomography, and gallium scanning. Because involvement can be focal, spleens and lymph nodes removed for staging must be sectioned at 3- to 5-mm intervals and carefully examined. Currently, surgery and lymphangiography are no longer used to stage HL because of potential infectious complications in these im-

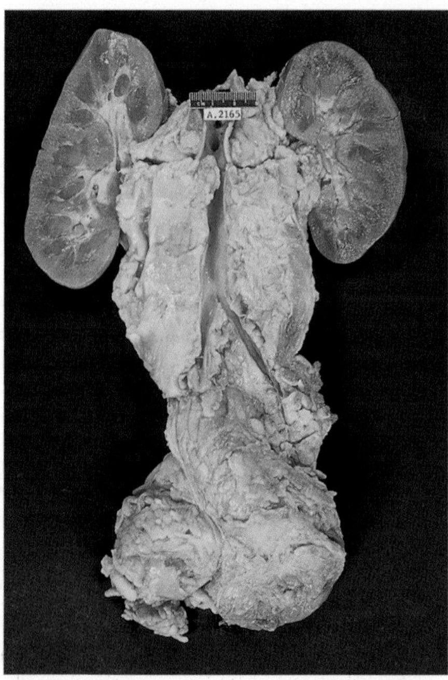

FIGURE 57.6. Paraaortic lymph nodes massively involved by Hodgkin lymphoma encasing and compressing the aorta and iliac vessels. Autopsy of a case of Hodgkin lymphoma performed in 1963 at the Francis Delafield Hospital in New York.

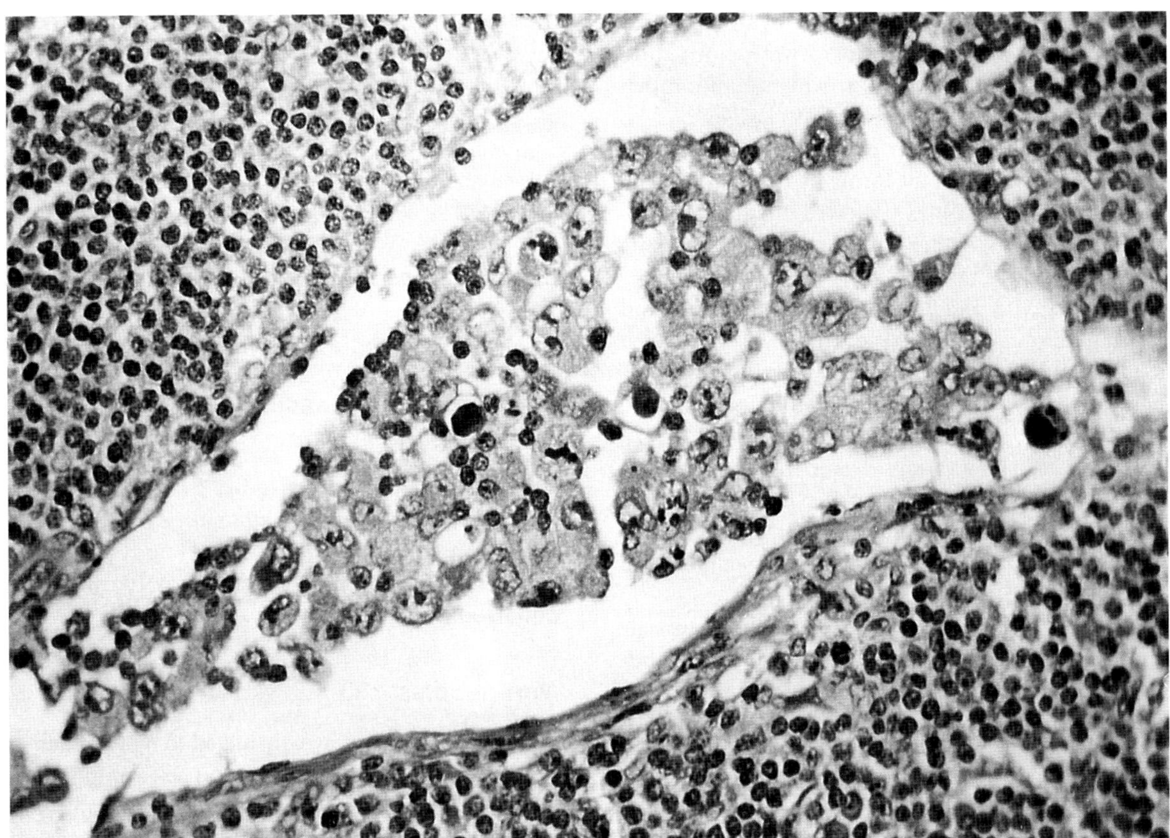

FIGURE 57.7. Vascular invasion in Hodgkin lymphoma. Mixed cellularity infiltrate including predominantly Hodgkin and Reed-Sternberg cells obliterates the vascular lumen. Hematoxylin, phloxine, and saffron stain.

mune-deficient patients. Advanced radiologic techniques and successful treatments for all stages have lessened the need for exhaustive staging. When the histologic types of HL are correlated with clinical stages, LP is strongly associated with clinical stages I and II, NS predominantly with stage II, and lymphocyte depletion (LD) primarily with clinical stages III and IV (9). MC is seen in all clinical stages without any strong associations. Thus, the histologic subtypes may help predict the stage, as in a reported series of 900 staged cases, in which the number of cases with early-stage disease was highest in the patients with LP and decreased progressively from NS to MC to LD (13). Male sex and advanced age were associated with advanced stage and unfavorable histologic type. Massive involvement of lymph nodes and viscera, which were common before modern combined treatment (Fig. 57.6), are rarely seen at the present time.

TABLE 57.2. ANN ARBOR STAGING CLASSIFICATION FOR HODGKIN DISEASE (AS MODIFIED AT COTSWOLDS)

Stage I	Involvement of a single lymph node region (I) or a single extralymphatic organ or site (I_E)
Stage II	Involvement of two or more lymph node regions on the same side of the diaphragm (II) or localized involvement of an extralymphatic organ or site (II_E)
Stage III	Involvement of lymph node regions on both sides of the diaphragm (III) or localized involvement of an extralymphatic organ or site (III_E) or spleen (III_S) or both (III_{SE})
	III_1: With or without splenic hilar, celiac, or portal nodes
	III_2: With paraaortic, iliac, or mesenteric nodes
Stage IV	Diffuse or disseminated involvement of one or more extralymphatic organs with or without associated lymph node involvement

CLINICAL SYNDROME

Most patients with HL first seek medical attention for enlarged lymph nodes (33). They are not usually painful or tender and so are noticed by chance. The growth of lymph nodes may be rapid or slow, but the rate generally correlates with the intensity of constitutional symptoms. The adoption of the Rye classification, based on the histologic subtypes described by Lukes and Butler (41), has made it possible to study large series of cases and establish clinicopathologic correlations. Thus, in a series of 659 patients with HL, the mediastinal lymph nodes were more commonly involved with lesions of NS, whereas abdominal lymph nodes were more often affected by lesions of MC (42). The cervical and supraclavicular lymph nodes were most commonly involved in all forms of HL, particularly NS. One-fourth of the cases of LP showed inguinal involvement. As in other series, earlier stages (I and II) were more often associated with LP and NS, whereas advanced stages (III and IV) had MC and LD lesions. The tonsils and Waldeyer ring are rarely involved in HL. In HIV-infected patients, HL may occur in unusual sites, and the bone marrow may be involved in the absence of lymph node involvement (43).

Patients with HL show various degrees of immune deficiency. Lymphocytopenia and a functional impairment of T lymphocytes are common and result in an increased susceptibility to some types of viral, bacterial, and fungal infections (44)

"B" symptoms include fever (>38°C for 3 days consecutively), night sweats (sometimes considerable as a consequence of nocturnal defervescence), pruritus, anorexia, fatigue, generalized weakness, and weight loss. Their presence and intensity generally correlate with the pathologic stage (33). The most frequent site of involvement is the cervical lymph nodes, followed by the inguinal lymph nodes. NS is the type that occurs most often in female patients and is commonly located in the mediastinum, suggesting a regional form of HL (11). The MC type is seen more often in middle-aged patients, who present in stages II and III, and LD, the most aggressive form of HL, affects predominantly elderly men, involving subdiaphragmatic lymph nodes and showing at autopsy a high rate of vascular invasion and extranodal spread.

As noted above, many centers now treat patients without laparotomy staging. Young age, female sex, few sites of involvement, absence of B symptoms, and favorable histology are the factors that identify patients who can be treated without prior laparotomy (45).

HISTOPATHOLOGY

The cell populations of HL are heterogeneous, including neoplastic and non-neoplastic reactive cells. Varying proportions of neoplastic and non-neoplastic cells give rise to multiple histologic patterns.

The Rye classification (Table 57.1), a simplified four-category version of the original six-category classification of Lukes and Butler (41), was formerly used worldwide and offered clinical relevance and high reproducibility (39). It has been replaced by the new WHO classification of HL; this system separates LP from classic HL, which includes all other histologic types (28) (Table 57.3).

TABLE 57.3. HODGKIN LYMPHOMA: WORLD HEALTH ORGANIZATION CLASSIFICATION

Lymphocyte predominance, nodular
Classic Hodgkin lymphoma
Nodular sclerosis
Lymphocyte-rich
Mixed cellularity
Lymphocyte depletion
Unclassifiable

Cell Types of Classic Hodgkin Lymphoma

Unlike the NHLs, which comprise a homogeneous population of tumor cells, the HLs are composed of mixed infiltrates of neoplastic and inflammatory cells, the latter forming the vast majority (Fig. 57.8). The R-S cells and their variants may be from 10% to as few as 1% of the entire cell population (46).

Non-neoplastic Cells

Non-neoplastic cells are considered to represent an immune cellular reaction to the neoplastic cell component of HL. Their morphologic features are indistinguishable from those of their normal counterparts, and their respective numbers vary in relation to the histologic subtypes of HL. *Lymphocytes,* which are small with round nuclei and rare mitoses, are the predominant cell type. The majority of lymphocytes are T cells, mostly of CD4+ (helper) type (47). The ratio of CD4+ to CD8+ T cells is within normal range. Admixed with the lymphocytes are occasional *immunoblasts, plasma cells, neutrophils,* and particularly *eosinophils.* These are a constant and characteristic component of the NS and MC

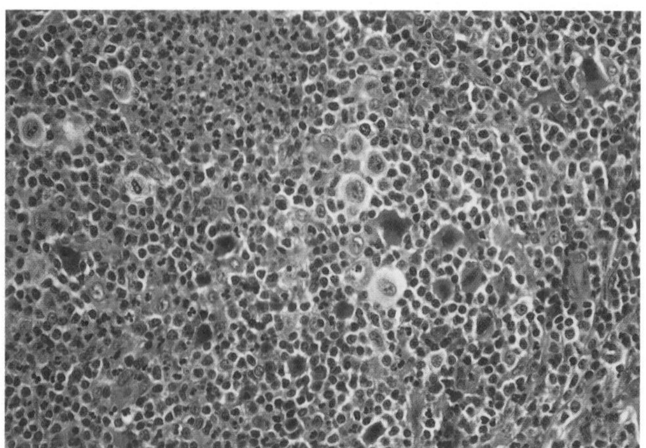

FIGURE 57.8. Mixed cellular population in Hodgkin lymphoma with various inflammatory cells, Reed-Sternberg cells, lacunar cells, and mummified cells. Hematoxylin, phloxine, and saffron stain.

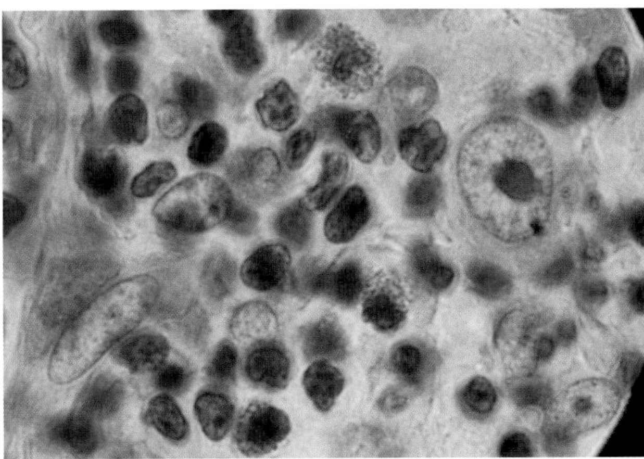

FIGURE 57.9. Hodgkin lymphoma, mixed cellularity type. Hodgkin cell (*upper right*) with abundant cytoplasm has a large round nucleus with a thick membrane and a huge, hyperchromatic nucleolus. Frequent eosinophils, lymphocytes, and histiocytes comprise the background cell population. Hematoxylin, phloxine, and saffron stain.

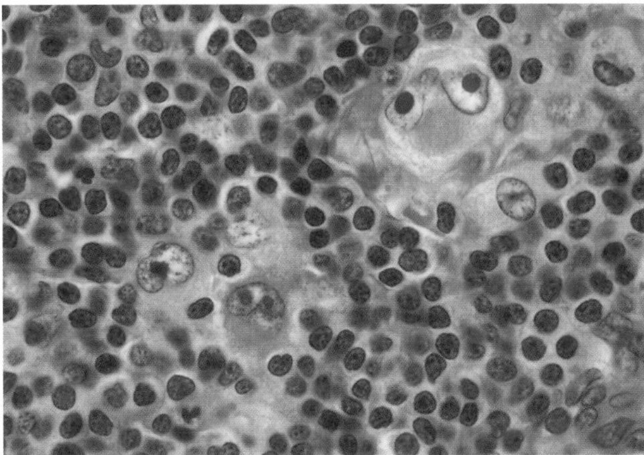

FIGURE 57.10. Hodgkin cells and Reed-Sternberg cells with bilobate, mirror image nuclei and "owl's eye" nucleoli. Hematoxylin, phloxine, and saffron stain.

types (Fig. 57.9). The number of eosinophils may be very great, and they sometimes form eosinophilic microabscesses. In one case, a 68-year-old man had a peripheral leukocyte count of 120,000/mm^3 with 92% eosinophils, which led to an initial diagnosis of eosinophilic leukemia (17). At autopsy in such cases, the lymph nodes and most other organs show infiltrates of MC in which the eosinophils are the predominant cell type. Neutrophils, when present, usually surround the foci of necrosis.

Histiocytes and *fibroblasts* are commonly noted. *Epithelioid cell granulomas* are occasionally present in the involved or uninvolved lymph nodes of patients with HL and have been described repeatedly (38,48–50). The incidence of this finding was 9% in a survey of 608 patients (49) and 16.7% in a study of 185 patients (48). The granulomas are randomly distributed in the nodal parenchyma and comprise epithelioid histiocytes, a few multinucleated giant cells of Langhans or foreign body type, and scattered lymphocytes and plasma cells. Central necrosis is minimal or lacking, and asteroid bodies are not seen. Some authors have reported longer survival for patients with epithelioid granulomas (49); however, the relation of epithelioid granulomas to HL is not understood. HL with a high content of epithelioid cells is classified with the MC type (50).

Neoplastic Cells

Reed-Sternberg Cells

Reed-Sternberg cells are considered the pathognomonic feature of HL, and it is generally understood that no positive histologic diagnosis of this disease should be made in their absence. However, R-S cells show great morphologic variability, and cells of striking similarity have been observed in several benign, probably unrelated, conditions, such as infectious mononucleosis (51–53), toxoplasmosis (53), postvaccinial lymphadenitis (54), and various unrelated neoplasms (55). Therefore, to avoid such pitfalls of interpretation, only the typical variants of R-S cells are considered to be diagnostic of HL (Figs. 57.10 and 57.11).

The diagnostic R-S cell is large, from 20 to 60 μm in diameter, with a variable amount of cytoplasm that is eosinophilic or amphophilic. The nuclei are large with thick nuclear membranes. Two nuclei may be present, sometimes symmetric with a "mirror image" appearance (Figs. 57.10 and 57.11; see 57.21); at other times, the nuclei may be multiple and interconnected, as shown by electron microscopy studies (see Fig. 57.22). Each nucleus or nuclear lobe has a single, prominent eosinophilic nucleolus that often resembles a nuclear inclusion. The presence of typical R-S cells (Figs. 57.10 and 57.11) and Hodgkin cells (Fig. 57.9), the mononucleated variant of the former, is

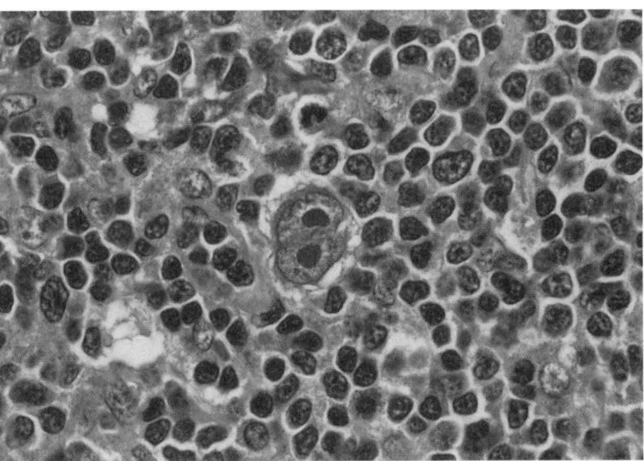

FIGURE 57.11. Reed-Sternberg cell with mirror image nuclei and prominent, eosinophilic, inclusion-like nucleoli. Hematoxylin, phloxine, and saffron stain.

considered a *sine qua non* for the diagnosis of HL. However, R-S–like cells, which are in fact activated or transformed lymphocytes, are often seen in benign, non-Hodgkin processes in addition to malignant ones. Furthermore, a number of R-S variants, some of which result from apoptosis or are artifacts of fixation, can be recognized in HL.

Previously, the R-S cell was considered an end-term cell. This is probably not the case because multipolar mitoses of these cells have been observed (17) (Fig. 57.12), and R-S and Hodgkin cells in tissue cultures have been shown to incorporate tritiated thymidine and synthesize DNA (56).

The origin of the R-S cells and their variants was for a long time a subject of debate. It was initially postulated that they derive by successive stages of transformation from histiocytes or reticulum cells of the lymph nodes and spleen (38). The capacity of Hodgkin and R-S cells for phagocytosis *in vivo* and *in vitro,* the presence of Fc and C3b receptors, and the absence of lymphocyte markers seemed to favor a histiocytic/macrophagic origin (47,57). Further evidence in favor of histiocytes or dendritic cells as precursors of the R-S cells was their expression of markers considered specific for those cells, such as fascin (58) and CD21 (59). The opposite opinion, that R-S cells derive from activated T or B lymphocytes, also referred to as *immunoblasts,* was originally proposed by Lukes et al. (51) and was further supported by new findings (60) and results of studies of single R-S cells isolated by micromanipulation (61). By means of Southern blot hybridization, immunoglobulin (Ig) rearrangements were identified in 10% to 20% of cases of classic HL (62,63). The patterns of Ig rearrangements were different from those observed in HL of LP type (64). Some studies of R-S cells detected both monoclonal and polyclonal Ig rearrangements and obtained conflicting results in regard to frequency and clonality (65). Through the technique of PCR analysis of single R-S cells isolated by micromanipulation, Ig chain gene rearrangements could be studied directly (61,66). Thus, the detection of Ig rearrangements in 96% of classic HD cases investigated in recent studies indicates that the R-S cells are of B-cell origin and represent a clonal expansion of cells from follicular germinal centers (66). Studies of composite lymphomas with features of both HL and follicular or small lymphocytic lymphoma in which the R-S cells coexpress CD15 and CD20 markers and exhibit EBV RNA support these conclusions (67,68). Similarly, when classic HL and NHL coexisted in the same patient, a somatic mutation typical of germinal center B cells was identified in single cells of both tumors isolated by micromanipulation, indicating a common precursor (69). Finally, the detection of EBV in R-S cells (19) also indicates a B-cell origin because in humans the B cells are the usual host for EBV (68).

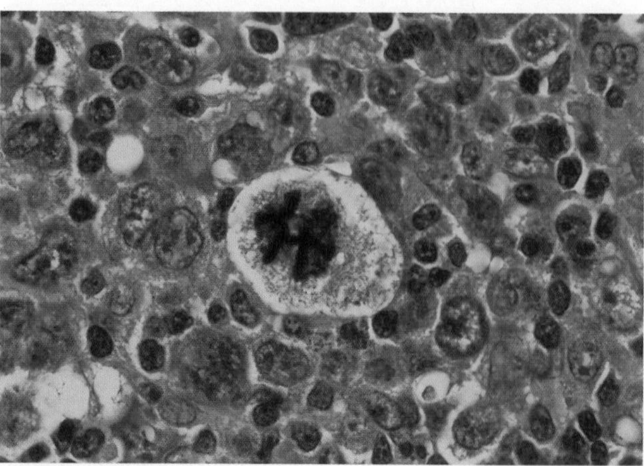

FIGURE 57.12. Mitosis of Reed-Sternberg cell. Hematoxylin, phloxine, and saffron stain.

The most peculiar feature of HL is that the neoplastic cellular component often comprises no more than 1% to 3% of the tumor volume. Nonetheless, the R-S cells and their variants, derived from the B cells of the germinal center and harboring EBV, are like many other types of lymphomas able in very small numbers to produce the distinctive signs and symptoms of HL (70). The explanation is the unique functionality of the R-S cells, which can produce more than 12 cytokines with a broad biologic spectrum (71). Among these are interleukin 5 (causing eosinophilia), transforming growth factor-β and platelet-derived growth factor (causing sclerosis), tumor necrosis factor (causing lymphopenia in the LD form), interleukin 1, interleukin 6, and others, which account for the constitutional symptoms of the syndrome (71).

Reed-Sternberg Cell Variants

In addition to the so-called diagnostic R-S cell (Figs. 57.10 and 57.11), characterized by its huge, inclusion-like nucleoli and excessive nuclear pleomorphism, several variants of this cell have been recognized as commonly associated with classic HL.

Hodgkin cells are sometimes referred to as *mononuclear R-S cell variants.* They are characterized by a large size, ovoid shape, indistinct cell borders, and a large, round, vesicular nucleus with a thick nuclear membrane and a single huge, hyperchromatic, intensely acidophilic nucleolus (Figs. 57.9 and 57.13). These cells, possibly the precursors of R-S cells, constitute the basic components of the neoplastic infiltrates in classic HL. Their origin and functions are considered similar to those of the R-S cells.

The *lacunar cell variant of the R-S cell* is characteristic of the NS type of HL. Lacunar cells have abundant, lightly acidophilic or water-clear cytoplasm, lobulated nuclei, and small nucleoli (41) (Fig. 57.14). The nuclear-to-cytoplasmic ratio is smaller than that of the typical R-S cells, the chromatin is coarser, and the nucleoli are larger than those in the LP-type cells. The lacunar effect is produced when formalin fixation causes the cytoplasm to collapse, creating an artifactual space between the retracted cytoplasm and the sharply demarcated peripheral cell margin (72). The shrinkage of the cytoplasm gives the impression of a nucleus lying within a clear space or lacuna. In Zenker-fixed tissues without the shrinkage artifact, the cytoplasm is finely granular and faintly acidophilic. In specimens fixed in glutaraldehyde

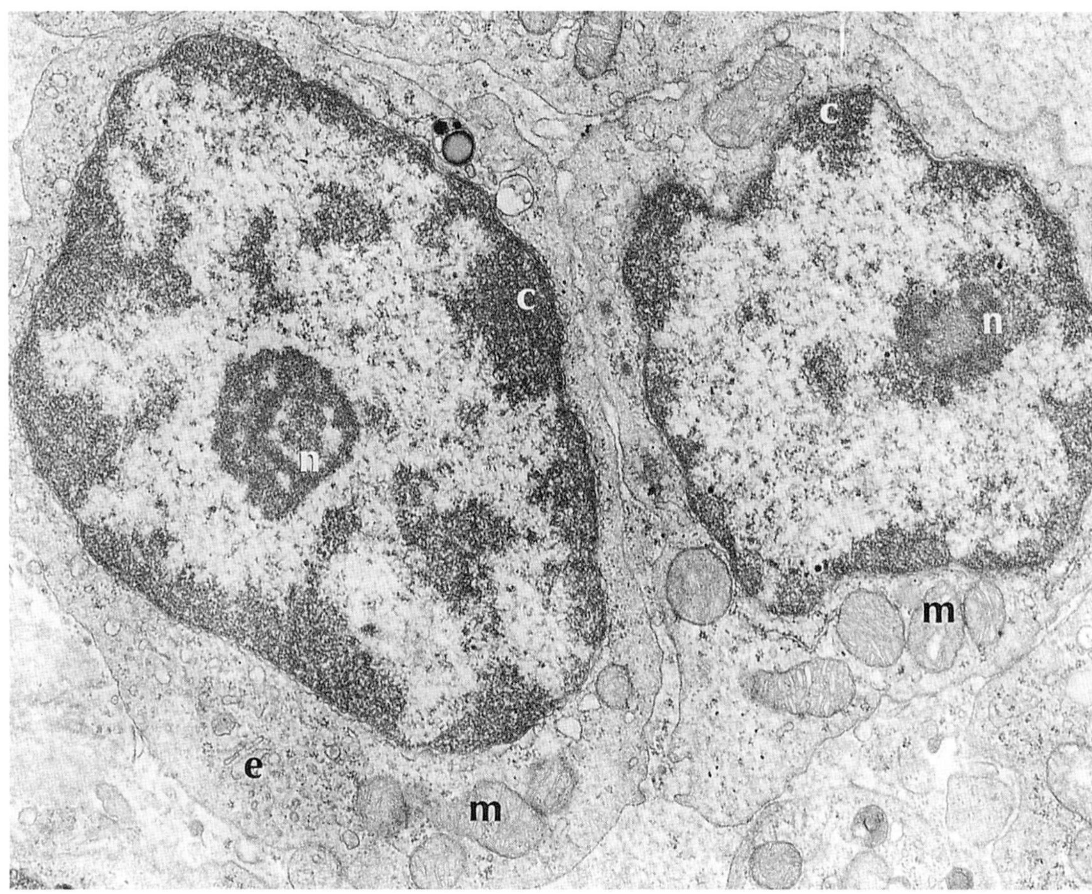

FIGURE 57.13. Hodgkin cells (neoplastic mononuclear cells) with multiple mitochondria (*m*), abundant endoplasmic reticulum (*e*), and huge nuclei with heterochromatin (*c*) and reticulated nucleoli (*n*). ×14,000.

and embedded in Epon for ultrastructural studies, the lacunar effect is inapparent. It is generally accepted that lacunar cells represent a variant of R-S cells, and recent ultrastructural and immunocytochemical studies have attempted to show that both originate in the activated small lymphocyte (72). The lacunar cells may be few and scattered between the lymphoid cells or very numerous and arrayed in clusters or sheets (36) with occasional necrotic foci, a pattern resembling metastatic carcinoma or histiocytic lymphoma (Fig. 57.15).

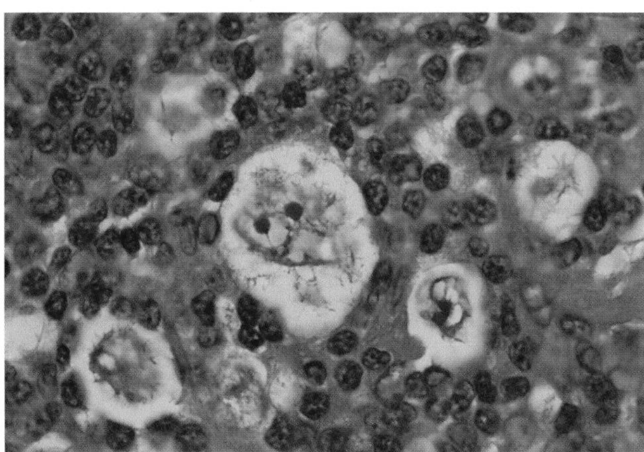

FIGURE 57.14. Lacunar cells (variants of Reed-Sternberg cells) with clear, partially collapsed cytoplasm and large nuclei with one or several prominent nucleoli. Hematoxylin, phloxine, and saffron stain.

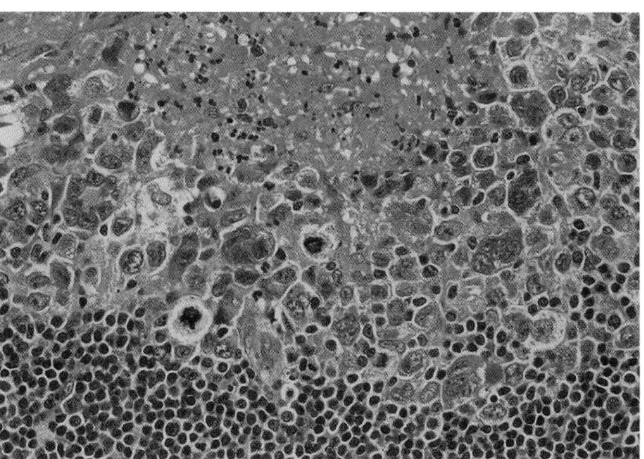

FIGURE 57.15. Island of Reed-Sternberg cells, Hodgkin cells, lacunar cells, frequent apoptotic cells, and area of tissue necrosis. Hematoxylin, phloxine, and saffron stain.

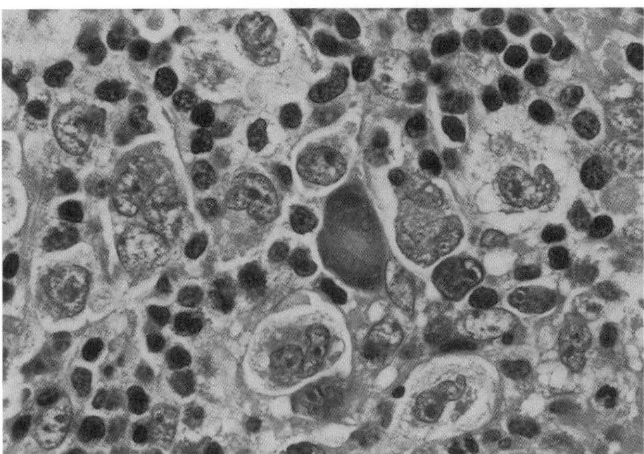

FIGURE 57.16. Reed-Sternberg cells, Hodgkin cells, and lacunar cells admixed with eosinophils and lymphocytes. Large mummified cell (*center*) with darkly staining eosinophilic cytoplasm and two nuclei. Hematoxylin, phloxine, and saffron stain.

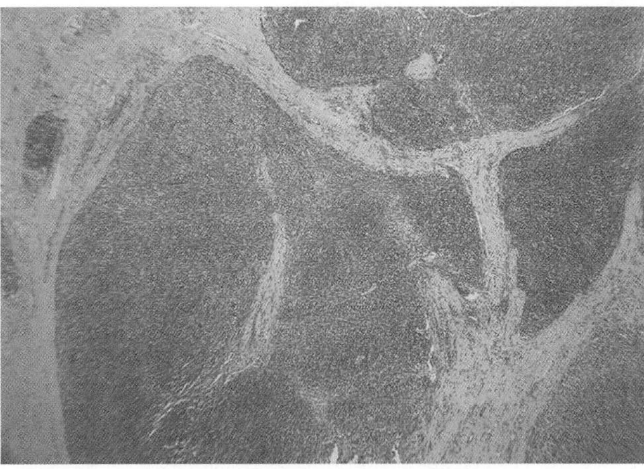

FIGURE 57.17. Hodgkin lymphoma, nodular sclerosis. Broad bands of fibrosis dissect the lymph node into nodules of various sizes and shapes. Hematoxylin, phloxine, and saffron stain.

The *mummified cell variant of the R-S cell* is a degenerated or apoptotic cell that may be seen singly or in clusters (in which case they are strongly indicative of HL) (Fig. 57.8). These cells are large, with darkly staining eosinophilic cytoplasm and a dense pyknotic nucleus that sometimes has a visible nucleolus (Fig. 57.16).

The *anaplastic variant of the R-S cell* is commonly seen in the LD type. These cells are large and highly pleomorphic; features of coarse chromatin and hyperchromatic, bizarre, polyploid nuclei with prominent nucleoli entail a differential diagnosis with anaplastic large cell lymphoma, anaplastic carcinoma, and sarcoma.

Histologic Patterns of Classic Hodgkin Lymphoma

Nodular Sclerosis

In developed countries, NS is the most common histologic form of HL, representing 40% to 70% of all cases (46). It is associated predominantly with clinical stage II (9), is the most common type in young women (8–10), usually affects mediastinal (41) or cervical lymph nodes or both, and shows a predilection for contiguous spread (38). The prognosis is consistently favorable (8–10,33,41).

The diagnosis of HL, NS type, as defined by Lukes and Butler (41), is based on three characteristic features: lacunar cells, diagnostic R-S cells, and bands of fibrosis. At least two of the three features must be present. The lacunar cells may occur singly, scattered within the nodules of lymphoid tissue, or in large sheets that may resemble metastatic seminoma, embryonal carcinoma, or histiocytic lymphoma (36). The number of R-S cells in NS is variable. When they are more numerous, they suggest progressive disease and possibly the classification of MC.

Sclerosis is a defining feature of NS. Broad, interconnecting bands of collagen originate in the thickened capsule of a lymph node and dissect it into nodules of various sizes and shapes (Figs. 57.17 and 57.18). The collagen in NS is laid down in parallel bundles that appear birefringent under polarized light. This characteristic feature distinguishes the organized sclerosis of NS from the disorderly fibrosis of LD, which is characterized by thin, non-birefringent fibers of connective tissue. The number of collagen bands varies from case to case and also between lymph nodes in an individual case. Even focal areas of bands of fibrosis strongly suggest NS (46). Reticulin staining reveals cellular nodules separated by fibrosis (Fig. 57.19). The extremes are a few bands of collagen with an abundance of lacunar cells, the *cellular phase* of NS, and extensive sclerosis with scarce cellularity, the *fibrotic phase* of NS. In the cellular phase, the lacunar

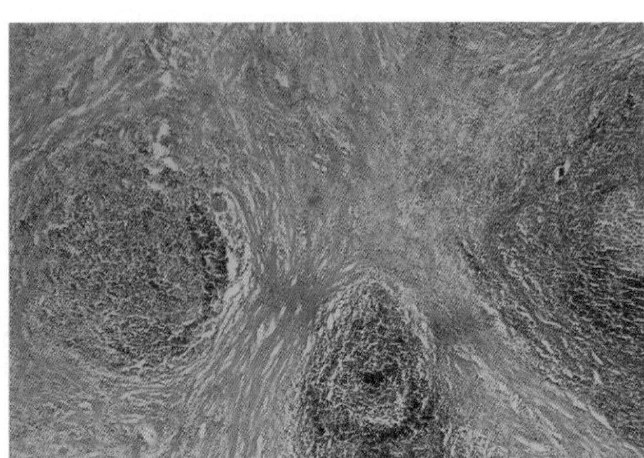

FIGURE 57.18. Hodgkin lymphoma, nodular sclerosis. Broad bands of collagen replace lymphoid tissues and separate nodules of remaining tissues. Hematoxylin, phloxine, and saffron stain.

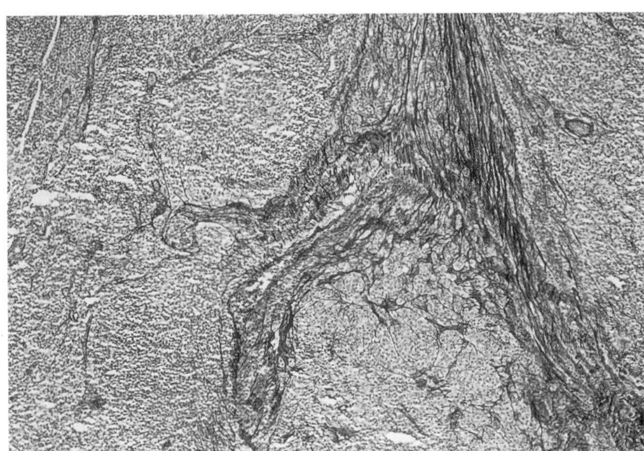

FIGURE 57.19. Hodgkin lymphoma, nodular sclerosis. Reticulin staining reveals bands of fibrosis and cellular nodules.

cells tend to congregate in the center of tumor nodules. Sometimes, they undergo focal necrosis and are associated with abundant and varied inflammatory reactions that include large numbers of eosinophils and mummified cells. It is believed that the cellular phase of NS indicates increased disease aggressiveness, and some authors recommend that such cases be classified as MC (72). Typical diagnostic R-S cells are usually present, but their numbers vary greatly from case to case and from area to area.

The *syncytial variant of NS* is an unusual morphologic manifestation of HL that probably occurs in fewer than 5% of cases (73) (Fig. 57.20). It is in fact an extreme form of the cellular phase of NS, in which numerous Hodgkin cells and R-S cells of classic and variant types are arranged in cohesive clusters or sheets, producing the appearance of metastatic carcinoma or melanoma (Fig. 57.15). Necrosis may be present in the center of cords and sheets (Fig. 57.20). The aggregates of large cells with highly atypical nuclei and prominent nucleoli may even occupy the trabecular sinuses, but rarely the subcapsular sinuses of lymph nodes (73). Birefringent bands of collagen surround the abnormal cellular areas, although in limited numbers.

The British National Lymphoma Investigation group has proposed grading NS according to the number of R-S cells: grade 1, few R-S cells; grade 2, highly anaplastic R-S cells in more than 25% of the nodules (74). However, the new WHO classification recommends that HL not be graded in routine diagnosis (28).

Lymphocyte-Rich Pattern

The lymphocyte-rich pattern of HL is defined as a few R-S and Hodgkin cells within a mass of lymphocytes and only a few eosinophils and neutrophils (Fig. 57.21). It is distinguished from the LP diffuse type, in which the cells scattered among the lymphocytes are lymphocytic and histiocytic cells (L & H), not R-S cells. For this reason, it is believed that these cases belong to the classic rather than the LP category of HL. The incidence of lymphocyte-rich classic HL is about 6%, similar to that of nodular LP. The prognosis is worse, closer to that of the classic forms. Because presently no studies are available, this subtype of HL was initially included in the classification as a provisional entity (28).

Mixed Cellularity

The MC type comprises a heterogeneous group of lesions in the central portion of the spectrum ranging from the L & H type to the LD type. It is the most common type in underdeveloped countries and in very young persons, the elderly, and patients with AIDS. Together, the MC and NS types account for 80% of all cases of HL. MC involves the whole or large areas of lymph nodes, which exhibit a total loss of architecture and occasional foci of necrosis.

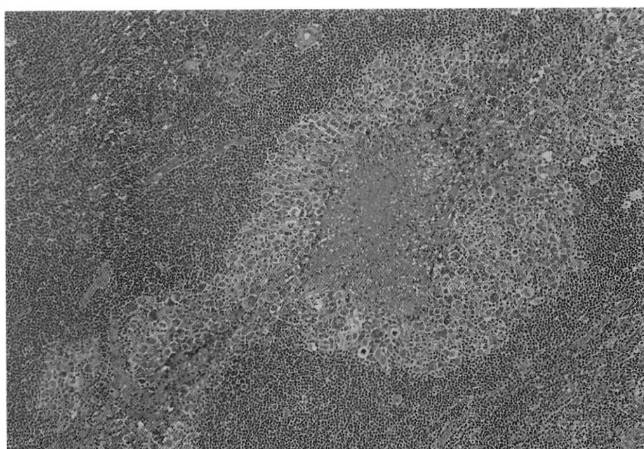

FIGURE 57.20. Hodgkin lymphoma, nodular sclerosis, syncytial variant. Solid sheets of Reed-Sternberg, Hodgkin, lacunar, and mummified cells with central area of necrosis. Hematoxylin, phloxine, and saffron stain.

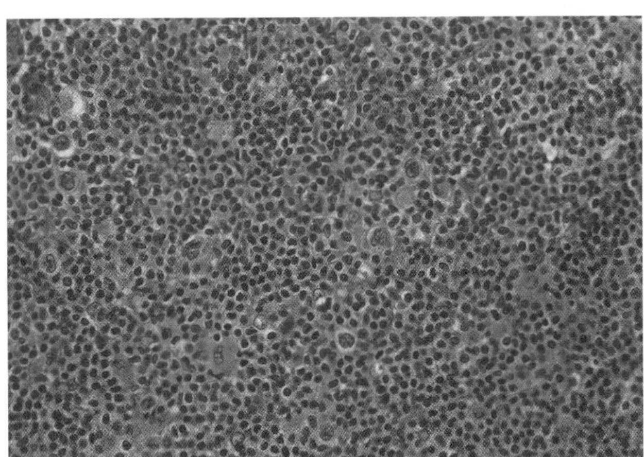

FIGURE 57.21. Hodgkin lymphoma, lymphocyte-rich type. Few Reed-Sternberg cells or variants within a mass of lymphocytes. Hematoxylin, phloxine, and saffron stain.

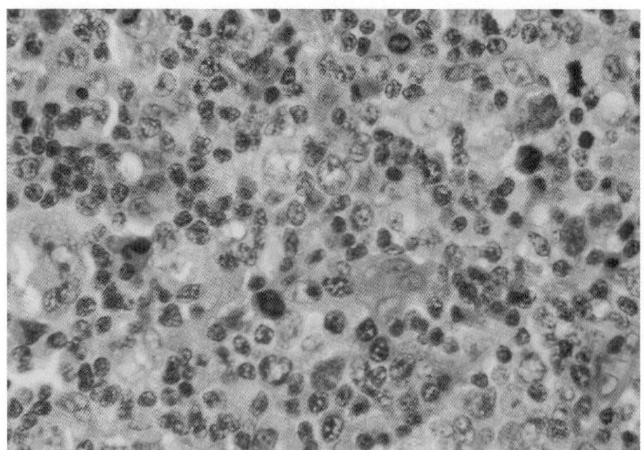

FIGURE 57.22. Hodgkin lymphoma, mixed cellularity. Reed-Sternberg cells and their variants within a mixture of eosinophils, lymphocytes, and neutrophils. Hematoxylin, phloxine, and saffron stain.

The process is diffuse rather than nodular, and the MC infiltrates include lymphocytes, plasma cells, histiocytes, eosinophils (sometimes in remarkably large numbers), occasional neutrophils, and numerous typical, diagnostic Hodgkin cells and R-S cells, which are present in almost every low-power microscopic field (Fig. 57.22). Moderate diffuse fibrosis is also present, but without collagen bands or nodular patterns.

In addition to the typical cases, Lukes and Butler recommend classifying as MC type those cases of NS that show lacunar cells but entirely lack bands of fibrosis. It is assumed that the coexistence of two histologic types indicates progressive disease. To separate the various histologic types better, some quantitative criteria have been proposed, as follows: MC is defined as between 5 and 15 diagnostic R-S and Hodgkin cells per high-power field (HPF), LP as fewer than 5 cells per HPF, and LD as more than 15 cells per HPF (75).

Lymphocyte Depletion

The LD type comprises fewer than 5% of cases of HL (46) and includes the subtypes of reticular and diffuse fibrosis of the original classification of Lukes and Butler (41). The incidence has decreased because with the use of immunohistochemistry, many cases have been reclassified as large cell NHL (76). The LD type is the most aggressive form of HL, occurring predominantly in older persons and commonly associated with clinical stages III and IV of disease. It has been proposed that the LD type of Hodgkin disease represents, by its characteristic clinical presentation, pathologic distribution, and short median survival (4.3 months from diagnosis), a distinct clinicopathologic entity (77). However, others oppose this view, pointing out that although this form of the disease occasionally runs a fulminating course, most cases still conform to the classic presentation of Hodgkin disease, and that modern chemotherapy is effective in inducing remissions and lengthening the median survival to 25.1 months (35).

The *diffuse fibrosis subtype* is more commonly found at autopsy, developing spontaneously or as a result of radiation or chemotherapy. It is characterized by lymph nodes that are poorly cellular and structureless. The normal parenchyma is replaced by fibrous tissue, including scattered R-S cells and few residual lymphocytes (Fig. 57.23). The broad bands of collagen seen in NS are absent in LD, in which the fibrous tissue involving the lymph nodes consists of fibrillar reticulin and deposits of amorphous proteinaceous material. Spindle cells make up the bulk of the tissue; a few bizarre giant cells may be recognized as R-S cells (71).

The *reticular subtype of LD* is characterized by hypercellularity. The lymph node architecture is similarly obliterated, not by fibrosis but by large numbers of pleomorphic neoplastic cells. These cells are either typical diagnostic R-S cells or bizarre variants thereof; they form sheets of large tumor cells with hyperchromatic, irregularly shaped nuclei with prominent nucleoli and frequent atypical mitoses. Usually, more than 15 cells per HPF are seen (75). This subtype of LD is hard to distinguish from pleomorphic large cell NHL. Infiltration by eosinophils, neutrophils, and macrophages may be present. Foci of tumor necrosis, minimal fibrosis, and invasion of the capsule and perinodal adipose tissue are characteristic. The resulting morphologic picture is similar to that of histiocytic lymphoma, sarcoma, or metastatic anaplastic carcinoma, so that the distinction between these different tumors is one of the most difficult in surgical pathology. Nonetheless, the proper diagnosis of the aggressive forms of Hodgkin disease is clinically important because some trials of combination chemotherapy have resulted in unexpectedly long remissions (35,36).

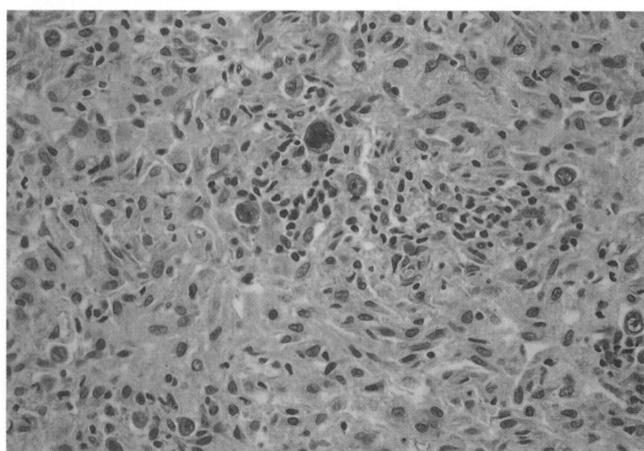

FIGURE 57.23. Hodgkin lymphoma, lymphocyte depletion. Large cells with anaplastic hyperchromatic nuclei and few lymphocytes, histiocytes, and fibroblasts. Hematoxylin, phloxine, and saffron stain.

Unclassifiable

All lesions that could not be classified as one of the definite histologic types were designated as MC by Butler (26). Rappaport and Neiman (36), however, preferred the term *Hodgkin disease, unclassifiable* for those lesions that do not conform with any histologic type. The present WHO classification maintains the category of *unclassifiable* for cases that cannot be defined by combined morphologic, immunohistochemical, and genetic examination (28).

ELECTRON MICROSCOPY

The diagnostic R-S cell usually in fact contains a single nucleus, clearly seen by *electron microscopy* (Fig. 57.24). The impression of multiple nuclei is created by an extreme degree of nuclear cleavage and indentation, in which the nucleus is fragmented into several segments interconnected by thin nuclear bridges (78) (Figs. 57.24 and 57.25).

The nuclear and nucleolar structure of diagnostic R-S cells is similar to that of Hodgkin cells (Fig. 57.25). The

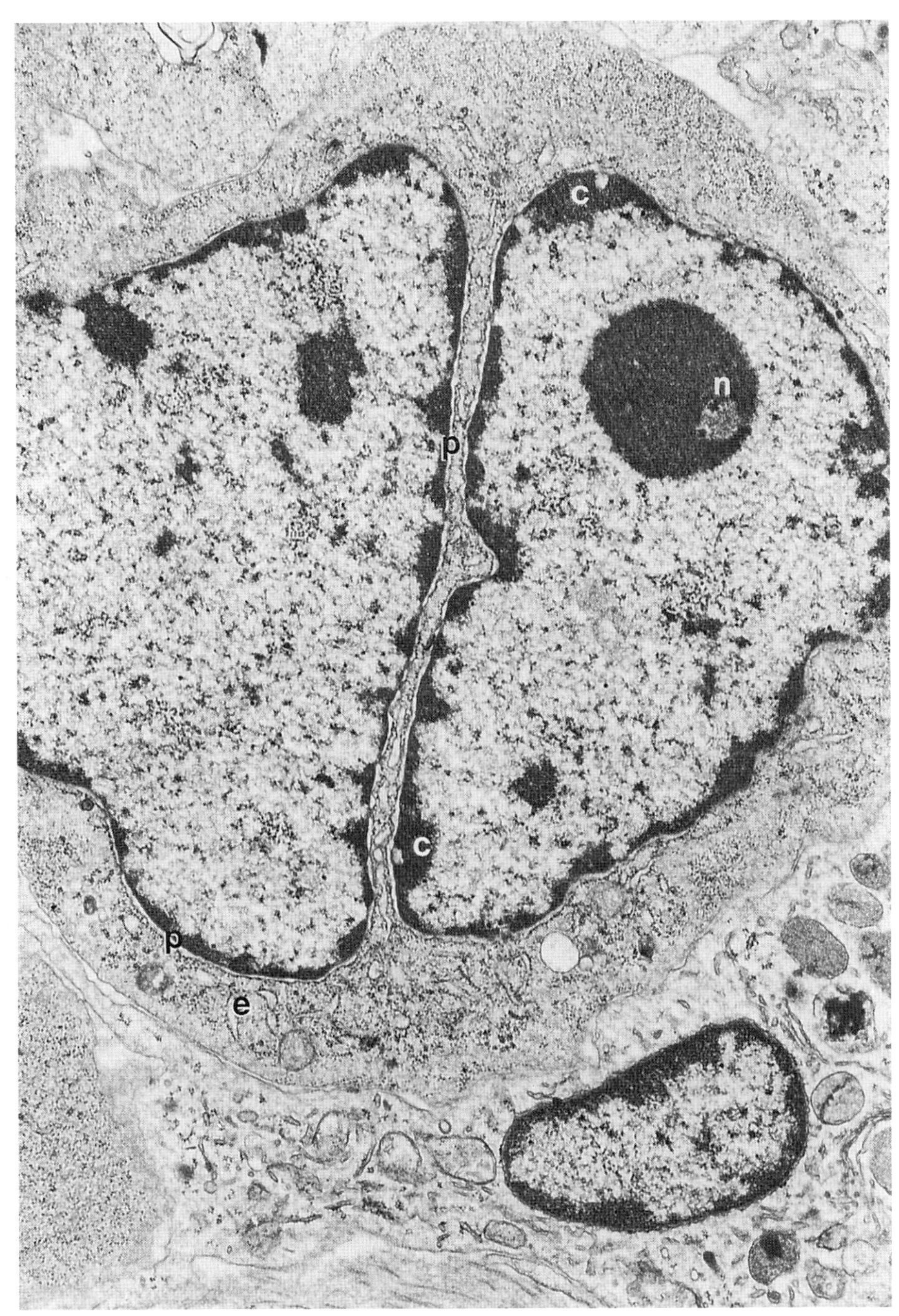

FIGURE 57.24. Reed-Sternberg cells with a deeply indented and convoluted nucleus appear binucleated. Huge, dense nucleolus (*n*) and heterochromatin (*c*). Dilated perinuclear cisternae and well-differentiated rough endoplasmic reticulum. ×12,000.

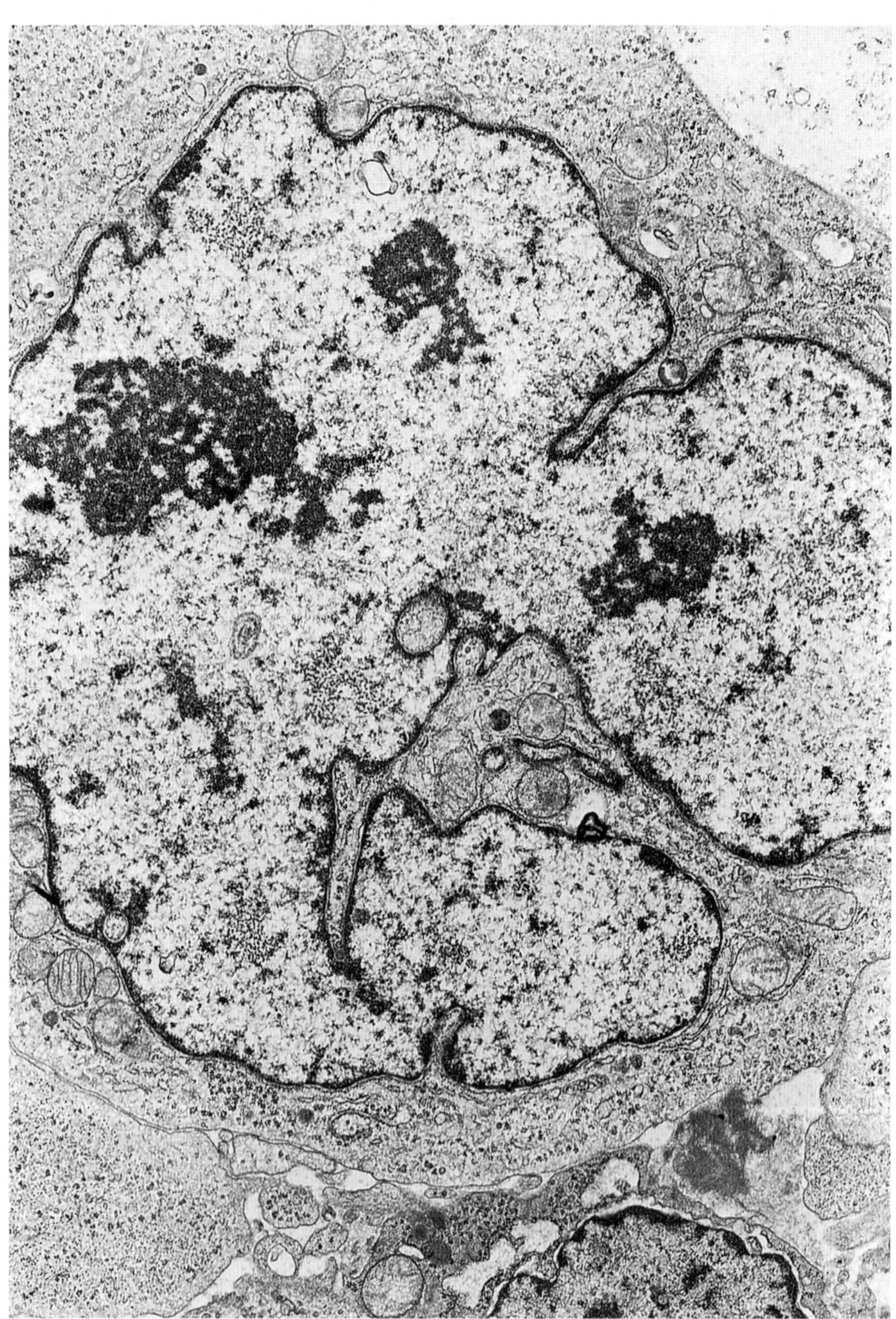

FIGURE 57.25. Reed-Sternberg cells with convoluted polylobate nucleus, heterochromatin, and large, reticulated nucleoli. Cytoplasm includes mitochondria, endoplasmic reticulum, and polyribosomes. ×8,800.

chromatin is either marginated or clustered into dense areas, appearing under the electron microscope as "spotted nuclei" (79). The nucleoplasm is less electron-dense than in the other cells of the lymph node (80). Two or three very large nucleoli with a condensed structure containing abundant RNA material are usually present in the nucleus. The typical nucleolus is spherical, 3 to 4 μm in diameter (the size of an erythrocyte), and sharply demarcated and resembles an inclusion body. The cytoplasm contains a fairly large number of organelles (78,80), including round or rod-shaped mitochondria, disseminated free ribosomes, a well-developed Golgi body, and occasional tubular arrays within the endoplasmic reticulum (81). The cell is commonly surrounded by lymphocytes, and their tight apposition suggests immune interactions between these elements (82).

IMMUNOHISTOCHEMISTRY

The background population of lymphocytes in HL is generally of the CD4+ (helper) T-cell phenotype; these cells often form rosettes around the R-S cells (47,83,84). The R-S cells and their variants react with a fairly large number of antibodies and lectins, some of which are more effective in frozen sections and others well adapted for paraffin-embedded tissues. Flow cytometry is not useful for making a positive diagnosis of HL because the characteristic R-S cells are a very small proportion of the total cell population, but it may be helpful in ruling out HL in cases of NHL. The characteristic immunophenotype for R-S and Hodgkin cells, CD15+, CD30+, CD45−, can be routinely and predictably obtained with formalin (Bouin, B5)-fixed, paraffin-embedded tissues. The antibody most commonly used to characterize the neoplastic cells of HL is directed against the *CD15* or *Leu-M1* antigen, which is primarily a myelomonocytic antigen (84–89). Therefore, the granules of polynuclear leukocytes stain for Leu-M1 and so provide a useful built-in control. R-S cells and variants express CD15 in 85% to 90% of cases of classic HL (89) (Fig. 57.26). In a characteristic Leu-M1 staining pattern, the cell membrane and Golgi area are stained in the form of a prominent paranuclear globule (Fig. 57.27). However, Leu-M1 is also present in 21% to 67% of peripheral T-cell lymphomas (86,89), 4% of B-cell lymphomas (89), and a variety of nonhematopoietic neoplasms, including many adenocarcinomas (86), reactive histiocytes (85), and cytomegalovirus-infected cells (90). A second antibody highly effective in the identification of Hodgkin and R-S cells is directed against the CD30 antigen. In a review of HL cases, R-S cells expressed the *CD30* antigen in 89% of cases (91). The antibodies for CD30 are Ki-1 in frozen tissues and Ber-H2 on paraffin-embedded tissues. CD30 is also not entirely specific for R-S cells; it is also expressed by anaplastic large cell lymphoma and some carcinomas, mainly embryonal carcinoma (92), and occasionally by immunoblasts, histiocytes, and plasma cells (93). *CD45,* the leukocyte common antigen (LCA), is detected in only about 7% of R-S cells, mostly in frozen sections (94), whereas it is detected in most cells of B-cell large cell lymphomas and in most lymphocytic and histiocytic ("popcorn") cells of lymphocyte predominance (LP)-type HL. Therefore, the combination of CD15+, CD30+, and CD45− is the diagnostic immunophenotype of R-S cells and their variants. CD45 expression does not exclude the presence of R-S cells when CD15 and CD30 are also expressed; however, CD45+ in association with CD15− and CD30− is not consistent with a diagnosis of classic HL. *Epithelial membrane antigen* (EMA) reactivity is present in 60% of cases of LP-type HL but absent in more than 90% of cases of classic HL (84). *Fascin,* a marker of dendritic cells, vimentin, and *CD74* may be expressed in R-S cells, but not constantly (Fig. 57.28). *CD20* and *CD79a,* which are B-cell markers, may be expressed in the cells of classic HL in up to 30% of cases (95). The distinction between LP-type HL and classic HL is largely based on their different immunophenotypic profiles. In the classic types of

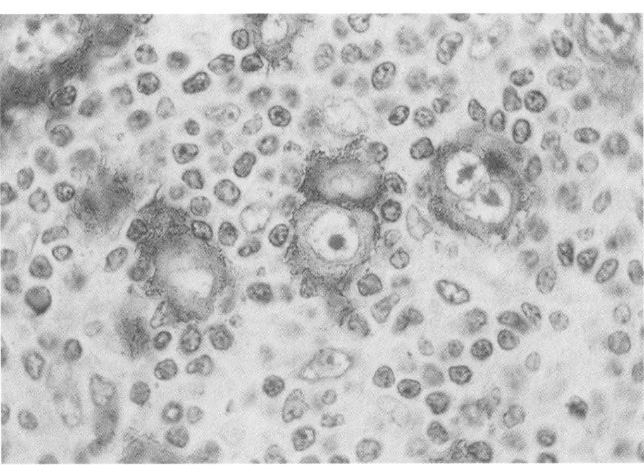

FIGURE 57.27. Reed-Sternberg and Hodgkin cells with selective membrane and Golgi area immunostainings. Anti-Leu-M1/peroxidase stain.

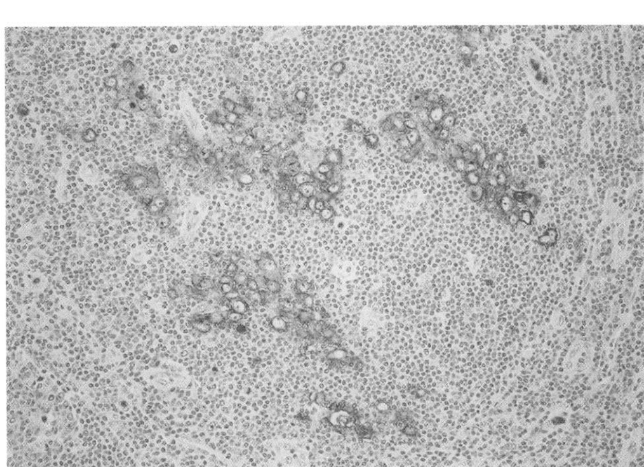

FIGURE 57.26. Reed-Sternberg and Hodgkin cells selectively immunostained for CD15 marker. The staining is membranous and paranuclear. Anti-Leu-M1/peroxidase stain.

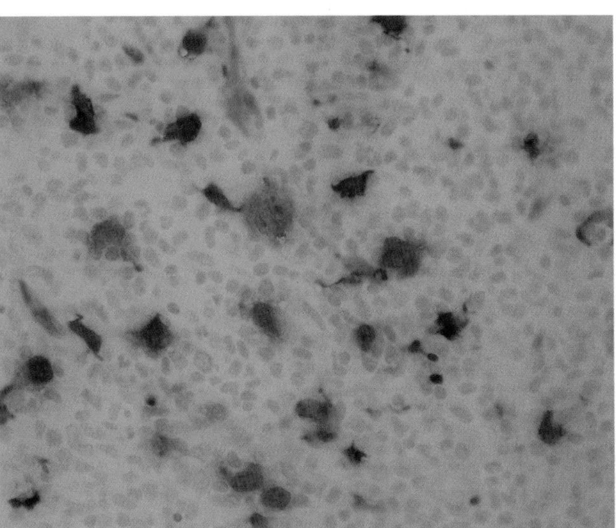

FIGURE 57.28. Reed-Sternberg and Hodgkin cells stained for fascin. Antifascin/peroxidase stain.

HL, the R-S cells and their variants stain for CD15 and CD30 and do not stain for CD45, CD20, and EMA (84,88,96). In HL of the LP nodular type, the neoplastic cells consistently express B-cell markers such as CD20 and CD79a, indicating the B-cell origin of this form; in contrast, in the three other forms, the R-S cells have been shown variously to express T-cell markers, B-cell markers, neither, or both (96). The difference in immunophenotypes supports the belief that LP-type HL is in fact a kind of B-cell lymphoma rather than a variant of HL. When difficult problems of differential diagnosis must be solved, as in deciding between the syncytial variant of HL and anaplastic carcinomas or melanomas, panels of multiple antibodies must be used. Thus, a combination of Leu-M1 (CD15), Ber-H2 (CD30), and LCA (CD45); CD20 or CD79a (for B-cell markers); CD3 (for T-cell markers); cytokeratins (high- and low-molecular-weight) to rule out carcinoma; S100 (to rule out melanoma); and lysozyme (muramidase) to rule out histiocytic lymphoma is indicated.

Phenotype

HODGKIN/R-S CELLS
CD15+, CD30+, fascin+
CD45−, CD20−/+, CD79a−/+
LYMPHOCYTES
CD3+

FLOW CYTOMETRY

Flow cytometry is not an appropriate method for the diagnosis of HL because the proportion of neoplastic cells is small; however, it is useful in ruling out NHL.

MOLECULAR BIOLOGY AND CYTOGENETICS

Molecular analysis of HL has yielded variable results because the neoplastic cells (Hodgkin and R-S cells) in most cases represent only a very small amount of the tissues analyzed. Most of the cells in HL tumor masses are reactive normal cells, and consequently studies of clonal rearrangements of HL have frequently ended by showing mostly germline configurations of the Ig and T-cell receptor (TCR) genes (97,98). Therefore, only lesions of HL that are rich in neoplastic cells, usually NS or LD, can be expected to yield conclusive results. In one study, six of seven cases of HL selected for the presence of numerous R-S cells showed clonal rearrangements for an Ig gene and no rearrangements for the TCR gene (99). In other studies, Ig rearrangements were identified by Southern blot hybridization in 10% to 20% of cases of HL (63,64). These results suggested a B-cell origin for the R-S cells; however, they could not identify the cells containing the rearranged genes. This was achieved by PCR studies of single R-S cells isolated by micromanipulation, which confirmed the clonal Ig rearrangements (61,62). Rearrangements of TCR chain genes were not convincingly demonstrated. Mutations of the p53 gene were demonstrated by PCR analysis of R-S cells (100). Cytogenetic studies entail difficulties of working with few cells and infrequent mitoses. So far, the chromosomal aberrations observed have not proved to be nonrandom and consistent. The bcl-6 gene is absent. Rearrangements of bcl-2 are rarely observed. The t(14:18) and t(2:5) translocations are not seen in HL.

DIFFERENTIAL DIAGNOSIS

Because of the morphologic diversity of HL, different diagnostic options must be considered for each histologic type.

Nodular Sclerosis

- Nodular LP: Lymphocytic and histiocytic cells present with CD20+, CD45+, CD15−, CD30− immunophenotype; R-S cells rare; fibrosis absent.
- Lymphocyte-rich classic type: Abundant lymphocytes, absence of eosinophils, R-S variants, and fibrosis.
- Infectious mononucleosis lymphadenitis and other viral lymphadenitides: The clinical symptoms are different, results of serologic tests are positive, and atypical Downey cells may be found in the peripheral blood. Histologically, the lymph node architecture is preserved and the sinuses are patent. Numerous immunoblasts, abundant apoptosis, and tingible-body macrophages are seen in infectious mononucleosis, but not in HL. The immunoblasts may resemble Hodgkin cells, and R-S–like cells may be present. However, they express T-cell markers and are CD15− and CD30−. Moreover, eosinophils and bands of sclerosis are not present.
- Large B-cell lymphoma, immunoblastic type: The large cells with pleomorphic nuclei and nucleoli may resemble NS-type HL; however, sclerosis is usually missing (Fig. 57.29). The atypical cells, large and small, show a B-cell phenotype and are CD45+, CD20+ and CD15−, CD30− (Fig. 57.30). The presence of Igs within large lymphoma cells does not necessarily rule out HL because R-S cells can phagocytose Igs; therefore, their identity should be confirmed by additional markers. A special case is mediastinal large B-cell lymphoma, which is more common in young, female patients, tends to involve the upper mediastinum, and is characterized by marked, intersecting bands of fibrosis. All these features are also usually displayed by HL of NS type. The differential diagnosis is often made by examining small biopsy specimens obtained at laparoscopy, in which the determination of cellular immunophenotype becomes of essential importance.

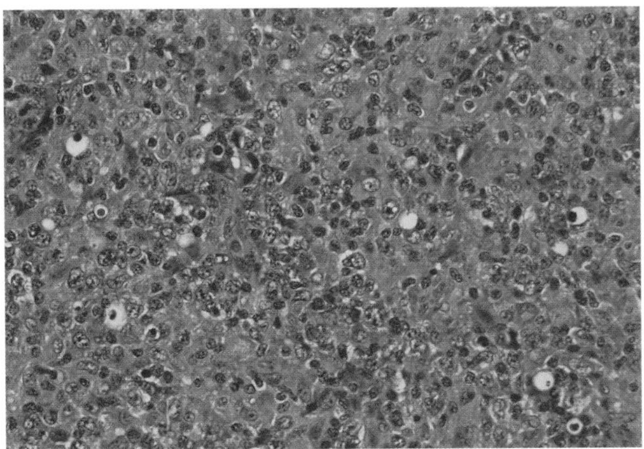

FIGURE 57.29. Hodgkin-like and Reed-Sternberg–like cells within a population of lymphocytes closely resembling Hodgkin lymphoma. Hematoxylin, phloxine, and saffron stain.

- Peripheral T-cell NHL may show numerous highly atypical cells that have large, pleomorphic nuclei admixed with small reactive lymphocytes and eosinophils. The distinction from HL is difficult and depends in many cases on a thorough immunohistochemical analysis that shows the large cells to be positive for Leu-Ml (CD15) and negative for LCA (CD45), whereas the lymphocytes are positive for pan-T-cell markers in the case of HL. The presence of birefringent sclerosis also favors HL.
- Anaplastic large cell lymphoma: Resembles NS-type HL, particularly the syncytial variant; cohesive cells are arranged in solid cords and sheets. The histologic distinction is subtle and often difficult, with some cases overlapping the two entities. In anaplastic large cell lymphoma, the tumor cells are often within the lymph node sinuses. Usually, fibrosis is absent and an inflammatory reaction is minimal or absent, whereas NS-type HL has bands of fibrosis and infiltrates of eosinophils, neutrophils, and plasma cells. The immunophenotype of R-S cells is CD15+, CD30+, EMA+, and CD45−, whereas that of anaplastic large cell lymphoma is basically one of B-cell type, with CD15−, CD30+, EMA−, CD45+, and CD20+. An important distinctive marker is anaplastic lymphoma kinase (ALK) protein, which is present in anaplastic large cell lymphoma and negative in HL.

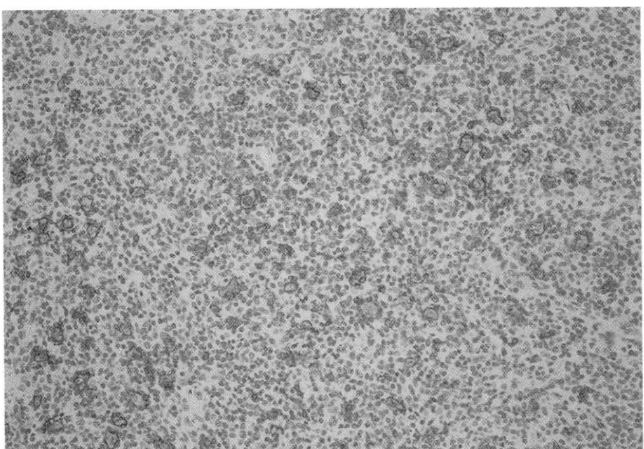

FIGURE 57.30. Same lesion as in Fig. 57.29 shows immunostaining of Hodgkin/Reed-Sternberg–like cells for CD20 (B-cell marker), indicating that the lesion is a large B-cell non-Hodgkin lymphoma. Anti-CD20/peroxidase stain.

- Metastatic anaplastic carcinoma, seminoma, embryonal carcinoma, and nasopharyngeal carcinoma may simulate the syncytial form of NS-type HL. Metastatic carcinomas usually invade the marginal sinuses, which is not a feature of HL. Carcinomas can best be distinguished by their positivity for cytokeratins and negative staining for the Leu-M1 (CD15) antigen, although some rare positive cases have been reported (101).
- Metastatic melanoma may resemble R-S cells in that the cells have large nuclei with prominent nucleoli. It differs in that it has more eosinophilic cytoplasm and frequent pseudonuclear inclusions. The difficulty can be resolved by demonstrating positivity for S100 antigen and HMB45 (negative in HL) and negativity for Leu-M1 (CD15) (positive in HL).

Lymphocyte-Rich Classic Type

- LP diffuse type is similar in that a large number of small lymphocytes comprise the tumor mass. However, in the classic type, R-S cells and their variants are scattered throughout the lymphocytes, whereas lymphocytic and histiocytic cells are seen in the LP type.

Mixed Cellularity

- Because of the characteristic cellularity of this type of HL, fewer problems of differential diagnosis arise. The classic R-S cells lie within a mixed population of non-neoplastic cells that are not homogeneous on histologic examination and not monoclonal on immunohistochemical study. Granulomatous lesions may sometimes raise problems of differential diagnosis, but if strict morphologic and immunohistochemical criteria for the recognition of R-S cells are followed, these can be avoided.

Lymphocyte Depletion

- NHL large cell polymorphic tumors of B- or T-cell type may closely resemble the reticular subtype of LD. The criteria for differential diagnosis based on immunohistochemistry are similar to those mentioned above (see criteria for NS).
- Malignant fibrous histiocytoma may be considered in the differential diagnosis of the diffuse fibrosis subtype of LD. Markers for lymphoid cell lineage such as LCA (CD45) must be used. On occasion, the distinction is impossible, and the diagnosis rests with the history and an earlier diagnosis of a less advanced stage of HL.

DIAGNOSTIC REPRODUCIBILITY

The histologic diagnosis of HL may be self-evident in some cases and quite difficult in others. The difficulties of HL diagnosis were well-known to Symmers (102), who before the advent of immunohistochemistry stated that HL presents more diagnostic difficulties than is usually realized; he advised, "The differential histologic diagnosis should be considered in every case in considerably greater depth than is used." He reviewed a series of 600 cases with a histologic diagnosis of Hodgkin disease and confirmed it in only 317 cases (53%). In the remaining 283 cases, he considered the

Checklist

HODGKIN LYMPHOMA

Nodular sclerosis
Most common type in developed countries
Young, female patients
Clinical stage II
Mediastinum frequently involved
Birefringent collagen bands
Nodular cellular areas
Syncytial variant
R-S cells
Hodgkin cells
Lacunar cells
Mummified cells
Eosinophils
Plasma cells, neutrophils
Lymphocytes (CD4+ T cells)
Immunophenotype: CD15+, CD30+, EMA+, CD45−, CD20−, EBV+

Lymphocyte-rich type
R-S cells and variants
Sheets of lymphocytes

Mixed cellularity
Most common type in underdeveloped countries
Children, elderly
HIV-infected patients
Clinical stages III and IV
Architecture obliterated
Necrosis
Fibrosis diffuse
R-S cells (5 to 15 cells per HPF)
Leu-MI (CD15)+, Ki-I (CD30)+, LCA (CD45)−
Hodgkin cells, mummified cells
Eosinophils, plasma cells, neutrophils
Epithelioid cells, occasional granulomas

Lymphocyte depletion
Elderly
Clinical stages III and IV
Reticular or diffuse fibrosis types
Necrosis
R-S cells (>15 cells per HPF)
High degree of nuclear pleomorphism
Few lymphocytes
Diffuse fibrillar reticulin

diagnosis of Hodgkin disease to be mistaken. The condition most frequently confused with Hodgkin disease was chronic nonspecific lymphadenitis. Other lesions often mistaken for Hodgkin disease were reticulum cell sarcoma, metastatic tumors, infectious mononucleosis, dermatopathic lymphadenopathy, and toxoplasmosis. In a different study, a panel of experts reviewed 186 cases of Hodgkin disease registered in the Southwest Oncology Group clinical trials and confirmed the histologic diagnosis in 175 cases (94%) (103). When the same material was compared in relation to diagnosis of histologic types and subtypes (classification of Lukes and Butler), the panel's diagnosis and the initial diagnosis were in agreement in only 66% of cases, with the best agreement in NS (68%) and the least in LD types (36%). In a study reported by Keller and co-workers (11), 179 biopsies were reviewed by three pathologists according to the criteria of the Rye classification; all three pathologists agreed in 120 cases (67%), and two of three agreed in 165 cases (92%). The results of these earlier studies indicate the difficulties inherent in the histologic diagnosis and typing of HL.

The introduction of immunohistochemistry, with the use of antibodies to antigenic markers of the cells of HL, has improved to a great extent the accuracy of diagnosis. Notwithstanding, some cases of lymphoma at the interface between HL and NHL may still prove difficult or impossible to classify. Hodgkin-like variants of large cell lymphomas with antigenic profiles of large B-cell lymphoma (Figs. 57.29 and 57.30) or anaplastic large cell lymphoma are not infrequent and have been a subject of controversy (104). Some authors believe that Hodgkin-like lymphomas with a B-cell phenotype are probably cases of HL with an abundance of neoplastic cells (104), whereas others conceive of a continuous morphologic and immunophenotypic spectrum between HL and NHL (105).

Fortunately, the advances made in the treatment of HL can diminish the effects of diagnostic uncertainties. Whereas HL was uniformly fatal at the turn of the century, it is now curable in three of every four patients, and the current 5-year survival rate is about 90% (106). As a consequence of highly effective chemotherapy, the differences in survival between stages are gradually diminishing. In the detection of aortic lymph nodes, lymphangiography is still considered to be more sensitive (85% to 98%) than computed tomography (40% to 65%); however, surgical staging, including splenectomy, is now rarely performed (107). Moreover, because of the efficiency of the chemotherapy regimens presently applied, histologic subtyping has lost some of its prognostic importance. Thus, the primary role of the pathologist is not to determine the histologic subtype but to distinguish HL from other lymphoproliferative processes (107).

REFERENCES

1. Correa P, O'Conor GT. Geographic pathology of lymphoreticular tumors: summary of survey from the Geographic Pathology Committee of the International Union against Cancer. J Natl Cancer Inst 1973;50:1609–1617.
2. Doll R, Muir C, Waterhouse J, eds. Cancer incidence in five continents, vol 2. Berlin: Springer-Verlag, 1970.
3. Young JL Jr, Percy C, Asire AJ, et al. Cancer incidence and mortality in the United States. NCI Monogr 1981;57:72–84.
4. Wakasa H. Hodgkin's disease in Asia, particularly in Japan. NCI Monogr 1973;36:15–23.
5. Greenlee RT, Hill-Harmon MB, Murray T, et al. Cancer Statistics 2001. CA Cancer J Clin 2001;51:15–36.
6. Correa P, O'Conor GT. Epidemiologic patterns of Hodgkin's disease. Int J Cancer 1971;8:192–201.
7. MacMahon B. Epidemiology of Hodgkin's disease. Cancer Res 1966;26:1189–1200.
8. Gough J. Hodgkin's disease: a correlation of histopathology with survival. Int J Cancer 1970;5:273–281.
9. Berard CW, Thomas LB, Axtell LM, et al. The relationship of histopathological subtype to clinical stage of Hodgkin's disease at diagnosis. Cancer Res 1971;31:1776–1785.
10. Dorfman RF. Relationship of histology to site in Hodgkin's disease. Cancer Res 1971;31:1786–1793.
11. Keller AR, Kaplan HS, Lukes RJ, et al. Correlation of histopathology with other prognostic indicators in Hodgkin's disease. Cancer 1968;22:487–499.
12. Cole P, MacMahon B, Aisenberg A. Mortality from Hodgkin's disease in the United States. Lancet 1968;2:1371–1376.
13. Desforges JF, Rutherford CJ, Piro A. Hodgkin's disease. N Engl J Med 1979;301:1212–1222.
14. Ioachim HL, Dorsett B, Cronin W, et al. Acquired immunodeficiency syndrome-associated lymphomas: clinical, pathologic, immunologic and viral characteristics of 111 cases. Hum Pathol 1991;22:659–673.
15. Ioachim HL. Immune deficiency: opportunistic tumors. In: Encyclopedia of cancer, vol 2. Bertino JR, ed. San Diego, CA: Academic Press, 1997:901–915.
16. Beral V, Newton R. Overview of the epidemiology of immunodeficiency-associated cancer. J Natl Cancer Inst 1998;23:1–6.
17. Ioachim HL. New vistas in Hodgkin's disease. Pathol Annu 1975;10:419–459.
18. Kvale G, Hoiby EA, Pederson E. Hodgkin's disease in patients with previous infectious mononucleosis. Int J Cancer 1979;23: 593–597.
19. Weiss LM, Movahed LA, Warnke RA, et al. Detection of Epstein-Barr viral genomes in Reed-Sternberg cells of Hodgkin's disease. N Engl J Med 1989;320:502–506.
20. Herbst H, Niedobitek G, Kneba M, et al. High incidence of Epstein-Barr virus genomes in Hodgkin's disease. Am J Pathol 1990;137:13–18.
21. Weiss LM, Chen YY, Lin X, et al. Epstein-Barr virus and Hodgkin's disease: a correlative *in situ* hybridization and polymerase chain reaction study. Am J Pathol 1991;139:1259.
22. Jarrett RF, Gallagher A, Jones DB, et al. Detection of Epstein-Barr virus genomes in Hodgkin's disease: relation to age. J Clin Pathol 1991;44:844.
23. Herndier BG, Sanchez HC, Chang KL, et al. High prevalence of Epstein-Barr virus in the Reed-Sternberg cells of HIV-associated Hodgkin's disease. Am J Pathol 1993;142:1073.
24. Masih A, Weisenburger D, Duggan M, et al. Epstein-Barr viral genome in lymph nodes from patients with Hodgkin's disease may not be specific to Reed-Sternberg cells. Am J Pathol 1991; 139:37–43.
25. Jackson H Jr, Parker F Jr. Hodgkin's disease. I. General considerations. N Engl J Med 1944;230:1–8.
26. Lukes RJ, Butler JJ. The pathology and nomenclature of Hodgkin's disease. Cancer Res 1966;26:1063–1083.
27. Mason DY, Banks PM, Chan J, et al. Nodular lymphocyte predominance Hodgkin's disease. A distinct clinicopathological entity. Am J Surg Pathol 1994;18:526–530.

28. Harris NL, Jaffe ES, Stein H, et al. A revised European-American classification of lymphoid neoplasms: a proposal from the International Lymphoma Study Group. Blood 1994;84:1361–1392.
29. Harris NL, Jaffe ES, Deibold J, et al. WHO classification of neoplastic diseases of the hematopoietic and lymphoid tissues: report of the clinical advisory committee meeting, Airlie House, Virginia, November 1997. J Clin Oncol 1999;17:3835–3849.
30. Ioachim HL, Pearse A, Keller SE. Patterns of metastases in hemopoietic neoplasms: immunologic correlations. In: Day SB, Myers WPL, Stansly P, eds. Cancer invasion and metastasis: biologic mechanisms and therapy. New York: Raven Press, 1977: 333–345.
31. Strum SB, Rappaport H. Significance of focal involvement of lymph nodes for the diagnosis and staging of Hodgkin's disease. Cancer 1970;25:1314–1319.
32. Kadin ME, Glatstein E, Dorfman RF. Clinicopathologic studies of 117 untreated patients subjected to laparotomy for the staging of Hodgkin's disease. Cancer 1971;27:1277–1294.
33. Kaplan HS. Hodgkin's disease. Cambridge, MA: Harvard University Press, 1972.
34. Rappaport H, Strum SB, Hutchison G, et al. Clinical and biological significance of vascular invasion in Hodgkin's disease. Cancer Res 1971;31:1794–1798.
35. Bearman RM, Pangalis GA, Rappaport H. Hodgkin's disease lymphocyte depletion type. A clinicopathologic study of 39 patients. Cancer 1978;41:293–302.
36. Neiman RS. Current problems in the histopathologic diagnosis and classification of Hodgkin's disease. Pathol Annu 1978;13 [Part 2]:289–328.
37. Strum SB, Rappaport H. Interrelations of the histologic types of Hodgkin's disease. Arch Pathol Lab Med 1971;91:127–134.
38. Rappaport H. Tumors of the hematopoietic system. In: Atlas of tumor pathology. Washington, DC: Armed Forces Institute of Pathology, 1966:188–193 (fascicle 8).
39. Rosenberg SA, Lukes RJ. Report of the Committee on the Staging of Hodgkin's Disease. Report of the Nomenclature Committee. Cancer Res 1966;26:1310–1311.
40. Lister TA, Crowther D, Sutcliffe SB, et al. Report of a committee convened to discuss the evaluation and staging of patients with Hodgkin's disease: Cotswolds meeting. J Clin Oncol 1989; 7:1630–1636.
41. Lukes RJ. Criteria for involvement of lymph node, bone marrow, spleen and liver in Hodgkin's disease. Cancer Res 1971;31: 1755–1767.
42. Colby TV, Hoppe RT, Warnke RA. Hodgkin's disease: a clinicopathologic study of 659 cases. Cancer 1982;49:1848–1858.
43. Ioachim HL. Pathology of AIDS. Textbook and atlas. Philadelphia: JB Lippincott Co, 1989.
44. Levy R, Kaplan HS. Impaired lymphocyte function in untreated Hodgkin's disease. N Engl J Med 1974;290:1181–1186.
45. Mauch P, Tarbell N, Weinstein H, et al. Supradiaphragmatic Hodgkin's disease: prognostic factors in surgically staged patients treated with mantle and paraaortic irradiation. J Clin Oncol 1988;6:1576–1583.
46. Warnke RA, Weiss LM, Chan JK, et al. Classic Hodgkin's disease. In: Atlas of tumor pathology. Series III, fascicle 14: Tumors of the lymph nodes and spleen. Washington, DC: Armed Forces Institute of Pathology, 1995:277–304.
47. Poppema S, Bhan AK, Reinherz EL, et al. *In situ* immunologic characterization of cellular constituents in lymph nodes and spleens involved by Hodgkin's disease. Blood 1982;59:226–232.
48. Kadin ME, Donaldson SS, Dorfman RF. Isolated granulomas in Hodgkin's disease. N Engl J Med 1970;283:859–861.
49. Sacks EL, Donaldson SS, Gordon J, et al. Epithelioid granulomas associated with Hodgkin's disease. Cancer 1978;41:562–567.
50. Patsouris E, Noel H, Lennert K. Cytohistologic and immunohistochemical findings in Hodgkin's disease, mixed cellularity type, with a high content of epithelioid cells. Am J Surg Pathol 1989;13:1014–1022.
51. Lukes RJ, Tindle BH, Parker JW. Reed-Sternberg–like cells in infectious mononucleosis. Lancet 1969;2:1003–1004.
52. McMahon JN, Gordon HW, Rosen RB. Reed-Sternberg cells in infectious mononucleosis. J Dis Child 1970;120:148–150.
53. Tindle BH, Parker JW, Lukes RJ. "Reed-Sternberg" cells in infectious mononucleosis? Am J Clin Pathol 1972;58:607–617.
54. Hartsock RJ. Postvaccinial lymphadenitis. Cancer 1968;21: 632–649.
55. Strum SB, Park JK, Rappaport H. Observations of cells resembling Reed-Sternberg cells in conditions other than Hodgkin disease. Cancer 1970;26:176–190.
56. Kadin ME, Asbury AK. Long-term cultures of Hodgkin's tissue: a morphologic and radioautographic study. Lab Invest 1973;28: 181–184.
57. Kadin ME, Stites DP, Levy R, et al. Exogenous immunoglobulin and the macrophage origin of Reed-Sternberg cells in Hodgkin's disease. N Engl J Med 1978;299:1208–1214.
58. Pinkus GS, Pinkus JL, Longhoff E, et al. Fascin, a sensitive new marker for Reed-Sternberg cells of Hodgkin's disease: evidence for a dendritic or B cell derivation? Am J Pathol 1997;150: 543–621.
59. Nakamura S, Nagahama M, Kagami Y, at al. Hodgkin's disease expressing follicular-dendritic cell marker CD21 without any other B-cell marker. A clinicopathologic study of nine cases. Am J Surg Pathol 1999;23:363–376.
60. Stein H, Mason DY, Gerdes J, et al. The expression of the Hodgkin's disease-associated antigen Ki-l in reactive and neoplastic lymphoid tissue: Evidence that Reed-Sternberg cells and histiocytic malignancies are derived from activated lymphoid cells. Blood 1985;66:848–858.
61. Kuppers R, Rajewsky K, Zhao M, et al. Hodgkin's disease: Hodgkin and Reed-Sternberg cells picked from histological sections show clonal immunoglobulin gene rearrangements and appear to be derived from B-cells at various stages of development. Proc Natl Acad Sci U S A 1994;91:10962–10966.
62. Brinker MGL, Poppema S. Buys CHCM, et al. Clonal immunoglobulin gene rearrangements in tissues involved by Hodgkin's disease. Blood 1987;70:186.
63. Weiss LM, Strickler JG, Hu E, et al. Immunoglobulin gene rearrangements in Hodgkin's disease. Hum Pathol 1986;17:1009.
64. Brauninger A, Kuppers R, Strickler J, et al. Hodgkin and Reed-Sternberg cells in lymphocyte predominant Hodgkin's disease represent clonal populations of germinal center-derived tumor cells. Proc Natl Acad Sci U S A 1997;94:9337.
65. Hummel M, Ziemann K, Lammert H, et al. Hodgkin's disease with monoclonal and polyclonal populations of Reed-Sternberg cells. N Engl J Med 1995;333:901.
66. Marafioti, T, Hummel M, Foss H-D, et al. Hodgkin and Reed-Sternberg cell represent an expansion of a single clone originating from a germinal center B-cell with functional immunoglobulin gene rearrangements but defective immunoglobulin transcription. Blood 2000;95:1443–1450.
67. Momose H, Jaffe ES, Shin SS, et al. Chronic lymphocytic leukemia/small lymphocytic lymphoma with Reed-Sternberg–like cells and possible transformation to Hodgkin's disease. Am J Surg Pathol 1992;16:859–867.
68. Jaffe ES. The elusive Reed-Sternberg cell. N Engl J Med 1989; 320:529–531.

69. Brauninger A, Hansmann M-L, Strickler JG, et al. Identification of common germinal-center B-cell precursors in two patients with both Hodgkin's disease and non-Hodgkin's lymphoma. N Engl J Med 1999;340:1239–1247.
70. Schwartz RS. Hodgkin's disease—time for a change. N Engl J Med 1997;337:495–496.
71. Gruss H-J, Pinto A, Duyster J, et al. Hodgkin's disease: a tumor with disturbed immunological pathways. Immunol Today 1997;18:156–163.
72. Anagnostou D, Parker JW, Taylor CR, et al. Lacunar cells of nodular sclerosing Hodgkin's disease. Cancer 1977;39:1032–1043.
73. Strickler JG, Michie SA, Warnke R, et al. The "syncytial variant" of nodular sclerosing Hodgkin's disease. Am J Surg Pathol 1986;10:470–477.
74. MacLennan KA, Bennett MH, Tu A, et al. Relationship of histopathologic features to survival and relapse in nodular sclerosing Hodgkin's disease. A study of 1659 patients. Cancer 1989;64:1686–1693.
75. Mann RB, Jaffe ES, Berard CW. Malignant lymphomas: a conceptual understanding of morphologic diversity. Am J Pathol 1979;94:105–192.
76. Kant JA, Hubbard SM, Longo DL. The pathologic and clinical heterogeneity of lymphocyte-depleted Hodgkin's disease. J Clin Oncol 1986;4:284–294.
77. Neiman RS, Rosen PJ, Lukes RJ. Lymphocyte depletion Hodgkin's disease: a clinicopathologic entity. N Engl J Med 1973;288:751–755.
78. Ioachim HL. Lymph nodes and spleen. In: Johannessen JV, ed. Electron microscopy in human medicine, vol 5. New York: McGraw-Hill, 1981:384–464.
79. Bernhard W. Some problems of fine structure in tumor cells. Prog Exp Tumor Res 1963;3:1–34.
80. Mori Y, Lennert K. Electron microscopic atlas of lymph node cytology and pathology. Berlin: Springer-Verlag, 1969.
81. Dorfman RF, Rice DF, Mitchell AD, et al. Ultrastructural studies of Hodgkin's disease. NCI Monogr 1973;36:221–238.
82. Frenster JH, Papalian MM, Masek MA, et al. Electron microscopic analysis of lymph node cellular activity in Hodgkin's disease. J Natl Cancer Inst 1979;63:331–335.
83. Forni M, Hofman FM, Parker JW, et al. B- and T-lymphocytes in Hodgkin's disease. An immunohistochemical study utilizing heterologous and monoclonal antibodies. Cancer 1985;55:728–737.
84. Chittal SM, Caverivière P, Schwarting R, et al. Monoclonal antibodies in the diagnosis of Hodgkin's disease. Am J Surg Pathol 1988;12:9–21.
85. Pinkus GS, Thomas P, Said JW. Leu-M1—a marker for Reed-Sternberg cells in Hodgkin's disease. An immunoperoxidase study of paraffin-embedded tissues. Am J Pathol 1985;119:244–252.
86. Sheibani K, Battifora H, Burke JS, et al. Leu-M1 antigen in human neoplasms. An immunohistologic study of 400 cases. Am J Surg Pathol 1986;10:227–236.
87. Hsu SM, Yang K, Jaffe ES. Phenotypic expression of Hodgkin's and Reed-Sternberg cells in Hodgkin's disease. Am J Pathol 1985;118:209–217.
88. Dorfman RF, Gatter KC, Pulford KAF, et al. An evaluation of the utility of anti-granulocyte and anti-leukocyte monoclonal antibodies in the diagnosis of Hodgkin's disease. Am J Pathol 1986;123:508–519.
89. Arber DA, Weiss LM. CD15: a review. Appl Immunohistochem 1993;1:17.
90. Rushin JM, Riordan GP, Heaton RB et al. Cytomegalovirus-infected cells express Leu-Ml antigen: a potential source of diagnostic error. Am J Pathol 1990;136:989.
91. Chang KL, Arber DA, Weiss LM. CD30: a review. Appl Immunohistochem 1993;1:244.
92. Pallesen G, Hamilton-Dutoit SJ. Ki-1 (CD30) antigen is regularly expressed by tumor cells of embryonal carcinoma. Am J Pathol 1988;133:446.
93. Andreesen R, Brugger W, Lohr GW, et al. Human macrophages can express the Hodgkin-cell-associated antigen Ki-1 (CD30). Am J Pathol 1989;134:187.
94. Strauchen J. Leucocyte common antigen in the differential diagnosis of Hodgkin's disease. Hematol Oncol 1989;7:149.
95. Schmid C, Pan L, Diss T, et al. Expression of B-cell antigens by Hodgkin's and Reed-Sternberg cells. Am J Pathol 1991;139:701.
96. Stein H, Herbst H, Anagnostopoulos I, et al. The nature of Hodgkin and Reed-Sternberg cells, their association with EBV, and their relationship to anaplastic large-cell lymphoma. Ann Oncol 1991;2[Suppl 2]:33–38.
97. Knowles DM, Neri A, Pellici PG, et al. Immunoglobulin and T-cell receptor beta-chain gene rearrangement analysis of Hodgkin's disease: implication for lineage determination and differential diagnosis. Proc Natl Acad Sci U S A 1986;83:7942–7946.
98. Chen Y-T, Godwin TA, Mouradian JA. Immunohistochemistry and gene rearrangement studies in the diagnosis of malignant lymphomas: a comparison of 152 cases. Hum Pathol 1991;22:1249–1257.
99. Weiss LM, Strickler JG, Hu E, et al. Immunoglobulin gene rearrangements in Hodgkin's disease. Hum Pathol 1986;17:1009–1014.
100. Trumper H, Brady G, Bragg A, et al. Single cell analysis of Hodgkin's and Reed-Sternberg cells: molecular heterogeneity of gene expression and p53 mutations. Blood 1993;81:3097– 3115.
101. Sheibani K, Battifora H, Burke JS, et al. Leu-M1 antigen in human neoplasms. An immunohistologic study of 400 cases. Am J Surg Pathol 1986;10:227–236.
102. Symmers W St C Sr. Survey of the eventual diagnosis in 600 cases referred for a second histological opinion after an initial biopsy diagnosis of Hodgkin's disease. J Clin Pathol 1968;21:650–653.
103. Jones SE, Butler JJ, Byrne GE, et al. Histopathologic review of lymphoma cases from the Southwest Oncology Group. Cancer 1977;39:1071–1076.
104. Chittal SM, Del Sol G. The interface of Hodgkin's disease and anaplastic large cell lymphoma. Cancer Surv 1997;30:87.
105. Leoncini L, del Vecchio MT, Kraft R, et al. Hodgkin's disease and CD30-positive anaplastic large cell lymphomas—a continuous spectrum of malignant disorders. Am J Pathol 1990;137:104–157.
106. Rosenberg SA. Hodgkin's disease: challenges for the future. Cancer Res 1989;49:767–769.
107. Urba WJ, Longo DL. Hodgkin's disease. N Engl J Med 1992;326:678–687.

58

HODGKIN LYMPHOMA

NODULAR LYMPHOCYTE PREDOMINANCE

DEFINITION

Nodular lymphoproliferation with clinicopathologic features of both Hodgkin lymphoma and low-grade B-cell lymphoma.

SYNONYM

Hodgkin lymphoma: paragranuloma

EPIDEMIOLOGY

The nodular lymphocyte predominance (NLP) type represents 2% to 6% of all cases of Hodgkin lymphoma (HL) (1).

PATHOGENESIS

Nodular lymphocyte predominance has been included as a distinct type of Hodgkin disease since the early classifications (2–4) and was considered to represent a first stage in the progression of the disease. Like other forms of HL, it is characterized by a small number of neoplastic cells scattered within a mass of reactive inflammatory cells; however, the characteristic Reed-Sternberg (R-S) cells are not part of the process. With the introduction of immunohistochemistry, it came to be realized that the immunophenotype of NLP is dissimilar to those of the other histologic types of HL, resembling more that of a low-grade B-cell lymphoma (5–7). Because of its distinctive histologic and immunophenotypic picture, it was decided to treat NLP as a separate clinicopathologic entity (8); however, because some features resemble those of HL, it continues to be classified with the HLs (9), at least until the etiology and pathogenesis are better understood.

CLINICAL SYNDROME

Nodular lymphocyte predominance/Hodgkin lymphoma (NLPHL) is manifested as an isolated lymph node enlargement that is usually unaccompanied by general symptoms. The lymph nodes involved are cervical, axillary, or inguinal; they are rarely pelvic or paraaortic and almost never mediastinal or mesenteric (4). The course of the disease is indolent and slow regardless of treatment. Involvement of the thymus and bone marrow is uncommon. NLPHL is more common in men than in women and may occur at any age. In contrast to classic HL, in which two age peaks occur, NLPHL is characterized by one age peak, in the fourth decade (4). Patients with NLPHL have frequent relapses that are independent of the stage of disease or treatment. The relapses tend to occur locally at equal intervals of up to 10 years without affecting survival, which remains long (10). Like other lymphomas, some NLPHLs during the course of the disease transform into a lymphoma of higher grade. In most cases reported, the transformation has been to a large cell lymphoma of B-cell type, which supports the concept that NLPHL is of B-cell origin (7,8,11).

The prognosis in NLPHL is always very good, and for stages I and II, survival is not affected (12).

HISTOPATHOLOGY

In the original classification, Lukes and Butler (13) distinguished between a nodular and a diffuse type.

Nodular Lymphocyte Predominance

The lymph node architecture is replaced by large lymphocytic nodules that compress the remaining lymphoid tissues toward the periphery (Fig. 58.1). The nodules vary in size, but most of them are larger than the reactive lymphoid follicles or the nodules of follicular lymphomas (Fig. 58.2). The contours are vague but appear sharper with a reticulin stain. Unlike the nodules of follicular lymphomas, the nodules of NLPHL are entirely composed of small lymphocytes without centroblasts or tingible-body macrophages. However, larger, clearer cells are scattered throughout (Fig. 58.3). These are the characteristic lymphocytic/histiocytic (L&H) cells and

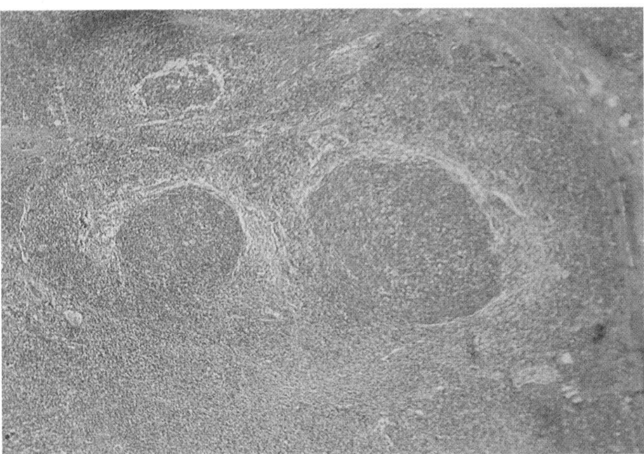

FIGURE 58.1. Hodgkin lymphoma, lymphocyte predominance. Architecture effaced by multiple nodules of various sizes and shapes. Hematoxylin, phloxine, and saffron stain.

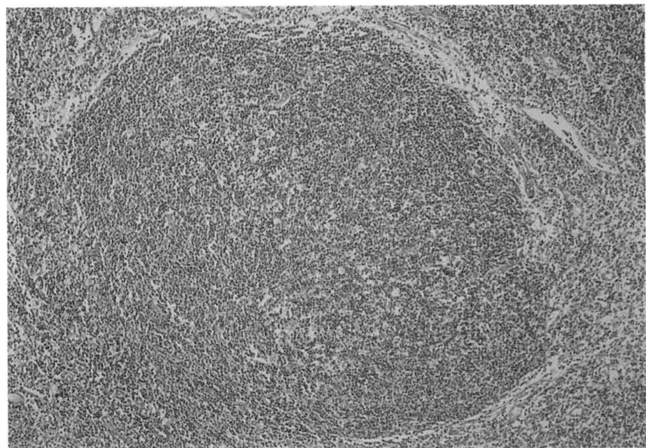

FIGURE 58.2. Hodgkin lymphoma, lymphocyte predominance. Nodule larger than lymphoid follicles, with vague contour and lack of germinal center and mantle zone. Hematoxylin, phloxine, and saffron stain.

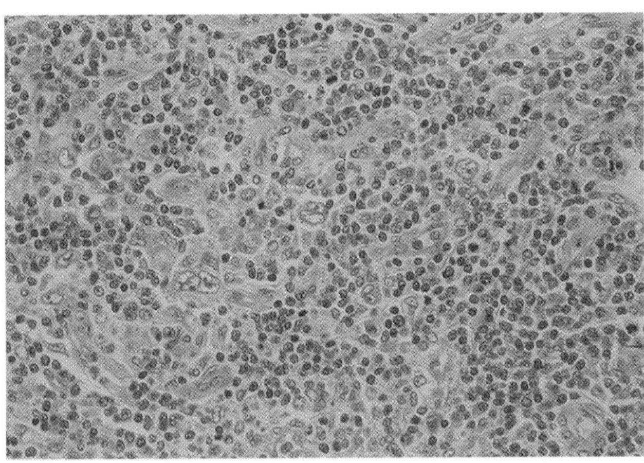

FIGURE 58.3. Hodgkin lymphoma, lymphocyte predominance. Within the nodules are lymphocytes with scattered lymphocytic/histiocytic cells. Hematoxylin, phloxine, and saffron stain.

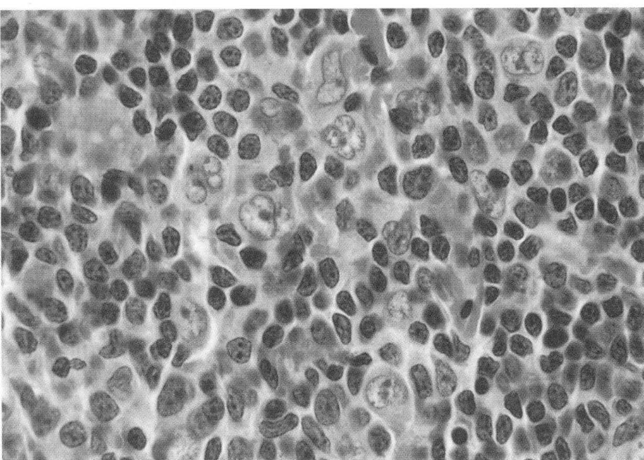

FIGURE 58.4. Hodgkin lymphoma, lymphocyte predominance. Lymphocytic/histiocytic (popcorn) cells and lymphocytes, no Reed-Sternberg or Hodgkin cells. Hematoxylin, phloxine, and saffron stain.

occasional clusters of epithelioid cells. The L&H cells, termed by Lukes and Butler, are considered variants of R-S cells. They are fairly large with a moderate amount of pale cytoplasm and characteristic vesicular, multilobate nuclei—hence the descriptive name of "popcorn" cells (Fig. 58.4). The nuclear membrane is thin, the chromatin finely dispersed, and the nucleoli small and nonprominent (Fig. 58.5). Mitoses are uncommon. Classic R-S cells are sometimes present; however, if relatively numerous, they indicate a different diagnosis. Epithelioid histiocytes may be present singly, in small clusters, or sometimes forming a wreath or circle at the periphery of the nodules. The background consists entirely of small lymphocytes. Eosinophils, neutrophils, plasma cells, and bands of fibrosis are not part of the picture.

In about 20% of cases, nodules of a particular form of reactive hyperplasia, known as *progressive transformation of germinal centers* (PTGC) (see Chapter 35), coexist with

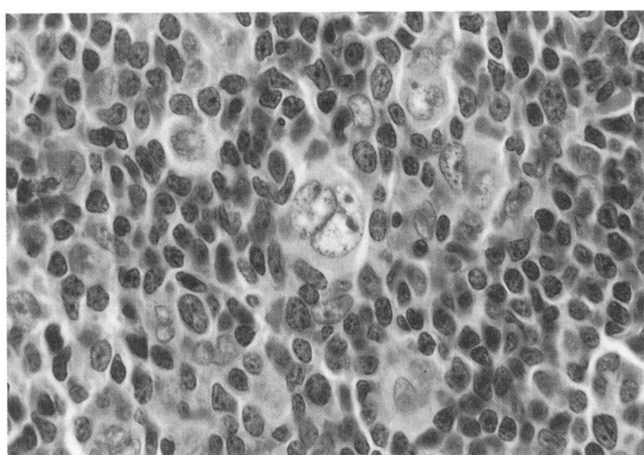

FIGURE 58.5. Hodgkin lymphoma, lymphocyte predominance. Lymphocytic/histiocytic (popcorn) cells with multilobate vesicular nuclei and conspicuous nucleoli not as prominent as those of Reed-Sternberg cells. Hematoxylin, phloxine, and saffron stain.

NLPHL. These are enlarged follicles with numerous B-cells of mantle zone type. The uninvolved lymph node tissues appear compressed between the enlarged proliferating nodules. The observation that PTGC in children and adolescents occasionally precedes NLPHL supported the idea that PTGC represents an early form of LP-type HL (4).

Diffuse Lymphocyte Predominance

In some cases with a diffuse pattern, L&H cells are scattered throughout sheets of small lymphocytes without forming distinct nodules (14). Sometimes, a few nodules are still present, which suggests that the diffuse pattern represents an advanced form of NLPHL.

IMMUNOHISTOCHEMISTRY

The L&H cells of NLP have a characteristic immunophenotype different from that of R-S cells (5–7,14–16). The L&H cells are CD45+ (positive for leukocyte common antigen) and express the full panel of pan-B-cell markers: CD19, CD20, CD22, CD75, and CD79a (Fig. 58.6). They do not express T-cell markers. The cells are also positive for epithelial membrane antigen (EMA) and negative for CD15 and CD30 (markers of R-S cells). Moreover, in a study of 19 cases of NLPLH, a κ light chain restriction was detected in the L&H cells in 68% of them (6). The majority of L&H cells also contained J chain and immunoglobulin G (IgG) heavy chain. All these features are consistent with the postulated B-cell origin of NLPHL and can be used to differentiate this form of HL from the classic types of HL and also from benign lymphadenopathies and other types of non-Hodgkin lymphomas. The background small lymphocytes in NLPHL, although polyclonal, are different from those in the classic types of HL. These lymphocytes are predominantly T-cell types, whereas in NLPHL, the majority express membrane IgM and IgD and thus are similar to the B-cell lymphocytes of the mantle area of the lymphoid follicles (17). In diffuse LP, the cell immunophenotypes are the same as in the nodular form of LP.

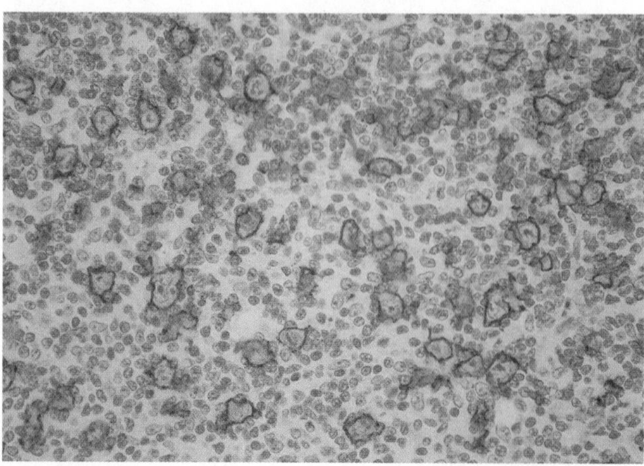

FIGURE 58.6. Hodgkin lymphoma, lymphocyte predominance. Lymphocytic/histiocytic cells stain for CD20, a B-cell marker. L26/peroxidase stain.

Phenotype

L&H (POPCORN) CELLS
CD45+, CD19+, CD20+, CD22+, CD75+, CD79a+
EMA+
CD15−, CD30−,

DIFFERENTIAL DIAGNOSIS

- Infectious mononucleosis and other viral lymphadenitides have diffuse patterns with a mottled or starry sky appearance. Large atypical cells are of T-cell type. Acute clinical symptoms, Downey cells in the peripheral blood, and positive serologic test results.
- Reactive lymphoid hyperplasia and atypical lymphoid hyperplasia: The nodules are smaller, centered on the lymph node follicles with distinctive germinal centers containing centroblasts and tingible-body macrophages. Mantle zones surround the follicles.
- PTGC: The pattern resembles that of reactive follicular hyperplasia, with prominent germinal centers, and L&H cells are not present.
- Classic HL: The histologic patterns are different, usually lacking nodules. The R-S cells have a different immunophenotype. If the R-S cells are more than very rare, the diagnosis of NLPHL becomes questionable (1).
- Follicular lymphoma has a nodular pattern; however, the nodules are smaller, composed of atypical cells with cleaved nuclei. They are of B-cell phenotype, expressing membrane monoclonal Ig. The cells forming the nodules and those spilling out around them are positive for bcl-2. The patients are elderly.
- T cell-rich B-cell lymphoma lacks nodularity; however, it can resemble the diffuse form of NLPHL. The difference is in the clustering and the nuclear atypia of the large cells of the lymphoma.

MOLECULAR PATHOLOGY

Genotypic analysis of HL has yielded variable results because the neoplastic cells (Hodgkin and Reed-Sternberg cells) in most cases represent only a very small amount of the tissues analyzed. Most of the cells in HL tumor masses are reactive normal cells, and consequently, studies of clonal rearrangements of HL have frequently ended by showing mostly germ line configurations of the Ig and T-cell recep-

Checklist

HODGKIN LYMPHOMA: LYMPHOCYTE PREDOMINANCE

Asymptomatic younger patients
Single peripheral lymph nodes enlarged
Frequent relapses
Very good prognosis
Nodular form more frequent
Large cellular nodules
L&H (popcorn) cells
CD45+, CD19+, CD20+, CD22+, EMA+
CD15−, CD30−
Small lymphocytes express B-cell markers
Epithelioid histocytes
R-S cells absent or rare
Necrosis and fibrosis absent
PTGC sometimes associated

tor genes (18). The analysis of Ig heavy chain rearrangements by PCR showed clonal VDJ rearrangement with somatic mutations in the VH genes (19).

REFERENCES

1. Warnke RA. Nodular lymphocyte predominance Hodgkin's disease. In: Atlas of tumor pathology. Series III, fascicle 14: Tumors of the lymph nodes and spleen. Washington, DC: Armed Forces Institute of Pathology, 1995:305–314.
2. Jackson H Jr, Parker F Jr. Hodgkin's disease. I. General considerations. N Engl J Med 1944;230:1–8.
3. Lukes RJ, Butler JJ. The pathology and nomenclature of Hodgkin's disease. Cancer Res 1966;26:1063–1083.
4. Poppema S, Kaiserling E, Lennert K. Hodgkin's disease with lymphocyte predominance, nodular type (nodular paragranuloma) and progressively transformed germinal centres: a cytohistologic study. Histopathology 1979;3:295–308.
5. Pinkus GS, Said JW. Hodgkin's disease, lymphocyte predominance type, nodular: further evidence for a B cell derivation. L&H variants of Reed-Sternberg cells express L26, a pan-B-cell marker. Am J Pathol 1988;133:211–217.
6. Schmid C, Sargent C, Isaacson PG. L&H cells of nodular lymphocyte predominance Hodgkin's disease show immunoglobulin light-chain restriction. Am J Pathol 1991;139:1281–1289.
7. Chittal SM, Alard C, Rossi J-F, et al. Further phenotypic evidence that nodular, lymphocyte-predominant Hodgkin's disease is a large B-cell lymphoma in evolution. Am J Surg Pathol 1990; 14:1024–1035.
8. Mason DY, Banks PM, Chan J, et al. Nodular lymphocyte predominance Hodgkin's disease. A distinct clinicopathological entity. Am J Surg Pathol 1994;18:526–530.
9. Harris NL, Jaffe ES, Deibold J, et al. WHO classification of neoplastic diseases of the hematopoietic and lymphoid tissues: report of the clinical advisory committee meeting, Airlie House, Virginia, November 1997. J Clin Oncol 1999;17:3835–3849.
10. Hansmann ML, Zwingers T, Boske A, et al. Clinical features of nodular paragranuloma (Hodgkin's disease, lymphocyte predominance type, nodular). J Cancer Res Clin Oncol 1984;108:321–330.
11. Miettenen M, Franssila KO, Saxen E. Hodgkin's disease, lymphocytic predominance nodular: increased risk for subsequent non-Hodgkin's lymphomas. Cancer 1983;51:2293–2300.
12. Regula DP, Hoppe RT, Weiss LM. Nodular and diffuse types of lymphocyte predominance Hodgkin's disease. N Engl J Med 1988;318:214–219.
13. Lukes RJ. Criteria for involvement of lymph node, bone marrow, spleen and liver in Hodgkin's disease. Cancer Res 1971;31:1755–1767.
14. Hansmann M-L, Stein H, Dallenbach F, et al. Diffuse lymphocyte-predominant Hodgkin's disease (diffuse paragranuloma). A variant of the B-cell-derived nodular type. Am J Pathol 1991;138: 29–36.
15. von Wasielewski R, Werner M, Fischer R., et al. Lymphocyte-predominant Hodgkin's disease. An immunohistochemical analysis of 208 reviewed Hodgkin's disease cases from the German Hodgkin Study Group. Am J Pathol 1997;150:793–803.
16. Rudiger T, Ott G, Ott MM, et al. Differential diagnosis between classic Hodgkin's lymphoma, T cell-rich B-cell lymphoma, and paragranuloma by paraffin immunohistochemistry. Am J Surg Pathol 1998;22:1184–1191.
17. Timens W, Visser L. Poppema S. Nodular lymphocyte predominance type of Hodgkin's disease is a germinal center lymphoma. Lab Invest 1986;54:457–461.
18. Knowles DM, Neri A, Pellici PG, et al. Immunoglobulin and T-cell receptor beta-chain gene rearrangement analysis of Hodgkin's disease: implication for lineage determination and differential diagnosis. Proc Natl Acad Sci U S A 1986;83:7942–7946.
19. Chen Y-T, Godwin TA, Mouradian JA. Immunohistochemistry and gene rearrangement studies in the diagnosis of malignant lymphomas: a comparison of 152 cases. Hum Pathol 1991;22: 1249–1257.

PART V

SECTION THREE

PRECURSOR B-CELL AND T-CELL NEOPLASMS

59

PRECURSOR B- AND T-LYMPHOBLASTIC LEUKEMIA/LYMPHOMA

DEFINITION

Diffuse lymphoma of immature or precursor lymphocytes, predominantly of T-cell phenotype. The World Health Organization (WHO) classification considers the precursor lymphoid lesions as one disease with different clinical manifestations: lymphoblastic lymphoma (LL) represents solid tumors, and acute lymphoblastic leukemia (ALL) represents bone marrow and blood involvement (1). The French– American–British cytologic categories L1, L2, and L3 have been discarded, but the term *acute lymphoblastic leukemia* has been retained for the leukemic phase of B- or T-precursor neoplasms (1). Because genetic alterations greatly influence the prognosis of precursor B-lymphoblastic malignancies, they should be incorporated in the diagnosis (1).

CLASSIFICATION

Precursor B-lymphoblastic leukemia/lymphoma (WHO)
Precursor T-lymphoblastic lymphoma/leukemia (WHO)
Precursor B-cell acute lymphoblastic leukemia (WHO) (cytogenetic subgroups)
  t(9;22)(q34;q11), BCR/ABL
  t(v;11q23), MLL rearranged
  t(12;21)(p13;q22), TEL/AML1 (ETV/CBFα)
  t(1;19)(q23;p13), E2A/PBX1
Precursor T-cell ALL (WHO) (1)
Burkitt cell leukemia (WHO) (1)

SYNONYMS

Lymphoma of convoluted nuclei
Lymphoma of precursor lymphocytes
Lymphoma of immature lymphocytes
Thymic lymphoma

PATHOGENESIS

Lymphoblastic lymphoma is a neoplasm of blast cells, which are immature or precursor lymphocytes indistinguishable from those of ALL (2,3). The cells have characteristic convoluted nuclei and a T-cell phenotype in 70% to 80% of cases (4). In most cases of T-cell LL, the supradiaphragmatic lymph nodes are involved (a mediastinal mass is present in 50% to 75% of cases), with eventual infiltration of the bone marrow and development of a leukemic phase identical to ALL (2–4). In older patients, LL less frequently involves the mediastinum, brain, or gonads, and leukemia is less commonly associated (5). The male-to-female ratio is approximately 2.5:1 at all ages (5). Fewer than 5% of adult but one-third to one-half of pediatric non-Hodgkin lymphomas can be classified as LL (6–8). The frequent location of LL in the anterior mediastinum, the young age of patients, and the expression of terminal deoxynucleotidyl transferase (TdT), characteristic of thymocytes, suggest that most LLs are of thymic or precursor T-cell origin.

CLINICAL SYNDROME

T-cell LL predominantly affects men in the third decade of life, causing a mediastinal mass or enlarged lymph nodes above the diaphragm or in the neck, supraclavicular, or axillary regions (9,10). The clinical course is particularly aggressive, characterized by progression, frequent relapses, and short survival. In a series of 92 patients, 91% were in stage III or IV, and 51% had generalized lymphadenopathy (5). Dissemination to other organs is common, particularly the central nervous system, where most relapses occur. LL infiltrates organs rarely involved by other types of lymphoma: skin, testes, eyes, kidneys, breast, and lungs (2). The abdominal lymph nodes are rarely involved, and intestinal involvement has not been reported, as it is in Burkitt lymphoma. The bone marrow is infiltrated early, and lymphoblasts circulate in the peripheral blood. Poor prognostic factors in adult LL include a high level of lactate dehydrogenase, involvement of the bone marrow and central nervous system (11), age above 30 years, and failure to achieve a complete response (12).

Only 10% of LLs express a B-precursor phenotype. In a series of 23 patients with B-precursor LL who did not have leukemia at presentation, the median age was 20 years (range, 5 to 68 years) (13). Only 3 of 23 cases primarily involved lymph nodes (13). Most B-precursor LLs presented in extranodal sites: skin, bones, soft tissue, breast, stomach and colon, mediastinum, and salivary gland (13,14). All cases expressed B-cell markers and TdT; three-fourths had CD10 (common acute lymphoblastic leukemia antigen, or CALLA) and one-half had CD20 (13). Leukemia was unusual at presentation (13) and rarely developed later (14). The clinical behavior of B-precursor LL differs from that of T-precursor LL, in which lymph node or mediastinal involvement and leukemia are frequent.

B-precursor LL is rare in adults and may pursue a clinically aggressive course (15). Adult patients with B-precursor LL present with nodal and extranodal disease that usually does not involve the mediastinum or bone marrow, and they achieve complete remission more often than those with T-precursor LL (16,17). B-LL should be distinguished from the blastoid variant of mantle cell lymphoma (MCL) (15–17) (see Chapter 66).

Acute lymphoblastic leukemia occurs more often in children than in adults; peripheral adenopathy and an enlarged mediastinum are uncommon. In children, the incidence is about 3 cases per 100,000 population; three-fourths are younger than 15 years, the peak age incidence is 2 to 5 years, and boys are more often affected than girls (18). Association with Down syndrome (19), other genetic diseases, and radiation (18) have been noted. Immunophenotypic studies predict the best prognosis for B-precursor ALL and an increasingly worse prognosis for T-cell and pre-B-cell ALL (20–22). Paradoxically, modern intensive therapy appears to have eliminated the immunophenotypic effect in childhood ALL with bulky extramedullary disease (23).

HISTOPATHOLOGY

Lymphoblastic lymphoma infiltrates multiple lymph nodes, diffusely replacing the normal architecture. LL involves the lymph node capsule in a single-file arrangement, the blood vessel walls, and perinodal adipose tissue (5) (Fig. 59.1). Although usually diffuse, the pattern sometimes appears demarcated when thin strands of collagen form compartments within the tumor (24,25) (Fig. 59.2). Such pseudonodules differ in size, shape, and particularly type of component cells from the nodules of follicular lymphoma (24) (see Chapter 64). Alternatively, LL infiltrates the paracortical T zone, leaving residual follicles (Fig. 59.3 A–F), "naked" germinal centers (Fig. 59.4 A–D), or lymphoid islands (5). The lymphoblasts infiltrate diffusely, are packed closely, and although not cohesive appear monomorphic with indistinct cytoplasm and a high nuclear-to-cytoplasmic ratio (Fig. 59.5). A "starry sky" pattern, like that of Burkitt lymphoma, occurs at least focally in one-fourth of cases (5) (Figs. 59.3 B,C and 59.4 B,C). Thin sections and smears reveal indentations and convolutions in most nuclei. The LL chromatin structure is fine and delicate or dusty, and the nucleoli are inconspicuous, cytologically indistinguishable from those of ALL. Mitoses are numerous (5) (Fig. 59.5). Crush artifact is frequent. In the nonconvoluted type, the nuclei are round or ovoid and show little variation in size and shape (2). Convoluted versus nonconvoluted lymphoblasts do not predict any clinical difference (5,26).

Lymphoblastic lymphoma with eosinophilic infiltration (27) (Fig. 59.3 A–F) suggests a specific clinicopathologic syndrome: LL, mostly in male patients, involving peripheral lymph nodes but not mediastinum; eosinophilia; and a

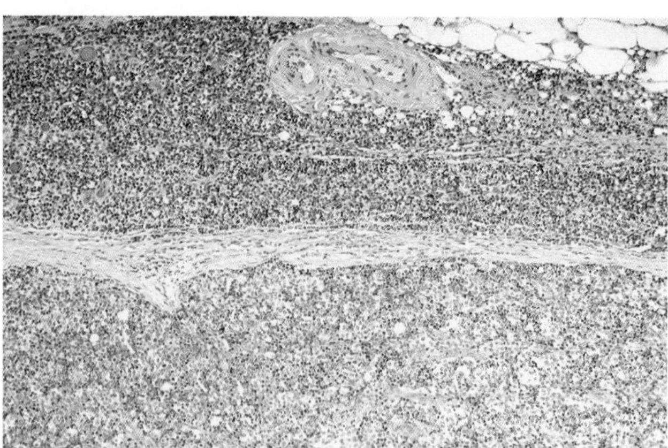

FIGURE 59.1. Lymphoblastic lymphoma in enlarged supraclavicular lymph node of a 66-year-old woman. Lymphoblasts infiltrate through lymph node capsule in a single-file pattern and into perinodal adipose tissue. Hematoxylin and eosin stain.

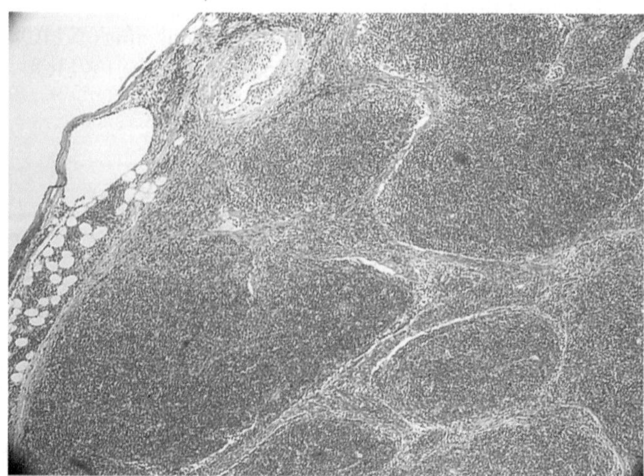

FIGURE 59.2. Lymphoblastic lymphoma in cervical lymph node of a 24-year-old woman. Compartmentalization of diffuse sheets of lymphoma cells by thin strands of collagen results in a pseudonodular pattern. Hematoxylin, phloxine, and saffron stain.

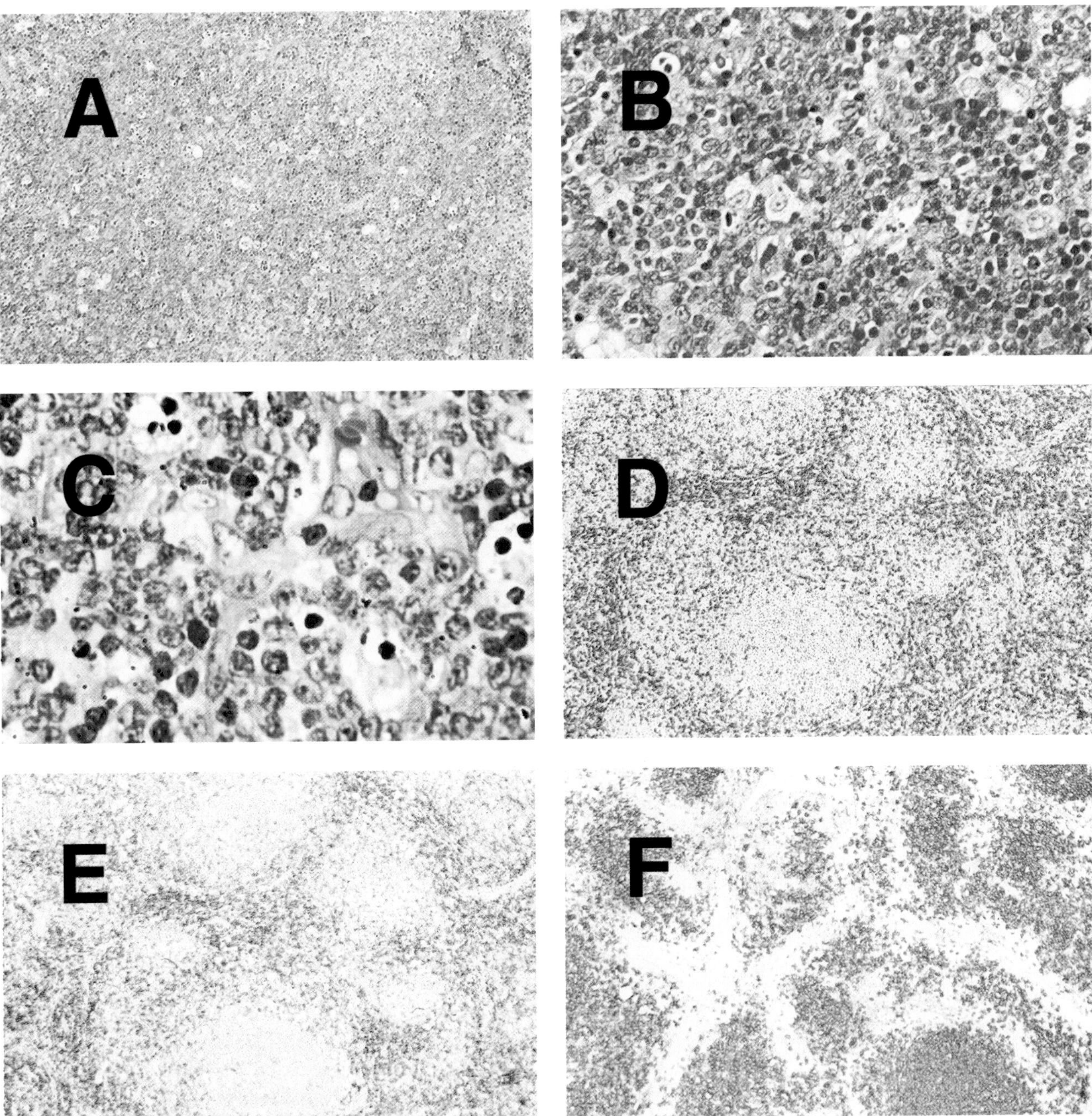

FIGURE 59.3. Lymphoblastic lymphoma in cervical lymph node of a 5-year-old boy. **A:** Scanning magnification reveals partially preserved follicles overrun by lymphoblasts. Hematoxylin and eosin stain. **B:** Lymphoblasts mixed with phagocytic histiocytes ("starry sky" pattern) and mature eosinophils. Hematoxylin and eosin stain. **C:** Same specimen as in B at higher magnification shows lymphoblasts, histiocytes, and mature eosinophils. Hematoxylin and eosin stain. **D:** Anti-CD3 stains interfollicular T lymphoblasts. Immunoperoxidase stain. **E:** Anti-CD99 (mic-2) stains interfollicular T lymphoblasts. Same distribution as in D. Immunoperoxidase stain. **F:** Anti-CD20 stains non-neoplastic, residual B-cell follicles. Immunoperoxidase stain.

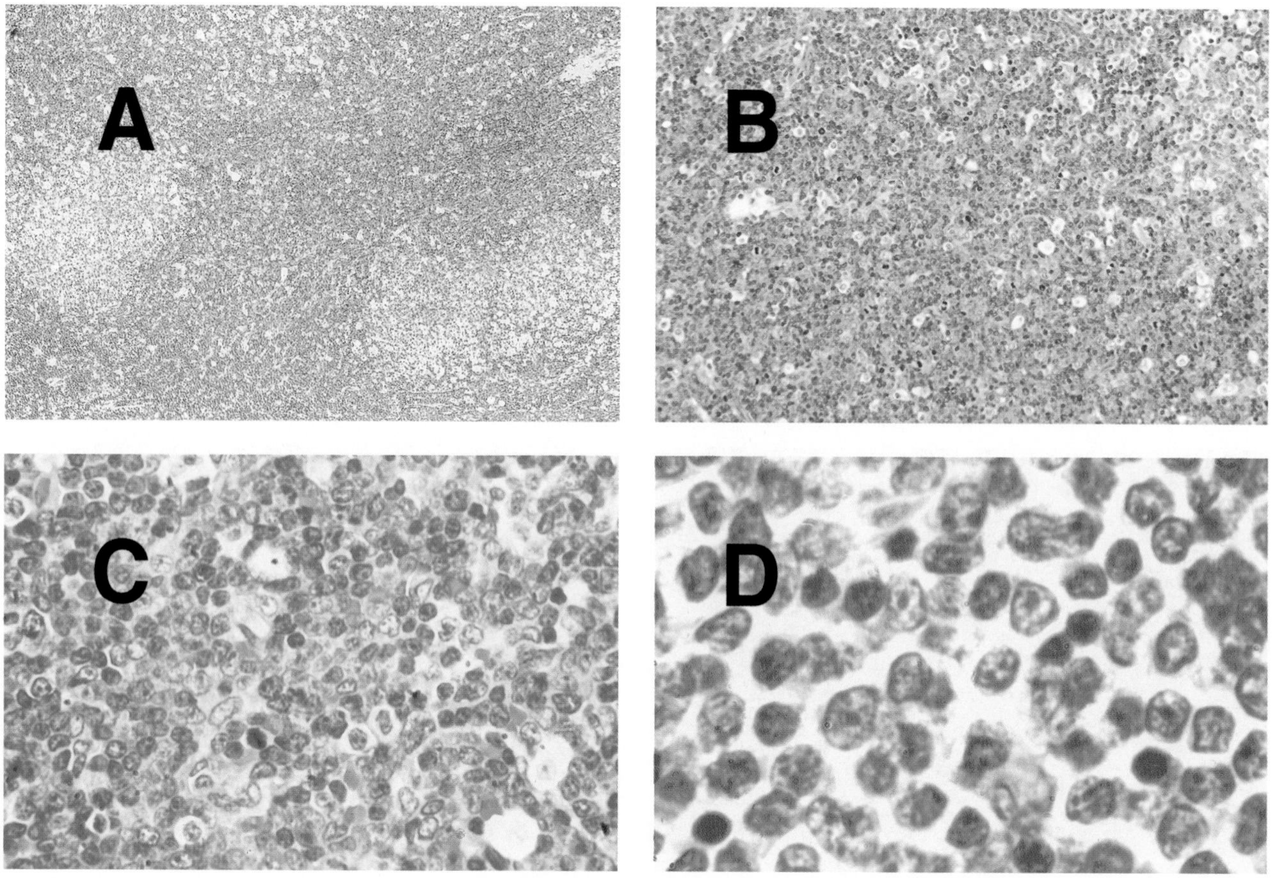

FIGURE 59.4. Same lymph node as in Fig. 59.1. **A:** "Naked" germinal centers surrounded by lymphoblasts. Hematoxylin and eosin stain. **B:** "Starry sky" pattern of phagocytic histiocytes interspersed among lymphoblasts. Residual "naked" germinal center (*right*). Hematoxylin and eosin stain. **C:** The diameter of medium-sized lymphoblasts equals the nuclear diameter of histiocytes. **D:** Lymphoblasts with fine and delicate nuclear chromatin, inconspicuous nucleoli, and scant cytoplasm. Scattered small, dark, apoptotic nuclei. Hematoxylin and eosin stain.

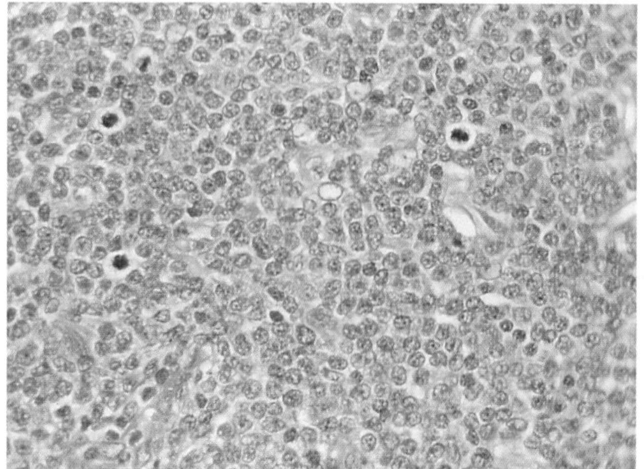

FIGURE 59.5. Lymphoblastic lymphoma of mediastinal lymph node of a 19-year-old woman. Normal architecture effaced; closely packed cells with uniform round nuclei, inconspicuous nucleoli, and numerous mitoses. Hematoxylin, phloxine, and saffron stain.

myeloproliferative disorder, myeloid hyperplasia or acute myeloblastic leukemia (AML), associated with t(8;13)(p11; q11) (28). This translocation combines fibroblast growth factor receptor 1 and fused in myeloproliferative (FIM) disorder genes to yield a chimeric protein with constitutive tyrosine kinase activity (29).

ELECTRON MICROSCOPY

On electron microscopy, the cells are of medium size, mostly round, with smooth surfaces and no cytoplasmic processes (Fig. 59.6). Non-T-cell, non-B-cell cases tend to have round or folded nuclei; T-cell cases tend to have nuclear irregularities (30). The scarce cytoplasm includes few mitochondria, strands of endoplasmic reticulum, free ribosomes, and perinuclear filaments and microtubules. Cells with filament bundles are common in blood but rare in lymph nodes (31). The nuclei are irregularly shaped, with

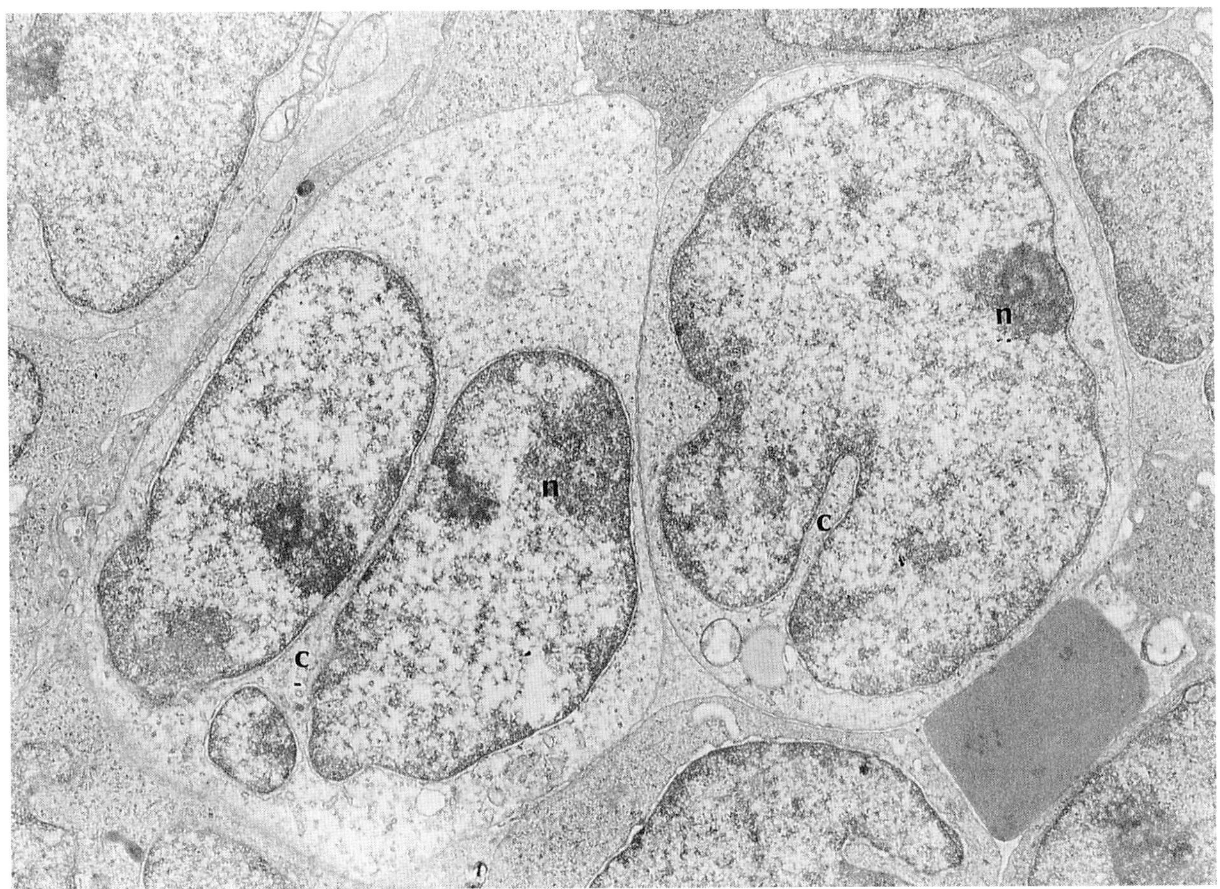

FIGURE 59.6. Lymphoblastic lymphoma in cervical lymph node. Cells have a high nuclear-to-cytoplasmic ratio, a small amount of cytoplasm with few organelles, and convoluted nuclei with deep indentations that sometimes create the appearance of multinucleated cells (*left*); fine chromatin (*c*) structure with peripheral nucleoli (*n*). ×16,000.

frequent deep fissures and convolutions (32), but without the serpentine or cerebriform configurations that characterize Sézary cells (31). The chromatin is evenly dispersed, with peripheral condensation. The nucleoli are dense and always adjacent to the nuclear membrane.

CYTOCHEMISTRY

A positive dotlike acid phosphatase reaction or a fluoride-resistant nonspecific esterase reaction in the paranuclear Golgi zone characterizes T-lymphoblasts (33). In about 80% of cases of T- or B-lineage LL/ALL, staining with periodic acid–Schiff (PAS) shows a discrete, blocklike pattern (34). For diagnosing ALL versus AML, PAS alone was 52% sensitive and 81% specific (34).

IMMUNOHISTOCHEMISTRY

T-precursor and B-precursor LLs express the nuclear enzyme TdT, which generates diversity in T-cell antigen receptors and immunoglobulin (Ig) genes (35) (Fig. 59.7) (see Chapter 8). Besides TdT, LLs often express CD34 and CD99 (35) (Fig. 59.3E). Mature non-Hodgkin lymphomas lack these markers, but some small, round cell tumors of childhood express CD99 (mic-2). TdT expression distinguishes CD99+/CD45− (leukocyte common antigen-negative) LL of bone from Ewing sarcoma (36). A minority of AMLs expresses TdT or CD99.

The majority (90%) of LLs derive from immature T cells, and the rest originate from B-cell precursors (4,13,37) (see Chapters 6 and 7). T-precursor LL corresponds to prethymic and intrathymic maturation stages, lacking CD4 and CD8 or sometimes coexpressing CD4 and CD8 (38). Many T-precursor LLs express cytoplasmic, but not surface, CD3. CD43 is a sensitive, but not specific, T-cell marker. For detecting immature B cells, CD79a is more sensitive than CD20. LL/ALL expressing CD45 dimly by flow cytometry analysis may be undetectable immunohistochemically. Cases positive for surface Igs with blastic morphology should be distinguished from Burkitt lymphoma and the blastoid variant of MCL.

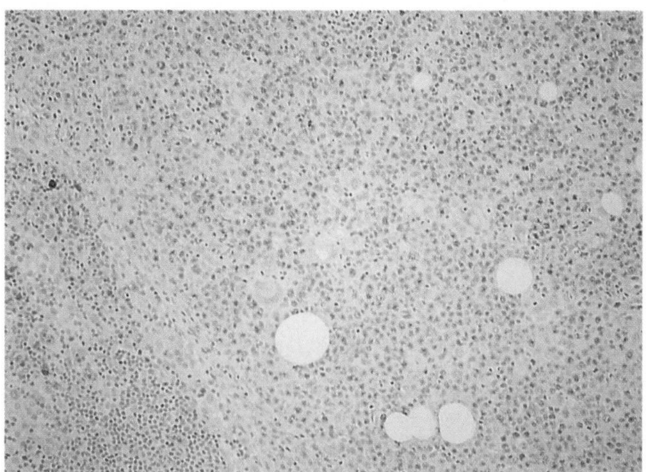

FIGURE 59.7. Lymphoblastic lymphoma in mediastinal lymph node. Results of nuclear immunostaining for terminal deoxynucleotidyl transferase (TdT) enzyme are positive in all lymphoma cells. Immunoperoxidase stain.

Phenotype

T-PRECURSOR LL	B-PRECURSOR LL
CD1a+/−	CD10+/−
CD2+/−	CD19+
Cytoplasmic CD3+, usually	CD20+/−
Surface CD3+/−	CD22+/−
CD4+/CD8+ or CD4−/CD8− or CD4+/CD8− or CD4−/CD8+	Cytoplasmic CD22+
CD5+/−	CD43+
CD7+/−	CD79a+
CD10+/−	CD99+
CD34+	TdT+
CD38+	Surface Ig−
CD43+	HLA-DR+
CD99+	
TdT+	
HLA-DR+/−	

CYTOGENETICS

The most common abnormalities seen in LL involve 14q11, 7q35, and 7p15 (39). The t(8;13)(p11;q11) is associated with eosinophilia and a specific syndrome (28) (see above).

In childhood ALL, numeric and structural cytogenetic abnormalities are assigned to prognostic risk groups as follows: (a) good: hyperdiploidy, more than 50 chromosomes; t(12;21)(p13;q22), TEL/AML1; (b) intermediate: t(1;19)(q23;p13), E2A/PBX1; (c) poor: t(9;22)(q34;q11), BCR/ABL; t(v;11q23), MLL rearranged; or hypodiploidy, fewer than 45 chromosomes (18). The effect of age on prognosis is probably related to the association of specific genetic abnormalities: infants less than 1 year frequently have rearranged MLL; 70% of patients 1 to 9 years old have hyperdiploidy or TEL/AML1 fusion. Older children and adults more often have rearranged MLL or BCR/ABL (18). E2A/PBX1 is associated with a pre-B-cell phenotype (cytoplasmic μ).

MOLECULAR DIAGNOSIS

TEL/AML1, the most frequent translocation of childhood B-precursor ALL, occurs in about 25% of cases. Molecular studies, but not cytogenetics, usually demonstrate the fusion of TEL at 12p13 to AML1 at 21q22 as part of t(12;21) (40). Only 5% of childhood, but 30% of adult, ALLs have the t(9;22) translocation; occasionally BCR/ABL can be detected only molecularly (40).

Cross-lineage T-cell receptor and Ig gene rearrangements and continuing or secondary gene rearrangements are common in ALL (41). Therefore, the assignment of a cell lineage should be based on immunophenotype, not on DNA alterations.

DIFFERENTIAL DIAGNOSIS

A correct diagnosis of LL is important, particularly because of the rapid progression and high malignant potential of these tumors, which require aggressive chemotherapy.

- Burkitt lymphoma also occurs in children and presents with a diffuse pattern and immature lymphoid cells; however, Burkitt lymphoma cells are about the size of a histiocyte nucleus, slightly larger than lymphoblasts; they have round, nonconvoluted nuclei with two to five prominent nucleoli and basophilic cytoplasm. On smears, cytoplasmic vacuoles containing lipid stain with oil red-O. The histologic pattern is characterized by a "starry sky" appearance, because of the presence of numerous scattered macrophages, and by many mitoses. The cells express surface Ig and mature B-cell markers; they are negative for TdT. Both LL and Burkitt lymphoma frequently express CD10 (CALLA) and have a "starry sky" appearance. In contrast, LL expresses TdT, CD34, and CD99 (35).
- B-cell chronic lymphocytic leukemia/small lymphocytic lymphoma occurs in the elderly. The cells are small and uniform, the nuclei are round, and mitoses are rare. The cells exhibit a CD5+ mature B-cell phenotype and usually a pseudofollicular pattern. TdT is negative.
- Follicular lymphoma: The architecture is that of sharply demarcated round nodules not separated by collagen fibers, as in the compartmentalized LLs. The small cleaved cells of both follicular and diffuse lymphomas have, in contrast to the LL cells, irregularly shaped nuclei with condensed chromatin. Mitoses are less frequent. The

Checklist

LYMPHOBLASTIC LYMPHOMA

CD34+, CD99+, TdT+
Children and adolescents
Male predominance
Supradiaphragmatic polylymphadenopathy
Mediastinal mass (50% to 75%)
Early bone marrow involvement
Acute lymphocytic leukemia, T-cell type (82% to 100%)
Relentless course, short survival
Relapse in central nervous system
Diffuse or pseudonodular pattern
Monomorphic cell population
Lymphoblasts
Convoluted nuclei (53%)
Dusty chromatin
Inconspicuous nucleoli
High mitotic index
Acid phosphatase, focal staining
T-cell markers: CD1, CD2, cytoplasmic CD3, CD5, CD7, CD4/CD8 double-negative or double-positive, HLA-DR, CD10 variable
B-cell markers: CD10, CD19, cytoplasmic CD22, CD79a, HLA-DR, cytoplasmic μ (pre-B cell)

cells express surface Ig and mature B-cell markers. TdT is negative.

- The blastoid variant of MCL morphologically simulates LL but has a typical CD5+, surface Ig+, mature B-cell phenotype and expresses nuclear bcl-1 (cyclin D1); TdT is negative. Patients with MCL are usually significantly older than those with LL (15–17).

REFERENCES

1. Harris NL, Jaffe ES, Diebold J, et al. The World Health Organization classification of hematological malignancies report of the clinical advisory committee meeting, Airlie House, Virginia, November 1997. Mod Pathol 2000;13:193–207.
2. Nathwani BN, Kim H, Rappaport H. Malignant lymphoma, lymphoblastic. Cancer 1976;38:964–983.
3. Jaffe ES, Berard CW. Lymphoblastic lymphoma, a term rekindled with new precision. Ann Intern Med 1978;89:415–417.
4. Cossman J, Chused TM, Fisher RI, et al. Diversity of immunological phenotypes of lymphoblastic lymphoma. Cancer Res 1983;43:4486–4490.
5. Nathwani BN, Diamond LW, Winberg CD, et al. Lymphoblastic lymphoma: a clinicopathologic study of 95 patients. Cancer 1981;48:2347–2357.
6. National Cancer Institute-sponsored study of classifications of non-Hodgkin's lymphomas: summary and description of a working formulation for clinical usage. The Non-Hodgkin's Lymphoma Pathologic Classification Project. Cancer 1982;49:2112–2135.
7. Murphy SB. Classification, staging and end results of treatment of childhood non-Hodgkin's lymphomas: dissimilarities from lymphomas in adults. Semin Oncol 1980;7:332–339.
8. The Non-Hodgkin's Lymphoma Classification Project. A clinical evaluation of the International Lymphoma Study Group classification of non-Hodgkin's lymphoma. Blood 1997;89:3909–3918.
9. Streuli RA, Kaneko Y, Variakojis D, et al. Lymphoblastic lymphoma in adults. Cancer 1981;47:2510–2516.
10. Picozzi VJ Jr, Coleman CN. Lymphoblastic lymphoma. Semin Oncol 1990;17:96–103.
11. Coleman CN, Picozzi VJ Jr, Cox RS, et al. Treatment of lymphoblastic lymphoma in adults. J Clin Oncol 1986;4:1628–1637.
12. Slater DE, Mertelsmann R, Koziner B, et al. Lymphoblastic lymphoma in adults. J Clin Oncol 1986;4:57–67.
13. Lin P, Jones D, Dorfman DM, et al. Precursor B-cell lymphoblastic lymphoma: a predominantly extranodal tumor with low propensity for leukemic involvement. Am J Surg Pathol 2000;24:1480–1490.
14. Schwob VS, Weiner L, Hudes G, et al. Extranodal non-T-cell lymphoblastic lymphoma in adults. A report of two cases. Am J Clin Pathol 1988;90:602–605.
15. Cheng AL, Su IJ, Tien HF, et al. Characteristic clinicopathologic features of adult B-cell lymphoblastic lymphoma with special emphasis on differential diagnosis with an atypical form probably of blastic lymphocytic lymphoma of intermediate differentiation origin. Cancer 1994;73:706–710.

16. Soslow RA, Zukerberg LR, Harris NL, et al. BCL-1 (PRAD-1/cyclin D-1) overexpression distinguishes the blastoid variant of mantle cell lymphoma from B-lineage lymphoblastic lymphoma. Mod Pathol 1997;10:810–817.
17. Soslow RA, Baergen RN, Warnke RA. B-lineage lymphoblastic lymphoma is a clinicopathologic entity distinct from other histologically similar aggressive lymphomas with blastic morphology. Cancer 1999;85:2648–2654.
18. Pui CH. Acute lymphoblastic leukemia. Pediatr Clin North Am 1997;44:831–846.
19. Watson MS, Carroll AJ, Shuster JJ, et al. Trisomy 21 in childhood acute lymphoblastic leukemia: a Pediatric Oncology Group study (8602). Blood 1993;82:3098–3102.
20. Dowell BL, Borowitz MJ, Boyett JM, et al. Immunologic and clinicopathologic features of common acute lymphoblastic leukemia antigen-positive childhood T-cell leukemia. A Pediatric Oncology Group Study. Cancer 1987;59:2020–2026.
21. Crist W, Boyett J, Jackson J, et al. Prognostic importance of the pre-B-cell immunophenotype and other presenting features in B-lineage childhood acute lymphoblastic leukemia: a Pediatric Oncology Group study. Blood 1989;74:1252–1259.
22. Pullen J, Shuster JJ, Link M, et al. Significance of commonly used prognostic factors differs for children with T-cell acute lymphocytic leukemia (ALL), as compared to those with B-precursor ALL. A Pediatric Oncology Group (POG) study. Leukemia 1999;13:1696–1707.
23. Steinherz PG, Gaynon PS, Breneman JC, et al. Treatment of patients with acute lymphoblastic leukemia with bulky extramedullary disease and T-cell phenotype or other poor prognostic features: randomized controlled trial from the Children's Cancer Group. Cancer 1998;82:600–612.
24. Ioachim HL, Finbeiner JA. Pseudonodular pattern of T-cell lymphoma. Cancer 1980;45:1370–1378.
25. Schwartz JE, Grogan TM, Hicks MJ, et al. Pseudonodular T cell lymphoblastic lymphoma. Am J Med 1984;77:947–949.
26. Pangalis GA, Nathwani BN, Rappaport H, et al. Acute lymphoblastic leukemia: the significance of nuclear convolutions. Cancer 1979;43:551–557.
27. Abruzzo LV, Jaffe ES, Cotelingam JD, et al. T-cell lymphoblastic lymphoma with eosinophilia associated with subsequent myeloid malignancy [see Comments]. Am J Surg Pathol 1992;16:236–245.
28. Inhorn RC, Aster JC, Roach SA, et al. A syndrome of lymphoblastic lymphoma, eosinophilia, and myeloid hyperplasia/malignancy associated with t(8;13)(p11;q11): description of a distinctive clinicopathologic entity [see Comments]. Blood 1995; 85:1881–1887.
29. Popovici C, Adelaide J, Ollendorff V, et al. Fibroblast growth factor receptor 1 is fused to FIM in stem-cell myeloproliferative disorder with t(8;13). Proc Natl Acad Sci U S A 1998;95:5712–5717.
30. Glick AD, Vestal BK, Flexner JM, et al. Ultrastructural study of acute lymphocytic leukemia: comparison with immunologic studies. Blood 1978;52:311–322.
31. Palutke M, Patt DJ, Weise R, et al. T cell leukemia-lymphoma in young adults. Am J Clin Pathol 1977;68:429–439.
32. Ioachim HL. The lymph nodes. In: Johannessen JV, ed. Electron microscopy in human medicine, vol 5. New York: McGraw-Hill, 1981:384–438.
33. Rosenthal NS, Farhi DC. Special stains in the diagnosis of acute leukemia. Clin Lab Med 2000;20:29–38, viii.
34. Snower DP, Smith BR, Munz UJ, et al. Reevaluation of the periodic acid–Schiff stain in acute leukemia with immunophenotypic analyses. Arch Pathol Lab Med 1991;115:346–350.
35. Soslow RA, Bhargava V, Warnke RA. MIC2, TdT, bcl-2, and CD34 expression in paraffin-embedded high-grade lymphoma/ acute lymphoblastic leukemia distinguishes between distinct clinicopathologic entities. Hum Pathol 1997;28:1158–1165.
36. Lucas DR, Bentley G, Dan ME, et al. Ewing sarcoma vs lymphoblastic lymphoma. Am J Clin Pathol 2001;115:11–17.
37. Sheibani K, Nathwani BN, Winberg CD, et al. Antigenically defined subgroups of lymphoblastic lymphoma. Relationship to clinical presentation and biologic behavior. Cancer 1987;60:183–190.
38. Roper M, Crist WM, Metzgar R, et al. Monoclonal antibody characterization of surface antigens in childhood T-cell lymphoid malignancies. Blood 1983;61:830–837.
39. Kaneko Y, Frizzera G, Shikano T, et al. Chromosomal and immunophenotypic patterns in T cell acute lymphoblastic leukemia (T ALL) and lymphoblastic lymphoma (LBL). Leukemia 1989;3: 886–892.
40. Farhi DC, Rosenthal NS. Acute lymphoblastic leukemia. Clin Lab Med 2000;20:17–28, vii.
41. Szczepanski T, Pongers-Willemse MJ, Langerak AW, et al. Unusual immunoglobulin and T-cell receptor gene rearrangement patterns in acute lymphoblastic leukemias. Curr Top Microbiol Immunol 1999;246:205–213.

PART V

SECTION FOUR

MATURE B-CELL NEOPLASMS

60

B-CELL CHRONIC LYMPHOCYTIC LEUKEMIA/SMALL LYMPHOCYTIC LYMPHOMA

DEFINITION

Lymphoma of small, inactive, mature-appearing lymphocytes with a diffuse pattern; the disseminated counterpart is chronic lymphocytic leukemia. These are two stages of the same disease.

SYNONYMS

Malignant lymphoma, diffuse, well-differentiated lymphocytic type (Rappaport)

Lymphoma, lymphocytic/chronic lymphocytic leukemia (Kiel)

Malignant lymphoma, diffuse, small lymphocytic type consistent with chronic lymphocytic leukemia (Working Formulation)

B-cell chronic lymphocytic leukemia/small lymphocytic lymphoma (Revised European-American Lymphoma Classification)

B-cell chronic lymphocytic leukemia/small lymphocytic lymphoma (World Health Organization)

GRADE

Low-grade lymphoma.

EPIDEMIOLOGY

Small lymphocytic lymphoma (SLL) and B-cell chronic lymphocytic leukemia (B-CLL) are neoplasms of late adult life, peaking in the sixth or seventh decade (1–4). They almost never occur before the age of 20 years and are very rare before 40 (3–5). After 40 years, the incidence increases linearly with age (3,4). Men outnumber women about 2:1 and fare worse clinically (6,7). B-CLL is the most common form of leukemia in the Western world; however, in Asia it is extremely infrequent (8,9). Although CLL represents only 2% of all leukemias in Japan, the CD5+ lymphoproliferative disorders have an exceptionally poor prognosis (10).

B-cell chronic lymphocytic leukemia develops more often in first-degree relatives of patients with B-CLL than in the general population, but the genetic basis is poorly understood (11). In familial B-CLL, offspring in whom disease develops two decades earlier than in their affected parent manifest anticipation (12). Sporadic and familial B-CLL, two epidemiologically distinct types of B-CLL, share similar immunoglobulin heavy chain variable genes and frequency of somatic mutation, which implies a common cellular origin and pathogenesis (13).

PATHOGENESIS

The World Health Organization classifies B-CLL and SLL as different stages of the same type of lymphoma, not as two unique diseases (14). Further, the recognition of plasmacytoid features (lymphoplasmacytoid immunocytoma according to the Kiel classification) is insufficient to diagnose a separate pathologic entity (14). It remains to be proved whether B-CLL/SLL with plasmacytoid features predicts a worse prognosis.

The cytologic diagnosis of CLL is based on a persistent absolute lymphocytosis of more than 5×10^9 cells per liter, bone marrow lymphocytosis of more than 30%, or both (15). Lymphocytosis of between 4,000 and 15,000 cells per cubic millimeter is considered to be an early low count (16). The blood and bone marrow in classic CLL should not contain more than 10% prolymphocytes or cells with irregular, cleaved, or convoluted nuclei (16). CLL morphologic variants include a mixed cell type (>10% and <55% prolymphocytes) and a pleomorphic type that is not clearly specified (17). The lymphomas and leukemias of small lymphocytic type are a heterogeneous group comprising several subtypes that differ clinically, morphologically, and immunologically. The French–American–British group has proposed a classification of CLL with 10 subtypes (17). The more common ones are the following:

- B-CLL is the main type and by far the most common, particularly in Europe and North America. The cell of origin is the small, inactive lymphocyte.
- T-cell chronic lymphocytic leukemia (T-CLL) is very rare, representing only 2% of all CLLs. It is now called *T-cell prolymphocytic leukemia* to reflect its clinical aggressiveness (14,18).
- Lymphosarcoma cell leukemia represents the disseminated stage or leukemic phase of follicular lymphoma (see Chapters 64 and 65). Most CD5− B-cell lymphoproliferative disorders involving blood or bone marrow are non-Hodgkin lymphomas in leukemic phase (19).
- Prolymphocytic leukemia involves a transformed or activated lymphocyte, suggested by the prominent nucleolus and the bright surface immunoglobulin (Ig).
- Macroglobulinemia of Waldenström is associated with a monoclonal gammopathy of the IgM class that can produce hyperviscosity (1,20).
- Other chronic leukemias, such as hairy cell leukemia (see Chapter 62) and Sézary syndrome (see Chapter 72), are described separately.

CLINICAL SYNDROME

The clinical course of B-CLL/SLL is highly variable. Some patients have only asymptomatic lymphadenopathy or splenomegaly; others present with fever, fatigue, night sweats, and breathlessness as a result of bone marrow involvement with anemia and thrombocytopenia. The lymphadenopathy is usually generalized (8). The lymph nodes involved are firm, discrete, and mobile. The bone marrow pattern (nodular, interstitial, or diffuse) in B-CLL/SLL indicates tumor burden but does not predict the clinical behavior better than does the clinical stage (21). The presence of a monoclonal gammopathy, usually IgM with κ or λ light chains (the former by far more common), reflects secretory activity (20). In a significant number of patients with B-CLL/SLL, a leukemic phase may not develop, even after long periods (1). The median survival time is approximately 8 years (22).

The clinical conversion of low-grade B-CLL/SLL to high-grade, usually large cell or immunoblastic, lymphoma is known as *Richter syndrome.* An aggressive lymphoma developed in approximately 39 of 1,374 patients (3%) with CLL at a single institution (23). The high-grade lymphoma is almost always clonally derived from the original low-grade B-CLL/SLL; rarely, a new clone appears. Transformation occurs in 11 to 240 months, with a mean interval of 63 months; survival is about 6 months after this event (24). Some B-CLL/SLL cases transform to Hodgkin disease (25). The Reed-Sternberg cells have essentially the same Ig heavy chain variable (IgH V) gene DNA sequence as the preceding B-CLL/SLL, which proves their clonal identity (26), and contain Epstein-Barr virus, especially after fludarabine treatment (27).

HISTOPATHOLOGY

The lymph node architecture is totally obscured by diffuse, monotonous sheets of mostly small lymphocytes that lack any recognizable histologic pattern. They obliterate the follicles and sinuses and spread through the capsule into the surrounding adipose tissue (Fig. 60.1). The cells are small, round, and uniform, resembling inactive, mature lymphocytes (Figs. 60.2 and 60.3). The nucleus is condensed and the nucleoli are inconspicuous. Intranuclear inclusions, such as Dutcher bodies, and plasmacytic differentiation are absent. Cytoplasm is scant. Mitoses are rare.

Pale, poorly defined areas, called *indistinct nodular areas* (28) or *pseudofollicular proliferation centers* (29), are scattered throughout the sea of small lymphocytes (Fig. 60.2 A–D). These terms distinguish pseudonodules with vague outlines ("pseudofollicles") in B-CLL/SLL from sharply circumscribed nodules ("true follicles") in reactive follicular hyperplasia and follicular lymphoma (see Chapter 64). During scanning magnification, decreasing the light intensity of the microscope enhances contrast and pseudofollicle visibility. The pseudofollicles appear pale because they contain numerous large cells with dispersed chromatin, and the distances between these cells are greater than between the surrounding, more densely packed small lymphocytes, so that hematoxylin staining is reduced in the pseudofollicles (Fig. 60.2 A,B). Pseudofollicles can be found in most cases of B-CLL/SLL if the tissue sections are technically perfect.

The pseudofollicles contain a mixture of small lymphocytes, medium-sized prolymphocytes with dispersed chromatin and a single nucleolus, and larger paraimmunoblasts

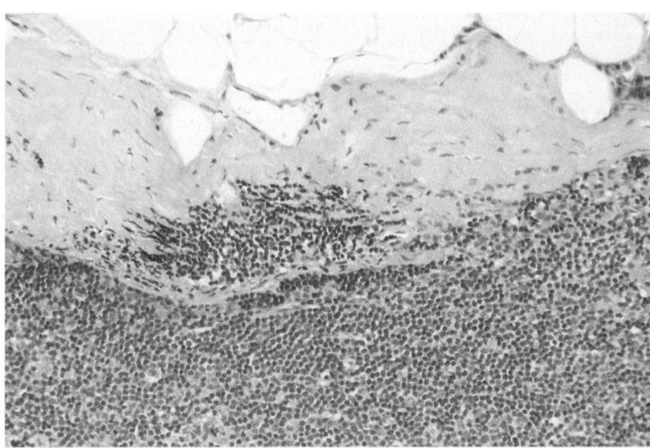

FIGURE 60.1. B-cell chronic lymphocytic leukemia/small lymphocytic lymphoma in lymph node. Homogeneous population of small lymphocytes effaces lymph node architecture, replacing follicles and infiltrating capsule and perinodal adipose tissue. Hematoxylin, phloxine, and saffron stain.

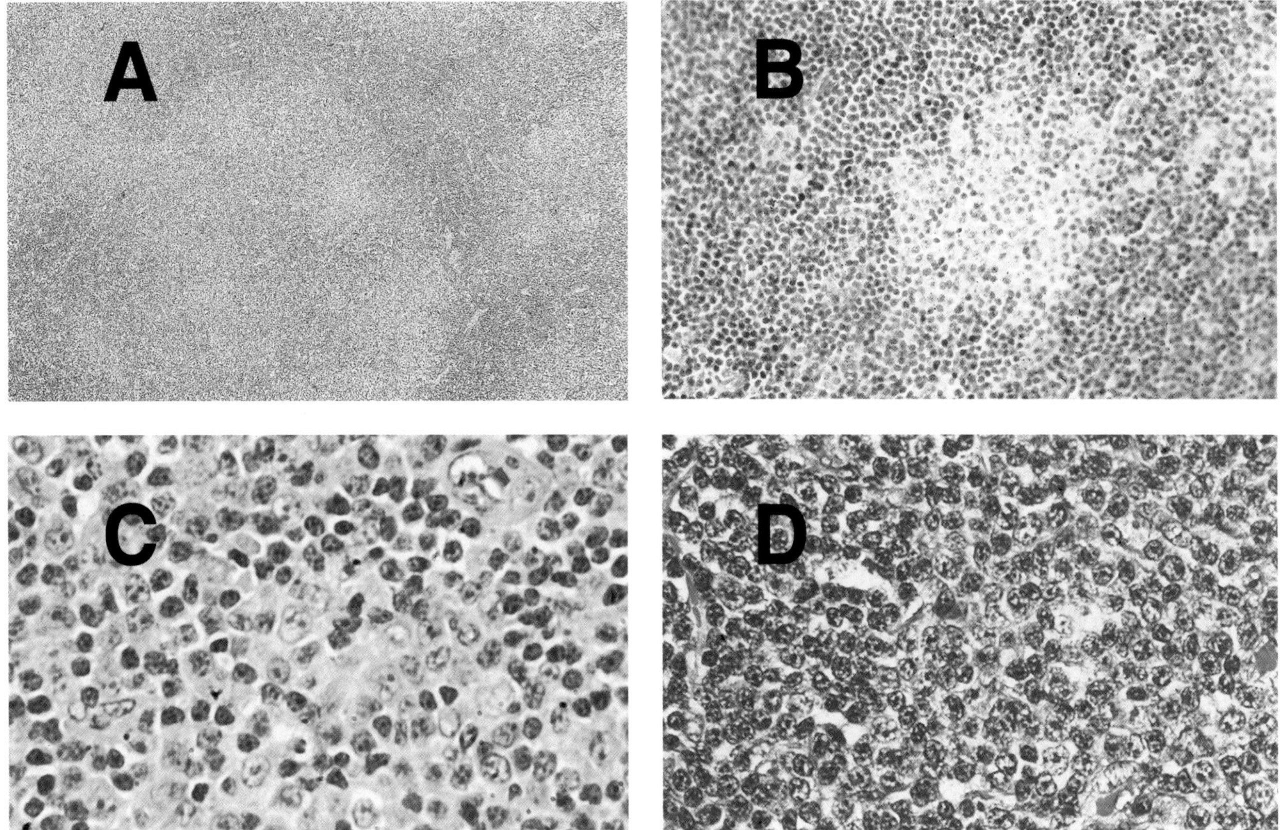

FIGURE 60.2. B-cell chronic lymphocytic leukemia/small lymphocytic lymphoma in lymph node. **A:** Large, pale, almost confluent "pseudofollicles." These can be confused with diffuse large B-cell lymphoma. Hematoxylin and eosin stain. **B:** Small "pseudofollicle." Hematoxylin and eosin stain. **C:** Specimen in A at higher magnification. Numerous prolymphocytes, paraimmunoblasts, and widely separated small, mature lymphocytes explain pale staining seen at scanning magnification. **D:** Same specimen as in **B**. Dark, small, mature-appearing lymphocytes (*left*). Scattered prolymphocytes and paraimmunoblasts in "pseudofollicle" (*right*). Hematoxylin and eosin stain.

with vesicular chromatin, a prominent central nucleolus, and relatively abundant cytoplasm (Fig. 60.2 C,D). Mitoses are more frequent in the pseudofollicles than in the rest of the lymph node. Pseudofollicles should be discriminated from the germinal centers of normal reactive follicles and the neoplastic nodules of follicular lymphomas. Prominent pseudofollicles must not be confused with diffuse large B-cell lymphoma, particularly in lymph nodes infiltrated by atypical CLL (30). Whether prominent pseudofollicles or abundant large cells predict a shortened survival remains controversial (28,30,31).

FLOW CYTOMETRY

The National Cancer Institute Working Group defines B-CLL by three phenotypic parameters: a major population expressing B-cell markers (CD19, CD20, and CD23) plus CD5 without other T-cell antigens; surface Ig κ or λ light chain monoclonality; and low-density surface Ig (15) (see Chapter 7). CD20 and CD22 are dim. In most cases of B-CLL/SLL, the Igs on the cell membrane are identified as IgM (Fig. 60.4), with or without IgD, more often with κ than with λ light chains (32). The idiotypes of the IgM and IgD molecules on the same cell are identical.

The immunofluorescent staining of surface Ig differs in B-CLL/SLL, prolymphocytic leukemia (PL), and follicular lymphoma (FL) (32). Whereas the cells of PL and FL show bright fluorescence on their surface, the cells of B-CLL/SLL show very faint surface fluorescence because they display a relatively smaller number of surface Ig molecules, approximately 9,000 per cell (8). Because the B-cell receptor complex is necessary for the expression of surface Ig, mutations of the B29 portion (CD79b) of the B-cell receptor yield low to undetectable levels of surface Ig and diminished B-cell receptor signaling in B-CLL/SLL (33).

The majority of CD5− lymphoproliferative disorders involving blood or bone marrow represent the leukemic phase of non-Hodgkin lymphomas: hairy cell leukemia, hairy cell leukemia variant, follicular lymphoma, lymphoplasmacytic lymphoma, and splenic marginal zone lymphoma (19). Any CD5− lymphoproliferative disorder that

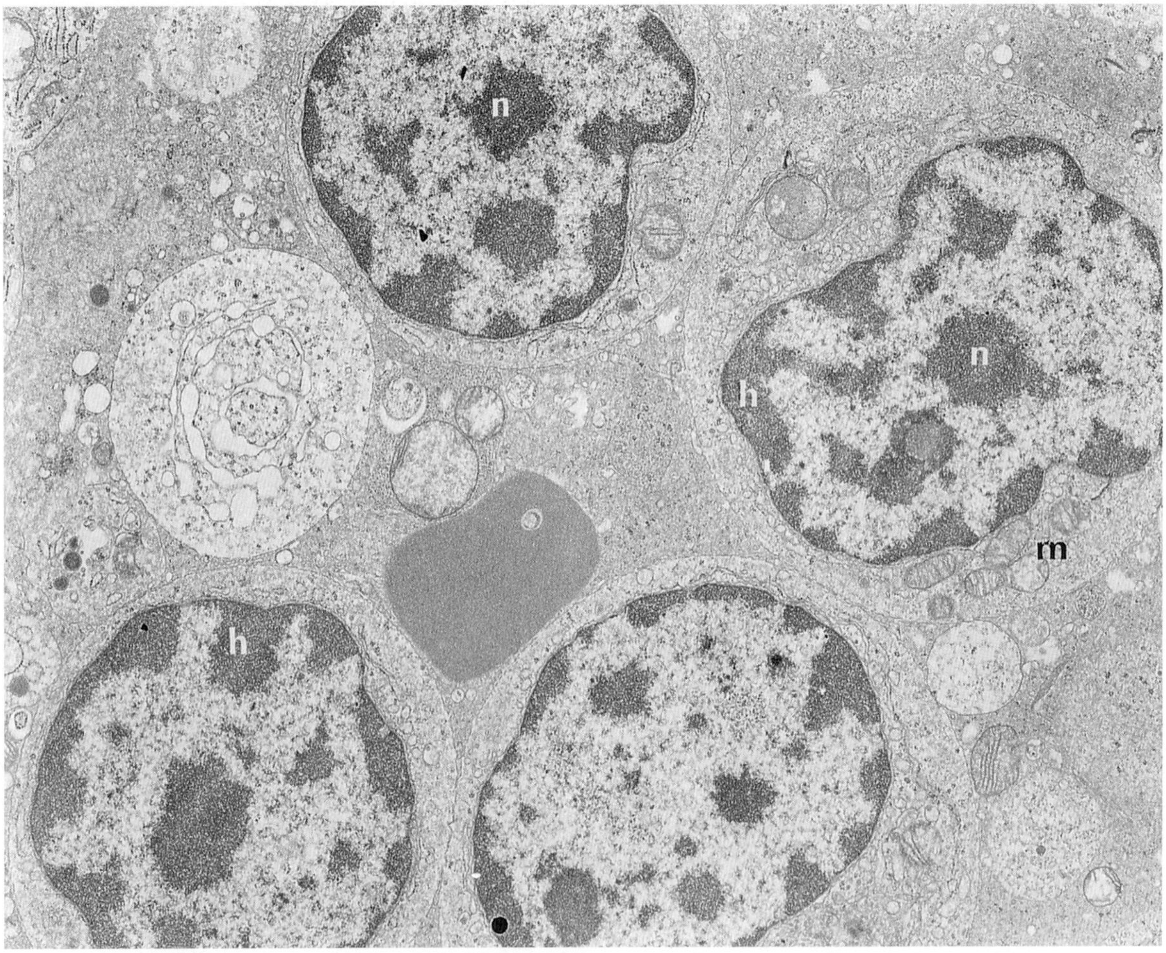

FIGURE 60.3. Cells of B-cell chronic lymphocytic leukemia/small lymphocytic lymphoma with scarce cytoplasm. Few polar mitochondria (*m*) and round, noncleaved nuclei with heterochromatin (*h*) and multiple nucleoli (*n*). ×10,200.

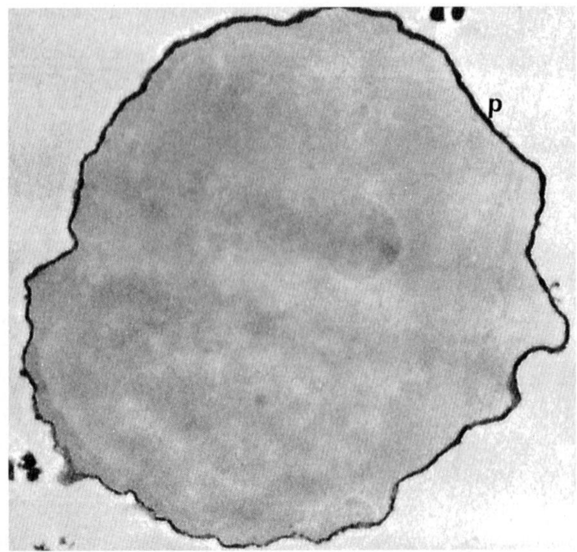

FIGURE 60.4. Cell of B-cell chronic lymphocytic leukemia/small lymphocytic lymphoma showing membrane deposits of peroxidase (*p*), indicating the presence of surface immunoglobulin M (IgM). Immunoelectron microscopy with peroxidase-labeled anti-human IgM serum. ×12,000.

morphologically, immunologically (except for CD5 expression), and clinically corresponds to CLL should be called *CD5− CLL variant* (34).

IMMUNOHISTOCHEMISTRY

Studies of B-CLL/SLL, particularly on frozen tissue sections with panels of monoclonal antibodies, show that all cases express monotypic Igs (Fig. 60.4); the HLA-DR (Ia) class II histocompatibility antigen; B-cell antigens CD19, CD20, and CD23; and CD5, a marker usually expressed by normal T-cells (35,36) (see Chapter 6). The "pseudofollicular proliferation centers" stain for the transferrin receptor, an activation marker, and Ki-67, a nuclear antigen associated with proliferating cells (35,36). The immune architecture of "pseudofollicles" resembles that of "true follicles" because both contain three follicle-defining cell types: B-cells, T-cells, and follicular dendritic reticulum cells (DRCs). In "pseudofollicles," some of the B-cells are mitotically active, the T-cells are more concentrated than in the surrounding small lymphocytic infiltrate, and the follicular DRC meshwork is attenuated (37–39). Follicular DRCs associated with "pseudofollicles" probably do not derive from preexisting germinal centers (37).

In paraffin sections, B-CLL/SLL is usually positive for the following markers: CD5, CD23 (most), and CD43 (most) (40). Markers for which negativity is important include CD10 and cyclin D1 (bcl-1 protein) (40). The detection of CD5 in tissue sections can be enhanced by using a biotinylated tyramide amplification method (41) or newer antibodies (42). Expression of the low-affinity IgE Fc receptor discriminates B-CLL/SLL, which is CD23+, from mantle cell lymphoma (MCL), which is CD23− (43). In addition, persistent CD23 expression separates CD23+ B-CLL/SLL blastic transformation from CD23− MCL blastic transformation in nearly all cases (43,44). Both B-CLL/SLL and MCL tend to express CD5 and CD43, but follicular lymphoma and marginal zone lymphoma generally do not (45).

The T-cells in B-CLL/SLL sometimes congregate near the "pseudofollicles" (38) but usually appear scattered (38,45). In contrast, the T-cells in MCL tend to localize around the B-cell nodules (45).

Phenotype

CD5+
CD10−
CD19+
CD20+ (dim)
CD22+ (dim)
CD23+
CD43+
CD79a+
Monoclonal surface Ig+ (dim)
FMC7−

CYTOGENETICS

The cytogenetic features of B-CLL/SLL that may be associated with adverse clinical outcome include the following: structural abnormalities of 11q22–23, 13q14, and 14q32 and trisomy 12 (46–48). In addition, deletion of 6q23–24 occurs in B-CLL/SLL and many other malignant lymphomas (49). The incidence of trisomy 12 is greater in patients with atypical CLL with CLL/PL morphology, stronger expression of surface Ig and FMC7, advanced stage, and possibly worse prognosis (50). Aberrations of p53 (tumor suppressor localized to 17p) predict a worse prognosis in CLL/PL but do not occur with trisomy 12 (51). Complex rearrangements and 17p translocations with various chromosomal partners are frequent in chronic B-lymphoid disorders (52).

The "paraimmunoblastic variant of small lymphocytic lymphoma" frequently carries t(11;14)(q13;q32), yielding a bcl-1/IgH fusion gene. Because this chromosomal translocation is characteristic of MCL, the "paraimmunoblastic variant of SLL" and MCL may represent variants of the same disease (53,54).

MOLECULAR DIAGNOSIS

Two separate maturational stages give rise to B-CLL cells; based on the mutational status of the IgH V gene, cases of B-CLL can be classified as unmutated, probably arising from pregerminal center naïve B lymphocytes, and mutated, likely originating from postgerminal center "memory" B-cells (55). A high level of CD38 expression may be a useful surrogate marker for unmutated IgH V genes, which predict a poor chemotherapeutic response and shorter survival (56).

DIFFERENTIAL DIAGNOSIS

- Lymphoplasmacytic lymphoma: Plasmacytoid cells and plasma cells are present; periodic acid-Schiff staining may identify Dutcher bodies and Russell bodies. Monoclonal gammopathy frequently associated.
- FL: The neoplastic nodules are sharply circumscribed and the component cells have angulated, cleaved shapes; absence of "pseudofollicles"; bright staining of surface Ig; CD5−, CD10+, CD43−.
- MCL: Cell population is composed of round to slightly irregular small lymphocytes in a mantle zone; vaguely nodular or diffuse pattern; no "pseudofollicular proliferation centers," although some atrophic germinal centers may be present; many cycling cells; CD23−, cyclin D1 (bcl-1 protein)+.
- Precursor lymphoblastic lymphoma: Patients are young. Cells are medium-sized, nuclei round or convoluted with fine and delicate chromatin, numerous mitoses. T-cell markers are present in most cases.
- Lymphocyte predominance Hodgkin lymphoma: The lymphocytic background may be similar; however, polyploid lymphocytic/histiocytic variants ("popcorn" cells) are present. The lymphocytic/histiocytic cells are CD20+. Patients with Hodgkin lymphoma are generally younger. Monoclonality supports the diagnosis of B-CLL/SLL.

Checklist

SMALL LYMPHOCYTIC LYMPHOMA

Elderly patients
More frequent in men (2.5:1)
Generalized lymphadenopathy
Bone marrow commonly involved
Hepatic, splenic involvement in late stages
Monoclonal gammopathy occasionally associated
Lymph node architecture effaced
Sinuses obliterated, perinodal infiltration
Diffuse cellular proliferation
Monomorphic cell population
Small, mature, inactive lymphocytes
Small, round nuclei
Rare mitoses
"Pseudofollicular proliferation centers" with activated lymphocytes
B-cell phenotype
Monoclonal surface Igs (low density)
CD5+, CD10−, CD19+, CD20+, CD23+, FMC7−
bcl-1 protein−, bcl-2 protein+
Low grade
Long survival (median, 8 years)
Conversion to high-grade large cell lymphoma (Richter syndrome) in 3% of cases

REFERENCES

1. Pangalis GA, Nathwani BN, Rappaport H. Malignant lymphoma, well-differentiated lymphocytic: its relationship with chronic lymphocytic leukemia and macroglobulinemia of Waldenstrom. Cancer 1977;39:999–1010.
2. Evans HL, Butler JJ, Youness EL. Malignant lymphoma, small lymphocytic type: a clinicopathologic study of 84 cases with suggested criteria for intermediate lymphocytic lymphoma. Cancer 1978;41:1440–1455.
3. Ries L, Miller B, Hankey B, et al. SEER cancer statistics review 1973–1991: tables and graphs. NIH publication No. 94-2789. Bethesda, MD: National Cancer Institute, National Institutes of Health, 1994.
4. Rai KR. Chronic lymphocytic leukemia in the elderly population. Clin Geriatr Med 1997;13:245.
5. Montserrat E, Gomis F, Vallespi T, et al. Presenting features and prognosis of chronic lymphocytic leukemia in younger adults [see Comments]. Blood 1991;78:1545–1551.
6. Mandelli F, De Rossi G, Mancini P, et al. Prognosis in chronic lymphocytic leukemia: a retrospective multicentric study from the GIMEMA group. J Clin Oncol 1987;5:398–406.
7. Catovsky D, Fooks J, Richards S. Prognostic factors in chronic lymphocytic leukaemia: the importance of age, sex and response to treatment in survival. A report from the MRC CLL 1 Trial. MRC Working Party on Leukaemia in Adults. Br J Haematol 1989;72:141–149.
8. Gale RP, Foon KA. Chronic lymphocytic leukemia. Recent advances in biology and treatment. Ann Intern Med 1985;103: 101–120.
9. Rai K, Patel D. Chronic lymphocytic leukemia. In: Hoffman R, Benz E, Shattil S, et al., eds. Hematology: basic principles and practice. New York: Churchill Livingstone, 1995:1308.
10. Kamihara S, Hirakata Y, Atogami S, et al. CD5-expressing B-cell lymphomas/leukemias: relatively high frequency of CD5+ B-cell lymphomas with an overall poor prognosis in Nagasaki Japan. Leuk Lymphoma 1996;22:137–142.
11. Bevan S, Catovsky D, Marossy A, et al. Linkage analysis for ATM in familial B cell chronic lymphocytic leukaemia. Leukemia 1999;13:1497–1500.
12. Yuille MR, Houlston RS, Catovsky D. Anticipation in familial chronic lymphocytic leukaemia. Leukemia 1998;12:1696–1698.
13. Sakai A, Marti GE, Caporaso N, et al. Analysis of expressed immunoglobulin heavy chain genes in familial B-CLL. Blood 2000; 95:1413–1419.
14. Harris NL, Jaffe ES, Diebold J, et al. The World Health Organization classification of hematological malignancies: report of the clinical advisory committee meeting, Airlie House, Virginia, November 1997. Mod Pathol 2000;13:193–207.
15. Cheson BD, Bennett JM, Grever M, et al. National Cancer Institute-sponsored Working Group guidelines for chronic lymphocytic leukemia: revised guidelines for diagnosis and treatment. Blood 1996;87:4990–4997.
16. Dick FR. Small lymphocytic malignancies and related immunoproliferative disorders. In: Jaffe ES, ed. Surgical pathology of the lymph nodes and related organs. Philadelphia: WB Saunders, 1985:146–164.
17. Bennett JM, Catovsky D, Daniel MT, et al. Proposals for the classification of chronic (mature) B and T lymphoid leukaemias. French–American–British (FAB) Cooperative Group. J Clin Pathol 1989;42:567–584.

18. Pileri SA, Milani M, Fraternali-Orcioni G, et al. From the R.E.A.L. classification to the upcoming WHO scheme: a step toward universal categorization of lymphoma entities? Ann Oncol 1998;9:607–612.
19. Huang JC, Finn WG, Goolsby CL, et al. CD5− small B-cell leukemias are rarely classifiable as chronic lymphocytic leukemia. Am J Clin Pathol 1999;111:123–130.
20. Pangalis GA, Angelopoulou MK, Vassilakopoulos TP, et al. B-chronic lymphocytic leukemia, small lymphocytic lymphoma, and lymphoplasmacytic lymphoma, including Waldenström's macroglobulinemia: a clinical, morphologic, and biologic spectrum of similar disorders. Semin Hematol 1999;36:104–114.
21. Zengin N, Kars A, Sungur A, et al. The significance of the bone marrow biopsy pattern in chronic lymphocytic leukemia: a prognostic dilemma. Am J Hematol 1999;62:208–211.
22. A clinical evaluation of the International Lymphoma Study Group classification of non-Hodgkin's lymphoma. The Non-Hodgkin's Lymphoma Classification Project. Blood 1997;89:3909–3918.
23. Robertson LE, Pugh W, O'Brien S, et al. Richter's syndrome: a report on 39 patients. J Clin Oncol 1993;11:1985–1989.
24. Lukes RJ, Collins RD. Tumors of the hematopoietic system. Washington, DC: Armed Forces Institute of Pathology, 1992: series II, fascicle 28.
25. Fayad L, Robertson LE, O'Brien S, et al. Hodgkin's disease variant of Richter's syndrome: experience at a single institution. Leuk Lymphoma 1996;23:333–337.
26. Ohno T, Smir BN, Weisenburger DD, et al. Origin of the Hodgkin/Reed-Sternberg cells in chronic lymphocytic leukemia with "Hodgkin's transformation." Blood 1998;91:1757–1761.
27. Shields DJ, Byrd JC, Abbondanzo SL, et al. Detection of Epstein-Barr virus in transformations of low-grade B-cell lymphomas after fludarabine treatment. Mod Pathol 1997;10:1151–1159.
28. Dick FR, Maca RD. The lymph node in chronic lymphocytic leukemia. Cancer 1978;41:283–292.
29. Lennert K, Mohri N, Stein H, et al. The histopathology of malignant lymphomas. Br J Haematol 1975;31[Suppl]:193–203.
30. Bonato M, Pittaluga S, Tierens A, et al. Lymph node histology in typical and atypical chronic lymphocytic leukemia. Am J Surg Pathol 1998;22:49–56.
31. Ben-Ezra J, Burke JS, Swartz WG, et al. Small lymphocytic lymphoma: a clinicopathologic analysis of 268 cases. Blood 1989;73:579–587.
32. Aisenberg AC, Bloch KJ. Immunoglobulins on the surface of neoplastic lymphocytes. N Engl J Med 1972;287:272–276.
33. Thompson AA, Talley JA, Do HN, et al. Aberrations of the B-cell receptor B29 (CD79b) gene in chronic lymphocytic leukemia. Blood 1997;90:1387–1394.
34. Shapiro JL, Miller ML, Pohlman B, et al. CD5− B-cell lymphoproliferative disorders presenting in blood and bone marrow. A clinicopathologic study of 40 patients. Am J Clin Pathol 1999;111:477–487.
35. Spier CM, Grogan TM, Fielder K, et al. Immunophenotypes in "well-differentiated" lymphoproliferative disorders, with emphasis on small lymphocytic lymphoma. Hum Pathol 1986;17:1126–1136.
36. Medeiros LJ, Strickler JG, Picker LJ, et al. "Well-differentiated" lymphocytic neoplasms. Immunologic findings correlated with clinical presentation and morphologic features. Am J Pathol 1987;129:523–535.
37. Mori N, Oka K, Kojima M. DRC antigen expression in B-cell lymphomas. Am J Clin Pathol 1988;89:488–492.
38. Ratech H, Sheibani K, Nathwani BN, et al. Immunoarchitecture of the "pseudofollicles" of well-differentiated (small) lymphocytic lymphoma: a comparison with true follicles [published erratum appears in Hum Pathol 1988;19:495]. Hum Pathol 1988;19:89–94.
39. Schmid C, Isaacson PG. Proliferation centres in B-cell malignant lymphoma, lymphocytic (B-CLL): an immunohistochemical study. Histopathology 1994;24:445–451.
40. Swerdlow SH. Small B-cell lymphomas of the lymph nodes and spleen: practical insights to diagnosis and pathogenesis. Mod Pathol 1998;12:125–140.
41. Luo JH, Matsushima AY, Chen R, et al. Detection of CD5 antigen on B cell lymphomas in fixed, paraffin-embedded tissues using signal amplification by catalyzed reporter deposition. Eur J Histochem 1998;42:31–39.
42. Dorfman DM, Shahsafaei A. Usefulness of a new CD5 antibody for the diagnosis of T-cell and B-cell lymphoproliferative disorders in paraffin sections. Mod Pathol 1997;10:859–863.
43. Kumar S, Green GA, Teruya-Feldstein J, et al. Use of CD23 (BU38) on paraffin sections in the diagnosis of small lymphocytic lymphoma and mantle cell lymphoma. Mod Pathol 1996;9:925–929.
44. Dunphy CH, Wheaton SE, Perkins SL. CD23 expression in transformed small lymphocytic lymphomas/chronic lymphocytic leukemias and blastic transformations of mantle cell lymphoma. Mod Pathol 1997;10:818–822.
45. Singh N, Wright DH. The value of immunohistochemistry on paraffin wax-embedded tissue sections in the differentiation of small lymphocytic and mantle cell lymphomas. J Clin Pathol 1997;50:16–21.
46. Raghoebier S, Kibbelaar RE, Kleiverda JK, et al. Mosaicism of trisomy 12 in chronic lymphocytic leukemia detected by non-radioactive *in situ* hybridization. Leukemia 1992;6:1220–1226.
47. Stilgenbauer S, Dohner H, Bulgay-Morschel M, et al. High frequency of monoallelic retinoblastoma gene deletion in B-cell chronic lymphoid leukemia shown by interphase cytogenetics. Blood 1993;81:2118–2124.
48. Dohner H, Stilgenbauer S, James MR, et al. 11q deletions identify a new subset of B-cell chronic lymphocytic leukemia characterized by extensive nodal involvement and inferior prognosis. Blood 1997;89:2516–2522.
49. Zhang Y, Weber-Matthiesen K, Siebert R, et al. Frequent deletions of 6q23–24 in B-cell non-Hodgkin's lymphomas detected by fluorescence *in situ* hybridization. Genes Chromosomes Cancer 1997;18:310–313.
50. Matutes E, Oscier D, Garcia-Marco J, et al. Trisomy 12 defines a group of CLL with atypical morphology: correlation between cytogenetic, clinical and laboratory features in 544 patients. Br J Haematol 1996;92:382–388.
51. Lens D, Dyer MJ, Garcia-Marco JM, et al. p53 abnormalities in CLL are associated with excess of prolymphocytes and poor prognosis. Br J Haematol 1997;99:848–857.
52. Callet-Bauchu E, Salles G, Gazzo S, et al. Translocations involving the short arm of chromosome 17 in chronic B-lymphoid disorders: frequent occurrence of dicentric rearrangements and possible association with adverse outcome. Leukemia 1999;13:460–468.
53. Pugh WC, Manning JT, Butler JJ. Paraimmunoblastic variant of small lymphocytic lymphoma/leukemia. Am J Surg Pathol 1988;12:907–917.
54. Grosso LE, Kelley PD. bcl-1 translocations are frequent in the paraimmunoblastic variant of small lymphocytic lymphoma. Mod Pathol 1998;11:6–10.
55. Naylor M, Capra JD. Mutational status of Ig V(H) genes provides clinically valuable information in B-cell chronic lymphocytic leukemia [Comment]. Blood 1999;94:1837–1839.
56. Damle RN, Wasil T, Fais F, et al. Ig V gene mutation status and CD38 expression as novel prognostic indicators in chronic lymphocytic leukemia [see Comments]. Blood 1999;94:1840–1847.

61

LYMPHOPLASMACYTIC LYMPHOMA

DEFINITION

Lymphoplasmacytic lymphoma (LPL) is a usually CD5−, small cell lymphoma of B-cell origin with plasmacytic differentiation that cannot be classified as any other lymphoma type. LPL expresses surface membrane and cytoplasmic immunoglobulin (Ig), which is often secreted as a monoclonal paraprotein. When LPL produces large amounts of monoclonal IgM detectable in the serum, it is associated with Waldenström macroglobulinemia (WM).

SYNONYMS

Immunocytoma

Malignant lymphoma, small lymphocytic, plasmacytoid (A) (Working Formulation)

Lymphoplasmacytic/lymphoplasmacytoid lymphoma (Kiel) (1)

Lymphoplasmacytic lymphoma (World Health Organization)

CLINICAL SYNDROME

Lymphoplasmacytic lymphoma and B-cell chronic lymphocytic leukemia/small lymphocytic lymphoma (B-CLL/SLL) have a similar age distribution, predominantly affecting elderly persons. The median age of patients with LPL is 63 years, and men are affected slightly more frequently than women (2,3). Depending on anatomic localization, extent of disease, and amount of Ig secreted, a wide clinical spectrum may result: (a) widely disseminated disease in lymph nodes, bone marrow, or both (4); (b) infrequent peripheral blood involvement with cell counts lower than those in B-CLL/SLL ($<4 \times 10^9$/L) (5); (c) complications of paraproteinemia (6); association with hepatitis C virus infection and mixed cryoglobulinemia (7,8).

About 60% of patients with LPL have mild lymphocytosis with circulating small lymphocytes and lymphoplasmacytoid cells (1,2,5). Paraproteinemia, in the form of a monoclonal increase in Ig levels, is seen in 36% of patients (9), usually IgM (Fig. 61.1), occasionally IgG, and rarely IgA, IgE, or light chains or heavy chains only (heavy chain disease) (1).

Lymphoplasmacytic lymphoma is frequently associated with WM. In approximately 15% of patients with WM, levels of monoclonal IgM above 3.0 g/dL are associated with hyperviscosity syndrome (6): a high erythrocyte sedimentation rate with rouleaux formation in the blood, visual disturbances resulting from blockage of retinal vessels, Raynaud phenomenon, and various symptoms caused by venous thrombosis in other organs. Patients also experience dizziness, bleeding from mucous membranes, fatigue, weight loss, anemia, and repeated pulmonary infections.

Earlier reports indicated that LPL developed in patients with long-standing autoimmune disease, Sjögren syndrome, or Hashimoto thyroiditis (1,10). It is possible that these cases were called LPL because of the presence of monoclonal plasma cells, but they might have been classified as marginal zone lymphoma in modern nomenclature.

The overall 5-year survival for LPL is 59% (3). Like other small B-cell lymphomas, LPL may undergo the blastic transformation known as *Richter syndrome* (1) (see Chapter 60). The result is usually a diffuse large B-cell lymphoma or a high-grade immunoblastic lymphoma. As in the original B-cell lymphoma, the surface Ig markers are in most cases identical to the monoclonal serum Ig (11,12).

HISTOPATHOLOGY

The lymph nodes are only moderately enlarged (average size, 9 × 13 mm) (13), but lymphoid infiltration of the capsule and perinodal fibrofatty tissues is usually present (Fig. 61.2). The architecture is effaced by a diffuse proliferation of uniform small lymphoid cells that replace all structures except a few peripheral follicles and the lymph node sinuses. Proliferation centers, such as those in B-CLL/SLL, are not seen in LPL (1,9). Despite the extensive cellular infiltration, silver staining shows a fairly well-preserved reticulin framework (13). Blood vessels and sinuses are prominent, and sometimes sinuses appear cavernously dilated. This is particularly evident with the periodic acid-Schiff (PAS) stain

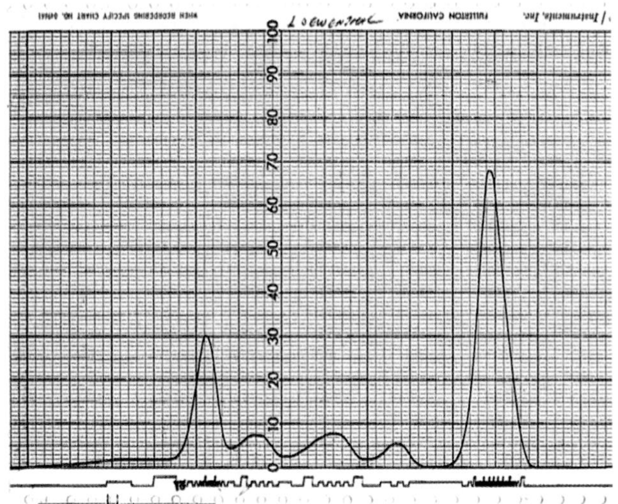

FIGURE 61.1. Monoclonal immunoglobulin M spike in serum of patient with lymphoplasmacytic lymphoma and Waldenström macroglobulinemia.

(14) because of the large amount of hexose-rich IgM in the serum (15). The staining of other Ig classes is paler because they are relatively poor in carbohydrate. Hemosiderin is common, especially in sinuses, and mast cells can be numerous (1,9).

The cellular infiltrate comprises small mature lymphocytes, plasmacytoid lymphocytes, and occasional mature plasma cells. Mitoses are infrequent (Fig. 61.3). The plasmacytoid lymphocyte (Fig. 61.3), a transitional cell form between a lymphocyte and a plasma cell, has a nucleus slightly larger than that of a lymphocyte with dispersed chromatin and ample PAS-positive cytoplasm. The typical cartwheel nuclei and paranuclear clear region (Golgi zone, hof) of plasma cells are lacking (16). The characteristic feature of LPL is the presence of intracellular inclusions (Fig. 61.4). These are round, strongly PAS-positive globules located in the cytoplasm, where they are called *Russell bodies,* or the nucleus, where they are referred to as *Dutcher bodies.* In a series of 78 biopsies of WM, intranuclear, PAS-positive inclusions were present in 77.5% (17). Russell bodies or amorphous paraprotein masses deposit between the tumor cells, on occasion inducing the formation of a few foreign body giant cells. Some LPLs contain abundant epithelioid histiocytes that can be confused with other types of lymphoma or with sarcoidosis (18,19).

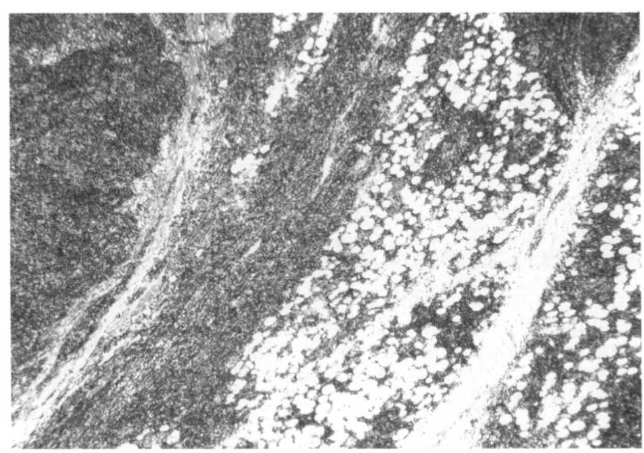

FIGURE 61.2. Lymphoplasmacytic lymphoma diffusely infiltrating lymph node parenchyma, capsule, and perinodal adipose tissue. Hematoxylin and eosin stain.

It is easier to recognize basophilic lymphoplasmacytoid cells in lymph node touch imprints stained with Giemsa than in tissue sections stained with hematoxylin and eosin. Giemsa or methyl green pyronin enhances their visibility by highlighting RNA-rich cytoplasm (1). Alternatively, immunohistochemical staining to demonstrate cytoplasmic Ig in tissue sections reliably reveals lymphoplasmacytoid cells in paraffin-embedded tissue sections (1).

Usually, transformed lymphocytes are scarce in LPL. Numerous immunoblasts indicate an increased proliferation rate. These cases have been called *LPL with a high content of blast cells* (1) or designated as *large cell-rich immunocytoma* (20) because the polymorphic LPL subtype has been discarded in the updated Kiel classification (1). Increased numbers of transformed lymphocytes predict a more aggressive clinical course.

CYTOCHEMISTRY

Cytochemically, the inclusions stained by PAS are not decolorized by diastase treatment, which indicates that they are composed of neutral polysaccharides and do not contain glycogen (17). The occurrence of nuclear inclusions is not specific for WM; similar intracytoplasmic and intranuclear bodies have been observed in various lymphomas (with or without dysproteinemia), multiple myeloma, and even immunoblastic lymphadenopathy (21). The histologic differences between monoclonal gammopathies of different Ig classes are not appreciable (21).

ELECTRON MICROSCOPY

Electron microscopy (Fig. 61.5) shows that the nuclear inclusions are membrane-bound, representing a dilation of the perinuclear cisterna or an intranuclear invagination of distended endoplasmic reticulum (17,22). The contents in both are a flocculent accumulation of Ig. Multiple inclusions can be present in a nucleus, which appears greatly distorted by their large number (Fig. 61.5). Although in most cases the distended cisterna filled with accumulated Ig is only invaginated into the nucleus, the inclusion body occasionally finally breaks its connection and become truly intranuclear (23).

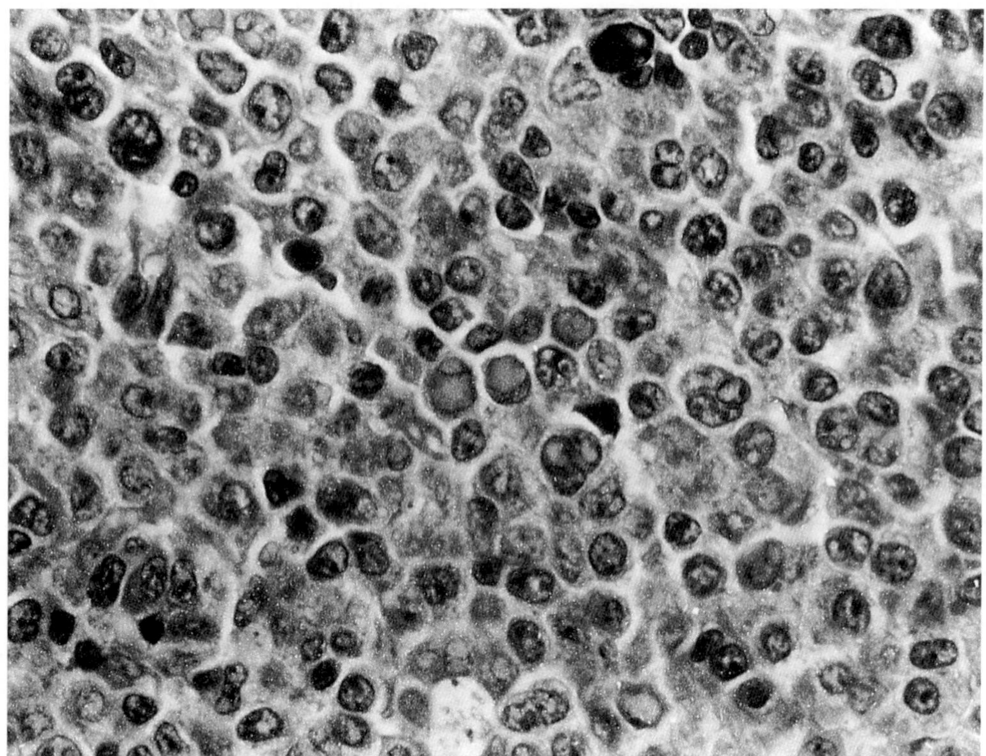

FIGURE 61.3. Lymphoplasmacytic lymphoma. Lymph node architecture effaced by diffuse proliferation of lymphocytes and plasmacytoid lymphocytes, some with intracytoplasmic and intranuclear inclusions (Dutcher bodies, *center*). Hematoxylin, phloxine, and saffron stain.

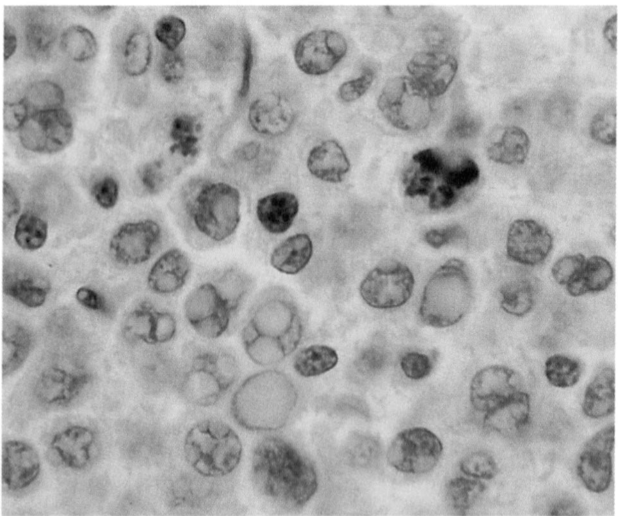

FIGURE 61.4. Lymphoplasmacytic lymphoma in inguinal lymph node and Waldenström macroglobulinemia. Numerous lymphoplasmacytoid lymphocytes with intracytoplasmic Russell bodies and intranuclear Dutcher bodies. Hematoxylin, phloxine, and saffron stain.

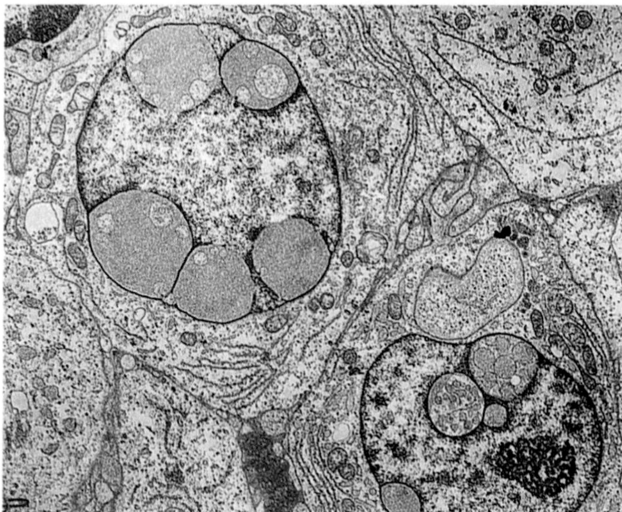

FIGURE 61.5. Two lymphoplasmacytoid lymphocytes with well-developed endoplasmic reticulum and intranuclear invaginations of perinuclear cisternae filled with immunoglobulin M (Dutcher bodies). One lymphoma cell (*right*) has a prominent reticulated nucleolus. ×8,600.

IMMUNOPATHOLOGY

Monoclonal Ig spikes detected on serum or urine electrophoresis usually indicate the presence of lymphoma, particularly LPL, WM, or multiple myeloma (Fig. 61.1). In one study of 1,682 patients, IgM spikes occurred in 4.5% of diffuse lymphomas, a prevalence 100 times greater than that observed in cancer-free control subjects or patients with other types of tumors (23). In the same study, 2.3% of patients with lymphomas and leukemias had an IgG spike (23). Both κ and λ Ig light chains may be associated with the monoclonal IgM of lymphomas; however, κ is present about twice as frequently as λ (23). On occasion, cryoglobulins, cold agglutinins, or both are associated with the 19S IgM of LPL.

IMMUNOHISTOCHEMISTRY

Plasmacytoid lymphocytes are intermediate between lymphocytes, which have high levels of surface Igs, and plasma cells, which have none (16). The monoclonality of membrane Igs in support of a diagnosis of B-cell lymphoma is best demonstrated on frozen sections. In the case of plasmacytoid lymphoma, because cytoplasmic Igs are present in addition to membrane Igs, paraffin-embedded sections can also be used with satisfactory results (1). When the immunoperoxidase method was used, cytoplasmic monoclonal Igs were detected in 93% of cases in one study (24), showing good correlation with serum immunoelectrophoresis findings. Whenever a monoclonal Ig was demonstrable in the lymph node sections, 30% to 85% of the cells were positive, and the intracytoplasmic Ig was easily recognized under light microscopy. The monoclonal intracytoplasmic Igs are revealed equally well in frozen sections immunostained with fluorescein isothiocyanate (FITC)-labeled antibodies and examined under the fluorescent microscope (Fig. 61.6), and in paraffin-embedded sections immunostained with peroxidase-labeled antibodies and examined under the light microscope (Fig. 61.7).

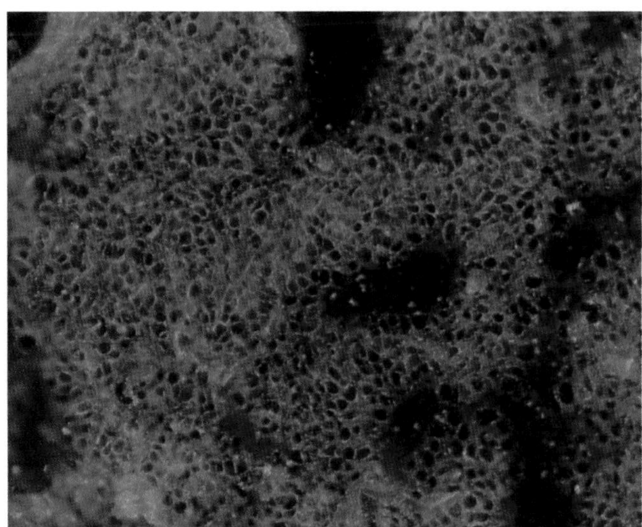

FIGURE 61.6. Lymph node in Waldenström macroglobulinemia shows abundant intracytoplasmic immunoglobulin M after staining with fluorescein-labeled antihuman immunoglobulin M. Immunofluorescence.

Phenotype

CD5−/+
CD10−
CD19+
CD20+
CD23−
CD43−/+
CD79a+
CD103−
Monoclonal surface and cytoplasmic IgM+
IgD−
HLA-DR+

The majority of LPLs stain with antibodies to the pan-B-cell markers CD19 and CD20, surface and cytoplasmic IgM, and HLA-DR; they do not express CD5, CD10, CD23, or IgD (25–28).

CYTOGENETICS

Approximately half of LPLs have a t(9;14)(p13;q32) chromosomal translocation as the sole aberration (29). Other translocations involving 9p13 and multiple other loci occur (30). Rare cases of WM have t(8;14)(q24:q32) with trisomy 3 (31) or bcl-2 rearrangements simultaneously involving variant cluster region (vcr) and major breakpoint region (mbr) breakpoints (32).

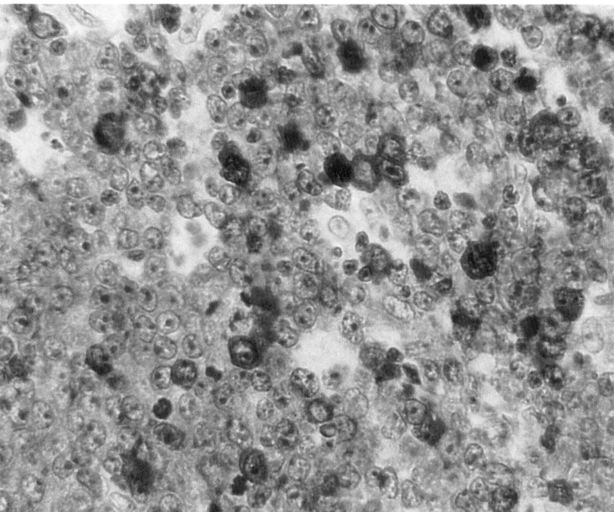

FIGURE 61.7. Lymphoplasmacytic lymphoma in cervical lymph node showing membrane and intracytoplasmic λ light chain immunoglobulin. Immunoperoxidase stain.

Checklist

LYMPHOPLASMACYTIC LYMPHOMA

Patients elderly (mean age, 63 years)
Lymph nodes moderately enlarged
Architecture effaced
Reticulin pattern preserved
Few or no follicles and germinal centers
Sinuses patent
Capsule and perinodal fat infiltrated
Diffuse cellular proliferation
Polymorphic cell population
Small, mature lymphocytes
Plasmacytoid lymphocytes, plasma cells
Infrequent mitoses
B-cell surface markers
Cytoplasmic monoclonal Igs
Dutcher bodies, Russell bodies
Darkly staining plasma in blood vessels
Monoclonal spike on electrophoresis, usually IgM
Associated with WM

MOLECULAR DIAGNOSIS

The t(9;14)(p13;q32) chromosomal translocation juxtaposes the PAX5 gene (9p13) and the immunoglobulin heavy chain (IgH) locus (14q32) in the opposite direction to transcription (33). PAX5, also called *B-cell lineage specific activator protein* (BSAP) (34), is a transcription factor specific to B cells that is involved in the proliferation and differentiation of pro-B cells, pre-B cells, and mature B cells, but not plasma cells (35). The PAX5 gene was identified in breakpoints involving LPL, α heavy chain disease, and a large cell lymphoma cell line (33). Because the breakpoints map to 5′ noncoding regions, the complete protein-coding portion of PAX5 is transcribed at increased levels, which can down-regulate p53 (33,35). Fluorescence *in situ* hybridization with a YAC clone containing PAX5 successfully identifies PAX5 rearrangements that are too dispersed to be detected by conventional Southern analysis (33).

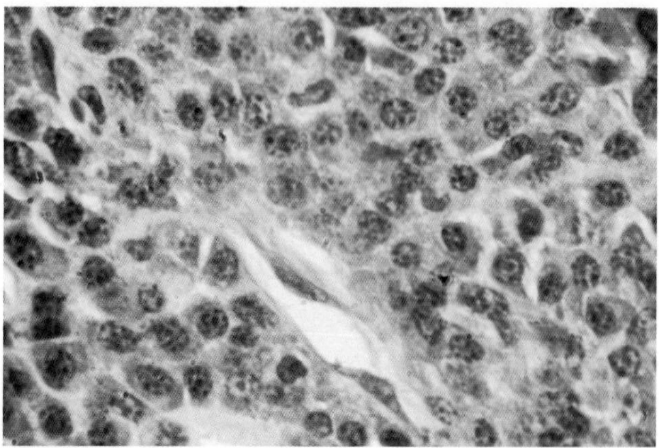

FIGURE 61.8. Plasmacytoma with sheets of monotonous, well-differentiated plasma cells. Some are binucleated.

DIFFERENTIAL DIAGNOSIS

- B-CLL/SLL: Most frequently considered in the differential diagnosis. Lacks the following features: intracytoplasmic Igs, Dutcher bodies, serum Ig spikes, plasmacytoid cells and plasma cells.
- Follicular lymphoma: Lacks plasmacytoid features and secretion of Igs (as above).
- Hairy cell leukemia: Lacks plasmacytoid features. Typical cells with reniform to oval nuclei and clear cytoplasm.
- Sézary syndrome: Infiltration of T-cell regions, T-cell markers, lack of plasmacytoid features.
- Hodgkin lymphoma, lymphocyte predominance: Contains Reed-Sternberg cells of lymphocytic/histiocytic type. No plasmacytoid cell features.
- Plasmacytoma (Fig. 61.8), multiple myeloma: Component cells are larger, often binucleated or with pleomorphic nuclei; monoclonal IgG more frequent than IgM; Bence Jones light chains and osteolytic lesions in multiple myeloma.

- Diffuse lymphoid hyperplasia: Sinuses not obliterated but evenly dilated and filled with lymphocytes. No predominance of B cells, as in plasmacytoid lymphomas.
- Sarcoidosis: Plasma cells are polyclonal. Distinguish from LPL with a high content of epithelioid histiocytes.

REFERENCES

1. Lennert K, Feller AC. Lymphoplasmacytic/lymphoplasmacytoid lymphoma (immunocytoma). Histopathology of non-Hodgkin's lymphomas (based on the updated Kiel classification). Berlin: Springer-Verlag, 1992:64–75.
2. Engelhard M, Brittinger G, Heinz R, et al. Chronic lymphocytic leukemia (B-CLL) and immunocytoma (LP-IC): clinical and prognostic relevance of this distinction. Leuk Lymphoma 1991; [Suppl]:161–173.
3. A clinical evaluation of the International Lymphoma Study Group classification of non-Hodgkin's lymphoma. The Non-Hodgkin's Lymphoma Classification Project. Blood 1997;89: 3909–3918.
4. Papamichael D, Norton AJ, Foran JM, et al. Immunocytoma: a retrospective analysis from St. Bartholomew's Hospital—1972 to 1996. J Clin Oncol 1999;17:2847–2853.
5. Pangalis GA, Boussiotis VA, Kittas C. Malignant disorders of small lymphocytes. Small lymphocytic lymphoma, lymphoplasmacytic lymphoma, and chronic lymphocytic leukemia: their clinical and laboratory relationship. Am J Clin Pathol 1993;99: 402–408.
6. Dimopoulos MA, Alexanian R. Waldenström's macroglobulinemia. Blood 1994;83:1452–1459.
7. Silvestri F, Barillari G, Fanin R, et al. Hepatitis C virus infection among cryoglobulinemic and non-cryoglobulinemic B-cell non-Hodgkin's lymphomas. Haematologica 1997;82:314–317.
8. Vallisa D, Berte R, Rocca A, et al. Association between hepatitis C virus and non-Hodgkin's lymphoma, and effects of viral infection on histologic subtype and clinical course. Am J Med 1999; 106:556–560.
9. Lennert K, Tamm I, Wacker H-H. Histopathology and immunocytochemistry of lymph node biopsies in chronic lymphocytic leukemia and immunocytoma. Leuk Lymphoma 1991; [Suppl]:157–160.
10. Stansfeld AG. Non-Hodgkin's lymphomas: low grade B-cell lymphomas. In: Stansfeld AG, ed. Lymph node biopsy interpretation. New York: Churchill Livingstone, 1985:228–277.
11. Leonhard SA, Muhleman AF, Hurtubise PE, et al. Emergence of immunoblastic sarcoma in Waldenström's macroglobulinemia. Cancer 1980;45:3102–3107.
12. Abe M, Takahashi K, Mori N, et al. "Waldenström's macroglobulinemia" terminating in immunoblastic sarcoma. A case report. Cancer 1982;49:2580–2586.
13. Harrison CV. The morphology of the lymph node in the macroglobulinaemia of Waldenström. J Clin Pathol 1972;25:12–16.
14. Brunning RD, Parkin J. Intranuclear inclusions in plasma cells and lymphocytes from patients with monoclonal gammopathies. Am J Clin Pathol 1976;66:10–21.
15. Dutcher TF, Fahey JL. The histopathology of the macroglobulinemia of Waldenström. J Natl Cancer Inst 1959;22:887–917.
16. Lidonnici KR, Becker JL, Engellener W. Plasmacytoid lymphocytes in a peripheral blood smear. Lab Med 1992;23:789–792.
17. Diebold J, Reynes M, Kalifat R, et al. Intranuclear inclusions in Waldenström's disease. Their biological significance and diagnostic value [in French]. Nouv Presse Med 1974;3:1067–1070.
18. Patsouris E, Noel H, Lennert K. Lymphoplasmacytic/lymphoplasmacytoid immunocytoma with a high content of epithelioid cells. Histologic and immunohistochemical findings. Am J Surg Pathol 1990;14:660–670.
19. Karakantza M, Matutes E, MacLennan K, et al. Association between sarcoidosis and lymphoma revisited. J Clin Oncol 1996; 49:208–212.
20. Warnke RA. Morphologic, immunologic and genetic features of B cell CLL/SLL and immunocytoma. In: Mason D, Harris NL, eds. Human lymphoma: clinical implications of the REAL classification, vol 1. New York: Springer-Verlag, 1999.
21. Kim H, Heller P, Rappaport H. Monoclonal gammopathies associated with lymphoproliferative disorders: a morphologic study. Am J Clin Pathol 1973;59:282–294.
22. Ioachim HL. Lymph nodes and spleen. In: Johannessen JV, ed. Electron microscopy in human medicine, vol 5. New York: McGraw-Hill, 1981:384–464.
23. Alexanian R. Monoclonal gammopathy in lymphoma. Arch Intern Med 1975;135:62–66.
24. Pangalis GA, Nathwani BN, Rappaport H. Detection of cytoplasmic immunoglobulin in well-differentiated lymphoproliferative diseases by the immunoperoxidase method. Cancer 1980;45: 1334–1339.
25. Harris NL, Bhan AK. B-cell neoplasms of the lymphocytic, lymphoplasmacytoid, and plasma cell types: immunohistologic analysis and clinical correlation. Hum Pathol 1985;16:829–837.
26. Zukerberg LR, Medeiros LJ, Ferry JA, et al. Diffuse low-grade B-cell lymphomas. Four clinically distinct subtypes defined by a combination of morphologic and immunophenotypic features [see Comments]. Am J Clin Pathol 1993;100:373–385.
27. Huang JC, Finn WG, Goolsby CL, et al. CD5− small B-cell leukemias are rarely classifiable as chronic lymphocytic leukemia. Am J Clin Pathol 1999;111:123–130.
28. Shapiro JL, Miller ML, Pohlman B, et al. CD5− B-cell lymphoproliferative disorders presenting in blood and bone marrow. A clinicopathologic study of 40 patients. Am J Clin Pathol 1999; 111:477–487.
29. Offit K, Parsa NZ, Filippa D, et al. t(9;14)(p13;q32) denotes a subset of low-grade non-Hodgkin's lymphoma with plasmacytoid differentiation. Blood 1992;80:2594–2599.
30. Offit K, Parsa NZ, Jhanwar SC, et al. Clusters of chromosome 9 aberrations are associated with clinico-pathologic subsets of non-Hodgkin's lymphoma. Genes Chromosomes Cancer 1993;7:1–7.
31. Chong YY, Lau LC, Lui WO, et al. A case of t(8;14) with total and partial trisomy 3 in Waldenström macroglobulinemia. Cancer Genet Cytogenet 1998;103:65–67.
32. Merup M, Spasokoukotskaja T, Einhorn S, et al. Bcl-2 rearrangements with breakpoints in both vcr and mbr in non-Hodgkin's lymphomas and chronic lymphocytic leukaemia. Br J Haematol 1996;92:647–652.
33. Iida S, Rao PH, Nallasivam P, et al. The t(9;14)(p13;q32) chromosomal translocation associated with lymphoplasmacytoid lymphoma involves the PAX-5 gene. Blood 1996;88:4110–4117.
34. Adams B, Dorfler P, Aguzzi A, et al. Pax-5 encodes the transcription factor BSAP and is expressed in B lymphocytes, the developing CNS, and adult testis. Genes Dev 1992;6:1589–1607.
35. Barr FG. Chromosomal translocations involving paired box transcription factors in human cancer. Int J Biochem Cell Biol 1997; 29:1449–1461.

62

HAIRY CELL LEUKEMIA

DEFINITION

Chronic lymphoid neoplasm of mature B cells with characteristic cytoplasmic projections.

SYNONYM

Leukemic reticuloendotheliosis

PATHOGENESIS

In hairy cell leukemia (HCL), originally called *leukemic reticuloendotheliosis* (1,2), the characteristic hairy cells display elongated processes (filopodia) if observed via phase-contrast microscopy (3). The nonretractable cell surface projections may be explained by selective cytoskeletal union or by surplus manufacture of pp52 (LSP1), the F-actin–binding, leukocyte-specific phosphoprotein (4). An uncommon neoplasm, HCL accounts for only 2% of adult leukemias (5). Various cells of origin were suggested, including B cells, T cells, monocytes, reticulum cells, and cells with both lymphocytic and monocytic features. Clonally rearranged immunoglobulin (Ig) genes definitively proved a B-cell origin (6,7). HCL has a late maturation-stage B-cell phenotype (pre-plasma cell), frequently containing cytoplasmic Igs and expressing plasma cell antigens (8–10).

CLINICAL SYNDROME

Hairy cell leukemia is primarily a disease of middle-aged men, and no cases have been reported in children (10). In a recent survey based on 725 cases of the Italian Cooperative Group, the male-to-female ratio was 3.9:1, and the mean age was 54 years (range, 23 to 85 years) (11).

The disease runs a chronic course, similar to that of chronic lymphocytic leukemia, and the common presenting symptoms are fatigue, weakness, moderate weight loss, sometimes fever, and sometimes abdominal pain resulting from splenomegaly. The major physical findings are splenomegaly in 78% (2) to 90% (5) of patients, hepatomegaly in 50% (2), lymphadenopathy in 13% to 25% (11–13), and petechiae and ecchymoses in 33% (2). The spleen may reach massive proportions (up to 4,650 g; mean, 1,809 g) (5) and frequently contributes to the pancytopenia of these patients (hence the favorable results obtained by splenectomy). The bone marrow is commonly involved, and the replacement of hematopoietic cells by tightly attached hairy cells surrounded by increased reticulin fibers explains the dry taps commonly obtained at bone marrow aspiration, in addition to the severe anemia, leukopenia, and thrombocytopenia of patients with HCL. Some 10% to 25% of patients are asymptomatic. At diagnosis, an absence of palpable splenomegaly and circulating hairy cells is exceptional (<6%) (11).

In older series, the lymph nodes were involved at the time of diagnosis in about 25% of cases, when they appeared only slightly enlarged (12). Occasionally, however, massive lymphadenopathy was reported in HCL (12–14), sometimes after removal of the spleen (5,13,15) or during relapse, especially in the abdomen (15). More recently, the rate of initial lymph node involvement has been 5% to 8%, probably because of earlier diagnosis of HCL in the bone marrow (16,17). In a modern study, 85 of 634 patients (13%) had enlarged peripheral lymph nodes or abdominal lymph nodes detectable by computed tomography (11).

In an autopsy study of HCL, the internal lymph nodes, including retroperitoneal, abdominal, and mediastinal groups, were consistently involved, even without peripheral lymphadenopathy (18). The same study showed frequent infiltration of the lungs by hairy cells.

During the last 25 years, the number of patients with HCL who have marked anemia or massive splenomegaly and the presenting stage of disease has declined (11). Five-year survivals have been reported as follows: 34.4%, untreated; 58.8%, chemotherapy, steroids, or other drugs; 64.1%, splenectomized; 88.9%, interferon alfa (11). Purine analogues, 2′-deoxycoformycin and 2-chlorodeoxyadenosine, appear to be at least as effective as interferon alfa and cause less toxicity, and these are now the preferred drugs (19). Although splenectomy for HCL has been surpassed by

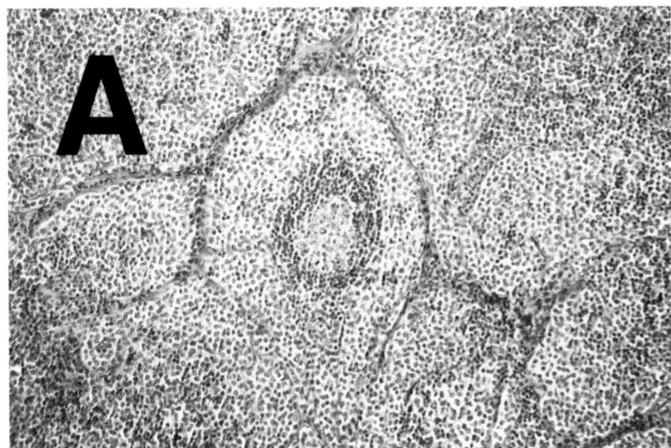

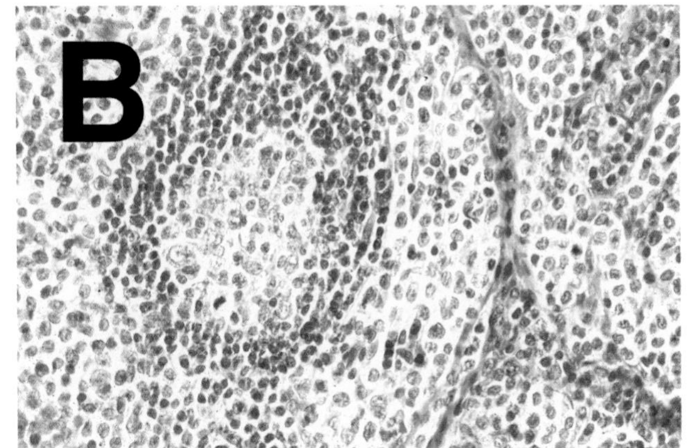

FIGURE 62.1. Lymph node with hairy cell leukemia. **A:** Architecture effaced by monotonous cell population with honeycomb ("fried egg") pattern. Residual island of non-neoplastic lymphocytes includes a thin mantle zone and germinal center. This pattern is nearly identical to that seen in nodal marginal zone B-cell lymphoma. **B:** Large cells with bland, oval nuclei and abundant clear cytoplasm. Hematoxylin and eosin stain. (Courtesy of Jerome S. Burke, M.D.)

other therapies (20), it may improve the peripheral blood counts in 40% to 70% of patients for a median of 20 months (19) and still has a role in antepartum control of HCL (21).

Second malignancies are increased among patients with HCL, possibly related to treatment with interferon alfa (22). Most second cancers develop several years after the inception of HCL, and the majority is nonhematopoietic (11).

HISTOPATHOLOGY

The lymph nodes are of moderate size, rarely exceeding 2 cm in diameter (12,13). The nodal architecture is partially preserved, although infiltration of neoplastic cells in the nodal parenchyma may be extensive. The hairy cells fill and distend the subcapsular and medullary sinuses and infiltrate the cortex and medulla diffusely; however, residual islands of lymphocytes are preserved (5) (Fig. 62.1). The pericapsular fat is often infiltrated, even when the peripheral sinus is still patent. The neoplastic cells in the spleen are located particularly in the red pulp, which is markedly expanded; in the liver, in the hepatic sinuses; and in the bone marrow diffusely, replacing hematopoietic and adipose tissues.

The population of cells infiltrating these various organs is remarkably homogeneous (Fig. 62.1), forming sheets of moderately large cells with abundant clear cytoplasm and distinct cell borders. The nuclei are monomorphic, with bland chromatin and inconspicuous nucleoli. Mitoses are not present. Necrosis and fibrosis are not noted. Plasma cells are often present in small scattered foci (18).

In blood smears and imprints stained with Giemsa stain, hairy cells can be recognized by their pale blue cytoplasm and characteristic fine, filamentous cytoplasmic projections (3) (Figs. 62.2 and 62.3). The cells are larger than lymphocytes, 10 to 15 μm in diameter. The nuclei are central and may be round, indented, or convoluted, with lacy chromatin and fine nucleoli. Cytoplasmic projections resembling hairs or ruffles are motile. The mitotic rate is low. Because of the clear cytoplasm and sharply defined borders of the hairy cells, their infiltrates have a characteristic appearance variably described as "honeycomb," "sponge," or "fried egg" (10).

ELECTRON MICROSCOPY

Hairy cells observed under the scanning electron microscope show broad-based ruffles with undulating edges; their

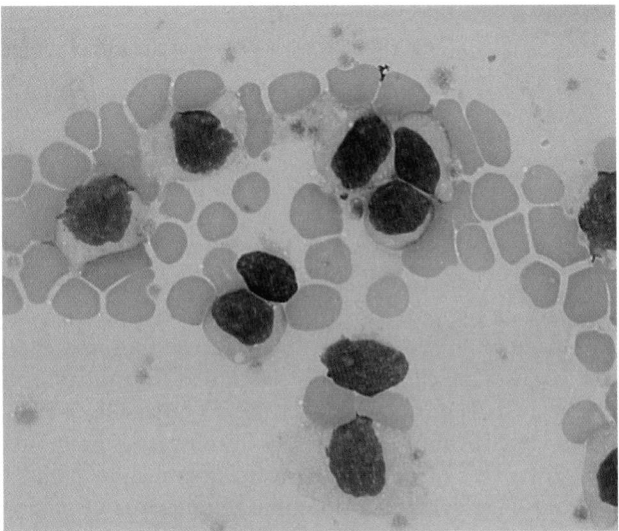

FIGURE 62.2. Hairy cells in tissue imprint show abundant, pale blue cytoplasm and uniform, ovoid, dense nuclei with inconspicuous nucleoli. Cell processes not visible on fixed specimens. Giemsa stain.

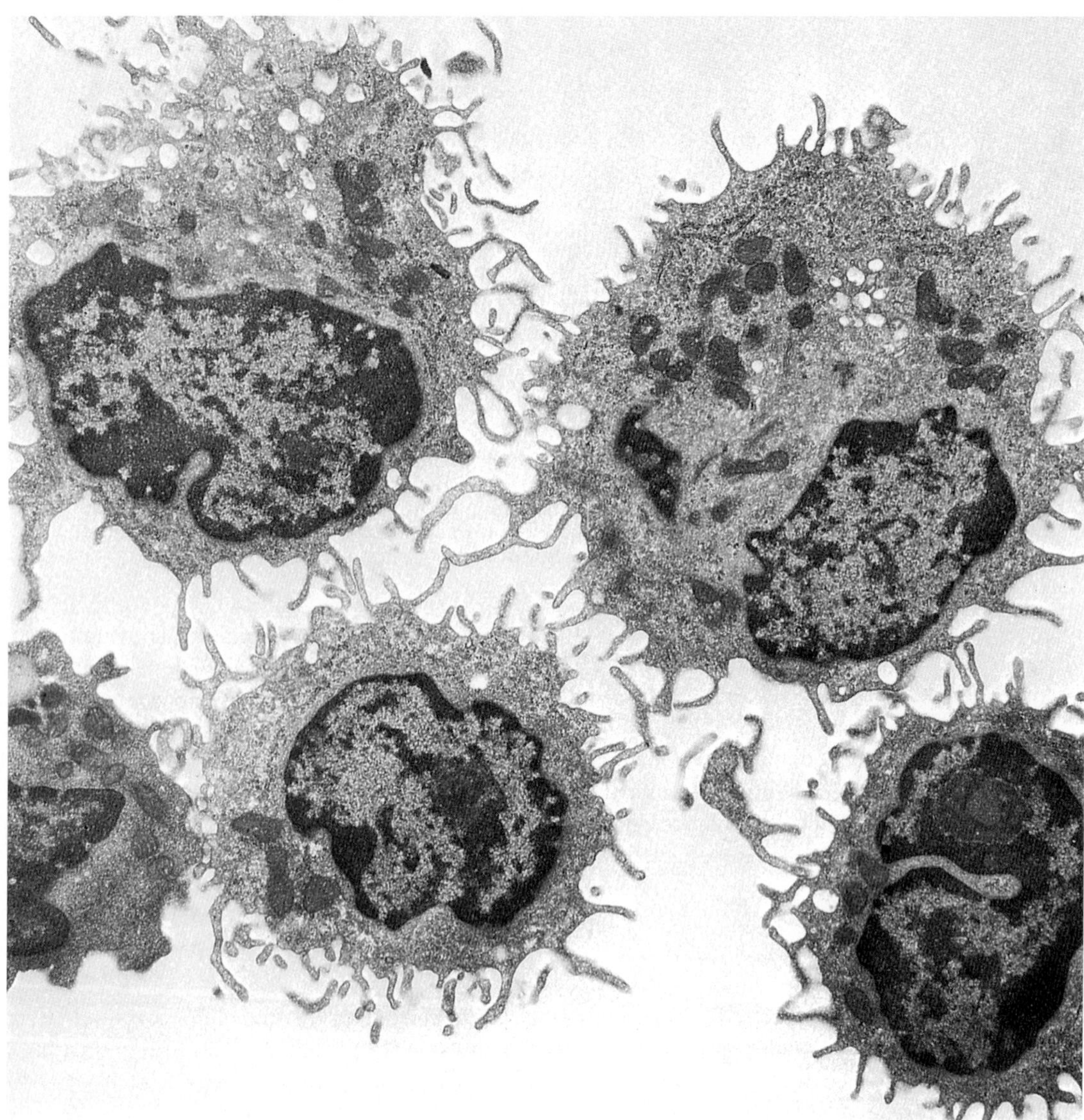

FIGURE 62.3. Hairy cells in suspension display the characteristic cytoplasmic processes. ×10,200.

surfaces are unlike the surfaces of lymphocytes (23) (Fig. 62.3).

Under the transmission electron microscope, hairy cells in tissue sections are closely apposed (Fig. 62.4), and their projections interdigitate (24). The cytoplasm contains a moderate number of mitochondria, free ribosomes, and few profiles of endoplasmic reticulum. In addition, a characteristic (although not exclusive) organelle, a ribosome–lamella complex, is present in most cases examined (24–26). This structure, comprising multiple parallel lamellae lined by rows of ribosome granules, has been seen only in tissues of hematologic malignancies, in 50% of all HCLs and about 10% of others. The lamellae form hollow cylinders (26) or sheetlike structures, and their nature is entirely obscure. Evidence of phagocytic activity is not noted.

CYTOGENETICS

Various abnormal chromosomal numbers and structures have been reported in cases of HCL, including abnormalities of chromosomes 1, 5, 6, 7, 8, and 17 (27–29). Recurrent imbalances involve chromosomes 5 and 7q22-q35 (29). One-third of patients with HCL have abnormalities involving band 5q13.3, which contains candidate tumor suppressor genes (30). Although HCL overexpresses cyclin D1, it does not contain the t(11;14)(q13;q32) translocation typically seen in mantle cell lymphoma (see Chapters 8 and 66).

CYTOCHEMISTRY

Hairy cell leukemia characteristically produces acid phosphatase isoenzyme 5 (31). The isoenzyme is resistant to tartaric acid, and this feature can be used as a marker for the identification of hairy cells. The majority of tartrate-resistant acid phosphatase (TRAP)-positive HCL cells stain bright red in a diffuse or granular cytoplasmic pattern (see Chapter 5). In a study of 29 cases of HCL, 22 were strongly positive for TRAP, 6 were intermediately positive, and only 1 was negative (32). Positive TRAP reactions may occasionally be seen in chronic lymphocytic leukemia, Sézary syndrome, and other disorders. An anti-TRAP monoclonal antibody that works in B5- and formalin-fixed tissues stained 80 of 86 cases of HCL and 2 of 3 cases of marginal zone lymphoma (33). The anti-TRAP antibody also detected Gaucher disease and mastocytosis (33).

IMMUNOHISTOCHEMISTRY

A long controversy about the origin of HCL, whether monocytic or lymphocytic, has now been settled. HCL is a B-cell disorder that expresses abundant B-cell antigens: CD19, CD20, CD22, and FMC7, but not CD5 or CD21 (10,34,35). CD103, an antigen found on mucosa-associated T-cells, is a sensitive HCL marker (35,36). CD11c, a myelomonocyte-related antigen, and CD25, the interleukin 2 receptor, are weakly expressed by B-cell chronic lymphocytic leukemia but strongly expressed by HCL (34,35). Both mantle cell lymphoma and HCL express cyclin D1 in the nucleus; expression is strong and uniform in the former but weak and spotty in the latter (37).

DBA.44, a fixation-resistant monoclonal antibody, helps diagnose HCL on tissue sections. It cannot be considered specific because, in addition to HCL, DBA.44 recognizes normal mantle zone cells and mantle cell lymphoma (38,39). Nodal marginal zone B-cell lymphoma (monocytoid B-cell lymphoma, marginal zone lymphoma) and B-cell chronic lymphocytic leukemia are usually DBA.44− (38, 39). Neoplastic monocytoid B cells differ from those of HCL; nodal marginal zone lymphoma does not express cyclin D1 and CD25 but does express CD21, CD35, and muscle-specific actin (40–42).

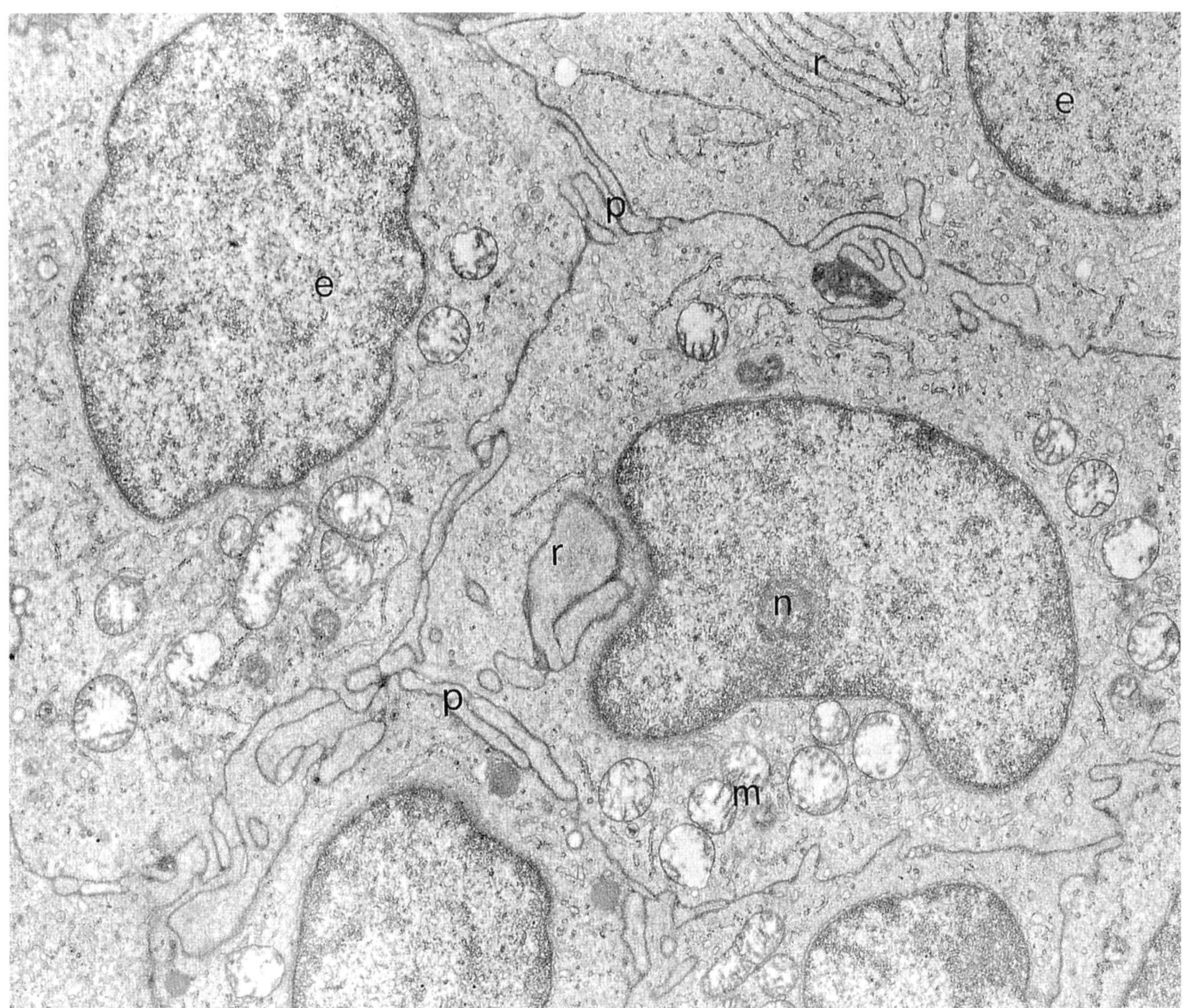

FIGURE 62.4. Hairy cells have interdigitated cytoplasmic processes (*p*), abundant cytoplasm with mitochondria (*m*), few profiles of endoplasmic reticulum (*r*), slightly indented nuclei, euchromatin (*e*), and small nucleoli (*n*). ×12,000.

Checklist

HAIRY CELL LEUKEMIA

Patients middle-aged, predominantly men
Fatigue, weakness, weight loss
Splenomegaly (90%), hepatomegaly (50%)
Lymphadenopathy (8% to 25%)
Bone marrow, dry tap
Leukopenia, thrombocytopenia, anemia
Hairy cells in peripheral blood
Lymph node architecture partially preserved
Homogeneous cell population
Honeycomb pattern
Distinct cell borders, clear cytoplasm
Monomorphic nuclei
Small nucleoli, no mitoses
Ruffles and villi
Ribosome–lamella complexes
Phagocytosis not present
Positive for TRAP
Bright monoclonal surface Ig
B-cell markers (CD19, CD20, CD22) plus CD11c, CD25, and CD103
Protracted course, long survival

Phenotype

B-cell antigens: CD19+, CD20+, CD22+
Clonal surface Ig+ (bright)
CD5−
CD11c+ (bright)
CD23−
CD25+
CD103+
DBA.44+
FMC7+
Cyclin D1+ (weak, not uniform)
TRAP+

DIFFERENTIAL DIAGNOSIS

- Chronic lymphocytic leukemia is associated with leukocytosis, HCL with leukopenia.
- Small lymphocytic non-Hodgkin lymphoma has sheets of tightly packed, uniformly hyperchromatic nuclei, not the honeycomb pattern with widely separated nuclei characteristic of HCL; cells are negative for TRAP.
- Nodal marginal zone B-cell lymphoma (monocytoid B-cell lymphoma) has cytologic and histologic patterns similar to those of HCL, but the cells are negative for interleukin 2 receptor (CD25), whereas they are positive in HCL.
- Large cell lymphomas have large pleomorphic nuclei, low nuclear-to-cytoplasmic ratios, prominent nucleoli.

REFERENCES

1. Bouroncle BA, Wiseman BK, Doan CA. Leukemic reticuloendotheliosis. Blood 1958;13:609–630.
2. Naeim F, Smith GS. Leukemic reticuloendotheliosis. Cancer 1974;34:1813–1821.
3. Schrek R, Donnelly WJ. "Hairy cells" in blood in lymphoreticular neoplastic disease and "flagellated" cells of normal lymph nodes. Blood 1966;27:199–211.
4. Miyoshi EK, Stewart PL, Kincade PW, et al. Aberrant expression and localization of the cytoskeleton-binding pp52 (LSP1) protein in hairy cell leukemia. Leuk Res 2001;25:57–67.
5. Burke JS, Byrne GE Jr, Rappaport H. Hairy cell leukemia (leukemic reticuloendotheliosis). I. A clinical pathologic study of 21 patients. Cancer 1974;33:1399–1410.
6. Cleary ML, Wood GS, Warnke R, et al. Immunoglobulin gene rearrangements in hairy cell leukemia. Blood 1984;64:99–104.
7. Foroni L, Catovsky D, Luzzatto L. Immunoglobulin gene rearrangements in hairy cell leukemia and other chronic B cell lymphoproliferative disorders. Leukemia 1987;1:389–392.
8. Hsu SM, Yang K, Jaffe ES. Hairy cell leukemia: a B-cell neoplasm

with a unique antigenic phenotype. Am J Clin Pathol 1983;80:421–428.
9. Anderson KC, Boyd AW, Fisher DC, et al. Hairy cell leukemia: a tumor of pre-plasma cells. Blood 1985;65:620–629.
10. Chang KL, Stroup R, Weiss LM. Hairy cell leukemia. Current status. Am J Clin Pathol 1992;97:719–738.
11. Frassoldati A, Lamparelli T, Federico M, et al. Hairy cell leukemia: a clinical review based on 725 cases of the Italian Cooperative Group (ICGHCL). Italian Cooperative Group for Hairy Cell Leukemia. Leuk Lymphoma 1994;13:307–316.
12. Turner A, Kjeldsberg CR. Hairy cell leukemia: a review. Medicine (Baltimore) 1978;57:477–499.
13. Orringer EP, Varia MA. A role for radiation in the treatment of hairy cell leukemia complicated by massive lymphadenopathy: a case report. Cancer 1980;45:2047–2050.
14. Budman DR, Koziner B, Arlin Z, et al. Massive lymphadenopathy mimicking lymphoma in leukemic reticuloendotheliosis. Am J Med 1979;66:160–162.
15. Mercieca J, Matutes E, Moskovic E, et al. Massive abdominal lymphadenopathy in hairy cell leukaemia: a report of 12 cases. Br J Haematol 1992;82:547–554.
16. Bartl R, Frisch B, Hill W, et al. Bone marrow histology in hairy cell leukemia. Identification of subtypes and their prognostic significance. Am J Clin Pathol 1983;79:531–545.
17. Flandrin G, Sigaux F, Sebahoun G, et al. Hairy cell leukemia: clinical presentation and follow-up of 211 patients. Semin Oncol 1984;11:458–471.
18. Vardiman JW, Variakojis D, Golomb HM. Hairy cell leukemia: an autopsy study. Cancer 1979;43:1339–1349.
19. Tallman MS, Peterson LC, Hakimian D, et al. Treatment of hairy-cell leukemia: current views. Semin Hematol 1999;36:155–163.
20. Baccarani U, Terrosu G, Donini A, et al. Splenectomy in hematology. Current practice and new perspectives. Haematologica 1999;84:431–436.
21. Stiles GM, Stanco LM, Saven A, et al. Splenectomy for hairy cell leukemia in pregnancy. J Perinatol 1998;18:200–201.
22. Kampmeier P, Spielberger R, Dickstein J, et al. Increased incidence of second neoplasms in patients treated with interferon alpha 2b for hairy cell leukemia: a clinicopathologic assessment. Blood 1994;83:2931–2938.
23. Braylan RC, Jaffe ES, Triche TJ, et al. Structural and functional properties of the "hairy" cells of leukemic reticuloendotheliosis. Cancer 1978;41:210–227.
24. Burke JS, Mackay B, Rappaport H. Hairy cell leukemia (leukemic reticuloendotheliosis) II. Ultrastructure of the spleen. Cancer 1976;37:2267–2274.
25. Katayama I, Li CY, Yam LT. Ultrastructural characteristics of the "hairy cells" of leukemic reticuloendotheliosis. Am J Pathol 1972;67:361–370.
26. Rosner MC, Golomb HM. Ribosome–lamella complex in hairy cell leukemia. Ultrastructure and distribution. Lab Invest 1980;42:236–247.
27. Sucak GT, Ogur G, Topal G, et al. del(17)(q25) in a patient with hairy cell leukemia: a new clonal chromosome abnormality. Cancer Genet Cytogenet 1998;100:152–154.
28. Sole F, Woessner S, Florensa L, et al. Cytogenetic findings in five patients with hairy cell leukemia. Cancer Genet Cytogenet 1999;110:41–43.
29. Ostergaard M, Andersen CL, Pedersen B, et al. Recurrent imbalances involving chromosome 5 and 7q22-q35 in hairy cell leukemia: a comparative genomic hybridization study. Genes Chromosomes Cancer 2001;30:218–219.
30. Wu X, Ivanova G, Merup M, et al. Molecular analysis of the human chromosome 5q13.3 region in patients with hairy cell leukemia and identification of tumor suppressor gene candidates. Genomics 1999;60:161–171.
31. Yam LT, Li CY, Lam KW. Tartrate-resistant acid phosphatase isoenzyme in the reticulum cells of leukemic reticuloendotheliosis. N Engl J Med 1971;284:357–360.
32. Katayama I, Yang JP. Reassessment of a cytochemical test for differential diagnosis of leukemic reticuloendotheliosis. Am J Clin Pathol 1977;68:268–272.
33. Hoyer JD, Li CY, Yam LT, et al. Immunohistochemical demonstration of acid phosphatase isoenzyme 5 (tartrate-resistant) in paraffin sections of hairy cell leukemia and other hematologic disorders. Am J Clin Pathol 1997;108:308–315.
34. Robbins BA, Ellison DJ, Spinosa JC, et al. Diagnostic application of two-color flow cytometry in 161 cases of hairy cell leukemia. Blood 1993;82:1277–1287.
35. DiGiuseppe JA, Borowitz MJ. Clinical utility of flow cytometry in the chronic lymphoid leukemias. Semin Oncol 1998;25:6–10.
36. Moller P, Mielke B, Moldenhauer G. Monoclonal antibody HML-1, a marker for intraepithelial T cells and lymphomas derived thereof, also recognizes hairy cell leukemia and some B-cell lymphomas. Am J Pathol 1990;136:509–512.
37. Miranda RN, Briggs RC, Kinney MC, et al. Immunohistochemical detection of cyclin D1 using optimized conditions is highly specific for mantle cell lymphoma and hairy cell leukemia [In Process Citation]. Mod Pathol 2000;13:1308–1314.
38. Hounieu H, Chittal SM, al Saati T, et al. Hairy cell leukemia. Diagnosis of bone marrow involvement in paraffin-embedded sections with monoclonal antibody DBA.44. Am J Clin Pathol 1992;98:26–33.
39. Ohsawa M, Kanno H, Machii T, et al. Immunoreactivity of neoplastic and non-neoplastic monocytoid B lymphocytes for DBA.44 and other antibodies [published erratum appears in J Clin Pathol 1994;47:1058]. J Clin Pathol 1994;47:928–932.
40. Burke JS, Sheibani K. Hairy cells and monocytoid B lymphocytes: are they related? Leukemia 1987;1:298–300.
41. Stroup R, Sheibani K. Antigenic phenotypes of hairy cell leukemia and monocytoid B-cell lymphoma: an immunohistochemical evaluation of 66 cases. Hum Pathol 1992;23:172–177.
42. Nathwani BN, Drachenberg MR, Hernandez AM, et al. Nodal monocytoid B-cell lymphoma (nodal marginal-zone B-cell lymphoma). Semin Hematol 1999;36:128–138.

63

NODAL MARGINAL ZONE B-CELL LYMPHOMA

DEFINITION

Uncommon, indolent B-cell lymphoma, probably originating from marginal zone B lymphocytes or a B-cell with diverse potential. The three subtypes have different natural histories according to their anatomic distribution: mucosa-associated lymphoid tissue (MALT), lymph nodes, or spleen (1).

SYNONYMS

- Monocytoid B-cell lymphoma (2,3)
- Parafollicular B-cell lymphoma (4,5)
- Marginal zone lymphoma (Revised European-American Lymphoma Classification)
  - Extranodal (MALT type +/− monocytoid B cells)
  - Provisional subtype: nodal (+/− monocytoid B cells)
  - Provisional entity: splenic marginal zone lymphoma (+/− villous lymphocytes)
- Marginal zone B-cell lymphoma (World Health Organization)
  - Marginal zone B-cell lymphoma of mucosa-associated lymphoid tissue (MALT) type (+/− monocytoid B-cells)
  - Nodal marginal zone B-cell lymphoma (+/− monocytoid B cells)
  - Splenic marginal zone lymphoma (+/− villous lymphocytes)

EPIDEMIOLOGY

Marginal zone lymphoma (MZL) accounts for approximately 8% of lymphomas worldwide, and 80% of patients survive 8 years (6). Three clinically distinct MZL variants are known: extranodal MALT type, nodal, and splenic (1). Nodal MZL (monocytoid B-cell lymphoma) presents at a median age of between 51 and 65 years and affects more women than men (3,7–9). A high prevalence of infection with hepatitis C virus (HCV) in patients with nodal MZL (monocytoid B-cell lymphoma) in the United States suggests a possible pathogenic role for chronic HCV infection (10).

PATHOGENESIS

Monocytoid B cells are reactive lymphoid cells found in various lymphadenitides, particularly those associated with toxoplasmosis (see Chapter 30), cat-scratch disease (see Chapter 18), and HIV infection (see Chapter 15) (11–15). Originally, they were given various descriptive names suggestive of a histiocytic/monocytic derivation: monocytoid cells (11,12), immature sinus histiocytes (13), and clear cells (15). Subsequent immunohistochemical studies showed the monocytoid cells to be polyclonal B lymphocytes (13,16, 17). Some considered these cells to originate from the marginal zone of follicles, representing a late stage in the differentiation of antibody-forming cells (18). Others believed that they represented parafollicular B cells reactive to infections and differentiating toward plasma cells (5). A strong cytologic resemblance to the cells of hairy cell leukemia (see Chapter 62) raised the question of a common cell of origin for both neoplasms (19); however, they do not express the same immunophenotype (7).

Molecular studies reveal immunoglobulin heavy chain variable gene somatic mutations typical of postgerminal center memory B cells (20,21). Continuing somatic mutation with intraclonal divergence could possibly be a consequence of chronic antigen stimulation or follicle center cell mechanisms (22).

CLINICAL SYNDROME

The clinical course of nodal MZL is indolent, similar to that of other low-grade B-cell lymphomas, with a small minority of cases transforming to a large cell type (23). Purely nodal MZL (monocytoid B-cell lymphoma), not involving mucosa and not combined with follicular lymphoma (FL), clearly does exist (8,24). Nodal MZL presents as localized or widespread lymphadenopathy, without leukemia or extranodal disease (3,7,9,25). Fever, weight loss, and other constitutional signs are usually absent (3). Paraproteinemia or Coomb's-positive hemolytic anemia is common (26). Nodal MZL, but not MALT-type MZL, frequently involves peripheral (axillary/inguinal/femoral) or paraaortic lymph nodes (p <.001) (9). A large mass (>5 cm) occurs in only 31% of cases of nodal MZL but in 68% of cases of MALT-type MZL (p = .03) (9). No statistical difference in bone marrow, liver, or spleen infiltration is noted (9). MALT-type MZL commonly but nodal MZL rarely involves the gastrointestinal tract (8,9). All patients with nodal MZL require staging to exclude occult extranodal MALT-type disease (27).

The 10-year estimated overall survival and failure-free survival were worse for 19 patients with MALT-type MZL than for 21 patients with nodal MZL (21% vs. 53%, p = .007; and 21% vs. 46%, p = .009) (8). These data appear to differ from those in patients presenting with advanced-stage (III and IV) disease; the 5-year overall survival and failure-free survival for 20 patients with nodal MZL were inferior to the survival rates for 73 patients with MALT-type MZL (56% vs. 81%, p = .09; and 28% vs. 65%, p = .01) (9).

Infection or autoimmune disease may be associated with MALT-type MZL involving extranodal anatomic sites: *Helicobacter pylori* and stomach, Sjögren syndrome and salivary gland, Hashimoto thyroiditis and thyroid gland (28). The clinical course remains indolent. Most patients achieve complete remission, although recurrences or progression to a large cell lymphoma can occur. If MALT-type MZL disseminates, it spreads to other extranodal MALT sites and to regional draining lymph nodes (9).

HISTOPATHOLOGY

Marginal zone lymphoma that surrounds reactive follicles containing a germinal center and a mantle zone creates a distinct third layer, referred to as a *marginal zone pattern.* MZL infiltrating from the marginal zone inward to the germinal center, in an apparently centripetal pattern of spread, causes follicular colonization. When MZL encircles "naked" germinal centers, the germinal centers appear dark and the outer zone of neoplastic monocytoid B cells appears light; this is called an *inverse follicular pattern.* Alternatively, MZL surrounds a germinal center with a mantle zone (29) (Fig. 63.1).

Large aggregates of the characteristic MZL cells (neoplastic monocytoid B cells) may form patches or fill and distend the lymph nodes sinuses (Fig. 63.1). Early, the lymph node architecture is maintained as the proliferation extends around the sinuses and parafollicular areas (2,3,7) (Fig. 63.1). Eventually, sinusoidal, parasinusoidal, parafollicular, marginal zone, and inverse follicular patterns appear as MZL replaces different lymph node compartments (7,29, 30).

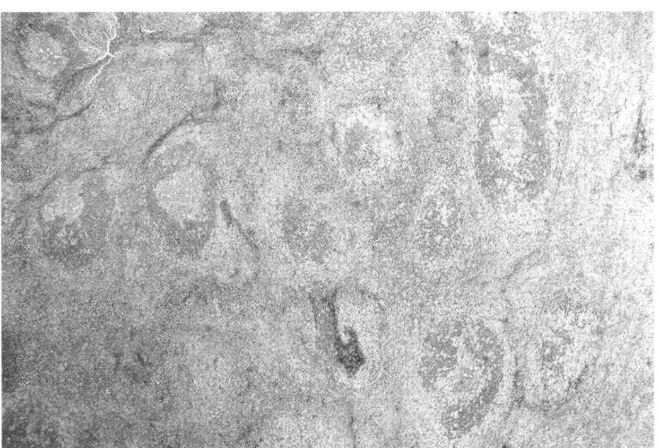

FIGURE 63.1. Nodal marginal zone lymphoma in inguinal lymph node from a 52-year-old man. Markedly distorted lymph node with nodular architecture shows lymphomatous, pale, monocytoid cells expanding the marginal zone (outer = light) that surrounds a non-neoplastic residual mantle zone (middle = dark) and a non-neoplastic residual germinal center (inner = light). Some follicles have only two layers, a so-called reverse follicle pattern (outer = light and inner = dark). Monocytoid cells also fill up sinuses. Although most of the lymph node cells were B cells, flow cytometry analysis could not demonstrate a restricted immunoglobulin light chain expression because of the abundance of contaminating reactive B cells from the non-neoplastic mantle zones and germinal centers. However, Southern blot analysis did reveal a clonal immunoglobulin heavy chain gene rearrangement. H&E stain.

Two MZL cytologic types are noted: a standard cell variant of small, lymphoid cells with slightly irregular nuclear contours and scant cytoplasm, and a clear cell variant of medium cells with plentiful pale cytoplasm, called *monocytoid B cells* (23,29,31,32). Some MZLs contain both (23). The monocytoid B cells have a bland, uniform appearance with abundant, entirely clear cytoplasm and well-defined

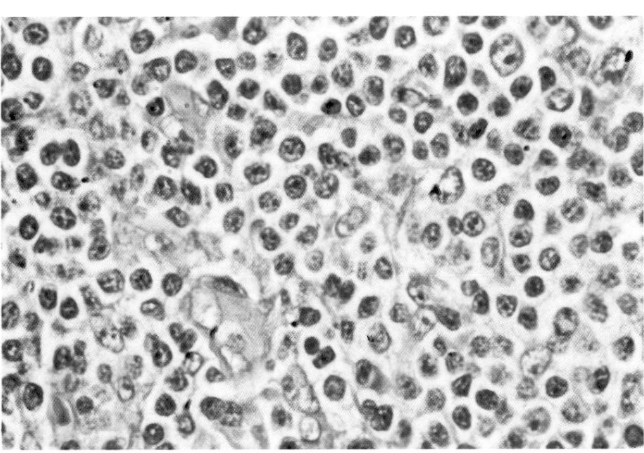

FIGURE 63.2. Same case of nodal marginal zone lymphoma as in Fig. 63.1. The marginal zone B cells (monocytoid B cells) have a bland, uniform appearance with abundant, entirely clear cytoplasm and well-defined cell borders. H&E stain.

cell borders (Fig. 63.2). The nuclei are small, round or slightly indented, and moderately hyperchromatic, with inconspicuous nucleoli and no or rare mitoses (2–4,7,27,33). In Giemsa-stained touch imprints, the nuclei show clumped chromatin with one to three small nucleoli and gray cytoplasm (34).

Compared with non-neoplastic monocytoid B cells in reactive lymph nodes, MZL cells grow in confluent sheets and have more irregular nuclei and higher mitotic rates (29). Neutrophils are usually associated with monocytoid cells, both benign and malignant (29). Plasmacytoid differentiation and plasma cells belonging to the same clone can be present (5,29,34–36). MZL is rarely histologically homogeneous.

Extranodal MALT-type MZL spreads to regional draining lymph nodes; monocytoid B cells infiltrate in a perivascular, parasinusoidal or parafollicular distribution that is indistinguishable from that of primary nodal MZL (27, 34–36) (Fig 63.3). Splenic MZL infiltrates hilar and rarely peripheral lymph nodes; the normal lymph node architecture is effaced while the dilated sinuses are retained, and a histologic pattern typically seen in spleen is reproduced. Nodular "bull's-eye" reactive follicular centers are surrounded by wide zones containing a mixture of small lymphocytes and monocytoid B-cells and a sprinkling of large transformed lymphocytes at the periphery; mantle cuffs are attenuated or absent (37–39). Uncommonly, nodal MZL has splenic histologic features without splenic disease (25).

ELECTRON MICROSCOPY

The monocytoid B cells have abundant cytoplasm with scattered ribosomes, interdigitating processes, and an irregular nuclear membrane. Ribosomal–lamellar complexes have not been noted (3).

IMMUNOHISTOCHEMISTRY

Most nodal MZLs express monoclonal surface immunoglobulins (usually IgM) and B-cell antigens CD19,

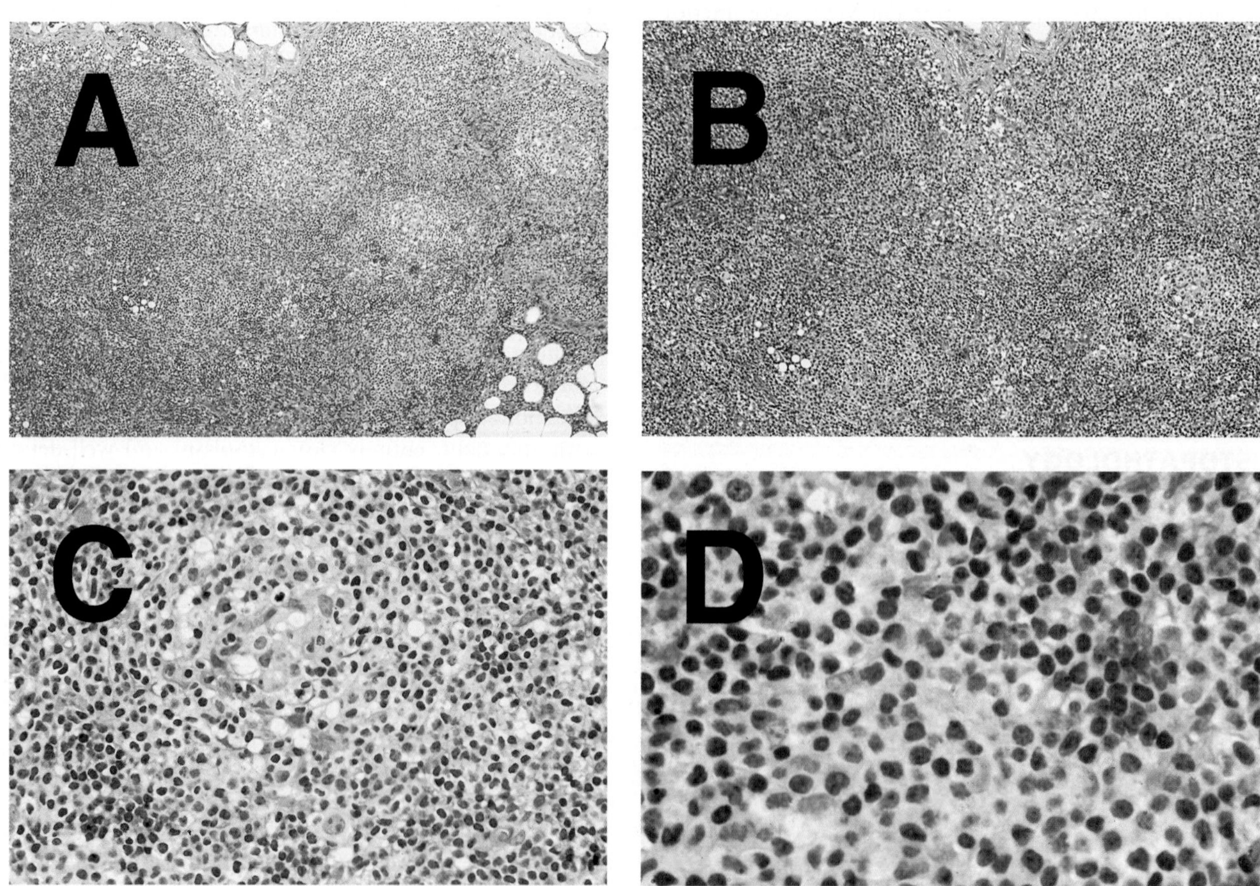

FIGURE 63.3. Draining gastric lymph node secondarily involved by extranodal marginal zone B-cell lymphoma of mucosa-associated lymphoid tissue type that originated in the stomach. **A,B:** Nodular pattern is seen at low magnification. Monocytoid cells expand sinuses and infiltrate perinodal adipose tissue. **C:** Monocytoid cells overrun follicle ("follicular colonization"). **D:** Monotonous population of monocytoid lymphoid cells with bland, small, dark nuclei and abundant pale cytoplasm are morphologically indistinguishable from nodal marginal zone lymphoma.

CD20, CD22, CD24, LN-1, and bcl-2 protein; they do not express CD5, CD10, CD11c, CD21, CD23, CD25, CD35, CD38, or cyclin D1 (bcl-1 protein); CD43 is variably expressed (34,40,41). In some cases of MZL, the neoplastic monocytoid cells infiltrate only the outer portion of the follicle, the zone theoretically reserved for marginal zone cells (34). The absence of CD5, CD10, and CD23 is most helpful in distinguishing MZL from other small B-cell lymphomas, such as B-cell chronic lymphocytic leukemia/small lymphocytic lymphoma (B-CLL/SLL), mantle cell lymphoma (MCL), and FL (26,42). However, rare CD5+ MZLs with localized presentation do occur (43). Splenic MZL and nodal MZL with splenic histologic features simultaneously express both IgM and IgD: this is in contrast to the majority of nodal MZLs and extranodal MZLs of MALT type, which express only IgM (25,39).

Phenotype

CD5−
CD10−
CD11c−
CD19+
CD20+
CD21−
CD22+
CD23−/+
CD25−
CD43−/+
CD79a+
Monoclonal surface Ig
IgM+
IgD− (usually) in nodal and MALT types

CYTOGENETICS

Extranodal, nodal, and splenic MZLs all have recurring complete or partial trisomy 3 (44) and trisomy 18 in addition to structural abnormalities involving breakpoints 1q21 and 1p34 (26). The t(11;18)(q21;q21) chromosomal translocation yielding *API2-MALT-1* fusion transcripts occurs exclusively in extranodal MZL of MALT type without a large cell component (45,46); it does not occur in nodal or splenic MZL (45,47). The observation that nodal MZL consistently lacks t(11;18)(q21;q21) (45,47) challenges the hypothesis that undetected extranodal MZL of MALT type is the source of most nodal MZL (34–36). Another, less common translocation restricted to MALT-type MZL involves bcl-10 on chromosome 1 and the Ig heavy chain, t(1;14)(p22;q32) (48). Interestingly, nuclear expression of bcl-10 protein often occurs in MALT lymphomas, even in the absence of the translocation (49).

MOLECULAR DIAGNOSIS

The simultaneous occurrence of nodal MZL and FL in the same lymph node has frequently been reported (3,7,8,29, 50,51). Could follicular colonization in MZL have been misinterpreted as FL (5,52)? The t(14;18) chromosomal translocation or the bcl-2 gene rearrangement characterizing FL is not detected in every MZL with a component of FL (7,30). Cases of MZL with a nodular growth pattern and lacking a BCL-2 gene rearrangement should not be called a composite lymphoma; they should be recognized as part of the MZL morphologic continuum. MZLs do not have chromosomal translocations of the BCL-1, BCL-2, BCL-3, BCL-6, or C-MYC genes (26).

DIFFERENTIAL DIAGNOSIS

- Reactive monocytoid B-cell hyperplasia exhibits patches of monocytoid cells entirely similar to those of MZL. Confluent sheets of cells, irregular nuclei, and the presence of mitoses are indicative of lymphoma; however, unless obvious signs of destructive expansion are present, the two entities cannot be reliably distinguished on morphologic grounds alone. The clonal nature of the monocytoid cells can be proved by the presence of Ig light chain restriction or Ig gene rearrangements. Alternatively, most MZLs express bcl-2 protein, but reactive monocytoid B cells do not (41).
- Secondary extranodal marginal zone B-cell lymphoma involving lymph nodes cannot be distinguished from primary nodal marginal zone B-cell lymphoma on histologic grounds alone. Clinicopathologic correlation is essential. Furthermore, MALT-type MZLs have unique cytogenetic findings such as t(11:18)(q21;q21) and t(1;14)(p22; q32) and tend to express bcl-10 protein in the nucleus (49).
- FL must be distinguished from follicular colonization of MZL. The reactive germinal center infiltrated by MZL is negative for bcl-2 protein and has a proliferative fraction that is highly positive for Ki-67. In contrast, FL has bcl-2 protein–positive nodules with a low proliferative fraction. FL has a t(14;18) chromosomal translocation and BCL-2 gene rearrangement.
- Hairy cell leukemia: Bone marrow, peripheral blood, and spleen are regularly affected, whereas lymph nodes are only rarely involved (19). Exceptions occur. Cytology is similar for hairy cells and monocytoid cells. Staining for tartrate-resistant acid phosphatase, DBA.44, bcl-1 protein (cyclin D1), and CD25 (interleukin 2 receptor) is positive in HCL but negative in MZL (2,53).
- MCL grows around "naked" follicle centers, creating a micronodular pattern somewhat similar to that of MZL at low magnification (2,39). However, the cytologic features are different. MCL cells have only scarce amounts of cy-

Checklist

NODAL MARGINAL ZONE LYMPHOMA

Patients elderly
Female predominance
Indolent course, long survival
Peripheral lymph nodes
Patches of monocytoid cells in sinuses and parafollicular areas
Follicular colonization
Monomorphic, bland cells with abundant clear cytoplasm and small round or slightly irregular nuclei
Monoclonal B cells expressing IgM and pan-B-cell markers but not CD5, CD10, or CD23

toplasm and no transformed lymphocytes. MCL expresses CD5, CD43, and bcl-1 protein; MZL is usually negative for these markers.

- Ki-1 anaplastic large cell lymphoma may resemble the sinus pattern of some MZLs at low magnification (2), but the cytologic and immunophenotypic features are entirely different.
- Growth along marginal zone outlines is neither necessary nor sufficient for diagnosing MZL because other diseases mimic a marginal zone (or pseudomantle zone) pattern: early stage B-CLL/SLL (54), T-cell lymphoma (23), and mast cell disease (55).

REFERENCES

1. Harris NL, Jaffe ES, Diebold J, et al. The World Health Organization classification of hematological malignancies: report of the clinical advisory committee meeting, Airlie House, Virginia, November 1997. Mod Pathol 2000;13:193–207.
2. Sheibani K, Sohn CC, Burke JS, et al. Monocytoid B-cell lymphoma. A novel B-cell neoplasm. Am J Pathol 1986;124:310–318.
3. Sheibani K, Burke JS, Swartz WG, et al. Monocytoid B-cell lymphoma. Clinicopathologic study of 21 cases of a unique type of low-grade lymphoma. Cancer 1988;62:1531–1538.
4. Cousar JB, McGinn DL, Glick AD, et al. Report of an unusual lymphoma arising from parafollicular B-lymphocytes (PBLs) or so-called "monocytoid" lymphocytes. Am J Clin Pathol 1987;87:121–128.
5. Davis GG, York JC, Glick AD, et al. Plasmacytic differentiation in parafollicular (monocytoid) B-cell lymphoma. A study of 12 cases. Am J Surg Pathol 1992;16:1066–1074.
6. The Non-Hodgkin's Lymphoma Classification Project. A clinical evaluation of the International Lymphoma Study Group classification of non-Hodgkin's lymphoma. Blood 1997;89:3909–3918.
7. Ngan BY, Warnke RA, Wilson M, et al. Monocytoid B-cell lymphoma: a study of 36 cases [see Comments]. Hum Pathol 1991;22:409–421.
8. Fisher RI, Dahlberg S, Nathwani BN, et al. A clinical analysis of two indolent lymphoma entities: mantle cell lymphoma and marginal zone lymphoma (including the mucosa-associated lymphoid tissue and monocytoid B-cell subcategories): a Southwest Oncology Group study. Blood 1995;85:1075–1082.
9. Nathwani BN, Anderson JR, Armitage JO, et al. Marginal zone B-cell lymphoma: a clinical comparison of nodal and mucosa-associated lymphoid tissue types. J Clin Oncol 1999;17:2486–2492.
10. Zuckerman E, Zuckerman T, Levine AM, et al. Hepatitis C virus infection in patients with B-cell non-Hodgkin lymphoma [see Comments]. Ann Intern Med 1997;127:423–428.
11. Stansfeld AG. The histological diagnosis of toxoplasmic lymphadenitis. J Clin Pathol 1961;14:565–573.
12. Dorfman RF, Remington JS. Value of lymph-node biopsy in the diagnosis of acute acquired toxoplasmosis. N Engl J Med 1973;289:878–881.
13. Stein H, Lennert K, Mason DY, et al. Immature sinus histiocytes. Their identification as a novel B-cell population. Am J Pathol 1984;117:44–52.
14. Sohn CC, Sheibani K, Winberg CD, et al. Monocytoid B lymphocytes: their relation to the patterns of the acquired immunodeficiency syndrome (AIDS) and AIDS-related lymphadenopathy. Hum Pathol 1985;16:979–985.
15. Ioachim HL, Cronin W, Roy M, et al. Persistent lymphadenopathies in people at high risk for HIV infection. Clinicopathologic correlations and long-term follow-up in 79 cases. Am J Clin Pathol 1990;93:208–218.
16. Sheibani K, Fritz RM, Winberg CD, et al. "Monocytoid" cells in reactive follicular hyperplasia with and without multifocal histiocytic reactions: an immunohistochemical study of 21 cases including suspected cases of toxoplasmic lymphadenitis. Am J Clin Pathol 1984;81:453–458.
17. Cardoso de Almeida P, Harris NL, Bhan AK. Characterization of immature sinus histiocytes (monocytoid cells) in reactive lymph nodes by use of monoclonal antibodies. Hum Pathol 1984;15:330–335.
18. van den Oord JJ, de Wolf-Peeters C, De Vos R, et al. Immature sinus histiocytosis. Light- and electron-microscopic features, immunologic phenotype, and relationship with marginal zone lymphocytes. Am J Pathol 1985;118:266–277.
19. Burke JS, Sheibani K. Hairy cells and monocytoid B lymphocytes: are they related? Leukemia 1987;1:298–300.

20. Kuppers R, Hajadi M, Plank L, et al. Molecular Ig gene analysis reveals that monocytoid B cell lymphoma is a malignancy of mature B cells carrying somatically mutated V region genes and suggests that rearrangement of the kappa-deleting element (resulting in deletion of the Ig kappa enhancers) abolishes somatic hypermutation in the human. Eur J Immunol 1996;26:1794–1800.
21. Klein U, Kuppers R, Rajewsky K. Evidence for a large compartment of IgM-expressing memory B cells in humans. Blood 1997; 89:1288–1298.
22. Bahler DW, Miklos JA, Swerdlow SH. Ongoing Ig gene hypermutation in salivary gland mucosa-associated lymphoid tissue-type lymphomas. Blood 1997;89:3335–3344.
23. Nathwani BN, Hernandez AM, Deol I, et al. Marginal zone B-cell lymphomas: an appraisal [see Comments]. Hum Pathol 1997;28:42–46.
24. Grogan TM. Does nodal marginal zone lymphoma exist? In: Mason DY, Harris NL, eds. Human lymphoma: clinical implications of the REAL classification. London: Springer-Verlag, 1999:18.1–18.5.
25. Campo E, Miquel R, Krenacs L, et al. Primary nodal marginal zone lymphomas of splenic and MALT type. Am J Surg Pathol 1999;23:59–68.
26. Dierlamm J, Pittaluga S, Wlodarska I, et al. Marginal zone B-cell lymphomas of different sites share similar cytogenetic and morphologic features [see Comments]. Blood 1996;87:299–307.
27. Cogliatti SB, Lennert K, Hansmann ML, et al. Monocytoid B cell lymphoma: clinical and prognostic features of 21 patients. J Clin Pathol 1990;43:619–625.
28. Burke JS. Are there site-specific differences among the MALT lymphomas—morphologic, clinical? Am J Clin Pathol 1999;111: S133–S143.
29. Nathwani BN, Mohrmann RL, Brynes RK, et al. Monocytoid B-cell lymphomas: an assessment of diagnostic criteria and a perspective on histogenesis. Hum Pathol 1992;23:1061–1071.
30. Hernandez AM, Nathwani BN, Nguyen D, et al. Nodal benign and malignant monocytoid B cells with and without follicular lymphomas: a comparative study of follicular colonization, light chain restriction, bcl-2, and t(14;18) in 39 cases. Hum Pathol 1995;26:625–632.
31. Isaacson PG, Spencer J. Malignant lymphoma of mucosa-associated lymphoid tissue. Histopathology 1987;11:445–462.
32. Isaacson PG, Spencer J. Monocytoid B-cell lymphomas [Comment]. Am J Surg Pathol 1990;14:888–891.
33. Nathwani BN, Drachenberg MR, Hernandez AM, et al. Nodal monocytoid B-cell lymphoma (nodal marginal-zone B-cell lymphoma). Semin Hematol 1999;36:128–138.
34. Nizze H, Cogliatti SB, von Schilling C, et al. Monocytoid B-cell lymphoma: morphological variants and relationship to low-grade B-cell lymphoma of the mucosa-associated lymphoid tissue. Histopathology 1991;18:403–414.
35. Ortiz-Hidalgo C, Wright DH. The morphological spectrum of monocytoid B-cell lymphoma and its relationship to lymphomas of mucosa-associated lymphoid tissue. Histopathology 1992;21: 555–561.
36. Mollejo M, Menarguez J, Cristobal E, et al. Monocytoid B cells. A comparative clinical pathological study of their distribution in different types of low-grade lymphomas. Am J Surg Pathol 1994;18:1131–1139.
37. Isaacson PG, Matutes E, Burke M, et al. The histopathology of splenic lymphoma with villous lymphocytes. Blood 1994;84: 3828–3834.
38. Hammer RD, Glick AD, Greer JP, et al. Splenic marginal zone lymphoma. A distinct B-cell neoplasm. Am J Surg Pathol 1996; 20:613–626.
39. Mollejo M, Lloret E, Menarguez J, et al. Lymph node involvement by splenic marginal zone lymphoma: morphological and immunohistochemical features. Am J Surg Pathol 1997;21:772–780.
40. Harris NL. Low-grade B-cell lymphoma of mucosa-associated lymphoid tissue and monocytoid B-cell lymphoma. Related entities that are distinct from other low-grade B-cell lymphomas [Editorial; Comment]. Arch Pathol Lab Med 1993;117:771–775.
41. Lai R, Arber DA, Chang KL, et al. Frequency of bcl-2 expression in non-Hodgkin's lymphoma: a study of 778 cases with comparison of marginal zone lymphoma and monocytoid B-cell hyperplasia. Mod Pathol 1998;11:864–869.
42. Swerdlow SH. Small B-cell lymphomas of the lymph nodes and spleen: practical insights to diagnosis and pathogenesis. Mod Pathol 1999;12:125–140.
43. Ballesteros E, Osborne BM, Matsushima AY. CD5+ low-grade marginal zone B-cell lymphomas with localized presentation. Am J Surg Pathol 1998;22:201–207.
44. Brynes RK, Almaguer PD, Leathery KE, et al. Numerical cytogenetic abnormalities of chromosomes 3, 7, and 12 in marginal zone B-cell lymphomas. Mod Pathol 1996;9:995–1000.
45. Rosenwald A, Ott G, Stilgenbauer S, et al. Exclusive detection of the t(11;18)(q21;q21) in extranodal marginal zone B cell lymphomas (MZBL) of MALT type in contrast to other MZBL and extranodal large B cell lymphomas. Am J Pathol 1999;155:1817–1821.
46. Baens M, Maes B, Steyls A, et al. The product of the t(11;18), an API2-MLT fusion, marks nearly half of gastric MALT type lymphomas without large cell proliferation. Am J Pathol 2000;156: 1433–1439.
47. Remstein ED, James CD, Kurtin PJ. Incidence and subtype specificity of API2-MALT1 fusion translocations in extranodal, nodal, and splenic marginal zone lymphomas. Am J Pathol 2000;156:1183–1188.
48. Willis TG, Jadayel DM, Du MQ, et al. Bcl10 is involved in t(1;14)(p22;q32) of MALT B cell lymphoma and mutated in multiple tumor types [see Comments]. Cell 1999;96:35–45.
49. Ye H, Dogan A, Karran L, et al. BCL10 expression in normal and neoplastic lymphoid tissue. Nuclear localization in MALT lymphoma. Am J Pathol 2000;157:1147–1154.
50. Slovak ML, Weiss LM, Nathwani BN, et al. Cytogenetic studies of composite lymphomas: monocytoid B-cell lymphoma and other B-cell non-Hodgkin's lymphomas. Hum Pathol 1993;24: 1086–1094.
51. Plank L, Hell K, Hansmann ML, et al. Reactive versus neoplastic monocytoid B-cell proliferations. *In situ* hybridization study of immunoglobulin light chain mRNA. Am J Clin Pathol 1995; 103:330–337.
52. Isaacson PG, Wotherspoon AC, Diss T, et al. Follicular colonization in B-cell lymphoma of mucosa-associated lymphoid tissue. Am J Surg Pathol 1991;15:819–828.
53. Hoyer JD, Li CY, Yam LT, et al. Immunohistochemical demonstration of acid phosphatase isoenzyme 5 (tartrate-resistant) in paraffin sections of hairy cell leukemia and other hematologic disorders. Am J Clin Pathol 1997;108:308–315.
54. Ellison DJ, Nathwani BN, Cho SY, et al. Interfollicular small lymphocytic lymphoma: the diagnostic significance of pseudofollicles. Hum Pathol 1989;20:1108–1118.
55. Travis WD, Li CY. Pathology of the lymph node and spleen in systemic mast cell disease. Mod Pathol 1988;1:4–14.

64

FOLLICULAR LYMPHOMA

DEFINITION

Lymphomas composed of cleaved and noncleaved B cells recapitulating the germinal centers of lymphoid follicles and growing in a nodular pattern.

SYNONYMS

Brill-Symmers disease
Nodular lymphosarcoma
Germinal center lymphoma
Nodular (and/or diffuse) lymphoma, poorly differentiated lymphocytic (Rappaport)
Nodular (and/or diffuse) lymphoma, mixed poorly differentiated lymphocytic and histiocytic (Rappaport)
Nodular (and/or diffuse) lymphoma, histiocytic (Rappaport)
Centroblastic–centrocytic lymphoma (Kiel)
Follicular centroblastic lymphoma (Kiel)
Follicular lymphoma (FL), predominantly small cleaved cell (Working Formulation)
FL, mixed small and large cell (Working Formulation)
FL, predominantly large cell (Working Formulation)
Follicle center lymphoma, follicular (Revised European-American Lymphoma Classification, or REAL)
- Grade 1
- Grade 2
- Grade 3

Follicle center lymphoma, diffuse, small cell (REAL; provisional)
Follicular lymphoma (World Health Organization, or WHO)
- Grade 1
- Grade 2
- Grade 3

Follicle center lymphoma, diffuse (WHO)

SUBTYPES

The Rappaport classification (1) and the Working Formulation (2) traditionally subclassify FLs into three groups according to the proportion of small cleaved lymphoid cells (poorly differentiated lymphocytes, centrocytes) and large lymphoid cells (histiocytic cells, centroblasts). The term *histiocytic* in the Rappaport classification refers to large lymphoid cells or centroblasts. The REAL (3) and WHO (4) classifications equate cytologic subtype with tumor grade because abundant large cells imply a worse overall survival. Although most pathologists can reproducibly recognize a follicular pattern, they do not always agree on the number of large cells (5). Therefore, the WHO classification recommends counting large cells in 10 to 20 high-power fields (HPFs) from various follicles, not just those with many large cells: *Grade 1,* 0 to 5 centroblasts per HPF; *Grade 2,* 6 to 15 centroblasts per HPF; *Grade 3,* more than 15 centroblasts per HPF (4,6). Diffuse areas should be recognized: predominantly follicular, more than 75% follicular; follicular and diffuse, 25% to 75% follicular; predominantly diffuse, less than 25% follicular (4). However, grade 3 FL with diffuse regions should be reported as FL, grade 3/3 with diffuse large B-cell lymphoma (DLBCL) and the percentages of the areas noted (4). On a practical level, the ability of pathologists to recognize follicular pattern and sheets of large cells reproducibly will probably yield just two clinically meaningful categories: FL, grades 1 and 2 versus FL, grade 3 (4). Among the subtypes of FL, grade 1 is the most common (2).

EPIDEMIOLOGY

After DLBCL, FL is the next most common lymphoma; it represented 22% of 1,378 non-Hodgkin lymphomas in a multiinstitutional study (7). FL is uncommon in Japan and other parts of Asia.

The male predominance noted in most lymphomas is not observed in FL (2). FL is distinctly a tumor of older age (2); it affects only 1% to 2% of lymphoma patients before the age of 20 years (8–10). FL in children is usually limited to lymph nodes or tonsils. It pursues an indolent clinical course, rarely progressing to a higher grade or a diffuse pattern, and unlike FL in adults, it can be cured with conservative therapy (9,10).

PATHOGENESIS

A germinal center origin, low proliferation rate, and nodular growth pattern characterize FLs. The complex architectural relationship between FL cells and accompanying nonneoplastic T cells and follicular dendritic reticulum cells (DRCs) suggests a continuing response to local signals. Although the t(14;18) chromosomal translocation is associated with overexpression of anti-apoptotic bcl-2 protein in most FLs, it is not sufficient to produce lymphomagenesis, as demonstrated by the finding of t(14;18) in lymphocytes from normal persons (11). In addition to bcl-2 protein, FLs express other death suppressor proteins belonging to the bcl-2 family (12), such as bcl-x_L and mcl1 (13). FLs, unlike germinal center B-cells, produce very low or undetectable amounts of the death-promoting proteins bax and bad (13). Activated CD40 maintains the synthesis of bcl-x_L, promoting FL cell survival (13). Because CD40 ligand-positive (CD40L+) T cells reside in reactive secondary follicles and in FLs (14), the microenvironment can inhibit FL cell death (13). FL cell and follicular DRC interactions also can contribute to preventing cell death (15,16).

CLINICAL SYNDROME

Follicular lymphoma is an indolent disease in which "B" symptoms are noted by only 20% of patients (17). Because of its insidious onset, about two-thirds to three-fourths of patients are already in stage III or IV at the time of diagnosis (2,17,18). FL is less likely than the diffuse lymphomas to involve extranodal primary sites; however, it is almost always disseminated at the time of diagnosis, often involving bone marrow, liver, and abdominal lymph nodes. The incidence of bone marrow disease rises with the number of involved lymph node groups (19). Only a minority of patients present in clinical stage I or II (2,17,18). Cervical and inguinal lymph nodes are involved most often. Mediastinal lymph nodes are very rarely a primary location. The proportion of patients with FL, grade 1 who have stage IV disease is greater than the proportion of those with grades 2 and 3 who have stage IV disease (2,17,18).

The Ann Arbor staging system predicts long-term prognosis poorly in FL because many patients already have widely disseminated disease at diagnosis and lymphoma cells occur in the peripheral blood (18). Factors that adversely affect complete remission and survival include the following: increased number of involved lymph node groups, constitutional symptoms, splenomegaly, and older age (19).

The survival curves for all histologic subtypes of FL have a similar shape without a plateau, which suggests that current therapy has no curative potential (2,17,18). Among patients presenting with stage III or IV FL, the estimated 10-year overall survival is approximately 35% to 40% (18). In contrast, patients with early-stage FL, especially if young, can have a good result after radiation therapy (20). The spectrum of clinical outcomes in FL is broad; about one-fifth of patients die within 2 years, and about one-fifth are alive 15 years after diagnosis (18). The FL histologic subtype should be supplemented by clinical information, such as the International Prognostic Index (IPI) (21), when clinical behavior is predicted (22). The overall and failure-free survival of FL patients with a high IPI is poor (7).

HISTOPATHOLOGY

The normal lymph node architecture is obliterated by numerous nodules (Fig. 64.1) of fairly uniform size and shape that involve the cortex and medulla and frequently penetrate the perinodal fibroadipose tissues (Fig. 64.2). The neoplastic nodules may occupy the lymph node totally or partially. When partially occupied, the lymph node areas lacking the nodular pattern represent either residual, uninvolved parenchyma or lymphoma of diffuse pattern resulting from the progression of nodular lymphoma (23).

In contrast to the enlarged lymphoid follicles of reactive follicular hyperplasia (RFH), which vary greatly in size and shape and frequently coalesce, the nodules of FL are round, isolated, and uniform (Fig. 64.3 A–C). Sometimes, the neoplastic nodules of FL lack a mantle zone, so that the borders are blurred (Fig. 64.3 A–C), but usually the nodules are sharply circumscribed. Sometimes, a "cracking" artifact highlights the neoplastic nodules (Fig. 64.4). In comparison with the follicles of RFH, the nodules of FL are more numerous and closer to each other, with very little uninvolved tissue left between them (Figs. 64.1 and 64.3). The nodules are not restricted to subcapsular areas but also involve the deep cortex and medulla (Figs. 64.1 and 64.3).

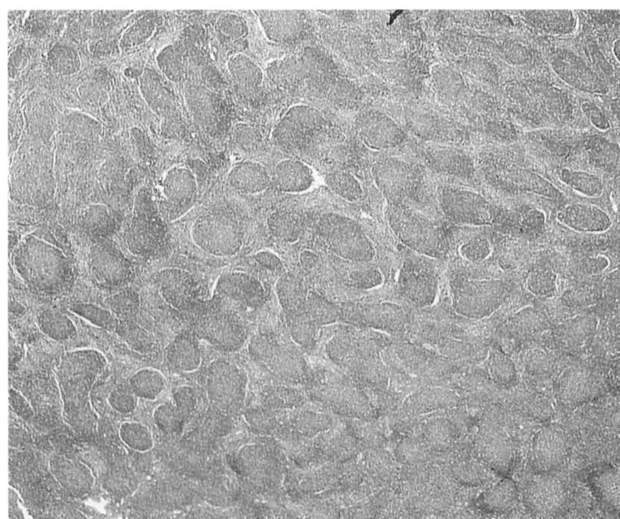

FIGURE 64.1. Follicular lymphoma showing characteristic pattern of closely packed nodules with some variation in size and shape. Hematoxylin, phloxine, and saffron stain.

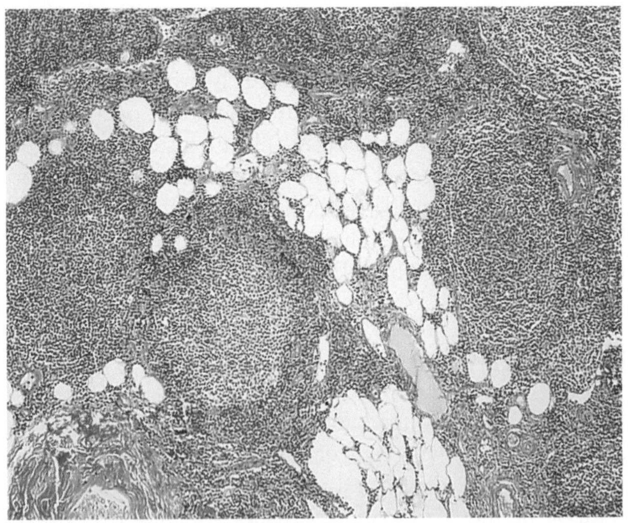

FIGURE 64.2. Follicular lymphoma: extension of neoplastic nodules into the perinodal adipose tissue. Hematoxylin, phloxine, and saffron stain.

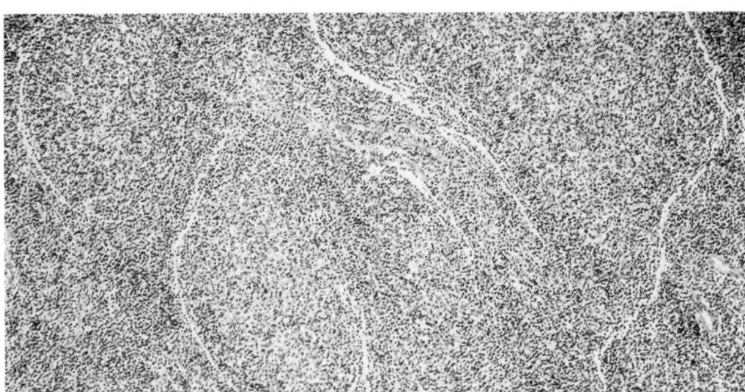

FIGURE 64.4. Follicular lymphoma. Artifactual cracking around nodules is a clue that neoplastic follicles are not intrinsically part of the lymph node architecture. H&E stain.

The cells in the nodules are similar to each other, representing a monotonous, monoclonal population (Fig. 64.3D). Mitoses are infrequent and no macrophages containing nuclear debris are seen, as they are in the hyperplastic follicles of reactive lymphadenopathies. Between the expanding neoplastic nodules, residual lymphocytes and sinus histiocytes appear compressed (Figs. 64.1 and 64.3), whereas vessels and reticulin fibers are distorted, as clearly shown by silver staining. Most characteristic of FLs is their tendency to form nodular structures, even outside the lymph nodes in the tissues they invade (Fig. 64.2).

Cytologically, the nodules of FL comprise neoplastic cells recapitulating the germinal centers of lymphoid follicles.

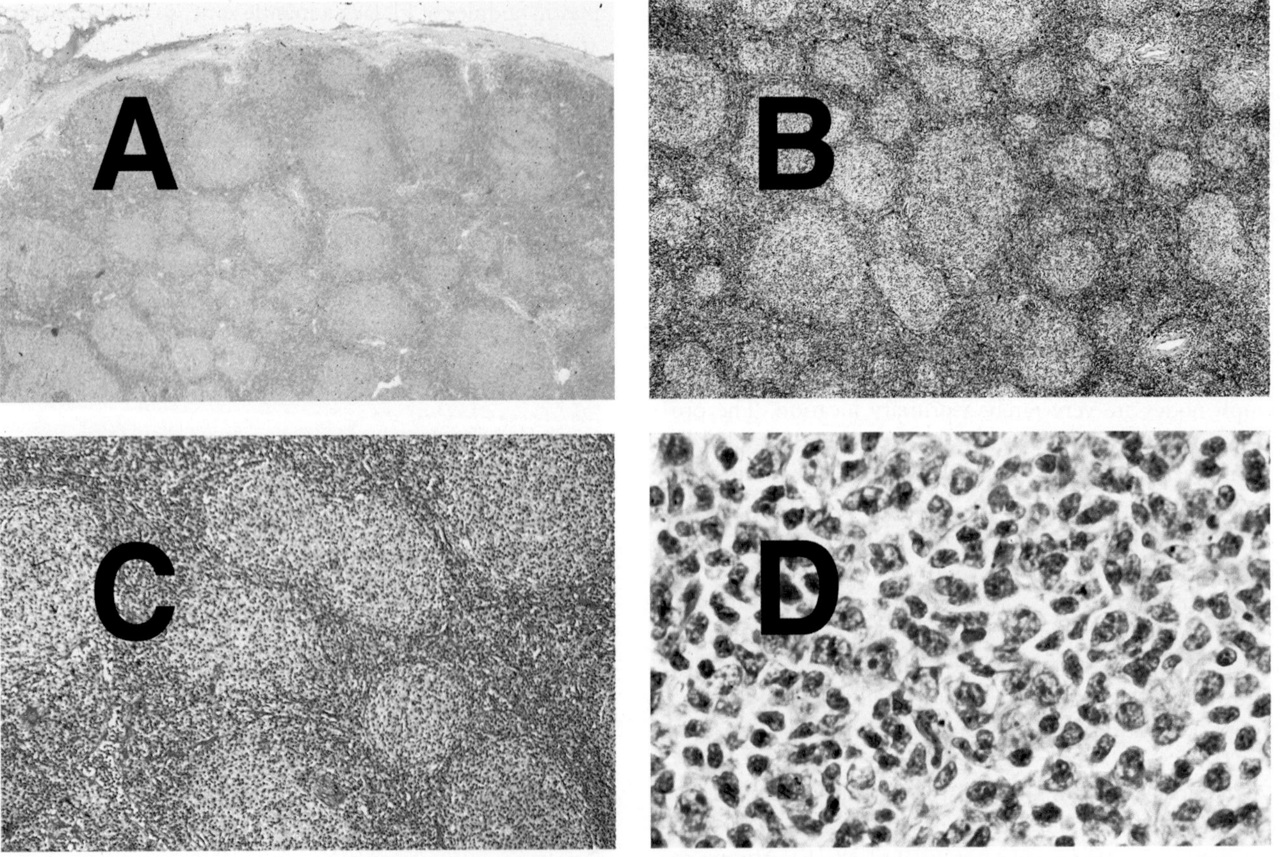

FIGURE 64.3. Follicular lymphoma, grade 1/3. **A:** Back-to-back follicles in cortex, deep cortex, and medulla. **B:** Interfollicular zone compressed by lymphoma nodules. **C:** Close apposition and fusion of neoplastic follicles. **D:** Homogeneous population of small cleaved lymphocytes without tingible-body macrophages; twisted, angulated, and raisin-shaped nuclei. H&E stain.

Normally, the germinal centers include a spectrum of B-lymphoid cells characterized by cleaved nuclei and varying from small to large. In addition, the normal germinal centers include small and large activated noncleaved B cells, a large number of T (mostly helper) lymphocytes, and a population of supportive, desmosome-connected follicular DRCs. Variable proportions of small and large cleaved and noncleaved neoplastic B lymphocytes compose FL.

Follicular lymphoma, grade 1 (Table 64.1), predominantly small cleaved cell type (Fig. 64.3), is characterized by cells the size of normal lymphocytes or slightly larger; their irregularly twisted "string bean"-shaped or "raisin"-shaped nuclei have indented or cleaved nuclear membranes and linear streaks representing nuclear infoldings. The nucleoli are small to inconspicuous, multiple, and peripherally apposed to the nuclear membrane.

Follicular lymphoma, grade 3 (Table 64.1), predominantly large cell type, is characterized by cells two to three times larger than normal lymphocytes; these have vesicular nuclei, a thick nuclear membrane, and two to three prominent ("snake bite") nucleoli. The cytoplasm is acidophilic and fairly abundant. Mitoses are frequent, reflecting a higher rate of cellular turnover, and nuclear pleomorphism may be marked, indicating a higher grade of tumor malignancy. Internodular and intercellular reticulin is more abundant, appearing as a well-developed fibrillar network on the silver stain.

Follicular lymphoma, grade 2 (Table 64.1), mixed small cleaved and large cell types, usually is composed of a mixture of small and large neoplastic germinal center cells.

Admixed with the neoplastic cells in FL are a variable but substantial number of non-neoplastic cells that represent residual cells of the involved follicles and cells reactive to neoplasia. T lymphocytes, mostly CD4+ helper cells, may comprise as much as 30% to 60% of the total cell population. Their presence must be kept in mind when the results of immunohistochemical staining are interpreted, to avoid misinterpretation. Follicular RDCs usually persist, but histiocytes do not; therefore, FLs lack tingible-body macrophages and "starry sky" patterns, which distinguishes them from RFH. Sclerosis is present in 40% of FLs (24) and is more common in the nodular than in the diffuse forms. It begins near the lymph node capsule and spreads both outside and within the areas of lymphoma, showing a pronounced tendency to hyalinization. Sometimes, sclerosis replaces large areas of lymph nodes, forming dense bands of hyaline tissue and exhibiting marked similarity to the nodular sclerosis type of Hodgkin lymphoma.

Circulating FL cells have the morphologic features of small cleaved cells, also known as *lymphosarcoma leukemia cells,* or *"buttock" cells* (25). The blood cell count remains within normal range or slightly increased for a long time.

TABLE 64.1. FOLLICULAR LYMPHOMAS: GRADING AND VARIANTS

Follicular lymphoma
- Grades
  - Grade 1: 0–5 centroblasts/HPF
  - Grade 2: 6–15 centroblasts/HPF
  - Grade 3: >15 centroblasts/HPF
    - 3a: >15 centroblasts, but centrocytes still present
    - 3b: centroblasts form solid sheets with no residual centrocytes

Variants
- Cutaneous follicle center lymphoma
- Diffuse follicle center lymphoma
  - Grade 1: 0–5 centroblasts/HPF
  - Grade 2: 6–15 centroblasts/HPF

HPF, high-power field.
Adapted from Harris NL, Jaffe ES, Diebold J, et al. The World Health Organization classification of hematological malignancies: report of the clinical advisory committee meeting, Airlie House, Virginia, November 1997. Mod Pathol 2000; 13:193–207.

CYTOLOGY

Aggregates of uniform cells bound by follicular DRCs and the absence of tingible-body macrophages are helpful clues for diagnosing FL by fine needle aspiration (26).

TRANSFORMATION

The process in which FL is converted to aggressive diffuse lymphoma is called *transformation* (27,28). Depending on the time of clinical follow-up, number of additional biopsies, and postmortem study, the frequency of FL transformation ranges between 10% and 70% (29,30). To avoid misinterpreting cases presenting with discordant histologies, at least 6 months must elapse between the initial biopsy and disease progression (27,28). FL that evolves from grade 1 to grade 2 to grade 3 and maintains a follicular pattern represents histologic progression, which does not have the same clinical significance as transformation. An initial FL, grade 3 must on a second biopsy show completely diffuse expansion by large cells to qualify as a transformation.

In a study of 220 patients with FL whose median follow-up time was 9 years, the overall incidence of transformation was 24% (31). The FL of patients who did not achieve complete remission after initial therapy was more likely to transform (31). However, not all investigators observed this (32,33). A poor outcome was associated with late-stage disease, older age, bone marrow involvement, systemic "B" symptoms, high levels of lactate dehydrogenase, high β_2-microglobulin levels, and number of prior treatments (34). In a multiparametric analysis, only β_2-microglobulin levels were significant in predicting freedom from transformation (31). Transformation tends to occur early in the clinical course of FL; the probability was 22% at 5 years and 31% at 10 years (31). The transformed diffuse aggressive histologic types included diffuse large cell lymphoma, immunoblastic lymphoma, diffuse mixed lymphoma, and Burkitt lymphoma (31). After transformation, the median survival time was 7 months, and transformation was responsible for 44% of deaths (31). A longer post-transformation survival period reported from Stanford is likely explained by the inclusion of many patients with early-stage disease (32).

Molecular alterations that appear to affect the risk for FL transformation include p53 mutation (35,36), C-MYC-translocation (37), deletions of tumor suppressor genes p15 and p16 (cyclin-dependent kinase inhibitors) (38,39), and chromosomal 6q23–26 and 17p aberrations (40).

SIGNET RING CELL LYMPHOMA (LYMPHOMA WITH INTRACELLULAR IMMUNOGLOBULINS)

Signet ring cell lymphoma, a rare variant of FL, is characterized by the presence of intracellular immunoglobulins (Igs) (41,42). The histologic pattern is nodular or combined nodular and diffuse (41). The predominant cell type resembles signet ring cells because of the presence of large clear vacuoles and eccentric, indented nuclei (Fig. 64.5). Some cells contain intracytoplasmic inclusions similar to Russell bodies or intranuclear inclusions (Fig. 64.6) such as the Dutcher bodies seen in Waldenström macroglobulinemia. These should be differentiated from the signet ring cells of mucinous adenocarcinomas. Signet ring cell lymphomas do not stain with mucicarmine; the vacuole contents and inclusion bodies are diastase-resistant and periodic acid–Schiff-positive (41). The vacuoles contain Igs. About 20 reported signet ring cell lymphomas contained monoclonal IgM, IgG, or IgA (41,42).

ELECTRON MICROSCOPY

The ultrastructure of FL is consistent with its germinal center origin, as suggested by light microscopy (43–45). Most FLs include a fairly uniform population of cells characterized by irregularly shaped, deeply indented nuclei with thick nuclear membranes, highly condensed and peripherally located chromatin, and occasional nuclear blebs (43). The nucleoli are multiple, relatively small, and apposed to the nuclear membrane. The cytoplasm includes a few mitochondria characteristically clustered in one area, a poorly developed Golgi body, and scattered ribosomes with rare formation of polysomes. Reticular or dendritic cells, normally seen in germinal centers, are always present. They appear

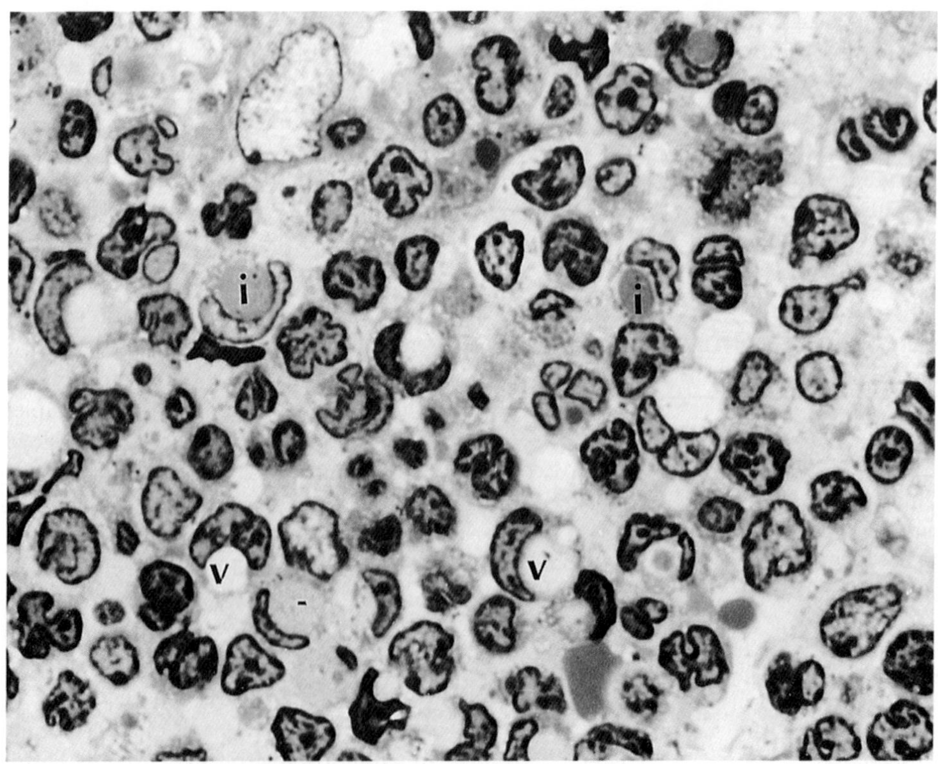

FIGURE 64.5. Follicular lymphoma, signet ring cell type. Cleaved lymphoid cells of germinal center type frequently have cytoplasmic vacuoles (*v*) or large inclusions (*i*) that stain with periodic acid–Schiff and eccentric, indented nuclei. ×1,700. (From Vernon S, Voet RL, Naeim F, et al. Nodular lymphoma with intracellular immunoglobulin. Cancer 1979;44:1273–1279, with permission.)

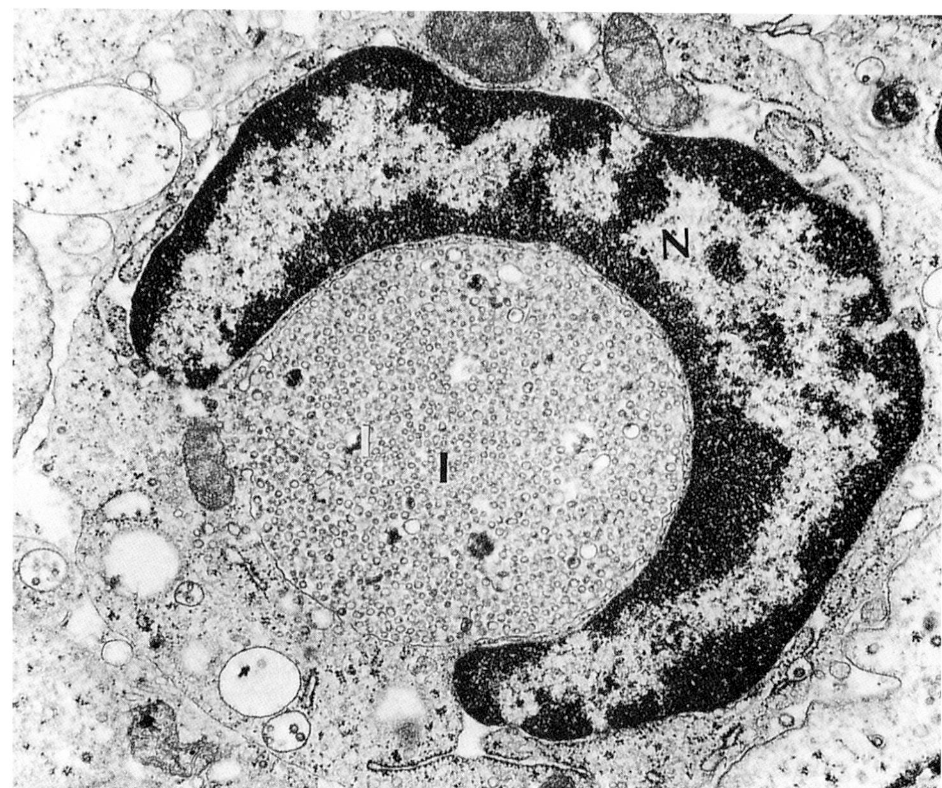

FIGURE 64.6. Follicular lymphoma, signet ring cell type, showing kidney-shaped nucleus (*N*) and large cytoplasmic inclusion (*i*) with fine microvesicular structure. ×9,400. (From Vernon S, Voet RL, Naeim F, et al. Nodular lymphoma with intracellular immunoglobulin. Cancer 1979;44:1273–1279, with permission.)

darkly stained and irregularly shaped, and their long processes are interconnected by desmosomes and inserted between the lymphoma cells.

Electron microscopy of signet ring cell lymphomas (Fig. 64.6) shows the intracytoplasmic inclusion bodies to be composed of electron-dense, homogeneous, flocculent material located in a vacuole that represents a distended cisterna of endoplasmic reticulum (41,42).

IMMUNOHISTOCHEMISTRY

Follicular lymphomas typically express monoclonal surface Ig, CD10, and pan-B-cell markers CD19, CD20 (Fig. 64.7A), CD22, and CD79a; they do not express CD5 or CD23 (3). Most are CD43−, except for rare cases of FL, grade 3 that have a DLBCL component (46). Both follicles and interfollicular zones contain clonally restricted B cells (47). Unlike reactive germinal centers, which are negative for bcl-2 protein, the overwhelming majority (about 90%) of FLs, grade 1 overexpress bcl-2 protein (Fig. 64.7B); slightly lower percentages of FLs, grades 2 and 3 have detectable bcl-2 protein (48). In addition to mimicking the growth pattern of reactive follicles, FLs contain comparable populations of non-neoplastic T cells (Fig. 64.7C) and follicular DRCs. Follicular DRC meshworks in FL and RFH are similar in diameter (49). Follicular DRCs in FL and RFH express CD21 and CD35; follicular DRCs in FL, but not in RFH, lack expression of fascin (50).

Phenotype

CD5−
CD10+/−
CD19+
CD21+
CD20+
CD22+
CD23−/+
CD43−
CD79a+
Monoclonal sIg+ (bright)

FLOW CYTOMETRY

Follicular lymphomas express brightly fluorescent monoclonal surface Igs and receptors for the third component of complement (CD21) (51). Most FLs express surface IgM,

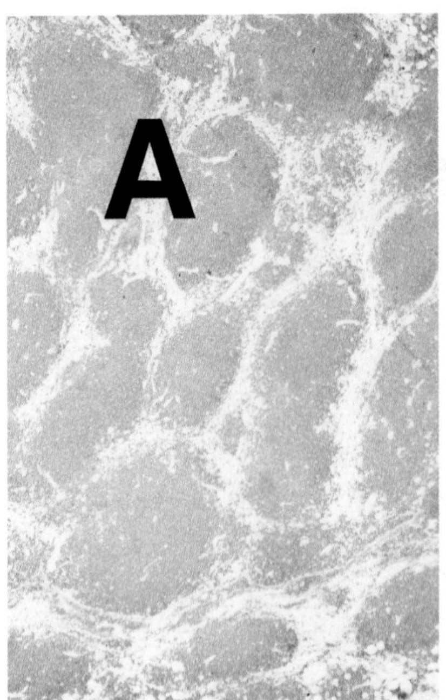

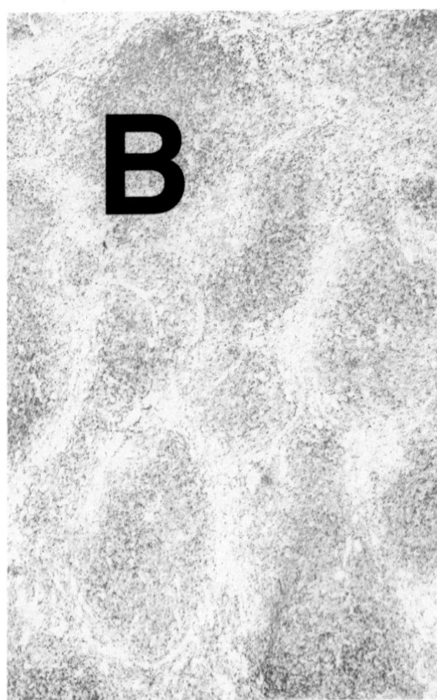

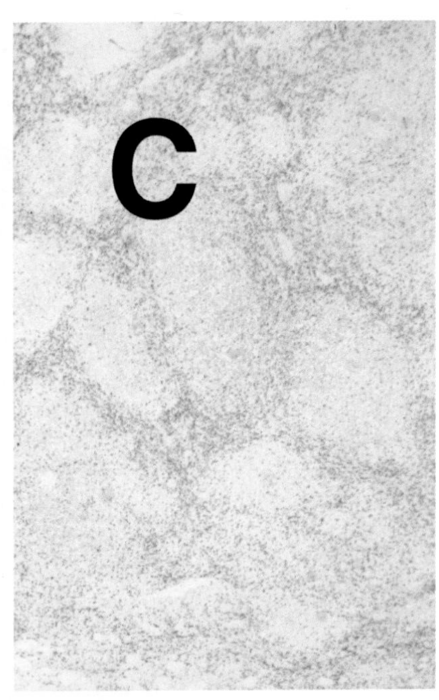

FIGURE 64.7. A: Neoplastic follicles express B-cell marker CD20 (stained with L26 antibody). Immunoperoxidase stain. **B:** Neoplastic follicles overexpress bcl-2 protein. Immunoperoxidase stain. **C:** CD3 highlights non-neoplastic, interfollicular T cells. Immunoperoxidase stain. The patterns in A and C are similar to those of reactive follicular hyperplasia (*RFH*), but the pattern in B is not. Germinal centers in RFH do not express bcl-2 protein, except in a few scattered T cells (see Chapter 33).

with or without surface IgD (52). IgG or IgA isotypes are more frequently found than in other low-grade B-cell lymphomas. The intensity of CD10 detected on FL cells is much greater than the intensity of that on reactive follicular B-cells (53).

CYTOGENETICS

The BCL-2 gene on chromosome 18q21 is deregulated by its juxtaposition with the Ig heavy chain locus on chromosome 14q32. The t(14;18)(q32;q21) chromosomal translocation (see Chapter 8) confers a survival advantage to the affected B cells because they overexpress bcl-2 protein, an apoptosis inhibitor (Fig. 64.7B).

Normally, bcl-6 protein is restricted to reactive germinal center B cells and rare interfollicular T cells (54). Some FLs carry both BCL-2 and BCL-6 rearrangements (55). In about 14% of FLs, the BCL-6 gene located on chromosome 3q27 translocates adjacent to various heterologous promoters from other chromosomes, so that an aberrantly persistent pattern of BCL-6 gene expression is obtained (56). Rearrangement of BCL-6 is detected more often in FLs with an increased number of large cells (57).

MOLECULAR DIAGNOSIS

See Chapter 8.

DIFFERENTIAL DIAGNOSIS

- RFH: A common hyperplastic reaction of lymph nodes in response to a variety of viruses, bacteria, drugs, and undetermined antigens produces histologic patterns closely resembling those of FL. Differentiation of these non-neoplastic lesions from their malignant counterparts is frequently difficult and sometimes impossible without special techniques. The patient's age is an important clue; children and young adults present often with lymph node RFH but only exceptionally with FL. Morphologically, the lymphoid follicles are large and irregularly shaped, often coalescing and forming bizarre, dumbbell shapes. In comparison with those of FL, the follicles of benign hyperplasia are less numerous, farther apart, and more restricted to the cortex. The germinal centers are prominent, and the periphery is sharply demarcated by a mantle of small mature lymphocytes. The cell population of the germinal centers is not uniform but varies and includes frequent mitoses and tingible-body macrophages. In a comparative study of 80 patients, the parameters commonly used to distinguish FL from RFH were evaluated to determine which are most valuable (58). In decreasing order of importance, the most reliable histologic features for diagnosing FL were the following: (a) a follicular pattern, because the neoplastic follicles, regardless of their size, are evenly distributed throughout the lymph

Checklist

FOLLICULAR LYMPHOMA

High incidence in Western industrialized countries
Patients elderly; cases rare before the age of 20 years
Equal sex distribution
Indolent course, long survival
Lymph node architecture obliterated
Round, numerous nodules in close proximity
Cracking artifact around nodules
Whole lymph node and perinodal fat involved
Perinodular lymphocyte mantles diminished to absent
Tingible-body macrophages absent
Nodular cell population monomorphic, closely packed
Nuclei cleaved, small, intermediate or large
Cells with similar cleaved nuclei in internodular areas
B cells monoclonal, with surface κ or λ light chain
CD10 and pan-B-cell markers, but not CD5 or CD43
t(14;18) translocation associated with bcl-2 deregulation

node and have a back-to-back arrangement with little intervening tissue; (b) a large number of follicles per unit area; (c) cells in the interfollicular areas with the same cytologic features as those in the follicles; and (d) an absence of histiocytes with phagocytic activity within the follicles (58).

- Progressive transformation of germinal centers can mimic a "floral" variant of FL, grade 3 (59). However, lymph node replacement by progressive transformation of germinal centers is partial. In contrast, all nodules in "floral" FL are involved by a uniform population of large transformed lymphocytes that are infiltrated by small lymphocytes; no residual reactive germinal center cells or phagocytic histiocytes are seen.
- Mantle cell lymphoma: A nodular pattern occurs in both mantle cell lymphoma and FL, but mantle cell lymphomas have less deeply invaginated nuclei, and they express CD5 and CD43 plus pan-B cell markers but not CD10; they also express bcl-1 protein (cyclin D1) associated with chromosomal translocation t(11;14).
- Primary nodal marginal zone lymphoma of splenic type: Follicular colonization can simulate FL, but the presence of residual bcl-2 protein-negative germinal center cells, IgD expression, and the absence of chromosomal translocation t(14;18) favor marginal zone lymphoma (60).
- Pseudonodular lymphomas: Some lymphomas show distinct compartmentalization by fine bands of fibrocollagen that may imitate the nodularity of FLs (61); however, the components of such lymphomas are not cells of follicle center type but usually contain convoluted nuclei and carry T-cell markers.
- Mucinous adenocarcinoma of signet ring cell type can be differentiated from signet ring lymphoma by mucicarmine and cytokeratin staining and the absence of CD45 and B-cell and Ig markers.

REFERENCES

1. Rappaport H. Tumors of the hematopoietic system. In: Atlas of tumor pathology. Washington, DC: Armed Forces Institute of Pathology, 1966.
2. National Cancer Institute-sponsored study of classifications of non-Hodgkin's lymphomas: summary and description of a working formulation for clinical usage. The Non-Hodgkin's Lymphoma Pathologic Classification Project. Cancer 1982;49:2112–2135.
3. Harris NL, Jaffe ES, Stein H, et al. A revised European-American classification of lymphoid neoplasms: a proposal from the International Lymphoma Study Group [see Comments]. Blood 1994; 84:1361–1392.
4. Harris NL, Jaffe ES, Diebold J, et al. The World Health Organization classification of hematological malignancies: report of the clinical advisory committee meeting, Airlie House, Virginia, November 1997. Mod Pathol 2000;13:193–207.
5. Metter GE, Nathwani BN, Burke JS, et al. Morphological subclassification of follicular lymphoma: variability of diagnoses among hematopathologists, a collaborative study between the Repository Center and Pathology Panel for Lymphoma Clinical Studies. J Clin Oncol 1985;3:25–38.
6. Mann R, Berard C. Criteria for the cytologic subclassification of follicular lymphomas: a proposed alternative method. Hematol Oncol 1982;1:187–192.
7. The Non-Hodgkin's Lymphoma Classification Project. A clinical evaluation of the International Lymphoma Study Group classification of non-Hodgkin's lymphoma. Blood 1997;89:3909–3918.

8. Winberg CD, Nathwani BN, Bearman RM, et al. Follicular (nodular) lymphoma during the first two decades of life: a clinicopathologic study of 12 patients. Cancer 1981;48:2223–2235.
9. Ribeiro RC, Pui CH, Murphy SB, et al. Childhood malignant non-Hodgkin lymphomas of uncommon histology. Leukemia 1992;6:761–765.
10. Atra A, Meller ST, Stevens RS, et al. Conservative management of follicular non-Hodgkin's lymphoma in childhood. Br J Haematol 1998;103:220–223.
11. Limpens J, Stad R, Vos C, et al. Lymphoma-associated translocation t(14;18) in blood B cells of normal individuals. Blood 1995; 85:2528–2536.
12. Yang E, Korsmeyer SJ. Molecular thanatopsis: a discourse on the BCL2 family and cell death. Blood 1996;88:386–401.
13. Ghia P, Boussiotis VA, Schultze JL, et al. Unbalanced expression of bcl-2 family proteins in follicular lymphoma: contribution of CD40 signaling in promoting survival. Blood 1998;91:244–251.
14. Carbone A, Gloghini A, Gruss HJ, et al. CD40 ligand is constitutively expressed in a subset of T-cell lymphomas and on the microenvironmental reactive T cells of follicular lymphomas and Hodgkin's disease. Am J Pathol 1995;147:912–922.
15. Petrasch S, Kosco M, Schmitz J, et al. Follicular dendritic cells in non-Hodgkin lymphoma express adhesion molecules complementary to ligands on neoplastic B cells. Br J Haematol 1992;82: 695–700.
16. Lindhout E, Mevissen ML, Kwekkeboom J, et al. Direct evidence that human follicular dendritic cells (FDC) rescue germinal centre B cells from death by apoptosis. Clin Exp Immunol 1993;91: 330–336.
17. Martin AR, Weisenburger DD, Chan WC, et al. Prognostic value of cellular proliferation and histologic grade in follicular lymphoma. Blood 1995;85:3671–3678.
18. Miller TP, LeBlanc M, Grogan TM, et al. Follicular lymphomas: do histologic subtypes predict outcome? Hematol Oncol Clin North Am 1997;11:893–900.
19. Denham JW, Denham E, Dear KB, et al. The follicular non-Hodgkin's lymphomas—II. Prognostic factors: what do they mean? Eur J Cancer 1996;32A:480–490.
20. MacManus MP, Hoppe RT. Is radiotherapy curative for stage I and II low-grade follicular lymphoma? Results of a long-term follow-up study of patients treated at Stanford University. J Clin Oncol 1996;14:1282–1290.
21. The International Non-Hodgkin's Lymphoma Prognostic Factors Project. A predictive model for aggressive non-Hodgkin's lymphoma [see Comments]. N Engl J Med 1993;329:987–994.
22. Bastion Y, Coiffier B. Is the International Prognostic Index for aggressive lymphoma patients useful for follicular lymphoma patients? [Editorial; Comment]. J Clin Oncol 1994;12:1340–1342.
23. Warnke RA, Kim H, Fuks Z, et al. The coexistence of nodular and diffuse patterns in nodular non-Hodgkin's lymphomas: significance and clinicopathologic correlation. Cancer 1977;40: 1229–1233.
24. Bennett MH. Sclerosis in non-Hodgkin's lymphomata. Br J Cancer 1975;31[Suppl 2]:44–52.
25. Come SE, Jaffe ES, Andersen JC, et al. Non-Hodgkin's lymphomas in leukemic phase: clinicopathologic correlations. Am J Med 1980;69:667–674.
26. Suh YK, Shabaik A, Meurer WT, et al. Lymphoid cell aggregates: a useful clue in the fine-needle aspiration diagnosis of follicular lymphomas. Diagn Cytopathol 1997;17:467–471.
27. Hubbard SM, Chabner BA, DeVita VT Jr, et al. Histologic progression in non-Hodgkin's lymphoma. Blood 1982;59:258–264.
28. Oviatt DL, Cousar JB, Collins RD, et al. Malignant lymphomas of follicular center cell origin in humans. V. Incidence, clinical features, and prognostic implications of transformation of small cleaved cell nodular lymphoma. Cancer 1984;53: 1109–1114.
29. Garvin AJ, Simon RM, Osborne CK, et al. An autopsy study of histologic progression in non-Hodgkin's lymphomas. One hundred ninety-two cases from the National Cancer Institute. Cancer 1983;52:393–398.
30. Ersboll J, Schultz HB, Pedersen-Bjergaard J, et al. Follicular low-grade non-Hodgkin's lymphoma: long-term outcome with or without tumor progression. Eur J Haematol 1989;42:155–163.
31. Bastion Y, Sebban C, Berger F, et al. Incidence, predictive factors, and outcome of lymphoma transformation in follicular lymphoma patients. J Clin Oncol 1997;15:1587–1594.
32. Yuen AR, Kamel OW, Halpern J, et al. Long-term survival after histologic transformation of low-grade follicular lymphoma. J Clin Oncol 1995;13:1726–1733.
33. Brice P, Bastion Y, Lepage E, et al. Comparison in low-tumor-burden follicular lymphomas between an initial no-treatment policy, prednimustine, or interferon alfa: a randomized study from the Groupe d'Étude des Lymphomes Folliculaires. Groupe d'Étude des Lymphomes de l'Adulte. J Clin Oncol 1997;15: 1110–1117.
34. Coiffier B, Bastion Y, Berger F, et al. Prognostic factors in follicular lymphomas. Semin Oncol 1993;20:89–95.
35. Sander CA, Yano T, Clark HM, et al. p53 mutation is associated with progression in follicular lymphomas. Blood 1993;82:1994–2004.
36. Lo Coco F, Gaidano G, Louie DC, et al. p53 mutations are associated with histologic transformation of follicular lymphoma. Blood 1993;82:2289–2295.
37. Yano T, Jaffe ES, Longo DL, et al. MYC rearrangements in histologically progressed follicular lymphomas. Blood 1992;80: 758–767.
38. Pinyol M, Cobo F, Bea S, et al. p16(INK4a) gene inactivation by deletions, mutations, and hypermethylation is associated with transformed and aggressive variants of non-Hodgkin's lymphomas. Blood 1998;91:2977–2984.
39. Elenitoba-Johnson KS, Gascoyne RD, Lim MS, et al. Homozygous deletions at chromosome 9p21 involving p16 and p15 are associated with histologic progression in follicle center lymphoma. Blood 1998;91:4677–4685.
40. Tilly H, Rossi A, Stamatoullas A, et al. Prognostic value of chromosomal abnormalities in follicular lymphoma. Blood 1994;84:1043–1049.
41. Kim H, Dorfman RF, Rappaport H. Signet ring cell lymphoma. A rare morphologic and functional expression of nodular (follicular) lymphoma. Am J Surg Pathol 1978;2:119–132.
42. Vernon S, Voet RL, Naeim F, et al. Nodular lymphoma with intracellular immunoglobulin. Cancer 1979;44:1273–1279.
43. Levine GD, Dorfman RF. Nodular lymphoma: an ultrastructural study of its relationship to germinal centers and a correlation of light and electron microscopic findings. Cancer 1975;35:148–164.
44. Mori Y, Lennert K. Electron microscopy atlas of lymph node cytology and pathology. New York: Springer-Verlag, 1969:189–201.
45. Ioachim HL. Lymph nodes and spleen. In: Johannessen JV, ed. Electron microscopy in human medicine, vol 5. New York: McGraw-Hill, 1981:384–463.
46. Lai R, Weiss LM, Chang KL, et al. Frequency of CD43 expression in non-Hodgkin lymphoma. A survey of 742 cases and further characterization of rare CD43+ follicular lymphomas. Am J Clin Pathol 1999;111:488–494.
47. Dogan A, Du MQ, Aiello A, et al. Follicular lymphomas contain a clonally linked but phenotypically distinct neoplastic B-cell population in the interfollicular zone. Blood 1998;91:4708–4714.

48. Swerdlow SH. Small B-cell lymphomas of the lymph nodes and spleen: practical insights to diagnosis and pathogenesis. Mod Pathol 1999;12:125–140.
49. Ratech H, Sheibani K, Nathwani BN, et al. Immunoarchitecture of the "pseudofollicles" of well-differentiated (small) lymphocytic lymphoma: a comparison with true follicles [published erratum appears in Hum Pathol 1988;19:495]. Hum Pathol 1988;19:89–94.
50. Said JW, Pinkus JL, Shintaku IP, et al. Alterations in fascin-expressing germinal center dendritic cells in neoplastic follicles of B-cell lymphomas. Mod Pathol 1998;11:1–5.
51. Jaffe ES, Shevach EM, Frank MM, et al. Nodular lymphoma—evidence for origin from follicular B lymphocytes. N Engl J Med 1974;290:813–819.
52. Leech JH, Glick AD, Waldron JA, et al. Malignant lymphomas of follicular center cell origin in man. I. Immunologic studies. J Natl Cancer Inst 1975;54:11–21.
53. Almasri NM, Iturraspe JA, Braylan RC. CD10 expression in follicular lymphoma and large cell lymphoma is different from that of reactive lymph node follicles. Arch Pathol Lab Med 1998;122: 539–544.
54. Ree HJ, Kadin ME, Kikuchi M, et al. Bcl-6 expression in reactive follicular hyperplasia, follicular lymphoma, and angioimmunoblastic T-cell lymphoma with hyperplastic germinal centers: heterogeneity of intrafollicular T cells and their altered distribution in the pathogenesis of angioimmunoblastic T-cell lymphoma. Hum Pathol 1999;30:403–411.
55. Skinnider BF, Horsman DE, Dupuis B, et al. Bcl-6 and Bcl-2 protein expression in diffuse large B-cell lymphoma and follicular lymphoma: correlation with 3q27 and 18q21 chromosomal abnormalities. Hum Pathol 1999;30:803–808.
56. Chen W, Iida S, Louie DC, et al. Heterologous promoters fused to BCL6 by chromosomal translocations affecting band 3q27 cause its deregulated expression during B-cell differentiation. Blood 1998;91:603–607.
57. Muramatsu M, Akasaka T, Kadowaki N, et al. Rearrangement of the BCL6 gene in B-cell lymphoid neoplasms: comparison with lymphomas associated with BCL2 rearrangement. Br J Haematol 1996;93:911–920.
58. Nathwani BN, Winberg CD, Diamond LW, et al. Morphologic criteria for the differentiation of follicular lymphoma from florid reactive follicular hyperplasia: a study of 80 cases. Cancer 1981; 48:1794–1806.
59. Osborne BM, Butler JJ. Follicular lymphoma mimicking progressive transformation of germinal centers. Am J Clin Pathol 1987;88:264–269.
60. Campo E, Miquel R, Krenacs L, et al. Primary nodal marginal zone lymphomas of splenic and MALT type [see Comments]. Am J Surg Pathol 1999;23:59–68.
61. Ioachim HL, Finkbeiner JA. Pseudonodular pattern of T-cell lymphoma. Cancer 1980;45:1370–1378.

65

DIFFUSE FOLLICLE CENTER CELL LYMPHOMA

DEFINITION

Diffusely growing, germinal center-derived lymphomas containing predominantly small cleaved B cells or a mix of small cleaved and large B cells; the diffuse counterpart of follicular (nodular) lymphomas showing some indication of originating from the follicle center, such as bcl-2 gene rearrangement or CD10 immunophenotype.

SYNONYMS

Diffuse poorly differentiated lymphocytic lymphoma (Rappaport) (1)

Diffuse small cleaved follicle center cell lymphoma (Lukes and Collins) (2)

Diffuse centrocytic or centroblastic–centrocytic lymphoma (Kiel) (3)

Malignant lymphoma, diffuse, predominantly small cleaved cell (Working Formulation) (4)

Follicle center lymphoma (FCL), diffuse, predominantly small cell (provisional subtype, Revised European-American Lymphoma Classification, or REAL) (5)

Follicular lymphoma variant: diffuse FCL [World Health Organization (WHO)] (6)

SUBTYPES

Follicle center B-cell lymphomas have been divided according to cell size and shape into three categories (7). The REAL and WHO systems introduce a three-tier grading system to emphasize that these are not distinct entities but only different grades of a single disease.

- Poorly differentiated lymphocytic; mixed lymphocytic/histiocytic; histiocytic (1)
- Small and large cleaved cell; small and large noncleaved cell (2)
- Centrocytic, small; centrocytic, small and large; centrocytic, large (3)
- Lymphocytic small cell; mixed small and large cell; large cell (8)
- Small lymphoid; mixed small and large lymphoid; large lymphoid (9)
- Prolymphocytic; prolymphocytic and lymphoblastic; lymphoblastic (10)
- Small cleaved cell; mixed, small and large cell; large cell (4)
- FCL, follicular; provisional cytologic grades 1 (predominantly small cell), 2 (mixed small and large cell), and 3 (predominantly large cell) (5)
- Follicular lymphoma: grade 1, 0 to 5 centroblasts per high-power field (HPF); grade 2, 6 to 15 centroblasts per HPF; grade 3, more than 15 centroblasts per HPF (6)

All classifications acknowledge the existence of three subtypes, characterized by a predominance of small, atypical lymphoid cells, a predominance of large atypical lymphoid cells, or a mixture of small and large atypical lymphoid cells. Diffuse FCLs are characterized by growth pattern and nuclear size. They are regarded as cellular variants of a single neoplastic process. Nuclear size, a major criterion for lymphoma classification with prognostic significance, is measured according to the size of histiocytic nuclei. Lymphomas with nuclei smaller than those of histiocytes are small cell type; lymphomas with nuclei larger than those of histiocytes are large cell type; lymphomas with a nuclear diameter approximately the same size as that of histiocytes are medium-sized. For a discussion of B-cell lymphomas retaining a nodular pattern, see Chapters 63, 64, and 66. For a discussion of B-cell lymphomas with diffusely arranged large cells, see Chapters 67 and 68.

EPIDEMIOLOGY

Morphologic mimics of diffuse FCL contaminate some older clinicopathologic studies. For example, the Rappaport category equivalent to diffuse FCL, diffuse poorly differentiated lymphocytic lymphoma, has yielded two clinically aggressive lymphomas: lymphoblastic lymphoma (11) (see

Chapter 59) and mantle cell lymphoma (see Chapter 66). Older reports of diffuse poorly differentiated lymphocytic lymphoma in children, with mediastinal masses of T-cell phenotype or other masses of non–T-cell, non–B-cell phenotype, and with a tendency to develop leukemia, likely refer to lymphoblastic lymphoma (12–14). Historical studies of diffuse poorly differentiated lymphocytic lymphoma in adults, with a higher relapse rate and worse prognosis than those of follicular (nodular) lymphoma, a leukemic phase, and more frequent extranodal disease, probably describe mantle cell lymphoma (15–18).

PATHOGENESIS

Follicle center lymphomas constitute most non-Hodgkin lymphomas in the United States and, at the time of diagnosis, may present in nodular or diffuse form. Follicular (nodular) lymphomas, as previously mentioned (see Chapter 64), almost never occur in children and are rarely seen before the age of 20 years. About 30% of nodular lymphomas change during their course to a diffuse pattern, and at autopsy, about 70% appear as diffuse lymphomas (19). Therefore, the diffuse lymphomas of cleaved cell type partly represent the progression of former follicular (nodular) lymphomas and partly lymphomas growing in a diffuse pattern from inception. Lymphosarcoma cell leukemia represents the disseminated phase of FCLs, follicular or diffuse, and results from the involvement of the bone marrow and peripheral blood.

The term *FCL, diffuse* in the WHO classification refers to a rare form of FCL. It grows diffusely and contains a majority of centrocytes and few centroblasts. In addition, some sign of follicle center origin, such as bcl-2 gene rearrangement or CD10 immunophenotype, is generally present (6).

CLINICAL SYNDROME

Follicular lymphoma (FL), grade 1 (WHO) and FL, grade 2 (WHO) behave more like each other than like FL, grade 3 (WHO) (6). Multiple biopsy specimens from the same patient indicate frequent histologic transitions between FL, grade 1 and FL, grade 2 but rarely between FL, grade 1 and FL, grade 3. Furthermore, a trend for earlier relapse is noted in patients with FL, grade 3 versus patients with FL, grade 1 or 2 (6). Many oncologists maintain that it is valuable to indicate in the pathologic diagnosis when a predominantly diffuse growth pattern is present, although it is not always obvious how this information will influence specific therapy (6). Nevertheless, the WHO classification recommends that diffuse areas should be pointed out according to the REAL classification criteria: predominantly follicular (75% follicular), follicular and diffuse (25% to 75% follicular), and predominantly diffuse (<25% follicular) (5,6).

The clinical presentation, as in other types of lymphoma, is nonspecific and may include anorexia, malaise, weight loss, fevers, and night sweats. In general, systemic symptoms are more frequent in diffuse than in nodular lymphomas (20). Localized extralymphatic involvement is also more common in diffuse than in nodular lymphomas (20). In one early study, the 5-year survival rate was 74% for patients with follicular (nodular) lymphoma and only 28% for those with diffuse lymphoma, both of cleaved cell type (21). Lymphomas with follicular and diffuse patterns may not behave significantly differently from those with an exclusively follicular pattern (22). Nevertheless, in the large cell or "histiocytic" subtype, the presence of diffuse areas indicates a poor prognosis and requires more aggressive chemotherapy.

The noncleaved (centroblastic) cell type of both nodular and diffuse lymphomas has a significantly worse prognosis than does the small cleaved (centrocytic) cell type. The cell size has important prognostic implications. Thus, lymphomas of large cell types, both nodular and diffuse, are characterized by a far more aggressive clinical course and a significantly worse prognosis than are the corresponding lymphomas of small cell types. However, despite their highly malignant behavior, large cell lymphomas initially disseminate less extensively than their small cell counterparts (see Chapters 67 and 68).

HISTOPATHOLOGY

Diffuse Follicle Center Lymphoma, Grade 1

The lymph node architecture is partially or totally obliterated (Fig. 65.1) by a diffuse and monotonous proliferation of atypical lymphocytes. These lymphocytes (Figs. 65.2 and 65.3) resemble some of the cellular components of normal germinal centers and are similar to the cells of nodular lymphomas of small cleaved cell type. The cytoplasm is inconspicuous, and the nuclei are irregularly shaped and angular, with indentations and infoldings. The nucleoli are small, multiple, and peripheral. The nuclear pleomorphism contrasts sharply with the nuclear uniformity of small lymphocytic lymphoma. Also, the general staining is weaker and more grayish than that of the well-differentiated lymphocytic lymphomas, which have darker, denser nuclei. Mitoses are more common. Reticulin fibers are scarce. No proliferation centers are seen, as they are in small lymphocytic lymphoma, and only residual nodules are present when the follicular (nodular) type has preceded the diffuse type.

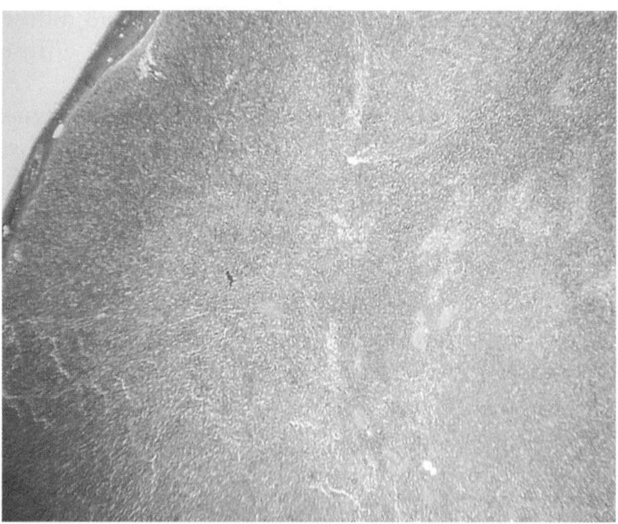

FIGURE 65.1. Diffuse follicle center cell lymphoma (diffuse, small cleaved cell; poorly differentiated non-Hodgkin lymphoma) in inguinal lymph node with complete effacement of nodal architecture. Hematoxylin, phloxine, and eosin stain.

Diffuse Follicle Center Lymphoma, Grade 2

These diffuse lymphomas consist of a mixture of nearly equal numbers of small cells with cleaved nuclei and large cells with vesicular nuclei containing conspicuous nucleoli (Fig. 65.4). They are infrequent and probably represent an advanced stage of their nodular counterparts.

Diffuse Follicle Center Lymphoma, Grade 3

The WHO classification considers diffuse areas in FL, grade 3 as representing diffuse large B-cell lymphoma (DLBCL) (6). These cases should not be called *FL, grade 3, follicular and diffuse* (6). Instead, they must be designated according to the portion replaced, such as *FL, grade 3/3 (75%) with DLBCL (25%)* (6). In DLBCL, sheets of atypical large lymphoid cells infiltrate and replace lymph node structure. A purely diffuse large cleaved cell type is uncommon (Fig. 65.5). Occasional foci of necrosis and fibrocollagen bands may divide tumor areas. Because the large cells contain greater amounts of cytoplasm, the nuclei are more widely separated. As a result, DLBCL appears more lightly stained because the large lymphoid cells are widely separated, unlike the closely packed small lym-

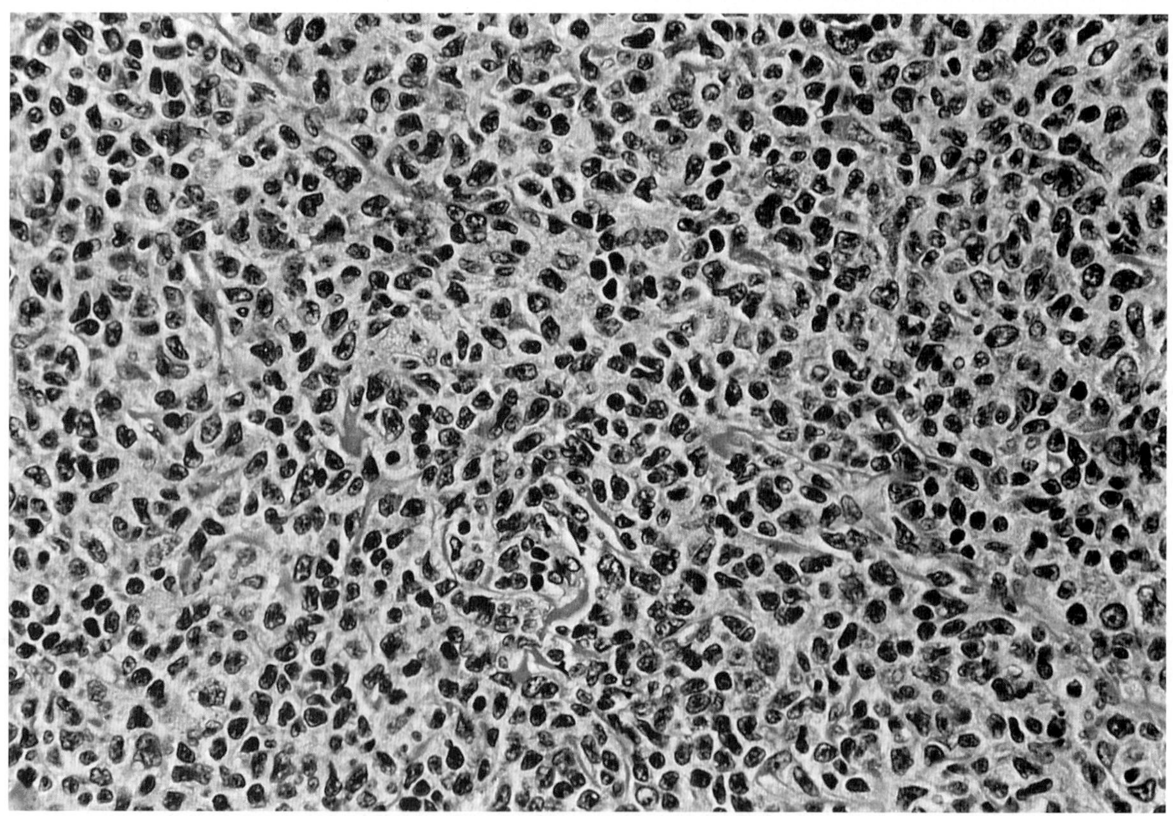

FIGURE 65.2. Diffuse follicle center cell lymphoma Grade 1. Nodal parenchyma replaced by uniform population of small, closely packed lymphoid cells with angular or cleaved nuclei. Hematoxylin, phloxine, and eosin stain.

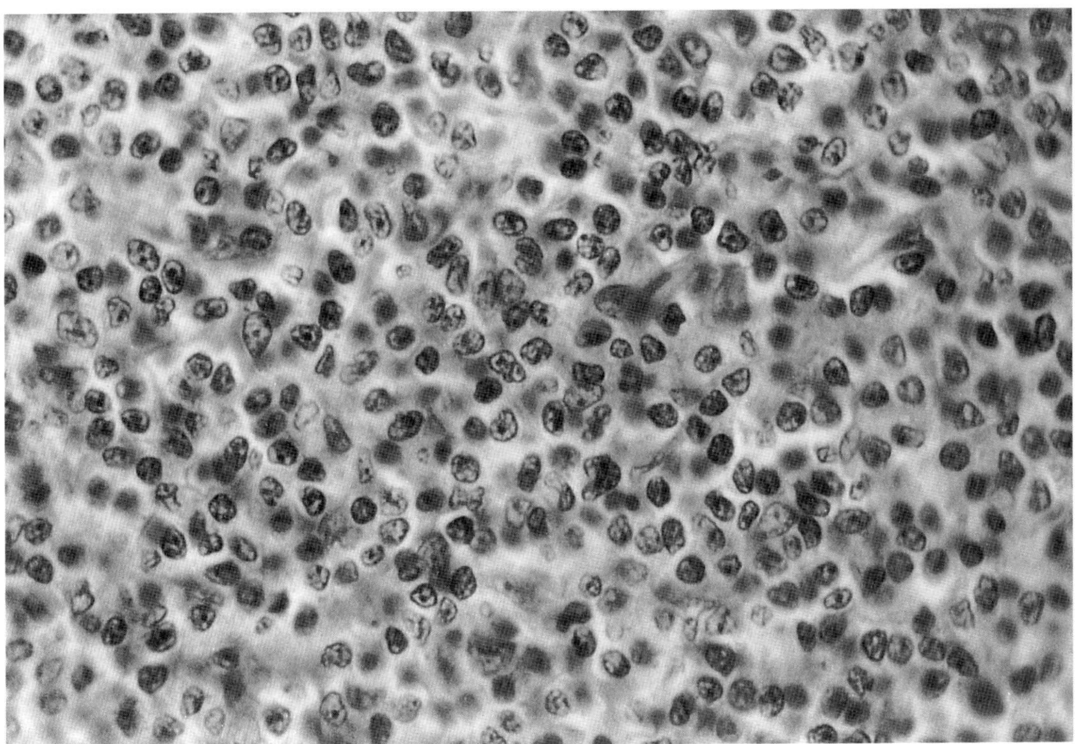

FIGURE 65.3. Diffuse follicle center cell lymphoma Grade 1. Sheets of small lymphoid cells with angular or cleaved nuclei containing conspicuous nucleoli. Hematoxylin, phloxine, and eosin stain.

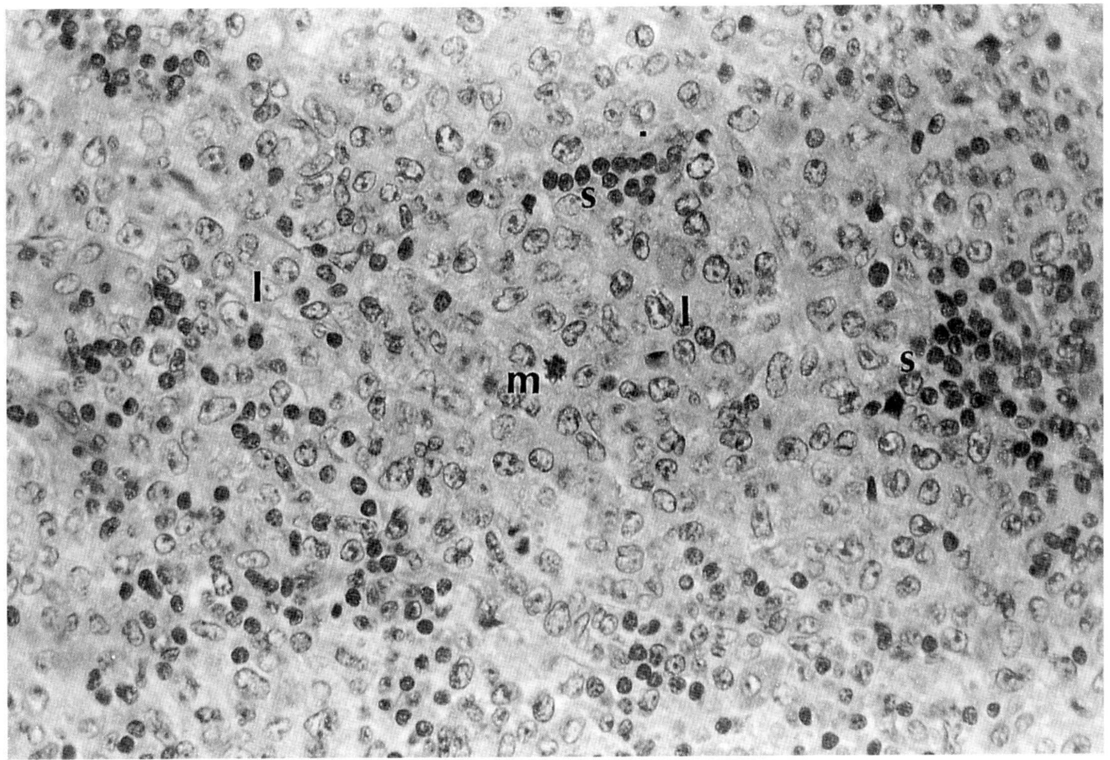

FIGURE 65.4. Diffuse, mixed small and large cleaved cell lymphoma Grade 2 in axillary lymph node. Nodal architecture obliterated by mixture of large (*l*) and small (*s*) lymphoid cells with cleaved nuclei and occasional mitoses (*m*). Hematoxylin, phloxine, and eosin stain.

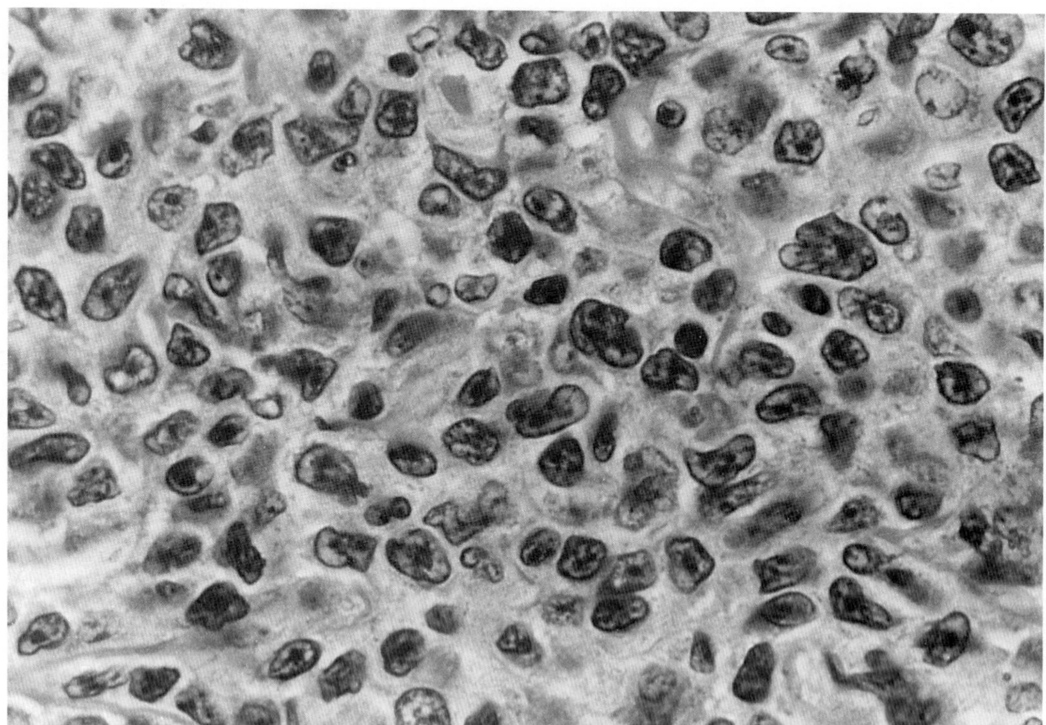

FIGURE 65.5. Diffuse, large cleaved cell lymphoma Grade 3 in supraclavicular lymph node. Population of lymphoid cells with fairly abundant cytoplasm, large cleaved nuclei, and multiple conspicuous nucleoli. Hematoxylin, phloxine, and eosin stain.

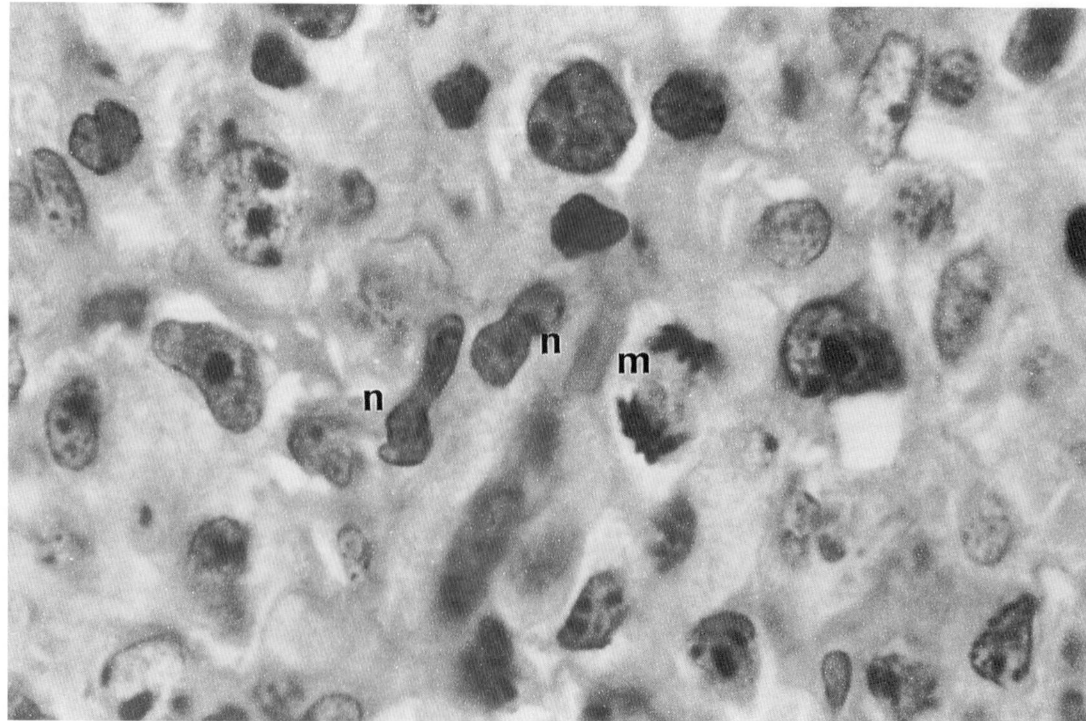

FIGURE 65.6. Diffuse large cleaved cell lymphoma Grade 3 (which still had areas of residual follicular non-Hodgkin lymphoma). Large cells with abundant cytoplasm and irregularly shaped, large, occasionally cleaved nuclei (*n*) with prominent nucleoli and frequent mitoses (*m*). Hematoxylin, phloxine, and eosin stain.

phocytes found in small cell lymphomas or normal lymph nodes (Fig. 65.6). DLBCL nuclei are round to oval, noncleaved or cleaved, with vesicular nuclear chromatin and 2 to 3 prominent nucleoli located near thick nuclear membranes. Mitoses may be numerous and sometimes atypical. Gene expression analysis has identified two distinct molecular types of DLBCL, mimicking either "germinal center B-like" or "activated B-like" gene profiles (23). See Chapter 67 for a discussion of DLBCL subtypes.

ELECTRON MICROSCOPY

The cytoplasm of cleaved small (Fig. 65.7) and large (Fig. 65.8) lymphoma cells contains few organelles. These include mitochondria, typically located at one pole of the cell, usually near the nuclear cleavage, endoplasmic reticulum with often distended cisternae, and a well-developed Golgi body. The absence of lysosomes and phagosomes indicates that the large lymphoma cells are not of histiocytic origin. Similarly, the coarse chromatin structure of the nucleus and peripheral large nucleoli are further indications that large cleaved lymphoma cells represent transformed lymphocytes rather than histiocytes (24). The large cells have processes that are often interlocked, which may explain their relatively high degree of cellular cohesion and diminished propensity to disseminate and involve peripheral blood.

IMMUNOHISTOCHEMISTRY

Like the cells of FL, the cells of diffuse FCL are of follicle center cell origin and therefore express abundant monoclonal surface membrane immunoglobulin (Ig), CD10, and B-cell antigens (see Chapter 64).

MOLECULAR DIAGNOSIS

In FLs, the BCL-2 gene is typically juxtaposed to the Ig heavy chain gene (see Chapter 8). In about 20% to 50% of

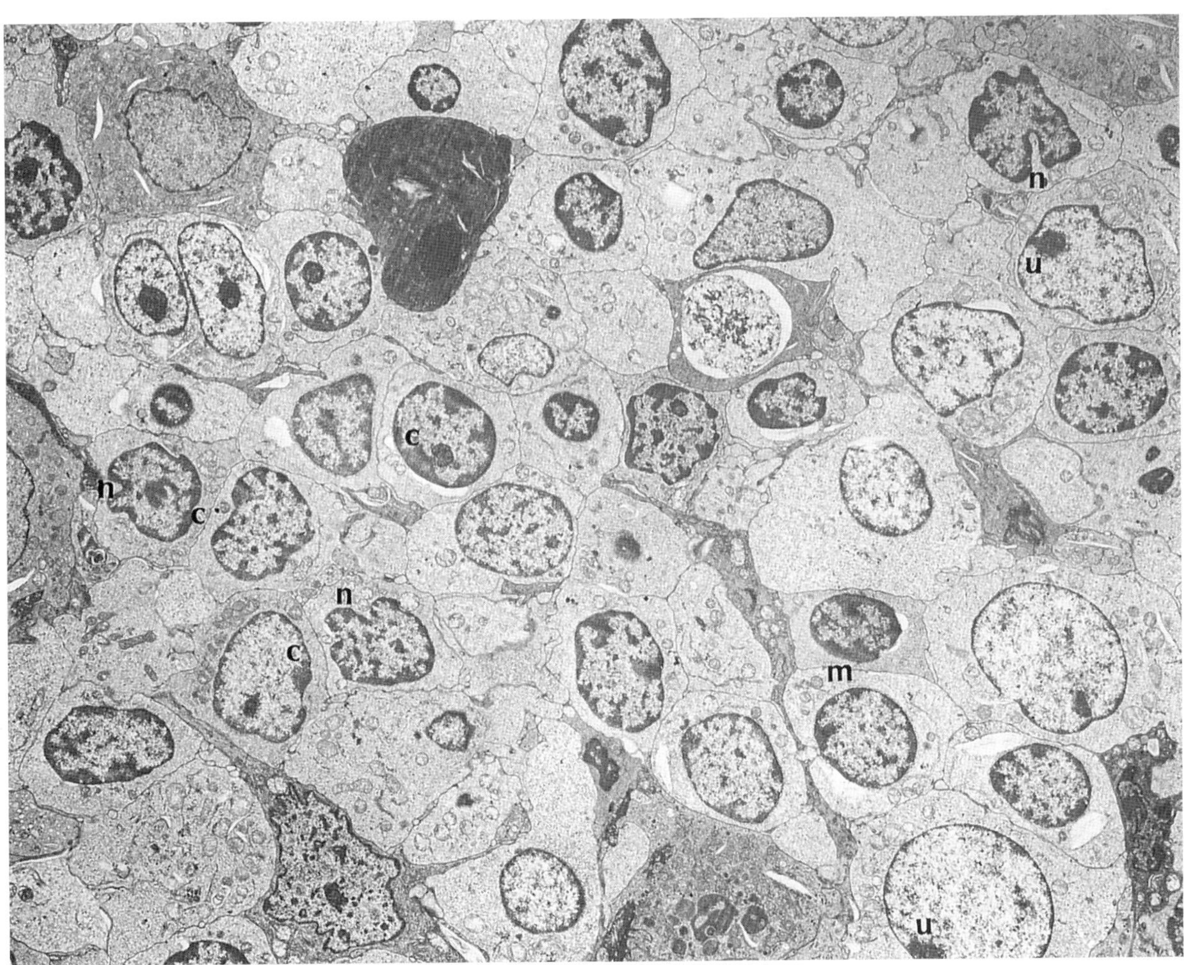

FIGURE 65.7. Diffuse follicle center cell lymphoma (diffuse, small cleaved cell non-Hodgkin lymphoma Grade 1) in cervical lymph node. Nuclei are irregular in shape and size, with occasional cleavages (*n*). Chromatin is clumped and peripheral (*c*). Nucleoli are frequently apposed to the nuclear membrane (*u*). Cytoplasm in moderate amount includes polar mitochondria (*m*). ×2,600.

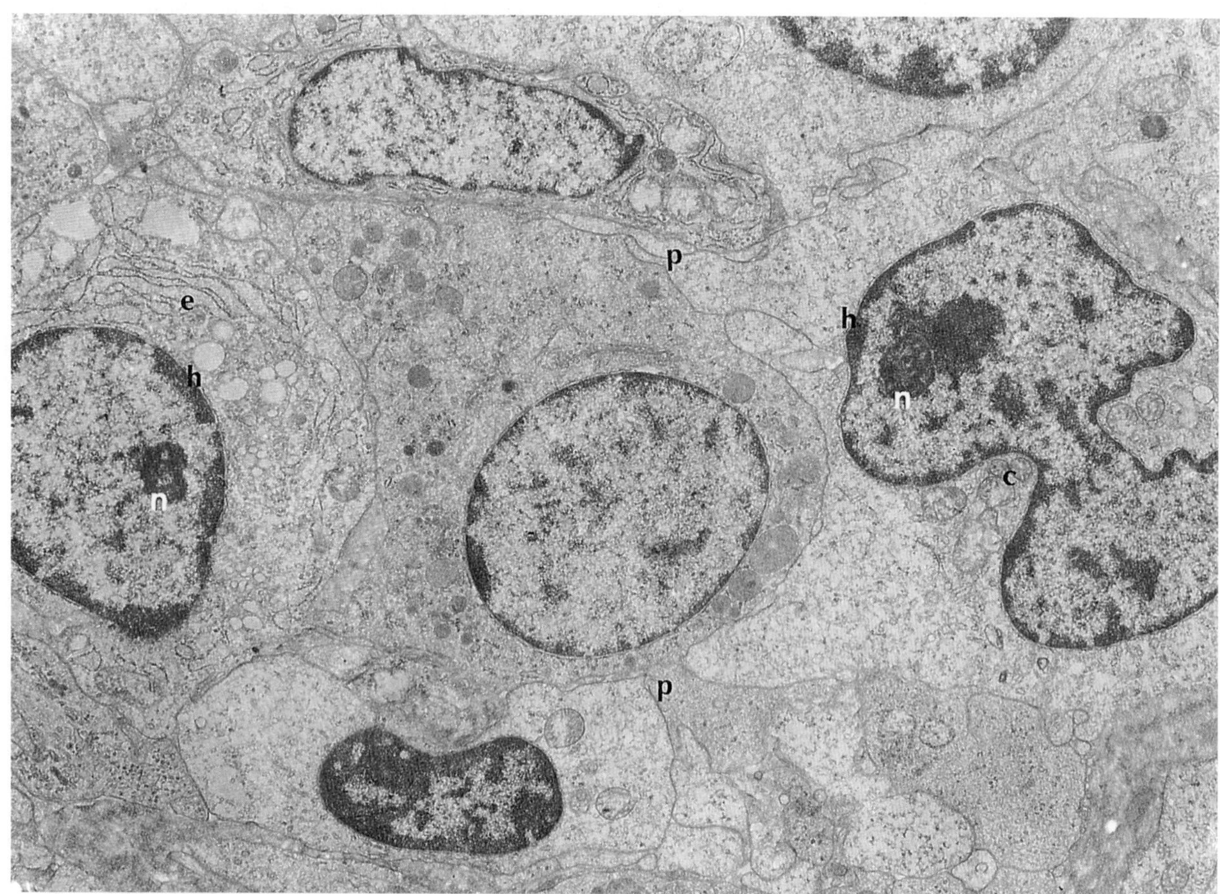

FIGURE 65.8. Diffuse follicle center cell lymphoma (diffuse, large cleaved cell non-Hodgkin lymphoma Grade 3) in abdominal lymph node. Large neoplastic cells have abundant cytoplasm and interlocking processes (*p*). Endoplasmic reticulum (*e*) is well developed with dilated cisternae, as in transformed lymphocytes. Nuclei are cleaved (*c*) and contain heterochromatin (*h*) and prominent nucleoli (*n*). The nuclear structure is of lymphocytic, not histiocytic, type. ×8,000.

cases of diffuse FCL, the BCL-2 gene is rearranged in an identical fashion (25,26). In one study comparing morphology and molecular alterations, four patients with diffuse FCL and BCL-2 rearrangement had a median survival of 56 months, whereas seven patients with diffuse FCL without BCL-2 rearrangement had a median survival of only 17 months (26). Occasionally, cases of diffuse FCL have been reported to rearrange the BCL-1 (cyclin D1) gene (26,27), so that mantle cell lymphoma may be mistakenly classified as diffuse FCL (see Chapters 8 and 66).

DIFFERENTIAL DIAGNOSIS

- Follicular (nodular) lymphomas of grade 1 (small), grade 2 (mixed), or grade 3 (large cleaved cells): The cytologic appearance is similar for each respective subtype. The nodular pattern should be present in 25% to 75% of the area.
- Small lymphocytic lymphoma: The cell population is monomorphic with pseudoproliferation centers, the nuclei are round, and the nucleoli are inconspicuous. Mitoses are fewer. The surface Ig stain is less accentuated and appears dimmer in immunofluorescence. Chronic lymphocytic leukemia is frequently associated.
- Lymphoplasmacytic lymphoma: A polymorphic cell population is composed of small lymphocytes and plasmacytoid lymphocytes. Intracytoplasmic and intranuclear inclusions (Dutcher bodies) stain with periodic acid–Schiff.
- Burkitt lymphoma: Monotonous cell population with medium-sized round vesicular nuclei, multiple prominent nucleoli, numerous mitoses, and starry sky pattern with frequent macrophages.
- Lymphoblastic lymphoma: Monomorphic cell population, convoluted or nonconvoluted medium-sized nuclei, fine nucleoli, scant cytoplasm, high mitotic index. Acute lymphoblastic leukemia or mediastinal tumor, or both, are frequently associated. Cell markers are usually of T-cell type with a mediastinal mass.
- Mantle cell lymphoma: nodular, mantle cell or diffuse pattern, small lymphocytes with slightly irregular nuclear contours (in between small lymphocytic lymphoma and FL, grade 1), condensed nuclear chromatin, inconspicu-

Checklist

DIFFUSE FOLLICLE CENTER LYMPHOMA

Patients middle-aged or elderly
Extranodal involvement common
Lymph node architecture effaced
Sinuses obliterated
Reticulin network disrupted
Nodular and diffuse patterns may coexist
CD5−, CD10+, B-cell markers
Monoclonal surface Igs
Rearrangement of BCL-2 gene
Tendency to early dissemination

ous nucleoli, and scant cytoplasm. CD5+, CD10−, moderately bright monoclonal surface Ig B-cell phenotype. The BCL-1 gene is rearranged; the BCL-2 gene is germline.

- Hodgkin lymphoma, lymphocyte predominance type: Reed-Sternberg cells of lymphocytic/histiocytic type are present. Lymphocytes are small and mature. Nuclei are not cleaved.
- Reactive lymphoid hyperplasia: Diffuse patterns are seen in lymphadenitides of viral origin (see Part III) and dermatopathic lymphadenopathy (see Chapter 42). The cell population is mixed and includes plasma cells, immunoblasts, and macrophages, so that a mottled appearance results. The surface Igs of lymphoid cells are polyclonal.
- Peripheral T-cell lymphoma: Diffuse pattern with a spectrum of cell size and irregular nuclear contours. Loss of pan-T-cell antigens and clonal T-cell receptor gene rearrangement.
- Lymphosarcoma cell leukemia represents the leukemic phase of small cleaved cell lymphoma; thus, involved lymph nodes appear identical.

REFERENCES

1. Rappaport H. Tumors of the hematopoietic system. In: Atlas of tumor pathology. Washington, DC: Armed Forces Institute of Pathology, 1966: section III, fascicle 8.
2. Lukes RJ, Collins RD. New approaches to the classification of the lymphomata. Br J Cancer 1975;31[Suppl 2]:1–28.
3. Lennert K. Histopathology of non-Hodgkin's lymphomas. Berlin: Springer-Verlag, 1981.
4. The Non-Hodgkin's Lymphoma Pathologic Classification Project. National Cancer Institute-sponsored study of classifications of non-Hodgkin's lymphomas: summary and description of a working formulation for clinical usage. Cancer 1982;49:2112–2135.
5. Harris NL, Jaffe ES, Stein H, et al. A revised European-American classification of lymphoid neoplasms: a proposal from the International Lymphoma Study Group [see Comments]. Blood 1994; 84:1361–1392.
6. Harris NL, Jaffe ES, Diebold J, et al. The World Health Organization classification of hematological malignancies: report of the clinical advisory committee meeting, Airlie House, Virginia, November 1997. Mod Pathol 2000;13:193–207.
7. Nathwani BN. A critical analysis of the classifications of non-Hodgkin's lymphomas. Cancer 1979;44:347–384.
8. Bennett M, Farrar-Brown G, Henry K, et al. Classification of non-Hodgkin's lymphomas [Letter]. Lancet 1974;2:405–406.
9. Dorfman RF. The non-Hodgkin's lymphomas. In: Rebuck JS, Berard CW, Abell MR, eds. The reticulo-endothelial system, vol 16. Baltimore: Williams & Wilkins, 1975:262–281.
10. Mathé G, Rappaport H, O'Connor GT, et al. Histological and cytological typing of neoplastic diseases of hematopoietic and lymphoid tissues. In: WHO International Histological Classification of Tumors, vol 14. Geneva: World Health Organization, 1976.
11. Nathwani BN, Kim H, Rappaport H. Malignant lymphoma, lymphoblastic. Cancer 1976;38:964–983.
12. Sullivan MP. Treatment of lymphoma. Cancer 1975;35:991–995.
13. Bloomfield CD, Kersey JH, Brunning RD, et al. Prognostic significance of lymphocytic surface markers and histology in adult non-Hodgkin's lymphoma. Cancer Treat Rep 1977;61:963–970.
14. Castella A, Neuberg RW, Kurec AS, et al. Non-Hodgkin's lymphoma with immunologic phenotype similar to non-T, non-B acute lymphocytic leukemia. Hum Pathol 1982;13:777–779.
15. McKelvey EM, Moon TE. Curability of non-Hodgkin's lymphomas. Cancer Treat Rep 1977;61:1185–1190.
16. Anderson T, DeVita VT Jr, Simon RM, et al. Malignant lymphoma. II. Prognostic factors and response to treatment of 473 patients at the National Cancer Institute. Cancer 1982;50:2708–2721.
17. Fram RJ, Skarin AT, Rosenthal DS, et al. Clinical, pathologic and immunologic features of patients with non-Hodgkin's lymphoma in a leukemic phase. A retrospective analysis of 34 patients. Cancer 1983;52:1220–1228.

18. Al-Katib A, Koziner B, Kurland E, et al. Treatment of diffuse, poorly differentiated lymphocytic lymphoma. An analysis of prognostic variables. Cancer 1984;53:2404–2412.
19. Garvin AJ, Simon RM, Osborne CK, et al. An autopsy study of histologic progression in non-Hodgkin's lymphomas. One hundred ninety-two cases from the National Cancer Institute. Cancer 1983;52:393–398.
20. Jones SE, Fuks Z, Bull M, et al. Non-Hodgkin's lymphomas. IV. Clinicopathologic correlation in 405 cases. Cancer 1973;31:806–823.
21. Butler JJ, Stryker JA, Shullenberger CC. A clinicopathological study of stages I and II non-Hodgkin's lymphomata using the Lukes-Collins classification. Br J Cancer 1975;31[Suppl 2]:208– 216.
22. Warnke RA, Kim H, Fuks Z, et al. The coexistence of nodular and diffuse patterns in nodular non-Hodgkin's lymphomas: significance and clinicopathologic correlation. Cancer 1977;40: 1229–1233.
23. Alizadeh AA, Eisen MB, Davis RE, et al. Distinct types of diffuse large B-cell lymphoma identified by gene expression profiling [see Comments]. Nature 2000;403:503–511.
24. Ioachim HL. Lymph nodes and spleen. In: Johannessen JV, ed. Electron microscopy in human medicine, vol 5. New York: Mc-Graw-Hill, 1981:384–464.
25. Aisenberg AC, Wilkes BM, Jacobson JO. The bcl-2 gene is rearranged in many diffuse B-cell lymphomas. Blood 1988;71:969–972.
26. Leith CP, Willman CL, Spier CM, et al. The presence of bcl-1 and bcl-2 gene rearrangements in diffuse small cleaved-cell lymphoma. A disease with diverse molecular and immunophenotypic findings. Diagn Mol Pathol 1994;3:178–183.
27. Rimokh R, Berger F, Cornillet P, et al. Break in the BCL1 locus is closely associated with intermediate lymphocytic lymphoma subtype. Genes Chromosomes Cancer 1990;2:223–226.

66

MANTLE CELL LYMPHOMA

DEFINITION

CD5+ B-cell malignant lymphoma with chromosomal translocation t(11;14), rearranged BCL-1 gene, cyclin D1 (bcl-1 protein) overexpression, and cytologic features intermediate between those of B-cell chronic lymphocytic leukemia/small lymphocytic lymphoma (B-CLL/SLL) and follicular lymphoma (FL). Probable origin from primary follicles or mantle zone of secondary follicles.

SYNONYMS

Mantle zone lymphoma (1)
Intermediate lymphocytic lymphoma (2)
Lymphocytic lymphoma of intermediate differentiation (3)
Centrocytic lymphoma (Kiel)
Malignant lymphoma, diffuse, small cleaved cell or malignant lymphoma, follicular, small cleaved cell (Working Formulation)
Mantle cell lymphoma (MCL) (Revised European-American Lymphoma Classification, or REAL; World Health Organization, or WHO)

VARIANTS

Mantle zone
Nodular
Diffuse
Blastic/blastoid

PATHOGENESIS

The t(11;14)(q13;q32) reciprocal chromosomal translocation yielding cyclin D1 (bcl-1 protein) overexpression characterizes MCL. In the United States, 2% to 8% of non-Hodgkin lymphomas are classified as MCLs, which originate from a CD5+ B-cell population in the mantle zones of secondary follicles (4,5). They grow in widened mantles surrounding nonlymphomatous, residual germinal centers, in vague nodules, or in diffuse sheets (1,2,6). However, the mantle zone pattern is not MCL-specific; lymphomas of other kinds can also enlarge follicular mantle zones (7). MCL expresses CD5, but not CD23, and coexpresses bright surface immunoglobulin M (IgM) and IgD. Absent or minimal somatic mutation of the rearranged Ig heavy chain variable genes indicate that MCL derives from antigen-naïve, pregerminal center B cells (8,9). On the other hand, MCL with blastoid transformation contains numerous somatic mutations, suggesting antigen selection (10).

CLINICAL SYNDROME

Mantle cell lymphoma is uncommon before the age of 50 years; the median age of patients at presentation is between 60 and 65 years (11–13). The male-to-female ratio is high, varying between 2:1 and 5:1 (2,11,12,14). Generalized lymphadenopathy is common and usually accompanies at least one "B" symptom, such as weight loss, fever, or night sweats. Like B-CLL/SLL, MCL disseminates early. Thus, at the time of diagnosis, most patients have stage III or IV disease, bone marrow involvement, and splenomegaly (2,11–14). Hepatomegaly and massive splenomegaly are frequent (15).

Primary extranodal presentations occur in spleen, Waldeyer ring, gastrointestinal tract, salivary gland, orbit, and other anatomic sites; node-based MCL infiltrates extranodal tissues (besides bone marrow) in approximately one-fourth of patients (2,11,12,14). Occasionally, monoclonal Ig spikes can be detected by serum protein electrophoresis (12,13). Many patients may be leukemic initially or become leukemic during the course of the disease. Because the median survival time is between 3 and 4 years (11,12,14), MCL behaves clinically as an intermediate-grade lymphoma (4).

A high proliferation rate, leukemic phase at diagnosis (but not bone marrow involvement), p53 mutation and overexpression, p16 inactivation, and blastoid transformation indicate a poor prognosis (2,11–14,16,17). Some investigators report that a mantle zone or nodular pattern may portend a better prognosis because fewer mitoses are present and the S fraction is lower than in the diffuse pattern

(2,18,19). In two studies, patients who had MCL with either a nodular or a diffuse pattern did worse than those with a mantle zone pattern (20,21). The predictive value of pattern is still controversial because some investigators report similar overall survival rates for all histologic types (11,14).

HISTOPATHOLOGY

Common or classic MCL exhibits intermediate features of both B-CLL/SLL and FL: small to medium-sized atypical lymphocytes with slightly irregular nuclear contours, condensed chromatin, inconspicuous nucleoli, and scant cytoplasm (2) (Fig. 66.1D). The nuclei are neither round as in B-CLL/SLL nor deeply indented as in FL. In some MCLs, a mixture of round and cleaved small cells, neither of which represent more than 30% of the total population, may coexist with cells with intermediate morphologic features (2). Larger cells of immunoblastic type are rare to absent. The mitotic rate is highly variable but usually moderate. Some cases contain venules with hyalinized vessel walls, non-neoplastic plasma cells, and scattered epithelioid histiocytes, but not tingible-body macrophages or granulomas (6).

Mantle cell lymphoma grows in three architectural patterns:

- The *mantle zone pattern* (Fig. 66.1 A–C) is characterized by lymphoma cells of intermediate type that form vague nodules by widening the mantle zones around small, non-neoplastic germinal centers. Coalescent nodules and diffuse areas may coexist without becoming predominant.
- The *nodular pattern* is otherwise similar to the mantle zone pattern, except that no residual, non-neoplastic follicle centers are seen within the nodules.
- The *diffuse pattern* entirely obliterates the normal lymph node architecture. Sometimes, naked residual germinal centers or lymphoid follicles persist in the midst of the lymphomatous proliferation (Fig. 66.2). The diffuse pattern may represent the progression of the mantle zone pattern, so that some authors suggested the term *mantle zone lymphoma* be used for both types of MCL (4,22).

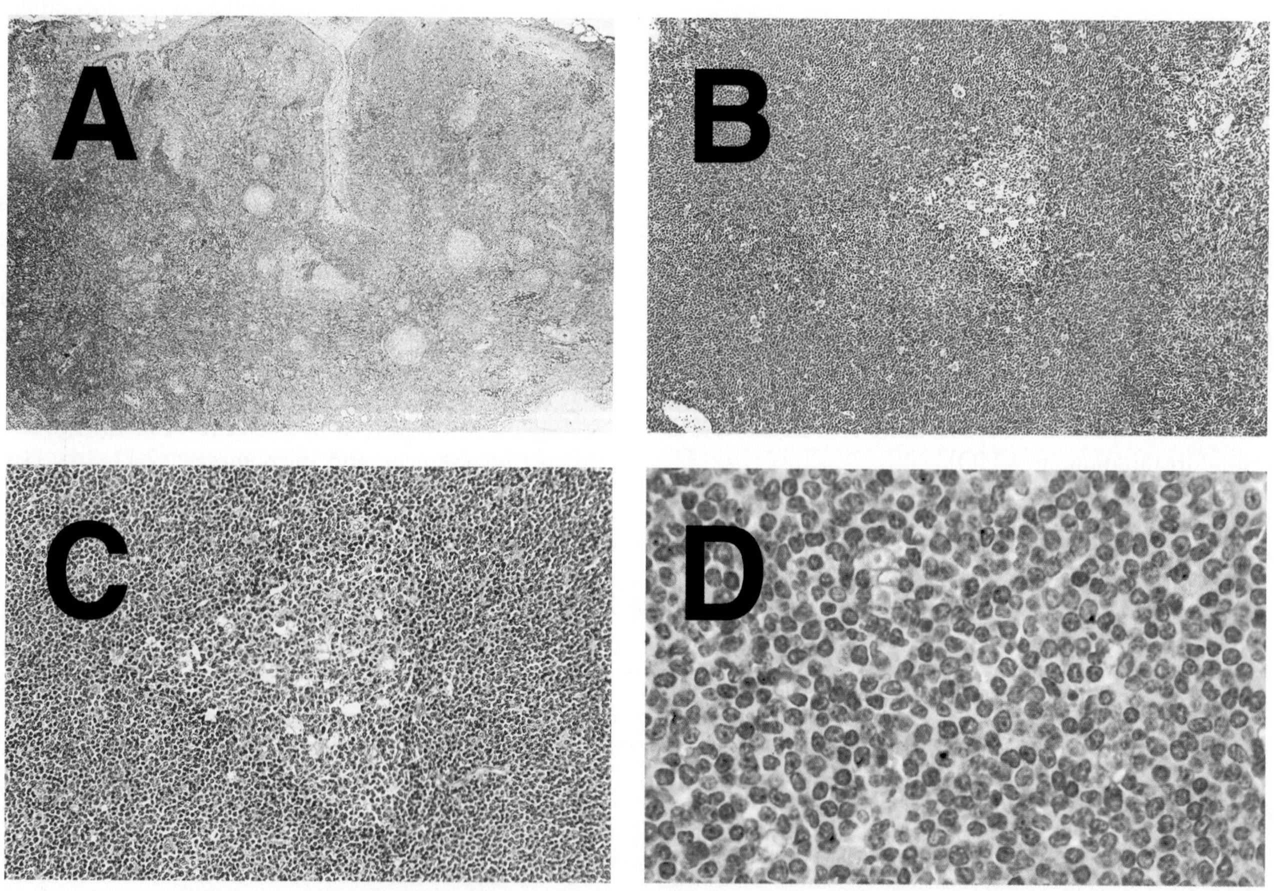

FIGURE 66.1. Mantle cell lymphoma in cervical lymph node from a 62-year-old man. **A:** Vague nodules centered on residual, non-neoplastic, atrophic germinal centers suggest an expanded interfollicular zone. **B:** Neoplastic mantle zone wider than non-neoplastic germinal center. **C:** Tingible-body macrophages in reactive, atrophic germinal center. **D:** Neoplastic lymphoid cells in widened mantle zone are small, with condensed nuclear chromatin, slightly irregular nuclear contours, inconspicuous nucleoli, and scant cytoplasm.

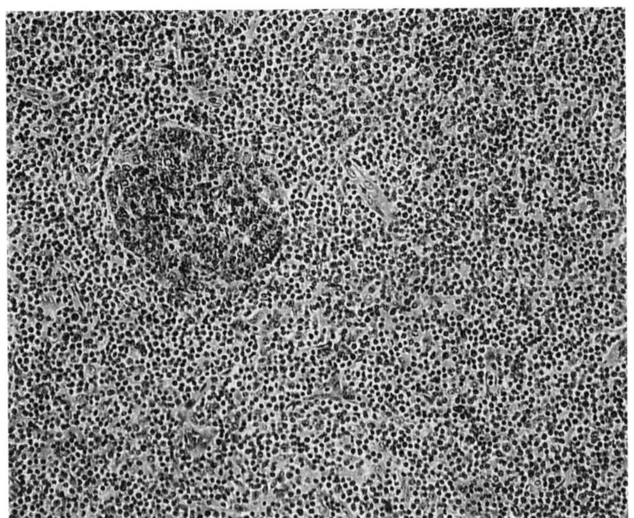

FIGURE 66.2. Mantle zone non-Hodgkin lymphoma in cervical lymph node of 60-year-old woman. Diffuse proliferation of intermediate lymphocytes effacing the normal architecture. Residual naked germinal center in the midst of the lymphomatous proliferation. Hematoxylin, phloxine, and saffron stain.

Against this proposal is the argument that the two subtypes may manifest different degrees of malignant behavior, with mantle zone lymphoma having fewer mitoses and behaving less aggressively (18).

Rearrangement of BCL-1 gene, cyclin D1 (bcl-1 protein) overexpression, or both identify several clinically aggressive "blastic" MCL variants (23) with uncommon morphologic subtypes: pleomorphic or anaplastic (24,25), large cell and blastoid (11,17,26). The WHO classification does not recommend subclassifying/grading MCL according to cytology or pattern for clinical purposes, although such grading may be of some value for research (27). Blastoid mantle cell lymphoma may occur in morphologic variants resembling lymphoblasts or a pleomorphic variety with prominent nucleoli (23–26).

ULTRASTRUCTURE

Features of MCL are an indented nucleus, evenly distributed heterochromatin, a relatively low nuclear-to-cytoplasmic ratio, and organelle-rich cytoplasm (28). In contrast, FL has more pronounced nuclear clefts, more condensed chromatin, a higher nuclear-to-cytoplasmic ratio, and fewer cytoplasmic organelles (28).

CYTOLOGY

Fine needle aspirates, smears, or imprints of MCL show a monotonous population of small to medium-sized lymphoid cells with slightly irregular or indented nuclei, chromatin lighter than that of B-CLL/SLL, up to three inconspicuous nucleoli, and scant cytoplasm (29). The nuclear contours of MCL appear less round than those of B-CLL/SLL and less angulated than those of FL. No paraimmunoblasts, as in "pseudofollicular proliferation centers" of B-CLL/SLL, or centroblasts, as in FL (29), are seen. Cytologically distinguishing MCL from FL requires support from the characteristic MCL immunophenotype: CD5+, CD10−, CD23−, and CD43+ (30). Although the Ki-67+ proliferation fraction is greater than 15% in MCL more often than it is in FL, the difference is not statistically significant (30). Cytokinetic study cannot separate MCL with a mantle zone pattern from MCL with a diffuse growth pattern; histologic evaluation is required (29).

IMMUNOHISTOCHEMISTRY

Surface Ig immunofluorescent staining appears brighter in MCL than in B-CLL/SLL but dimmer than in FL. In contrast to the lymphoma cells in the mantles, nodules, or diffuse sheets, which are monoclonal, the remaining atrophic germinal centers are polyclonal, which indicates that they are not part of the neoplastic growth. MCLs express a variety of B-cell antigens: CD19, CD20, CD22, CD24, IgM, IgD and HLA-DR. They also express the T cell-associated markers CD5 and CD43 (6). They do not stain for CD10 (common acute lymphoblastic leukemia antigen, or CALLA) or for CD23, but they do stain strongly for CD5 (6). Because both B-CLL/SLL and MCL express CD5, the presence or absence of CD23 can help to distinguish them. (see Chapter 7). In addition, the proliferative rate of B-CLL/SLL is low to negligible, whereas the proliferative rate of MCL is moderate. Cyclin D1 (bcl-1) nuclear expression is one of the most specific immunohistochemical markers for diagnosing MCL (Fig. 66.3), but the determination can be technically challenging to perform.

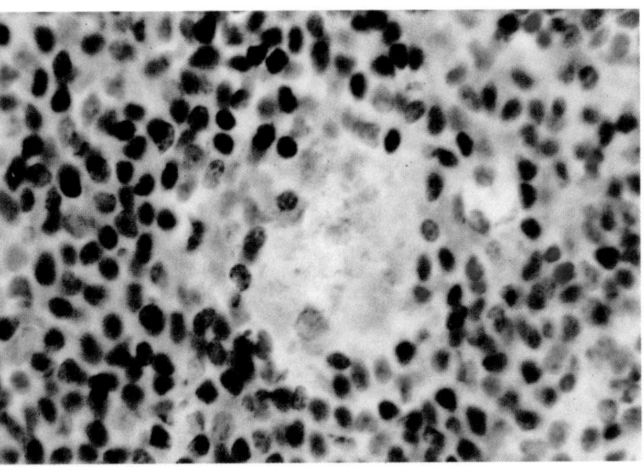

FIGURE 66.3. Mantle cell lymphoma aberrantly expresses bcl-1 protein (cyclin D1) in a nuclear pattern as a consequence of t(11;14)(q13;q32).

Phenotype

CD5+
CD10−
CD19+
CD20+
CD23− (some partially CD23+)
CD43+
CD79a+
Monoclonal surface Ig+ (brighter than B-CLL)

CYTOGENETICS

The t(11;14)(q13;q32) reciprocal chromosomal translocation characterizing MCL involves the BCL-1 locus encoding cyclin D1 (bcl-1 protein) and the Ig heavy chain gene (Fig. 66.4) (see Chapter 8). MCL blastoid transformation and aggressive variants may become tetraploid (26).

MOLECULAR DIAGNOSIS

See Chapter 8.

DIFFERENTIAL DIAGNOSIS

- Reactive follicular hyperplasia usually has thinner mantles composed of small, round, mature lymphocytes with a polyclonal immunophenotype surrounding prominent polyclonal germinal centers.
- Castleman disease, hyaline vascular type, presents usually as a large localized mass in a young person. The architecture is not entirely effaced, the lymphocytes are concentrically layered in a target pattern, and the germinal center is atrophic and partly hyalinized. The component lymphocytes are polyclonal.
- FL is composed of sharply circumscribed nodules containing small lymphoid cells with cleaved nuclei. FL cells express bright monoclonal surface Ig and CD10, but not CD5 or CD43. In the Kiel classification, centrocytic lymphoma included MCL.
- B-CLL/SLL usually shows diffusely effaced lymph node architecture, "pseudofollicular proliferation centers," and a monotonous population of small lymphocytes with round, darkly stained nuclei. The neoplastic B cells express dim surface Ig, are CD5+ and CD23+, but do not produce cyclin D1 (bcl-1 protein).
- Marginal zone B-cell lymphoma (monocytoid B-cell lymphoma) may simulate a "monocytoid B cell-like" MCL variant, containing cells with abundant pale cytoplasm that sometimes surround germinal centers (31), particularly in spleen (31,32). Splenic marginal zone lymphoma does not express cyclin D1 (33).
- B-lineage lymphoblastic lymphoma histologically mimics "blastic" MCL, with medium-sized cells, evenly dispersed nuclear chromatin, a diffuse growth pattern, a very high mitotic index, and sometimes a "starry sky" background (34). Patients with "blastic" MCL are significantly older than those with lymphoblastic lymphoma (34). Lymphoblastic lymphoma expresses terminal deoxynucleotidyl transferase; MCL expresses cyclin D1.

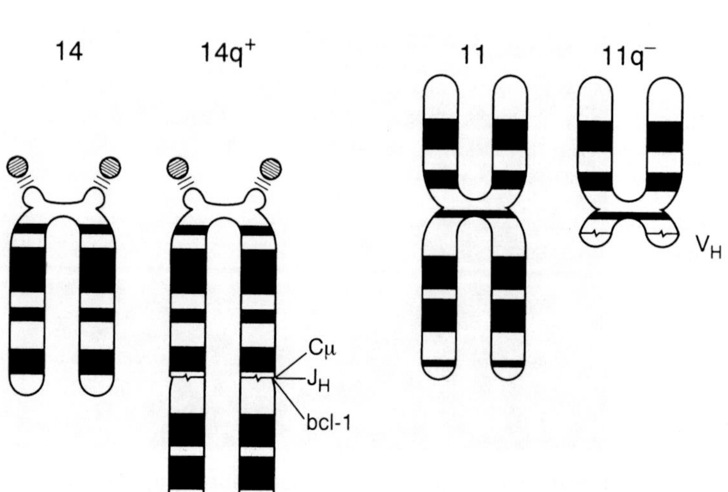

FIGURE 66.4. Chromosome translocation in mantle cell lymphoma, t(11;14)(q13;q32), by which oncogene BCL-1 from chromosome 11 is brought into juxtaposition with the immunoglobulin heavy chain locus (C-μ JH) on chromosome 14. (From Croce CM, Tsujimoto Y, Erikson J, et al. Chromosome translocations and B cell neoplasia. Lab Invest 1984;51:258–267, with permission.)

Checklist

MANTLE CELL LYMPHOMA

Patients elderly
Male predominance
Generalized lymphadenopathy
Early dissemination with bone marrow, spleen, and peripheral blood involvement
Subtypes
- Mantle zone
- Nodular
- Diffuse
- Blastoid transformation

Cell type intermediate between B-CLL/SLL and FL
Nuclei slightly irregular
Moderate numbers of mitoses
Reciprocal chromosomal translocation t(11;14)(q13;q32)
Cyclin D1 (bcl-1 protein) nuclear expression
CD5+, CD10−, CD19+, CD20+, CD23−, CD43+ immunophenotype
Monoclonal B cells in widened mantles, nodules, and diffuse sheets
Polyclonal B cells in residual, atrophic germinal centers
Median survival of 3 to 4 years

REFERENCES

1. Weisenburger DD, Kim H, Rappaport H. Mantle-zone lymphoma: a follicular variant of intermediate lymphocytic lymphoma. Cancer 1982;49:1429–1438.
2. Weisenburger DD, Nathwani BN, Diamond LW, et al. Malignant lymphoma, intermediate lymphocytic type: a clinicopathologic study of 42 cases. Cancer 1981;48:1415–1425.
3. Berard CW, Dorfman RF. Histopathology of malignant lymphomas. Clin Haematol 1974;3:39–76.
4. Banks PM, Chan J, Cleary ML, et al. Mantle cell lymphoma. A proposal for unification of morphologic, immunologic, and molecular data [see Comments]. Am J Surg Pathol 1992;16:637–640.
5. Abe M, Tominaga K, Wakasa H. Phenotypic characterization of human B-lymphocyte subpopulations, particularly human CD5+ B-lymphocyte subpopulation within the mantle zones of secondary follicles. Leukemia 1994;8:1039–1044.
6. Kurtin PJ. Mantle cell lymphoma. Adv Anat Pathol 1998;5:376–398.
7. Harris NL, Bhan AK. Mantle-zone lymphoma. A pattern produced by lymphomas of more than one cell type. Am J Surg Pathol 1985;9:872–882.
8. Hummel M, Tamaru J, Kalvelage B, et al. Mantle cell (previously centrocytic) lymphomas express VH genes with no or very little somatic mutations like the physiologic cells of the follicle mantle. Blood 1994;84:403–407.
9. Du MQ, Diss TC, Xu CF, et al. Ongoing immunoglobulin gene mutations in mantle cell lymphomas [see Comments]. Br J Haematol 1997;96:124–131.
10. Pittaluga S, Tierens A, Pinyol M, et al. Blastic variant of mantle cell lymphoma shows a heterogeneous pattern of somatic mutations of the rearranged immunoglobulin heavy chain variable genes. Br J Haematol 1998;102:1301–1306.
11. Argatoff LH, Connors JM, Klasa RJ, et al. Mantle cell lymphoma: a clinicopathologic study of 80 cases. Blood 1997;89:2067–2078.
12. Samaha H, Dumontet C, Ketterer N, et al. Mantle cell lymphoma: a retrospective study of 121 cases. Leukemia 1998;12:1281–1287.
13. Bosch F, Lopez-Guillermo A, Campo E, et al. Mantle cell lymphoma: presenting features, response to therapy, and prognostic factors. Cancer 1998;82:567–575.
14. Norton AJ, Matthews J, Pappa V, et al. Mantle cell lymphoma: natural history defined in a serially biopsied population over a 20-year period. Ann Oncol 1995;6:249–256.
15. Pittaluga S, Verhoef G, Criel A, et al. "Small" B-cell non-Hodgkin's lymphomas with splenomegaly at presentation are either mantle cell lymphoma or marginal zone cell lymphoma. A study based on histology, cytology, immunohistochemistry, and cytogenetic analysis. Am J Surg Pathol 1996;20:211–223.
16. Greiner TC, Moynihan MJ, Chan WC, et al. p53 mutations in mantle cell lymphoma are associated with variant cytology and predict a poor prognosis. Blood 1996;87:4302–4310.
17. Pinyol M, Hernandez L, Cazorla M, et al. Deletions and loss of expression of p16INK4a and p21Waf1 genes are associated with aggressive variants of mantle cell lymphomas. Blood 1997;89:272–280.
18. Weisenburger DD, Duggan MJ, Perry DA, et al. Non-Hodgkin's lymphomas of mantle zone origin. Pathol Annu 1991;26:139–158.
19. Segal GH, Masih AS, Fox AC, et al. CD5-expressing B-cell non-Hodgkin's lymphomas with bcl-1 gene rearrangement have a relatively homogeneous immunophenotype and are associated with an overall poor prognosis. Blood 1995;85:1570–1579.

20. Lardelli P, Bookman MA, Sundeen J, et al. Lymphocytic lymphoma of intermediate differentiation. Morphologic and immunophenotypic spectrum and clinical correlations. Am J Surg Pathol 1990;14:752–763.
21. Majlis A, Pugh WC, Rodriguez MA, et al. Mantle cell lymphoma: correlation of clinical outcome and biologic features with three histologic variants. J Clin Oncol 1997;15:1664–1671.
22. Jaffe ES, Bookman MA, Longo DL. Lymphocytic lymphoma of intermediate differentiation—mantle zone lymphoma: a distinct subtype of B-cell lymphoma. Hum Pathol 1987;18:877–880.
23. Campo E, Raffeld M, Jaffe ES. Mantle-cell lymphoma. Semin Hematol 1999;36:115–127.
24. Swerdlow SH, Habeshaw JA, Murray LJ, et al. Centrocytic lymphoma: a distinct clinicopathologic and immunologic entity. A multiparameter study of 18 cases at diagnosis and relapse. Am J Pathol 1983;113:181–197.
25. Ott MM, Ott G, Kuse R, et al. The anaplastic variant of centrocytic lymphoma is marked by frequent rearrangements of the bcl-1 gene and high proliferation indices. Histopathology 1994;24: 329–334.
26. Ott G, Kalla J, Ott MM, et al. Blastoid variants of mantle cell lymphoma: frequent bcl-1 rearrangements at the major translocation cluster region and tetraploid chromosome clones. Blood 1997;89:1421–1429.
27. Harris NL, Jaffe ES, Diebold J, et al. The World Health Organization classification of hematological malignancies: report of the clinical advisory committee meeting, Airlie House, Virginia, November 1997. Mod Pathol 2000;13:193–207.
28. Resnitzky P, Matutes E, Hedges M, et al. The ultrastructure of mantle cell lymphoma and other B-cell disorders with translocation t(11;14)(q13;q32). Br J Haematol 1996;94:352–361.
29. Wojcik EM, Katz RL, Fanning TV, et al. Diagnosis of mantle cell lymphoma on tissue acquired by fine needle aspiration in conjunction with immunocytochemistry and cytokinetic studies. Possibilities and limitations. Acta Cytol 1995;39:909–915.
30. Rassidakis GZ, Tani E, Svedmyr E, et al. Diagnosis and subclassification of follicle center and mantle cell lymphomas on fine-needle aspirates: a cytologic and immunocytochemical approach based on the Revised European-American Lymphoma (REAL) classification. Cancer 1999;87:216–223.
31. Swerdlow SH, Zukerberg LR, Yang WI, et al. The morphologic spectrum of non-Hodgkin's lymphomas with BCL1/cyclin D1 gene rearrangements. Am J Surg Pathol 1996;20:627–640.
32. Piris MA, Mollejo M, Campo E, et al. A marginal zone pattern may be found in different varieties of non-Hodgkin's lymphoma: the morphology and immunohistology of splenic involvement by B-cell lymphomas simulating splenic marginal zone lymphoma. Histopathology 1998;33:230–239.
33. Savilo E, Campo E, Mollejo M, et al. Absence of cyclin D1 protein expression in splenic marginal zone lymphoma. Mod Pathol 1998;11:601–606.
34. Soslow RA, Baergen RN, Warnke RA. B-lineage lymphoblastic lymphoma is a clinicopathologic entity distinct from other histologically similar aggressive lymphomas with blastic morphology. Cancer 1999;85:2648–2654.

67

DIFFUSE LARGE B-CELL LYMPHOMA

DEFINITION

Non-Hodgkin diffuse lymphoma of large B cells.

SYNONYMS

Lymphoma, diffuse, histiocytic (Rappaport) (1)
Lymphoma, large cell, cleaved, noncleaved, and immunoblastic (Lukes-Collins) (2)
Lymphoma, centroblastic and immunoblastic (Kiel) (3)
Lymphoma, large cell, cleaved, noncleaved, immunoblastic, and polymorphous (Working Formulation) (4)

INCIDENCE

Large B-cell lymphomas constitute 30% to 40% of adult non-Hodgkin lymphomas (NHLs) (4,5). Like other types of highly aggressive lymphomas, they account for a relatively large proportion of lymphomas in underdeveloped countries and in people with immune deficiencies, particularly AIDS. Forty percent of large cell B-cell lymphomas are extranodal, but in patients with AIDS or induced immunosuppression, these tumors may originate in internal organs in more than 60% of cases (6). The age range of patients with large cell lymphomas is wide; they are more common in adults and older persons, but children are occasionally affected. Large cell lymphoma of T-cell type, described in the chapter on peripheral T-cell lymphoma (see Chapter 73), is far less common in the Western hemisphere than its B-cell counterpart (3,7).

PATHOGENESIS

Diffuse large B-cell lymphoma was defined as a category of lymphoma in the 1994 Revised European-American Lymphoma (REAL) classification (5), which in a slightly modified form became the official World Health Organization (WHO) classification (8). The category of diffuse large B-cell lymphoma, as defined in this classification, comprises the lymphomas for which synonyms are listed above; these were considered to be individual entities in earlier classifications. The proponents of the REAL classification unified these entities because (a) subclassifying large cell lymphomas was difficult and resulted in poor reproducibility and (b) all cases of large B-cell lymphomas are treated similarly (5). The two subtypes of large B-cell lymphoma included in the unified category are *centroblastic* (cleaved and noncleaved) and *immunoblastic,* as described by Lukes and Collins (2) and Lennert and Mohri. (3). Because of the large size and irregular shape of these cells, they were earlier thought to originate from reticulum cells or histiocytes (1). When immunohistochemical methods were introduced, it could be demonstrated that the large lymphoma cells are of lymphocytic origin and that the category of large cell lymphoma is morphologically and immunologically heterogeneous.

Centroblastic lymphomas include large cell lymphomas derived from the cells of germinal centers (centroblasts) and extrafollicular areas of lymph nodes. According to concepts introduced by Lukes and Collins (2) and Lennert and Mohri (3), large cell lymphomas, like small cell lymphomas, can originate from cleaved (resting) or noncleaved (proliferating) lymphocytes, and also from lymphocytes that are being activated by antigen. Such activated or transformed lymphocytes, also known as *immunoblasts,* are the source of a particular form of large cell NHL, the immunoblastic lymphoma (IBL) of B-cell or T-cell type (9–11).

The IBLs of T-cell type are commonly located in lymph nodes; their course is usually aggressive, and patients have a poor prognosis (7,10,12). In more recent classifications, they are included in the category of peripheral T-cell lymphomas (see Chapter 73).

Immunoblastic lymphomas of B-cell type show characteristic features of immunoglobulin (Ig) synthesis and plasmacytic differentiation (2,3,9,10). They often arise in extranodal locations, and patients frequently have a history of an immune disorder. In a series of patients with IBL, prior immune disease was noted in 36% of IBLs of B-cell type and 16% of IBLs of T-cell type, whereas a lymphoproliferative condition was recorded in 26% of IBLs of T-cell type and 13% of IBLs of B-cell type (7). Among the autoimmune diseases that have been noted to precede IBL are systemic lupus erythematosus, rheumatoid arthritis, Hashimoto thyroiditis, Sjögren syndrome, celiac disease, and various drug allergies (13,14). Benign or low-grade lymphoproliferative conditions that have preceded IBL are angioimmunoblastic lymphadenopathy, chronic lymphocytic leukemia, Waldenström macroglobulinemia, and well-differentiated lymphocytic lymphoma (15,16). IBL has also developed in patients with congenital immune deficiencies and in immunosuppressed recipients of renal transplants (17–19). More recently, IBL of B-cell type has developed in unprecedentedly high proportions among patients with AIDS, accounting for more than 30% of the NHLs that are becoming increasingly prevalent in these patients (6, 20,21). The presence of Epstein-Barr viral antigens in some of these cases indicates an etiologic role for the virus (22). The documented relationship between altered immunity and IBL supports the concepts of Lukes and Collins, who first described IBL. In their view, IBL may represent the development of a malignant clone of immunoblasts in immunodeficient organisms exposed to prolonged immunologic stimulation (10,23). Thus, various abnormal immune conditions associated with an increased incidence of lymphomas, particularly IBLs, may be "prelymphomatous states," possibly a result of alterations in the control mechanisms of lymphocyte transformation.

Most large cell lymphomas arise *de novo*; however, some, after variable periods of time, follow lymphomas of a lower grade, treated or untreated (24). Among the preceding lymphomas are follicular lymphoma (FL), B-cell chronic lymphocytic leukemia (B-CLL), lymphoplasmacytoid lymphoma, mucosa-associated lymphoid tissue (MALT) lymphoma, and even some forms of Hodgkin lymphoma (24–27). The transformation of CLL into large cell lymphoma is known as the *Richter syndrome* (see Chapter 60). In 20% to 30% of cases, diffuse large B-cell lymphoma evolves from a preceding FL (24). The diffuse pattern of growth succeeding the follicular pattern usually signals acceleration and increased aggressiveness of the tumor. Sometimes, the two patterns coexist, whereas in others, the first is entirely replaced. The large cell lymphomas associated with FL are usually of the *centroblastic type,* with cleaved or noncleaved nuclei.

The major subtypes of diffuse large B-cell lymphomas, *centroblastic* and *immunoblastic,* may appear as clearly distinguishable histologically or a mixture of a variety of large B cells. In one study attempting to differentiate between the variants of large B-cell lymphoma, 85 cases were reviewed by a panel of hematopathologists (28). Based on agreement of two of three observers, the cases were classified as 60 diffuse large cell (16 large cleaved, 36 large noncleaved, and 8 unclassified), 19 immunoblastic, and 6 unclassifiable. All patients were treated comparably with modern chemotherapy. A retrospective analysis showed no significant differences in prognosis between the histologic variants. Based on this and several other studies with similar results (29,30), the subtypes of diffuse large B-cell lymphomas were not included in the newly adopted classifications (5,8).

CLINICAL SYNDROME

The age distribution of large B-cell lymphomas is bimodal. The largest number of cases occur in persons 65 to 69 years old; a smaller peak in persons 35 to 39 years old mainly represents the high incidence of this type of lymphoma in patients with AIDS (31). The sex distribution is equal, or a slight male predominance may be noted (4).

Large cell lymphomas grow rapidly and form bulky tumors in nodal or extranodal sites, the latter affected particularly often in cases of immune deficiency. About 30% of patients have fever, night sweats, or weight loss ("B" symptoms) (32). Bone marrow involvement is less frequent (10% to 20% of cases) than in small cell lymphomas and does not occur before lymph node involvement (33). The peripheral blood is involved only in a terminal phase. Patients who report a previous allergic disorder, autoimmune disease, or lymphoid neoplasm present in more than 60% of cases with advanced disease and systemic symptoms, and 70% already have stage III or IV disease (13,14). Most reported cases have been in elderly patients, who show marked lymphopenia ($<1,000/mm^3$ in 45% of cases), anemia, fever, weight loss, and skin rashes. Hypergammaglobulinemia, monoclonal or polyclonal, is present in 44% of cases (13). Lymph nodes in various locations are involved, either in isolation or in association with visceral lymphomas in intestine, lung, skin, testis, or salivary gland. Not infrequently, the affected organs were the site of the previous disorder. Survival time for untreated patients with IBL is generally short, with a median of 17 months in a study of 35 cases (7). In a retrospective study of 51 cases followed for 14 to 28 years, patients with T-cell IBL fared significantly worse than those with B-cell disease (12). AIDS patients with IBL, usually of B-cell type, succumb even sooner, in 6 to 12 months.

Combination chemotherapy has changed the prognosis of patients with aggressive large cell lymphomas; what was formerly a fatal disease is now in most cases curable (34). Particularly patients with early-stage disease treated with effective chemotherapy and adjuvant radiotherapy are able to achieve long-term disease-free survival (35).

HISTOPATHOLOGY

The normal architectural features of the involved lymph nodes, including the follicles and sinuses, are replaced by sheets of large lymphoma cells. Sometimes, the lymph nodes are only partially involved, and the lymphoma cells are aggregated in nodular confluent areas (Fig. 67.1). Such neoplastic nodules differ from lymph node follicles in size

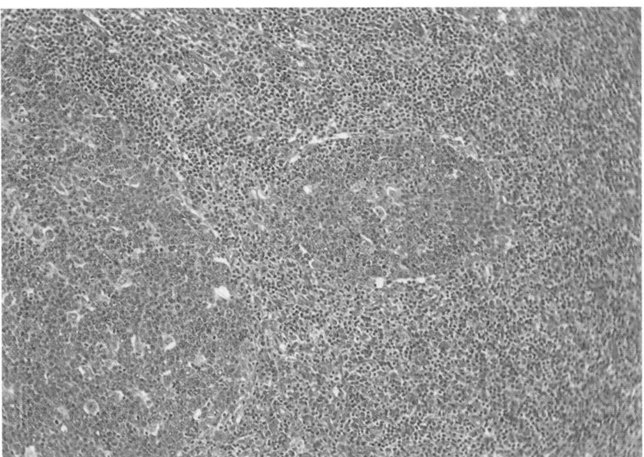

FIGURE 67.1. Diffuse large B-cell lymphoma. Nodular aggregates of large cell lymphoma replace areas of lymph node parenchyma. Hematoxylin, phloxine, and saffron stain.

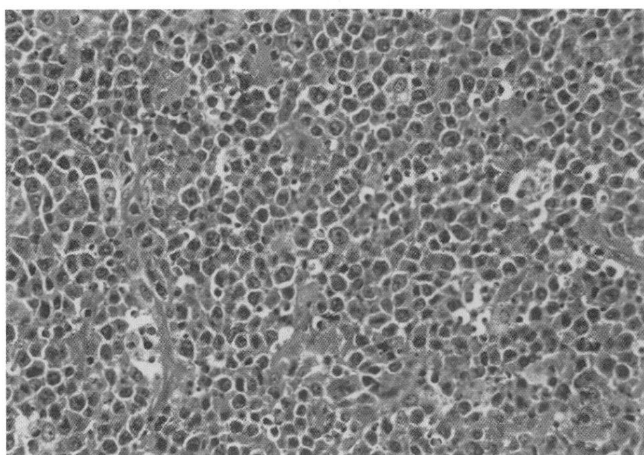

FIGURE 67.2. Diffuse large B-cell lymphoma, centroblastic subtype. Sheets of large lymphoma cells with foci of cell necrosis, apoptotic cells, and tingible-body macrophages. Hematoxylin, phloxine, and saffron stain.

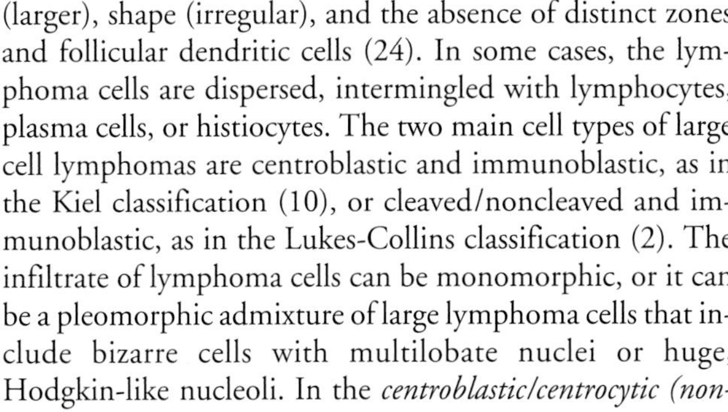

(larger), shape (irregular), and the absence of distinct zones and follicular dendritic cells (24). In some cases, the lymphoma cells are dispersed, intermingled with lymphocytes, plasma cells, or histiocytes. The two main cell types of large cell lymphomas are centroblastic and immunoblastic, as in the Kiel classification (10), or cleaved/noncleaved and immunoblastic, as in the Lukes-Collins classification (2). The infiltrate of lymphoma cells can be monomorphic, or it can be a pleomorphic admixture of large lymphoma cells that include bizarre cells with multilobate nuclei or huge, Hodgkin-like nucleoli. In the *centroblastic/centrocytic (noncleaved/cleaved)* subtype (Figs. 67.2 and 67.3), the cells resemble their normal counterparts in the reactive germinal centers. The nuclei are either round and centrally located, with multiple small nucleoli (centroblastic/noncleaved) (Figs. 67.2 and 67.4), or smaller, irregular, and angulated (centrocytic/cleaved) (Figs. 67.3 and 67.5). The nucleus is sometimes vesicular, with chromatin clumped or condensed under the nuclear membrane. The cytoplasm is occasionally entirely clear. In the *immunoblastic* subtype (Figs. 67.6–67.8), the nuclei are round, with thick nuclear membranes and single, centrally located, prominent nucleoli that often

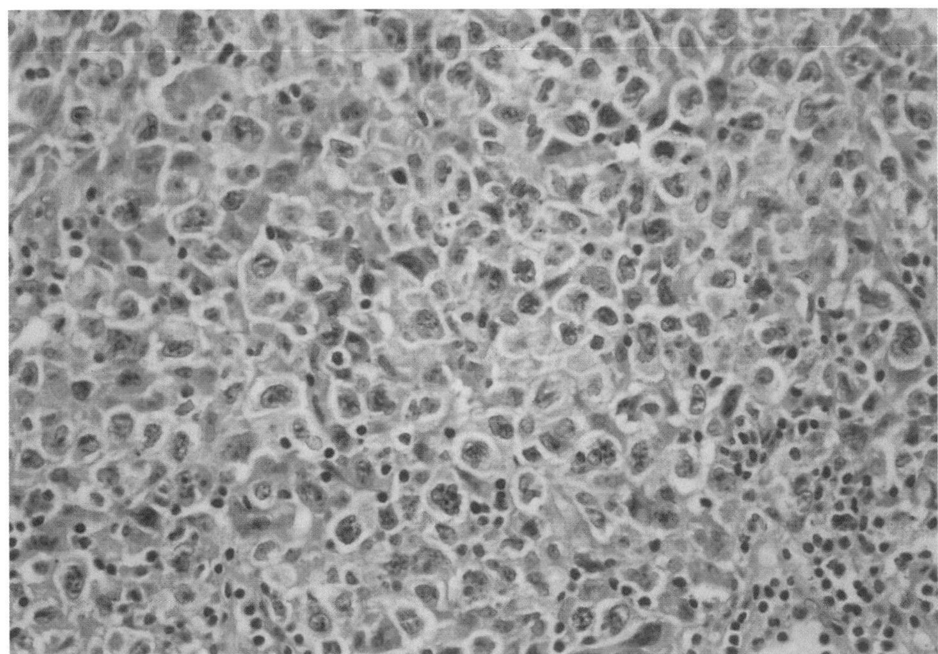

FIGURE 67.3. Diffuse large B-cell lymphoma. The lymphoma cells are large, with relatively abundant cytoplasm and irregular cleaved nuclei. Hematoxylin, phloxine, and saffron stain.

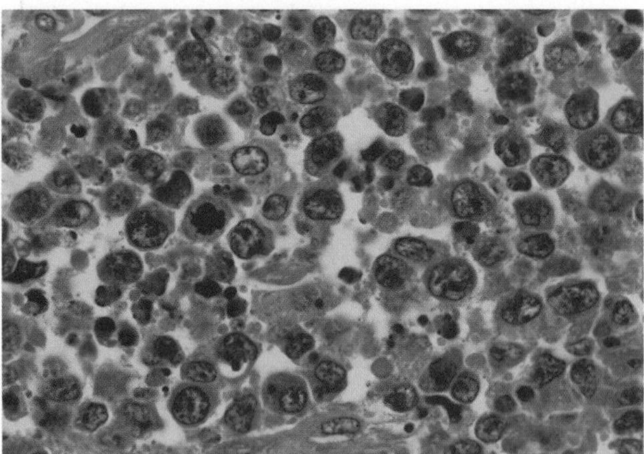

FIGURE 67.4. Same slide as in Fig. 67.2. The lymphoma cells, which resemble centroblasts, have a moderate amount of cytoplasm and large, round nuclei with multiple nucleoli. Numerous mitoses and cells in apoptosis. Hematoxylin, phloxine, and saffron stain.

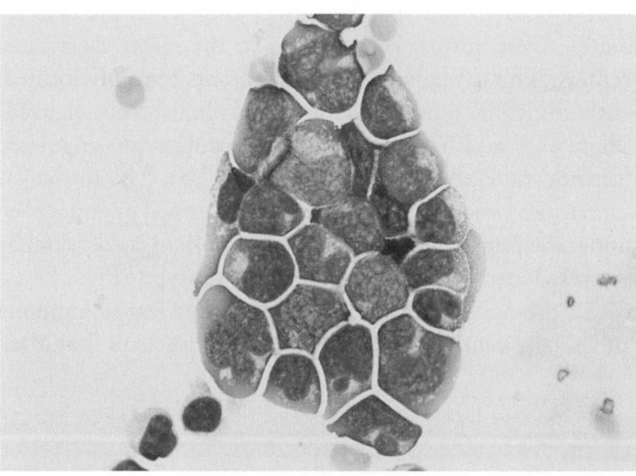

FIGURE 67.5. Large B-cell lymphoma, smear of spinal fluid. Cells with deep blue cytoplasm and large, cleaved nuclei with multiple nucleoli. Giemsa stain.

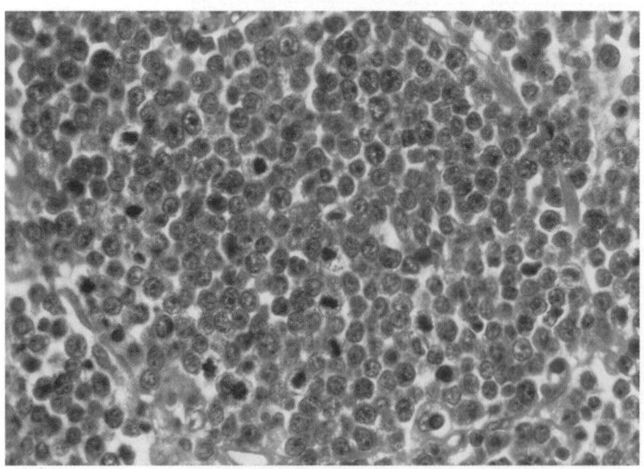

FIGURE 67.6. Diffuse large B-cell lymphoma, immunoblastic subtype. Lymphoma cells are fairly monomorphic, with numerous cells in mitosis. Hematoxylin, phloxine, and saffron stain.

resemble those of Hodgkin cells (Fig. 67.9). The cytoplasm is abundant, strongly pyroninophilic, amphophilic on hematoxylin and eosin stain, and deep blue on Giemsa stain (Fig. 67.5). It also stains strongly with periodic acid–Schiff (16). Often, the cells have a plasmacytoid appearance with an eccentric nucleus. In all large cell lymphomas, mitoses, both typical and atypical, are frequent. In the classification of lymphomas known as the *Working Formulation* (4), four histologic subtypes are described: plasmacytoid, clear cell, polymorphous, and with an epithelioid cell component. These subtypes are no longer in use. *T cell-rich large B-cell lymphoma* (Fig. 67.9) is a special type of large cell lymphoma in which a large number of T lymphocytes are admixed with and sometimes obscure the lymphoma cells (36–39). The T lymphocytes are small, reactive, nonlymphomatous lymphocytes. They should comprise at least 50% of the cell population; some authors require that 90% of the cell population be T lymphocytes for this definition (36,37). T cell-rich large B-cell lymphoma is not important because of its clinical features; the course and prognosis do not differ from those of the more typical large cell lymphomas. However, because of the abundance of small lymphocytes, it can be confused with other types of lymphomas, particularly Hodgkin lymphoma, lymphocyte predominance type.

Large B-cell lymphomas with multilobate nuclei (40,41), signet ring large cell lymphoma (42,43), and various other subtypes with pleomorphic nuclei have been described. Because their unusual histologic features do not correlate with any differences in clinical behavior, they have been included, at least temporarily, in the now expanded category of large B-cell lymphoma. The only two types of large B-cell lymphomas considered to be distinct clinicopathologic entities are mediastinal large B-cell lymphoma (see Chapter 68) and anaplastic large cell lymphoma, B-cell type (see Chapter 75), which are described separately.

ELECTRON MICROSCOPY

Under the electron microscope, the cells of immunoblastic lymphoma (Figs. 67.10 and 67.11) have large, round, sometimes indented nuclei with coarse chromatin and one to three prominent nucleoli. A rough endoplasmic reticulum with dilated cisternae and prominent Golgi apparatus is also apparent. The degree to which these features are present reflects the cellular degree of plasmacytoid differentiation (Fig. 67.10).

IMMUNOHISTOCHEMISTRY

Of the diffuse large cell lymphomas, 65% to 85% are of B-cell type and 15% to 35% are of T-cell type. A few are of null cell type, without marker expression, or coexpress B and T cells (28,44–47). Diffuse large B-cell lymphomas ex-

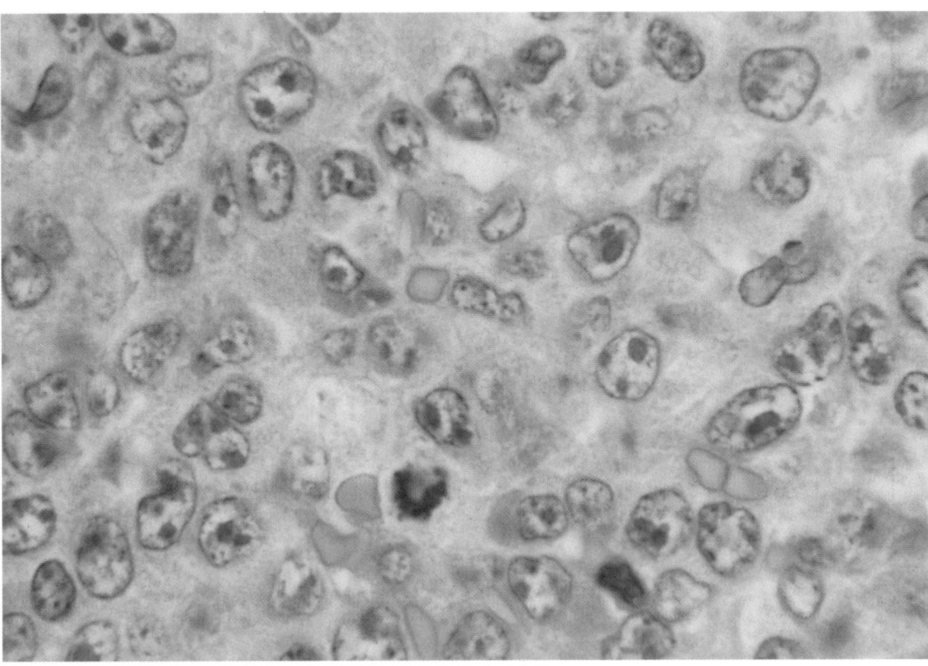

FIGURE 67.7. Diffuse large B-cell lymphoma, immunoblastic subtype. Large vesicular nuclei with thick nuclear membranes, prominent and sometimes huge nucleoli, and frequent atypical mitoses. Hematoxylin, phloxine, and saffron stain.

press the pan-B-cell markers CD19, CD20, CD22, and CD79a (Figs. 67.8, 67.12, and 67.13). One or more of these may be missing (48). The incidental small T lymphocytes, sometimes present in large numbers, as in the T cell-rich variant, show the usual pan-T-cell markers (CD3) (Fig. 67.14). Diffuse large B-cell lymphomas express monoclonal Ig light chains on the cell surface and in the cytoplasm (Fig 67.12), although less frequently than small B-cell NHLs. In an immunohistochemical study of 345 cases of B-cell NHL, Ig expression was recorded in 59% of large cell lymphomas but in as many as 100% of small cell lymphomas (49). IBLs, particularly those with plasmacytoid features, are more likely to show cytoplasmic Igs, most often IgM followed by IgG (48) (Fig. 67.13). The lymphomas are usually HLA-DR+ and may also express activation markers such as CD25 and CD30. Aberrant expression of CD5, CD10, and CD21 has been reported (48,50). About 20% to 30% of large B-cell lymphomas are CD10+, perhaps those of cen-

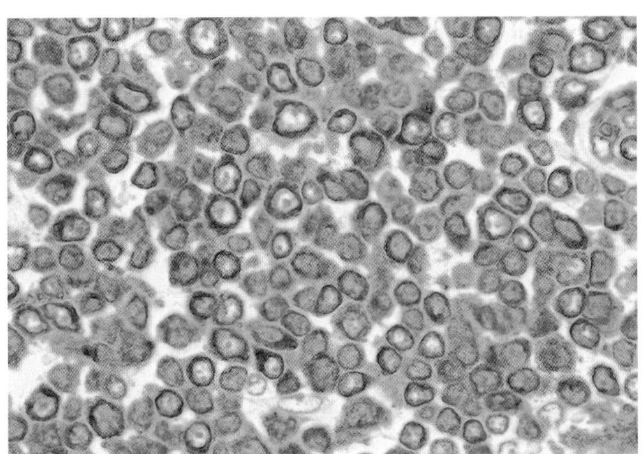

FIGURE 67.8. Diffuse large B-cell lymphoma, immunoblastic type. Distinct membrane staining for CD20, a pan-B-cell marker. L26/peroxidase immunostaining.

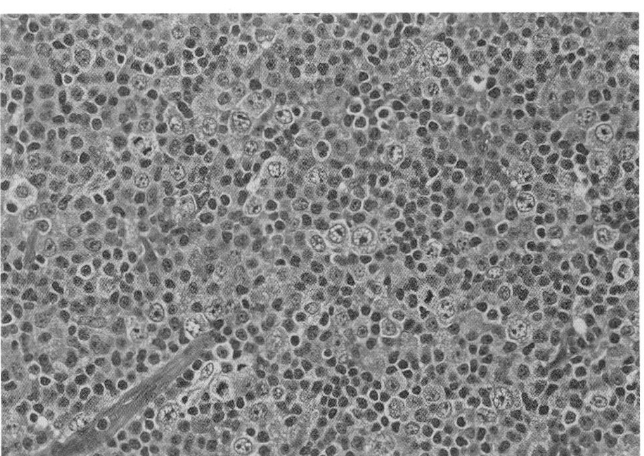

FIGURE 67.9. T cell-rich large B-cell lymphoma. Large vesicular nuclei with prominent nucleoli in the background partly obscured by the predominant reactive T-lymphocytes. Hematoxylin, phloxine, and saffron stain.

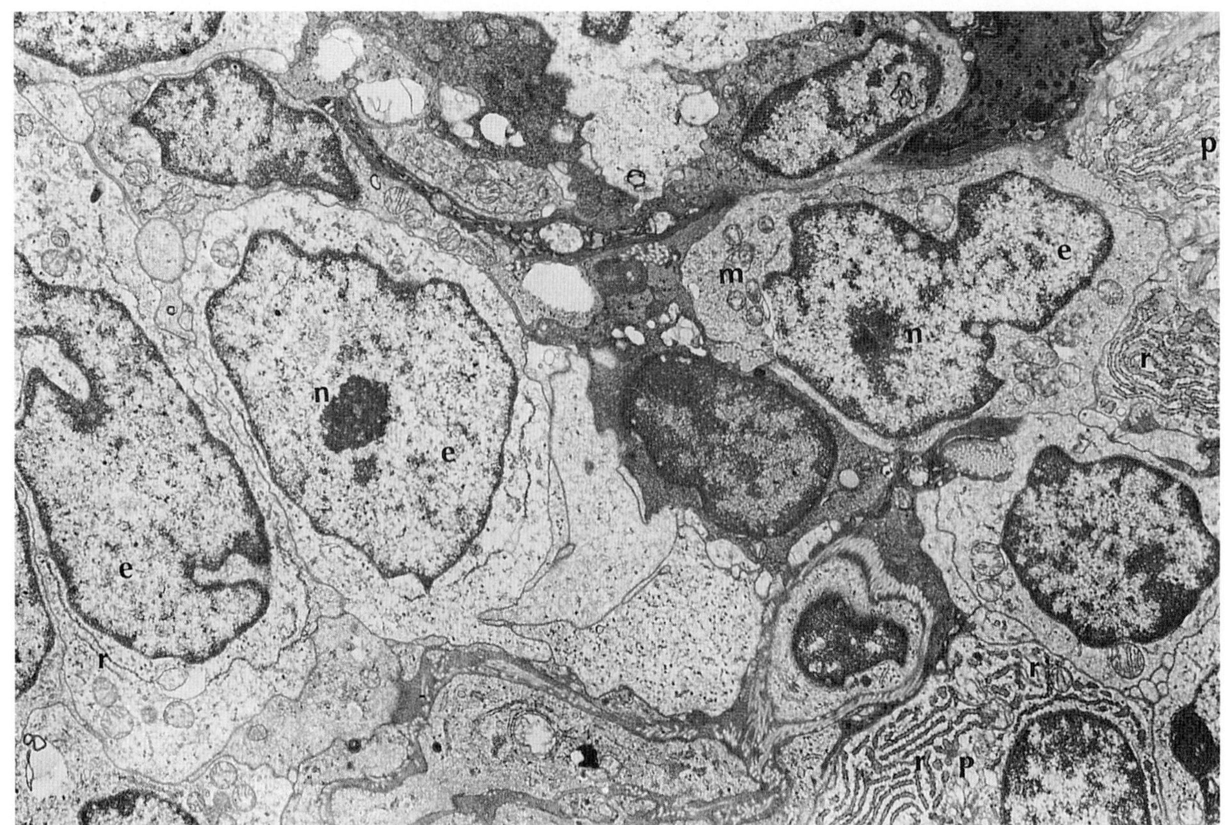

FIGURE 67.10. B-cell immunoblastic non-Hodgkin lymphoma. Large cells with irregularly shaped nuclei containing euchromatin (e) and prominent nucleoli (*n*). Cytoplasm includes polysomes, endoplasmic reticulum (*r*), and clustered mitochondria (*m*). Plasma cells (*P*) with abundant granular endoplasmic reticulum and plasmacytoid lymphocytes (*p*). × 8,200.

troblastic origin, as FLs are usually CD10+ (51). Recent studies have suggested that expression of CD10, CD5, or both correlates with a poor prognosis (52). Proliferation markers such as Ki-67 and p53 protein are more commonly present in large cell than in small cell lymphomas, indicating the higher aggressiveness of the large cell tumors (24). The proliferative index, measured by Ki-67, is a prognostic factor, with 80% or higher indicative of a poor prognosis (53). Overexpression of p53 also indicates a poor prognosis (54).

The category of diffuse large B-cell lymphoma is not well defined at the present time, and its heterogeneity is reflected

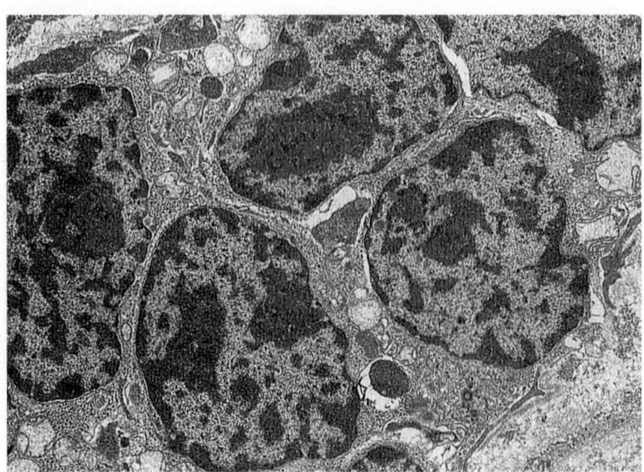

FIGURE 67.11. Large cell immunoblastic non-Hodgkin lymphoma. High nuclear-to-cytoplasmic ratios, large noncleaved nuclei with heterochromatin and a single, central, prominent nucleolus. ×9,600.

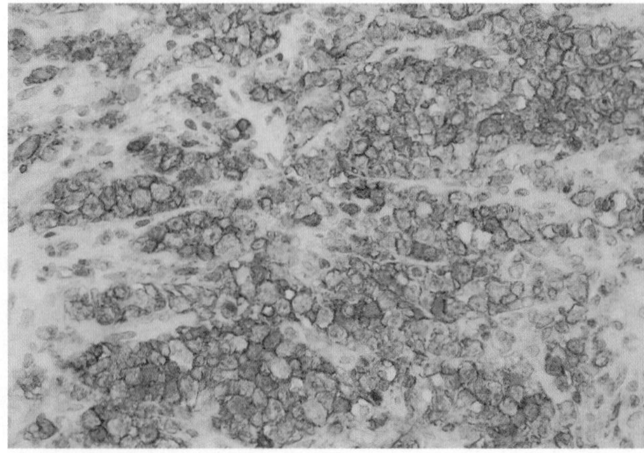

FIGURE 67.12. Diffuse large B-cell lymphoma, immunoblastic subtype, with plasmacytoid cells. The relatively abundant cytoplasm, which appears clear with the usual stains, is CD20+. L26/peroxidase immunostaining.

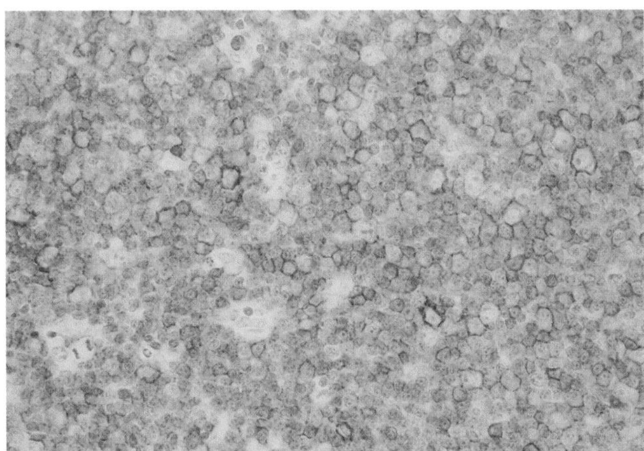

FIGURE 67.13. Diffuse large B-cell lymphoma. Membrane staining for CD20, a pan-B-cell marker, in all lymphoma cells. L26/peroxidase immunostaining.

by variable clinical behavior. Thus, 50% to 60% of patients with diffuse large cell lymphoma can be cured with anthracycline chemotherapy, whereas 40% to 50% of cases are resistant (52). To identify and characterize the subtypes of large cell lymphomas better, it is important to continue the search for prognostic markers in these neoplasms.

Phenotype

Cd19+, Cd20+, Cd22+, Cd79a+
CD45+/−, CD5−/+, CD10−/+
Surface Ig+/−, cytoplasmic Ig+/−
HLA-DR+, CD30+/−, p53+, Ki-67+
CD3+ (for the small lymphocytes in T cell-rich B-cell NHL)
bcl-2+ (20% to 30%); bcl-6+ (30%); c-myc+ (10% to 20%)

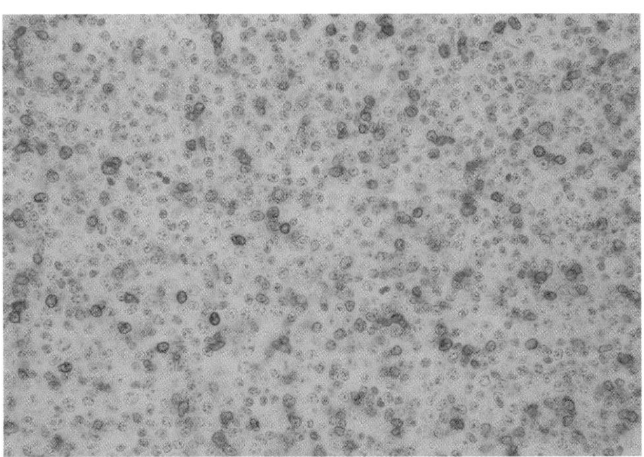

FIGURE 67.14. Same slide as in Fig. 67.9. Membrane staining of incidental lymphocytes for CD3, a pan-T-cell marker. CD3/peroxidase immunostaining.

MOLECULAR AND GENETIC ASSAYS

Diffuse large B-cell lymphoma is a heterogeneous category, and consequently the genetic features are also varied (24).

Immunoglobulin heavy and light chain genes usually exhibit rearrangements in one or both alleles in the large cell lymphomas with a B-cell immunophenotype (55).

Chromosomal translocation of the bcl-2 gene related to t(14;18), characteristic of FLs, occurs in 20% to 30% of diffuse large B-cell lymphomas, which suggests that these tumors evolve from FLs (24).

The bcl-6 gene (also known as *LAZ3*) is rearranged in about one-third of diffuse large B-cell lymphomas, more commonly in the extranodal lymphomas (56). Except in a small proportion of FLs, bcl-6 is rarely rearranged in other types of lymphoma. It is located at the breakpoint on 3q27, where a reciprocal translocation with other chromosomes occurs in 10% to 12% of diffuse large B-cell lymphomas (57). Because bcl-6 and bcl-1 rearrangements are mutually exclusive in diffuse large B-cell lymphoma, it is probable that the rearrangement of bcl-6 is an important change underlying the formation *de novo* of diffuse large B-cell lymphoma (24). About 10% to 20% of diffuse large B-cell lymphomas also show translocation of the oncogene c-myc (58).

DIFFERENTIAL DIAGNOSIS

- Infectious mononucleosis lymphadenitis may resemble the immunoblastic type of large cell lymphoma by its immunoblasts and Hodgkin-like cells. In infectious mononucleosis, T cells predominate; in Burkitt lymphoma, B cells predominate. Light chain restriction studies, cell rearrangement studies, or both may be necessary.
- Hodgkin lymphoma, classic type, particularly in some syncytial forms, closely resembles large cell lymphoma, whereas lymphocyte predominance Hodgkin lymphoma resembles T cell-rich large B-cell lymphoma. The large lymphoma cells are CD15− and CD30− and express B-cell markers.
- Large cell lymphoma of T-cell type, particularly of immunoblastic subtype, is more likely to contain lymphoma cells with clear cytoplasm and polylobate nuclei; the reactive cellular infiltrate includes eosinophils rather than the plasma cells that characterize the IBLs of B-cell type. Nevertheless, no morphologic criteria reliably differentiate the T-cell and B-cell types of IBL. The immunophenotypes must be determined by immunohistochemistry or clonal rearrangement studies.
- Granulocytic sarcoma (chloroma) has intracytoplasmic granules visible by light and electron microscopy. Results of studies with chloroacetate esterase, lysozyme, myeloperoxidase, and CD68 are positive.
- Anaplastic large cell lymphoma exhibits cords of cohesive anaplastic cells with pleomorphic nuclei and numerous

Checklist

DIFFUSE LARGE B-CELL LYMPHOMA

Highly aggressive, poor prognosis
Wide age range, elderly predominant
History of immune disorder
Lymph nodes markedly enlarged
Extranodal in 60% of cases
Two major subtypes
  Centroblastic
  Immunoblastic
Follows small cell type lymphoma or arises *de novo*
Neoplastic centroblasts/centrocytes (cleaved/noncleaved)
Neoplastic immunoblasts
Large nuclei with multiple nucleoli
Large vesicular nuclei with prominent nucleoli
B-cell surface (sometimes cytoplasmic) markers
Activation and proliferation markers
Ig light chain restriction
Ig gene rearrangements
Centroblastic bcl-2+
Immunoblastic bcl-6+
Plasmacytoid lymphocytes, plasma cells
T cell-rich large B-cell lymphoma

mitoses. It expresses anaplastic lymphoma kinase protein and epithelial membrane antigen (EMA).

- Histiocytic lymphoma: Nonspecific esterase staining, and expression of CD11b, CD11c, CD14, and CD68.
- Undifferentiated carcinoma may be morphologically similar. Some large cell lymphomas seem to form cords and islands. T cell-rich B-cell lymphoma may closely resemble lymphoepithelial carcinoma. In all cases, the diagnosis is determined by immunohistochemistry, results of which are positive for cytokeratin and negative for CD45 (leukocyte common antigen). Staining for EMA is not reliable because IBL may express EMA (59).
- Melanoma: Amelanotic forms of melanomas may show noncohesive, highly pleomorphic cellularity, similar to that of IBL. Immunohistochemical analysis with S100 protein and HMB-45 versus CD45 (leukocyte common antigen) antibodies is necessary to make the distinction.

REFERENCES

1. Rappaport H. Tumors of the hematopoietic system. Washington, DC: Armed Forces Institute of Pathology, 1966 (Atlas of tumor pathology, series I, fascicle 8).
2. Lukes RJ, Collins RD. New approaches to the classification of the lymphomata. Br J Cancer 1975;31[Suppl 2]:1–28.
3. Lennert K, Mohri W. Histopathology and diagnosis of non-Hodgkin's lymphomas. In: Malignant lymphomas other than Hodgkin's disease. New York: Springer-Verlag, 1978.
4. National Cancer Institute. Summary and description of a working formulation for clinical usage. The non-Hodgkin's Lymphoma Pathologic Classification Project. Cancer 1982;49:2112–2135.
5. Harris NL, Jaffe ES, Stein H, et al. A revised European-American classification of lymphoid neoplasms: a proposal from the International Lymphoma Study Group. Blood 1994;84:1361–1392.
6. Ioachim HL, Dorsett B, Cronin W, et al. Acquired immunodeficiency syndrome-associated lymphomas: clinical, pathologic, immunologic, and viral characteristics of 111 cases. Hum Pathol 1991;22:659–673.
7. Levine AM, Taylor CR, Schneider DR, et al. Immunoblastic sarcoma of T-cell versus B-cell origin: I. Clinical features. Blood 1981;58:52–60.
8. Harris NL, Jaffe ES, Diebold J, et al. The World Health Organization classification of hematological malignancies: report of the clinical advisory committee meeting, Airlie House, Virginia, November, 1997. Mod Pathol 2000;13:193–207.
9. Lukes JR, Collins RD. Immunoblastic lymphoma B type. In: Tumors of the hematopoietic system. Washington, DC: Armed Forces Institute of Pathology, 1992:212–215 (Atlas of tumor pathology, series II, fascicle 28).
10. Schneider DR, Taylor CR, Parker JW, et al. Immunoblastic sarcoma of T- and B-cell types: morphologic description and comparison. Hum Pathol 1985;16:885–900.
11. Stansfeld AG, Diebold J, Noel H, et al. Updated Kiel classification for lymphomas. Lancet 1988;1:292–293.
12. Brown DC, Heyret A, Gatter KC, et al. The prognostic significance of immunophenotype in high-grade non-Hodgkin's lymphoma. Histopathology 1989;14:621–627.
13. Lichtenstein A, Levine AM, Lukes RJ, et al. Immunoblastic sarcoma: a clinical description. Cancer 1979;43:343–352.

14. Michel RP, Case BW, Moinuddin M. Immunoblastic lymphosarcoma. Cancer 1979;43:224–236.
15. Lukes RJ, Tindle BH. Immunoblastic lymphadenopathy: a hyperimmune entity resembling Hodgkin's disease. N Engl J Med 1975;292:1–8.
16. Fisher R, Jaffe ES, Braylan RC, et al. Immunoblastic lymphadenopathy: evolution into a malignant lymphoma with plasmacytoid features. Am J Med 1976;61:553–559.
17. Filipovich AH, Heinitz KJ, Robison LL, et al. The immunodeficiency cancer registry. A research resource. Am J Pediatr Hematol Oncol 1987;9:183–184.
18. Matas AJ, Hertel B, Rosai J, et al. Post-transplant malignant lymphoma. Am J Med 1976;61:716–720.
19. Ioachim HL. Neoplasms associated with immune deficiencies. Pathol Annu 1987;22:177–222.
20. Beral V, Peterman T, Berkelman R, et al. AIDS-associated non-Hodgkin's lymphoma. Lancet 1991;337:805–809.
21. Ioachim HL. Immune deficiency: opportunistic tumors. In: Encyclopedia of cancer, vol II. San Diego, CA: Academic Press, 1997:901.
22. Hamilton-Dutoit SJ, Pallesen G. A survey of Epstein-Barr virus gene expression in sporadic non-Hodgkin's lymphomas. Detection of Epstein-Barr virus in subset of peripheral T-cell lymphomas. Am J Pathol 1992;140:1315–1325.
23. Lukes RJ. The immunologic approach to the pathology of malignant lymphomas. Am J Clin Pathol 1979;72:657–669.
24. Warnke RA, Weiss LM, Chan JKC, et al. Tumors of the lymph nodes and spleen. Washington, DC: Armed Forces Institute of Pathology, 1995 (Atlas of tumor pathology, series III, fascicle 14).
25. Harousseau JL, Flandrin G, Tricot G, et al. Malignant lymphoma supervening in chronic lymphocytic leukemia and related disorders. Richter's syndrome: a study of 25 cases. Cancer 1981;48: 1302–1308.
26. York JC, Glick AD, Cousar JB, et al. Changes in the appearance of hematopoietic and lymphoid neoplasms: clinical, pathologic and biologic implications. Hum Pathol 1984;15:11–38.
27. Chan JK, Ng CS, Isaacson PG. Relationship between high-grade lymphoma and low-grade B-cell mucosa-associated lymphoid tissue lymphoma (MALToma) of the stomach. Am J Pathol 1990; 136:1153–1164.
28. Kwak LW, Wilson M, Weiss L, et al. Clinical significance of morphologic subdivision in diffuse large cell lymphoma. Cancer 1991;68:1988–1993.
29. Nathwani BN, Dixon DO, Jones SE, et al. The clinical significance of the morphological subdivision of diffuse "histiocytic" lymphoma: a study of 162 patients treated by the Southwest Oncology Group. Blood 1982;60:1068–1074.
30. Armitage JO, Dick FR, Platz CE, et al. Clinical usefulness and reproducibility of histologic subclassification of advanced diffuse histiocytic lymphoma. Am J Med 1979;67:929–934.
31. Greiner TC, Medeiros J, Jaffe ES. Non-Hodgkin's lymphoma. Cancer 1995;75:370–380.
32. Simon R, Durrelman S, Hoppe TR, et al. The Non-Hodgkin Lymphoma Pathologic Classification Project. Long-term follow-up of 1,153 patients with non-Hodgkin lymphomas. Ann Intern Med 1988;109:935–945.
33. Bain B, Matutes E, Robinson D, et al. Leukaemia as a manifestation of large cell lymphoma. Br J Haematol 1991;77:301–310.
34. Shipp MA. Prognostic factors in aggressive non-Hodgkin's lymphoma: who has "high-risk disease"? Blood 1994;83:1165–1173.
35. Longo DL. The REAL classification of lymphoid neoplasms: one clinician's view. Principles and Practice of Oncology 1995;9:1–12.
36. Winberg CD, Sheibani K, Burke JS, et al. T cell-rich lymphoproliferative disorders: morphologic and immunologic differential diagnoses. Cancer 1988;62:1539–1555.
37. Ramsay AD, Smith WJ, Isaacson PG. T cell-rich B-cell lymphoma. Am J Surg Pathol 1988;12:433–443.
38. Ng CS, Chan JK, Hui PK, et al. Large B-cell lymphomas with a high content of reactive T-cells. Hum Pathol 1989;20:1145–1154.
39. Chittal SM, Brousset P, Voigt JJ, et al. Large B-cell lymphoma rich in T-cells and simulating Hodgkin's disease. Histopathology 1991;19:211–220.
40. Chan JK, Ng CS, Tung S, et al. Multilobated B-cell lymphoma, a variant of centroblastic lymphoma. Report of four cases. Histopathology 1986;10:601–612.
41. Weiss RL, Kjeldsberg CR, Colby TV, et al. Multilobated B-cell lymphomas. A study of 7 cases. Hematol Oncol 1985;3:79–86.
42. Lennert K, Feller AC. Histopathology of the non-Hodgkin's lymphomas (based on the updated Kiel classification), 2nd ed. Berlin: Springer-Verlag, 1992:93.
43. Dardick I, Sriniavasan R. Signet-ring cell variant of large cell lymphoma. Ultrastruct Pathol 1983;5:195–200.
44. Cossman J, Jaffe ES, Fisher RI. Immunologic phenotypes of diffuse, aggressive, non-Hodgkin's lymphomas, correlation with clinical features. Cancer 1984;54:1310–1317.
45. Doggett RS, Wood GS, Horning S, et al. The immunologic characterization of 95 nodal and extranodal diffuse large cell lymphomas in 89 patients. Am J Pathol 1984;115:245–252.
46. Spier CM, Grogan TM, Lippman SM, et al. The aberrancy of immunophenotype and immunoglobulin status as indicators of prognosis in B-cell diffuse large cell lymphoma. Am J Pathol 1988;133:118–126.
47. Weiss LM, Picker LJ, Copenhaver CM, et al. Large-cell hematolymphoid neoplasms of uncertain lineage. Hum Pathol 1988; 19:967–973.
48. Picker LJ, Weiss LM, Medeiros LJ, et al. Immunophenotypic criteria for the diagnosis of non-Hodgkin's lymphoma. Am J Pathol 1987;128:181–201.
49. Strauchen JA, Mandeli JP. Immunoglobulin expression in B-cell lymphoma. Immunohistochemical study of 345 cases. Am J Clin Pathol 1991;95:692–695.
50. Slater DM, Krajewski AS, Cunningham S. Activation and differentiation antigen expression in B-cell non-Hodgkin's lymphoma. J Pathol 1988;154:209–222.
51. Fang JM, Finn WG, Hussong JW, et al. CD10 antigen expression correlates with the t(14;18)(q32;q21) major breakpoint region in diffuse large B-cell lymphoma. Mod Pathol 1999;12: 295–300.
52. Hsi ED. The search for meaningful prognostic markers in diffuse large B-cell lymphoma. Am J Clin Pathol 2001;115:481– 483.
53. Miller TP, Grogan TM, Dahlberg S, et al. Prognostic significance of the Ki-67-associated proliferative antigen in aggressive non-Hodgkin's lymphomas: a prospective Southwest Oncology Group trial. Blood 1994;83:1460–1466.
54. Piris MA, Pezzella F, Martinez-Montero JC, et al. p53 and bcl-2 expression in high-grade B-cell lymphomas: correlation with survival time. Br J Cancer 1994;69:337–341.
55. Cleary ML, Chao J, Warnke R, et al. Immunoglobulin gene rearrangement as a diagnostic criterion of B-cell lymphoma. Proc Natl Acad Sci U S A 1984;81:593–597.
56. Offit K, Lo Coco F, Louie DC, et al. Rearrangement of the bcl-6 gene as a prognostic marker in diffuse large-cell lymphoma. N Engl J Med 1994;331:74–80.
57. Lo Coco F, Ye BH, Lista F, et al. Rearrangements of the bcl-6 gene in diffuse large cell non-Hodgkin's lymphoma. Blood 1994;83:1757–1759.
58. Gaidano G, Dalla-Favera R. Protooncogenes and tumor suppressor genes. In: Knowles DM, ed. Neoplastic hematopathology. Baltimore: Williams & Wilkins, 1992:245–261.
59. Delsol G, Al Saati T, Gatter KC, et al. Coexpression of epithelial membrane antigen (EMA), Ki-1, and interleukin-2 receptor by anaplastic large cell lymphomas. Diagnostic value in so-called malignant histiocytosis. Am J Pathol 1988;130:59–70.

68

MEDIASTINAL LARGE B-CELL LYMPHOMA

DEFINITION

Large B-cell lymphoma originating in the anterior mediastinum.

INCIDENCE

Mediastinal large cell lymphomas represent about 6% of all lymphomas in adults (1) and 26% of all childhood non-Hodgkin lymphomas (2). Secondary involvement of the mediastinum by lymphomas in adults is far more common, estimated to occur in 15% to 25% of all lymph node lymphomas (1).

PATHOGENESIS

Large lymphomas arising in the anterior mediastinum exhibit distinctive clinicopathologic features, reported in studies of large series of cases (1,3–9). Because of its particular age and sex preference, location, and morphologic and immunophenotypic features, mediastinal large B-cell lymphoma has been listed separately in the new lymphoma classifications (10). Mediastinal large cell lymphomas are of B-cell type and believed to originate in the B cells of the thymus (6–9,11), which are normally located in the medulla and extraparenchymal septa (12).

CLINICAL SYNDROME

In a series of 29 cases (18 women and 11 men), the patients ranged in age from 15 to 73 years, with a median age of 32 years (6). In the largest series studied, 141 patients who had mediastinal large cell lymphoma were compared with 916 patients who had nonmediastinal large cell lymphoma (8). The mediastinal lymphomas showed a predilection for women (59%) and persons of relatively young age (37 years); of the patients with nonmediastinal lymphomas, 42% were female, and their mean age was 54 years. Mediastinal lymphomas are usually bulky and commonly extend to adjacent organs—pericardium, pleura, and lung (33% of cases in one series) (9). Superior vena cava syndrome may result from local invasion (8 of 29 patients in one series) (6). However, unlike most large cell lymphomas, mediastinal lymphomas rarely involve the bone marrow (2% vs. 17%) (8) or expand beyond the thoracic cavity. They very rarely involve the central nervous system, and a leukemic phase seldom develops (11). Levels of serum lactic dehydrogenase become much higher than in nonmediastinal lymphomas (8). Despite their high-grade histology and local aggressiveness, mediastinal large cell lymphomas respond well to various regimens of combination chemotherapy with or without radiotherapy. In an earlier series, 5-year survival was 57% (6). In a more recent large collaborative European study, 79% of patients achieved complete remission, in comparison with 68% of patients with large cell nonmediastinal lymphomas, and disease-free survival at 3 years was 61% (8).

HISTOPATHOLOGY

The mediastinal tumor infiltrates adipose tissues and other local structures and may include lymph nodes and remnants of thymus (5,13). The cell population may be monomorphic or diverse (Figs. 68.1–68.3). The predominant lymphoma cells are of follicular center type—centroblasts and centrocytes (cleaved and noncleaved) (Fig. 68.2). Immunoblasts are infrequently the predominant type; they are more often scattered and admixed with the centroblasts (5–8) (Fig. 68.3). Also described, although less often, are large cell lymphomas of clear cell type, in which the cells have abundant clear cytoplasm and resemble neoplastic "monocytoid" cells (8,9,14) (Fig. 68.2), and large cell lymphomas of pleomorphic type, in which the cells have bizarre sarcomatoid or multilobate nuclei (8,13). Foci of tumor necrosis may be present. Characteristic of this particular tumor is sclerosis, which was included in its earlier names

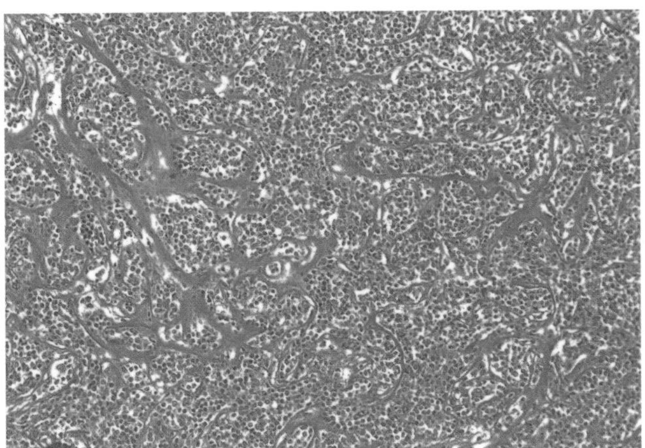

FIGURE 68.1. Mediastinal large B-cell lymphoma in a 32-year-old woman. Intersecting bands of fibrosis divide sheets of lymphoma cells. Hematoxylin, phloxine, and saffron stain.

(5,15). The sclerosis varies from fine fibrous strands to thick, broad bands of fibrosis that compartmentalize the tumor and clearly separate nests of cells (Figs. 68.1 and 68.2). In this respect, the tumor often resembles the nodular sclerosis type of classic Hodgkin lymphoma (see Chapter 57), which also shows a predilection for the mediastinum, so that a difficult problem of differential diagnosis arises. The tumor cells are locally aggressive, invading mediastinal organs and the thoracic wall (Fig. 68.4).

ELECTRON MICROSCOPY

In general, electron microscopy is not required for the diagnosis of mediastinal lymphoma; however, it may occasionally be useful in distinguishing it from other mediastinal tumors, such as thymoma, germ cell tumors, neuroendocrine tumors, Ewing sarcoma, and melanoma (11). In such cases, the absence of intercellular junctions, tonofilaments, "Chinese character" nuclei, annular lamellae, large lakes of glycogen, neurosecretory granules, sarcomeres, and melanosomes, established by electron microscopy, supports the diagnosis of lymphoma (11). Positive findings for lymphoma are abundant ribosomes and polysomes, rough endoplasmic reticulum, a prominent Golgi body, and a variable number of mitochondria.

IMMUNOHISTOCHEMISTRY

Mediastinal large cell lymphoma expresses a B-cell phenotype: CD19+, CD20+, CD22+, CD79a+ (Figs. 68.4 and 68.5), and CD3−. Most cases show immunoglobulin (Ig) heavy or light chain rearrangement by Southern blot analysis (6). A monotypic pattern of staining for IgG or IgA, κ or λ, is seen; some cases are Ig− (6). The tumor is CD45+ and HLA-DR+, and CD5− and CD10−. Negativity for the CD30 marker, characteristic of Hodgkin and Reed-Sternberg cells, was reported in earlier studies of mediastinal large B-cell lymphoma. However, in a recent study

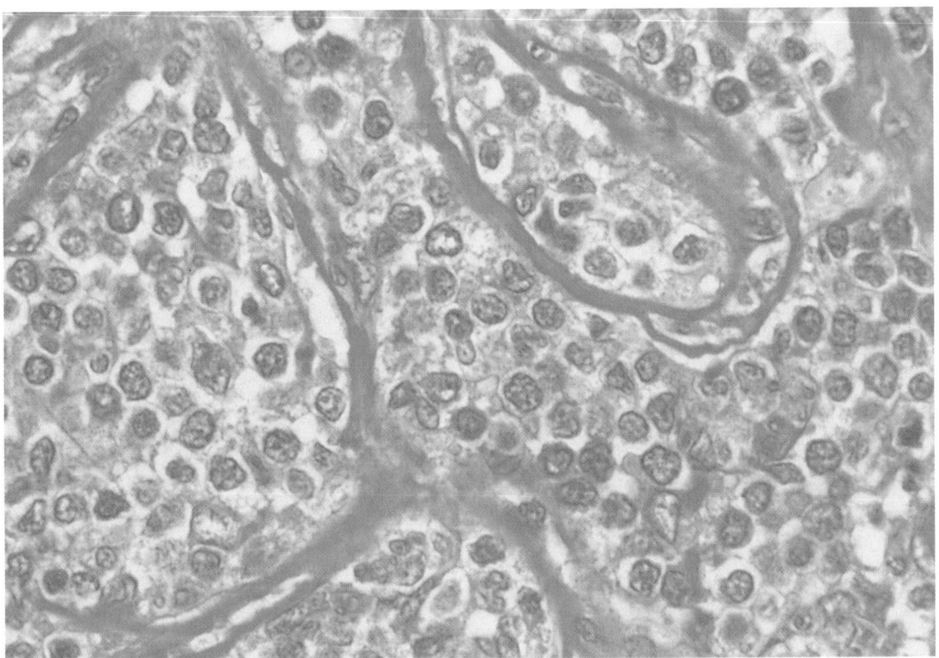

FIGURE 68.2. Same section as in Fig. 68.1. Bands of fibrosis compartmentalize the tumor, separating nests of cells. Some cells resemble centroblasts. Hematoxylin, phloxine, and saffron stain.

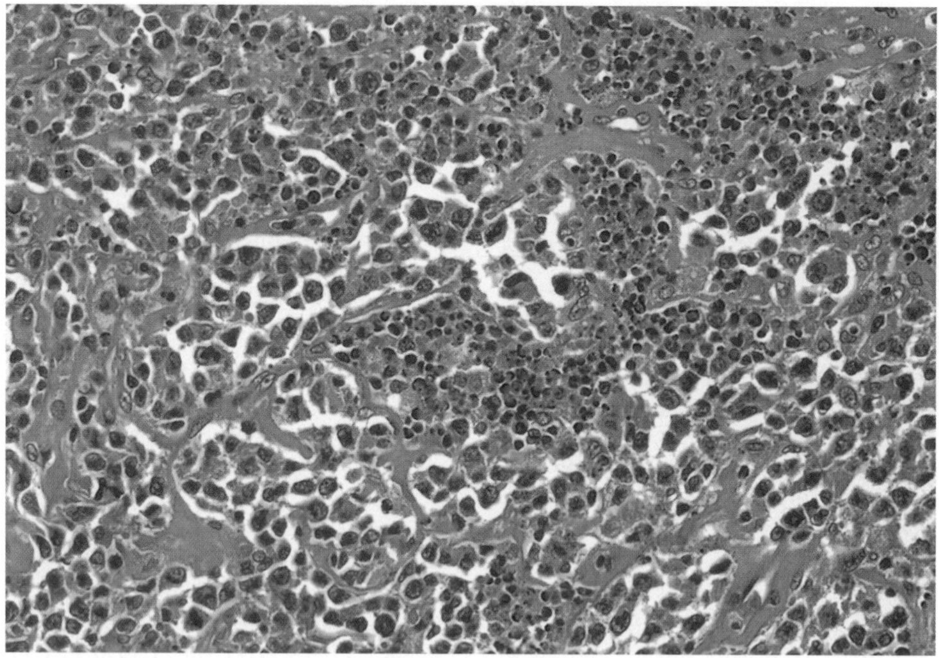

FIGURE 68.3. Mediastinal large B-cell lymphoma with nests of cells resembling centroblasts and immunoblasts. Hematoxylin, phloxine, and saffron stain.

in which the microwave technique for unmasking antigens was used, 69% of paraffin-embedded cases were strongly positive for the CD30 (Ki-1) marker (16). This finding is important because it shows that CD30 positivity, previously used to separate Hodgkin lymphoma (+) from mediastinal B-cell lymphoma (−), is likely to be present in both and therefore is not a reliable differential feature. It fact, it may reflect a close link between the two diseases that was previously unsuspected.

Phenotype

CD19+, CD20+, CD22+, CD79a+
CD45+, HLA-DR+, CD30+ (69%)
CD5−, CD10−
Ig heavy and light chains rearrangement
bcl-2+ (30%), bcl-6−, c-myc−, Epstein-Barr virus−

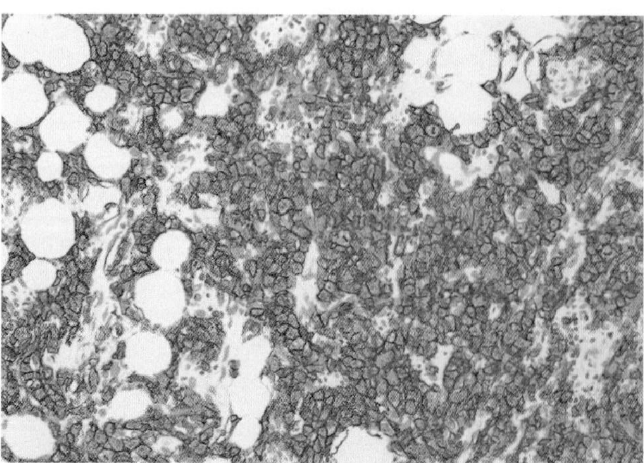

FIGURE 68.4. Mediastinal large B-cell lymphoma invading parietal pleura, adipose tissue, and pectoral muscle. L26/peroxidase immunostain.

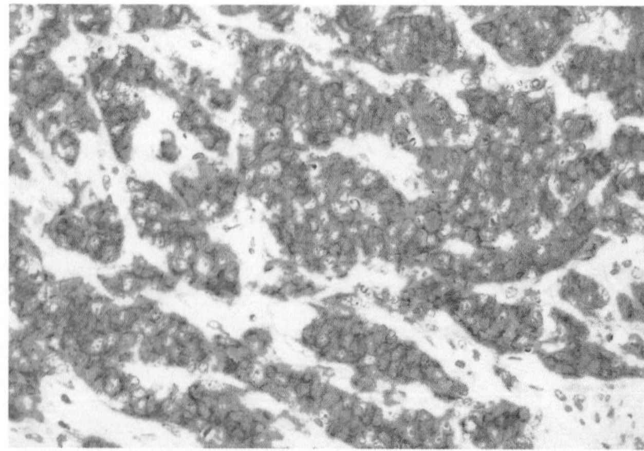

FIGURE 68.5. Same case as in Fig. 68.3. Large lymphoma cells express membrane C20 B-cell markers. L26/peroxidase immunostain.

Checklist

MEDIASTINAL LARGE B-CELL LYMPHOMA

Arises from B cells of medullary thymus
Tends to affect younger female patients
Extension to pericardium, pleura, lung
No leukemic phase or bone marrow involvement
Bulky tumor mass
Compartmentalizing sclerosis
Centroblasts/centrocytes (cleaved/noncleaved)
Clear cells, pleomorphic cells
CD19+, CD20+, CD79a+
CD5−, CD10−, CD30+
bcl-2+ (30%), bcl-6−, EBV−

MOLECULAR ASSAYS

In one study, bcl-2 was rearranged in a third of cases (8). Rearrangement of bcl-6, which occurs in up to 45% of diffuse nonmediastinal large cell lymphomas, was noted in only 1 of 16 cases (6%) of mediastinal large cell lymphoma (17). Epstein-Barr virus is not detected, and c-myc is not rearranged (9,17).

DIFFERENTIAL DIAGNOSIS

- Thymic carcinoma: Cells cohesive, nuclei round, blood vessels involved; cytokeratin+, CD45−.
- Hodgkin lymphoma classic type, nodular sclerosis: With nests of lacunar cells (syncytial variant) and intersecting bands of fibrosis, it may be difficult to separate. Typical features are Reed-Sternberg cells, CD45−, CD15+, CD30+, CD20−/+, and eosinophils.
- Diffuse large B-cell lymphoma may extend to the mediastinum from another location.
- Anaplastic large cell lymphoma, also occurring in younger persons: The component cells may be similarly large, with pleomorphic nuclei. Sclerosis is not a feature, and the immunophenotype is CD30+, anaplastic lymphokinase positive.
- Seminoma also may exhibit nests of clear cells; however, they contain glycogen and are positive for placental alkaline phosphatase and negative for CD45.

REFERENCES

1. Lichtenstein AK, Levine A, Taylor OR, et al. Primary mediastinal lymphoma in adults. Am J Med 1980;68:509–514.
2. Graham M. Non-Hodgkin's lymphoma. Pediatr Ann 1988;17: 192–203.
3. Levitt LJ, Aisenberg AC, Harris NL, et al. Primary non-Hodgkin's lymphoma of the mediastinum. Cancer 1982;50: 2486–2492.
4. Addis BJ, Isaacson PG. Large cell lymphoma of the mediastinum: a B-cell tumour of probable thymic origin. Histopathology 1986;10:379–390.
5. Perrone T, Frizzera G, Rosai J. Mediastinal diffuse large cell lymphoma with sclerosis: a clinicopathological study of 60 cases. Am J Surg Pathol 1986;10:176–191.
6. Lamarre L, Jacobsen JO, Aisenberg AC, et al. Primary large cell lymphoma of the mediastinum: a histologic and immunophenotypic study of 29 cases. Am J Surg Pathol 1989;13:730–739.
7. Davis RE, Dorfman RF, Warnke RA. Primary large-cell lymphoma of the thymus: a diffuse B-cell neoplasm presenting as primary mediastinal lymphoma. Hum Pathol 1990;21:1262– 1268.
8. Cazals-Hatem D, Lepage E, Brice P, et al. Primary mediastinal large B-cell lymphoma. A clinicopathological study of 141 cases compared with 916 nonmediastinal large B-cell lymphomas, a GELA (Groupe d'ÉEtude des Lymphomes de l'Adulte) study. Am J Surg Pathol 1996;20:877–888.
9. Paulli M, Strater J, Gianelli U, et al. Mediastinal B-cell lymphoma: a study of its histomorphologic spectrum based on 109 cases. Hum Pathol 1999;30:178–187.
10. Harris NL, Jaffe ES, Diebold J, et al. The World Health Organization classification of hematological malignancies: report of the clinical advisory committee meeting, Airlie House, Virginia, November, 1997. Mod Pathol 2000;13:193–207.
11. Payne CM, Grogan TM, Spier CM. Lymphomas of the mediastinum. Ultrastruct Pathol 1991;15:439–474.
12. Levine GD, Rosai J. Thymic hyperplasia and neoplasia: a review of current concepts. Hum Pathol 1978;9:495–515.
13. Suster S, Moran CA. Pleomorphic large cell lymphomas of the mediastinum. Am J Surg Pathol 1996;20:224–232.
14. Moller P, Lammler B, Eberlein-Gonska M, et al. Primary mediastinal clear cell lymphoma of B-cell type. Virchows Arch A Pathol Anat Histopathol 1986;409:79–92.
15. Scarpa A, Bonetti F, Menestrina F, et al. Mediastinal large-cell lymphoma with sclerosis. Virchows Arch A Pathol Anat Histopathol 1987;412:17–21.
16. Higgins JP, Warnke RA. CD30 expression is common in mediastinal large B-cell lymphoma. Am Clin Pathol 1999;112:241–247.
17. Tsang P, Cesarman E, Chadburn A, et al. Molecular characterization of primary mediastinal B cell lymphoma. Am J Pathol 1996;148:2017–2025.

69

BURKITT LYMPHOMA

DEFINITION

Non-Hodgkin B-cell lymphoma, small noncleaved cell type, associated with the Epstein-Barr virus (EBV).

SYNONYM

Small noncleaved cell lymphoma

VARIANTS

Small noncleaved cell, Burkitt type
Small noncleaved cell, non-Burkitt type

GRADE

High

EPIDEMIOLOGY

The tumor originally described by Burkitt in 1958 is endemic in Africa and in Papua, New Guinea (1–3). The geographic distribution depends on climatic factors, such as altitude and rainfall, and is similar to that of yellow fever; this observation led to the suggestion that Burkitt lymphoma (BL), like yellow fever, might be caused by a virus with an insect vector. Epidemiologic investigations have shown a high degree of geographic correlation between incidence of BL and degree of infestation with *Plasmodium falciparum* (1–3). Thus, BL occurs most commonly in areas where malaria is endemic. In Africa, in areas where temperature and humidity are high and malaria is endemic, BL is the most common malignant tumor in children, 10 times more frequent than Wilms tumor, the next most common malignancy (4). In such areas, the incidence reaches 5 to 10 cases per 100,000 children; in comparison, the same number of cases occurs per l million children in regions where BL is a sporadic malignancy (5). The lymphomas are associated with Epstein-Barr virus (EBV) in 90% of cases (6). In the United States and western Europe, Burkitt-like lymphomas, first reported in 1965, occur sporadically and account for about 2% of all lymphomas (7,8). They usually present as abdominal tumors and are associated with EBV in 20% of cases (6).

The AIDS epidemic has brought with it a fairly large number of cases of BL, apparently unrelated to the sporadic cases of BL that occur outside endemic areas. The incidence of lymphomas in patients with AIDS has gradually increased; lymphomas are currently associated with more than 3% of all cases. Almost a third of lymphomas associated with AIDS are of the Burkitt type (9,10) (see Chapter 81).

PATHOGENESIS

The search for an infectious agent as a possible cause of BL led to the discovery of EBV, a herpesvirus later found to be the cause of infectious mononucleosis. The virus is ubiquitous, infecting 70% to 100% of persons in all societies (11). In Uganda, where the prevalence of BL is high, most children have antibodies to EBV by their first birthday (3).

The lymphoma cells do not contain virus particles, which indicates that EBV is harbored in a latent state; however, the cells express specific viral antigens and produce viruses when cultured *in vitro.* Additional evidence for the etiologic relation between EBV and BL is provided by the high titers of anti-EBV antibodies in patients with BL, and by the ability of this virus to transform human B lymphocytes *in vitro* (12). Injected into marmosets, EBV produces an undifferentiated lymphoma (13). EBV DNA can be detected consistently by nucleic acid hybridization in about 95% of biopsy specimens from BLs in endemic African areas, but in only 15% to 20% of tumors in the rare American cases (2,5,11).

Immunologic studies have demonstrated membrane immunoglobulins (Igs) in BL cells, which are therefore of B-cell lineage. On this pathway, they appear to be further along in the differentiation process than immunoblastic lymphomas, which express cytoplasmic, but usually not membrane, Igs (3). The majority of BL cells also show a characteristic translocation between chromosome 8 at the site of the c-myc oncogene and chromosome 14 at the site of the Ig heavy chain gene (14).

The induction of BL proceeds in several steps: (a) immortalization of B lymphocytes by EBV in infected patients; (b) continuous stimulation of lymphocytes, including the EBV-bearing B cells, by malaria or other infections; and (c) reciprocal chromosomal translocation that leads to c-myc deregulation and the development of a malignant clone (15). An important part of this process is the suppression of T cells in malaria or HIV infection, which then fail to control the proliferation of EBV-bearing B cells (5). BL is a rapidly growing tumor with a very high growth fraction and short doubling time (5).

CLINICAL SYNDROME

In the regions of Africa where BL is endemic, the disease affects predominantly children. The mean age is 7 years (range, 2 to 16 years) and the male-to-female ratio about 2:1 (16,17). BL presents characteristically with jaw and orbital bone tumors (60% of cases); abdominal tumors, particularly of the ovaries and kidneys (25% of cases); or retroperitoneal or extradural tumors that cause paraplegia (15% of cases) (17). Central nervous system involvement is more often a manifestation of relapse after chemotherapy (2). Peripheral lymph nodes, mediastinal organs, and the spleen are rarely the primary site of endemic BL (8).

In contrast, the age range in the sporadic cases that occur in the United States is broad, within the first three decades; the median age of patients is 11 years (18,19). Men are affected more frequently than women, and blacks represent only 5% of all patients with BL (7). The abdomen is the most common localization, whereas the jaws are involved in only 25% to 33% of cases (Fig. 69.1). In addition to the abdominal lymph nodes, peripheral lymph nodes, particularly of the neck, may be involved; however, these are usually localized to one area, and generalized lymphadenopathy is very rare (18). Bone marrow involvement develops only in late stages and is sometimes associated with invasion of the meninges (20). Involvement of the bone marrow is more common in Americans (up to 30% of cases) than in Africans (about 8% of cases) (5,16). A leukemic phase is very rare, and only a few cases of BL cell leukemia have been reported. In the absence of treatment, the prognosis is very poor; however, various drugs, particularly cyclophosphamide and methotrexate, have been effective in inducing dramatic and complete tumor regression (17). The central nervous system may be involved, particularly in AIDS-associated lymphomas, most of which present as small noncleaved cell lymphomas of Burkitt or non-Burkitt type (10).

Among the sporadic cases of BL in the United States, the predominant histologic type is a Burkitt-like variant that has been described under the name of *small noncleaved lymphoma of non-Burkitt type* (21–23). It affects older patients more often than BL does (median age of 34 years vs. 10 years in a series of 66 cases) and more often involves the lymph nodes than the internal organs. Survival is marginally shorter with the non-Burkitt variant (21,22).

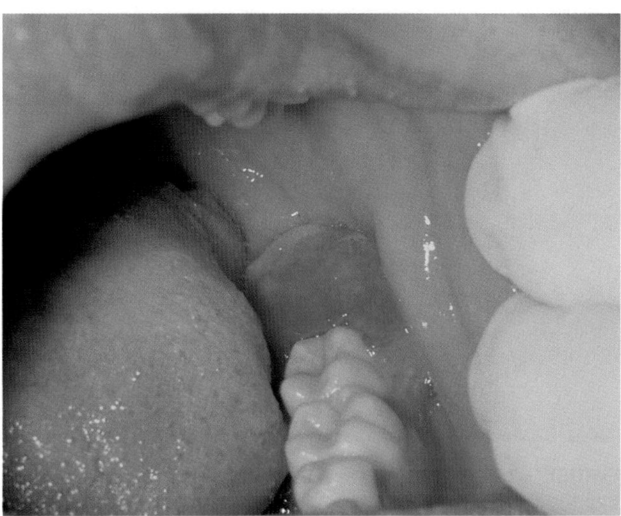

FIGURE 69.1. Burkitt lymphoma in left mandible of 18-year-old American man. The tumor fills the extraction molar wound. (Courtesy of Dr. E. Baden.)

HISTOPATHOLOGY

Whereas the clinical and epidemiologic features of the African and American forms of BL differ in many respects, the histopathology is similar in both, representing the unifying feature of the disease (23). The BL of AIDS patients is also similar histologically, immunologically, and cytogenetically to the typical forms of BL (10).

In the characteristic diffuse histologic (starry sky) pattern, sheets of monomorphic neoplastic lymphoid cells are evenly interspersed with histiocytes (Fig. 69.2). Usually, no residual normal structures are left, having been replaced by a population of tumor cells remarkably uniform in size and shape. The nuclei are round, without cleavages or deep indentations. They are smaller than the centroblasts of the germinal centers but larger than the usual lymphocytes (4). The cells have a thin rim of cytoplasm that is strongly basophilic. Small, round cytoplasmic vacuoles are present. These lipid droplets are better seen in Giemsa-stained tumor imprints (Fig. 69.3) or smears and can be stained with oil red-O. The cytoplasm also stains with methyl green-pyronine but not with periodic acid–Schiff (16). The nucleus contains clumped chromatin and several prominent basophilic nucleoli. Mitoses are very numerous and can be noted in about 4% of lymphoma cells (18) (Fig. 69.4). Kinetic studies indicate a doubling time of 24 to 48 hours, with the growth fraction approaching 100%, a proliferation rate matched by

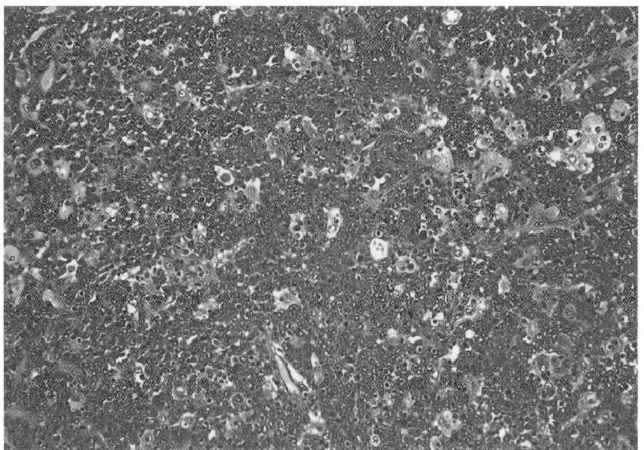

FIGURE 69.2. Burkitt lymphoma. Sheets of uniform cells with evenly interspersed tingible-body macrophages result in the characteristic "starry sky" pattern. Hematoxylin, phloxine, and saffron stain.

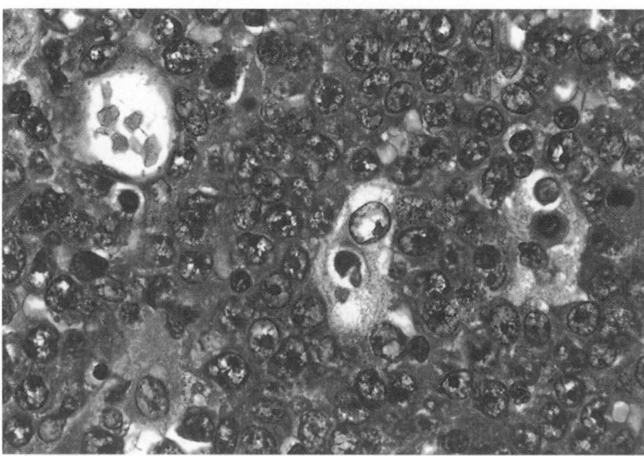

FIGURE 69.4. Same section as in Fig. 69.3. Burkitt lymphoma cells with round, noncleaved, basophilic nuclei, coarse chromatin, dense nucleoli, and frequent mitoses. Macrophages with engulfed pyknotic nuclei and nuclear debris. Hematoxylin, phloxine, and saffron stain.

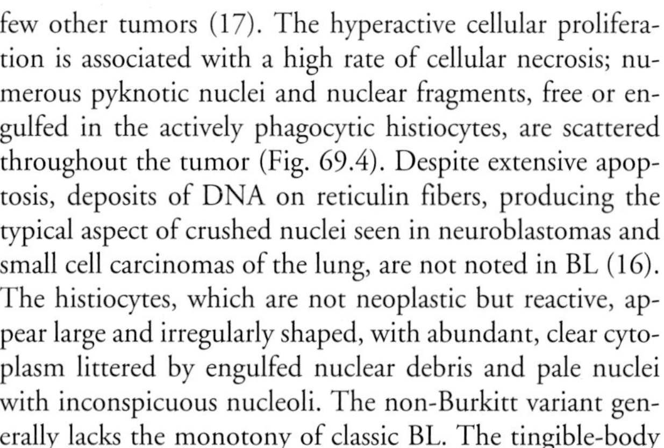

few other tumors (17). The hyperactive cellular proliferation is associated with a high rate of cellular necrosis; numerous pyknotic nuclei and nuclear fragments, free or engulfed in the actively phagocytic histiocytes, are scattered throughout the tumor (Fig. 69.4). Despite extensive apoptosis, deposits of DNA on reticulin fibers, producing the typical aspect of crushed nuclei seen in neuroblastomas and small cell carcinomas of the lung, are not noted in BL (16). The histiocytes, which are not neoplastic but reactive, appear large and irregularly shaped, with abundant, clear cytoplasm littered by engulfed nuclear debris and pale nuclei with inconspicuous nucleoli. The non-Burkitt variant generally lacks the monotony of classic BL. The tingible-body macrophages are fewer in number, and therefore the starry sky pattern is sometimes less evident. The size and shape of the nuclei vary moderately, and occasional cells have single prominent nucleoli (22). Although both Burkitt and non-Burkitt variants of small noncleaved cell lymphoma always exhibit diffuse patterns, the structure of their component cells and the expression of B-cell surface markers suggest that these lymphoma cells of germinal center type originate in the germinal centers of lymphoid follicles (24). Because of the round shape and relatively small size of Burkitt cells, Lukes and Collins even earlier proposed that they derive from the small noncleaved cells of the germinal centers (25).

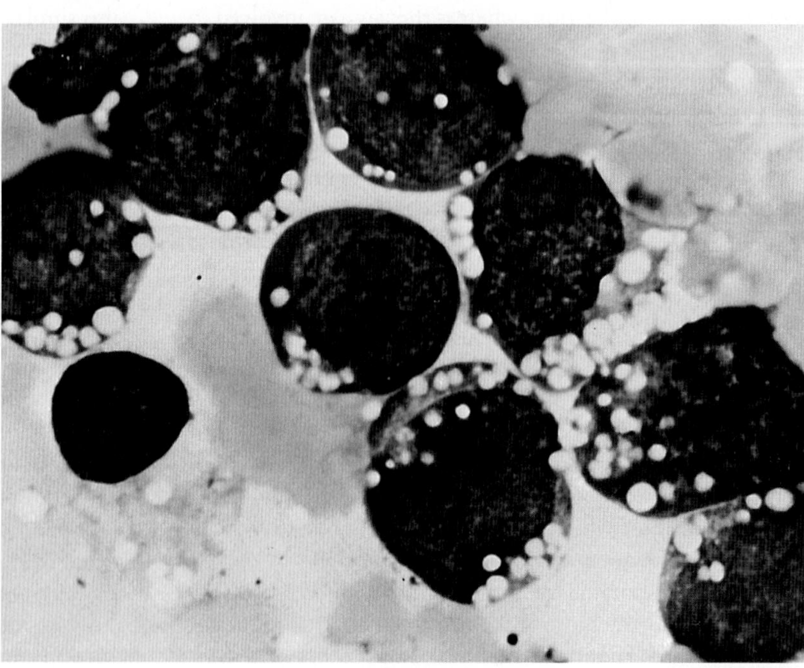

FIGURE 69.3. Burkitt lymphoma, Giemsa-stained imprint. Cells with round, strongly basophilic nuclei, high nuclear-to-cytoplasmic ratio, and multiple intracytoplasmic lipid droplets. Giemsa stain.

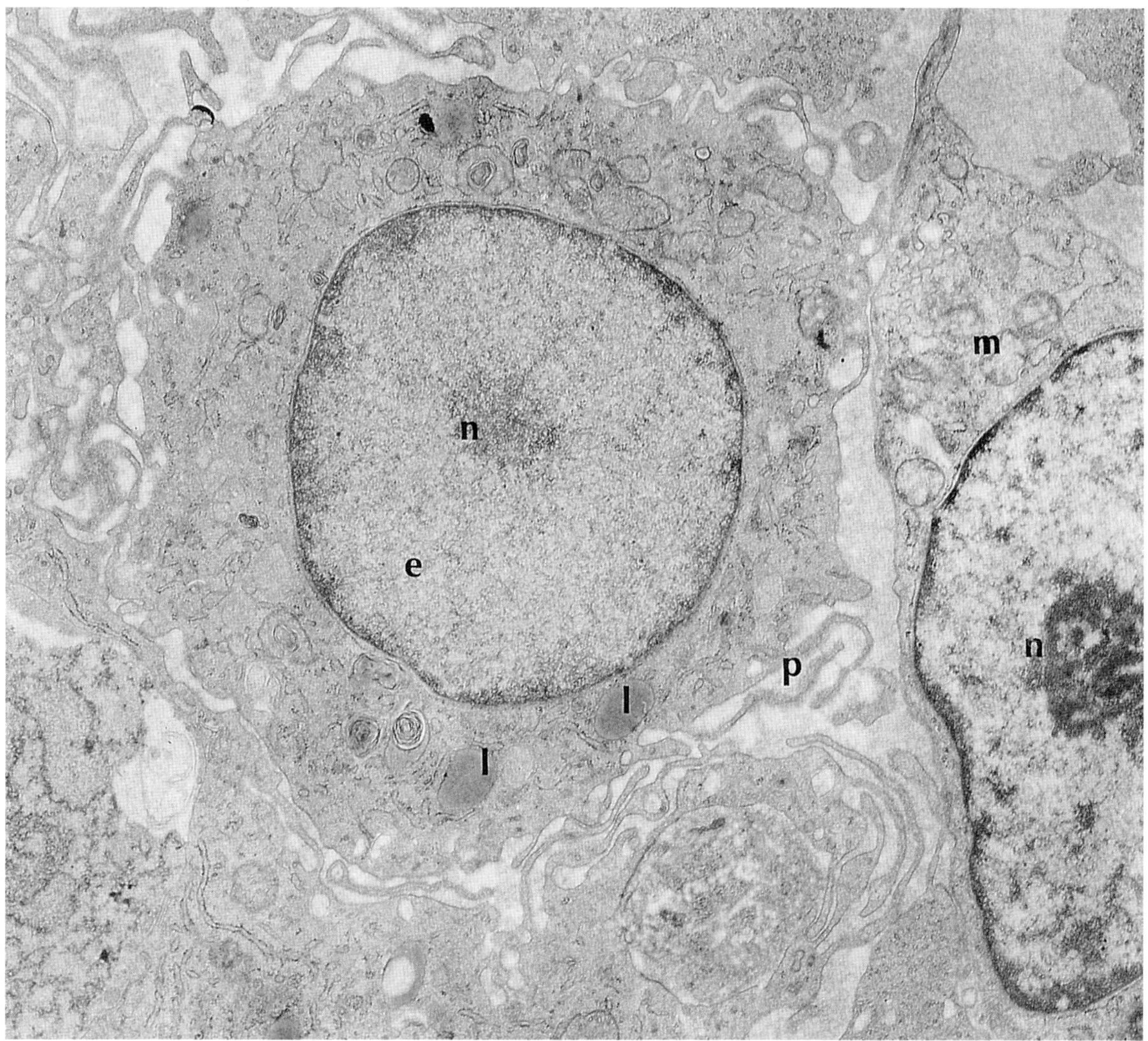

FIGURE 69.5. Burkitt lymphoma (case from the United States). Rounded cells with multiple processes (*p*), high nuclear-to-cytoplasmic ratio, cytoplasm with few polar mitochondria (*m*), endoplasmic reticulum, and lipid droplets (*l*). *e,* euchromatin; *n,* nucleolus. $\times$15,000. (Courtesy of B. Mackay, M.D.)

CYTOCHEMISTRY

The presence of large numbers of polyribosomes is one of the characteristic features of BL cells and is responsible for the strong basophilia of the cytoplasm (16). This can be demonstrated with methyl green-pyronine staining; BL cells typically exhibit a uniform cytoplasmic pyroninophilia. The cytoplasmic vacuoles, which appear empty after methyl alcohol or xylene treatment of sections and smears, contain abundant lipid droplets; in frozen sections, these can be stained with neutral fat stains. This feature is useful diagnostically because lymphocytic lymphomas do not contain lipids (16).

Burkitt lymphoma cells do not contain glycogen (23), and therefore staining with periodic acid–Schiff is not useful. Nonspecific esterases and acid phosphatase stain the interspersed non-neoplastic histiocytes.

ELECTRON MICROSCOPY

The typical BL cell (Fig. 69.5) is about 12 μm in diameter; the nucleus is round, oval, or slightly indented, the chromatin is finely dispersed, and the nucleoli are prominent and multiple. Endoplasmic reticulum and Golgi apparatus are poorly developed. Mitochondria are few and grouped at one pole of the cell. Lipid droplets are frequent, but glycogen granules are not seen. The most prominent cytoplasmic feature is the presence of large numbers of ribosomes that are frequently clustered, forming polysomes (26).

CYTOGENETICS

Like other high-grade lymphomas, BL shows a variety of random chromosomal aberrations (Fig. 69.6). Nevertheless,

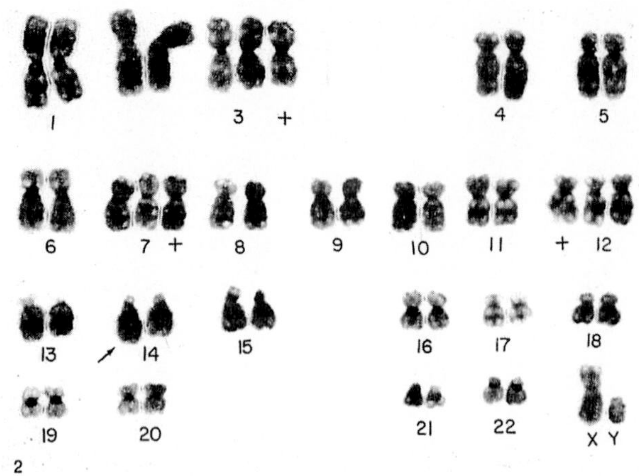

FIGURE 69.6. Burkitt lymphoma cell karyotype shows 49 chromosomes with trisomies of chromosomes 3, 7, and 12 and 14q translocation. (From Biggar RJ, Lee EC, Nkrmath FK, et al. Direct cytogenetic studies by needle aspiration of Burkitt's lymphoma in Ghana, West Africa. J Natl Cancer Inst 1981;67:769–776, with permission.)

BL was the first lymphoma in which a consistent nonrandom cytogenetic abnormality was observed. It consists of a reciprocal translocation that in more than 80% of BLs involves the q24 region on the terminal portion of chromosome 8 and q32 on chromosome 14—that is, t(8;14) (q24;q32) (5,27) (Fig. 69.7). In the remaining 20% of cases, one of two variants is seen: a reciprocal translocation of q24 of chromosome 8 with either p11 of chromosome 2 or q11 of chromosome 22. The breakpoint on chromosome 8, which is always involved, is at band q23, the location of the human c-myc protooncogene. As a consequence, the c-myc oncogene becomes translocated on chromosome 14 band q32, the site of heavy chain Igs; on chromosome 2 band q13, the site for κ light chain Igs; or on chromosome 22 band q13, the site for λ light chain Igs (5,27). Thus, a consistent feature of the translocation is that the c-myc oncogene is brought into association with a rearranged and transcriptionally active Ig gene, and inappropriate expression of the oncogene results. The product of the c-myc gene is a nuclear protein that affects the growth and differentiation of B cells. The c-myc translocations are less frequent in the sporadic forms of BL than in endemic BL (28). Rearrangements of bcl-2 are found in lymph node BLs but not in extranodal BLs (29). The cytogenetic data suggest that endemic BL arises in a pre-B-cell at the time that the Ig genes are rearranged, and that sporadic BL occurs at a later stage of B-cell differentiation (4). At any rate, although the nonrandom Ig translocations are the hallmark of BL, they are not the only cytogenetic abnormalities seen in this type of lymphoma, which displays additional aberrations in up to 70% of cases (28).

IMMUNOHISTOCHEMISTRY

The expression of surface-bound monoclonal Igs on Burkitt cells indicates the B-cell origin of these tumors. IgM is the Ig found in more than 90% of cases, in association with κ or λ light chains. (5).

Immunofluorescence staining is granular and bright, in contrast to the faint staining commonly seen in the well-differentiated lymphocytic lymphomas. BL cells also form rosettes with erythrocyte-antibody-complement (EAC)

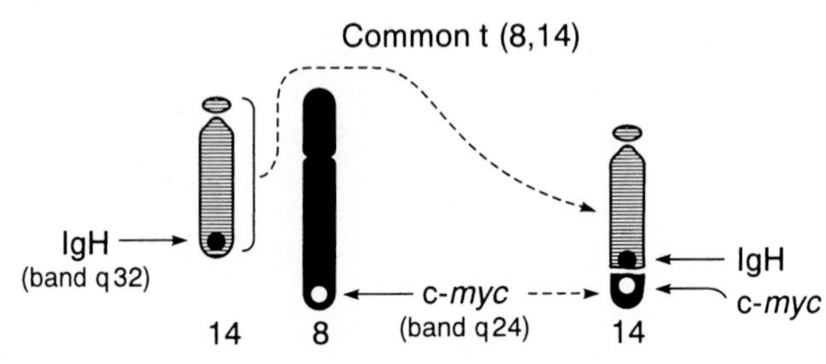

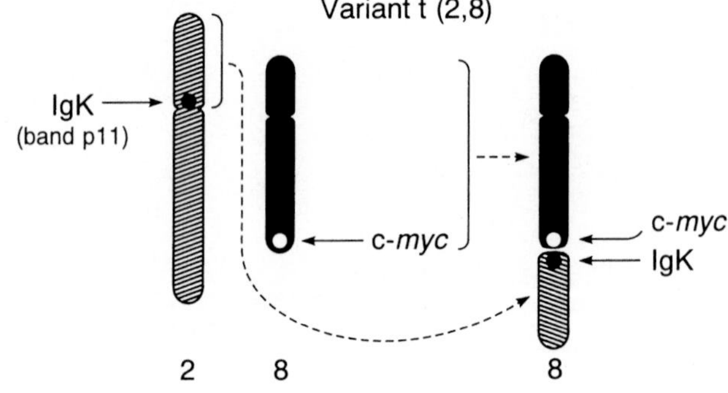

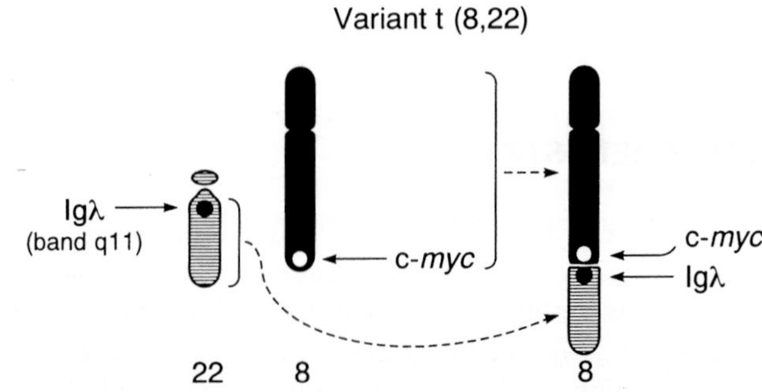

FIGURE 69.7. The common t(8;14) and variants t(2;8) and t(8;22) chromosomal translocations in Burkitt lymphoma; c-myc is indicated by *white dots,* and the immunoglobulin genes by *black dots.* The normal chromosomes are illustrated on the left, and the abnormal chromosomes bearing c-myc on the right. The second abnormal chromosome produced by each translocation (which may contain nonfunctional fragments of c-myc or immunoglobulin genes) is not represented, nor is the normal chromosome of each pair, which does not participate in the translocation. (From Croce CM, Tsujimoto Y, Erikson J. Chromosomal translocations and B-cell neoplasia. Lab Invest 1984;51:265, with permission.)

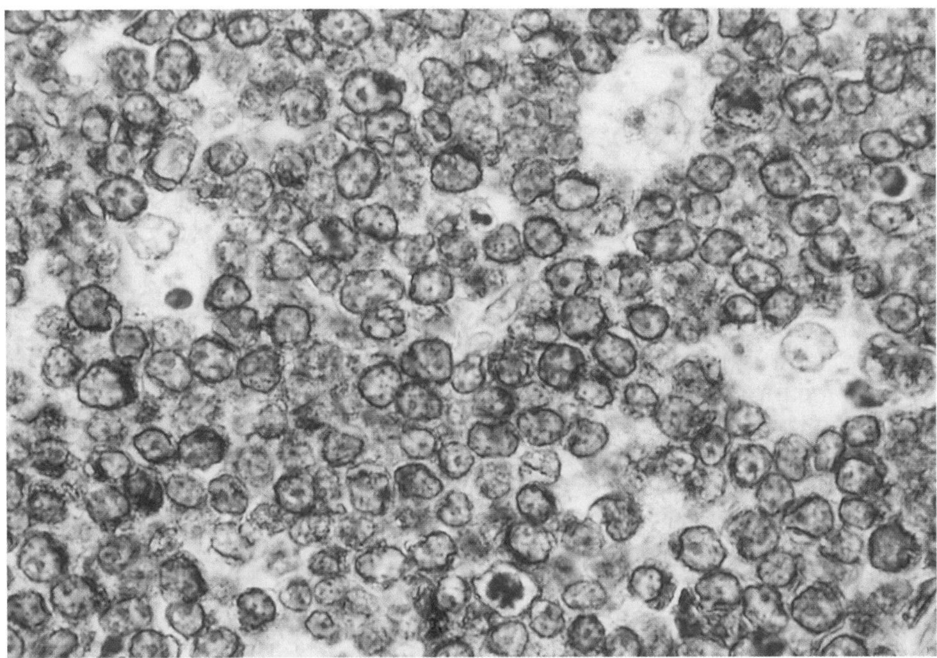

FIGURE 69.8. Burkitt lymphoma of cervical lymph node. Uniform immunostaining of Burkitt lymphoma cell membranes but not of tingible-body macrophages with anti-B-cell marker CD74 (LN-2). LN-2/peroxidase stain.

complexes and do not bear Fc or E receptors. Both BL and non-Burkitt variant cells express the common acute lymphoblastic leukemia antigen (CD10) in addition to a number of B-cell antigens, such as CD19, CD20, CD22, CD74, CD79a, and HLA-DR (4,5) (Fig. 69.8). Unlike the lymphoblastic lymphomas, neither of the two BL variants has the enzyme terminal deoxynucleotidyl transferase (TdT) (5). The presence of EBV is noted in about 30% of AIDS cases. BLs can be demonstrated by *in situ* hybridization for EBV-encoded RNAs (Fig. 69.9).

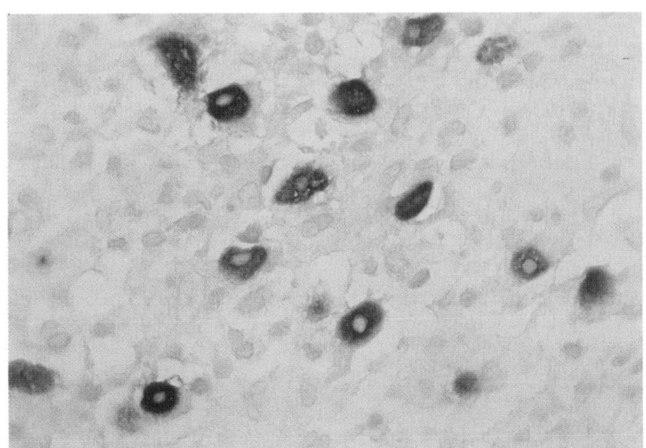

FIGURE 69.9. Burkitt lymphoma cells with positive reaction to *in situ* hybridization for Epstein-Barr virus RNA. Nuclear EBER staining. Nucleoli and cytoplasm unstained. EBER *in situ* hybridization.

DIFFERENTIAL DIAGNOSIS

- Small lymphocytic lymphoma affects elderly patients. The cells are lymphocytic and therefore smaller, with minimal cytoplasm, inconspicuous nucleoli, and virtually no mitoses. Phagocytic histiocytes are not present. Leukemia is frequently associated.
- Lymphoblastic lymphoma also occurs in children and adolescents; however, it is almost always mediastinal, whereas BL usually affects abdominal organs. It also has a diffuse pattern and immature, noncleaved cells with frequent mitoses. However, the nuclei are convoluted, the chromatin is fine and dusty, the nucleoli are small, and the cytoplasm is not as intensely basophilic as that of the BL cells. Lymphoblastic lymphomas are in most cases of T-cell type, and staining for TdT is positive. Further distinctions can be made by cytogenetic and molecular studies.
- Ewing sarcoma: Starry sky pattern absent; abundant intracytoplasmic glycogen.
- Neuroblastoma: Starry sky pattern absent; deposits of hematoxyphilic DNA material; rosette pattern; intracytoplasmic neurosecretory granules.
- Embryonal rhabdomyosarcoma: May occur in jaws and orbit; starry sky pattern absent; nuclei are spindle-shaped; intracytoplasmic striations sometimes visible.
- Small cell carcinoma of lung occurs in older patients, shows necrosis and deposits of hematoxyphilic DNA material.

Checklist

BURKITT LYMPHOMA

Endemic in tropical Africa and New Guinea; sporadic in other regions
Geographic distribution related to warm, humid climate
Most common in regions of endemic malaria
High incidence in AIDS patients
Immune deficiency (malaria, AIDS) contributing factor
Etiologic relation to EBV
Lymphoma of childhood (median age 7 years in Africa, 11 years in United States)
Male predominance
Predilection for jaws, gonads, abdominal viscera, central nervous system
Short survival without treatment
Good response to chemotherapy
Diffuse, starry sky pattern
Histiocytes with engulfed nuclear debris
Monomorphic, undifferentiated lymphoid cells
Small, round, noncleaved nuclei
Multiple prominent nucleoli
Numerous mitoses
Intensely basophilic cytoplasm
Polysomes, lipid droplets
Surface Igs (most commonly IgM with κ or λ light chains)
B-cell germinal center origin
B-cell-restricted antigens CD19, CD20, CD22, HLA-DR
Common acute lymphoblastic leukemia antigen (CD10)
Reciprocal chromosomal translocation (8;14) in 80% of cases; (8;2) or (8;22) in the rest
Juxtaposition of c-myc oncogene with Ig gene

- Granulocytic sarcoma (chloroma) also may involve the ovaries or orbital bones. The cells have amphophilic or eosinophilic cytoplasm, often with granules. Myeloperoxidase and nonspecific esterase can be demonstrated.
- Large cell lymphoma, immunoblastic type has larger cells, more abundant cytoplasm that is less basophilic, and nuclei with one prominent, centrally located nucleolus. Nuclear pleomorphism is seen, and the starry sky pattern is inapparent.

REFERENCES

1. Burkitt D, O'Connor GT. Malignant lymphoma in African children. I. A clinical syndrome. Cancer 1961;14:258–269.
2. Ziegler JL. Burkitt's lymphoma. J Natl Cancer Inst 1981;305: 735–745.
3. Wright DH. Pathogenesis of non-Hodgkin's lymphomas: clues from geography. In: Magrath IT, ed. The Non-Hodgkin's lymphomas. Baltimore: Williams & Wilkins, 1990:122–134.
4. Warnke RA, Weiss LM, Chan JKC, et al. Malignant lymphoma, small noncleaved cell. In: Tumors of the lymph nodes and spleen. Washington, DC: Armed Forces Institute of Pathology, 1994:221–232 (Atlas of tumor pathology, series III, fascicle 14).
5. Magrath I: Small noncleaved cell lymphoma. In: Magrath I, ed. The Non-Hodgkin's lymphomas. Baltimore: Williams & Wilkins, 1990: 256–278.
6. Cohen JI. Epstein-Barr virus infection. N Engl J Med 2000;343: 481–492.
7. Mann RB, Jaffe ES, Braylan RC, et al. Non-endemic Burkitt's lymphoma: a B-cell tumor related to germinal centers. N Engl J Med 1976;295:685–691.
8. Levine PH, Kamaraju LS, Connelly RR, et al. The American Burkitt's lymphoma registry. Eight years' experience. Cancer 1982;49:1016–1022.
9. Beral V, Peterman T, Berkelman R, et al. AIDS-associated non-Hodgkin's lymphoma. Lancet 1991;337:805–809.
10. Ioachim HL, Dorsett B, Cronin W, et al. Acquired immunodeficiency syndrome-associated lymphomas: clinical, pathologic, immunologic, and viral characteristics of 111 cases. Hum Pathol 1991;22:659–673.
11. De Thé G. Role of Epstein-Barr virus in human disease: infectious mononucleosis, Burkitt's lymphoma and nasopharyngeal

carcinoma. In: Klein G, ed. Viral oncology, vol 2. New York: Raven Press, 1980:769–797.
12. Henle W, Henle G. Evidence for an oncogenic potential of the Epstein-Barr virus. Cancer Res 1973;33:1419–1423.
13. Miller G, Shope T, Coope D, et al. Lymphoma in cotton-top marmosets after inoculation with Epstein-Barr virus. J Exp Med 1977;45:948–967.
14. Aisenberg AC. New genetics of Burkitt's lymphoma and other non-Hodgkin's lymphomas. Am J Med 1984;77:1083–1090.
15. Klein G. Lymphoma development in mice and man. Proc Natl Acad Sci U S A 1979;76:2442.
16. Wright DH. Burkitt's lymphoma: a review of the pathology, immunology and possible etiologic factors. Pathol Annu 1971;6: 336–363.
17. Ziegler JL, Magrath IT. Burkitt's lymphoma. Pathobiol Annu 1974;4:129–142.
18. Mann RB, Jaffe ES, Berard CW. Malignant lymphomas: a conceptual understanding of morphologic diversity. Am J Pathol 1979;94:105–192.
19. O'Conor GT, Rappaport H, Smith EB. Childhood lymphoma resembling "Burkitt's tumor" in the United States. Cancer 1965; 18:411–417.
20. Banks PM, Arseneau JC, Gralnick HR, et al. American Burkitt's lymphoma: a clinicopathologic study of 30 cases. II. Pathologic correlations. Am J Med 1975;58:322–329.
21. Miliauskas JR, Berard CW, Young RC, et al. Undifferentiated non-Hodgkin's lymphomas (Burkitt's and non-Burkitt's types). The relevance of making this histologic distinction. Cancer 1982;50:2115–2121.
22. Levine AM, Pavlova Z, Pockros AW, et al. Small, noncleaved follicular center cell (FCC) lymphoma: Burkitt and non-Burkitt variants in the United States. I. Clinical features. Cancer 1983; 52:1073–1079.
23. Berard CW, O'Conor GT, Thomas LB, et al. Histo-pathological definition of Burkitt's tumour. Bull World Health Organ 1969;40:601–607.
24. Lukes RJ, Collins RD. New approaches to the classification of the lymphomata. Br J Cancer 1975;31:1–28.
25. Kuppers R, Klein U, Hansmann M-L, et al. Cellular origin of human B-cell lymphomas. N Engl J Med 1999;341:1520–1529.
26. Achong BG, Epstein MA. Fine structure of the Burkitt tumor. J Natl Cancer Inst 1966;36:877–897.
27. Nowell PC, Croce CM. Chromosome translocations and oncogenes in human lymphoid tumors. Am J Clin Pathol 1990;94: 229–237.
28. Heim S, Mitelman F. Cancer cytogenetics. New York: Alan R Liss, 1987:203–206.
29. Yano T, van Krieken JHJM, Magrath IT, et al. Histogenetic correlations between subcategories of small noncleaved cell lymphomas. Blood 1992;79:1282–1290.

70

COMPOSITE LYMPHOMA

DEFINITION

In composite lymphoma, two or even three varieties of non-Hodgkin lymphoma (NHL), or Hodgkin lymphoma (HL) and NHL, coexist in the same organ or tissue, but their distinct histologic patterns and a zonal configuration are preserved (1). An intimate mixture of various malignant cell types does not qualify as composite lymphoma (1). Composite lymphoma should be distinguished from discordant histology, in which two types of lymphoma occur at separate anatomic sites (2,3), and from sequential lymphoma, in which two types of lymphoma occur at different times. In short, a composite lymphoma is an amalgam of multiple lymphoid neoplasms in a single anatomic space, each of which retains a separate morphologic identity regardless of its immunophenotypic and clonal connection to the other neoplastic component(s).

PATHOGENESIS

Although composite lymphomas were originally considered to be a coincidental coexistence of two different NHLs in the same anatomic site (4), some composite lymphomas have been shown to represent one neoplastic clone with dimorphic expression (5,6). Recent immunophenotypic and genotypic studies indicate that the pathogenesis of composite lymphoma appears analogous to that of Richter syndrome (Chapter 60), in which a neoplastic clone of B-cell chronic lymphocytic leukemia (B-CLL) progresses to diffuse large B-cell lymphoma (Chapter 67).

Most often, composite lymphomas comprise two separate types of NHL; however, HL may coexist with NHL (usually of B-cell type) (7). Such cases are of great interest because the two diseases traditionally were considered to be entirely separate entities. Nodular lymphocyte predominance Hodgkin lymphoma (NLPHL) is the HL subtype that most often accompanies NHL (7). Recently, the B-cell origin of NLPHL (8) and classic HL of nodular sclerosis or mixed cellularity type (9) was established in polymerase chain reaction studies demonstrating clonally rearranged immunoglobulin (Ig) VDJ genes in individual Reed-Sternberg (R-S) cells. DNA sequencing demonstrated a common B-cell precursor in a composite lymphoma in which classic HL and follicular lymphoma (FL) were together in the same lymph node (10). However, some combined HL and NHL composite lymphomas have different clonal rearrangements in their individual elements (11).

Reed-Sternberg cells typical of classic HL, expressing CD15 and CD30 and surrounded by T-cell rosettes, develop rarely in cases of B-CLL and FL (7,12,13). Epstein-Barr virus (EBV), found in the R-S cells, may transform B-CLL to composite lymphoma of combined B-CLL plus HL type (14).

Some composite lymphomas contain elements from different cells of origin; for example, B-cell NHL may coexist with T-cell NHL (15,16). In these cases, a more aggressive T-cell lymphoma develops in the presence of an indolent B-cell lymphoma. It remains speculative whether this phenomenon represents malignant transformation in a stem cell capable of dual evolution or two unrelated genetic events. In a case of peripheral T-cell lymphoma that developed during HL in relapse, the neoplastic T cells and the R-S cells contained different cytogenetic abnormalities, which proved that they arose from different clones (17).

CLINICAL SYNDROME

The lack of uniform criteria for diagnosing composite lymphoma makes epidemiologic comparisons difficult. In more than 1,000 cases of malignant lymphoma, the incidence of composite lymphoma varied between 1% and 4.7%, depending on the classification system (18). In other lymphoma series, the incidence of discordant histology varied between 9.3% and 33% (2,3) and was considerably greater than that of composite lymphoma.

Composite lymphoma sometimes appears in liver and spleen as well as in lymph nodes. Composite lymphoma includes various combinations of NHL, or HL with NHL. The age of patients ranges from 3 to 85 years; the median age of patients with composite NHL is in the sixth decade (4,19), and the median age of patients with combined NLPHL and NHL composite lymphoma is 37 years (7).

Patients with composite lymphoma in which NLPHL and diffuse large cell lymphoma are combined tend to have disease at an earlier stage and survive longer than patients with diffuse large B-cell lymphoma without NLPHL (20,21). In composite lymphomas, the component with the greatest malignant potential usually determines the overall clinical course and prognosis. When HL coexists with NHL, the NHL seems to have a greater influence, especially if it is an aggressive type. On the other hand, if an indolent NHL is combined with HL, then therapy should be directed to the HL (7).

HISTOPATHOLOGY

The histologic patterns are those of the types of lymphomas involved. The combination most frequently observed is follicular ("nodular") lymphoma and diffuse large cell lymphoma (1,22) (Fig. 70.1). The World Health Organization classification does not refer to these entities as composite lymphomas but does suggest quantifying the individual components (see Chapter 64). In such cases, both lymphomas usually express identical surface Ig light chains, an indication that they have arisen from the same B-cell clone. In a case of three coexisting patterns of NHL, they were well-differentiated lymphocytic, poorly differentiated lymphocytic, and nodular histiocytic (23). Nodal marginal zone B-cell lymphoma (low-grade monocytoid B-cell lymphoma) can accompany FL, but their clonal relationship has been controversial (24) (see Chapter 63). Cytogenetic analysis indicates that the marginal zone B-cell component exhibits the same abnormalities as the rest of the composite lymphoma and therefore probably represents a morphologic variation, not a separate clone (25).

The association of HL and NHL has been observed occasionally, mainly NLPHL with large cell NHL (7). In combined NHL and classic HL composite lymphoma, the R-S cells should be identifiable in a background typical of HL, even if some intermingling between the two components is noted (19,21).

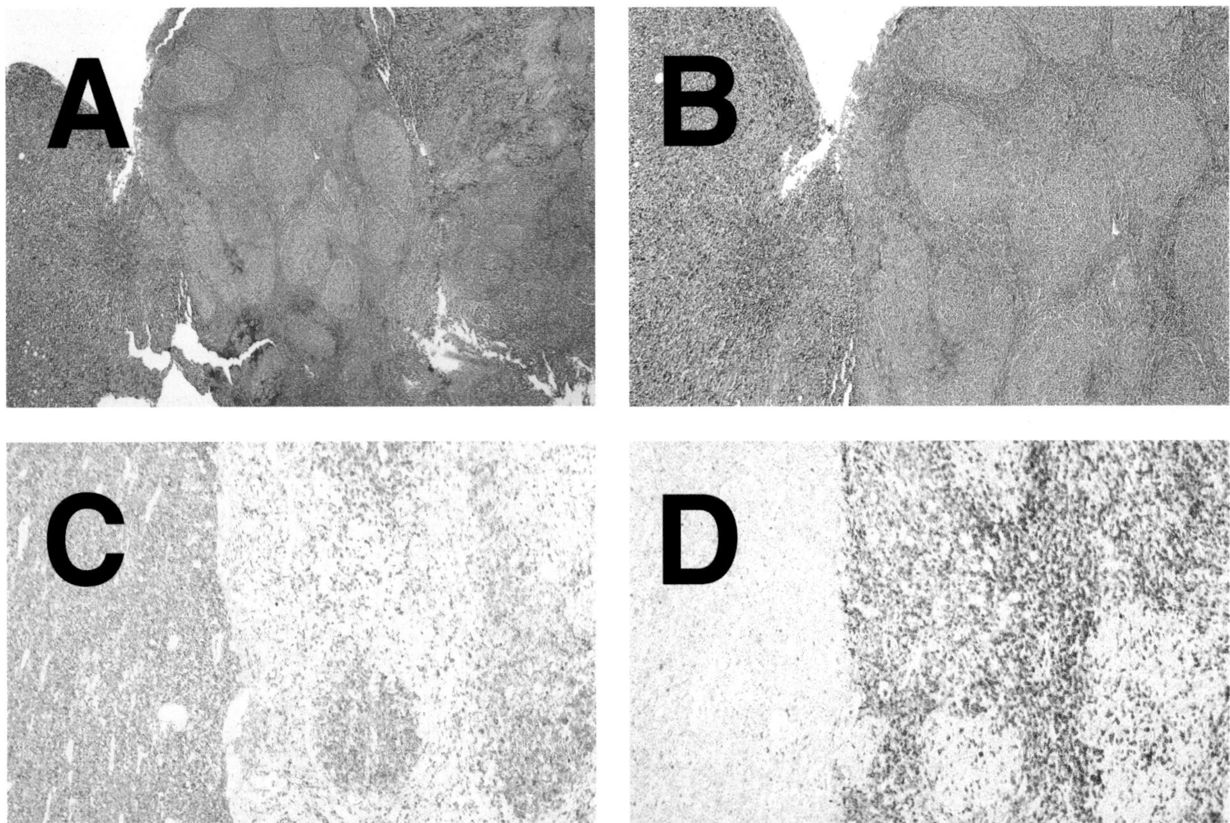

FIGURE 70.1. Composite lymphoma in submandibular lymph node from a 94-year-old woman. **A,B:** Diffuse pattern (*left*) and follicular pattern (*right*) sharply separate zones containing diffuse large B-cell lymphoma (*DLBCL*) and follicular lymphoma (*FL*). Hematoxylin and eosin stain. **C:** Almost all cells of DLBCL (*left*) and neoplastic follicles of FL (*right*) express CD20 (B-cell marker). Immunoperoxidase stain. **D:** CD3 (T-cell marker) is almost entirely absent from DLBCL (*left*) and highlights non-neoplastic, interfollicular T cells in FL (*right*). Immunoperoxidase stain. Ki-67 nuclear proliferation marker identified 10% of cells in FL and 80% to 90% of cells in DLBCL; both low- and high-grade components expressed CD10 (*not shown*).

When the diagnosis relies on either mediastinal fine needle aspiration (26) or abdominal laparoscopic biopsy (27), the diagnosis of composite lymphoma may be missed because of inadequate sampling.

IMMUNOHISTOCHEMISTRY

Immunophenotyping of the NHLs in composite lymphomas usually reveals similar markers (Fig. 1C), which suggests a common clonal origin. For example, identical Ig light chain restriction has been found in combined FL and nodal marginal zone B-cell lymphoma (28,29). In patients with HL and NHL composite lymphomas, the HL component was of various histologic subtypes, whereas the NHL component was always of B-cell type (19). On the other hand, multinucleated R-S–like cells expressing B-cell markers (CD15−, CD20+, CD30−, CD45+) that phenotypically resemble a pre-existing B-CLL, FL, or mantle cell lymphoma probably represent transformed B cells, which should not be confused with HL or composite lymphoma (30). Rare composite NHLs combining B- and T-cell NHL in the same lymph node have been reported (15,16). A review of the literature revealed no lymph node-based composite lymphomas with multiple T-cell components.

DIFFERENTIAL DIAGNOSIS

- Follicular lymphoma, grade 2/3 (mixed, small cleaved and large cell, follicular and diffuse lymphomas): The two cell types are intermingled without forming different and separate histologic patterns. Therefore, an important requirement for composite lymphoma is not met.
- Reed-Sternberg–like cells in indolent B-cell lymphomas, such as B-CLL or FL: If the R-S–like cells have the same B-cell phenotype as the pre-existing B-cell lymphoma, then they probably represent transformed B cells. In composite lymphoma of the combined HL and NHL type, the R-S cells express CD15 and CD30 and occur in a background appropriate for HL; in this instance, the R-S cells, but not the B-cell lymphoma, may contain EBV.

REFERENCES

1. Kim H. Composite lymphoma and related disorders. Am J Clin Pathol 1993;99:445–451.
2. Fisher RI, Jones RB, DeVita VT Jr, et al. Natural history of malignant lymphomas with divergent histologies at staging evaluation. Cancer 1981;47:2022–2025.
3. Mead GM, Kushlan P, O'Neil M, et al. Clinical aspects of non-Hodgkin's lymphomas presenting with discordant histologic subtypes. Cancer 1983;52:1496–1501.
4. Kim H, Hendrickson R, Dorfman RF. Composite lymphoma. Cancer 1977;40:959–976.
5. Woda BA, Knowles DMD. Nodular lymphocytic lymphoma eventuating into diffuse histiocytic lymphoma: immunoperoxidase demonstration of monoclonality. Cancer 1979;43:303–307.
6. De Jong D, Voetdijk BM, Beverstock GC, et al. Activation of the c-myc oncogene in a precursor-B-cell blast crisis of follicular lymphoma, presenting as composite lymphoma. N Engl J Med 1988;318:1373–1378.
7. Jaffe ES, Zarate-Osorno A, Kingma DW, et al. The interrelationship between Hodgkin's disease and non-Hodgkin's lymphomas. Ann Oncol 1994;5:7–11.
8. Ohno T, Stribley JA, Wu G, et al. Clonality in nodular lymphocyte-predominant Hodgkin's disease. N Engl J Med 1997;337: 459–465.
9. Kueppers R, Rajewsky K, Zhao M, et al. Hodgkin and Reed-Sternberg cells picked from histological sections show clonal immunoglobulin gene rearrangements and appear to be derived from B-cells at various stages of development. Proc Natl Acad Sci U S A 1994;91:10962–10966.
10. Brauninger A, Hansmann M-L, Strickler JG, et al. Identification of common germinal-center precursors in two patients with both Hodgkin's disease and non-Hodgkin's lymphoma. N Engl J Med 1999;340:1239–1247.
11. Kerl K, Girardet C, Borisch B. A common B-cell precursor in composite lymphomas [Letter]. N Engl J Med 1999;341:764–765.
12. Dunphy CH, Craver JL, Emerson WA. Demonstration of composite nodal B-cell lymphoma and subsequent Hodgkin's disease

Checklist

COMPOSITE LYMPHOMA

Combination of NHLs of different histologic type or different immunophenotype
Combinations of HL and NHL
Two or more different lymphoma patterns in one lymph node
Two or more different lymphoma patterns in lymph nodes and other lymphoid organs
Prognosis that of the most malignant histologic type

by flow cytometry and immunohistochemistry. Case report and review of the literature. Arch Pathol Lab Med 1997;121:637–640.

13. Thirumala S, Esposito M, Fuchs A. An unusual variant of composite lymphoma: a short case report and review of the literature. Arch Pathol Lab Med 2000;124:1376–1378.
14. Weiss LM, Movahed LA, Warnke RA, et al. Detection of Epstein-Barr viral genomes in Reed-Sternberg cells of Hodgkin's disease. N Engl J Med 1989;320:502–506.
15. York JCD, Cousar JB, Glick AD, et al. Morphologic and immunologic evidence of composite B- and T-cell lymphomas. A report of three cases developing in follicular center cell lymphomas. Am J Clin Pathol 1985;84:35–43.
16. Strickler JG, Amsden TW, Kurtin PJ. Small B-cell lymphoid neoplasms with coexisting T-cell lymphomas [see Comments]. Am J Clin Pathol 1992;98:424–429.
17. Wlodarska I, Delabie J, de Wolf-Peeters C, et al. T-cell lymphoma developing in Hodgkin's disease: evidence for two clones. J Pathol 1993;170:239–248.
18. Hoppe RT. Histologic variation in non-Hodgkin's lymphomas: commentary. Cancer Treat Rep 1981;65:935–939.
19. Gonzalez CL, Medeiros LJ, Jaffe ES. Composite lymphoma. A clinicopathologic analysis of nine patients with Hodgkin's disease and B-cell non-Hodgkin's lymphoma. Am J Clin Pathol 1991; 96:81–89.
20. Sundeen JT, Cossman J, Jaffe ES. Lymphocyte predominant Hodgkin's disease nodular subtype with coexistent "large cell lymphoma." Histological progression or composite malignancy? [see Comments]. Am J Surg Pathol 1988;12:599–606.
21. Hansmann M-L, Fellbaum C, Hui PK, et al. Morphological and immunohistochemical investigation of non-Hodgkin's lymphoma combined with Hodgkin's disease. Histopathology 1989;15:35–48.
22. Tezcan H, Vose JM, Bast M, et al. Limited stage I and II follicular non-Hodgkin's lymphoma: the Nebraska lymphoma study group experience. Leuk Lymphoma 1999;34:273–285.
23. Poon MC, Flint A, Miles GL. Composite lymphoma: report of a unique case. Cancer 1980;46:1676–1682.
24. Ngan BY, Warnke RA, Wilson M, et al. Monocytoid B-cell lymphoma: a study of 36 cases [see Comments]. Hum Pathol 1991;22:409–421.
25. Slovak ML, Weiss LM, Nathwani BN, et al. Cytogenetic studies of composite lymphomas: monocytoid B-cell lymphoma and other B-cell non-Hodgkin's lymphomas. Hum Pathol 1993;24: 1086–1094.
26. Hughes JH, Katz RL, Fonseca GA, et al. Fine-needle aspiration cytology of mediastinal non-Hodgkin's nonlymphoblastic lymphoma. Cancer (Cancer Cytopathol) 1998;84:26–35.
27. Strickler JG, Donohue JH, Porter LE, et al. Laparoscopic biopsy for suspected abdominal lymphoma. Mod Pathol 1998;11:831–836.
28. Schmid U, Cogliatti SB, Diss TC, et al. Monocytoid/marginal zone B-cell differentiation in follicle centre cell lymphoma. Histopathology 1996;29:201–208.
29. Siebert JD, Mulvaney DA, Vukov AM, et al. Utility of flow cytometry in subtyping composite and sequential lymphoma. J Clin Lab Anal 1999;13:199–204.
30. Shin SS, Ben-Ezra J, Burke JS, et al. Reed-Sternberg–like cells in low-grade lymphomas are transformed neoplastic cells of B-cell lineage. Am J Clin Pathol 1993;99:658–662.

PART V

SECTION FIVE

MATURE T-CELL NEOPLASMS

71

ADULT T-CELL LYMPHOMA/LEUKEMIA

DEFINITION

Lymphoma of mature (post-thymic) T lymphocytes caused by infection with the human T-cell lymphotropic virus type 1 (HTLV-1).

SYNONYMS

HTLV-1-associated T-cell lymphoma
Pleomorphic small, medium, and large cell types (HTLV-1+) (Kiel)
Adult T-cell lymphoma/leukemia (ATLL) (Revised European-American Lymphoma Classification, or REAL) (1)
Adult T-cell leukemia/lymphoma (HTLV-1+) (World Health Organization, or WHO) (2)
- Acute
- Lymphomatous
- Chronic
- Smoldering
- Hodgkin-like

EPIDEMIOLOGY

Adult T-cell leukemia/lymphoma and its associated retrovirus, HTLV-1, are endemic in southwestern Japan (3), the Caribbean basin, notably the West Indies (4), northern South America (5), the southeastern United States (6), and possibly some areas of Africa, the Middle East, and the South Pacific. The prevalence of HTLV-1 infection is high in endemic areas; approximately 20% of the adult population is seropositive in southwestern Japan (7). In a study of U.S. blood donors, 0.05% of volunteer blood donors were seropositive for HTLV, and two-thirds of these were infected with HTLV-2 (8). The HTLV-1+ donors came from endemic regions, whereas the HTLV-2+ donors used intravenous drugs (8). Immigrant populations from endemic areas living in London or New York City may carry HTLV-1 infection and acquire ATLL (4,9,10).

In Japan, ATLL occurs predominantly in the sixth decade, with a male-to-female ratio of 1.4:1. In the Caribbean, patients are much younger (range, 21 to 55 years), and the male-to-female ratio is 1:2 (4). In a U.S. study, the age range was 24 to 62 years (mean, 33 years) (6).

ETIOLOGY

The first oncogenic human virus to be discovered was HTLV-1. HTLV-1 transforms human T cells in culture, and HTLV-1 DNA is present in ATLL cells. ATLL develops in areas where HTLV-1 infection rates are high. Patients with ATLL have antibodies to HTLV-1. HTLV-1 is transmitted (a) in virus-bearing mononuclear cells in breast milk of infected mothers to suckling babies (11); (b) via lymphocytes in semen during sexual intercourse, most often from male to female (11); and (c) in transfused blood (12).

PATHOGENESIS

HTLV-1 is a C-type retrovirus (13) containing an RNA genome, the enzyme reverse transcriptase, and two special regulatory proteins: *tax* and *rex* (14). Many cellular genes are transcriptionally activated by tax, including the growth factor interleukin 2 (IL-2) and its high-affinity receptor α subunit (IL-2Rα; CD25). CD25 promotes autocrine stimulation and serves as an immunotherapeutic target (15). In addition, tax can alter genes controlling programmed cell death (16), inhibit tumor suppressor protein $p16^{INK4A}$ (17), and enhance random genomic mutations (18).

The ATLL cells contain HTLV-1 as a provirus integrated in the cellular DNA, which indicates that the virus is not simply a passenger but is present in the cell before neoplastic transformation. The site of integration varies from patient to patient and is not close to an oncogene; however, its constancy within each tumor proves a monoclonal origin (19). Monoclonality can also be demonstrated with probes that detect T-cell receptor gene rearrangements. The cells infected and transformed by HTLV-1 are the CD4+ (helper/inducer) T lymphocytes. Of persons infected by HTLV-1, ATLL eventually develops in only 1% to 2%, usually after a latency period that can be as long as 10 years. All Japanese patients with ATLL are seropositive for anti-HTLV-1 antibodies. In addition to ATLL, HTLV-1 may induce a severe myelopathy known as *tropical spastic paraparesis* (TSP)/*HTLV-1-associated myelopathy* (HAM) (20). Thus, HTLV-1 resembles HIV, another human retrovirus with strong tropisms for both CD4+ lymphocytes and nerve cells.

CLINICAL SYNDROME

Before ATLL develops, anti-HTLV-1 antibody titers rise (21). ATLL presents in a variety of clinical subtypes: smoldering (5.5%), chronic (18.6%), lymphomatous (19.1%), and acute (56.8%) (22). In the chronic form, lymphadenopathy and disease involving liver, spleen, skin, or lung may be features (22). The lymphomatous type, characterized by prominent lymphadenopathy, may progress to the acute form (23). More often, ATLL presents in its acute leukemic form, involving bone marrow and peripheral blood; the white blood cell count is high (T lymphocytosis of $>3.5 \times 10^9$/L), but often without significant anemia or thrombocytopenia (22). Eosinophilia and neutrophilia may be present. The lymph nodes are invariably infiltrated, although a mediastinal mass is less common than in peripheral T-cell lymphoma or lymphoblastic lymphoma (6). ATLL frequently produces a scaly and erythematous rash, cutaneous plaques, and nodules. The bone marrow is commonly involved, and most patients have leukemia (22). After the skin, the lungs, liver, gastrointestinal tract, and central nervous system (usually in the form of lymphomatous meningitis) are most frequently affected. Skin and lung lesions are less commonly observed in the lymphomatous type (22).

In most patients, ATLL is already in stage IV at presentation (22). ATLL cells secrete parathyroid hormone-related protein, which causes hypercalcemia and osteolytic bone lesions (24), more often in Caribbean than in Japanese patients (4,25). The hypercalcemia is refractory to treatment, and its absence is associated with a better prognosis. Immune deficiency in ATLL patients encourages opportunistic infections. The majority of ATLL patients have rapidly progressive disease; median survival time for the lymphomatous type is only 10.2 months (22). TSP/HAM accompanying ATLL results in various neurologic abnormalities, including paraparesis with spasticity, a gait disorder, and bladder dysfunction with incontinence (26).

HISTOPATHOLOGY

The lymph nodes in ATLL are morphologically heterogeneous (25,27–29). Initially, ATLL involves the paracortical T-cell zones, leaving the cortex or B-cell zones temporarily unaffected (27) (Fig. 71.1). In a later phase, the lymph node parenchyma is diffusely invaded (Figs. 71.2 and 71.3). The characteristic ATLL cells, which are about three times the size of normal lymphocytes, have pleomorphic, multilobate nuclei, which have been variously described as "walnut-shaped," "maple leaf," "cerebriform," or "flower" cells (Figs.

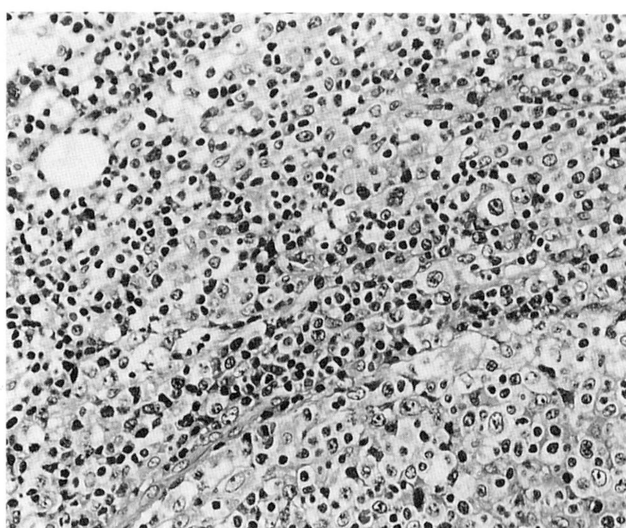

FIGURE 71.1. Adult T-cell lymphoma in lymph node of 53-year-old man with systemic lymphadenopathy. Parenchyma, capsule, and perinodal fibrofatty tissues invaded by sheets of large clear cells with irregularly shaped nuclei admixed with lymphocytes. (From Watanabe S, Shimosato Y, Shimoyama M, et al. Adult T-cell lymphoma with hypergammaglobulinemia. Cancer 1980;46: 2472– 2483, with permission.)

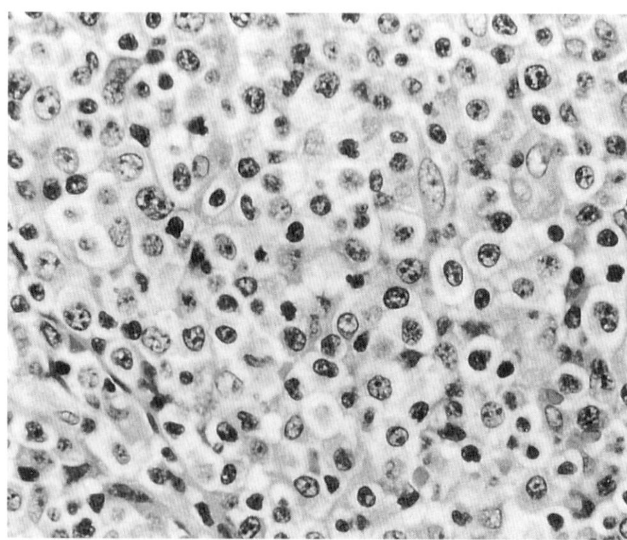

FIGURE 71.2. Adult T-cell lymphoma in lymph node of 42-year-old man with systemic lymphadenopathy. Sheets of large cells with distinct cell borders, clear cytoplasm, and lobulate nuclei. (From Watanabe S, Shimosato Y, Shimoyama M, et al. Adult T-cell lymphoma with hypergammaglobulinemia. Cancer 1980;46: 2472–2483, with permission.)

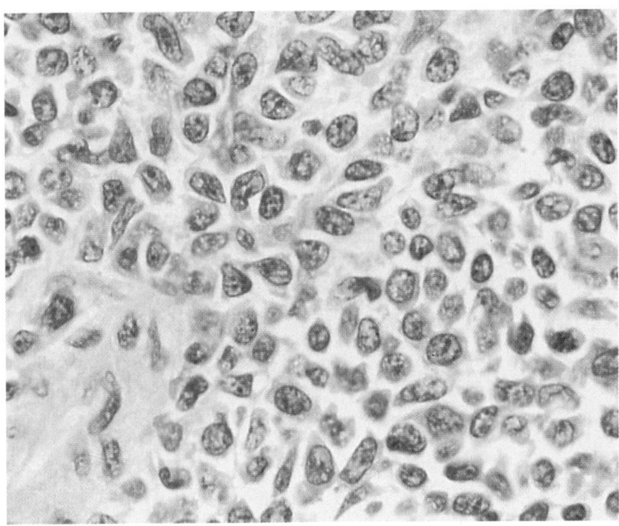

FIGURE 71.3. Adult T-cell lymphoma in HTLV-1-positive Caribbean woman. Lymph node architecture replaced by sheets of cells with high nuclear-to-cytoplasmic ratio and irregularly shaped nuclei. Hematoxylin, phloxine, and saffron stain.

71.4–71.6). Compared with the nuclei of mycosis fungoides or Sézary cells, the nuclei of ATLL cells are more lobulate and less gyriform; however, not all patients have the characteristic ATLL cells. In most cases of ATLL, the cells are more uniform in size and shape, with nuclei that are smaller, more hyperchromatic, and less pleomorphic (25,27–29). In about 20% of ATLL cases, the nuclei are larger, round or oval, strongly basophilic, and accompanied by cytoplasmic vacuoles (27). Prominent central nucleoli, peripheral chromatin, and small amounts of cytoplasm are seen. Atypical mitoses are numerous. The pattern of organ infiltration is diffuse, and the general histologic appearance is that of a large cell immunoblastic or pleomorphic non-Hodgkin lymphoma. ATLL with multinucleated lymphoma cells can mimic Hodgkin disease (30). Another type of lymphoma giant cell has nuclear convolutions, coarse chromatin, and multiple prominent nucleoli (31). ATLL involving skin resembles cutaneous T-cell lymphoma or anaplastic large cell lymphoma (27–29).

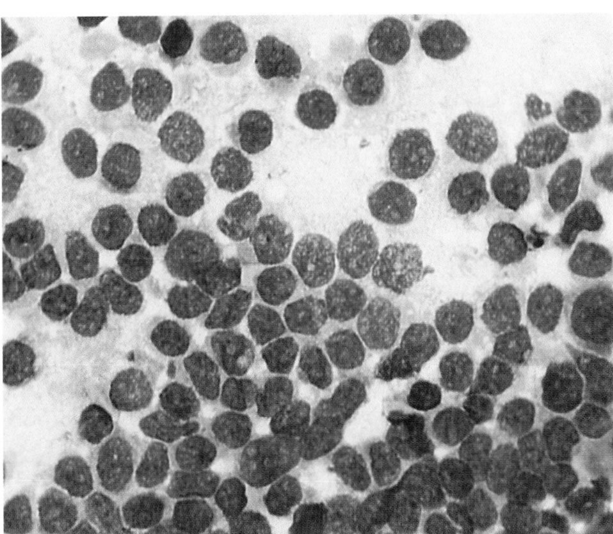

FIGURE 71.4. Adult T-cell lymphoma/leukemia in HTLV-1-positive Caribbean woman. Imprint of affected lymph node shows uniform population of large lymphoma cells with convoluted nuclei and prominent nucleoli. Giemsa stain.

CYTOLOGY

In tissue imprints and blood smears, ATLL shows large lymphoma cells with bizarre, multilobate nuclei, prominent nucleoli, and the characteristic morphology of flower cells (Figs. 71.4 and 71.5).

IMMUNOHISTOCHEMISTRY

CD7 is consistently lost (Fig. 71.7A); more than 90% of ATLL cases express a mature CD3+, CD4+, CD8− helper/inducer T-cell phenotype (Fig. 71.7B); other pan-T-cell markers (CD2, CD3, and CD5) are variably decreased or absent (28). ATLL cells characteristically express activation markers HLA-DR and especially CD25 (Fig. 71.7C) (28). UCHL-1 (CD45RO) stains T cells in tissue sections (Fig. 71.8). Patients with circulating lymphocytes expressing an intermediate level of CD45RO (CD45ROint) do better clinically than those without CD45ROint (32). CD95 (Fas/Apo-1) can induce programmed cell death. Mutations eliminating CD95 protein expression on ATLL cells may be associated with disease progression and drug resistance (33).

Phenotype

CD1a−
CD2+/−
CD3+/−
CD4+
CD5+/−
CD7−
CD8−
CD25+
CD45RO+
HLA-DR+
Terminal deoxynucleotidyl transferase−

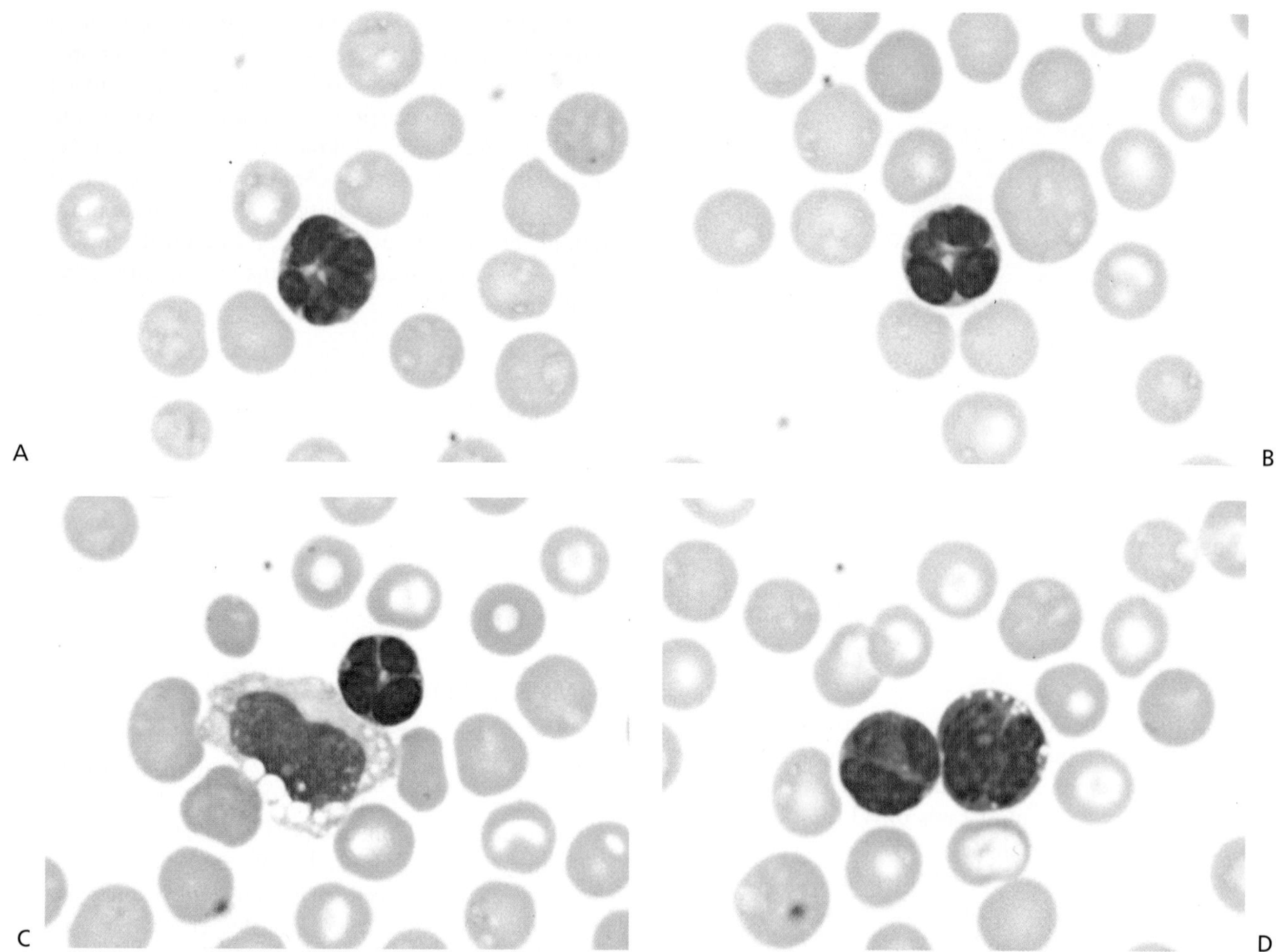

FIGURE 71.5. Peripheral blood smear from patient with adult T-cell lymphoma/leukemia. **A–D:** Four fields show "flower" cells with petal-like nuclear lobules connected by thin chromatin strands and deep blue cytoplasm. Monocyte with abundant pale gray cytoplasm at lower left. Giemsa stain.

CYTOGENETICS

HTLV-1 clonally integrates into genomic DNA in a random fashion (19). Complex karyotypic abnormalities of almost all chromosomes have been reported. Detailed mapping localizes a putative tumor suppressor gene to chromosome 6q15-21 (34). Comparative genomic hybridization reveals imbalances affecting 2p16-22, 7q21-36, and 14q32 (35). The TCL1 gene at 14q32 cannot contribute to lymphomagenesis because it is not transcribed in ATLL (36).

MOLECULAR DIAGNOSIS

Clonal T-cell receptor (TCR) β and γ gene rearrangements can be detected even though ATLL expresses only TCR αβ protein (see Chapter 8). The sites of provirus insertion vary from case to case but are constant within each case of ATLL (19).

DIFFERENTIAL DIAGNOSIS

- Lymphoblastic lymphoma: Cells uniform, nuclei round with fine chromatin, nucleoli inconspicuous, TdT+.
- Peripheral T-cell lymphoma: Elderly patients, frequently with preexisting illnesses, including angioimmunoblastic lymphadenopathy, Sjögren syndrome, or other autoimmune disorders. Leukemia, hypercalcemia, and HTLV-1 absent.
- Immunoblastic lymphoma: Preexisting autoimmune illnesses, B-cell markers. HTLV-1 and hypercalcemia absent.
- Mycosis fungoides: Characteristic skin lesions, mycosis or Sézary cells with cerebriform nuclei, HTLV-1−, CD25−.

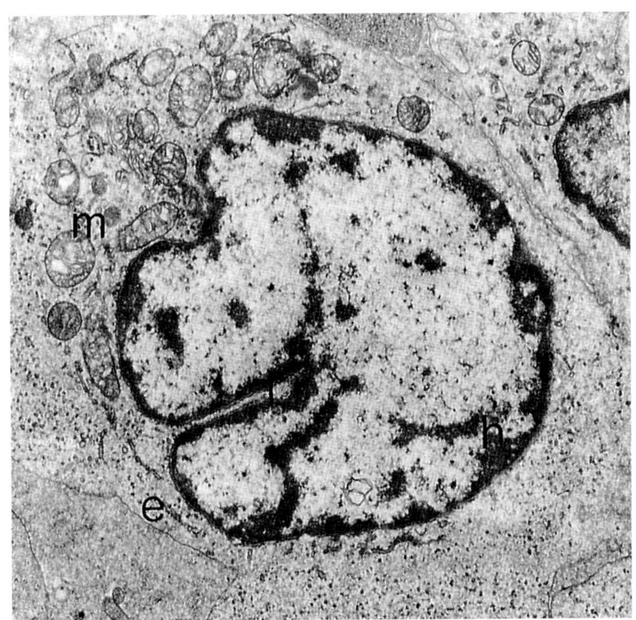

FIGURE 71.6. Adult T-cell lymphoma cell with lobulate nucleus, heterochromatin, polyribosomes, and mitochondria (*m*) aggregated at one pole of the cell. *e*, endoplasmic reticulum. ×10,000. (From Watanabe S, Shimosato Y, Shimoyama M, et al. Adult T-cell lymphoma with hypergammaglobulinemia. Cancer 1980;46: 2472–2483, with permission.)

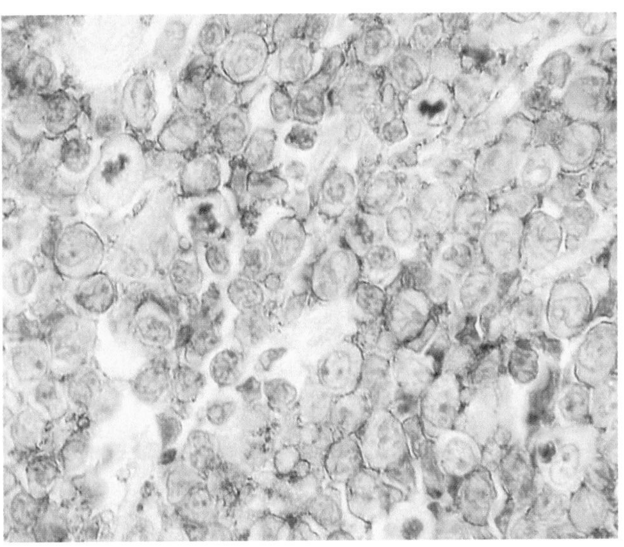

FIGURE 71.8. Adult T-cell lymphoma cells in supraclavicular lymph node of HTLV-1-positive patient showing strong expression of T-cell markers on immunostaining with UCHL-1 antibody. Immunoperoxidase stain.

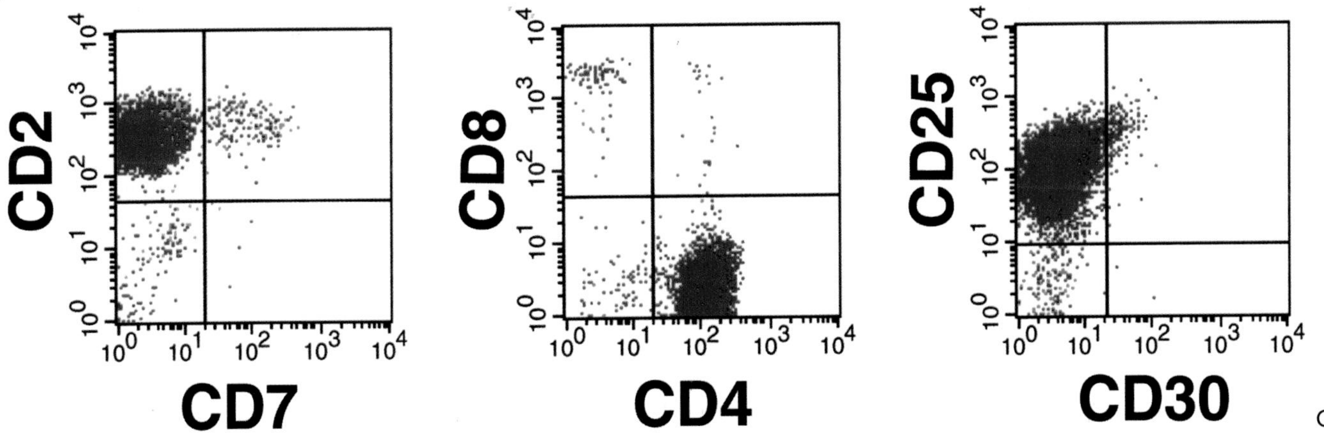

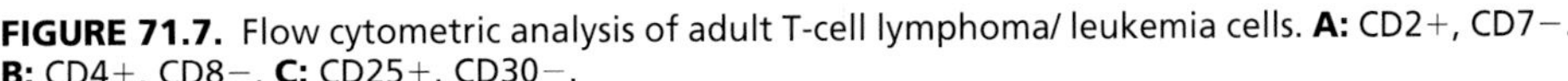

FIGURE 71.7. Flow cytometric analysis of adult T-cell lymphoma/ leukemia cells. **A:** CD2+, CD7−. **B:** CD4+, CD8−. **C:** CD25+, CD30−.

Checklist

ADULT T-CELL LYMPHOMA

Endemic to southwestern Japan, Caribbean
HTLV-1 infection
Immune deficiency
Lymphadenopathies
Skin, internal organs frequently involved
Hypercalcemia, osteolytic lesions
Bone marrow and peripheral blood involved in majority of cases
Tropical spastic paraparesis often associated
Lymphoma cells with multilobate nuclei ("flower" cells)
Peripheral (mature) T-cell immunophenotype
Positive for CD2, CD3, CD4 (helper/inducer), HLA-DR, and CD25 (IL-2Rα)
Aggressive, early dissemination and short survival

REFERENCES

1. Harris NL, Jaffe ES, Stein H, et al. A revised European-American classification of lymphoid neoplasms: a proposal from the International Lymphoma Study Group [see Comments]. Blood 1994;84:1361–1392.
2. Harris NL, Jaffe ES, Diebold J, et al. The World Health Organization classification of hematological malignancies: report of the clinical advisory committee meeting, Airlie House, Virginia, November 1997. Mod Pathol 2000;13:193–207.
3. Uchiyama T, Yodoi J, Sagawa K, et al. Adult T-cell leukemia: clinical and hematologic features of 16 cases. Blood 1977;50: 481–492.
4. Catovsky D, Greaves MF, Rose M, et al. Adult T-cell lymphoma-leukaemia in blacks from the West Indies. Lancet 1982;1:639–643.
5. Barbosa HS, Bittencourt AL, Barreto de Araujo I, et al. Adult T-cell leukemia/lymphoma in northeastern Brazil: a clinical, histopathologic, and molecular study. J Acquir Immune Defic Syndr Hum Retrovirol 1999;21:65–71.
6. Bunn PA Jr, Schechter GP, Jaffe E, et al. Clinical course of retrovirus-associated adult T-cell lymphoma in the United States. N Engl J Med 1983;309:257–264.
7. Hinuma Y, Komoda H, Chosa T, et al. Antibodies to adult T-cell leukemia virus-associated antigen (ATLA) in sera from patients with ATL and controls in Japan: a nation-wide sero-epidemiologic study. Int J Cancer 1982;29:631–635.
8. Lee HH, Swanson P, Rosenblatt JD, et al. Relative prevalence and risk factors of HTLV-1 and HTLV-2 infection in U.S. blood donors. Lancet 1991;337:1435–1439.
9. Chadburn A, Athan E, Wieczorek R, et al. Detection and characterization of human T-cell lymphotropic virus type 1 (HTLV-1)-associated T-cell neoplasms in an HTLV-1 nonendemic region by polymerase chain reaction. Blood 1991;77:2419–2430.
10. Levine PH, Dosik H, Joseph EM, et al. A study of adult T-cell leukemia/lymphoma incidence in central Brooklyn. Int J Cancer 1999;80:662–666.
11. Kajiyama W, Kashiwagi S, Ikematsu H, et al. Intrafamilial transmission of adult T-cell leukemia virus. J Infect Dis 1986;154: 851–857.
12. Inaba S, Okochi K, Sato H, et al. Efficacy of donor screening for HTLV-1 and the natural history of transfusion-transmitted infection. Transfusion 1999;39:1104–1110.
13. Taffarel M, Andrada-Serpa MJ. Electron microscopic observation of a Brazilian HTLV-1 isolated. J Submicrosc Cytol Pathol 1998;30:393–397.
14. Wong-Staal F, Gallo RC. Human T-lymphotropic retroviruses. Nature 1985;317:395–403.
15. Waldmann TA. T-cell receptors for cytokines: targets for immunotherapy of leukemia/lymphoma. Ann Oncol 2000;11:101–106.
16. Harhaj EW, Good L, Xiao G, et al. Gene expression profiles in HTLV-1-immortalized T cells: deregulated expression of genes involved in apoptosis regulation. Oncogene 1999;18:1341–1349.
17. Suzuki T, Kitao S, Matsushime H, et al. HTLV-1 Tax protein interacts with cyclin-dependent kinase inhibitor p16INK4A and counteracts its inhibitory activity towards CDK4. EMBO J 1996;15:1607–1614.
18. Miyake H, Suzuki T, Hirai H, et al. Trans-activator Tax of human T-cell leukemia virus type 1 enhances mutation frequency of the cellular genome. Virology 1999;253:155–161.
19. Ohshima K, Ohgami A, Matsuoka M, et al. Random integration of HTLV-1 provirus: increasing chromosomal instability. Cancer Lett 1998;132:203–212.
20. Taylor GP. Pathogenesis and treatment of HTLV-1-associated myelopathy. Sex Transm Infect 1998;74:316–322.
21. Hisada M, Okayama A, Shioiri S, et al. Risk factors for adult T-cell leukemia among carriers of human T-lymphotropic virus type 1. Blood 1998;92:3557–3561.
22. Shimoyama M. Diagnostic criteria and classification of clinical subtypes of adult T-cell leukaemia-lymphoma. A report from the Lymphoma Study Group (1984–87). Br J Haematol 1991;79: 428–437.
23. Yamaguchi K, Yoshioka R, Kiyokawa T, et al. Lymphoma type adult T-cell leukemia—a clinicopathologic study of HTLV related T-cell type malignant lymphoma. Hematol Oncol 1986; 4:59–65.
24. Watanabe T, Yamaguchi K, Takatsuki K, et al. Constitutive expression of parathyroid hormone-related protein gene in human

T cell leukemia virus type 1 (HTLV-1) carriers and adult T-cell leukemia patients that can be trans-activated by HTLV-1 tax gene. J Exp Med 1990;172:759–765.
25. Swerdlow SH, Habeshaw JA, Rohatiner AZ, et al. Caribbean T-cell lymphoma/leukemia. Cancer 1984;54:687–696.
26. Carvalho ES, Brites C, Badaro R. HTLV-1-associated myelopathy: clinical and epidemiological profile. Braz J Infect Dis 2000;4:126–130.
27. Jaffe ES, Blattner WA, Blayney DW, et al. The pathologic spectrum of adult T-cell leukemia/lymphoma in the United States. Human T-cell leukemia/lymphoma virus-associated lymphoid malignancies. Am J Surg Pathol 1984;8:263–275.
28. Suchi T, Lennert K, Tu LY, et al. Histopathology and immunohistochemistry of peripheral T-cell lymphomas: a proposal for their classification. J Clin Pathol 1987;40:995–1015.
29. Pinkus GS, O'Hara CJ, Said JW. Peripheral/post-thymic T-cell lymphomas: a spectrum of disease. Clinical, pathologic, and immunologic features of 78 cases. Cancer 1990;65:971–998.
30. Duggan DB, Ehrlich GD, Davey FP, et al. HTLV-1-induced lymphoma mimicking Hodgkin's disease. Diagnosis by polymerase chain reaction amplification of specific HTLV-1 sequences in tumor DNA. Blood 1988;71:1027–1032.
31. Kikuchi M, Mitsui T, Takeshita M, et al. Virus-associated adult T-cell leukemia (ATL) in Japan: clinical, histological and immunological studies. Hematol Oncol 1986;4:67–81.
32. Suzuki M, Matsuoka H, Yamashita K, et al. CD45RO expression on peripheral lymphocytes as a prognostic marker for adult T-cell leukemia. Leuk Lymphoma 1998;28:583–590.
33. Tamiya S, Etoh K, Suzushima H, et al. Mutation of CD95 (Fas/Apo-1) gene in adult T-cell leukemia cells. Blood 1998;91:3935–3942.
34. Hatta Y, Yamada Y, Tomonaga M, et al. Detailed deletion mapping of the long arm of chromosome 6 in adult T-cell leukemia. Blood 1999;93:613–616.
35. Ariyama Y, Mori T, Shinomiya T, et al. Chromosomal imbalances in adult T-cell leukemia revealed by comparative genomic hybridization: gains at 14q32 and 2p16-22 in cell lines. J Hum Genet 1999;44:357–363.
36. Takizawa J, Suzuki R, Kuroda H, et al. Expression of the TCL1 gene at 14q32 in B-cell malignancies but not in adult T-cell leukemia. Jpn J Cancer Res 1998;89:712–718.

72

MYCOSIS FUNGOIDES

DEFINITIONS

Primary cutaneous T-cell lymphoma (CTCL) refers to a heterogeneous group of skin-homing T-cell malignancies; they should be distinguished from systemic T-cell lymphomas secondarily involving skin (1). The European Organization for Research and Treatment of Cancer (EORTC) proposes a specific classification of mycosis fungoides based on clinical, histologic, and immunophenotypic features (2).

Mycosis fungoides (MF) is a CTCL with primary lesions of the skin and subsequent involvement of lymph nodes and internal organs.

Sézary syndrome (SS) is a rare condition (<5% of new cases of CTCL) (1) of primary erythroderma and circulating atypical lymphocytes secondarily involving lymph nodes (3).

Specific variants of MF (EORTC) are the following (2):

MF plus follicular mucinosis
Pagetoid reticulosis
Granulomatous slack skin

Mycosis fungoides/Sézary syndrome (World Health Organization)

SYNONYM

Cutaneous T-cell lymphoma

PATHOGENESIS

Only about 1,000 new cases of MF are diagnosed per year (4). MF affects African-Americans more often than Caucasians, and men more often than women (4). In most patients with MF, skin lesions first develop between the ages of 40 and 60 years; extracutaneous disease evolves in an older group (5). Palpable lymph nodes occur in 38% of patients with plaques and in 90% of patients with tumor-stage MF (6).

The histologic changes of MF lymph nodes encompass a broad spectrum ranging from benign dermatopathic lymphadenopathy (DL), a form of reactive hyperplasia, to melanin and other skin antigens (see Chapter 42), to frank, pleomorphic lymphoma (7). Distinguishing benign from malignant lymph node lesions in MF can be made difficult by overlapping histologic patterns. Nevertheless, the diagnostic distinction is clinically important because lymph node involvement indicates a worse prognosis (7).

It is possible that a defective or variant human T-cell lymphotropic virus (HTLV) has a pathogenic role in MF (8). Some studies have identified retroviral pol and tax genes in approximately 10% of MF cases (9); results of other studies have been negative (10). However, MF does not follow the geographic pattern of endemic HTLV-1 infection, and most patients with MF do not produce antibodies to HTLV-1 (7). Adult T-cell leukemia/lymphoma, which is caused by HTLV-1 infection (see Chapter 71), and MF are clinically and phenotypically distinct, even in Japan (11).

Molecular clues to the pathogenesis of MF are few. Alterations in p53 and p16^{INK4A} have been identified in the tumor stage (12,13). The p53 mutations resemble the DNA damage induced by ultraviolet B radiation (13).

CLINICAL SYNDROME

The median duration of skin symptoms before MF is diagnosed is 6 years (14). MF is clinically indolent but progressive, and late-stage disease is characterized by fever, weight loss, generalized lymphadenopathy, enlarged liver and spleen, peripheral blood eosinophilia, and atypical lymphocytosis. Survival time ranges from 3 to 18 months after the first diagnosed extracutaneous involvement (5).

Mycosis fungoides can be divided into three skin stages: erythematous patches, plaques, and eventually tumors, which asymmetrically involve hips, buttocks, lower trunk, groin, axillae, and breasts (7). The plaques thicken until tumors form, occasionally ulcerating. All three types of lesions can occur simultaneously. MF infiltrates lymph nodes in 75% of patients with extracutaneous disease (15). Even in patients without clinical hepatosplenomegaly, MF can microscopically involve liver and spleen (16).

Risk factors for disease progression include failure to respond to initial therapy and age above 60 years (17). The lymph nodes of patients with sparse plaques are uninvolved; patients with generalized skin disease tend to have infiltrated lymph nodes (18). Septicemia develops during the tumor stage, associated with necrosis and local infection (19).

Lymph nodes or other visceral organs were involved in 71% of 45 MF autopsies: lungs (66%), spleen (60%), and liver (53%) (20). The thyroid, parathyroids, pancreas, and thymus were more commonly infiltrated than in other types of lymphoma; the bone marrow was less frequently affected (20). In contrast to most lymph node-based lymphomas, MF principally involves the skin early, shows a strong predilection for epithelial tissues, and infiltrates the bone marrow late and less often (21).

The median time from initial MF diagnosis to large cell transformation is 6.5 years (22). The probability of transformation after 12 years is 39%, especially in patients with stages IIB through IV disease or with tumors (23). The percentage of large cells or CD30+ cells cannot predict transformation (22). The mean survival after transformation is 22 months (22). Large cell transformation can produce a dramatic increase in soluble interleukin 2 receptor levels (24).

HISTOPATHOLOGY

In the skin, MF produces a bandlike or patchy infiltrate in the upper dermis that involves the dermal papillae and extends to the basal layer of the epidermis. Single lymphocytes with halos infiltrate the epidermis, sometimes causing spongiosis but without microvesiculation or cytopathic keratinocyte changes. In a minority of patients, collections of lymphocytes within the epidermis form Pautrier microabscesses. Lymphocytic atypia occurs in 50% to 100% of cases. The papillary dermis may contain variable fibrosis, eosinophils, and plasma cells (25–27).

In the plaque stage, MF forms superficial, or superficial and deep, perivascular infiltrates mimicking inflammatory patterns (26). The cellular infiltrates in the skin, as in the other organs, consist of large and small MF cells admixed with eosinophils, lymphocytes, plasma cells, and melanophages, which may represent a reaction to the tumor cells or a response to chemokines. In late stages, cells with round large nuclei, prominent nucleoli, and scant cytoplasm, representing blastic transformation, replace the atypical lymphocytes. The blast cells may show loss of their T-cell markers but remain epidermotropic.

In early disease, the lymph nodes draining the skin lesions show features of DL: mottled paracortical expansion, histiocytic proliferation, and melanin deposition (28,29). These changes coexist with, and may obscure, early MF cells infiltrating the lymph nodes (28,29). DL may represent the reaction of draining regional lymph nodes to a benign skin disease, to the cutaneous lesions of MF, or to MF involving lymph node.

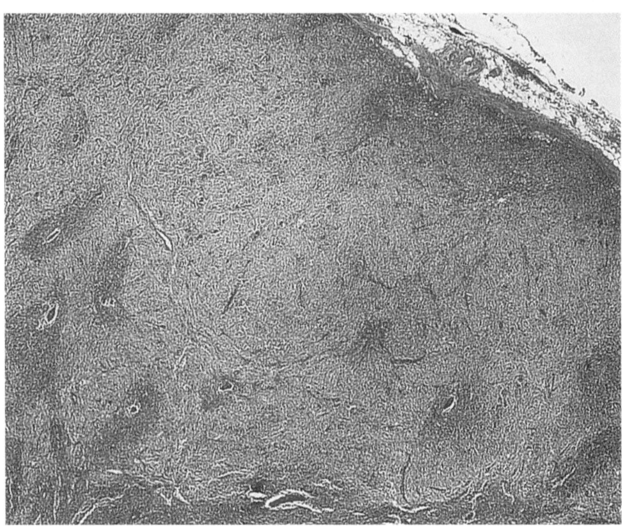

FIGURE 72.1. Mycosis fungoides involving inguinal lymph node. Cortex and paracortex replaced by sheets of mycosis fungoides cells with sparing of perivascular lymphocytic areas. Hematoxylin, phloxine, and eosin stain.

The lymph nodes involved by MF are large but not fused together, and except for occasionally in the retroperitoneum, they do not form large, matted masses (15). The nodal parenchyma may be partially or entirely replaced by the neoplastic infiltrate, which usually begins in the paracortical T zone (Figs. 72.1 and 72.2). Affected lymph nodes show partial or total architectural replacement by a relatively monomorphic infiltrate of atypical lymphoid cells that include large and small variants (30).

The large variant of MF cells is usually noted by clear or vesicular staining of the nuclei. In size (15 to 20 μm), they are equal to or larger than histiocytes but not as large as Reed-Sternberg cells. Multiple, deep nuclear indentations and convolutions result in a typical serpentine appearance of the nuclei. In three dimensions, the nuclei are cerebriform. The nucleoli are prominent but not acidophilic or as large as those of Reed-Sternberg cells. The small variant of MF cells in skin, lymph nodes, and other organs is morphologically equivalent to circulating Sézary cells in patients with SS (30). These cells (8 to 10 μm in diameter) resemble atypical lymphocytes; they have a thin cytoplasmic rim and nuclei with indentations not as deep as those of large Sézary cells. The serpentine nuclei can best be seen on thin sections under oil immersion with repeated focusing and, more distinctly, by electron microscopy. Both variants are typical but not specific. The nodal areas occupied by MF infiltrates may be focally necrotic, but fibrosis is usually lacking. Mitoses may be frequent. The capsule and perinodal fat are commonly infiltrated.

In an attempt to predict clinical outcome, lymph nodes from patients with MF have been graded as LN0, uninvolved; LN1, reactive node; LN2, dermatopathic node with small clusters (<6 cells per cluster) of convoluted cells;

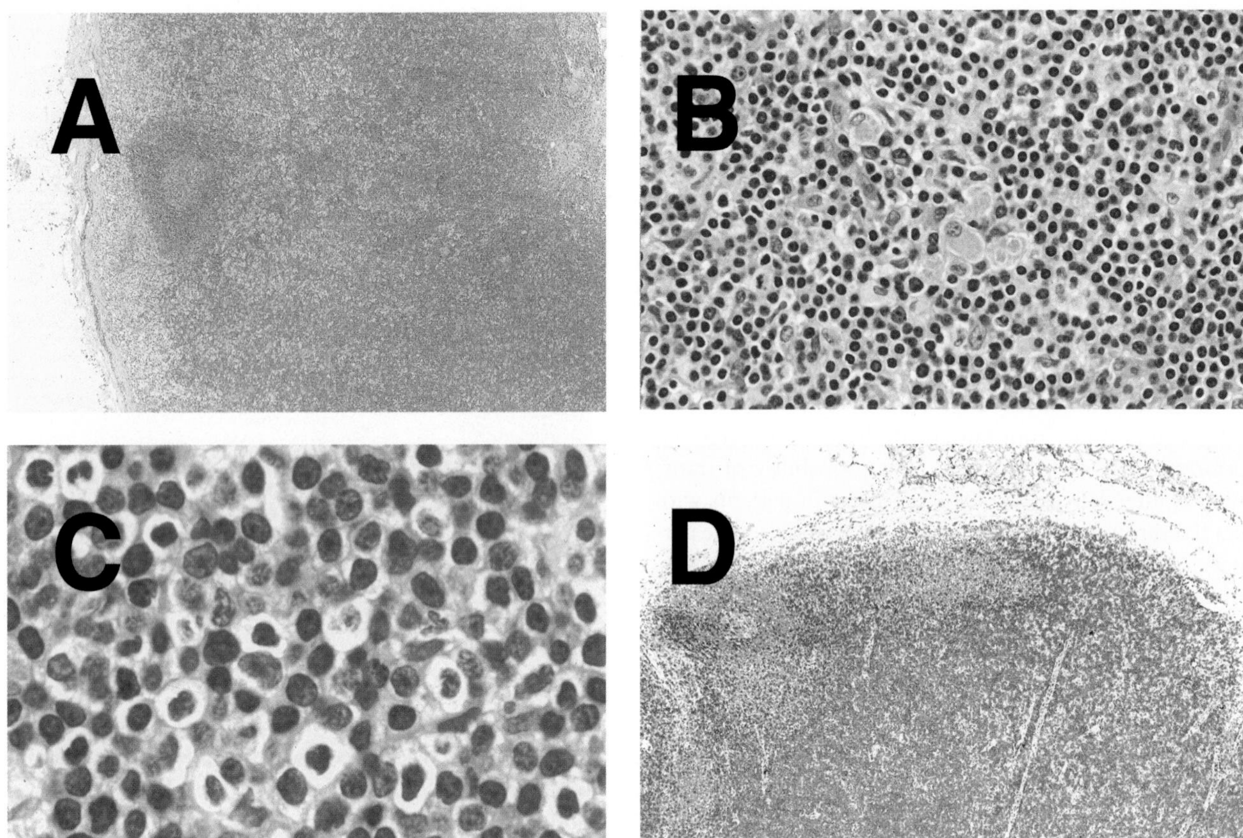

FIGURE 72.2. After 7 years of skin plaques, mycosis fungoides (*MF*) simulating dermatopathic lymphadenopathy in an axillary lymph node of a 60-year-old man. **A:** Thin capsule, a single reactive follicle, and a widened paracortical T zone with variegated color ("mottling") caused by histiocytes, interdigitating reticulum cells, small lymphocytes, and MF cells. Hematoxylin and eosin stain. **B:** Histiocytes containing melanin mimic dermatopathic lymphadenopathy. Hematoxylin and eosin stain. **C:** Individual and clustered large lymphoid cells with cerebriform nuclei and abundant clear cytoplasm. Hematoxylin and eosin stain. **D:** CD3+ T cells expand the paracortex. Immunoperoxidase stain. More than 50% of T cells lacked CD7 (*not shown*).

LN3, dermatopathic node with large clusters (>6 cells per cluster) of convoluted cells (Fig. 72.2); and LN4, lymph node effacement (31). However, the presence of cerebriform mononuclear cell clusters in lymph nodes does not reliably distinguish early MF from DL (3,28) (see Chapter 42). Accurately diagnosing MF in lymph nodes, especially histologic grades LN2 and LN3, requires a determination of T-cell clonality by molecular studies (32) (Fig. 72.3).

ELECTRON MICROSCOPY

The ultrastructure of MF and SS cells is similar whether the cells are obtained from skin, lymph nodes, spleen, or peripheral blood (33). The majority of these cells are larger than lymphocytes but smaller than histiocytes, and their nuclei show varying irregularities, ranging from slightly indented to highly convoluted or cerebriform (33). The MF cells have a diameter of about 15 μm and a high nuclear-to-

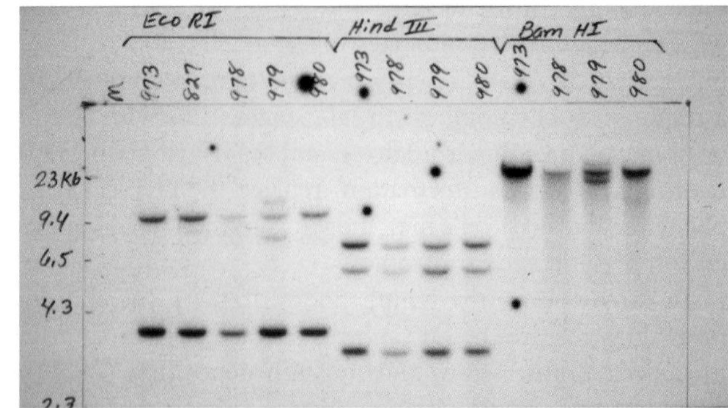

FIGURE 72.3. Southern blot analysis with T-cell receptor (*TCR*) β probe. Lanes 979 represent genomic DNA extracted from the lymph node in Fig. 72.2. Clonal TCR gene rearrangement is indicated by two novel bands after *Eco*RI digest and one novel band after *Bam*HI digest.

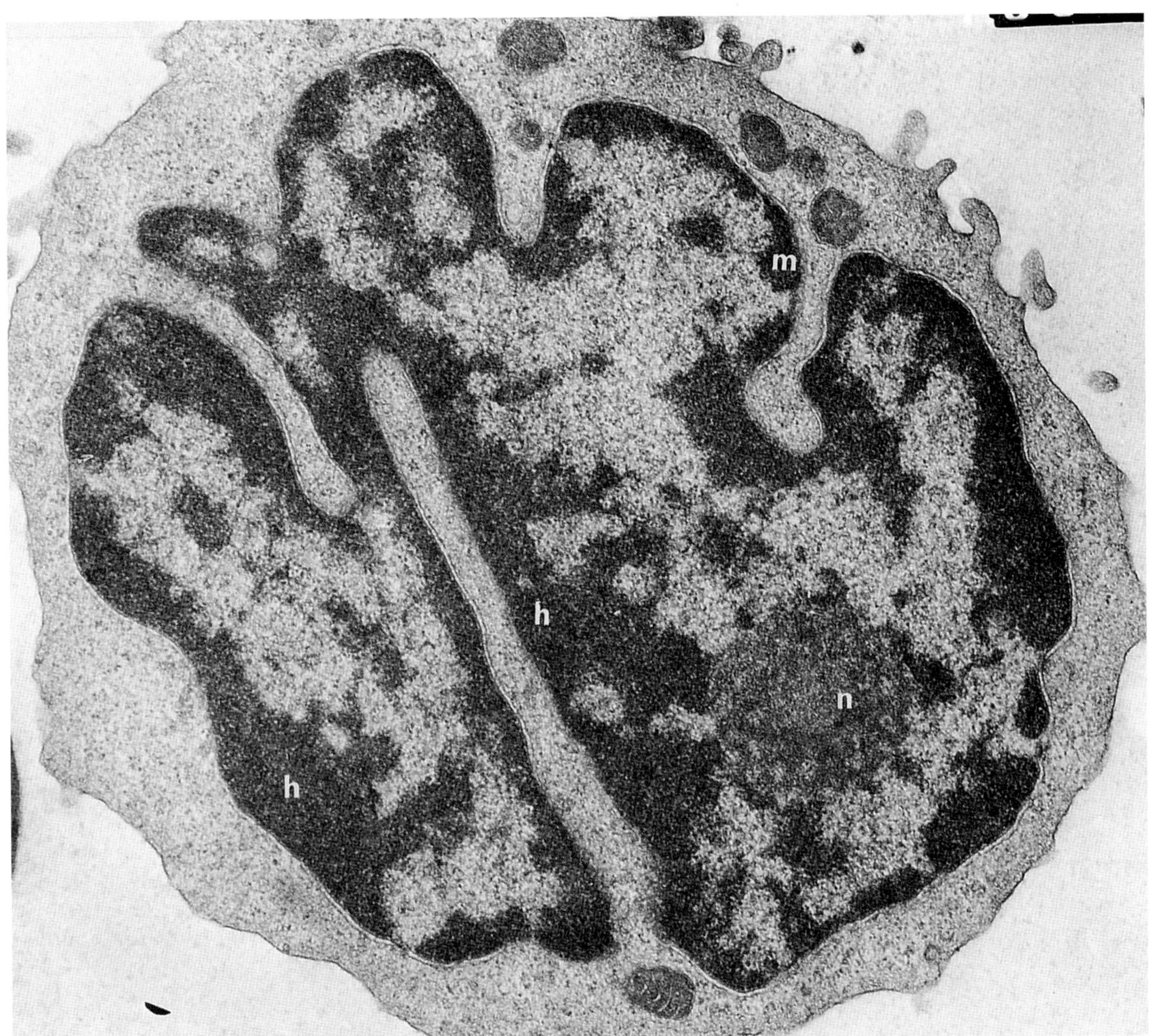

FIGURE 72.4. Large variant of Sézary cell with serpentine nucleus in patient with mycosis fungoides and circulating Sézary cells. Deeply convoluted nucleus with marginated heterochromatin (*h*) and large reticulated nucleolus (*n*). Cytoplasm with few mitochondria (*m*). ×28,200.

cytoplasmic ratio. The nuclei have a typical cerebriform appearance, with the serpentine shape and deep convolutions characteristic of Sézary cells (Fig. 72.4). The small MF cell variant, described by Lutzner and co-workers (30), has an average diameter of 11 μm, slightly larger than that of a normal lymphocyte, and a nucleus with grooves and indentations. These cells do not have the serpentine structure or complex cerebriform lobulation of typical Sézary cells.

IMMUNOPATHOLOGY

The cells of MF typically have a mature CD4+ helper/inducer T-cell phenotype; they variably express pan-T-cell markers CD2, CD3 (Fig 72.2D), and CD5 and delete CD7 (34,35). Unlike adult T-cell leukemia/lymphoma, MF does not overexpress CD25 (11). Rarely, a CD8+ suppressor/cytotoxic T-cell phenotype is associated with more aggressive disease. MF selectively localizes in lymph node paracortex and splenic periarteriolar sheath T-cell areas. The large immunoblastic cells of MF in the tumor stage tend to lose their T-cell antigens (2). Immunophenotypic studies could not distinguish between the T cells and histiocytes in DL versus DL with early MF (29).

MOLECULAR DIAGNOSIS

It is now well established that CTCL is a clonal T-cell malignancy at its earliest stage in skin (36). The finding of a clonal T-cell receptor gene rearrangement in the lymph nodes of a patient with MF (Fig. 72.3) overcomes the am-

Checklist

MYCOSIS FUNGOIDES

Patients elderly (mean age, 64 years)
Primary skin lesions (erythema, patch, plaque, tumor)
Lymph node involvement in 75%
Visceral involvement (lung, spleen, liver) in 60%
Leukemia–Sézary syndrome
Lymph nodes enlarged, not matted
Partial or total node replacement
Paracortical location of early lesions
Polymorphic infiltrate
Large MF or blast cells, serpentine, cerebriform nuclei
Small MF or SS cells, hyperchromatic, indented nuclei
MF/SS cells CD4+, CD25−
Eosinophils, lymphocytes, plasma cells, melanophages
Interdigitating reticulum cells
Focal necrosis
Fibrosis absent

biguous histologic changes of DL (see Chapter 42) and predicts a poor clinical outcome (32,37,38).

Phenotype

CD1a−
CD2+/−
CD3+/−
CD4+ (usually)
CD5+/−
CD7− (often)
CD8− (usually)
CD25−
CD45RO+
HLA-DR+
Terminal deoxynucleotidyl transferase−

DIFFERENTIAL DIAGNOSIS

- DL is the major differential diagnosis, particularly when it coexists with MF. In contrast to MF, which presents with partial or complete obliteration of nodal architecture by sheets of MF cells, DL shows only clusters of histiocytes containing lipid and melanin. However, early involvement by MF in the form of interfollicular foci of MF cells is difficult to determine.
- Hodgkin lymphoma may also involve the paracortex and exhibit confluent, pale-staining areas; however, MF cells are large and atypical in comparison with small lymphocytes, but smaller than Hodgkin and Reed-Sternberg cells. The nucleoli of MF cells are not acidophilic. Fibrosis, typical of Hodgkin lymphoma, is usually absent in MF.
- Systemic lymphomas associated with skin lesions involve the skin late in the course of widespread disease.

REFERENCES

1. Willemze R, Beljaards RC, Meijer CJ. Classification of primary cutaneous T-cell lymphomas [see Comments]. Histopathology 1994;24:405–415.
2. Willemze R, Kerl H, Sterry W, et al. EORTC classification for primary cutaneous lymphomas: a proposal from the Cutaneous Lymphoma Study Group of the European Organization for Research and Treatment of Cancer. Blood 1997;90:354–371.
3. Scheffer E, Meijer CJ, van Vloten WA, et al. A histologic study of lymph nodes from patients with the Sézary syndrome. Cancer 1986;57:2375–2380.
4. Weinstock MA, Horm JW. Mycosis fungoides in the United States. Increasing incidence and descriptive epidemiology. JAMA 1988;260:42–46.
5. Epstein EH Jr, Levin DL, Croft JD Jr, et al. Mycosis fungoides. Survival, prognostic features, response to therapy, and autopsy findings. Medicine (Baltimore) 1972;51:61–72.
6. Bunn PA Jr, Huberman MS, Whang-Peng J, et al. Prospective staging evaluation of patients with cutaneous T-cell lymphomas. Demonstration of a high frequency of extracutaneous dissemination. Ann Intern Med 1980;93:223–230.
7. Diamandidou E, Cohen PR, Kurzrock R. Mycosis fungoides and Sézary syndrome [see Comments]. Blood 1996;88:2385–2409.
8. Zucker-Franklin D, Pancake BA. The role of human T-cell lymphotropic viruses (HTLV-1 and -2) in cutaneous T-cell lymphomas. Semin Dermatol 1994;13:160–165.

9. Whittaker SJ, Luzzatto L. HTLV-1 provirus and mycosis fungoides [Letter; Comment]. Science 1993;259:1470; discussion 1471.
10. Bazarbachi A, Saal F, Laroche L, et al. HTLV-1 provirus and mycosis fungoides [Letter; Comment]. Science 1993;259:1470–1471.
11. Nagatani T, Miyazawa M, Matsuzaki T, et al. Comparative study of cutaneous T-cell lymphoma and adult T-cell leukemia/lymphoma. Semin Dermatol 1994;13:216–222.
12. McGregor JM, Crook T, Fraser-Andrews EA, et al. Spectrum of p53 gene mutations suggests a possible role for ultraviolet radiation in the pathogenesis of advanced cutaneous lymphomas. J Invest Dermatol 1999;112:317–321.
13. Navas IC, Ortiz-Romero PL, Villuendas R, et al. p16(INK4a) gene alterations are frequent in lesions of mycosis fungoides. Am J Pathol 2000;156:1565–1572.
14. Hoppe RT, Wood GS, Abel EA. Mycosis fungoides and the Sézary syndrome: pathology, staging, and treatment. Curr Probl Cancer 1990;14:293–371.
15. Rappaport H, Thomas LB. Mycosis fungoides: the pathology of extracutaneous involvement. Cancer 1974;34:1198–1229.
16. Griem ML, Moran EM, Ferguson DJ, et al. Staging procedures in mycosis fungoides. Br J Cancer 1975;31[Suppl 2]:362–367.
17. Kim YH, Jensen RA, Watanabe GL, et al. Clinical stage IA (limited patch and plaque) mycosis fungoides. A long-term outcome analysis. Arch Dermatol 1996;132:1309–1313.
18. Kim YH, Bishop K, Varghese A, et al. Prognostic factors in erythrodermic mycosis fungoides and the Sézary syndrome [see Comments]. Arch Dermatol 1995;131:1003–1008.
19. Posner LE, Fossieck BE Jr, Eddy JL, et al. Septicemic complications of the cutaneous T-cell lymphomas. Am J Med 1981;71: 210–216.
20. Thomas LB, Rappaport H. Mycosis fungoides and its relationship to other malignant lymphomas. In: Rebuck JR, Berard CW, Abell MR, eds. The reticulo-endothelial system. International Academy of Pathology Monograph No. 16. Baltimore: Williams & Wilkins, 1975:243–261.
21. Edelson RL, Kirkpatrick CH, Shevach EM, et al. Preferential cutaneous infiltration by neoplastic thymus-derived lymphocytes. Morphologic and functional studies. Ann Intern Med 1974;80: 685–692.
22. Vergier B, de Muret A, Beylot-Barry M, et al. Transformation of mycosis fungoides: clinicopathological and prognostic features of 45 cases. French Study Group of Cutaneous Lymphomas. Blood 2000;95:2212–2218.
23. Diamandidou E, Colome-Grimmer M, Fayad L, et al. Transformation of mycosis fungoides/Sézary syndrome: clinical characteristics and prognosis. Blood 1998;92:1150–1159.
24. Vonderheid EC, Zhang Q, Lessin SR, et al. Use of serum soluble interleukin-2 receptor levels to monitor the progression of cutaneous T-cell lymphoma. J Am Acad Dermatol 1998;38:207–220.
25. Nickoloff BJ. Light-microscopic assessment of 100 patients with patch/plaque-stage mycosis fungoides. Am J Dermatopathol 1988;10:469–477.
26. Shapiro PE, Pinto FJ. The histologic spectrum of mycosis fungoides/Sézary syndrome (cutaneous T-cell lymphoma). A review of 222 biopsies, including newly described patterns and the earliest pathologic changes. Am J Surg Pathol 1994;18:645–667.
27. Smoller BR, Bishop K, Glusac E, et al. Reassessment of histologic parameters in the diagnosis of mycosis fungoides. Am J Surg Pathol 1995;19:1423–1430.
28. Burke JS, Colby TV. Dermatopathic lymphadenopathy. Comparison of cases associated and unassociated with mycosis fungoides. Am J Surg Pathol 1981;5:343–352.
29. Burke JS, Sheibani K, Rappaport H. Dermatopathic lymphadenopathy. An immunophenotypic comparison of cases associated and unassociated with mycosis fungoides. Am J Pathol 1986;123:256–263.
30. Lutzner MA, Emerit I, Durepaire R, et al. Cytogenetic, cytophotometric, and ultrastructural study of large cerebriform cells of the Sézary syndrome and description of a small-cell variant. J Natl Cancer Inst 1973;50:1145–1162.
31. Sausville EA, Worsham GF, Matthews MJ, et al. Histologic assessment of lymph nodes in mycosis fungoides/Sézary syndrome (cutaneous T-cell lymphoma): clinical correlations and prognostic import of a new classification system. Hum Pathol 1985;16: 1098–1109.
32. Lynch JW Jr, Linoilla I, Sausville EA, et al. Prognostic implications of evaluation for lymph node involvement by T-cell antigen receptor gene rearrangement in mycosis fungoides. Blood 1992;79:3293–3299.
33. Payne CM. Ultrastructural morphometry in the diagnosis of mycosis fungoides and Sézary's syndrome. Clin Dermatol 1991;9: 187–203.
34. Wallace ML, Smoller BR. Immunohistochemistry in diagnostic dermatopathology. J Am Acad Dermatol 1996;34:163–183; quiz 184–186.
35. Izban KF, Hsi ED, Alkan S. Immunohistochemical analysis of mycosis fungoides on paraffin-embedded tissue sections. Mod Pathol 1998;11:978–982.
36. Veelken H, Wood GS, Sklar J. Molecular staging of cutaneous T-cell lymphoma: evidence for systemic involvement in early disease. J Invest Dermatol 1995;104:889–894.
37. Bakels V, Van Oostveen JW, Geerts ML, et al. Diagnostic and prognostic significance of clonal T-cell receptor beta gene rearrangements in lymph nodes of patients with mycosis fungoides. J Pathol 1993;170:249–255.
38. Kern DE, Kidd PG, Moe R, et al. Analysis of T-cell receptor gene rearrangement in lymph nodes of patients with mycosis fungoides. Prognostic implications [see Comments]. Arch Dermatol 1998;134:158–164.

73

PERIPHERAL T-CELL LYMPHOMA

DEFINITION

Peripheral T-cell lymphoma (PTL), not otherwise categorized, includes predominantly nodal non-Hodgkin lymphoma (NHL) of mature lymphocytic origin with heterogeneous morphology and post-thymic T-cell immunophenotype. It excludes specific entities, such as T-cell prolymphocytic leukemia, adult T-cell leukemia/lymphoma (HTLV-1+), mycosis fungoides, anaplastic large cell lymphoma, γδ T-cell lymphoma, and angiocentric or natural killer cell lymphoma.

SYNONYMS

- Immunoblastic sarcoma of T cells (1)
- Node-based T-cell lymphoma (2)
- T-cell lymphomas (Kiel) (3)
  - Pleomorphic small cell (Kiel)
  - T-zone lymphoma (Kiel)
  - Lymphoepithelioid cell (Kiel)
  - Pleomorphic medium and large cell (Kiel)
  - Immunoblastic (Kiel)
- PTL, unspecified (Revised European-American Classification, or REAL) (4)
  - Lymphoepithelioid cell (Lennert, REAL)
  - Medium-sized cell (provisional, REAL)
  - Mixed medium and large cell (provisional, REAL)
  - Large cell (provisional, REAL)
- PTL, not otherwise categorized (World Health Organization, or WHO) (5)
  - Lymphoepithelioid (Lennert) (variant, WHO)
  - T-zone lymphoma (variant, WHO)

PATHOGENESIS

In the Western hemisphere, about 10% to 15% of NHLs are of T-cell type (6). In Japan, depending on the district, 43% to 75% of NHLs express T-cell antigens (7). T-cell neoplasms arising from immature thymus and bone marrow precursors are called *lymphoblastic lymphomas* and *acute lymphoblastic leukemias* (see Chapter 59). Because node-based PTLs are morphologically heterogeneous, they have been described under a variety of names (see synonyms). T-cell neoplasms arising from mature post-thymic lymphocytes include a variety of NHLs: some in skin, such as mycosis fungoides (see Chapter 72), some in the upper respiratory tract, some associated with the human T-lymphotropic virus type 1 (HTLV-1) (see Chapter 71), and others. The majority originate in lymph nodes. Angioimmunoblastic lymphadenopathy with dysproteinemia (AILD)-like T-cell lymphoma is considered a special subtype of PTL and is separately described (see Chapter 74). Anaplastic large cell lymphoma carries the chromosomal translocation t(2;5)(p23;q35) and has a better prognosis than PTL (see Chapter 75). Angiocentric or natural killer lymphoma is primarily an extranodal lesion (8) and is therefore not included.

CLINICAL SYNDROME

The median age of patients with PTL is between 54 and 63.5 years (range, 4 to 97 years) (9–11). The male-to-female ratio varies from 1.5:1 to 2.8:1 (9–12). "B" symptoms occur in 56% to 67% of cases (9,10,12,13), and 72% to 82% of patients present in clinical stage III or IV (9–13), reflecting the highly aggressive behavior of this neoplasm. The lymph nodes are the main site of PTL, and in one study, generalized adenopathy was present in 69% of 42 cases (9). Extranodal involvement is frequent; it affects bone marrow in 28% to 41% of cases (9–12), lung in 11% (10), and liver in 13% to 29% (9,10,12). In one series, the spleen was involved in 43% of cases (9). The skin is involved in 9% to 13% of cases (10–12). Like B-cell lymphomas, PTLs of small cell histologic type more often involve bone marrow than do PTLs of large cell type (10). Leukemia is uncommon in PTL (10,12). Many patients with PTL have cytokine-related paraneoplastic syndromes causing plasmacytosis, hypergammaglobulinemia, constitutional "B" symptoms, eosinophilia, and hemophagocytosis (9,14–16).

Comparisons between PTLs and their B-cell counterparts have shown greater aggressiveness, shorter failure-free survival (FFS), and shorter overall survival (OS) for the T-

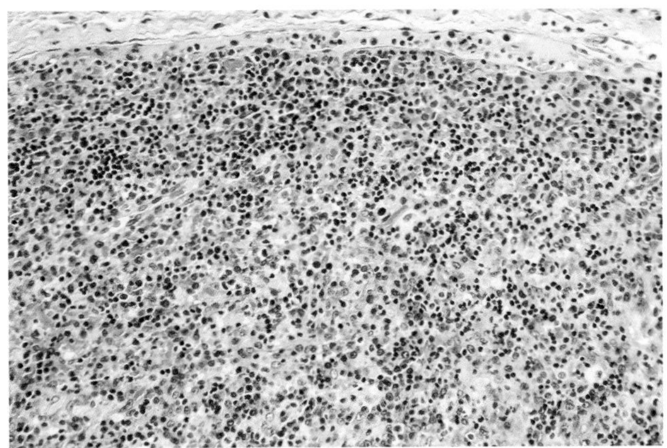

FIGURE 73.1. Peripheral T-cell lymphoma. Nodal architecture totally effaced by diffuse proliferation of medium-sized lymphoma cells admixed with numerous reactive histiocytes. Hematoxylin and eosin stain.

cell lymphomas (17,18). Some PTL cases are preceded by immunologic disorders, such as AILD, Hashimoto thyroiditis, immune thrombocytopenic purpura, and rheumatoid arthritis (9). The Kiel scheme categorizes PTLs according to the predominant cell size (3). However, because of poor interobserver reproducibility and lack of prognostic value, clinical stage is more useful than morphologic subclassification (19,20).

Poor prognostic factors in PTL include advanced stage of disease, poor performance status, and high levels of lactate dehydrogenase (21,22). The International Prognostic Index and T-cell phenotype are independent variables that predict FFS and OS (11,13).

HISTOPATHOLOGY

Peripheral T-cell lymphomas arise in the paracortical or T-zone areas of lymph nodes. By the time PTL is diagnosed, the lymph node architecture is usually obliterated (Fig. 73.1) and overrun by a diffuse cellular proliferation (Fig. 73.2A). If small uninvolved areas persist, they are usually cortical, showing small, compressed lymphoid follicles (23) (Fig. 73.3A). The neoplastic infiltrate is usually diffuse. However, thin strands of fibrocollagen sometimes irregularly divide the lymph node and create a pattern of compartmentalization that must not be confused with the round nodules of follicular lymphomas (24). Another characteristic feature of PTL is a prominent vascular component formed by the proliferation of postcapillary venules in a fine, interweaving fashion (23,24) (Fig. 73.3B). The lymphoid infiltrates consist of lymphoma cells intermingled with a large number of reactive non-neoplastic inflammatory cells (Fig. 73.3C). These include eosinophils, plasma cells, epithelioid histiocytes, and small, mature lymphocytes. Lymphokines secreted by the lymphoma cells are believed to be the cause of the abundant inflammatory reaction (25). The polymorphic cellular composition resembles that of Hodgkin lymphoma (HL), so that it is sometimes very difficult to distinguish between them (26). However, in contrast to the uniformly small, mature lymphocytes of HL, the PTL infiltrate consists of neoplastic lymphocytes in a range of cell sizes and nuclear configurations.

Morphologically, PTLs represent a spectrum of cytologic subtypes, from small atypical cells to large polymorphic cells. The small cells have spare cytoplasm, slightly irregular and crinkled but not cleaved nuclei, inconspicuous nucleoli, and rare mitoses (9,24) (Figs. 73.2B and 73.3C). The large cells have fairly abundant eosinophilic or entirely clear cytoplasm (Fig. 73.4). The nuclei are usually centrally placed and lobate, with distinct infolding (Figs. 73.2B and 73.3C). Nuclear pleomorphism is common, and bizarre forms may be seen, including giant multinucleated cells. Such cells often have prominent eosinophilic nucleoli, which increase their resemblance to Hodgkin and Reed-Sternberg cells. Mitoses are frequent. Multilobate nuclei and multinucleate

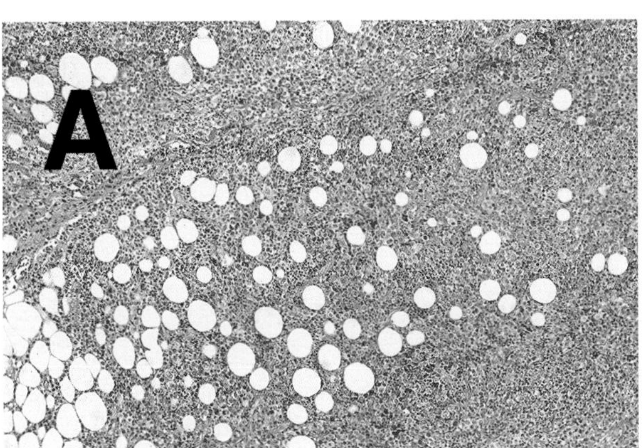

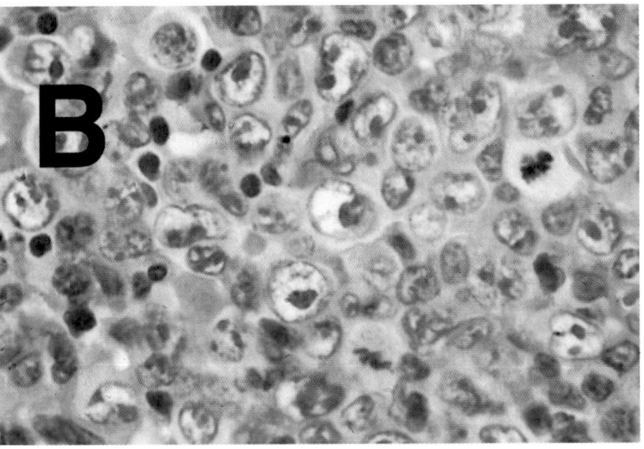

FIGURE 73.2. Peripheral T-cell lymphoma. **A:** Obliterates normal lymph node architecture, infiltrates lymph node capsule and perinodal adipose tissue. Hematoxylin and eosin stain. **B:** Small, medium, and large lymphoid cells with irregular nuclear contours. Numerous mitoses. Hematoxylin and eosin stain.

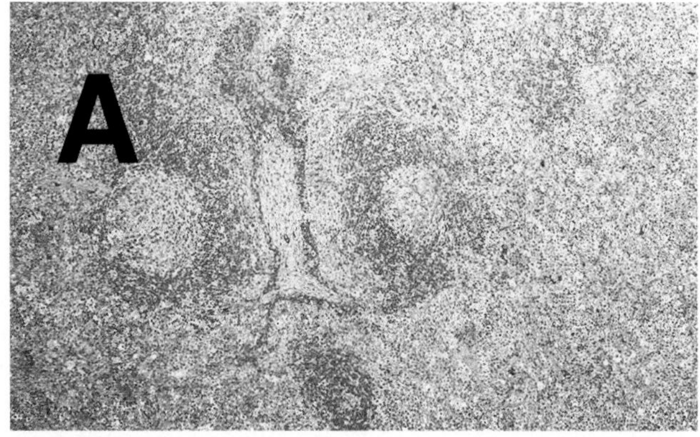

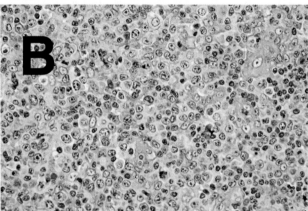

FIGURE 73.3. Peripheral T-cell lymphoma. **A:** Residual reactive follicles compressed by paracortical T-zone expansion. Hematoxylin and eosin stain. **B:** Prominent postcapillary venules and a mixed population of lymphocytes. Hematoxylin and eosin stain. **C:** Postcapillary venules (*top*). Lymphoid cells in a spectrum of sizes intermingled with small, round lymphocytes and an occasional plasma cell. Hematoxylin and eosin stain.

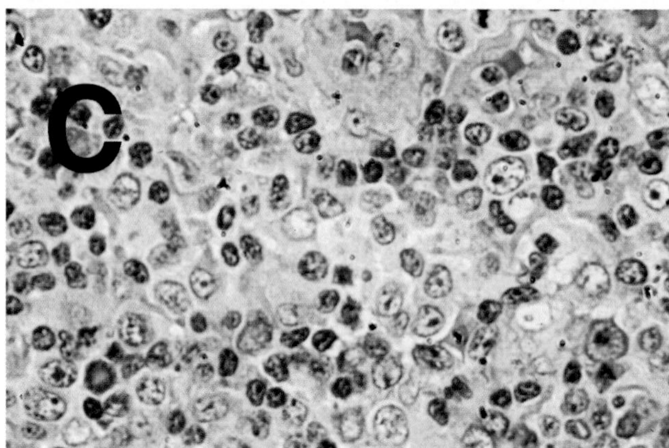

pleomorphic cells are not unique to large T-cell lymphomas. Similar aberrant forms can be seen in large B-cell lymphomas, which suggests that the histologic appearance of large cell lymphomas is not a reliable indicator of their immunophenotype (27).

It is not certain whether the T-zone PTL variant represents a disease phase or a distinct entity. The lymphoepithelioid variant (Lennert lymphoma) is not noticeably different clinically from other PTLs; it is not clearly defined, and many other PTL subtypes also contain epithelioid histiocytes (19,20,28).

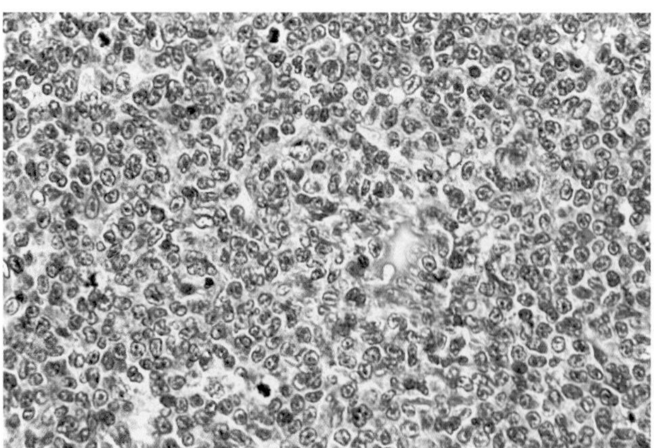

FIGURE 73.4. Peripheral T-cell lymphoma. Diffuse pattern of large lymphoid cells with vesicular nuclear chromatin. Hematoxylin and eosin stain. Peripheral T-cell lymphoma of this pattern cannot be distinguished from diffuse large B-cell lymphoma without immunophenotypic study.

CYTOLOGY

The most important cytologic features on fine needle aspiration include a spectrum of small, intermediate, and large lymphoid cells with irregular nuclear contours, epithelioid histiocytes, and atypical mononuclear cells (29) (Fig. 73.5). Flow cytometry can confirm a T-cell phenotype but does not reveal aneuploidy in most cases (29). Reactive granulomatous lymphadenitis and HL should be considered in the differential diagnosis.

ELECTRON MICROSCOPY

The ultrastructure of the large lymphoma cells reveals abundant cytoplasm with occasional lysosomal bodies, medium-sized mitochondria, and a few rough endoplasmic reticulum profiles. Interdigitating cell processes are seen. The nuclei are usually irregularly shaped and contain marginated heterochromatin and centrally placed nucleoli with an exagger-

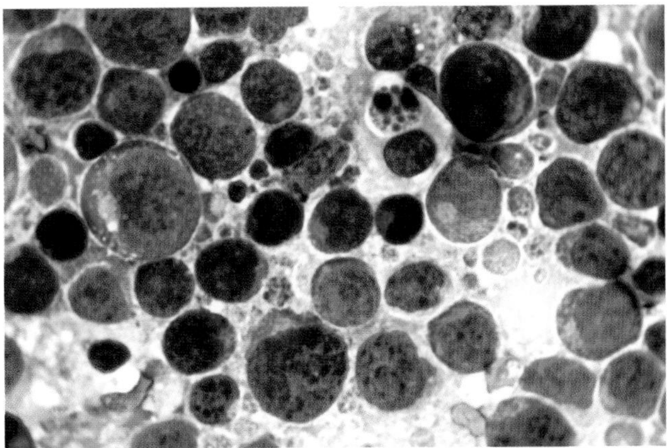

FIGURE 73.5. Peripheral T-cell lymphoma, touch imprint. Spectrum of cell sizes; small, intermediate, and large lymphoid cells with nuclear irregularities. Many lymphoglandular bodies in the background. Giemsa stain.

ated nucleolonema; they are sometimes indistinguishable from Hodgkin and Reed-Sternberg cells (24,30) (Fig. 73.6). Clear cell lymphomas have electron-lucent cytoplasm with few organelles (31).

IMMUNOHISTOCHEMISTRY

Peripheral T-cell lymphomas have the immunophenotype of post-thymic, mature, peripheral T cells (see Chapters 6 and 7). PTLs can express either CD4 (helper/inducer T cell) or CD8 (suppressor/cytotoxic T cell). They are negative for CD1a, CD99, and terminal deoxynucleotidyl transferase (TdT), which only precursor T-cells in the thymus or bone

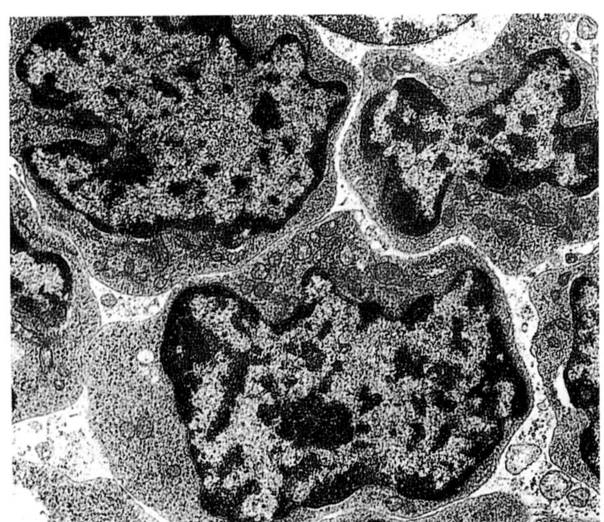

FIGURE 73.6. Peripheral T-cell non-Hodgkin lymphoma in axillary lymph node. Large cells with few intracytoplasmic organelles and irregularly shaped, lobate nuclei with heterochromatin and multiple nucleoli. ×9,600.

marrow produce. The majority of PTLs express CD4, a smaller proportion express CD8, and rare cases express both or neither (32). In PTL cells, expression of the common pan-T-cell antigens (CD2, CD3, CD5, CD7) is aberrantly decreased by 50% or more (33,34). An abnormal T-cell phenotype includes assorted pan-T-cell antigens in any combination. However, CD7 is most often lost, followed by CD5. Variable expression of the TCR β chain also occurs in PTLs (34). An aberrant T-cell phenotype does not prove clonality but is still a powerful clue for diagnosing post-thymic T-cell malignancy.

Phenotype

Usually CD4+/CD8−
Occasionally CD4−/CD8+
Rarely CD4+/CD8+ or CD4−/CD8−
Absence of one or more pan-T-cell markers: CD2, CD3, CD5, CD7
CD1a−
CD99−
TdT−

MOLECULAR DIAGNOSIS

Most PTLs show a good correspondence between T-cell immunophenotype and T-cell receptor (TCR) β or γ gene rearrangement (35) (see Chapter 8); they also rearrange TCR α (36) and delete TCR δ. Immunoglobulin loci usually remain germline (37). On the other hand, true natural killer cell lymphomas express CD16, CD56, or CD57 plus T-cell antigens CD2 and CD7, but not CD3 or CD5, and they do not rearrange TCRs (38).

CYTOGENETICS

Numeric abnormalities of chromosomes 7q and 13, alterations of 13q14 and 14, deletions of 6q, and other complex cytogenetic aberrations occur in PTLs (39,40). However, no recurrent cytogenetic abnormalities are noted (40).

DIFFERENTIAL DIAGNOSIS

- Adult T-cell lymphoma (HTLV-1+): Leukemia usually associated, hypercalcemia more common, inflammatory cellular reaction moderate or absent. Tropical spastic parapareisis HTLV-1+ lymphoma cells overexpress interleukin 2 receptor (CD25).
- Mycosis fungoides (cutaneous T-cell lymphoma): Skin lesions predominant, mycosis cells present, leukemia (Sézary syndrome) frequent.

Checklist

PERIPHERAL T-CELL LYMPHOMA

Patients elderly
Advanced stages at presentation
Lymph nodes major location
Extranodal locations common, leukemia infrequent
Paracortical or diffuse pattern, or both
Vascular hyperplasia
Inflammatory cellular reaction
Small, medium, and large lymphoma cells with irregular nuclei
Multilobate, bizarre nuclei
Post-thymic T-cell immunophenotypes
Loss of pan-T-cell markers, CD4+ predominant
HTLV-1−
Very aggressive, poor prognosis

- Immunoblastic lymphoma, B-cell type: Reactive inflammatory infiltrate less prominent, eosinophilia absent, B-cell markers present.
- Anaplastic large cell (Ki-1) lymphoma: Young adults, nodal sinuses involved, cohesive cell cords, pleomorphic wreathlike nuclei, CD30 (Ki-1, Ber-H2)+, t(2;5)(p23;q35).
- HL: Skin lesions and hypercalcemia absent, small lymphoid cells non-neoplastic. Because Reed-Sternberg cells may be seen in both PTL and HL, the background population of lymphocytes should be evaluated for a spectrum of cell sizes with nuclear irregularities in the former and uniformity of small, round lymphocytes in the latter.
- T cell-rich B-cell lymphoma: Few scattered, monoclonal, large neoplastic B cells; more than 70% polyclonal, background reactive small T cells (41).
- PTL that has a perifollicular growth pattern and medium-sized cells with clear cytoplasm can be confused with marginal zone lymphoma (42). Immunohistochemistry is useful to distinguish T-cell from B-cell proliferations.
- PTL that has a follicular growth pattern can be confused with follicular lymphoma. PTL phenotype is CD4+, CD8−, CD57−, bcl-6+, CD10−/+ (43).

REFERENCES

1. Lukes RJ, Collins RD. Immunologic characterization of human malignant lymphomas. Cancer 1974;34[Suppl]:1488–1503.
2. Collins RD, Waldron JA, Glick AD. Results of multiparameter studies of T-cell lymphoid neoplasms. Am J Clin Pathol 1979;72: 699–707.
3. Lennert K, Feller AC. Histopathology of non-Hodgkin's lymphomas (based on the updated Kiel classification). Berlin: Springer-Verlag, 1992:312.
4. Harris NL, Jaffe ES, Stein H, et al. A revised European-American classification of lymphoid neoplasms: a proposal from the International Lymphoma Study Group [see Comments]. Blood 1994;84:1361–1392.
5. Harris NL, Jaffe ES, Diebold J, et al. The World Health Organization classification of hematological malignancies: report of the clinical advisory committee meeting, Airlie House, Virginia, November 1997. Mod Pathol 2000;13:193–207.
6. The Non-Hodgkin's Lymphoma Classification Project. A clinical evaluation of the International Lymphoma Study Group classification of non-Hodgkin's lymphoma. Blood 1997;89:3909–3918.
7. Shimoyama M. Peripheral T-cell lymphoma in Japan: recent progress. Ann Oncol 1991;2[Suppl 2]:157–162.
8. Takeshita M, Akamatsu M, Ohshima K, et al. Angiocentric immunoproliferative lesions of the lymph node. Am J Clin Pathol 1996;106:69–77.
9. Greer JP, York JC, Cousar JB, et al. Peripheral T-cell lymphoma: a clinicopathologic study of 42 cases. J Clin Oncol 1984;2:788–798.
10. Armitage JO, Greer JP, Levine AM, et al. Peripheral T-cell lymphoma. Cancer 1989;63:158–163.
11. Ansell SM, Habermann TM, Kurtin PJ, et al. Predictive capacity of the International Prognostic Factor Index in patients with peripheral T-cell lymphoma. J Clin Oncol 1997;15:2296–2301.
12. Lopez-Guillermo A, Cid J, Salar A, et al. Peripheral T-cell lymphomas: initial features, natural history, and prognostic factors in a series of 174 patients diagnosed according to the R.E.A.L. Classification. Ann Oncol 1998;9:849–855.
13. Melnyk A, Rodriguez A, Pugh WC, et al. Evaluation of the Revised European-American Lymphoma Classification confirms the clinical relevance of immunophenotype in 560 cases of aggressive non-Hodgkin's lymphoma. Blood 1997;89:4514–4520.
14. Tamaki T, Katagiri S, Kanayama Y, et al. Helper T-cell lymphoma with marked plasmacytosis and polyclonal hypergammaglobulinemia. A case report. Cancer 1984;53:1590–1595.
15. Chott A, Augustin I, Wrba F, et al. Peripheral T-cell lymphomas: a clinicopathologic study of 75 cases. Hum Pathol 1990;21: 1117–1125.
16. Falini B, Pileri S, De Solas I, et al. Peripheral T-cell lymphoma associated with hemophagocytic syndrome [see Comments]. Blood 1990;75:434–444.

17. Coiffier B, Brousse N, Peuchmaur M, et al. Peripheral T-cell lymphomas have a worse prognosis than B-cell lymphomas: a prospective study of 361 immunophenotyped patients treated with the LNH-84 regimen. The GELA (Groupe d'Étude des Lymphomes Aggressives). Ann Oncol 1990;1:45–50.
18. Cabanillas F. Do lymphomas in the peripheral T cell (unspecified) category differ clinically from B cell lymphomas? In: Mason DY, Harris NL, eds. Human lymphoma: clinical implications of the REAL Classification. London: Springer-Verlag, 1999:28.1–28.4.
19. Noorduyn LA, van der Valk P, van Heerde P, et al. Stage is a better prognostic indicator than morphologic subtype in primary noncutaneous T-cell lymphoma [see Comments]. Am J Clin Pathol 1990;93:49–57.
20. Hastrup N, Hamilton-Dutoit S, Ralfkiaer E, et al. Peripheral T-cell lymphomas: an evaluation of reproducibility of the updated Kiel classification. Histopathology 1991;18:99–105.
21. Lippman SM, Miller TP, Spier CM, et al. The prognostic significance of the immunotype in diffuse large-cell lymphoma: a comparative study of the T-cell and B-cell phenotypes. Blood 1988;72:436–441.
22. Kwak LW, Wilson M, Weiss LM, et al. Similar outcome of treatment of B-cell and T-cell diffuse large-cell lymphomas: the Stanford experience. J Clin Oncol 1991;9:1426–1431.
23. Brisbane JU, Berman LD, Neiman RS. Peripheral T-cell lymphoma: a clinicopathologic study of nine cases. Am J Clin Pathol 1983;79:285–293.
24. Waldron JA, Leech JH, Glick AD, et al. Malignant lymphoma of peripheral T-lymphocyte origin: immunologic, pathologic, and clinical features in six patients. Cancer 1977;40:1604–1617.
25. Ohnishi K, Ichikawa A, Kagami Y, et al. Interleukin 4 and gamma-interferon may play a role in the histopathogenesis of peripheral T-cell lymphoma. Cancer Res 1990;50:8028–8033.
26. Quintanilla-Martinez L, Fend F, Moguel LR, et al. Peripheral T-cell lymphoma with Reed-Sternberg–like cells of B-cell phenotype and genotype associated with Epstein-Barr virus infection. Am J Surg Pathol 1999;23:1233–1240.
27. Jaffe ES, Strauchen JA, Berard CW. Predictability of immunologic phenotype by morphologic criteria in diffuse aggressive non-Hodgkin's lymphomas. Am J Clin Pathol 1982;77:46–49.
28. Nakamura S, Suchi T. A clinicopathologic study of node-based, low-grade, peripheral T-cell lymphoma. Angioimmunoblastic lymphoma, T-zone lymphoma, and lymphoepithelioid lymphoma. Cancer 1991;67:2566–2578.
29. Katz RL, Gritsman A, Cabanillas F, et al. Fine-needle aspiration cytology of peripheral T-cell lymphoma. A cytologic, immunologic, and cytometric study. Am J Clin Pathol 1989;91:120–131.
30. Said JW, Shintaku IP, Chien K, et al. Peripheral T-cell lymphoma (immunoblastic sarcoma of T-cell type): an immuno-ultrastructural study. Hum Pathol 1984;15:324–329.
31. Zhuang HG, Liang GZ, Li WC, et al. Clear cell lymphoma: a clinicopathological study of four cases. Hum Pathol 1988;19:760–765.
32. Nakamura S, Koshikawa T, Koike K, et al. Phenotypic analysis of peripheral T-cell lymphoma among the Japanese. Acta Pathol Jpn 1993;43:396–412.
33. Weiss LM, Crabtree GS, Rouse RV, et al. Morphologic and immunologic characterization of 50 peripheral T-cell lymphomas. Am J Pathol 1985;118:316–324.
34. Picker LJ, Weiss LM, Medeiros LJ, et al. Immunophenotypic criteria for the diagnosis of non-Hodgkin's lymphoma. Am J Pathol 1987;128:181–201.
35. Williams ME, Innes DJ Jr, Borowitz MJ, et al. Immunoglobulin and T-cell receptor gene rearrangements in human lymphoma and leukemia. Blood 1987;69:79–86.
36. Knowles DM. Immunophenotypic and antigen receptor gene rearrangement analysis in T-cell neoplasia. Am J Pathol 1989;134:761–785.
37. van Krieken JH, Elwood L, Andrade RE, et al. Rearrangement of the T-cell receptor delta chain gene in T-cell lymphomas with a mature phenotype. Am J Pathol 1991;139:161–168.
38. Emile JF, Boulland ML, Haioun C, et al. CD5− CD56+ T-cell receptor silent peripheral T-cell lymphomas are natural killer cell lymphomas [see Comments]. Blood 1996;87:1466–1473.
39. Sanada I, Ishii T, Matsuoka M, et al. Chromosomal abnormalities in non-Hodgkin lymphoma with peripheral T-cell type: effect of HTLV-1 infection. Hematol Oncol 1987;5:157–166.
40. Schlegelberger B, Himmler A, Godde E, et al. Cytogenetic findings in peripheral T-cell lymphomas as a basis for distinguishing low-grade and high-grade lymphomas. Blood 1994;83:505–511.
41. Rodriguez J, Pugh WC, Cabanillas F. T cell-rich B-cell lymphoma. Blood 1993;82:1586–1589.
42. Rudiger T, Ichinohasama R, Ott MM, et al. Peripheral T-cell lymphoma with distinct perifollicular growth pattern: a distinct subtype of T-cell lymphoma? Am J Surg Pathol 2000;24:117–122.
43. de Leval L, Savilo E, Longtine J, et al. Peripheral T-cell lymphoma with follicular involvement and a CD4+/bcl-6+ phenotype. Am J Surg Pathol 2001;25:395–400.

74

ANGIOIMMUNOBLASTIC T-CELL LYMPHOMA

DEFINITION

Angioimmunoblastic lymphadenopathy with dysproteinemia (AILD) (1,2), immunoblastic lymphadenopathy (IBL) (3), and lymphogranulomatosis X (LgX) (4), despite subtle differences (5), are indistinguishable from angioimmunoblastic lymphadenopathy (AIL)-like or IBL-like T-cell lymphoma (6–8). Molecular and cytogenetic analyses confirm that most cases histologically diagnosed as AILD (or IBL) are clonal disorders consistent with a subtype of peripheral T-cell lymphoma (6,7,9). Acute onset in the sixth or seventh decade, generalized lymphadenopathy, hepatosplenomegaly, fever, anemia, and polyclonal hypergammaglobulinemia characterize the clinical syndrome (9,10). A triad of features—diffuse architectural effacement, hyperplastic branching blood vessels, and proliferating immunoblasts—defines the lymph node histology (9,10).

SYNONYMS

Angioimmunoblastic lymphadenopathy with dysproteinemia

Immunoblastic lymphadenopathy

Lymphogranulomatosis X

Angioimmunoblastic lymphadenopathy-like T-cell lymphoma

Immunoblastic lymphadenopathy-like T-cell lymphoma

Lymphogranulomatosis X-like T-cell lymphoma

PATHOGENESIS

Early reports hypothesized that an autoimmune disorder with defective T-cell suppression, autoreactive B cells, and B-cell proliferation causes AILD (1,2), and that an abnormal systemic hyperimmune response to undetermined, possibly therapeutic, agents produces IBL (3). However, because the majority of AILDs and IBLs clonally rearrange their T-cell antigen receptors (11–14) and contain clonal cytogenetic abnormalities (15–17), it is now generally accepted that these disorders begin as a subtype of T-cell malignancy called *AIL-like T-cell lymphoma* or *IBL-like T-cell lymphoma.* Japanese investigators, who also speculated that, especially in early disease, small monoclonal T-cell populations might exist below the level of conventional Southern blot detection, first proposed this conceptual shift (6,18, 19). The CD4+ helper/inducer T-cell phenotype predominates (11,20,21), although some cases express a CD8+ suppressor/cytotoxic T-cell phenotype (6). Many of the paraneoplastic signs and symptoms associated with AIL-like T-cell lymphoma are caused by the release from neoplastic and non-neoplastic cells of interleukins 1 and 6, tumor necrosis factor, lymphotoxin, or other cytokines (22,23).

Although most malignant lymphomas with AIL-like histology express a T-cell phenotype, a few B-cell lymphomas crop up. The role of Epstein-Barr virus (EBV) is critical but difficult to assign precisely; EBV can infect both B cells and T cells in AILD (and AIL-like T-cell lymphoma) (24–26), and the number of EBV-infected cells varies widely in each lymph node (27,28). Frequent deaths from bacterial infection, and abnormal results of *in vitro* lymphocyte function studies, suggest an underlying immunologic deficit in many cases (29,30). It is likely that EBV participates in the development of B-cell immunoblastic lymphomas arising in an AIL-like histologic background (25,27,31,32); EBV promotes B-cell neoplastic transformation under immunosuppressive conditions (e.g., after transplantation and in AIDS-related lymphomas), and partial deletion or point mutations of EBV latent membrane protein 1 (LMP-1) enhance oncogenicity (31,32).

CLINICAL SYNDROME

Angioimmunoblastic lymphadenopathy-like T-cell lymphoma manifests protean clinical and laboratory abnormalities, so that a lymph node biopsy is required to distinguish "AIL-related lesions" from a hyperimmune reaction

(33,34). The disease more often affects middle-aged or older persons (median age is in the sixth or seventh decade) (2,3). The onset is usually rapid; symptoms develop within days or weeks and include fever, sweats, weight loss, generalized lymphadenopathy, hepatosplenomegaly, and changes in the bone marrow, lungs, and skin (9,10,35). The latter, consisting of maculopapular rashes, edema, and pruritus, may be related to drug hypersensitivity in some cases (2,3). In a few patients, withdrawal of the suspected drug causes the signs and symptoms to resolve (10). More frequently, however, the immune deficiency inherent in this syndrome facilitates infection. Some patients have ascites, effusions, or edema (29,35). The clinical spectrum varies between indolent disease with remission (about 25%) and rapid demise within about 2 years (21). Several groups report median survivals between 11 and 30 months (6,29,35–38). The long-term survival rate (>5 years) is about 20% (10). Retrospective studies suggest that patients with "AIL-related lesions" showing atypical nuclei and "clear" cell proliferation have a poor prognosis (16,36,38,39). Starting combination chemotherapy containing doxorubicin shortly after diagnosis may be beneficial (38). A contrary report indicates no predictive value for "clear" cells (8). Patients administered steroids or other chemotherapy who achieve a complete remission have an improved prognosis (8).

LABORATORY DATA

Hemolytic anemia with a positive Coombs test result is frequent (9). Also common is dysproteinemia manifested by polyclonal hypergammaglobulinemia (9) (Fig. 74.1), sometimes with cryoglobulinemia (40). During active disease, a decrease in the percentage of CD4+ T cells (41), an inverted ratio of CD4+ to CD8+ cells (41), and circulating clonal T cells (13) are seen in the peripheral blood.

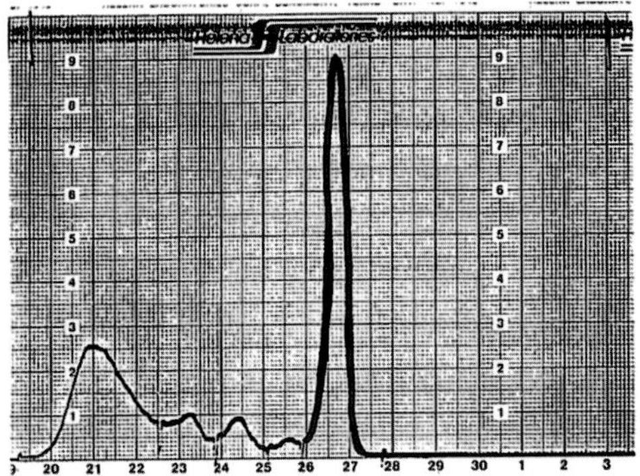

FIGURE 74.1. Electrophoresis of angioimmunoblastic lymphadenopathy-like T-cell lymphoma shows polyclonal hypergammaglobulinemia. Immunoglobulin (*Ig*) G, 3,460 mg/dL (normal range for age, 592–1,593); IgA, 690 (100–296); IgM, 330 (38–240).

HISTOPATHOLOGY

Initially, it was believed that subtle criteria, such as atypical nuclei and the number of "clear" or "pale" cells, could distinguish AILD (or IBL) from malignant lymphoma (5,42). Later, it was realized that morphology could not reliably separate AILD (or IBL) from AIL-like (or IBL-like) T-cell lymphoma because molecular and cytogenetic studies revealed clonality in both (6,8,11,20). The historical descriptions of AILD (1,2), IBL (3), and LgX (4,35) indicate identity in certain key morphologic features: diffusely effaced lymph node architecture without follicles and minimal to absent sinuses (Fig. 74.2 A,B); numerous arborizing blood vessels, the size of postcapillary venules, lined by hyperplastic endothelial cells (Fig. 74.2 B,C,E,F); and a mixed population of immunoblasts, plasmacytoid lymphocytes, and plasma cells (Fig. 74.2D). Some cases include numerous eosinophils; others contain clusters of epithelioid histiocytes without the formation of granulomas. Additional minor findings considered exclusive include the following: depleted lymphocytes in IBL; occasional burned-out and fibrosed germinal centers in one-third of AILDs and sometimes in LgX, but not in IBL; deposits of acidophilic, sludgy, periodic acid–Schiff (PAS)-positive proteinaceous material (Figs. 74.2 C,F) in all IBLs, but only sometimes in AILD and LgX. Rare cases deposit amyloid in the involved lymph nodes (43). Necrosis and fibrosis are not components of the process. Immunoblasts, previously referred to as *reticular cells,* are the predominant cell type, scattered throughout the lymph node or occurring in compact "clusters" and "islands" (5) (Fig. 74.3). The immunoblasts are 15 to 25 μm in size, about three times larger than small lymphocytes, with vesicular nuclear chromatin, prominent nucleoli, and strongly pyroninophilic cytoplasm. Mitoses are frequent. Occasionally, large immunoblasts with irregularly shaped, polylobate nuclei resembling Reed-Sternberg cells are present (3) (Fig. 74.3).

"AIL-related lesions" are systemic, often involving other organs in addition to lymph nodes. Extranodal locations include bone marrow in as many as 30% of cases (44), spleen, liver, lungs, and skin. The terms *AIL, AIL-like dysplasia,* and *AIL-like lymphoma* have been suggested for lymphoproliferative disorders with AIL histology, depending on immunophenotypic, cytogenetic, and genotypic evidence proving clonality (7).

A recently described AIL-like T-cell lymphoma histologic variant with hyperplastic germinal centers (AITL/GC) (Fig. 74.4) must be differentiated from a hyperimmune reaction (45). These cases progress to typical AIL-like T-cell lymphoma with either absent or "burned-out" germinal centers (45). AITL/GC has numerous tingible-body macrophages within hyperplastic germinal centers (Fig. 74.4A) and in the interfollicular region (Fig. 74.4 B,C); however, follicular dendritic cell hyperplasia is absent (45). In AITL/GC, the germinal center borders are not sharply circumscribed (Fig. 74.4A) (45,46).

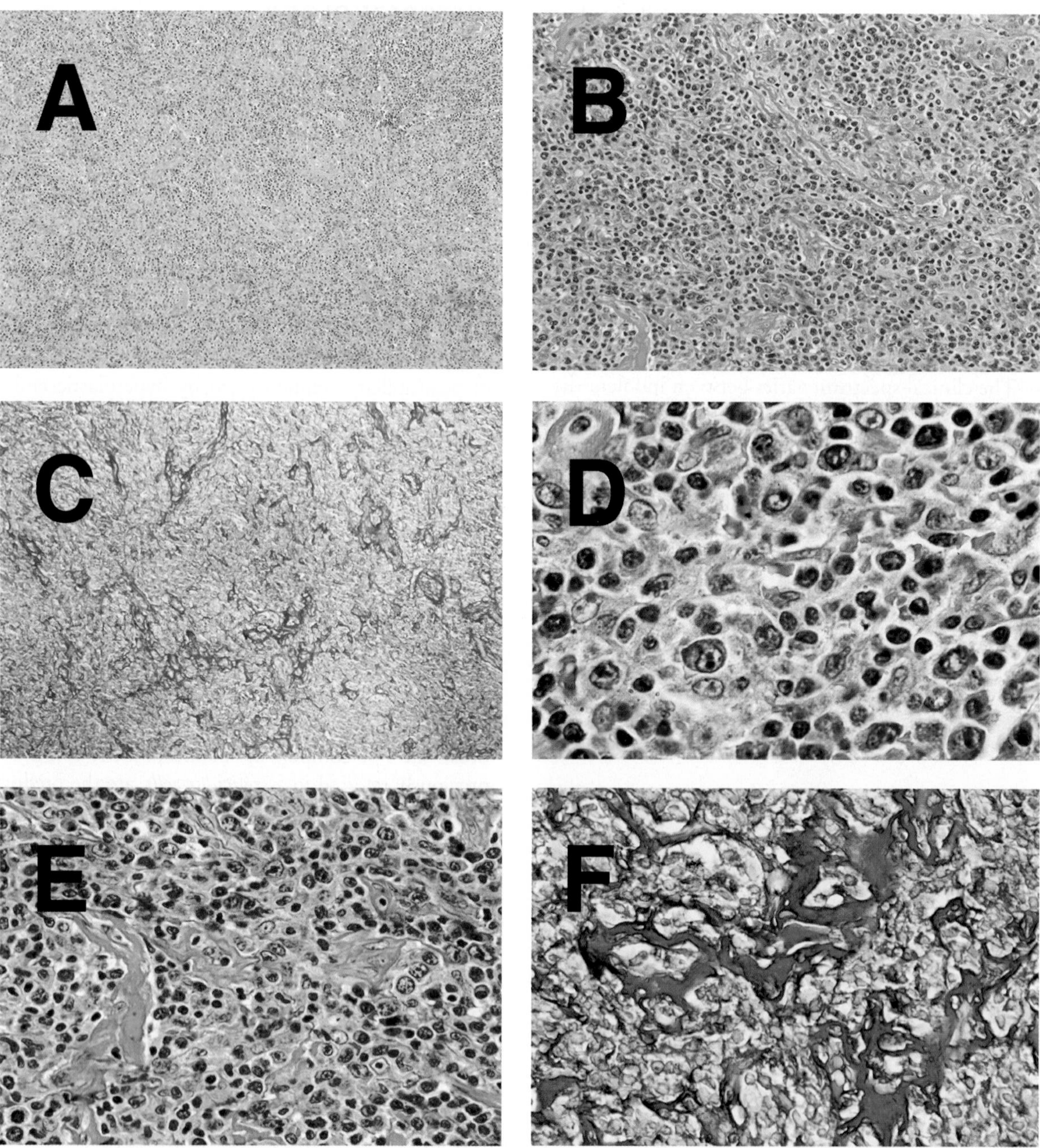

FIGURE 74.2. Angioimmunoblastic lymphadenopathy-like T-cell lymphoma. **A:** Diffuse nodal architectural effacement. **B,E:** Arborizing blood vessels. Hematoxylin and eosin stain. **C,F:** Arborizing blood vessels outlined by periodic acid–Schiff (*PAS*)-positive proteinaceous material. PAS stain. **D:** Mixed population of small and medium-sized lymphocytes, plasma cells, and plasmacytoid lymphocytes, plus larger immunoblasts.

IMMUNOHISTOCHEMISTRY

The CD4+ helper/inducer phenotype predominates in AIL-like T-cell lymphoma (20,47,48). Anti-dendritic cell staining reveals follicular structure remnants, and anti-collagen staining reveals intercellular collagen fibrils and blood vessels surrounded by basement membrane collagen (47).

Phenotype

Usually CD4+/CD8−
Occasionally CD4−/CD8+
Rarely CD4+/CD8+ or CD4−/CD8−
Absence of one or more pan-T-cell markers: CD2, CD3, CD5, CD7
CD1a−
CD99−
Terminal deoxynucleotidyl transferase− (TdT−)

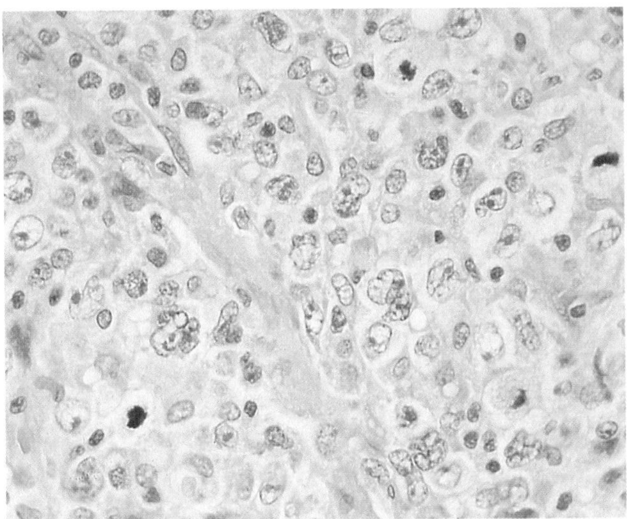

FIGURE 74.3. Angioimmunoblastic lymphadenopathy (*AIL*)-like T-cell lymphoma in paraaortic lymph node of 76-year-old man with so-called AIL dysproteinemia of 2 years' duration. Large cells with clear cytoplasm and bizarre vesicular nuclei containing prominent nucleoli. Numerous atypical mitoses, intermingled lymphocytes, blood vessel. Hematoxylin, phloxine, and saffron stain.

MOLECULAR DIAGNOSIS

Even before genotypic studies were generally available, a relationship between AILD (IBL) and AIL-like (IBL-like) T-cell lymphoma was suspected because of their essentially identical morphology and because many patients with AILD (IBL) progressed to AIL-like (IBL-like) T-cell lymphoma (18). The T-cell receptor (TCR) β gene is clonally rearranged in most (11,12,49,50), if not all (13,51), cases. Simultaneous rearrangement of the immunoglobulin (Ig) heavy chain locus occurs in fewer than 10% of cases, as in other peripheral T-cell lymphomas, and does not necessarily indicate the presence of an emerging B-cell clone. A report of transitory T-cell clones in AILD (13) has stimulated the hypothesis that unstable oligoclonal T cells eventually evolve into a neoplastic monoclonal T-cell population (7,9).

CYTOGENETICS

Cytogenetic studies demonstrate trisomies (3,5) and duplicated X chromosomes (15,52). Aberrant clones are detectable in nearly all cases of AIL-like T-cell lymphoma (32 of 36 patients, or 89%) when interphase and metaphase cytogenetic techniques are combined (17). A simultaneous, cytogenetically unrelated clone occurs more often in "AIL-related lesions" than in other hematologic malignancies, except for cutaneous T-cell lymphoma, which suggests an unstable genetic background (17,53,54). The presence of complex aberrant clones is a poor prognostic factor, trisomy 3 is neutral, and trisomy 5 is associated with longer survival (55).

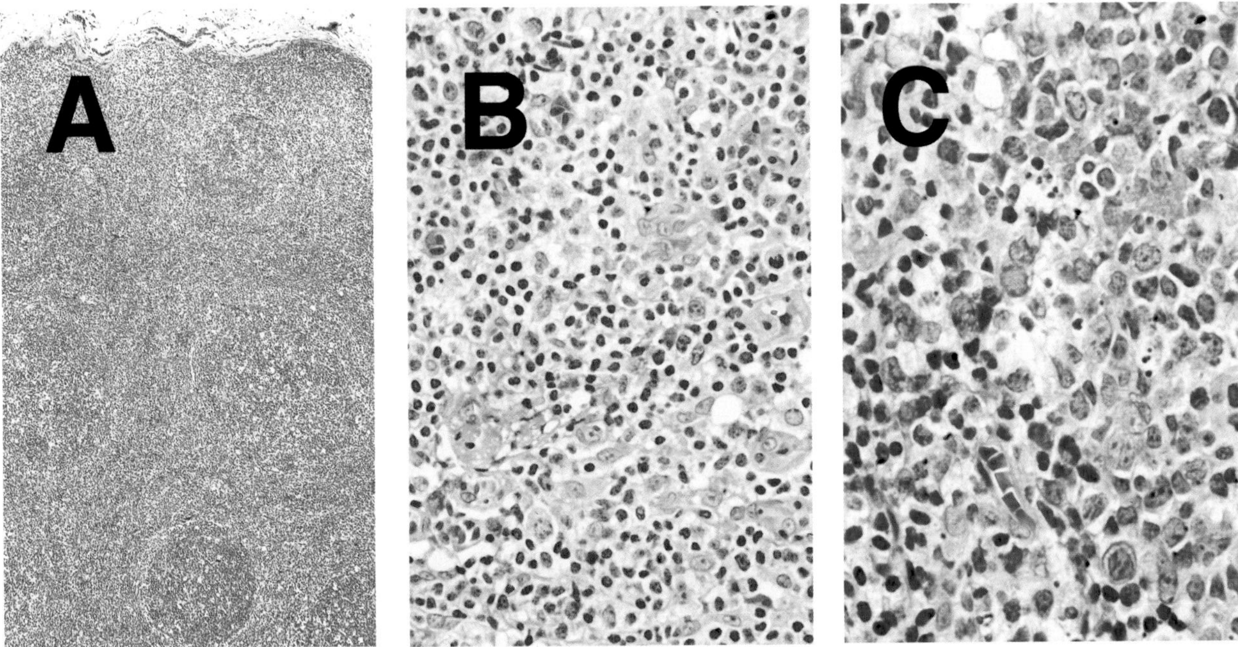

FIGURE 74.4. Angioimmunoblastic lymphadenopathy-like T-cell lymphoma histologic variant with hyperplastic germinal centers. **A:** Poorly demarcated germinal centers containing abundant tingible-body macrophages. Hematoxylin and eosin stain. **B:** Interfollicular region with increased numbers of blood vessels and many small to medium-sized lymphocytes. Hematoxylin and eosin stain. **C:** Interfollicular region showing numerous tingible-body macrophages and scattered immunoblasts. (Courtesy of Howe J. Ree, M.D.) Hematoxylin and eosin stain.

Checklist

ANGIOIMMUNOBLASTIC T-CELL LYMPHOMA

Middle-aged and elderly patients
Generalized lymphadenopathy
Polyclonal hypergammaglobulinemia
Hemolytic anemia
Effaced lymph node architecture
Diffuse cellular proliferation
Characteristic triad of (a) arborization, hyperplasia of small vessels; (b) immunoblasts, predominantly T-cell type; (c) PAS-positive material, clear cell immunoblasts, Reed-Sternberg–like cells
Plasma cells, eosinophils, epithelioid cells
Bone marrow, spleen, liver, lung may be involved

DIFFERENTIAL DIAGNOSIS

- Reactive lymphadenopathies of undetermined cause: Architecture is better preserved, lymphoid follicles are distinct, and germinal centers are hyperplastic.
- Hyperimmune reaction: Sharply circumscribed germinal centers and few tingible-body macrophages in the interfollicular zone help separate a hyperimmune reaction from AITL/GC.
- Infectious mononucleosis: Nodal architecture partially preserved, follicles with hyperplastic germinal centers, immunoblasts of mainly B-cell type, predominance of reactive CD8+ T cells.
- Castleman disease: Follicles are apparent and composed of an atrophic hyalinized center, penetrating arteriole, and concentric peripheral layers of lymphocytes.
- HIV lymphadenopathy (B or C type): Has in common marked vascular proliferation, but follicles are apparent and have the appearance described above for Castleman disease.
- Hodgkin lymphoma: Probably the most common diagnosis applied to AIL-like T-cell lymphoma before it was described because of the effacement of lymph node architecture and mixed proliferations of immunoblasts, plasma cells, eosinophils, and histiocytes. However, typical Reed-Sternberg cells, necrosis, and fibrosis are not noted in AIL-like T-cell lymphoma.
- Non-Hodgkin lymphoma, diffuse, small lymphocytic or small cleaved cell type: Has in common effacement of architecture, but the cell population is homogeneous and the gammopathy monoclonal.
- Peripheral T-cell lymphoma: Hypervascularity, eosinophils, plasma cells are absent. Large, irregularly shaped cells with convoluted bizarre nuclei and atypical mitoses are present.

REFERENCES

1. Frizzera G, Moran EM, Rappaport H. Angio-immunoblastic lymphadenopathy with dysproteinaemia. Lancet 1974;1:1070–1073.
2. Frizzera G, Moran EM, Rappaport H. Angio-immunoblastic lymphadenopathy. Diagnosis and clinical course. Am J Med 1975;59:803–818.
3. Lukes RJ, Tindle BH. Immunoblastic lymphadenopathy. A hyperimmune entity resembling Hodgkin's disease. N Engl J Med 1975;292:1–8.
4. Radaszkiewicz T, Lennert K. Immunoblastic adenopathy: clinical features, treatment and prognosis [in German; author's translation]. Dtsch Med Wochenschr 1975;100:1157–1163.
5. Nathwani BN, Rappaport H, Moran EM, et al. Malignant lymphoma arising in angioimmunoblastic lymphadenopathy. Cancer 1978;41:578–606.
6. Watanabe S, Sato Y, Shimoyama M, et al. Immunoblastic lymphadenopathy, angioimmunoblastic lymphadenopathy, and IBL-like T-cell lymphoma. A spectrum of T-cell neoplasia. Cancer 1986;58:2224–2232.
7. Frizzera G, Kaneko Y, Sakurai M. Angioimmunoblastic lymphadenopathy and related disorders: a retrospective look in search of definitions. Leukemia 1989;3:1–5.
8. Ch'ang HJ, Su IJ, Chen CL, et al. Angioimmunoblastic lymphadenopathy with dysproteinemia—lack of a prognostic value of clear cell morphology. Oncology 1997;54:193–198.
9. Freter CE, Cossman J. Angioimmunoblastic lymphadenopathy with dysproteinemia. Semin Oncol 1993;20:627–635.
10. Knecht H. Angioimmunoblastic lymphadenopathy: ten years' experience and state of current knowledge. Semin Hematol 1989; 26:208–215.
11. Weiss LM, Strickler JG, Dorfman RF, et al. Clonal T-cell populations in angioimmunoblastic lymphadenopathy and angioimmunoblastic lymphadenopathy-like lymphoma. Am J Pathol 1986;122:392–397.
12. O'Connor NT, Crick JA, Wainscoat JS, et al. Evidence for monoclonal T-lymphocyte proliferation in angioimmunoblastic lymphadenopathy. J Clin Pathol 1986;39:1229–1232.
13. Lipford EH, Smith HR, Pittaluga S, et al. Clonality of angioimmunoblastic lymphadenopathy and implications for its evolution to malignant lymphoma. J Clin Invest 1987;79:637–642.

14. Feller AC, Griesser H, Schilling CV, et al. Clonal gene rearrangement patterns correlate with immunophenotype and clinical parameters in patients with angioimmunoblastic lymphadenopathy. Am J Pathol 1988;133:549–556.
15. Godde-Salz E, Feller AC, Lennert K. Chromosomal abnormalities in lymphogranulomatosis X (LgrX)/angioimmunoblastic lymphadenopathy (AILD). Leuk Res 1987;11:181–190.
16. Kaneko Y, Maseki N, Sakurai M, et al. Characteristic karyotypic pattern in T-cell lymphoproliferative disorders with reactive "angioimmunoblastic lymphadenopathy with dysproteinemia-type" features. Blood 1988;72:413–421.
17. Schlegelberger B, Zhang Y, Weber-Matthiesen K, et al. Detection of aberrant clones in nearly all cases of angioimmunoblastic lymphadenopathy with dysproteinemia-type T-cell lymphoma by combined interphase and metaphase cytogenetics. Blood 1994;84:2640–2648.
18. Shimoyama M, Minato K, Saito H, et al. Immunoblastic lymphadenopathy (IBL)-like T-cell lymphoma. Jpn J Clin Oncol 1979;9[Suppl]:347–356.
19. Watanabe S, Ochi H, Mukai K. Immunoblastic lymphadenopathy and IBL-like T-cell lymphoma: a spectrum of T-cell neoplasia. In: Hanaoka M, ed. Lymphoid malignancy. New York: Field & Wood, 1987:147–154.
20. Namikawa R, Suchi T, Ueda R, et al. Phenotyping of proliferating lymphocytes in angioimmunoblastic lymphadenopathy and related lesions by the double immunoenzymatic staining technique. Am J Pathol 1987;127:279–287.
21. Steinberg AD, Seldin MF, Jaffe ES, et al. NIH conference. Angioimmunoblastic lymphadenopathy with dysproteinemia. Ann Intern Med 1988;108:575–584.
22. Hsu SM, Waldron JA Jr, Fink L, et al. Pathogenic significance of interleukin 6 in angioimmunoblastic lymphadenopathy-type T-cell lymphoma. Hum Pathol 1993;24:126–131.
23. Foss HD, Anagnostopoulos I, Herbst H, et al. Patterns of cytokine gene expression in peripheral T-cell lymphoma of angioimmunoblastic lymphadenopathy type. Blood 1995;85: 2862–2869.
24. Anagnostopoulos I, Hummel M, Finn T, et al. Heterogeneous Epstein-Barr virus infection patterns in peripheral T-cell lymphoma of angioimmunoblastic lymphadenopathy type. Blood 1992;80:1804–1812.
25. Abruzzo LV, Schmidt K, Weiss LM, et al. B-cell lymphoma after angioimmunoblastic lymphadenopathy: a case with oligoclonal gene rearrangements associated with Epstein-Barr virus. Blood 1993;82:241–246.
26. Ohshima K, Takeo H, Kikuchi M, et al. Heterogeneity of Epstein-Barr virus infection in angioimmunoblastic lymphadenopathy type T-cell lymphoma. Histopathology 1994;25:569–579.
27. Weiss LM, Jaffe ES, Liu XF, et al. Detection and localization of Epstein-Barr viral genomes in angioimmunoblastic lymphadenopathy and angioimmunoblastic lymphadenopathy-like lymphoma. Blood 1992;79:1789–1795.
28. Zhou XG, Hamilton-Dutoit SJ, Yan QH, et al. High frequency of Epstein-Barr virus in Chinese peripheral T-cell lymphoma [see Comments]. Histopathology 1994;24:115–122.
29. Cullen MH, Stansfeld AG, Oliver RT, et al. Angio-immunoblastic lymphadenopathy: report of ten cases and review of the literature. Q J Med 1979;48:151–177.
30. Pizzolo G, Vinante F, Agostini C, et al. Immunologic abnormalities in angioimmunoblastic lymphadenopathy. Cancer 1987;60: 2412–2418.
31. Knecht H, Martius F, Bachmann E, et al. A deletion mutant of the LMP1 oncogene of Epstein-Barr virus is associated with evolution of angioimmunoblastic lymphadenopathy into B immunoblastic lymphoma. Leukemia 1995;9:458–465.
32. Knecht H, Bachmann E, Brousset P, et al. Mutational hot spots within the carboxy terminal region of the LMP1 oncogene of Epstein-Barr virus are frequent in lymphoproliferative disorders. Oncogene 1995;10:523–528.
33. Koo CH, Nathwani BN, Winberg CD, et al. Atypical lymphoplasmacytic and immunoblastic proliferation in lymph nodes of patients with autoimmune disease (autoimmune disease-associated lymphadenopathy). Medicine (Baltimore) 1984;63:274–290.
34. Upara S, Ruchutrakool T, Sukpanichnant S. Lymph node pathology in patients with a clinical diagnosis of angioimmunoblastic lymphadenopathy with dysproteinemia (AILD): an analysis of 37 cases. Asian Pac J Allergy Immunol 1997;15:15–20.
35. Knecht H, Schwarze EW, Lennert K. Histological, immunohistological and autopsy findings in lymphogranulomatosis X (including angio-immunoblastic lymphadenopathy). Virchows Arch A Pathol Anat Histopathol 1985;406:105–124.
36. Pangalis GA, Moran EM, Nathwani BN, et al. Angioimmunoblastic lymphadenopathy. Long-term follow-up study. Cancer 1983;52:318–321.
37. Archimbaud E, Coiffier B, Bryon PA, et al. Prognostic factors in angioimmunoblastic lymphadenopathy. Cancer 1987;59:208–212.
38. Ohsaka A, Saito K, Sakai T, et al. Clinicopathologic and therapeutic aspects of angioimmunoblastic lymphadenopathy-related lesions. Cancer 1992;69:1259–1267.
39. Aozasa K, Ohsawa M, Fujita MQ, et al. Angioimmunoblastic lymphadenopathy. Review of 44 patients with emphasis on prognostic behavior. Cancer 1989;63:1625–1629.
40. Schultz DR, Yunis AA. Immunoblastic lymphadenopathy with mixed cryoglobulinemia. A detailed case study. N Engl J Med 1975;292:8–12.
41. Paloczi K, Suranyi P, Nemes Z, et al. A study of lymphocyte subsets in patients with angioimmunoblastic lymphadenopathy. Br J Haematol 1986;62:615–618.
42. Nathwani BN, Rappaport H, Moran EM, et al. Evolution of immunoblastic lymphoma in angioimmunoblastic lymphadenopathy. Recent Results Cancer Res 1978;64:235–240.
43. Madri JA, Fromowitz F. Amyloid deposition in immunoblastic lymphadenopathy. Hum Pathol 1978;9:157–162.
44. Pangalis GA, Moran EM, Rappaport H. Blood and bone marrow findings in angioimmunoblastic lymphadenopathy. Blood 1978;51:71–83.
45. Ree HJ, Kadin ME, Kikuchi M, et al. Angioimmunoblastic lymphoma (AILD-type T-cell lymphoma) with hyperplastic germinal centers. Am J Surg Pathol 1998;22:643–655.
46. Ree HJ, Kadin ME, Kikuchi M, et al. Bcl-6 expression in reactive follicular hyperplasia, follicular lymphoma, and angioimmunoblastic T-cell lymphoma with hyperplastic germinal centers: heterogeneity of intrafollicular T-cells and their altered distribution in the pathogenesis of angioimmunoblastic T-cell lymphoma. Hum Pathol 1999;30:403–411.
47. Knecht H, Odermatt BF, Maurer R, et al. Diagnostic and prognostic value of monoclonal antibodies in immunophenotyping of angioimmunoblastic lymphadenopathy/lymphogranulomatosis X. Br J Haematol 1987;67:19–24.
48. Cabecadas JM, Isaacson PG. Phenotyping of T-cell lymphomas in paraffin sections—which antibodies? Histopathology 1991;19: 419–424.
49. Suzuki H, Namikawa R, Ueda R, et al. Clonal T-cell population in angioimmunoblastic lymphadenopathy and related lesions. Jpn J Cancer Res 1987;78:712–720.
50. Tobinai K, Minato K, Ohtsu T, et al. Clinicopathologic, immunophenotypic, and immunogenotypic analyses of immunoblastic lymphadenopathy-like T-cell lymphoma. Blood 1988;72:1000–1006.

51. Griesser H, Feller A, Lennert K, et al. Rearrangement of the beta chain of the T-cell antigen receptor and immunoglobulin genes in lymphoproliferative disorders. J Clin Invest 1986;78:1179– 1184.
52. Schlegelberger B, Feller A, Godde E, et al. Stepwise development of chromosomal abnormalities in angioimmunoblastic lymphadenopathy. Cancer Genet Cytogenet 1990;50:15–29.
53. Heim S, Mitelman F. Cytogenetically unrelated clones in hematological neoplasms. Leukemia 1989;3:6–8.
54. Schlegelberger B, Himmler A, Godde E, et al. Cytogenetic findings in peripheral T-cell lymphomas as a basis for distinguishing low-grade and high-grade lymphomas. Blood 1994;83:505–511.
55. Schlegelberger B, Zwingers T, Hohenadel K, et al. Significance of cytogenetic findings for the clinical outcome in patients with T-cell lymphoma of angioimmunoblastic lymphadenopathy type [see Comments]. J Clin Oncol 1996;14:593–599.

75

ANAPLASTIC LARGE CELL LYMPHOMA

DEFINITION

Non-Hodgkin large cell anaplastic lymphoma with characteristic nuclear pleomorphism, sinus growth pattern, and expression of CD30 antigen.

SYNONYMS

Ki-1+ large cell lymphoma
Ki-1 lymphoma

VARIANTS

Anaplastic large cell natural killer (NK)/T-cell lymphoma
Anaplastic large cell B-cell lymphoma

EPIDEMIOLOGY

Anaplastic large cell lymphoma (ALCL) represents about 5% of all non-Hodgkin lymphomas (NHLs) (1,2); in children, it accounts for 30% to 40% of all large cell lymphomas (3–5). Patients of all races, with an age range of 3 to 72 years (mean, 22 years; median, 13.5 years) and a male-to-female ratio of 2.2:1, were reported in one study of 19 Ki-1 large cell NHLs (2). In another study, including 10 cases of large cell Ki-1+ lymphoma, all patients were in their early twenties or younger (6); in a third study, comprising 41 cases, the age distribution showed two broad peaks, at 20 and 50 years, and six patients were younger than 17 years (7). In the largest and most recent series, of 123 cases of ALCL, the ages ranged from 3 months to 92 years, with a mean age of 21.3 years (8). The male-to-female ratio was 1.3:1 in one study and 1.4:1 in another (7,8).

PATHOGENESIS

Anaplastic large cell lymphomas include a heterogeneous group of tumors with different clinical presentations and outcomes, various morphologic features, T-cell, B-cell, or null cell immunophenotypes, and dissimilar cytogenetic abnormalities (8–11). However, most cases of ALCL occur in a younger population, are of T-cell immunophenotype, and as a result of a t(2;5)(p23;q35) translocation express the NPM/ALK protein. The t(2;5) fuses a part of the nucleolar protein nucleophosmin (NPM) gene on chromosome 5q35 to a portion of the anaplastic lymphoma kinase (ALK) receptor gene on chromosome 2p23, so that a chimeric NPM/ALK protein forms (8,12,13). ALK is absent from normal lymphoid and other tissues; therefore, it is specific for ALCL. A monoclonal antibody, ALK-1, has been produced that can be used to detect ALK protein. More than two-thirds of ALCLs, most of them of T-cell type, exhibit the t(2;5) and NPM/ALK gene (14), whereas ALCLs of B-cell type generally do not (11,15). Some authors consider the NPM/ALK fusion gene the most characteristic feature of ALCL and probably the major etiologic factor, and they have suggested for this entity the name *ALK lymphomas* (8). Other unifying features of this group of lymphomas are large cells with a typical morphology and expression of the CD30 or Ki-1 antigen, which is the most common characteristic and the one first recognized in the initial description of ALCL (1).

CLINICAL SYNDROME

Anaplastic large cell lymphoma may be localized or systemic, nodal or extranodal. It may arise *de novo* or follow an earlier, usually low-grade lymphoma. In most cases, only the lymph nodes are involved, or occasionally other organs, particularly the skin (2,7). In one series of 19 cases, 5 presented with adenopathy, 6 with adenopathy and skin lesions, 4 with skin lesions only, and the rest with disease in other organs (2). The skin lesions may be solitary or multiple papules or nodules (16). The lungs, bones, gastrointestinal tract, and soft tissues have also been reported as primary sites of ALCL (10,17,18). In most cases, the lymphadenopathies are peripheral; however, mediastinal, abdominal, and retro-peritoneal lymph nodes may also be primarily involved (2,3). Constitutional symptoms were noted in 59% of patients in one study (7). Laboratory tests at presentation showed high levels of lactate dehydrogenase (>250 IU/L), anemia, and pancytopenia (7). Eosinophilia is only occasionally present, and the bone marrow is involved in only 30% of cases (7). A significant number of patients (55%), particularly among those with the anaplastic large cell type of ALCL, are still in stage I or II at presentation (7,9,19). The clinical course and response to therapy are variable, reflecting the heterogeneity of ALCL. In a series of 41 treated patients, the overall median survival time was 13 months. Age and stage generally predicted the clinical outcome (7); surprisingly, however, patients with the anaplastic large cell type had the best prognosis, particularly young patients with stage I or II disease at presentation (6,7,20). Spontaneous remissions and prolonged survival despite recurrences have been reported, clinical behavior that is totally unusual for high-grade lymphomas (20). One report details the histories of three patients with ALCL who experienced remission after single-agent chemotherapy or local irradiation and survived for an unusually long time, 14 to 25 years (20). Patients with the far less common ALCL of B-cell type, a tumor of older people (mean age of 63.2 years in one study), have a worse prognosis and a much shorter survival (11,15).

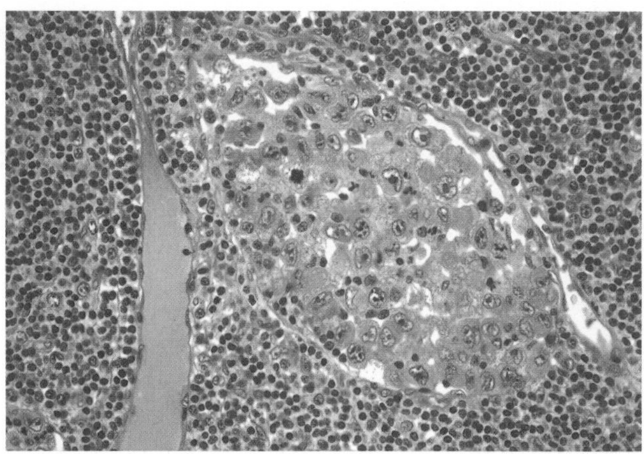

FIGURE 75.2. Anaplastic large cell lymphoma. Same section as in Fig. 75.1. Distended sinus filled with large pleomorphic cells. Hematoxylin, phloxine, and saffron stain.

HISTOPATHOLOGY

In 40% to 50% of cases, the affected lymph nodes are only partially involved by lymphoma (2,3). In the majority of cases, the T zones or paracortical areas are preferentially involved, with sparing of the lymphoid follicles and germinal centers (2) (Figs. 75.1–75.3). The large lymphoma cells may be cohesive, forming solid cords and sheets that resemble anaplastic carcinomas. In other lymph nodes or other areas of one node, the cells may be noncohesive. The sinuses may be preferentially involved, appearing largely distended by cords of attached cells, which, particularly in the peripheral sinuses, mimic the appearance of metastatic carcinoma (Figs. 75.1, 75.2, and 75.4). Some tumors, particularly the small cell variants, frequently exhibit a perivascular pattern (8). Areas of necrosis are seen. The lymph node capsule is thickened, and fibrous bands extend into the lymph node and divide it into nodules, creating a pattern that resembles nodular sclerosis Hodgkin lymphoma (HL).

The cellular morphology is striking for its pleomorphism (2) (Figs. 75.5–75.7). The cells are large and in various stages of transformation. The cytoplasm is abundant and amphophilic or deeply basophilic (Fig. 75.5), sometimes with a paranuclear pale-staining hof. The nuclei are round, lobulated, or bizarrely shaped (Figs. 75.6 and

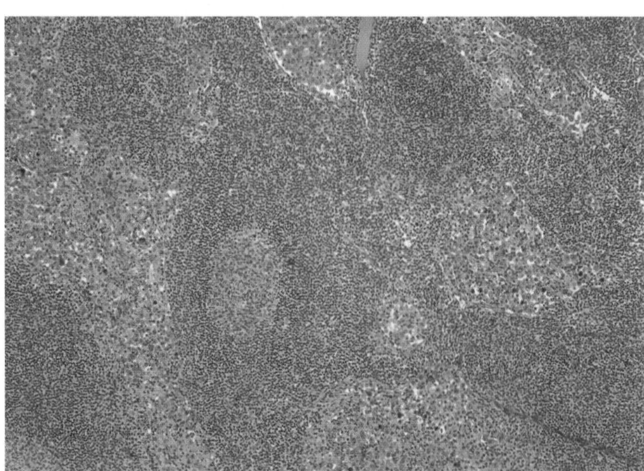

FIGURE 75.1. Anaplastic large cell lymphoma with typical sinus pattern. All sinuses are distended, filled by pleomorphic cells. Follicle (*center*) and surrounding lymphoid areas are spared. Hematoxylin, phloxine, and saffron stain.

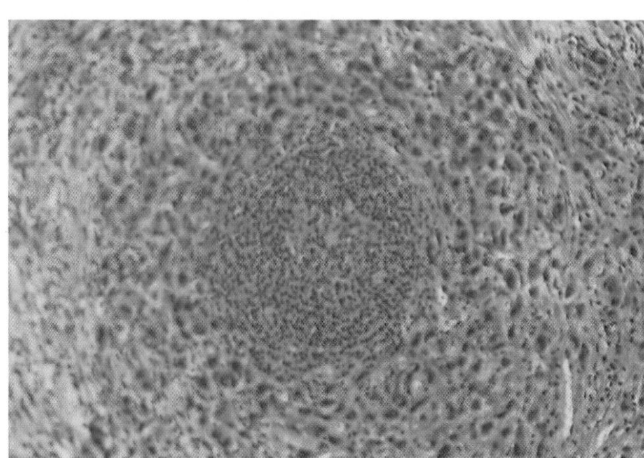

FIGURE 75.3. Anaplastic large cell lymphoma with perifollicular and perivascular distribution. Hematoxylin, phloxine, and saffron stain.

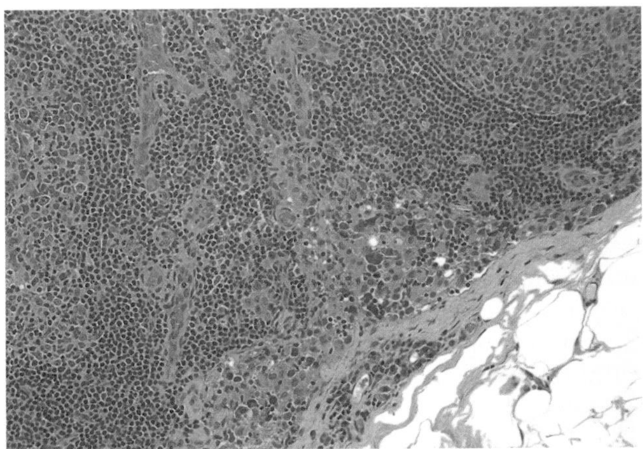

FIGURE 75.4. Anaplastic large cell lymphoma involving marginal and cortical sinuses, sparing the follicles and lymphoid tissues. Hematoxylin, phloxine, and saffron stain.

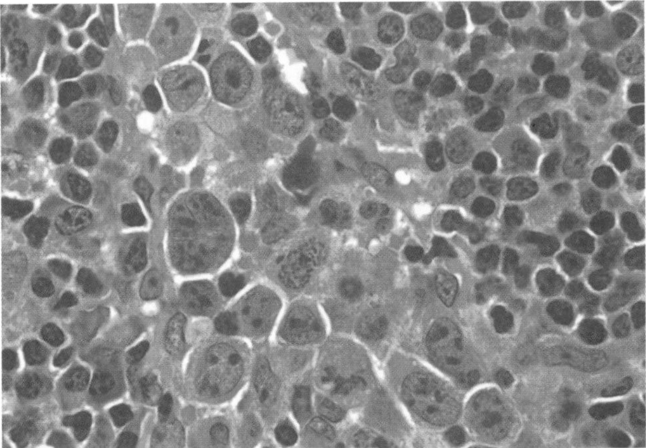

FIGURE 75.5. Anaplastic large cell lymphoma showing lymphoma cells with large or giant nuclei, several prominent nucleoli, and atypical mitoses within cortical sinus. Hematoxylin, phloxine, and saffron stain.

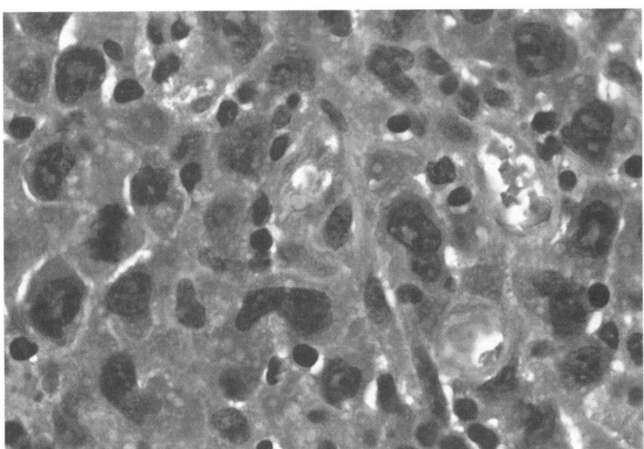

FIGURE 75.6. Anaplastic large cell lymphoma. Same section as in Fig. 75.3 showing extreme pleomorphism of tumor cell nuclei. Hematoxylin, phloxine, and saffron stain.

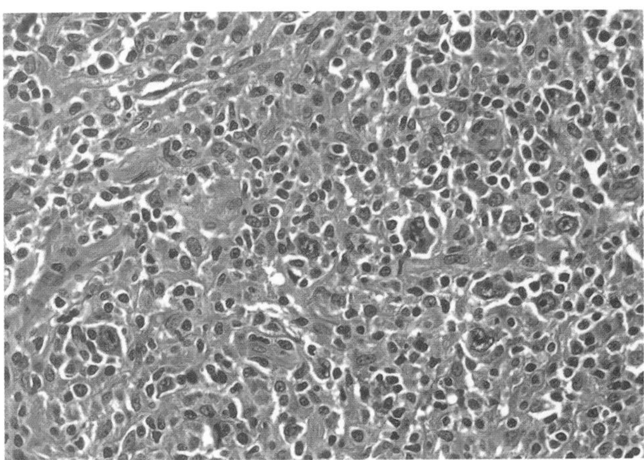

FIGURE 75.7. Anaplastic large cell lymphoma with highly pleomorphic cells, including Hodgkin-like and Reed-Sternberg–like cells. Hematoxylin, phloxine, and saffron stain.

75.7). Multinucleated giant cells are frequent, and wreathlike nuclei are sometimes noted (3). The nucleoli are prominent, resembling those of immunoblasts (2), or inclusion-like, giving the cells a Hodgkin-like or Reed-Sternberg–like appearance that can be observed in about half of the cases (3) (Fig. 75.7). The mitotic rate is uniformly high, ranging from 10 to 120 per 10 high-power fields (2). A large number of mitoses are atypical. Admixed with the large lymphoma cells are lymphocytes, plasma cells, and eosinophils, which may be numerous in some cases (2,3). Neutrophil-rich cases of ALCL, characterized by numerous neutrophils in the absence of necrosis, probably attracted by a particular cytokine, have been also described (21).

As noted in various studies, ALCLs are heterogeneous, not only clinically and immunologically but also morphologically (3,6,22). In addition to the characteristic anaplastic large cell type of CD20+ lymphomas are tumors that are composed of smaller, more uniform lymphoma cells and comprise fewer multinucleated giant cells (3,6). They do not include wreathlike nuclei, and the nucleoli are less prominent. Interestingly, this subtype of CD30+ NHL, designated *group B* (cf. *group A* of the anaplastic large cell type, previously described) is more common in elderly patients who present with advanced disease and have a significantly less favorable prognosis (3). An infrequent spindle cell variant resembling sarcoma has been also described (23).

In the skin, the infiltrates of CD30+ cells may be extensive, involving the dermis and subcutis but not the epidermis. The cytology of the cutaneous infiltrates is similar to that of the lymph nodes (2). The morphologic heterogeneity of ALCL may be related to the process of activation or dedifferentiation of the lymphoid cells, which results in variants with apparent clinical correlations in terms of response to treatment and survival (3,6,20).

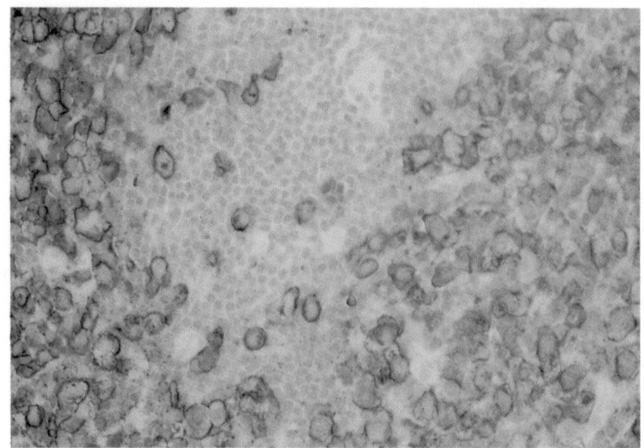

FIGURE 75.8. Anaplastic large cell lymphoma. Same lymph node as in Fig. 75.3. Strong CD30 staining of cell membranes. Anti-CD30/peroxidase stain.

CYTOLOGY

On imprints, the lymphoma cells have deeply basophilic cytoplasm with prominent vacuoles. The nuclei are round or lobate. Binucleated and multinucleated cells are common. The nuclear chromatin is clumped. Nucleoli are prominent (2).

ELECTRON MICROSCOPY

A study of 26 cases of high-grade, CD30+ (Ki-1+) lymphomas showed anaplastic nuclear and cytoplasmic changes similar or identical to those observed in HL (24). These changes suggest cellular activation; the unusual nuclear shapes are similar to those of lacunar, Hodgkin, or Reed-Sternberg cells. An immunohistochemical technique for labeling cells with gold was used to demonstrate CD30+ (Ki-1+) particles in the Golgi complex and occasionally in the cell membranes (24). In a different ultrastructural study, some of the anaplastic large cells with nuclear and nucleolar features of cell activation also exhibited long, slender, microvillus-like processes, similar to those of the cells of so-called anemone cell lymphomas (24–26). Like these, Ki-1+ (CD30+) lymphomas with microvilli were of the infrequent B-cell type (22).

IMMUNOHISTOCHEMISTRY

- CD30: In all cases examined [19 cases in one study (2) and 41 cases in another (7)], 80% to 100% of the large lymphoma cells expressed Ki-1/CD30 when stained with the Ki-1 monoclonal antibody against an HL tissue culture cell line (1) (Figs. 75.8 and 75.9). Similarly, on paraffin sections, most lymphoma cells expressed the Ki-1 marker when stained with Ber-112, a monoclonal antibody that recognizes a formalin-resistant epitope of Ki-1 (27). With the Ber-H2 antibody, the cells of CD30+ lymphomas exhibit strong membrane staining and frequently a paranuclear dotlike staining of the Golgi area (3) (Fig. 75.9). In the largest series of cases examined, virtually all ALCL cells strongly expressed CD30, and the staining pattern was as in the earlier studies with Ki-1 and Ber-142 antibodies, mainly on the cell membrane and in

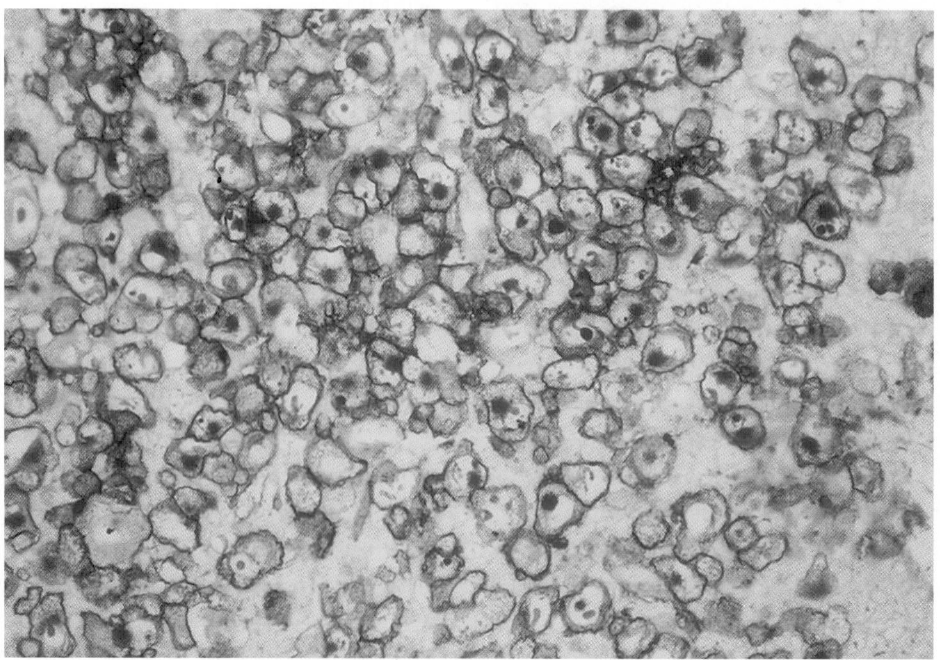

FIGURE 75.9. Anaplastic large cell lymphoma with strong CD30 membrane staining of tumor cells. Anti-CD30/peroxidase stain.

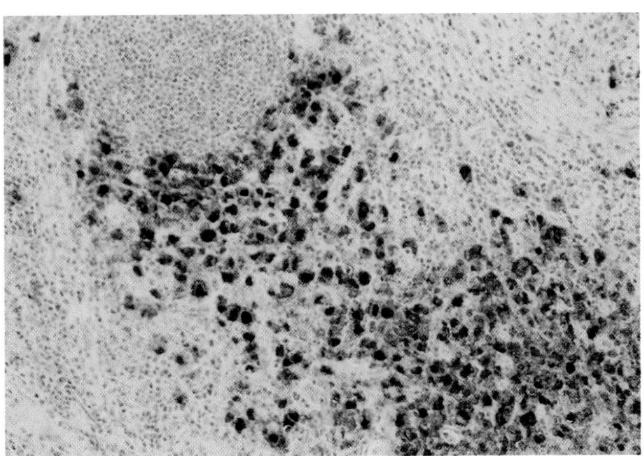

FIGURE 75.10. Anaplastic large cell lymphoma stained for anaplastic lymphoma kinase (*ALK*) protein. Both cytoplasm and nucleus are heavily stained. Anti-ALK protein/peroxidase stain.

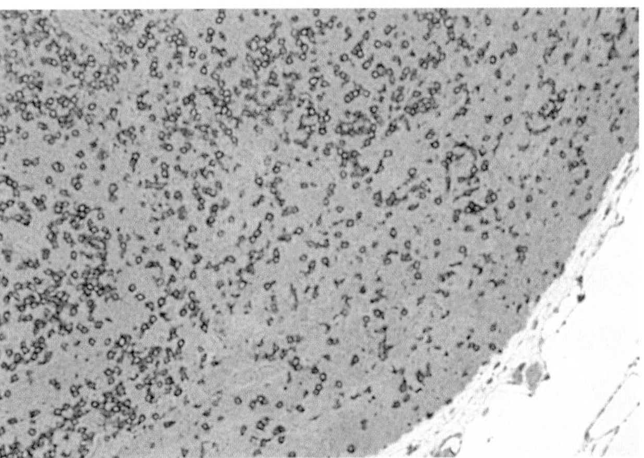

FIGURE 75.12. Anaplastic large cell lymphoma. Same section as in Fig. 75.10. CD3 staining of incidental small lymphocytes but not of lymphoma cells. Anti-CD3/peroxidase stain.

the Golgi area (8). The B-cell types of ALCL also expressed CD30 antigen (15), so that it is the most common marker for all variants of ALCL tumors.

- ALK protein: All 124 cases in the study mentioned above expressed ALK protein, with labeling of both cytoplasm and nucleus in 82% and only cytoplasmic staining in 16% (8). In the small cell variant of ALCL, some of the cells stained variably (8), whereas all B-cell cases of ALCL were negative for ALK (Fig. 75.10).
- Epithelial membrane antigen (EMA): In one study, all cases of large cell ALCL expressed EMA (8); in another series, only 58% did so (7).
- T-cell markers: A majority of cases (54% to 70%), including small cell and mixed variants, are of T-cell lineage. Some T-cell markers, such as CD3, may not be expressed; others (CD43) may more often be expressed (28) (Fig. 75.11). In 78% of cases, at least two of the common pan-T-cell antigens (CD2, CD3, CD5, CD7) are not expressed (7).
- B-cell markers: About 10% of cases express B-cell markers (Figs. 75.12 and 75.13), and 10% to 20% of cases, considered null, are negative for both T-cell and B-cell antigens (Figs. 75.14 and 75.15).
- CD15: The carbohydrate antigen typically labeling Reed-

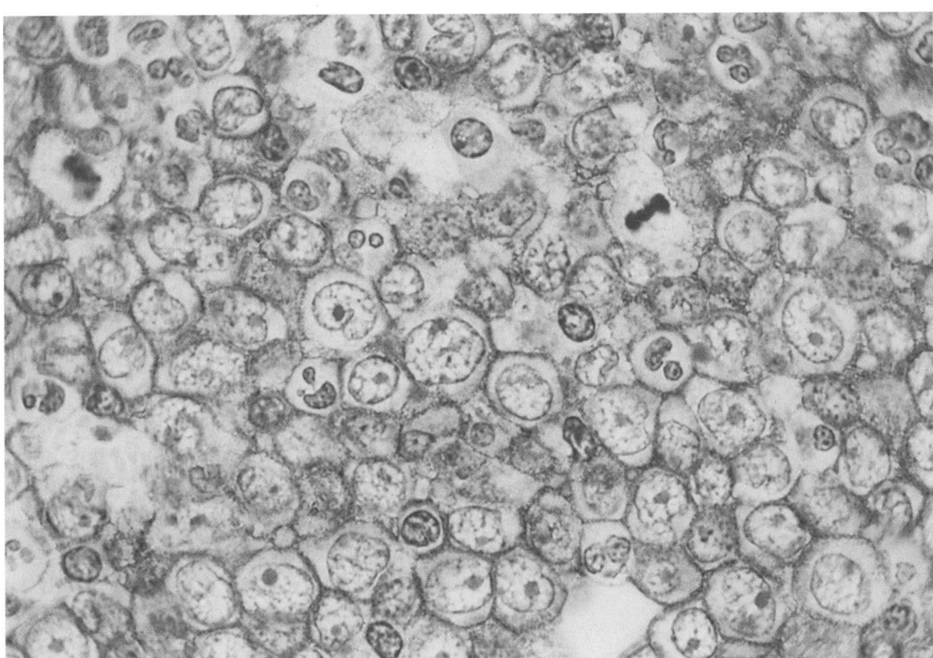

FIGURE 75.11. Anaplastic large cell lymphoma with large nuclei, prominent nucleoli, and multiple atypical mitoses; cellular membrane staining for CD43 indicates T-cell lineage. Anti-CD43/peroxidase stain.

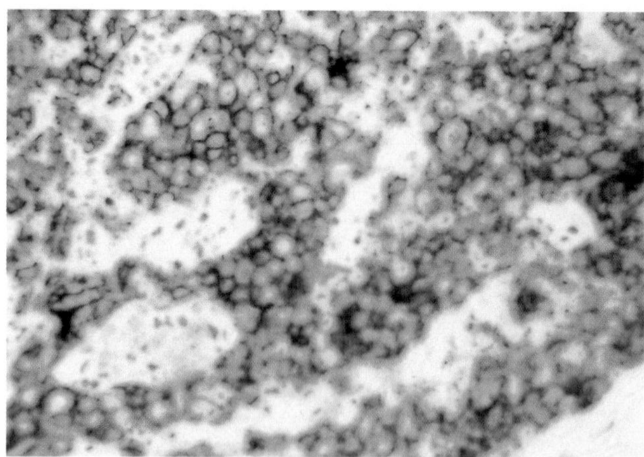

FIGURE 75.13. Anaplastic large cell lymphoma. Same section as in Fig. 75.10. Membrane staining of CD20 marker in tumor cells. B-cell lineage. Anti-CD20/peroxidase stain.

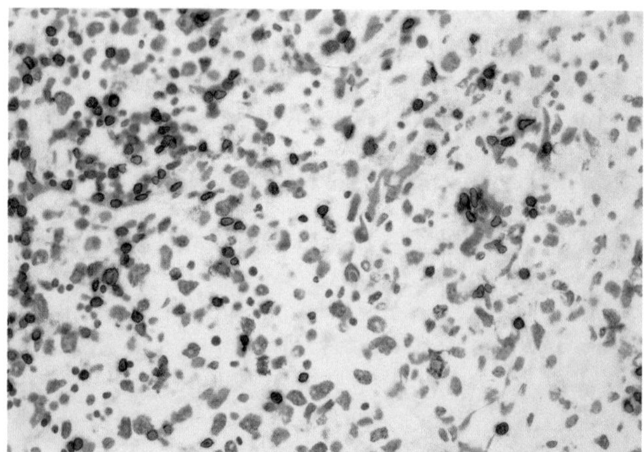

FIGURE 75.14. Anaplastic large cell lymphoma. Same lymph node as in Fig. 75.3. CD3 staining of incidental small lymphocytes, but not of lymphoma cells. Null cell lineage. Anti-CD3/peroxidase stain.

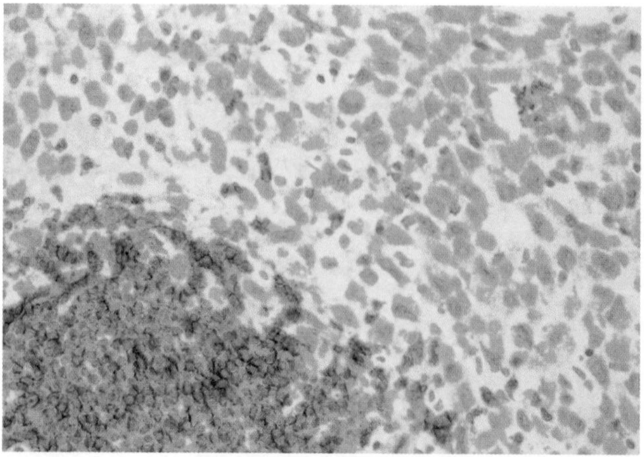

FIGURE 75.15. Anaplastic large cell lymphoma. Same lymph node as in Fig. 75.3. CD20 staining of uninvolved follicle but not of lymphoma cells. Null cell lineage. Anti-CD20/peroxidase stain.

Sternberg cells is not expressed, a feature that provides a reliable criterion in the differential diagnosis with HL.

- Leukocyte common antigen (LCA) is expressed in 54% of cases.
- Blood group-related antigens such as H and Y, detected by antibody BNH.9, are expressed in 80% of cases.
- Activation markers such as 1a (HLA-DR), TAC (interleukin 2) and T9 (transferrin) are often expressed (2).
- Lysozyme is not expressed.
- Epstein-Barr viral infection: No evidence has been found by *in situ* hybridization or immunostaining (8).

CYTOGENETICS

The t(2;5), in which the NPM gene on chromosome 5q35 is juxtaposed with the tyrosine kinase ALK gene on chromosome 2q23, is characteristic of ALCL. The result is aberrant production of the ALK fusion product (12). The t(2;5) occurs predominantly in ALCLs of T-cell or null cell type. B-cell ALCLs lack t(2;5) (11,15).

DIFFERENTIAL DIAGNOSIS

- Infectious mononucleosis lymphadenitis: Diffuse proliferation of activated (transformed) lymphoid cells is noted, mostly in the T-cell areas and sinuses. Immunoblasts with highly pleomorphic Reed-Sternberg–like nuclei may be present, some of which may be CD30+ (29). However, the cells in infectious mononucleosis do not form cohesive cords, and only isolated cells are CD30+.
- HL, nodular sclerosis type may present as a syncytial variant in which highly anaplastic cells, including Hodgkin cells and Reed-Sternberg cells, grow in sheets resembling ALCL (30). However, the immunophenotypes are different. The Hodgkin/Reed-Sternberg cells are LCA−, EMA−, negative for T-cell markers, BNH9−, CD15+, and CD30+. The ALCL cells are LCA+, EMA+, positive for T-cell markers (approximately 60%), BNH9+, CD15−, and CD30+.
- Large cell lymphoma may be morphologically similar to ALCL; the borderline between the two entities is not sharp. ALCL more often has a sinus pattern, and its cells are larger, with more pleomorphic and sometimes bizarre nuclei. The majority of large cell lymphomas are of B-cell type, whereas most ALCLs are of T-cell type. CD30 and ALK are expressed in ALCL, but not in large cell lymphoma.
- Microvillous (anemone cell) lymphoma: Microvilli on the surface of some ALCLs may resemble those of the microvillous lymphomas under electron microscopic examination. Histologically, both ALCL and microvillous lymphomas have features of large cell anaplastic transformed

Checklist

ANAPLASTIC LARGE CELL LYMPHOMA

Heterogeneous group of NHLs with CD30 markers
Large anaplastic cell type most common
Patients young adults
Peripheral lymph nodes affected
Partial nodal involvement
Paracortical areas (T zones) and sinuses involved (sinus pattern)
Follicles and germinal centers (B zones) spared
Skin occasionally involved
Cohesive cell cords and sheets
Anaplastic large cells
Pleomorphic, bizarre, wreathlike nuclei
Prominent nucleoli
Numerous atypical mitoses
T-cell phenotype predominant
Positive for CD30, LCA, EMA, BNH9
Positive for activation markers: HLA-DR, TAC, T9
Negative for CD15
T-cell markers positive (60%), B-cell markers positive (10%)
Translocation t(2;5)(p23;q35)
Chimeric protein NPM-ALK detected by antibody ALK-1

lymphocytes. The latter, however, are negative for Ki-1 and have in general a B-cell phenotype (9).

- Malignant histiocytosis is more common in children, is usually systemic, and has a rapidly fatal course (31). Histologically, sheets of atypical cells with aberrant nuclei and a sinusoidal pattern of lymph node growth are seen. However, in contrast to CD30+ lymphomas, the cells exhibit histiocytic features such as phagocytosis, including erythrophagocytosis. The malignant histiocytes are CD30−. α_1-Antitrypsin may stain cells of both malignancies and is therefore an unreliable criterion for the differential diagnosis (1).
- Metastatic carcinoma: The cohesive cords of anaplastic CD30+ lymphoma cells within the peripheral sinuses of lymph nodes may suggest metastatic anaplastic carcinoma, and a further cause of potential confusion is that both tumors stain for EMA (2). Cytokeratins and LCA antibodies are needed for the differential diagnosis. Both stainings are required because ALCL may occasionally be negative for the LCA marker.
- Metastatic melanoma may be also confused with ALCL because of the cohesive sheets of cells and the location in the marginal sinus. Immunostainings with LCA vs. HMB45 and S100 protein can resolve the differential diagnosis.

REFERENCES

1. Stein H, Mason DY, Gerdes J, et al. The expression of the Hodgkin's disease-associated antigen Ki-1 in reactive and neoplastic lymphoid tissue: Evidence that Reed-Sternberg cells and histiocytic malignancies are derived from activated lymphoid cells. Blood 1985;66:848–858.
2. Agnarsson BA, Kadin ME. Ki-1-positive large cell lymphoma. A morphologic and immunologic study of 19 cases. Am J Surg Pathol 1988;12:264–274.
3. Kadin ME, Sako D, Berliner N, et al. Childhood Ki-1 lymphoma presenting with skin lesions and peripheral lymphadenopathy. Blood 1986;68:1042–1049.
4. Kadin ME. Ki-1/CD30+ (anaplastic) large-cell lymphoma. Maturation of a clinicopathologic entity with prospects of effective therapy. J Clin Oncol 1994;12:884.
5. Sandlund JT, Pui C-H, Roberts WM, et al. Clinicopathologic features and treatment outcome of children with large cell lymphoma and the t (2;5)(p23; q35). Blood 1994;84:2467.
6. Bitter MA, Franklin WA, Larson RA, et al. Morphology in Ki-1 (CD3 0)-positive non-Hodgkin's lymphoma is correlated with clinical features and the presence of a unique chromosomal abnormality, t(2;5)(p23;q35). Am J Surg Pathol 1990;14:305–316.
7. Chott A, Kaserer K, Augustin 1, et al. Ki-1-positive large cell lymphoma. A clinicopathologic study of 41 cases. Am J Surg Pathol 1990;14:439–448.
8. Benharroch D, Meguerian-Bedoyan Z, Lamant L, et al. ALK-positive lymphoma: a single disease with a broad spectrum of morphology. Blood 1998;91:2076–2084.

9. Kinney MC, Greer JP, Glick AD, et al. Anaplastic large cell Ki-1 malignant lymphomas: recognition, biological and clinical implications. Pathol Annu 1991;26:1–24.
10. Penny RJ, Blaustein JC, Longtine JA, et al. Ki-1-positive large cell lymphomas, a heterogeneous group of neoplasms. Morphologic, immunophenotypic, genotypic and clinical features of 24 cases. Cancer 1991;68:362–373.
11. Delsol, G, Lamant L, Mariame B, et al. A new subtype of large B-cell lymphoma expressing the ALK kinase and lacking the 2;5 translocation. Blood 1997;89:1483–1490.
12. Morris SW, Kirstein MN, Valentine MB, et al. Fusion of a kinase gene, ALK, to a nucleolar protein gene, NPM, in non-Hodgkin's lymphoma. Science 1994;263:1281.
13. Pulford K, Lamant L, Morris SW, et al. Detection of anaplastic lymphoma kinase (ALK) and nucleolar protein nucleophosmin (NPM)-ALK proteins in normal and neoplastic cells with the monoclonal antibody ALKI. Blood 1997;89:1394.
14. Chan WC. The t(2;4) or NPM-ALK translocation in lymphomas. Diagnostic considerations. Adv Anat Pathol 1996;3: 396.
15. Lai R, Medeiros J, Dabbagh L, et al. Sinusoidal CD30-positive large B-cell lymphoma: a morphologic mimic of anaplastic large cell lymphoma. Mod Pathol 2000;13:223–228.
16. Beliaards RC, Kandewitz P, Berti E, et al. Primary cutaneous CD30-positive large cell lymphoma. Definition of a new type of cutaneous lymphoma with a favorable prognosis. Cancer 1993; 71:2097–2104.
17. Kanavaros P, Lavergne A, Galian A, et al. Primary gastric peripheral T-cell malignant lymphoma with helper/inducer phenotype. First case report with a complete histologic, ultrastructural and immunochemical study. Cancer 1988;61:1602–1610.
18. Chan JK, Ng CS, Hui PK, et al. Anaplastic large cell Ki-1 lymphoma of bone. Cancer 1991;68:2186–2191.
19. Hansmann ML, Fellbaum C, Bohm A. Large cell anaplastic lymphoma: evaluation of immunophenotype on paraffin and frozen sections in comparison with ultrastructural features. Virchows Arch A Pathol Anat Histopathol 1991;418:427–433.
20. Salhany KE, Collins RD, Greer JP, et al. Long-term survival in Ki-1 lymphoma. Cancer 1991;67:516–522.
21. Mann KP, Hall B, Kamino H, et al. Neutrophil-rich, Ki-1-positive anaplastic large cell malignant lymphoma. Am J Surg Pathol 1995;19:407–416.
22. Kinney MC, Glick AD, Stein H, et al. Comparison of anaplastic large cell Ki-1 lymphomas and microvillous lymphomas in their immunologic and ultrastructural features. Am J Surg Pathol 1990;14:1047–1060.
23. Chan JK, Buchanan R, Fletcher CD. Sarcomatoid variant of anaplastic large cell Ki-1 lymphomas. Report of a case. Am J Surg Pathol 1990;14:983–988.
24. Rivas C, Piris MA, Gamallo C, et al. Ultrastructure of 26 cases of Ki-1 lymphomas: morphoimmunologic correlation. Ultrastruct Pathol 1990;14:381–397.
25. Taxy JB, Almanaseer 1Y. "Anemone" cell (villiform) tumors: electron microscopy and immunohistochemistry of five cases. Ultrastruct Pathol 1984;7:143–150.
26. Sibley R, Rosai J, Froehlich W. A case for the panel: anemone cell tumor. Ultrastruct Pathol 1980;1:449–453.
27. Schwarting R, Gerdes J, Durkop H, et al. Ber-H2: a new anti-Ki (CD30) monoclonal antibody directed at a formol-resistant epitope. Blood 1989;74:1678–1689.
28. Macon WR, Casey TT, Kinney MC, et al. Leu 22 (L60) a more sensitive marker than UCHL-1 for peripheral T-cell lymphomas, particularly large cell types. Am J Clin Pathol 1991;95: 696–701.
29. Abbondanzo SL, Sato N, Straus SE, et al. Acute infectious mononucleosis: CD30 (Ki-1) antigen expression and histologic correlations. Am J Clin Pathol 1990;93:698–702.
30. Strickler JG, Michie SA, Warnke RA, et al. The "syncytial variant" of nodular sclerosing Hodgkin's disease. Am J Surg Pathol 1986;10:470–477.
31. Turner RR, Woods GS, Beckstead JC, et al. Histiocytic malignancies. Morphologic, immunologic, and enzymatic heterogeneity. Am J Surg Pathol 1984;8:485–500.

PART

VI

GRANULOCYTIC, HISTIOCYTIC, AND DENDRITIC CELL NEOPLASMS

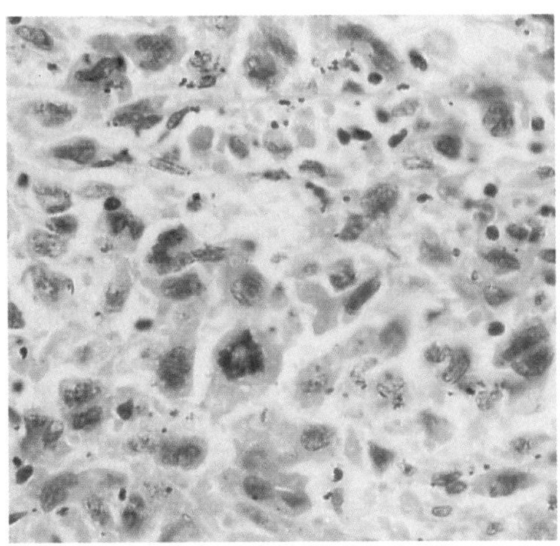

Like other lymphoid organs, lymph nodes comprise, in addition to the various populations of lymphocytes, cells derived from the monocytic lineage. These cells originate in the bone marrow from myelomonocytic progenitors and differentiate subsequently into various cell types, some circulating in the lymph and blood and others fixed in various tissues. They are generally referred to as the *mononuclear phagocyte system* and have been classified into various categories according to their morphology and function. Some of these mononuclear cells become macrophages, with the important role of removing and digesting particulate antigens. Others become antigen-presenting cells, with the main function of facilitating contact between foreign antigenic substances and the antigen-sensitive lymphoid cells. As organs specialized in the presentation and processing of antigens, the lymph nodes comprise all the variants of the mononuclear phagocyte system cells—histiocytes, macrophages, dendritic reticulum cells, and interdigitating reticulum cells. They are referred to as *accessory cells* because of their important role in the immune response, and they represent a major part of the lymph node structure. Occasionally, they are a source of neoplasms. However, in comparison with lymphoid neoplasms, which have a high incidence, the tumors of histiocytes and reticulum cells are rare.

Regarding their nomenclature, it must be kept in mind that the term *histiocytic lymphoma,* previously applied to all the large cell tumors of the lymphoid organs, is now restricted to those tumors in which the true histiocytic nature of cells can be demonstrated. This means that neoplasms of accessory cells must exhibit the morphologic and immune phenotypes associated with their lineage and may not have lymphoid gene rearrangements or express B- or T-cell markers. When these criteria are applied, very few tumors qualify as genuine neoplasms of accessory cells. Because of their small numbers, few studies have been conducted. Therefore, the neoplasms of accessory cells in the lymph nodes are not yet well characterized and clearly defined.

76

GRANULOCYTIC SARCOMA

DEFINITION

Neoplasm in which immature myeloid cells (acute myeloblastic leukemia) form a tumor in an extramedullary site.

SYNONYMS

Chloroma
Extramedullary myeloid cell tumor
Myeloblastoma

PATHOGENESIS

These tumors were originally called *chloromas* because of their greenish color, caused by the presence of myeloperoxidase; the color fades on exposure to air. Henry Rappaport renamed this tumor granulocytic sarcoma (GS) to emphasize the ability of immature myeloid cells to form "invasive and destructive tumor masses" (1). In modern usage, *GS* refers to either a tumor mass or a leukemic infiltration manifested by extramedullary acute myeloblastic leukemia (AML) (2,3). Although granulocytic precursors (i.e., myeloblasts and promyelocytes) proliferate in both GS and AML, GS is rare in comparison with AML. In two large studies, GS occurred in about 3% of patients with myeloid leukemias (4,5). After the atomic bomb explosions in Hiroshima and Nagasaki, GS developed in about 7% of patients with myeloid leukemia (6). In another series, which included 478 patients with myeloid leukemias, GS occurred in 3%—twice as often in patients with chronic myeloid leukemia as in those with AML (4).

Acute monoblastic leukemia predisposes to the development of GS (7). Chromosomal translocation t(8;21)(p22;q22) and expression of CD56 may have a synergistic effect and promote recurrent GS (8). When myeloblasts express T-cell markers, CD13, and CD14, patients have a greater incidence of GS (9,10).

CLINICAL SYNDROME

In a review of 61 GSs in 50 patients, the ages of the 29 male and 21 female patients ranged from 2 to 81 years (mean, 48 years) (2). In most series, a predominance of children and young adults is noted, and males outnumber females (1,4–6,11). In a literature review of 154 cases of primary GS, the male-to-female ratio was 1:1, and the median age was 36 years (7). In children up to age 16 presenting simultaneously with AML and GS, the orbit is the most common anatomic site (12). Primary GS (without bone marrow AML) involves, with decreasing frequency, skin, lymph nodes, spine, small intestine, orbit, bone, breast, cervix, nasal sinuses, mediastinum, and brain (7).

Granulocytic sarcoma occurs in three clinical settings, all related to myeloproliferative diseases: (a) before AML in nonleukemic patients, (b) during myelodysplastic or chronic myeloproliferative disorders (13), and (c) in association with AML (2,14). In a multiinstitutional study of GS, 22 tumors occurred in 15 patients with no known disease, 26 in 24 patients with a recognized myeloproliferative disorder, and 13 in 11 patients with AML (2). AML developed in the vast majority of nonleukemic patients within 1 to 49 months (mean interval, 10.5 months) (2). AML eventually develops in most untreated patients with GS. However, in one study, 66% of 154 patients presenting with GS who received chemotherapy did not progress to AML (7). AML recurring as GS portends eventual bone marrow relapse and should be treated (7). The appearance of GS in a patient with a chronic myeloproliferative disorder, such as polycythemia vera, myelofibrosis, or chronic myeloid leukemia, signifies a blastic crisis and a poor prognosis (2).

HISTOPATHOLOGY

Usually, GS replaces the lymph node architecture with sheets of myeloblasts, including foci of necrosis. Often, GS partially infiltrates lymph node sinuses, paracortex, and medulla, leaving residual germinal centers (14) (Fig. 76.1 A–D). The blasts have medium to large nuclei with multilobate, round, reniform, or folded contours, small to inconspicuous nucleoli, and a high nuclear-to-cytoplasmic ratio

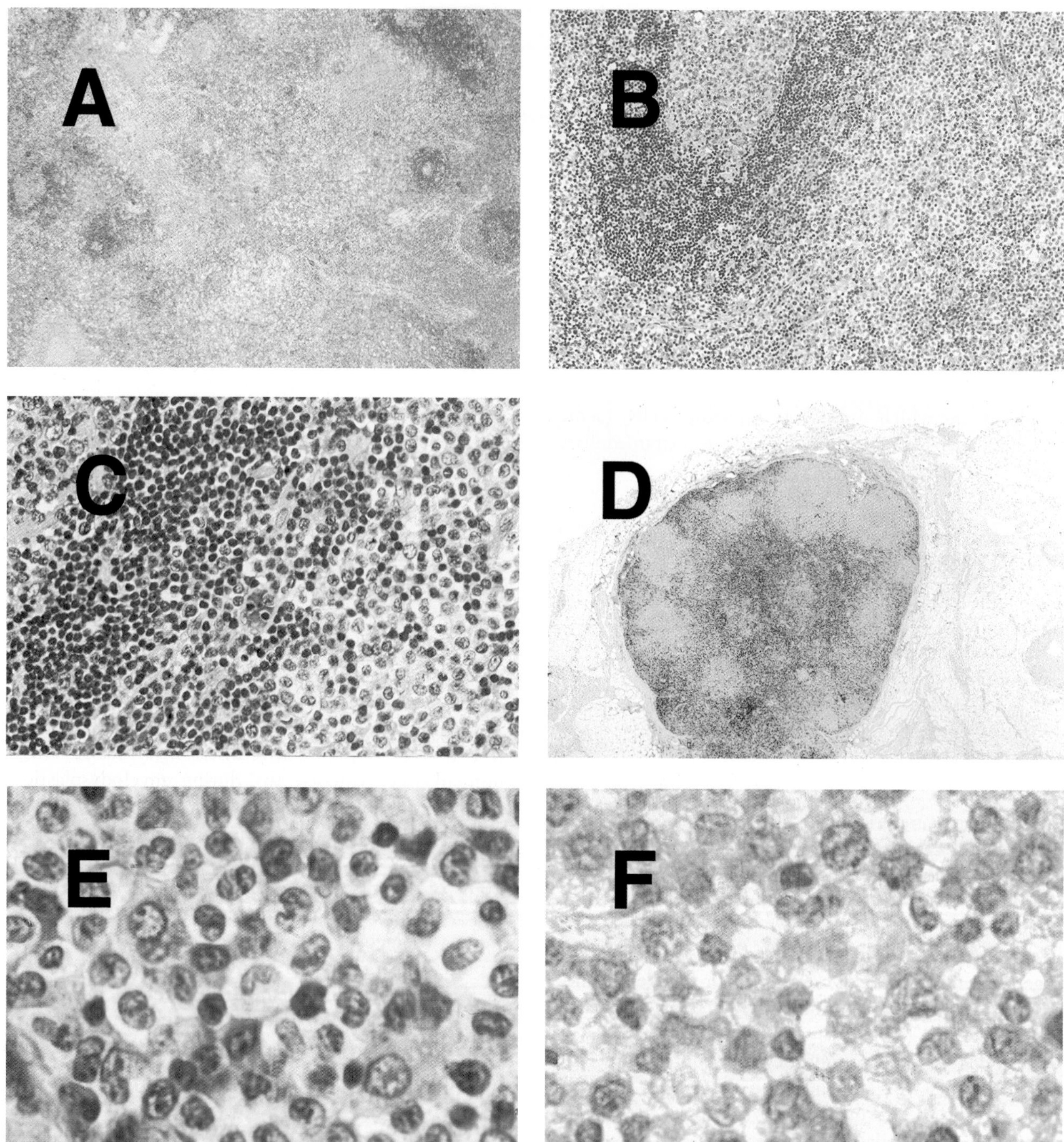

FIGURE 76.1. Granulocytic sarcoma (GS). Right cervical lymph node from a 78-year-old woman in whom acute myeloblastic leukemia had been diagnosed 1 year earlier. **A:** Scanning magnification reveals GS infiltrating lymph node paracortex and medulla. Hematoxylin and eosin stain. **B:** GS (*right*) does not invade residual reactive lymphoid follicle with germinal center or mantle zone (*left*). Hematoxylin and eosin stain. **C:** Sharp border between GS (*right*) and reactive lymphoid follicle (*left*). **D:** Anti-myeloperoxidase antibody stains GS (*brown*) in paracortex and medulla, exposing uninvolved follicles in cortex. Immunoperoxidase stain. **E:** Medium-sized GS blasts (myeloblasts) with fine and delicate nuclear chromatin, inconspicuous nucleoli, and scant cytoplasm. Some eosinophilic myelocytes are also seen. Hematoxylin and eosin stain. **F:** Many GS blasts (myeloblasts) retain chloroacetate esterase enzyme activity (*red*), even in formalin-fixed, paraffin-embedded tissue sections. Leder stain.

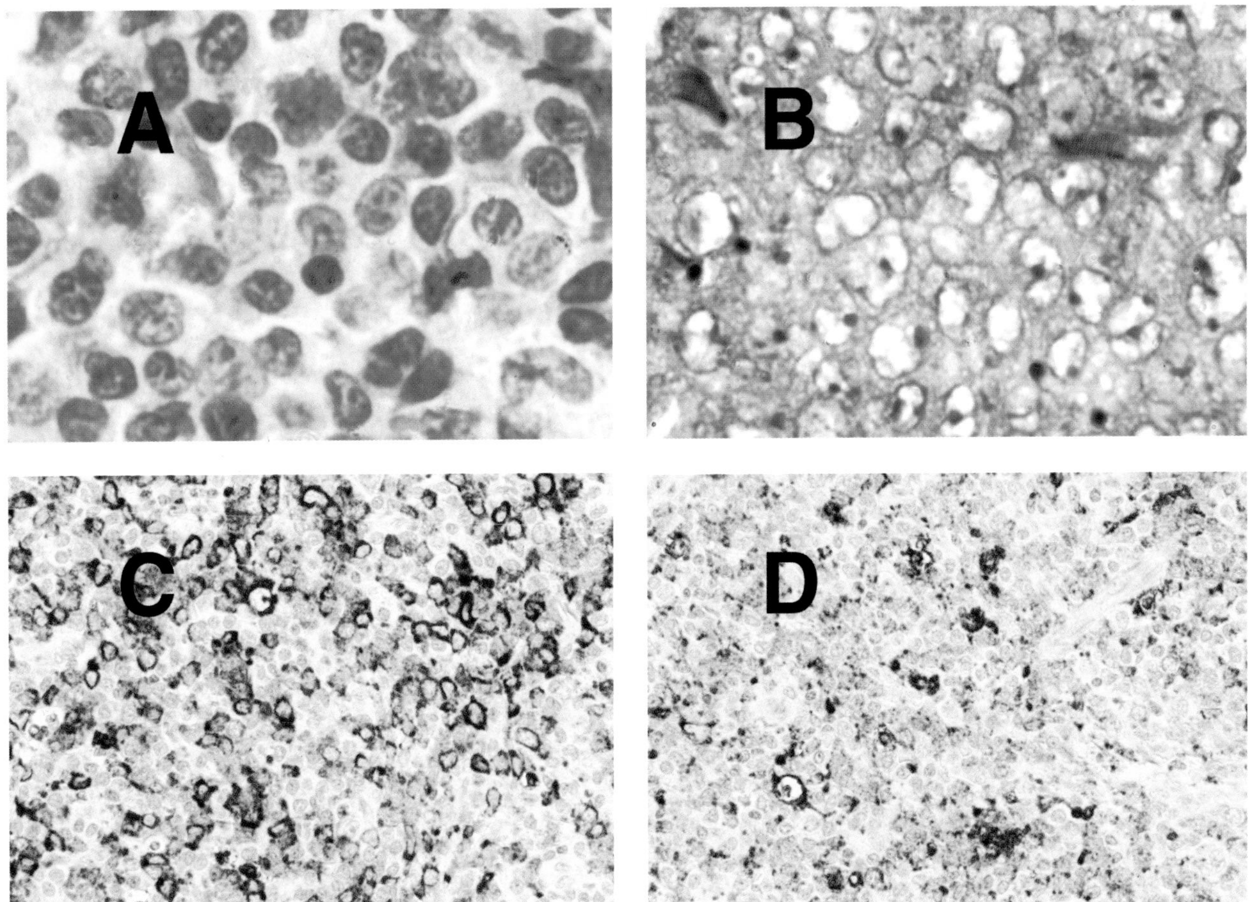

FIGURE 76.2. Granulocytic sarcoma. **A:** Inguinal lymph node from a 49-year-old man with no other disease. Sheets of myeloblasts and scattered eosinophilic myelocytes. **B:** Retroperitoneal mass in a 34-year-old woman whose bone marrow simultaneously contains acute myeloblastic leukemia. Large blasts with vesicular nuclear chromatin mimic a large cell lymphoma. These cells expressed myeloperoxidase, CD68, and lysozyme. **C:** Same specimen as in **A**. Anti-myeloperoxidase antibody stains about half of the blasts. Immunoperoxidase stain. **D:** Same specimen as in **A**. Anti-CD68 (KP-1) antibody faintly stains many blasts. The most intense reaction identifies scattered, non-neoplastic histiocytes. Immunoperoxidase stain.

(Figs. 76.1 E,F and 76.2 A,B). Auer rods are not visible in tissue sections stained with hematoxylin and eosin. Mitoses are frequent (2,14). GSs have been classified as *well differentiated* when numerous eosinophilic myelocytes could be seen in any section of a given case (Figs. 76.1E and 76.2A), *poorly differentiated* when only rare eosinophilic myelocytes were present, and *blastic* when no evidence of granulocytic differentiation was evident (Fig. 76.2 B) (2,15).

Granulocytic sarcomas, particularly those that are poorly differentiated or blastic, are often misdiagnosed as large cell lymphomas (Fig. 76.2B). Thus, 46% of 154 cases of GS were originally misdiagnosed (7). In some, GS displayed cleaved nuclei, like those in large cleaved cell lymphomas (2); in others, plasmacytoid features, as in plasmacytoma (16); and in still others, the blastic aspect of lymphoblastic lymphoma (2).

CYTOLOGY

The primitive myeloid cells that compose GS (i.e., myeloblasts, promyelocytes, and occasionally myelocytes) are best observed on Giemsa-stained imprints and smears. There, the cells exhibit the typical appearance of blast cells, with strongly basophilic cytoplasm, folded nuclei, and large nucleoli. The cytoplasm contains azurophilic (primary) granules and, in more mature cells, a few differentiated (secondary) granules. Among the more differentiated cells are eosinophilic myelocytes and metamyelocytes, the recognition of which is helpful in establishing the diagnosis of myeloid leukemia. Auer rods resulting from the fusion of azurophilic granules are also present. Fine needle aspiration in combination with flow cytometry yields an accurate diagnosis of GS (17).

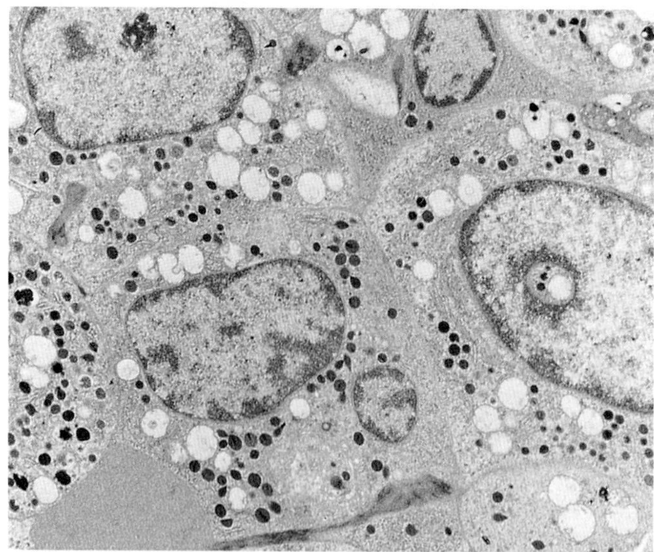

FIGURE 76.3. Chloroma in rat lymph node shows blast cells with large atypical nuclei and numerous intracytoplasmic electron-dense granules. ×6,000. (From Ioachim HL, Sabbath M, Anderson B, et al. Viral and chemical leukemia in the rat: comparative study. J Natl Cancer Inst 1971;47:161–177, with permission.)

ELECTRON MICROSCOPY

Examination of GS shows nuclei with dispersed heterochromatin and prominent nucleoli. The cytoplasm includes a distended endoplasmic reticulum, numerous ribosomes, and frequent membrane-bound, electron-dense granules (Fig. 76.3). The granules contain crystalline rectangular bars (Fig. 76.4); in cross-section, these exhibit cores composed of longitudinal arrays of dense bands, similar to those described in the granules of eosinophils (18) and in the chloromas of rats (19). The Auer rods (Fig. 76.4) are similar longer crystals bound by a membrane and showing a periodic internal structure. In AML M0 or M1 (French–American–British classification), a few granules are present, but no ferritin particles or rhopheocytosis (20,21). Intercellular junctions of opposing dense patches of the cytoplasmic plasmalemma were observed in a case of acute promyelocytic leukemia producing GS (22).

CYTOCHEMISTRY

Chloromas and chloroleukemias characteristically exhibit a green color that fades on exposure to air within 2 to 3 hours. It may be preserved by storing the tissues in glycerol and restored by applying hydrogen peroxide or sodium metabisulfite (1). The pigmentation is caused by myeloperoxidase (initially called *verdoperoxide*), a green peroxidative enzyme present in the cytoplasmic granules of chloroma cells. Myeloperoxidase is also present, although in smaller amounts, in normal granulocytes. Under ultraviolet light, the chloromatous tissues exhibit bright red fluorescence because of the presence of abundant protoporphyrins.

Chloroacetate esterase enzyme activity can be detected in neoplastic myeloblasts and promyelocytes in some cases of AML and GS, in the secondary granules of non-neoplastic myeloid cells, and in mast cells (23). The Leder stain, which uses naphthyl-ASD-chloroacetate as a substrate (NASD reaction), yields a red cytoplasmic precipitate that identifies granulocytes and their precursors in formalin-fixed, paraffin-embedded tissue sections (24) (Fig. 76.1F). The intensity of the NASD reaction (Leder stain) and the number of myeloid precursors that stain is generally adequate in well differentiated GS (14,15). Unfortunately, blastic or poorly differentiated GSs often fail to react with the Leder stain, so

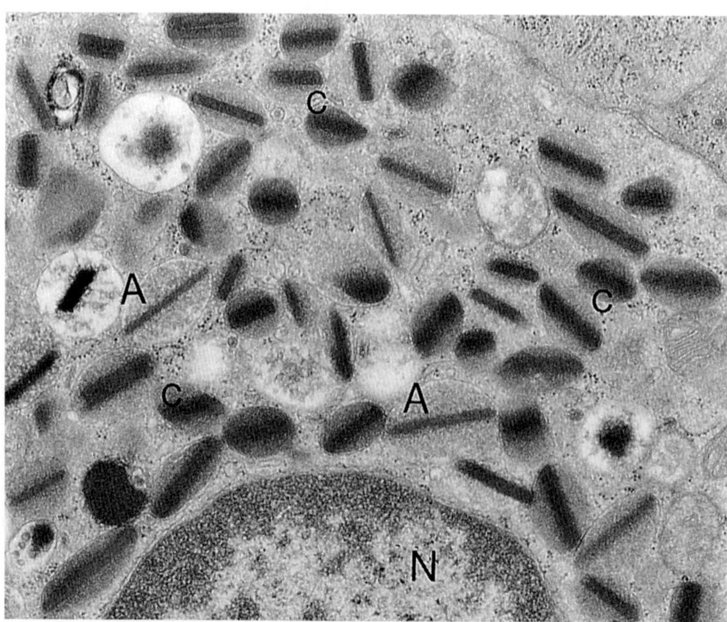

FIGURE 76.4. Chloroma in rat lymph node. Myeloblast with immature nucleus (*N*) and cytoplasm with numerous membrane-bound granules containing crystalline bars (*c*) and Auer rods (*A*). ×12,000. (From Ioachim HL, Sabbath M, Anderson B, et al. Viral and chemical leukemia in the rat: comparative study. J Natl Cancer Inst 1971;47: 161–177, with permission.)

that the sensitivity is low (2,3). Also, GS with monocytic differentiation evolving in patients with chronic myelomonocytic leukemia does not express chloroacetate esterase (13).

IMMUNOHISTOCHEMISTRY

Immunoperoxidase staining for elastase, CD15, CD43 (leukosialin), CD45 (leukocyte common antigen), myeloperoxidase (Figs. 76.1D and 76.2C), CD68 (Fig. 76.2D), and lysozyme detects GS in paraffin-embedded, tissue-sections (2,15). Staining for other myelomonocytic lineage markers, CD13 and CD33, works well in frozen tissue. Results of staining for CD30 are consistently negative (15,25) except for one case report (26). All well-differentiated GSs express elastase, CD15, and CD68; blastic GSs rarely express elastase or CD15 (15). CD43 is highly sensitive but not specific (15,25,27); CD34 stains about one-third of GSs (15). In one study of 26 GSs, 15% expressed CD99 (O13, MIC2) (25). Rarely, GS expresses B-lineage marker CD20 (15). A panel for diagnosing GS in paraffin-embedded tissue sections could include antibodies directed against CD43, CD68, myeloperoxidase, lysozyme, B-cell (CD79a) and T-cell (CD3) markers, plus the Leder stain (chloroacetate esterase) (2,15,25).

Lysozyme, a highly sensitive marker for GS, is sometimes unreliable owing to serum uptake by other tumor cell types. Although heavy metal fixation (Zenker, B5) or acid decalcification inhibits chloroacetate esterase enzyme activity (Leder stain) in paraffin-embedded tissue sections, it does not affect immunohistochemical staining for lysozyme (2).

Phenotype

CD13+ Chloroacetate esterase
CD15+ Elastase
CD33+ Lysozyme
CD34+ Myeloperoxidase
CD43+
CD45+
CD68+
CD99+/−

CYTOGENETICS

Patients with AML and t(8;21)(q22;q22) have an especially high incidence of GS (28,29).

DIFFERENTIAL DIAGNOSIS

- Large cell non-Hodgkin lymphomas, B- and T-cell types, may be very similar histologically. Large cell lymphoma causes tissue destruction and is associated with coagulative necrosis; GS infiltrates along tissue planes and tends to maintain the original tissue architecture (14). Well-differentiated GS contains eosinophilic myelocytes. GS, but not large cell lymphoma, expresses myeloperoxidase and CD68, and the NASD reaction is positive.
- Lymphoblastic lymphoma has convoluted or nonconvoluted nuclei and T- or B-cell markers. Intracytoplasmic granules are absent. The NASD reaction is negative; myeloperoxidase and lysozyme are absent. Terminal de-

Checklist

GRANULOCYTIC SARCOMA

Young patients
Acute myeloid leukemia often associated
Tumors of orbit, bones, kidneys
Lymph nodes frequently involved
Green discoloration of tissues
Blast cells
Folded nuclei
Large nucleoli
Numerous mitoses
Intracellular granules
Crystalline bars
Auer rods
Lysozyme
Myeloperoxidase
Chloroacetate esterase
CD68

oxynucleotidyl transferase and CD99 may be expressed in both lymphoblastic lymphoma and GS.

- Hairy cell leukemia has pale-staining cells, monomorphic nuclei, and rare mitoses. The NASD reaction is negative; the tartrate-resistant acid phosphatase reaction is positive.
- Undifferentiated carcinoma has no intracytoplasmic granules and expresses cytokeratin.
- Sarcomas (rhabdomyosarcoma, Ewing sarcoma) do not express myeloperoxidase or CD45 (leukocyte common antigen). The NASD reaction is negative. Ewing sarcoma and some GSs express CD99.

REFERENCES

1. Rappaport H. Tumors of the hematopoietic system. Washington, DC: Armed Forces Institute of Pathology, 1966:241–243 (Atlas of tumor pathology, series I, fascicle 8).
2. Neiman RS, Barcos M, Berard C, et al. Granulocytic sarcoma: a clinicopathologic study of 61 biopsied cases. Cancer 1981;48: 1426–1437.
3. Davey FR, Olson S, Kurec AS, et al. The immunophenotyping of extramedullary myeloid cell tumors in paraffin-embedded tissue sections. Am J Surg Pathol 1988;12:699–707.
4. Muss HB, Moloney WC. Chloroma and other myeloblastic tumors. Blood 1973;42:721–728.
5. Krause JR. Granulocytic sarcoma preceding acute leukemia: a report of six cases. Cancer 1979;44:1017–1021.
6. Liu PI, Ishimaru T, McGregor DH, et al. Autopsy study of granulocytic sarcoma (chloroma) in patients with myelogenous leukemia, Hiroshima-Nagasaki 1949–1969. Cancer 1973;31: 948–955.
7. Byrd JC, Edenfield WJ, Shields DJ, et al. Extramedullary myeloid cell tumors in acute nonlymphocytic leukemia: a clinical review. J Clin Oncol 1995;13:1800–1816.
8. Byrd JC, Weiss RB. Recurrent granulocytic sarcoma. An unusual variation of acute myelogenous leukemia associated with 8;21 chromosomal translocation and blast expression of the neural cell adhesion molecule. Cancer 1994;73:2107–2112.
9. Griffin JD, Davis R, Nelson DA, et al. Use of surface marker analysis to predict outcome of adult acute myeloblastic leukemia. Blood 1986;68:1232–1241.
10. Cross AH, Goorha RM, Nuss R, et al. Acute myeloid leukemia with T-lymphoid features: a distinct biologic and clinical entity. Blood 1988;72:579–587.
11. Wiernik PH, Serpick AA. Granulocytic sarcoma (chloroma). Blood 1970;35:361–369.
12. Shome DK, Gupta NK, Prajapati NC, et al. Orbital granulocytic sarcomas (myeloid sarcomas) in acute nonlymphocytic leukemia. Cancer 1992;70:2298–2301.
13. Elenitoba-Johnson K, Hodges GF, King TC, et al. Extramedullary myeloid cell tumors arising in the setting of chronic myelomonocytic leukemia. A report of two cases. Arch Pathol Lab Med 1996;120:62–67.
14. Meis JM, Butler JJ, Osborne BM, et al. Granulocytic sarcoma in nonleukemic patients. Cancer 1986;58:2697–2709.
15. Traweek ST, Arber DA, Rappaport H, et al. Extramedullary myeloid cell tumors. An immunohistochemical and morphologic study of 28 cases. Am J Surg Pathol 1993;17:1011–1019.
16. Carmichael GP Jr, Lee YT. Granulocytic sarcoma simulating "nonsecretory" multiple myeloma. Hum Pathol 1977;8:697–700.
17. Tao J, Wu M, Fuchs A, et al. Fine-needle aspiration of granulocytic sarcomas: a morphologic and immunophenotypic study of seven cases. Ann Diagn Pathol 2000;4:17–22.
18. Miller F, DeHarven E, Palade GE. The structure of eosinophil leukocyte granules in rodents and in man. J Cell Biol 1966;31: 349–362.
19. Ioachim HL, Keller S, Sabbath M, et al. Myeloperoxidase and crystalline bodies in the granules of DMBA-induced rat chloroma cells. Am J Pathol 1972;66:147–162.
20. Hamamoto K, Date M, Taniguchi H, et al. Heterogeneity of acute myeloblastic leukemia without maturation: an ultrastructural study. Ultrastruct Pathol 1995;19:9–14.
21. Villamor N, Zarco MA, Rozman M, et al. Acute myeloblastic leukemia with minimal myeloid differentiation: phenotypical and ultrastructural characteristics [see Comments]. Leukemia 1998;12:1071–1075.
22. Nihei K, Terashima K, Nito T, et al. An electron microscopic study of acute promyelocytic leukemia with chloroma. Acta Pathol Jpn 1984;34:159–168.
23. Yam LT, Li CY, Crosby WH. Cytochemical identification of monocytes and granulocytes. Am J Clin Pathol 1971;55:283–290.
24. Leder LD. Uber die selektive Ferment cytochemische Darstellung von Neutrophilen, myeloischen Zellen, und Gewebsmastzellen im Paraffinschnitt. Klin Wochenschr 1964;42:553.
25. Menasce LP, Banerjee SS, Beckett E, et al. Extra-medullary myeloid tumour (granulocytic sarcoma) is often misdiagnosed: a study of 26 cases. Histopathology 1999;34:391–398.
26. Fickers M, Theunissen P. Granulocytic sarcoma with expression of CD30. J Clin Pathol 1996;49:762–763.
27. Segal GH, Stoler MH, Tubbs RR. The "CD43 only" phenotype. An aberrant, nonspecific immunophenotype requiring comprehensive analysis for lineage resolution. Am J Clin Pathol 1992;97: 861–865.
28. Tallman MS, Hakimian D, Shaw JM, et al. Granulocytic sarcoma is associated with the 8;21 translocation in acute myeloid leukemia. J Clin Oncol 1993;11:690–697.
29. Felice MS, Zubizarreta PA, Alfaro EM, et al. Good outcome of children with acute myeloid leukemia and t(8;21)(q22;q22), even when associated with granulocytic sarcoma: a report from a single institution in Argentina. Cancer 2000;88:1939–1944.

77

HISTIOCYTIC SARCOMA

DEFINITION

Malignant neoplasm arising from histiocytic cells in lymphoid tissue. *Histiocyte* refers to two main cell types: monocytes/macrophages and dendritic cells. This chapter focuses on macrophage-like malignancies.

CLASSIFICATION

Macrophage/histiocytic neoplasm
Histiocytic sarcoma (World Health Organization classification)

SYNONYMS

Reticulum cell sarcoma
Reticulosarcoma
Histiocytic sarcoma (HS)
True histiocytic lymphoma

PATHOGENESIS

When the term *histiocytic lymphoma* was first introduced, all large cell lymphomas were assumed to originate from histiocytes (1). This heterogeneous group had earlier been named *reticulum cell sarcomas* or *reticulosarcomas* (2). Modern immunologic and molecular techniques proved that the vast majority of large cell lymphomas originate from transformed B or T lymphocytes. Fewer than 0.5% of lymph node malignancies derive from histiocytes; in other words, true HSs are rare (3–5).

Histiocytes belong to the mononuclear phagocyte and immunoregulatory effector (M-PIRE) system. Monocytes circulate in the peripheral blood, and histiocytes reside in tissues. Lymph node histiocytes include a heterogeneous population of specialized cells, such as macrophages in the sinuses and medulla, follicular dendritic reticulum cells in the germinal centers, and Langerhans cells and interdigitating reticulum cells in the paracortical T zone. Histochemical, ultrastructural, immunophenotypic, and molecular studies have been used to characterize benign and malignant histiocytic proliferations (3). HS presumably arises from the monocyte/macrophage cell series.

The differential diagnosis of HS includes clonal neoplasms, such as non-Hodgkin malignant lymphomas and Langerhans cell histiocytosis (6); it also includes various nonclonal, reactive histiocytoses, such as sinus histiocytosis with massive lymphadenopathy (Rosai-Dorfman disease; see Chapter 37) and hemophagocytic lymphohistiocytic syndrome (7,8).

Malignant histiocytosis (MH) refers to a systemic monocyte/macrophage disorder, occurring mainly in children and adolescents, that causes pancytopenia, adenopathy, hepatosplenomegaly, and wasting. When monoclonal antibodies were used to analyze cases of MH diagnosed before the era of immunophenotyping, MH essentially appeared not to exist. Hallmark atypical hemophagocytic cells could be found in several other conditions. Cases of so-called MH actually represented Ki-1 anaplastic large cell lymphoma, peripheral T-cell lymphoma, B-cell lymphoma, carcinoma, or virus-associated hemophagocytic syndrome (9–11).

CLINICAL SYNDROME

Histiocytic sarcoma manifests principally as localized lymph node disease in adults. The lymph nodes, often unilaterally located in the cervical region, are initially painless. In 37 patients with HS, the male-to-female ratio was 1.6:1 (3–5,12). In about 50% of cases, HS involved extranodal locations, such as skin, bone, spleen, and gastrointestinal tract (3–5,12–15). Except for tumor masses, patients are usually symptom-free, and results of laboratory tests are normal. The bone marrow is typically not involved. HS evolving to a leukemic phase with cytologic features of mature histiocytes (so-called French–American–British M5c) (16) has been reported in one patient (17).

Histiocytic sarcoma has developed following therapy as a second malignancy after indolent follicular lymphoma (18) and aggressive lymphoblastic lymphoma/acute lymphoblastic leukemia (19).

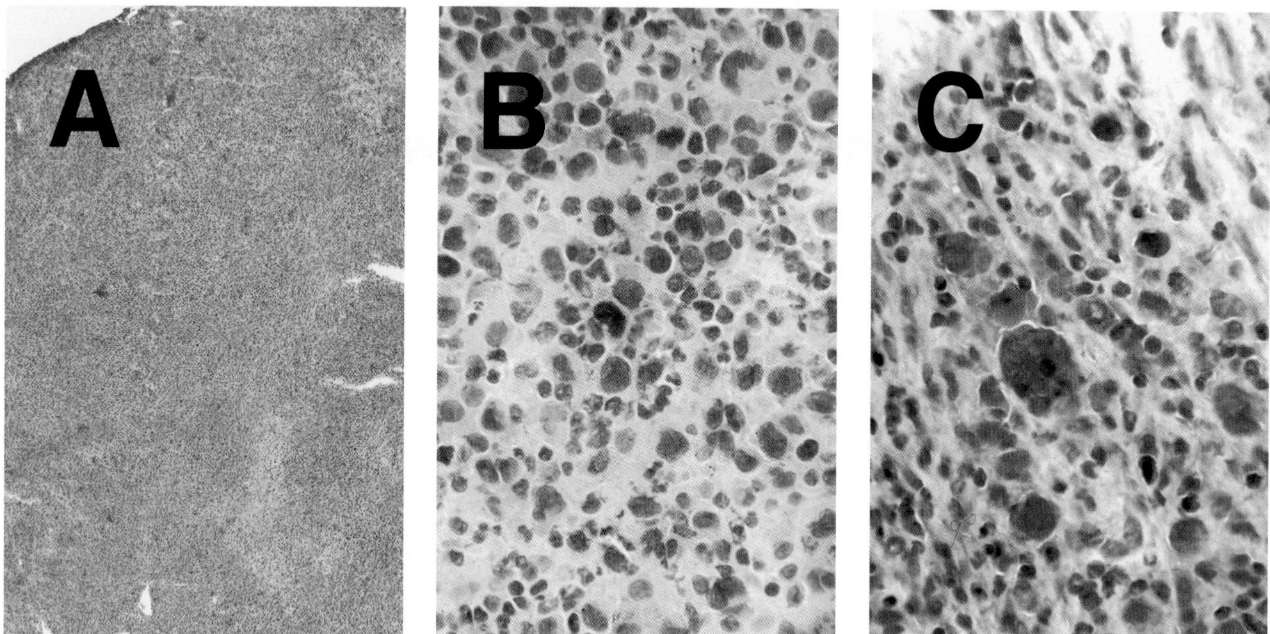

FIGURE 77.1. Histiocytic sarcoma, frozen tissue section. **A:** Diffusely effaced normal lymph node architecture. Hematoxylin and eosin stain. **B:** Medium-sized to giant tumor cells with rare intervening small lymphocytes. Hematoxylin and eosin stain. **C:** Neoplastic cells phagocytosing erythrocytes. Hematoxylin and eosin stain. (Courtesy of Glauco Frizzera, M.D.)

HISTOPATHOLOGY

Lymph nodes may be partially or totally replaced by sheets of pale, large cells distributed in a sinusoidal or diffuse pattern (3–5,12–14) (Fig. 77.1A). The tumor cells superficially resemble sinus histiocytes. The cell borders are indistinct, and the cytoplasm is abundant, pale, and acidophilic. The nuclei are fairly large, elongated, or irregularly shaped, with finely dispersed chromatin and two or more conspicuous but not very large nucleoli (Fig. 77.1B). Mitotic activity is moderate or intense. Multinucleated cells may be present (Fig. 77.1B). Occasionally, phagocytosis of erythrocytes, lymphocytes, or nuclear debris by the neoplastic histiocytes is seen (Fig. 77.1C).

Sometimes, the reticulin formation is obviously increased, and silver staining reveals a well-formed reticulin network with fine fibrils wrapped around individual cells. This pattern of pericellular growth of reticulin fibers is a valuable criterion for differentiating HS from carcinomas, in which the reticulin fibers delineate only cords and nests of tumor cells.

Extramedullary acute monoblastic leukemia infiltrates skin, lymph nodes, small intestine, and soft tissues; the same anatomic sites are commonly involved by HS (20). Also, acute monoblastic leukemia and HS share similar immunophenotypic markers (20). At least one author has asked, "Is HS an entity?" (20). Others claim that uniformly round or reniform nuclei and distinct nucleoli distinguish acute monoblastic leukemia in extramedullary tissues from HS, which appears cytologically pleomorphic (5).

ELECTRON MICROSCOPY

The electron microscopic examination is useful for differentiating large cell lymphomas. In HS (true histiocytic lymphoma) (Fig. 77.2), the neoplastic cells may be unusually large, with abundant cytoplasm and cellular processes. The nucleus is irregularly, sometimes bizarrely, shaped and includes mostly euchromatin and several fairly large, reticulated nucleoli (21). The cytoplasm contains lysosomes and

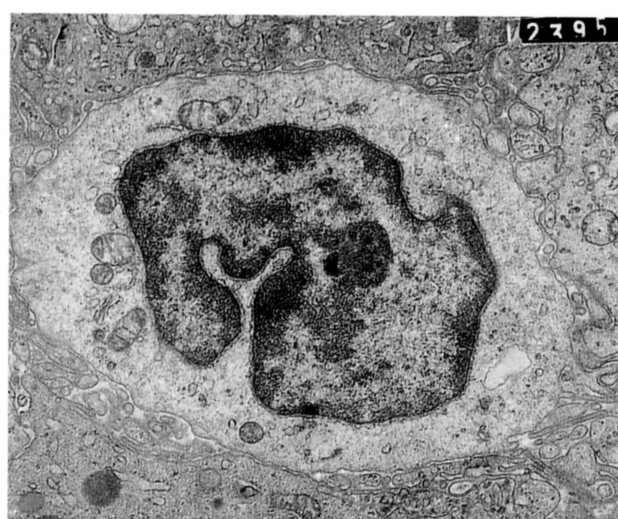

FIGURE 77.2. Histiocytic sarcoma. Large cell with abundant cytoplasm containing only a few mitochondria. Deeply indented nucleus with heterochromatin and huge nucleolus. ×10,000.

phagosomes. In contrast, large cell lymphomas have nuclei with a characteristic lymphoid structure in which the heterochromatin is predominant and peripheralized (21). HSs do not contain Birbeck granules.

CYTOCHEMISTRY

Histiocytes of the monocyte/macrophage lineage contain a variety of lysosomal enzymes (e.g., acid phosphatase and esterases) that can be cytochemically stained on air-dried smears and imprints. Fluoride inhibits nonspecific esterase enzyme activity, also called *α-naphthyl acetate esterase,* in monocyte/macrophage cells but not in myeloid cells (see Chapter 5).

IMMUNOHISTOCHEMISTRY

Histiocytic sarcoma expresses many antigens found on normal monocytes/macrophages and myeloid cells, such as CD4, CD11b, CD11c, CD13, CD14, and CD68, plus markers found on multiple cell lineages, CD43 and CD45RO (UCHL-1) (4,5,9,13,22,23) (Fig. 77.3). α_1-Antitrypsin and lysozyme are no longer considered reliable for diagnosing a histiocytic lineage because they can be detected in a variety of other tumor cell types, probably via uptake. HS does not react with antibodies for CD1a, CD30, or B- and T-cell lineage-specific antigens; HS variably stains for S100 protein (4,5,9,13,22,23).

MOLECULAR DIAGNOSIS

Histiocytic sarcoma does not show immunoglobulin or T cell-receptor gene rearrangements except in rare cases (22,23).

Phenotype

CD4+
CD11b+
CD11c+
CD13+
CD14+
CD43+
CD45RO+
CD68+
S100 protein+/−
CD1a−
CD30−
B-cell antigen−
T-cell antigen−

DIFFERENTIAL DIAGNOSIS

- Non-Hodgkin lymphoma, large B-cell cleaved or immunoblastic types: Cells with smaller amount of cytoplasm than in Hodgkin lymphoma. B-cell markers (CD19, CD20) and membrane immunoglobulins are expressed. Nonspecific esterase and acid phosphatase are not expressed.
- Histiocyte-rich B-cell lymphoma: B-cell lymphoma with predominant reactive histiocytic infiltrate may also have many reactive T cells (24).
- Non-Hodgkin lymphoma, large T-cell types: T-cell markers (CD2, CD3, CD5, CD7) are expressed. Nonspecific esterase is not expressed. Erythrophagocytosis may be present, but histiocytes are benign.
- Ki-1 anaplastic large cell lymphoma: Skin, lymph node, or systemic distribution; expression of CD30 (Ki-1) and T-cell markers; chromosomal t(2;5)(p23;q35), except in primary skin tumors.
- Langerhans cell histiocytosis: Complex nuclear contours.

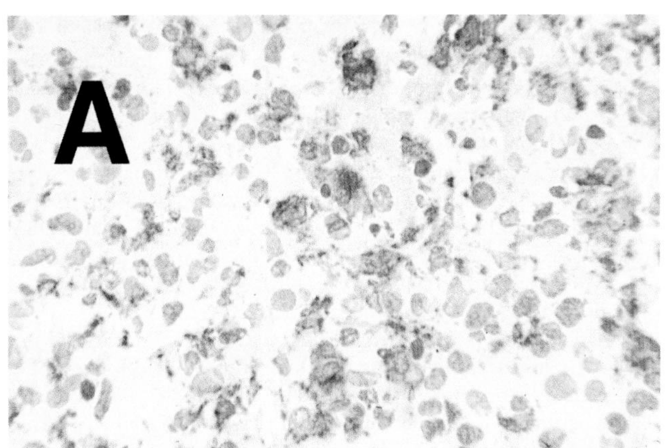

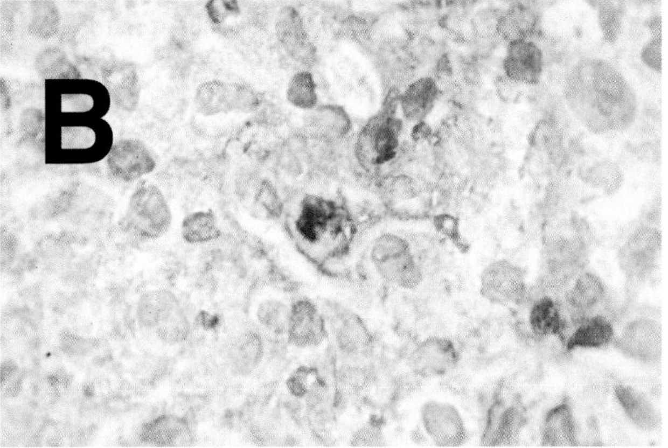

FIGURE 77.3. Histiocytic sarcoma, frozen tissue sections. **A:** Tumor cells express CD68 (Ki-M6). Immunoperoxidase stain. **B:** Tumor cells express CD11c (Ki-M1). Immunoperoxidase stain. (Courtesy of Glauco Frizzera, M.D.)

Checklist

HISTIOCYTIC SARCOMA

Fewer than 0.5% of all lymphomas
Patients middle-aged or elderly
Localized tumor
No peripheral blood involvement
Marked cellular pleomorphism
Large atypical histiocytes
Abundant eosinophilic cytoplasm
Irregular vesicular nuclei
Lysosomes
Cytoplasmic processes
Multinucleated cells
Phagocytosis
Well-developed reticulin network
Nonspecific esterase
α-Naphthyl acetate esterase
Acid phosphatase
CD4, CD11b, CD11c, CD13, CD14, CD68 (α_1-antitrypsin and lysozyme not reliable)
Absence of immunoglobulins
Absence of B- and T-cell markers
Absence of B- and T-cell receptor gene rearrangements

CD1a+, S100 protein+. Ultrastructural Birbeck granules present, typically in infancy or early childhood (25).

- Hodgkin lymphoma: Diagnostic Reed-Sternberg cells must be identified.
- Metastatic anaplastic carcinoma, particularly nasopharyngeal carcinoma: Cytokeratin markers must be used to identify the epithelial origin of anaplastic tumor cells. Nonspecific esterase and acid phosphatase are not expressed.
- Hemophagocytic lymphohistiocytosis: Benign histiocytic proliferation showing hemophagocytosis. Cellular morphology more monotonous, smaller, less hyperchromatic, with rare atypical nuclei. Prominent nucleoli and mitoses absent. Often associated with infections, especially Epstein-Barr viral infection, persistent fever, and cytopenia.

REFERENCES

1. Rappaport H. Tumors of the hematopoietic system. Washington, DC: Armed Forces Institute of Pathology, 1966 (Atlas of tumor pathology, series I, fascicle 8).
2. Oberling C. Les réticulosarcomes et les réticuloendotheliosarcomes de la moelle osseuse (sarcome d'Ewing). Bull Assoc Fr ÉEtude Cancer 1928;17:259–296.
3. Hanson CA, Jaszcz W, Kersey JH, et al. True histiocytic lymphoma: histopathologic, immunophenotypic and genotypic analysis. Br J Haematol 1989;73:187–198.
4. Ralfkiaer E, Delsol G, O'Connor NT, et al. Malignant lymphomas of true histiocytic origin. A clinical, histological, immunophenotypic, and genotypic study. J Pathol 1990;160:9–17.
5. Lauritzen AF, Delsol G, Hansen NE, et al. Histiocytic sarcomas and monoblastic leukemias. A clinical, histologic, and immunophenotypical study. Am J Clin Pathol 1994;102:45–54.
6. Willman CL, McClain KL. An update on clonality, cytokines, and viral etiology in Langerhans cell histiocytosis. Hematol Oncol Clin North Am 1998;12:407–416.
7. Cline MJ. Histiocytes and histiocytosis. Blood 1994;84:2840–2853.
8. Arceci RJ. The histiocytoses: the fall of the Tower of Babel. Eur J Cancer 1999;35:747–767; discussion 767–769.
9. Wilson MS, Weiss LM, Gatter KC, et al. Malignant histiocytosis. A reassessment of cases previously reported in 1975 based on paraffin section immunophenotyping studies. Cancer 1990;66:530–536.
10. Egeler RM, Schmitz L, Sonneveld P, et al. Malignant histiocytosis: a reassessment of cases formerly classified as histiocytic neoplasms and review of the literature. Med Pediatr Oncol 1995;25:1–7.
11. Mongkonsritragoon W, Li CY, Phyliky RL. True malignant histiocytosis. Mayo Clin Proc 1998;73:520–528.
12. van der Valk P, Meijer CJ, Willemze R, et al. Histiocytic sarcoma (true histiocytic lymphoma): a clinicopathological study of 20 cases. Histopathology 1984;8:105–123.
13. Miettinen M, Fletcher CD, Lasota J. True histiocytic lymphoma of small intestine. Analysis of two S-100 protein-positive cases with features of interdigitating reticulum cell sarcoma. Am J Clin Pathol 1993;100:285–292.
14. Boisseau-Garsaud AM, Vergier B, Beylot-Barry M, et al. Histio-

cytic sarcoma that mimics benign histiocytosis. J Cutan Pathol 1996;23:275–282.
15. Kimura H, Nasu K, Sakai C, et al. Histiocytic sarcoma of the spleen associated with hypoalbuminemia, hypogammaglobulinemia and thrombocytopenia as a possibly unique clinical entity—report of three cases. Leuk Lymphoma 1998;31:217–224.
16. Laurencet FM, Chapuis B, Roux-Lombard P, et al. Malignant histiocytosis in the leukaemic stage: a new entity (M5c-AML) in the FAB classification? Leukemia 1994;8:502–506.
17. Esteve J, Rozman M, Campo E, et al. Leukemia after true histiocytic lymphoma: another type of acute monocytic leukemia with histiocytic differentiation (AML-M5c)? Leukemia 1995;9:1389–1391.
18. Martin Rodilla C, Fernandez Acenero J, Pena Mayor L, et al. True histiocytic lymphoma as a second neoplasm in a follicular centroblastic–centrocytic lymphoma. Pathol Res Pract 1997;193: 319–322.
19. Soslow RA, Davis RE, Warnke RA, et al. True histiocytic lymphoma following therapy for lymphoblastic neoplasms. Blood 1996;87:5207–5212.
20. Elghetany MT. True histiocytic lymphoma: is it an entity? Leukemia 1997;11:762–764.
21. Ioachim HL. Lymph nodes and spleen. In: Johannessen JV, ed. Electron microscopy in human medicine, vol 5. New York: McGraw-Hill, 1981:417–495.
22. Kamel OW, Gocke CD, Kell DL, et al. True histiocytic lymphoma: a study of 12 cases based on current definition. Leuk Lymphoma 1995;18:81–86.
23. Copie-Bergman C, Wotherspoon AC, Norton AJ, et al. True histiocytic lymphoma: a morphologic, immunohistochemical, and molecular genetic study of 13 cases. Am J Surg Pathol 1998;22: 1386–1392.
24. Sun T, Susin M, Tomao FA, et al. Histiocyte-rich B-cell lymphoma. Hum Pathol 1997;28:1321–1324.
25. Huang F, Arceci R. The histiocytoses of infancy. Semin Perinatol 1999;23:319–331.

78

DENDRITIC CELL NEOPLASMS

DEFINITION

Neoplasms originating from the reticulum cells of the lymph node framework. Two main types occur as primary lymph node tumors: follicular dendritic cell sarcoma (FDCS), derived from antigen-presenting cells in the B-cell follicle, and interdigitating dendritic cell sarcoma (IDCS), derived from antigen-presenting cells in the paracortical T-zone.

CLASSIFICATION

Dendritic cell neoplasms (World Health Organization, or WHO)
- Langerhans cell histiocytosis
- Langerhans cell sarcoma
- Interdigitating dendritic cell sarcoma/tumor
- Follicular dendritic cell sarcoma/tumor

Dendritic cell sarcoma, not otherwise specified

SYNONYMS

Interdigitating reticulum cell sarcoma, or interdigitating dendritic cell sarcoma/tumor

Dendritic reticulum cell sarcoma, or follicular dendritic cell sarcoma/tumor

PATHOGENESIS

When all tumors unrelated to the reticulum cells of lymph nodes are discounted, only a small group of rare malignant neoplasms remains. Two morphologically similar but distinctive subtypes exist. They express complex immunophenotypes that do not include the usual T-cell or B-cell markers (1). Reticulum cell sarcomas arise from either the follicular dendritic cells (FDCs) of the germinal centers (2) or the interdigitating dendritic cells (IDCs) of the lymph node paracortex (3).

Follicular dendritic cells, possibly originating from mesenchyme, form a taut meshwork within primary B-cell follicles and within germinal centers of secondary follicles (2). Complex cell processes display complement receptors that trap antigen–antibody complexes, thereby helping to retain and present antigen to commence B-cell proliferation and differentiation.

Interdigitating dendritic cells, located in the T-zone of the nodal paracortex, arise from myeloid precursors induced by cytokines to follow a dendritic pathway (3). IDCs resemble the Langerhans cells of the skin, except that they lack ultrastructural Birbeck granules and CD1a. They present antigen to T lymphocytes.

Reported cases of FDCS and IDCS are few (1). They should be distinguished from other primary lymph node spindle cell neoplasms derived from histiocytes, fibroblasts, or endothelial cells; from lymph node metastases of sarcomas; and from Langerhans cell histiocytosis/sarcoma.

CLINICAL SYNDROME

Follicular Dendritic Cell Sarcoma

Follicular dendritic cell sarcoma is a rare tumor. Recent clinical reviews describe 13, 17, and 51 patients, with some overlap (1,4,5). FDCS usually occurs as a painless, slowly enlarging mass; the median age of patients is in the fifth decade, with a range of 17 to 76 years (1,4,5). The numbers of male and female patients are approximately equal (1,4,5). Cervical lymphadenopathy predominates, but axillary and mediastinal lymph nodes can also be involved. Inguinal disease has not been reported. A few patients have abdominal pain caused by intraabdominal tumors (5). In one-third of cases, FDCS involves extranodal sites, such as oral cavity, spleen, liver, small bowel, pancreas, and peritoneum (1).

Fever and weight loss are uncommon symptoms. Most patients survive for long periods, often with local recurrences, similar to patients with low-grade soft tissue sarcomas (4). However, metastases can develop and lead to death (1,6).

Rarely, hyaline-vascular Castleman disease (see Chapter 43) gives rise to unusual stromal cell proliferations in lymph nodes, mediastinum, retroperitoneum, or soft tissues (5–7).

FDCS developing in this setting can recur and metastasize, just like FDCS that arises *de novo* (5–7).

Interdigitating Dendritic Cell Sarcoma

The features of 21 cases of IDCS have been recently summarized (1). The median age of patients at presentation is 52 years, with a range of 8 to 74 years; males slightly outnumber females (1). Most have enlarged lymph nodes, but in about one-fourth, extranodal disease develops initially; systemic symptoms such as fever and night sweats are uncommon (1).

In a review, only 3 of 15 patients had bone marrow involvement, and a superior vena cava syndrome developed in two patients (1). Although variable, the clinical course of IDCS appears more aggressive than that of FDCS (1). IDCS, or closely related dendritic cell tumors, can rarely arise in lymph nodes or in skin as a second neoplasm after B-cell chronic lymphocytic leukemia (see Fig. 78.2 E,F) or after follicular lymphoma (8).

HISTOPATHOLOGY

Follicular Dendritic Cell Sarcoma

The lymph node architecture in FDCS is effaced by a proliferation of oval to spindle-shaped cells arranged in sheets, fascicles, or concentric whorls, as in meningioma, sometimes with storiform foci (1,5,9) (Fig. 78.1 A–C). Necrosis or cellular atypia is uncommon but indicates a poor prognosis. Characteristically, numerous small lymphocytes are interspersed between the tumor cells (Fig. 78.1 B,C) and form prominent cuffs around blood vessels (Fig 78.1A), as in a thymoma (1,5,9). The tumor cells have a moderate amount of pale eosinophilic cytoplasm, poorly defined cell outlines, elongated nuclei, inconspicuous nucleoli, and a moderate number of mitoses (Fig. 78.1D). Frequent multinucleated cells resemble Warthin-Finkeldey giant cells. Recurrent FDCS shows histologic progression to greater cytologic atypia (1,5,9).

Interdigitating Dendritic Cell Sarcoma

The proliferating tumor cells of IDCS similarly replace the normal architecture, growing in fascicles or nests (Fig. 78.2 A,B). Some reports note frequent infiltration of lymph node sinuses (10–13) (Fig. 78.2A). The cells are elongated and have eosinophilic cytoplasm, oval or irregularly shaped although generally folded nuclei, and inconspicuous nucleoli (11–14). Some reports describe the cells as large, with pleomorphic nuclei and frequent mitoses (Fig. 78.2C) (11,12). Unlike FDCSs, IDCSs do not have scattered small lymphocytes between tumor cells or vascular cuffing (9). Cytologic atypia appears greater than in FDCS (1,9).

ELECTRON MICROSCOPY

The FDCS cytoplasm contains poorly developed rough endoplasmic reticulum. The nuclei are plump and ovoid with peripherally marginated chromatin and one medium-sized or large nucleolus (1,5,9) (Fig. 78.3). The most characteristic feature is the presence of long, complex, undulating villous cell processes interconnected by desmosomes (1,5,9). Weibel-Palade bodies, tonofilaments, intracytoplasmic lumina, and basement membranes are absent.

The IDCS cytoplasm has scant organelles. Bizarre-shaped nuclei have finely dispersed chromatin. Birbeck granules are absent. Junctional complexes are characteristically absent, although early reports mentioned desmosomes (1).

CYTOCHEMISTRY

Interdigitating dendritic cell sarcoma exhibits adenosine triphosphatase (ATPase) enzyme activity (15). In contrast, FDCS expresses 5′-nucleotidase activity (1).

IMMUNOHISTOCHEMISTRY

Follicular Dendritic Cell Sarcoma

Follicular dendritic cell sarcomas have C3d and C3b complement receptors: CD21 (Fig. 78.1F) and CD35 (1,5,9). They express HLA-DR and characteristic antigens recognized by monoclonal antibodies R4/23, Ki-M4 (Fig. 78.1E), Ki-M4p, and Ki-FDC1p (1,5,9). FDCSs also express low-affinity nerve growth factor receptor (16) and CAN.42 (17). They do not stain for CD3 (T-cell) or CD20 (B-cell) lineage-specific markers, CD1a, cytokeratin, or vascular markers. FDCSs sometimes express desmoplakin, epithelial membrane antigen, muscle-specific actin, S100 protein, vimentin, CD14, CD45 (leukocyte common antigen), or CD68 (1,5,9). Epstein-Barr virus is rarely detected, except in liver FDCSs simulating inflammatory pseudotumors (9,18).

Phenotype

FOLLICULAR DENDRITIC CELL SARCOMA

CD21+
CD35+
HLA-DR+
R4/23+
Ki-M4+
Ki-M4p+
Ki-FDC1p+
Low-affinity nerve growth factor receptor+
CAN.42+

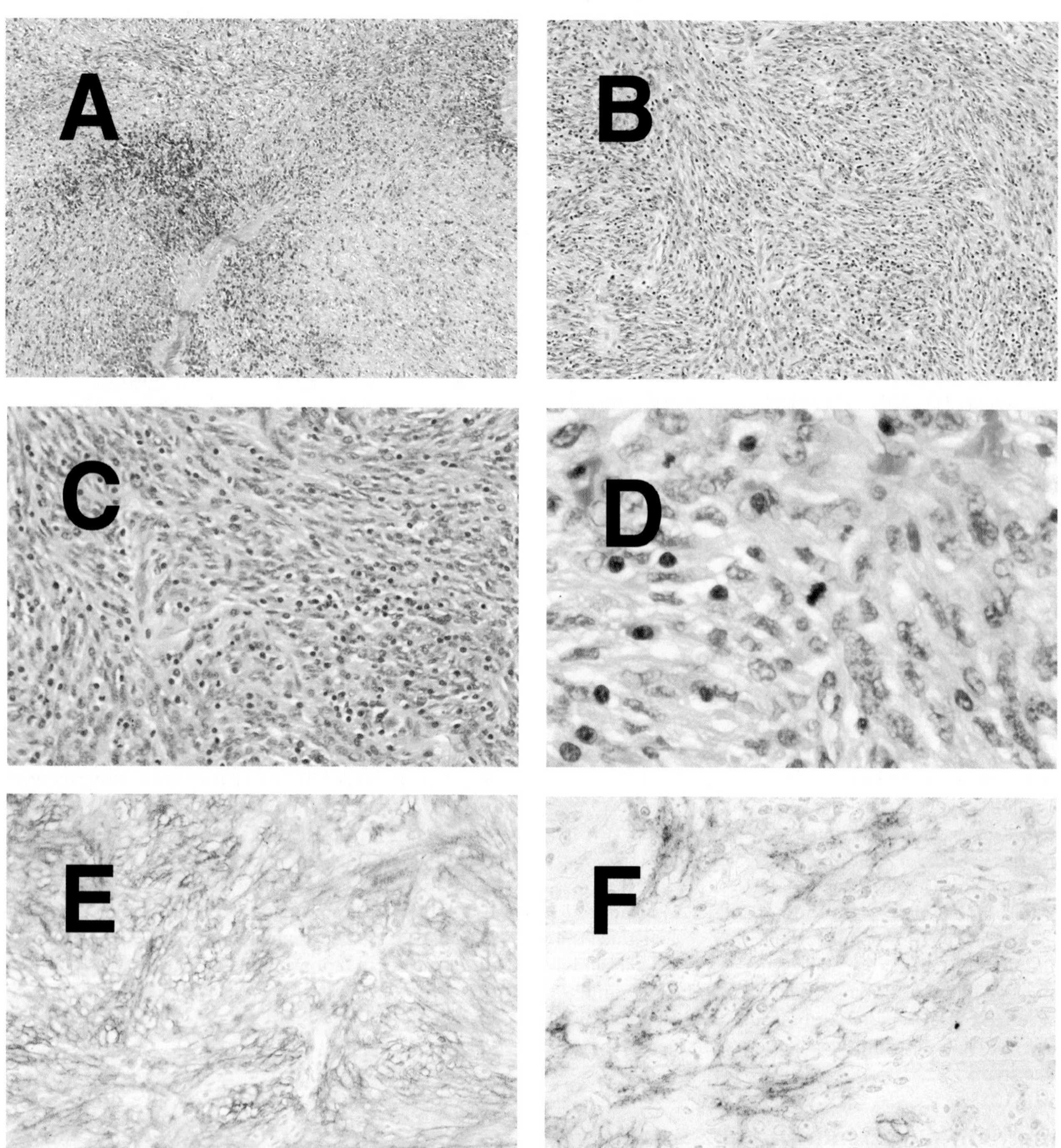

FIGURE 78.1. Follicular dendritic cell sarcoma. **A:** Perivascular lymphocytes. Hematoxylin and eosin stain. **B:** Fascicles and whorls of spindle cells. Hematoxylin and eosin stain. **C:** Numerous small lymphocytes interspersed between spindle cells. Hematoxylin and eosin stain. **D:** Tumor cells with moderately abundant pale eosinophilic cytoplasm, poorly defined cell borders, and elongated nuclei. Mitosis in center field. Hematoxylin and eosin stain. **E:** Spindle cells express Ki-M4. Immunoperoxidase stain. **F:** Spindle cells express CD21. Immunoperoxidase stain. (Courtesy of Glauco Frizzera, M.D.)

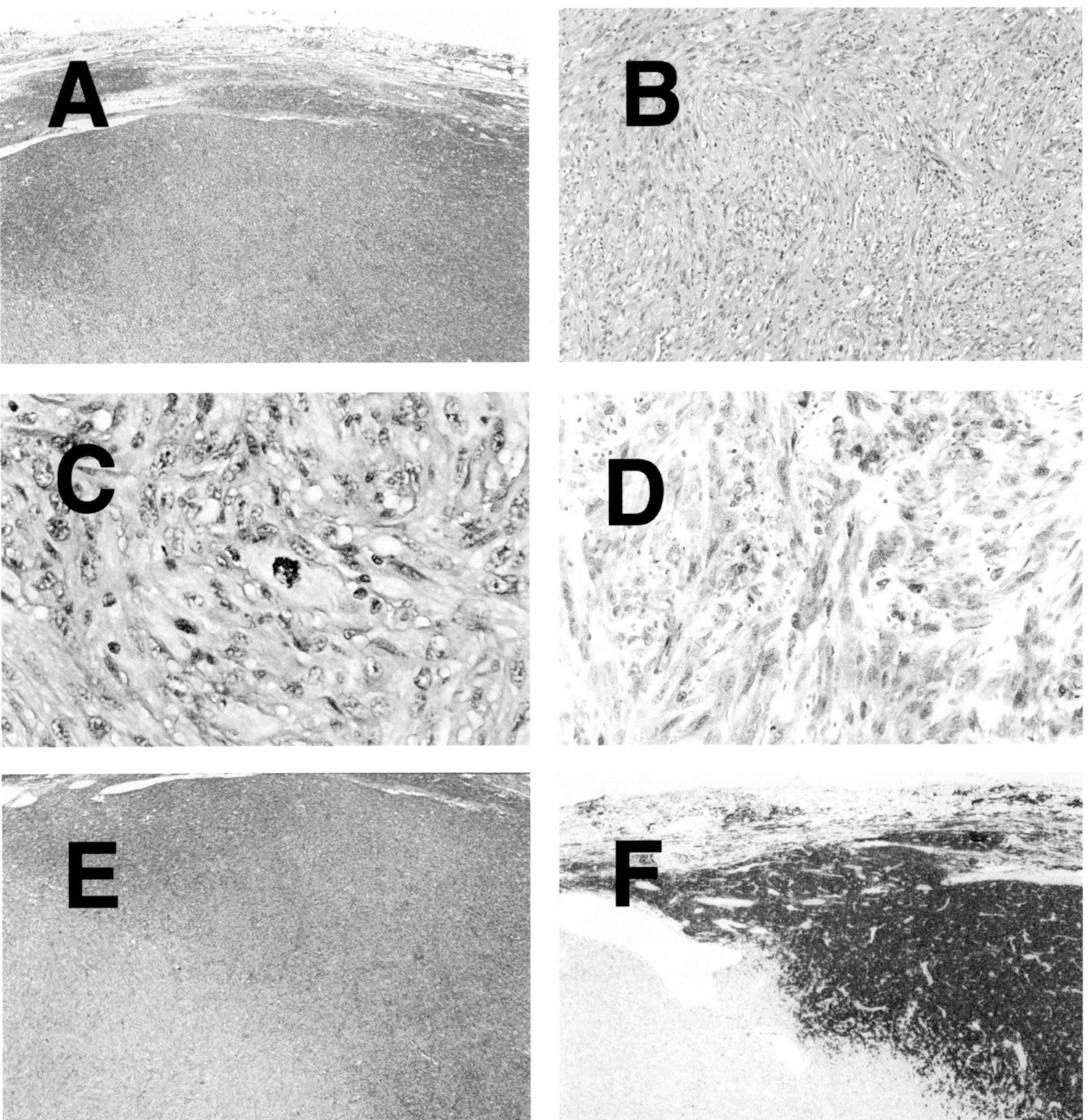

FIGURE 78.2. Interdigitating dendritic cell sarcoma (IDCS). **A:** Tumor cells replace lymph node architecture and infiltrate sinuses. Hematoxylin and eosin stain. **B:** Fascicles of spindle cells. Hematoxylin and eosin stain. **C:** Atypical mitosis in center field. Hematoxylin and eosin stain. **D:** Tumor cells stain positively for S100 protein. **E:** IDCS (*lower left*) replacing lymph node containing B-cell chronic lymphocytic leukemia (B-CLL) (*upper right*). Hematoxylin and eosin stain. **F:** Same lymph node as in **E**. B-CLL expressing CD20 B-cell marker (*upper right*) sharply demarcates edge of IDCS, which is CD20− (*lower left*). (Courtesy of Glauco Frizzera, M.D.)

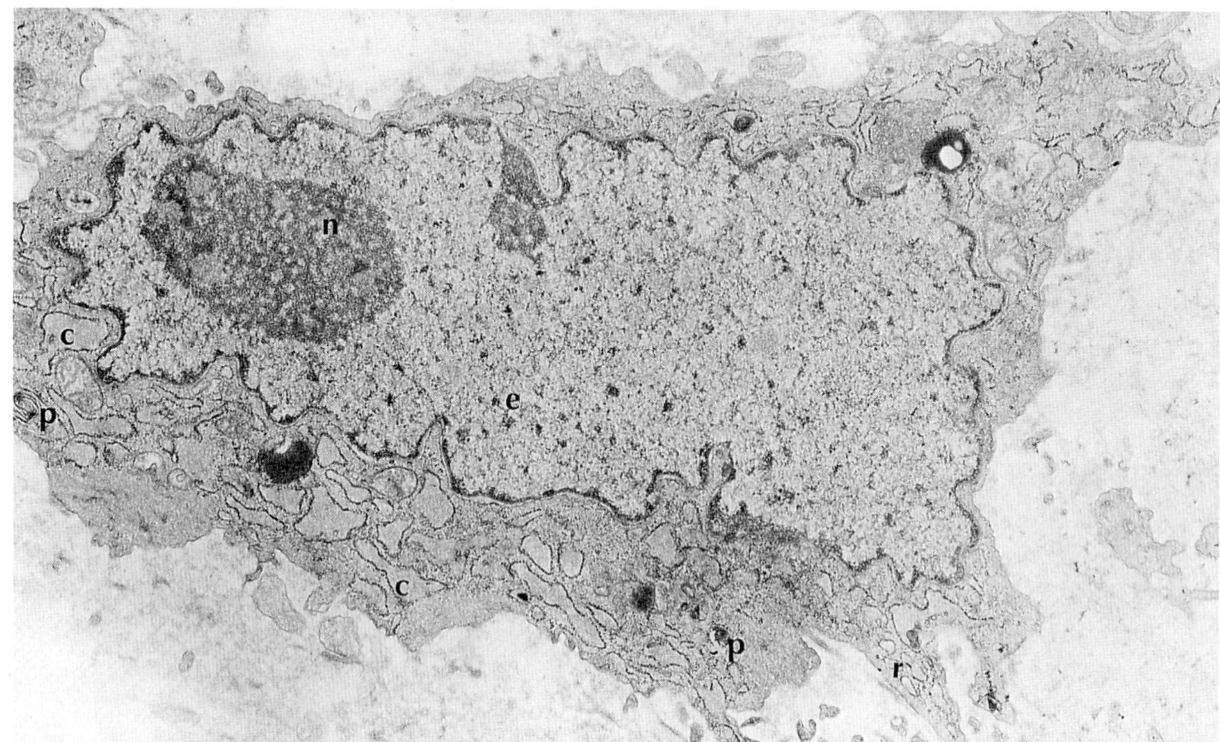

FIGURE 78.3. Follicular dendritic cell sarcoma. Large, stellate cell with multiple elongated processes and abundant cytoplasm containing well-developed granular endoplasmic reticulum with distended cisternae (*c*). Large nucleus, irregularly shaped with abundant euchromatin and very large reticulated nucleolus (*n*). ×15,600.

Interdigitating Dendritic Cell Sarcoma

Interdigitating dendritic cell sarcomas share immunophenotypic similarities with Langerhans cells, their normal counterparts in skin (1). In contrast to Langerhans cells, IDCs are CD1a− (1). IDCSs stain intensely for S100 protein (Fig. 78.2D), CD45, and HLA-DR, and inconstantly for CD4, CD11c, and CD15. IDCSs also react with two new monoclonal antibodies: HB15a/CD83 and CD-LAMP (19). Unlike FDCSs, IDCSs do not have complement receptors CD21 and CD35 (1,5,9).

Phenotype

INTERDIGITATING DENDRITIC CELL SARCOMA

S100 protein+
CD45+
HLA-DR+
HB15a/CD83+
CD-LAMP+
CD21−
CD35−

MOLECULAR DIAGNOSIS

Neither FDCS nor IDCS rearranges immunoglobulin or T-cell receptor genes. The human androgen receptor gene assay has proved the clonal nature of dendritic cell tumors (20).

DIFFERENTIAL DIAGNOSIS

- Palisaded myofibroblastoma: Benign spindle cell tumor, usually in inguinal lymph nodes. Presence of amyanthoid fibers.
- Inflammatory pseudotumor: Spindle cells, inflammation, and small vessels in lymph node capsule extending along trabeculae. No atypia.
- Histiocytic lymphoma: Stains for monocyte/macrophage markers but lacks CD21, CD35, and Ki-M4p.
- Large cell lymphoma: Can be morphologically mimicked by either FDCS (21) or IDCS (22).
- Hodgkin lymphoma, lymphocyte depletion type: Presence of diagnostic Reed-Sternberg cells, Leu-M1+, S100 protein−.
- Malignant fibrous histiocytoma: S100 protein−.
- Metastatic spindle cell carcinoma: Easily confused on fine needle aspiration biopsy (23). Cytokeratin+.
- Metastatic melanoma: Also S100 protein+, but in addition shows positivity for specific melanoma markers such as HMB-45.

Checklist

RETICULUM CELL SARCOMA

Localized tumor masses
Spindle or stellate cells
Fascicular, whorled patterns
Nuclear atypia, moderate mitoses

Follicular Dendritic Cell Sarcoma
CD21+, CD35+, Ki-M4p+, R4/23+; CD1a−; storiform foci; scattered small lymphocytes between tumor cells and vascular cuffing; long, complex, interconnected cell processes; desmosomes

Interdigitating Dendritic Cell Sarcoma
ATPase+, HLA-DR+, S100 protein+, CD45+, CD11c+; more cytologic atypia than FDCS; complement receptors absent

- Ectopic meningioma: Lacks CD21, CD35, and Ki-M4p.
- Ectopic thymoma: Cytokeratin+ epithelial cells and immature T cells.

REFERENCES

1. Fonseca R, Yamakawa M, Nakamura S, et al. Follicular dendritic cell sarcoma and interdigitating reticulum cell sarcoma: a review. Am J Hematol 1998;59:161–167.
2. Heinen E, Bosseloir A, Bouzahzah F. Follicular dendritic cells: origin and function. Curr Top Microbiol Immunol 1995;201:15–47.
3. Hart DN. Dendritic cells: unique leukocyte populations which control the primary immune response. Blood 1997;90:3245–3287.
4. Perez-Ordonez B, Erlandson RA, Rosai J. Follicular dendritic cell tumor: report of 13 additional cases of a distinctive entity. Am J Surg Pathol 1996;20:944–955.
5. Chan JK, Fletcher CD, Nayler SJ, et al. Follicular dendritic cell sarcoma. Clinicopathologic analysis of 17 cases suggesting a malignant potential higher than currently recognized. Cancer 1997;79:294–313.
6. Chan JK, Tsang WY, Ng CS. Follicular dendritic cell tumor and vascular neoplasm complicating hyaline-vascular Castleman's disease. Am J Surg Pathol 1994;18:517–525.
7. Lin O, Frizzera G. Angiomyoid and follicular dendritic cell proliferative lesions in Castleman's disease of hyaline-vascular type: a study of 10 cases [published erratum appears in Am J Surg Pathol 1998;22:39] [see Comments]. Am J Surg Pathol 1997;21:1295–1306.
8. Vasef MA, Zaatari GS, Chan WC, et al. Dendritic cell tumors associated with low-grade B-cell malignancies. Report of three cases. Am J Clin Pathol 1995;104:696–701.
9. Perez-Ordonez B, Rosai J. Follicular dendritic cell tumor: review of the entity. Semin Diagn Pathol 1998;15:144–154.
10. Feltkamp CA, van Heerde P, Feltkamp-Vroom TM, et al. A malignant tumor arising from interdigitating cells; light microscopical, ultrastructural, immuno- and enzyme-histochemical characteristics. Virchows Arch A Pathol Anat Histopathol 1981;393:183–192.
11. Nakamura S, Hara K, Suchi T, et al. Interdigitating cell sarcoma. A morphologic, immunohistologic, and enzyme-histochemical study. Cancer 1988;61:562–568.
12. Yamakawa M, Matsuda M, Imai Y, et al. Lymph node interdigitating cell sarcoma. A case report. Am J Clin Pathol 1992;97:139–146.
13. Rousselet MC, Francois S, Croue A, et al. A lymph node interdigitating reticulum cell sarcoma. Arch Pathol Lab Med 1994;118:183–188.
14. Weiss LM, Berry GJ, Dorfman RF, et al. Spindle cell neoplasms of lymph nodes of probable reticulum cell lineage. True reticulum cell sarcoma? Am J Surg Pathol 1990;14:405–414.
15. van den Oord JJ, de Wolf-Peeters C, de Vos R, et al. Sarcoma arising from interdigitating reticulum cells: report of a case, studied with light and electron microscopy and enzyme- and immunohistochemistry. Histopathology 1986;10:509–523.
16. Dorfman DM, Shahsafaei A, Chan JKC, et al. Dendritic reticulum cell (DRC) sarcomas are immunoreactive for low-affinity nerve growth factor receptor (LNGFR). Further evidence for DRC differentiation. Appl Immunohistochem 1996;4:249–258.
17. Raymond I, Al Saati T, Tkaczuk J, et al. CNA.42, a new monoclonal antibody directed against a fixative-resistant antigen of follicular dendritic reticulum cells. Am J Pathol 1997;151:1577– 1585.
18. Shek TW, Ho FC, Ng IO, et al. Follicular dendritic cell tumor of the liver. Evidence for an Epstein-Barr virus-related clonal proliferation of follicular dendritic cells. Am J Surg Pathol 1996;20:313–324.
19. Hyjek E, Tam W, Chadburn A, et al. Identification of interdigitating cell sarcoma (ICS) with the HB15/CD83 and CD-LAMP antibodies. Mod Pathol 2000;13:150A(abst).
20. Wu CD, Wickert RS, Williamson JE, et al. Using fluorescence-based human androgen receptor gene assay to analyze the clonality of microdissected dendritic cell tumors. Am J Clin Pathol 1999;111:105–110.
21. Fonseca R, Tefferi A, Strickler JG. Follicular dendritic cell sarcoma mimicking diffuse large cell lymphoma: a case report. Am J Hematol 1997;55:148–155.
22. Liu SM, Huang PH, Liu JM. Interdigitating reticulum cell tumor of lymph node: a case report and literature review. Pathol Int 1998;48:974–980.
23. Dusenbery D, Watson CG. Fine-needle aspiration biopsy findings in a case of follicular dendritic cell tumor. Am J Clin Pathol 1996;106:689–692.

PART

VII

LYMPHOPROLIFERATIVE DISORDERS ASSOCIATED WITH IMMUNE DEFICIENCY

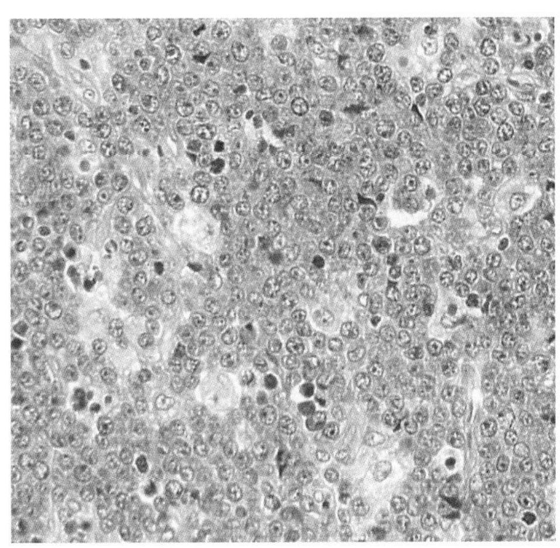

The immune system, comprising a multitude of interdependent cellular and humoral components, defends the body against environmental pathogens. Deficiencies in any part of this system expose the host to a greater risk for opportunistic infections and neoplasms. The opportunistic infections differ substantially from the infections common in the general population; their incidence is higher, and they are especially severe and exhibit unusual features. A relationship between immune deficiency and neoplasms has long been suspected, based on available clinical and experimental observations. Human neoplasms, particularly of the lymphoid system, are most prevalent in very old and very young persons, who are in the two periods of life when immunocompetence is weakest. Like the opportunistic infections, the neoplasms that develop in immunodeficient persons are characterized by an unusually high incidence and degree of severity and by specificity; thus, they can be called *opportunistic tumors.* The two major categories of immune deficiencies are primary and secondary. The primary group is defined by developmental deficits of various elements of the immune system; therefore, they are generally congenital and occur predominantly in children. The secondary or acquired immune deficiencies include those induced by immunosuppressant therapy, particularly in organ transplant recipients, and those caused by infection with HIV. Cancer registries started in the early 1970s in Minneapolis for tumors in persons with congenital immune deficiencies and in Denver and then Cincinnati for tumors in transplant recipients document prevalence rates for neoplasms far greater than those for age-matched segments of the general population.

The largest group of neoplasms associated with immune deficiencies of any kind are those of the lymphoid system. Regardless of the type and cause of immune deficiency, non-Hodgkin lymphomas are the prevailing tumors. Moreover, although the immune deficiencies with which they are associated represent a broad and heterogeneous spectrum, these lymphomas are fairly homogeneous in regard to high-grade histology, B-cell immunophenotype, occurrence in unusual sites, aggressiveness, and resistance to treatment. Also associated with immune deficiency are a variety of lymphoproliferative lesions, ranging from benign reactive hyperplasia to malignant lymphoma. Not infrequently, the distinction between benign and malignant lesions cannot be made solely on the basis of histologic features. Such lymphoid proliferations, encountered particularly in recipients of organ transplants, are generally described by the relatively ambiguous term of *post-transplant lymphoproliferative disorders.* Epstein-Barr virus has been demonstrated in the majority of such lesions. The lymphoproliferative disorders associated with congenital immune deficiencies are described in Chapter 79, and those associated with organ transplantation in Chapter 80. The lymphadenopathies associated with HIV infection are described in Chapter 15, and the lymphomas associated with AIDS in Chapter 81.

79

LYMPHOPROLIFERATIVE DISORDERS ASSOCIATED WITH CONGENITAL IMMUNE DEFICIENCIES

DEFINITION

Lymphadenopathies and lymphomas associated with congenital immune deficiencies.

PATHOGENESIS

Primary immune deficiencies (PIDs) are a large group of syndromes of great diversity that were initially named and classified in 1971 by a special committee of the World Health Organization (1). They are basically divided into cellular and humoral types, or T-cell and B-cell types, according to which major system is particularly affected; however, the many specific subtypes of each type result in a complex classification (2–4). Immune deficiencies involving the B-cell system, expressed as antibody immunodeficiencies, are the most common, representing 50% of all PIDs. About 40% of PIDs are of the T-cell system; three-fourths of these are associated with B-cell (i.e., antibody) deficiencies, such as severe combined immune deficiency (SCID), and are therefore far more severe. Disorders of the phagocytes (6%) and complement system (4%) account for the rest (2). Almost all PIDs are congenital, and many are hereditary.

In the early 1970s, strong evidence was produced in support of a relationship between PID and neoplasia (5). Accumulated data showed that the risk for development of a malignant tumor is 4% for persons with PID, a risk 10,000 times greater than that for normal healthy persons. The majority of tumors are lymphomas (58%) and leukemias (17%); by contrast, in the general childhood population, tumors such as neuroblastoma, Wilms tumor, and retinoblastoma are more common (5,6). Many of the PID syndromes develop at a very early age and cut life short because overwhelming infections ensue. In SCID, which has the shortest survival of all the PIDs, lymphomas and leukemias may develop in infancy; in sharp contrast, lymphomas are virtually absent in immunocompetent children of this age (7). Children with the Wiskott-Aldrich syndrome (WAS), caused by mutations in the X-linked WAS gene, are at high risk for malignancy; the risk actually increases as they live longer as a consequence of more efficient treatment of their infections. Of 71 cases of tumors in patients with WAS reported to the Immunodeficiency Cancer Registry by 1985, 62 were lymphomas or leukemias. Ataxia-telangiectasia (A-T), an autosomal recessive disorder associated with a mutant kinase gene, is characterized by profound immunologic abnormalities, systemic manifestations, and a predisposition for cancer. Of 150 tumors associated with A-T, 122 were leukemias or lymphomas (6) (Figs. 79.1 and 79.2). The histologic types are mostly high-grade malignancies (8), as are all other malignancies associated with immune deficiency (9). Also as in other types of immune deficiency, persistent, indolent, unexplainable lymphadenopathies frequently precede the lymphomas, sometimes by several years (10). Reactive lymphoid hyperplasia and atypical lymphoid hyperplasia, in addition to malignant lymphomas, are associated with PID. Epstein-Barr virus has frequently been identified by *in situ* hybridization in both benign and malignant lymphoid lesions (11). In the X-linked lymphoproliferative syndrome, which is transmitted by females and affects males exclusively, a specific congenital T-cell defect causes an inability to control B cells infected with Epstein-Barr virus. As a result, patients are affected by malignant lymphoproliferative diseases; in the original observation, six boys in the Duncan family all died within a 13-year period of severe forms of infectious mononucleosis and lymphomas (12) (see Chapter 9).

CLINICAL SYNDROME

The predominant symptoms are those of the PID clinical syndrome; they may vary from the triad of eczema, thrombocytopenia, and severe recurrent infections in WAS to the triad of progressive cerebellar ataxia, mucocutaneous telangiectasia, and sinopulmonary infections in A-T. The age distribution of the associated tumors follows the age at onset of

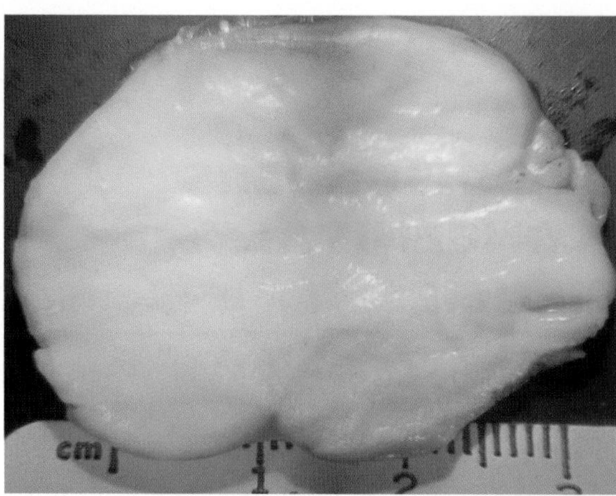

FIGURE 79.1. Non-Hodgkin lymphoma in abdominal lymph node of 12-year-old boy with ataxia-telangectasia. (Courtesy of Dr. Renate Dische.)

the PID. Thus, the peak incidence of lymphoma in SCID is before the age of 10 years, and in A-T it is before the age of 20 years. In common variable immune deficiency (CVID), which usually develops in adults after years of apparently normal immune function, lymphoid tumors may not arise until the patient is 50 to 60 years old (3,5). A male predominance is observed in all non-Hodgkin lymphomas (NHLs) related to PID, including A-T and CVID, which have an autosomal recessive inheritance (13).

In CVID, a block in the normal differentiation of B lymphocytes into plasma cells results in persistent hypogammaglobulinemia (14). Associated with CVID, as with other PIDs, are lymphoproliferative lesions, which range from benign reactive hyperplasia to malignant lymphoma. In a study of 11 cases of lymphoproliferative lesions associated with CVID, nine were benign and only two were malignant (11). In two cases of CVID observed by us, aggressive forms of NHL developed in both after an extended period. In one case, of a 63-year-old man with hereditary hemorrhagic telangiectasia (Osler-Weber-Rendu syndrome) and CVID, rapidly enlarging peripheral lymph nodes developed, and the patient died a month later of large cell immunoblastic lymphoma (Fig. 79.3) and multiple infections (4). In another case, of a woman who had had idiopathic thrombocytopenic purpura in addition to CVID as a child and had undergone a splenectomy, enlarged cervical lymph nodes developed when the patient was 24 years old that on histologic examination showed atypical lymphoid hyperplasia; when she was 36, a lymphoma with plasmacytoid differentiation developed, to which the patient succumbed at the age of 38 years (4) (Figs. 79.4 and 79.5).

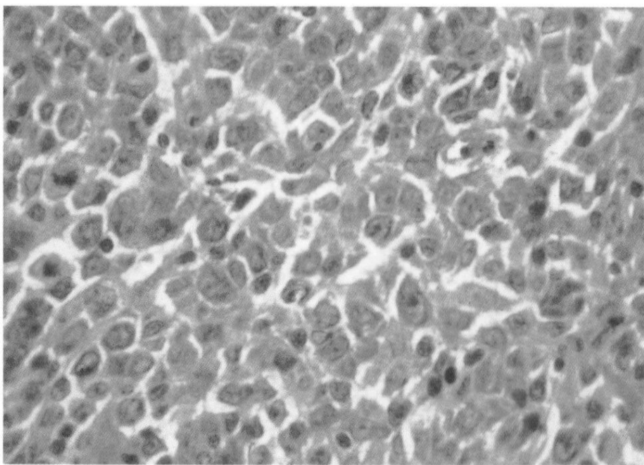

FIGURE 79.2. Specimen from case of ataxia-telangectasia in Fig. 79.1 showing histologic appearance of non-Hodgkin lymphoma, large cell B-cell type. Hematoxylin and eosin stain.

HISTOPATHOLOGY

The lymphadenopathies noted in children with PID may show atrophic follicles with hyalinized germinal centers and marked vascular proliferations, a picture reminiscent of Castleman disease. Depending on the type of PID, the lymph nodes may show depletion of the paracortex in predominantly T-cell deficiencies and involuted, atrophic follicles in predominantly B-cell deficiencies. In addition, activated lymphocytes or immunoblasts are seen in clusters or confluent sheets. These cells have large vesicular nuclei and one or several prominent nucleoli. Mitoses are present in variable numbers. Such lymphadenopathies, usually diagnosed as atypical lymphoid hyperplasias, occasionally have been misdiagnosed as lymphomas.

Lymphomas associated with PID, like those associated with acquired immune deficiencies, are far more commonly of non-Hodgkin than Hodgkin type and more frequently occur in extranodal locations than in lymph nodes (8,9). The histologic phenotypes of lymphomas associated with PID, particularly those in young children, are more commonly of high-grade, large cell, immunoblastic or Burkitt type. In older persons with less severe PID, NHL of lower grades may be seen (4).

IMMUNOPATHOLOGY

The NHLs associated with PIDs, like those associated with other immune deficiencies, are almost exclusively of B-cell type, probably as a result of a failure of T-cell immune surveillance over EBV-activated B cells (9). Therefore, the cells show membrane immunoglobulin restriction (Fig. 79.5) and express the common pan-B-cell markers (CD19, CD20, CD22).

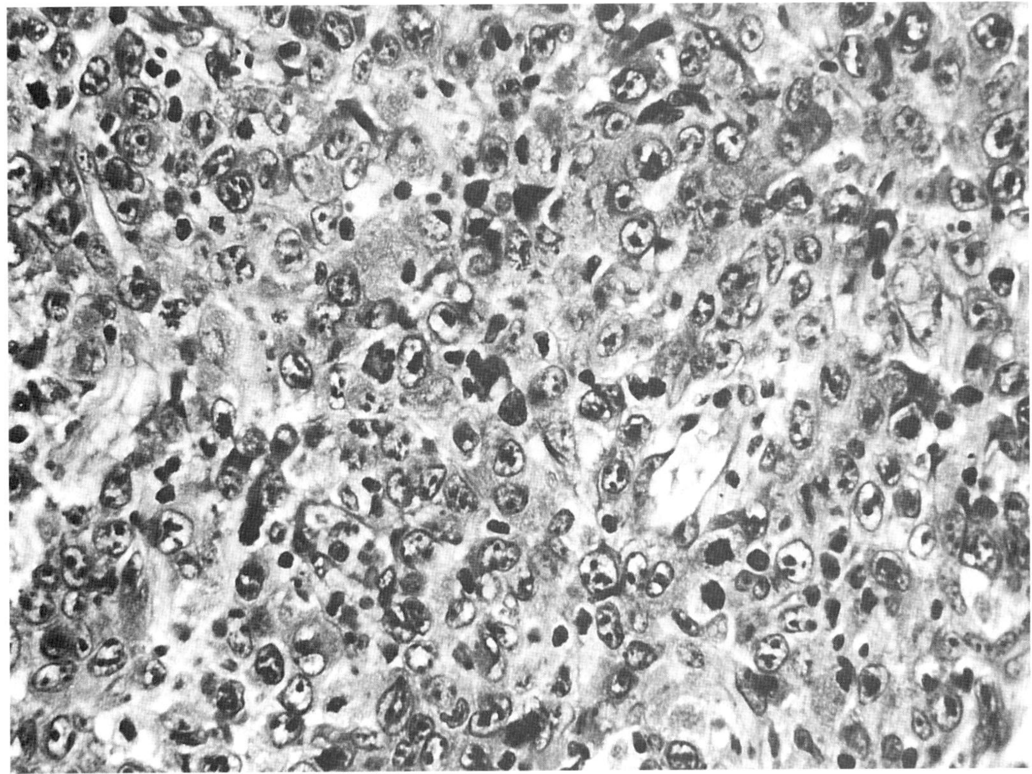

FIGURE 79.3. Non-Hodgkin lymphoma, large cell immunoblastic B-cell type, in 63-year-old man with common variable immune deficiency. Hematoxylin, phloxine, and saffron stain.

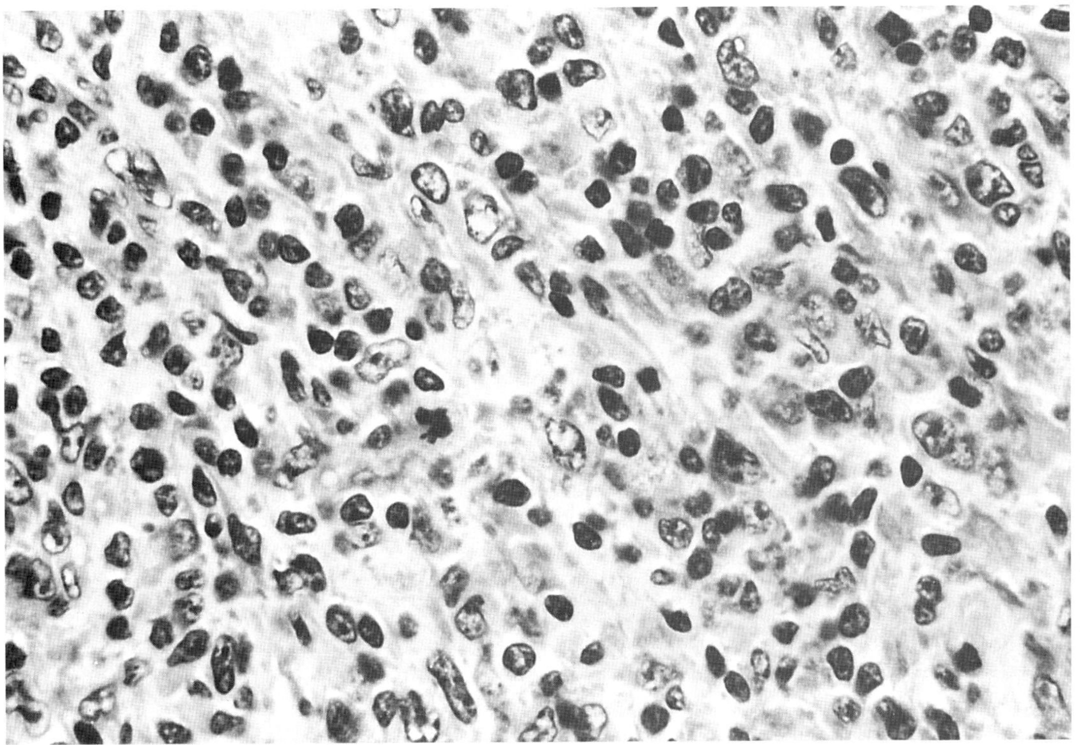

FIGURE 79.4. Cervical lymph node in 36-year-old woman with common variable immune deficiency. Mixed cell populations of small lymphocytes and large cells with vesicular nuclei representing activated lymphocytes and lymphoma cells. Hematoxylin, phloxine, and saffron stain.

Checklist

LYMPHOPROLIFERATIVE DISORDERS ASSOCIATED WITH CONGENITAL IMMUNE DEFICIENCIES

Congenital deficiency of one or more immune systems
Longer survival with opportunistic infections increases chances for development of lymphoma
Benign, indolent lymphadenopathy preceding malignancies
Atypical lymphoid hyperplasia
NHLs predominantly of large cell immunoblastic or Burkitt type
Extranodal sites prevalent
B-cell phenotype
Short survival

DIFFERENTIAL DIAGNOSIS

- Angioimmunoblastic lymphadenopathy: Histologic patterns may be similar, however, angioimmunoblastic lymphadenopathy occurs in elderly patients, whereas the lymphadenopathies associated with PID occur in the young.
- Castleman lymphadenopathy shows atrophic follicles and hypervascularity but not a florid proliferation of immunoblasts.
- Atypical lymphoid hyperplasia is difficult, sometimes impossible, to distinguish from NHL without the aid of clonal rearrangement analysis.
- NHLs of large cell immunoblastic or Burkitt type are not different histologically from their counterparts in the general population.

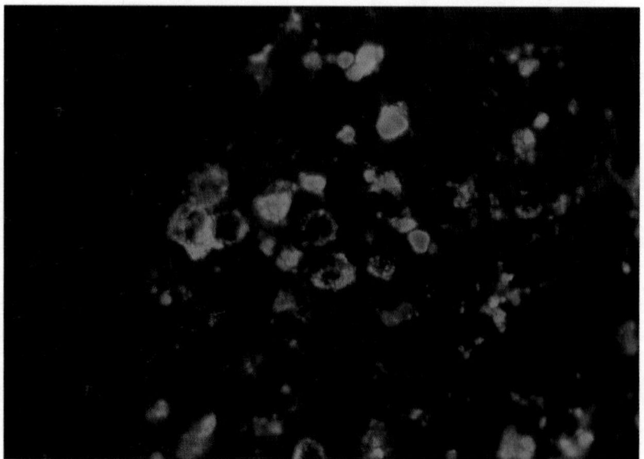

FIGURE 79.5. Cells from lymph node in Fig. 79.4 stained with fluorescein isothiocyanate-labeled anti-κ light chain show membrane immunoglobulin restriction, consistent with non-Hodgkin lymphoma, and plasmacytoid differentiation.

REFERENCES

1. Fudenberg H, Good RA, Goodman HC, et al. Primary immunodeficiencies. Pediatrics 1971;47:927.
2. Stiehm RE. Immunodeficiency disorders—general considerations. In: Stiehm RE, Fulginiti VA, eds. Immunologic disorders in infants and children. Philadelphia: WB Saunders, 1980:183–218.
3. Amman AJ, Hong R. In: Stiehm RE, Fulginiti VA, eds. Immunologic disorders in infants and children. Philadelphia: WB Saunders, 1980:291–297.
4. Ioachim HL. Neoplasms associated with immune deficiencies. Pathol Annu 1987;22:177–222.
5. Kersey JH, Spector BD, Good RA. Primary immunodeficiency diseases and cancer: the immunodeficiency cancer registry. Int J Cancer 1973;12:333.
6. Filipovich AH, Heinitz KJ, Robinson LL, et al. The immunodeficiency cancer registry, a research resource. Am J Pediatr Hematol Oncol 1987;9:183–184.
7. Waldman TA, Strober W, Blaese RM. Immunodeficiency disease and malignancy. Ann Intern Med 1972;77:605.
8. Frizzera G, Rosai J, Dehner LP, et al. Lymphoreticular disorders in primary immunodeficiencies: new findings based on an up-to-date histologic classification of 35 cases. Cancer 1980;46:692.
9. Ioachim HL. The opportunistic tumors of immune deficiency. Adv Cancer Res 1990;54:301–317.
10. Gatti RA, Good RA. Occurrence of malignancy in immunodeficiency disease. Cancer 1971;28:89.
11. Sander CA, Medeiros LJ, Weiss LM, et al. Lymphoproliferative lesions in patients with common variable immunodeficiency syndrome. Am J Surg Pathol 1992;16:1170–1182.
12. Purtilo DT, Cassel C, Yang JPS, et al. X-linked recessive progressive combined variable immunodeficiency (Duncan's disease). Lancet 1975;1:935.
13. Filipovich AH, Shapiro R, Robison L, et al. Lymphoproliferative disorders associated with immunodeficiency, In: Magrath IT, ed. The non-Hodgkin's lymphomas. Baltimore: Williams & Wilkins, 1990:134–154.
14. Rosen FS, Cooper MD, Wedgwood RJP. The primary immunodeficiencies (second of two parts). N Engl J Med 1984;311:300–310.

80

LYMPHOPROLIFERATIVE DISORDERS ASSOCIATED WITH ORGAN TRANSPLANTATION

DEFINITION

Lymphadenopathies and lymphomas affecting recipients of organ transplants.

SYNONYM

Post-transplant lymphoproliferative disorders

PATHOGENESIS

Malignant tumors occur three to four times more often in recipients of organ transplants than in the age-matched general population. The types of tumors, incidence, and times of occurrence vary with the transplanted organs and regimens of immunosuppression. Overall, neoplasms arise in 4% to 18%, an average of 6%, of organ transplant recipients (1,2). Of these tumors, lymphomas make up a disproportionately large percentage, 26%, in comparison with 3% to 4% of all tumors in the general population (1). The incidence of lymphomas in allograft recipients was estimated to be 350 times greater than that in normal controls. As the types of organs transplanted expanded and immunosuppressant regimens became more intensive, a considerable increase in the incidence of lymphoma was recorded. Kidney recipients have the lowest rate, 1.0%, and heart and lung recipients the highest rate, 9.4%, of lymphoproliferative disorders (3,4). These differences are most likely related to the intensity of immunosuppression, which increased greatly with the introduction of cyclosporin A and OKT3, a monoclonal antibody directed against CD3+ T cells (2–5). The latency period from the administration of treatment to the appearance of tumors is directly related to the immunosuppressive regimen used (6). It was considerably reduced, from 4 to 5 years with azathioprine to 5 to 7 months with cyclosporin A and OKT3 (2–6).

Post-transplantation lymphoid neoplasms affect approximately 2% of all organ allograft recipients (7) and encompass a variety of lymphoid proliferations, from benign reactive lymphoid hyperplasia at one end of the spectrum to high-grade malignant lymphoma at the other (5–8). Virtually all lesions are of B-cell type, and almost all are associated with a primary or reactivated Epstein-Barr viral (EBV) infection. The whole group is referred to as *post-transplantation lymphoproliferative disorders* (PTLDs). Extranodal locations in up to 70% of cases, and often the transplanted organs, liver or lung, may be the site of lymphomas. A unique feature of PTLDs is that some regress when the immunosuppressive treatment is reduced or discontinued (9). Others progress rapidly despite intensive treatment. The clinical behavior does not always correlate with the histologic appearance or clonality of the tumor. The presence of the EBV genome is demonstrated by immunohistochemical studies with antibodies to EBV nuclear antigen (EBNA), which demonstrate positive cells in 38% to 100% of cases, and *in situ* hybridization with a fragment of EBV DNA labeled with a radioactive isotope, which identifies EBV in most of the lymphoid lesions (8–12). In some cases of PTLD, the EBV genome cannot be identified; such EBV-negative tumors generally appear later and have a worse prognosis, although some may still regress after the discontinuation of immunosuppressive treatment (13). In general, the pathogenesis of PTLD seems to be an exaggerated proliferation of EBV-carrying B cells released from the control of immunosuppressed T cells. The B-cell proliferation progresses from polyclonal to monoclonal in a relatively short time, which explains the coexistence of hyperplastic and neoplastic histologic patterns and the difficulty of separating benign from malignant lesions (5,10,14).

CLINICAL SYNDROME

A PTLD may present soon after transplantation in the form of an indolent lymphadenopathy or as an infectious mononucleosis-like illness with mild or severe symptoms (3–5). Tumor masses, single or multiple, involving lymph nodes or the gastrointestinal tract may develop. In a 12-year-old boy with severe combined immunodeficiency, bone marrow transplantation was followed 80 days later by systemic disease and multiple lymphomas (15). Extranodal locations of PTLD predominate; with conventional immunosuppression, the gastrointestinal tract and brain are favored sites for atypical lymphoid proliferations and lymphomas (3,4,16). However, a change in the distribution of lesions, with lymph node involvement in more than 50% of cases, was recorded after OKT3 and cyclosporin A were introduced as immunosuppressants (5,17). The allograft itself may be the site of PTLD, as in a series of 54 patients with heart–lung implants, 60% of whose lesions developed in the transplanted lung (4). The prognosis of PTLD is related to the histopathologic diagnosis. The early lesions are generally reversible, whereas the monomorphic lesions that usually present in stages III or IV disease have a poor prognosis. The outcome of polymorphic lesions varies between regression following withdrawal of immune suppression or chemotherapy and uninterrupted progression.

HISTOPATHOLOGY

Lymph nodes involved by PTLD show effaced architecture and cellular infiltration of vessel walls, fibrous stroma, capsule, and even perinodal fibrofatty tissues (3,4,17).

A spectrum of histologic patterns ranges from one that resembles infectious mononucleosis, with a mottled paracortex containing a polymorphic mixture of large immunoblasts and small lymphocytes, to one that resembles large cell lymphoma, with a monomorphic population of large atypical immunoblasts containing pleomorphic nuclei and large nucleoli (3,17). The lymphoma-like lesions may include Reed-Sternberg–like cells, frequent mitoses, and focal areas of necrosis (4). To distinguish between benign and malignant lesions, some authors regard the absence or presence of necrosis and atypical immunoblasts as decisive criteria (17). Others consider polymorphic cell populations, including small and large, cleaved and noncleaved lymphocytes, immunoblasts, and plasma cells, as indicative of non-neoplastic disease, as opposed to the cellular monomorphism of lymphomas (3). Because of rapid progression of the lymphoid proliferation, frequently more than one pattern is found when multiple lesions are sampled at the same time (3,8). Sometimes, nodules of apparent lymphoma cells can be seen in a lymph node that otherwise shows a pattern of reactive or atypical hyperplasia. This unusual pattern has also been noted in other lymphoproliferative lesions associated with immune deficiencies.

In the new World Health Organization classification of hematologic malignancies, the PTLDs are divided into the following categories:

1. *Early lesions* include reactive plasmacytic hyperplasia and infectious mononucleosis-like lesions. These are benign reactive processes occurring in the adenoids, tonsils, lymph nodes, and occasionally the lung or gastrointestinal tract. Virtually all early lesions regress following a reduction in immunosuppression (3,18). The lymph node architecture is maintained, and the follicles are hyperplastic or diminished at a later time. The interfollicular area includes plasmacytoid lymphocytes and plasma cells with scattered immunoblasts of B- or T-cell type. The lesions are polyclonal, and some show the marks of EBV infection (3,18).

2. *Polymorphic PTLD.* In these lesions, the architecture is effaced by a polymorphic cell population that ranges from small and large cells with plasmacytoid differentiation to cells that are exclusively lymphoid and exhibit significant nuclear atypia. Some are highly pleomorphic, often resembling Reed-Sternberg cells. All cells are of B-cell origin. Foci or confluent areas of necrosis are often present (17,18) (Fig. 80.1). Because the cell populations are mixed and variable, a prognosis based on histopathology may be uncertain. Therefore, a trial withdrawal of immunosuppression is recommended before the inception of chemotherapy.

3. *Monomorphic PTLD.* These lesions include lymphomas and multiple myelomas that are no different from those typically seen in the general population. The lymphomas are of Burkitt (Fig. 80.2) or diffuse large B-cell types (Fig. 80.3). The cell populations are monomorphic and obliterate the architecture of the lymph nodes or other organs. In lymphomas, the cells are large, with vesicular nuclei, multiple or one prominent nucleolus, abundant cytoplasm, and numerous atypical mitoses (Fig. 80.4). In multiple myeloma, plasmacytoid immunoblasts and plasmablasts are often binucleated and atypical. The cells exhibit clonal

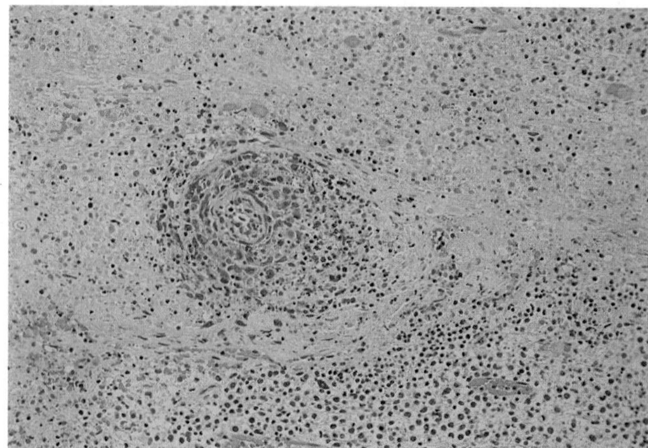

FIGURE 80.1. Cervical lymph node in 50-year-old man after transplantation of cord stem cells. Extensive tumor necrosis with tumor cells preserved around blood vessel and bottom area.

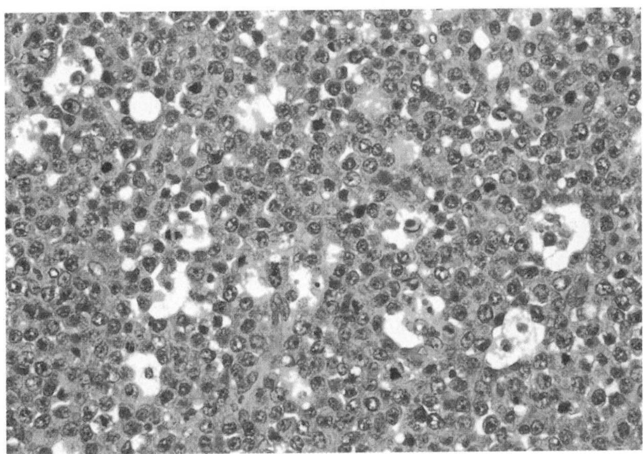

FIGURE 80.2. Large B-cell lymphoma with diffuse growth and numerous interspersed tingible-body macrophages in a 10-year-old girl following a heart transplant. The cells have plasmacytoid or immunoblastic features, with basophilic cytoplasm and ovoid nuclei that have prominent nucleoli.

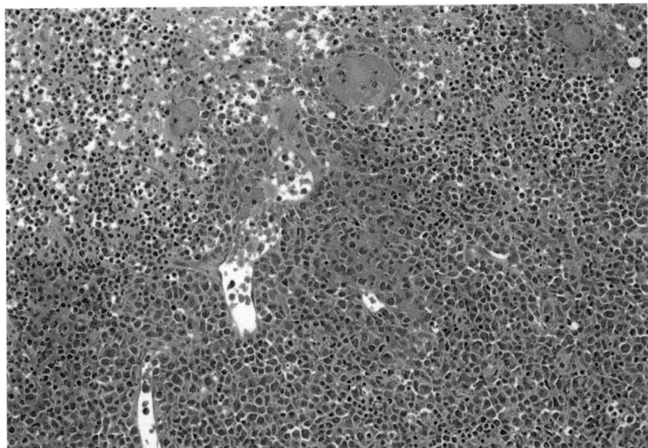

FIGURE 80.3. Same lymph node as in Fig. 80.2 entirely replaced by sheets of monomorphic large lymphoma cells, B-cell phenotype, with scattered small, incidental T cells.

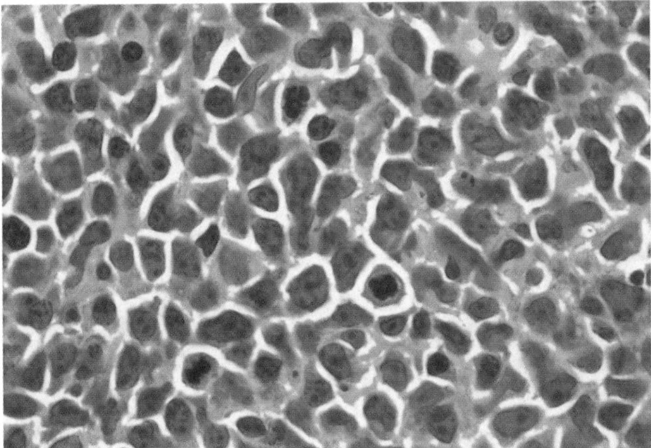

FIGURE 80.4. Lymphoma cells of previous figures are monomorphic and large, with abundant basophilic cytoplasm and large, angular, sometimes eccentric nuclei that have inconspicuous nucleoli and show frequent atypical mitoses.

immunoglobulin heavy and light chain gene rearrangements, and most show evidence of clonal EBV infection (10,18,19,20).

4. *T-cell PTLD.* These lesions are very rare, and only few cases have been reported (21,22). They tended to occur later after transplantation (after a median of 5 years vs. a median of 4.5 months) (14). They included cases of lymphoblastic lymphoma, peripheral T-cell lymphoma, and anaplastic large cell lymphoma. EBV was associated in only half of the cases of T-cell PTLD (14).

IMMUNOHISTOCHEMISTRY

Although the vast majority of PTLDs are of B-cell type, T-cell lymphomas occasionally have been reported, such as a case of non-Hodgkin lymphoma of T-cell type in the liver of a heart transplant patient (21). In the Cincinnati Transplant Tumor Registry, 86% of post-transplant lymphomas were of B-cell type, 14% of T-cell type, and 1% of null cell type (2). Monoclonality was demonstrated in most reported cases by light chain immunoglobulin restriction. B-cell origin was demonstrated by positivity for CD22, CD20, CD19, and HLA-DR, whereas T-cell lymphomas were CD4+ or CD8+ (5).

MOLECULAR PATHOLOGY

In contrast to lymphomas in general, which derive from the same clone, PTLD lesions frequently exhibit a variable clonal composition (18,19,20,23). Genotypic studies have shown that multiple clones may arise concomitantly in one or different organs during stimulation by EBV and in the absence of regulation by suppressed T cells (3,4,12,15). In a 15-year-old heart transplant recipient, 24 separate PTLD lesions in the colon exhibited different clonal immunoglobulin heavy chain gene rearrangements and evidence of different EBV infectious events (14). This determination is important because it shows that although some PTLD lesions in the same patient or even in the same location may regress when treatment is withheld, others, representing different clones, may advance uninhibited. Karyotypic abnormalities have been reported in PTLD, but consistent chromosomal aberrations have not been described. EBV can be detected in more than 90% of PTLDs with the use of Southern blot hybridization, *in situ* hybridization, or polymerase chain reaction techniques. The clonality of EBV can be determined with probes to the EBV terminal repeat region. It has been noted that polyclonal PTLDs are usually associated with multiple EBV infectious events, whereas monoclonal malignant lesions exhibit evidence of EBV infection before the clonal expansion of tumors (14,19,20, 23).

Checklist

POST-TRANSPLANT LYMPHOPROLIFERATIVE DISORDERS

Organ transplant recipients under immunosuppressive therapy
EBV infection, primary or reactivated
Spectrum of lymphoid lesions, from polyclonal benign to monoclonal malignant
Frequent regression after decrease or discontinuation of immunosuppression
Lymph nodes, extranodal locations, or both affected
Early lesions
  Reactive plasmacytic hyperplasia
  Infectious mononucleosis-like lesion
Polymorphic PTLD: mixed cell populations difficult to assess
Monomorphic PTLD
  Non-Hodgkin lymphoma
  Multiple myeloma
B-cell origin in vast majority of cases

DIFFERENTIAL DIAGNOSIS

- The two extremes of the PTLD spectrum, reactive hyperplasia and lymphoma, usually can be diagnosed by the general morphologic criteria. However, in the polymorphic PTLD, the distinction between atypical lymphoid hyperplasia and non-Hodgkin lymphoma is difficult to make and sometimes impossible without the aid of immunohistochemistry and clonal rearrangement analysis.

REFERENCES

1. Penn I. Lymphomas complicating organ transplantation. Transplant Proc 1983;15:2790–2797.
2. Penn I. The changing pattern of posttransplant malignancies. Transplant Proc 1991;23:1101–1103.
3. Nalesnik MA, Jaffe R, Starzl TE, et al. The pathology of posttransplant lymphoproliferative disorders occurring in the setting of cyclosporin A–prednisone immunosuppression. Am J Pathol 1988;133:173–192.
4. Yousem SA, Randhawa P, Locker J, et al. Posttransplant lymphoproliferative disorders in heart–lung transplant recipients: primary presentation in the allograft. Hum Pathol 1989;20:361–369.
5. Swerdlow SH. Post-transplant lymphoproliferative disorders: a morphologic, phenotypic and genotypic spectrum of disease. Histopathology 1992;20:373–385.
6. Swinnen LJ, Costanzo-Nordin MR, Fisher SC, et al. Increased incidence of lymphoproliferative disorders after immunosuppression with the monoclonal antibody OKT3 in cardiac transplant recipients. N Engl J Med 1990;323:1723–1728.
7. Nalesnik MA, Makowka L, Starzl TE. The diagnosis and treatment of posttransplant lymphoproliferative disorders. Curr Probl Surg 1988;25:367–472.
8. Hanto DW, Frizzera G, Gajl-Peczalska KJ, et al. Epstein-Barr virus immunodeficiency and B-cell lymphoproliferation. Transplantation 1985;39:461–472.
9. Starzl TE, Nalesnik MA, Porter KA, et al. Reversibility of lymphomas and lymphoproliferative lesions developing under cyclosporine–steroid therapy. Lancet 1984;1:584–587.
10. Cleary ML, Warnke R, Sklar J. Monoclonality of lymphoproliferative lesions in cardiac transplant recipients. Clonal analysis based on immunoglobulin gene rearrangements. N Engl J Med 1984;310:477–482.
11. Ho M, Miller G, Atchison RW, et al. Epstein-Barr virus infection and DNA hybridization studies in post-transplantation lymphoma and lymphoproliferative lesions: the role of primary infection. J Infect Dis 1985;152:876–886.
12. Randhawa P, Jaffe R, Demetris AJ, et al. The systemic distribution of Epstein-Barr virus genomes in fatal post-transplantation lymphoproliferative disorders. An *in situ* hybridization study. Am J Pathol 1991;138:1027–1033.
13. Nelson BP, Nalesnik MA, Bahler DW, et al. Epstein-Barr virus-negative post-transplant lymphoproliferative disorders. A distinct entity? Am J Surg Pathol 2000;24:375–385.
14. Chadburn A, Cesarman E, Knowles DM. Molecular pathology of posttransplantation lymphoproliferative disorders. Semin Diagn Pathol 1997;14:15–26.
15. Shearer WT, Ritz J, Finegold MJ, et al. Epstein-Barr virus-associated B-cell proliferations of diverse clonal origins after bone marrow transplantation in a 12-year-old patient with severe combined immunodeficiency. N Engl J Med 1985;312:1151–1159.
16. Weintraub J, Warnke RA. Lymphoma in cardiac allotransplant recipients. Clinical and histological features and immunological phenotype. Transplantation 1982;33:347–351.
17. Frizzera G, Hanto DW, Gajl-Peczalska KJ, et al. Polymorphic diffuse B-cell hyperplasias and lymphomas in renal transplant recipients. Cancer Res 1981;41:4262–4279.
18. Knowles DM, Cesarman E, Chadburn A, et al. Correlative morphologic and molecular genetic analysis demonstrates three dis-

tinct categories of posttransplantation lymphoproliferative disorders. Blood 1995;85:552–565.

19. Cleary ML, Nalesnik MA, Shearer WT, et al. Clonal analysis of transplant-associated lymphoproliferations based on the structure of the genomic termini of the Epstein-Barr virus. Blood 1988;72:349–352.
20. Kaplan MA, Ferry JA, Harris NL, et al. Clonal analysis of posttransplant lymphoproliferative disorders, using both Epstein-Barr virus and immunoglobulin genes as markers. Am J Clin Pathol 1994;101:590–596.
21. Kemnitz J, Cremer J, Gebel M, et al. T-cell lymphoma after heart transplantation. Am J Clin Pathol 1990;94:95–101.
22. Waller EK, Siemianska M, Bangs CD, et al. Characterization of posttransplant lymphomas that express T cell-associated markers: immunophenotypes, molecular genetics, cytogenetics and heterotransplantation in severe combined immunodeficient mice. Blood 1993;82:247–261.
23. Locker J, Nalesnik M. Molecular genetic analysis of lymphoid tumors arising after organ transplantation. Am J Pathol 1989;135: 977–987.

81

LYMPHOMAS ASSOCIATED WITH ACQUIRED IMMUNODEFICIENCY SYNDROME

DEFINITION

A heterogeneous group of Hodgkin lymphomas (HLs) and non-Hodgkin lymphomas (NHLs) arising in persons with severe AIDS induced by infection with HIV.

EPIDEMIOLOGY

Non-Hodgkin lymphomas in HIV-infected persons are considered AIDS-defining illnesses. They occur in 3% of patients with AIDS (1), whose risk for NHL is therefore 60 times greater than that of the general population (2). Recent studies show a continuing increase in the incidence of lymphomas among AIDS patients, who now survive longer because of antiretroviral and antifungal therapies. In patients on anti-HIV treatments for longer than 3 years, the incidence of NHL may be as high as 28% (3). In contrast to Kaposi sarcoma, which is far more common in homosexual AIDS patients than in other patients with AIDS, NHL affects all AIDS risk groups equally, including children (4). HL is also more frequent in AIDS patients, whose risk for this disease is 10 times greater than that of persons without AIDS (5).

PATHOGENESIS

The high incidence of NHLs in persons with AIDS parallels the increased frequency of these tumors in persons with congenital immune deficiencies (see Chapter 79) and in immunodepressed recipients of organ transplants (see Chapter 80) (6–9). The AIDS-associated NHLs are a group of heterogeneous neoplasms that are virtually all of B-cell type but differ in histologic type, location, and pathogenesis (9,10). The HIV that is at the origin of AIDS is not involved in the malignant transformation of B cells; no HIV sequences have been detected in lymphoma cells (11). However, HIV infection induces the production of a variety of cytokines and growth factors that play an important role in the activation and differentiation of B cells. The intense follicular hyperplasia of HIV lymphadenitis shows an active proliferation of B cells, which leads to cellular instability and molecular alterations such as mutations, translocations, and deletions of tumor suppressor genes (11–14). Thus, excessive stimulation of B cells, selection of B-cell clones carrying genetic alterations, and cellular immune deficiency with inactivation of immune surveillance are combined factors in the pathogenesis of AIDS-associated NHLs (11). In the case of Burkitt lymphoma, which accounts for 30% of AIDS-associated NHLs, the molecular pathway involves infection with Epstein-Barr virus (EBV), activation of the c-myc protooncogene, and inactivation of the p53 tumor suppressor gene (11–14).

CLINICAL SYNDROME

In contrast to the lymphomas that occur in the general population of young adults, which are more often HLs, the lymphomas of persons with AIDS are far more frequently NHLs. Also unlike the lymphomas in the general population, the lymphomas in AIDS patients more often originate in extranodal locations (15). In a study of 111 cases of AIDS-associated lymphomas, we found that 11 were HLs and 100 were NHLs (16). In the same study, of the 100 NHLs, 61 originated in various internal organs, whereas only 49 were initially located in lymph nodes. In the extranodal cases, the digestive tract, with 27 cases, and the central nervous system, with 15 cases, were the most common primary sites (16).

The lymph nodes within and around the salivary glands, particularly the parotid, are often involved in HIV infection presenting as unilateral or bilateral, often primary, lymphadenitis (17) (see Chapter 16). Like lymph nodes in other locations, the salivary gland lymph nodes may become the site of lymphomas. In both lymphadenitis and lymphoma, the salivary glands are not directly involved (17). Salivary gland lymphomas, as we previously reported, are associated with EBV infection and may be synchronous with or succeed an HIV salivary lymphadenitis (18). Regardless of their location, AIDS-associated lymphomas, which are in almost all cases of a high histologic grade, exhibit great clinical aggressiveness (4,16,19). HLs in AIDS more often present in late stages III and IV, with noncontiguous lymph node progression and involvement of internal organs, including bone marrow dissemination. NHLs in AIDS are invariably of a high histologic grade and highly aggressive; early dissemination, resistance to treatment, frequent relapses, and short survivals are typical (4,15,16,19–21).

HISTOPATHOLOGY

Lymphadenopathies, characteristic of HIV infection, may precede lymphomas in AIDS patients (16,21). They were noted in the histories of a third of 100 patients with AIDS-associated lymphomas and confirmed by lymph node biopsy in 14 of these cases (16). The histologic features of the preceding lymphadenopathies were characteristic of HIV infection. In the majority of cases, atrophic follicles, hyalinized germinal centers, and excessive vascular proliferation of the advanced stages of histologic patterns B and C were noted (22–24) (see Chapter 15). Sometimes, nodules of lymphoma cells can be seen in a lymph node that still shows a pattern of reactive hyperplasia (Fig. 81.1). This observation is consistent with the reported finding of monoclonal rearranged bands in HIV lymphadenopathies, possibly representing the emergence of lymphoma clones in lymph nodes that still have a benign histologic appearance (12).

Hodgkin lymphomas in AIDS patients are usually of the mixed cellularity and lymphocyte depletion types, which are

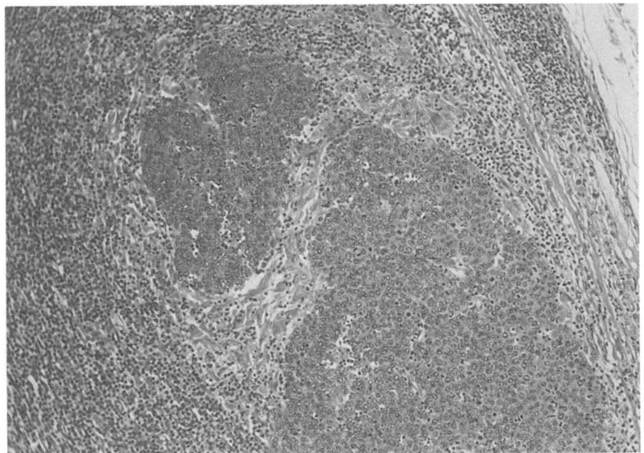

FIGURE 81.1. Non-Hodgkin lymphoma, diffuse large noncleaved cell type arising as confluent tumor nodules in the cortex of a supraclavicular lymph node with HIV lymphadenitis. Hematoxylin, phloxine, and saffron stain.

higher histologic grades that are otherwise infrequently seen in Europe and North America (5) (Fig. 81.2).

Lymph nodes are less often the primary location of HL in AIDS patients than in the general population. In the lymphomas that arise in lymph nodes, the distribution among the different groups of lymph nodes appears to be random. The lymph nodes of the salivary glands seem to be particularly affected by HIV infection and subsequently by lymphoma (17,18) (Fig. 81.3) (see Chapter 16). Histologically, the AIDS-associated NHLs are a heterogeneous group; about 30% of cases are Burkitt and Burkitt-like lymphomas (Fig. 81.4), and the remaining 70% of cases are diffuse large cell lymphomas (Fig. 81.5), divided almost equally between the immunoblastic and pleomorphic variants (11,16,21, 25). Rare cases of primary effusion lymphomas, related etiologically to human herpesvirus type 8 (Kaposi sarcoma-associated virus), have been more recently reported; however, they do not involve lymph nodes and are not further described (26).

Burkitt lymphoma is 1,000 times more common in HIV-infected people than in the population at large, where its frequency is only 1% of all lymphomas (27). In AIDS patients, Burkitt and Burkitt-like lymphomas are predominantly located in lymph nodes, whereas large cell lymphomas are more often in extranodal locations, particularly the central nervous system, where Burkitt lymphoma is infrequent (16,25). AIDS patients with the Burkitt type of NHL are usually younger, have higher levels of CD4+ T cells, and may not have had prior manifestations of AIDS, whereas patients with large cell lymphomas present with symptoms of advanced AIDS and CD4+ T-cell counts below 100/mm^3 (11). The histopathology of lymph nodes with NHL of Burkitt and diffuse large cell types in AIDS patients is similar to that previously described (see Chapters 67 and 69).

IMMUNOPATHOLOGY

Virtually all AIDS-associated lymphomas are of B-cell type and express monotypic surface immunoglobulins and pan-B-cell membrane antigens CD19, CD20, and CD22; they lack all T-cell antigens (28) (Fig. 81.6). The few exceptions reported as T-cell lymphomas are uncertain or related to the T-cell lymphotropic virus (HTLV-1) (29,30).

MOLECULAR BIOLOGY

Signs of EBV infection are found in about 30% of AIDS-associated Burkitt lymphomas and in more than 70% of AIDS-associated diffuse large cell lymphomas (11) (Fig. 81.7). Like all other Burkitt lymphomas, those associated with AIDS exhibit the 8;14 reciprocal translocation, in which juxtaposition of the protooncogene c-myc and the

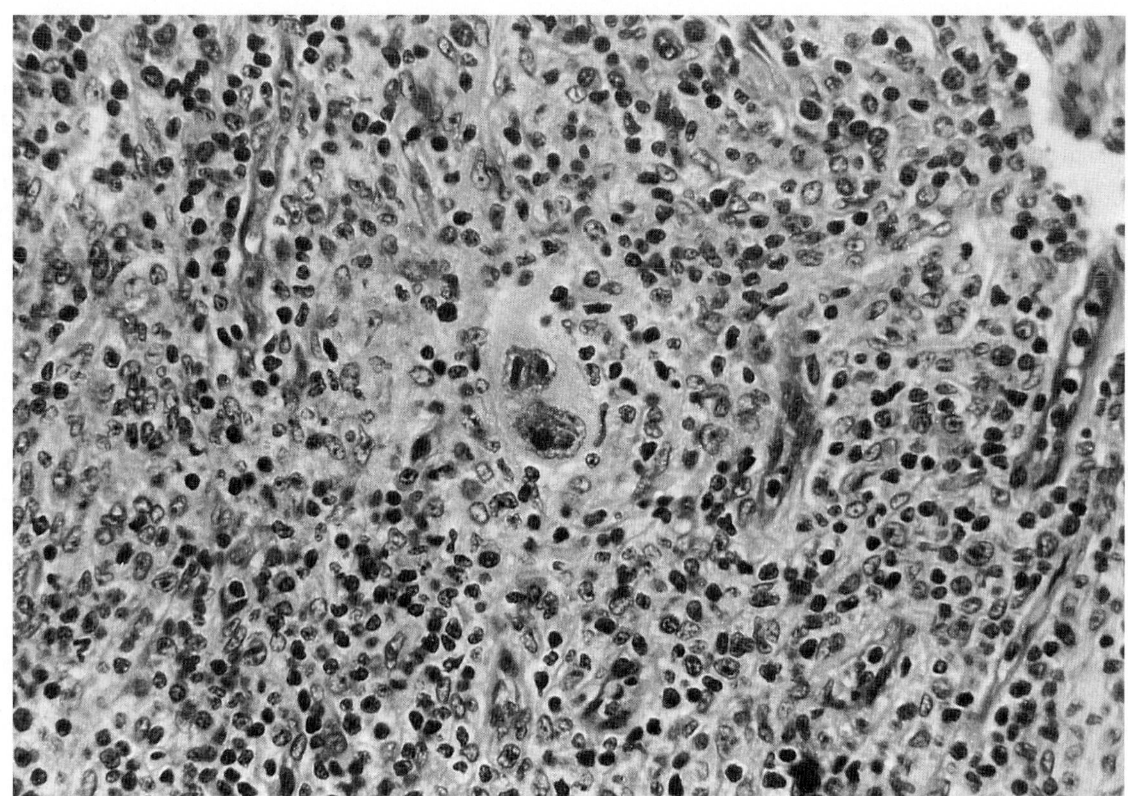

FIGURE 81.2. Hodgkin lymphoma, mixed cellularity type with diagnostic Reed-Sternberg cell in a depleted germinal center of a lymph node with HIV lymphadenitis. Numerous blood vessels surround the atrophic follicle. Hematoxylin, phloxine, and saffron stain.

immunoglobulin locus causes transcriptional deregulation. Other mutations and deletions result in inactivation of the p53 tumor suppressor gene (11,13). In diffuse large cell lymphomas and in HL, EBV-positive tumors express the transforming antigen latent membrane protein (LMP) and in some cases Epstein-Barr nuclear antigen 2 (EBNA-2). Deregulation of the protooncogene bcl-6 also occurs (11,14).

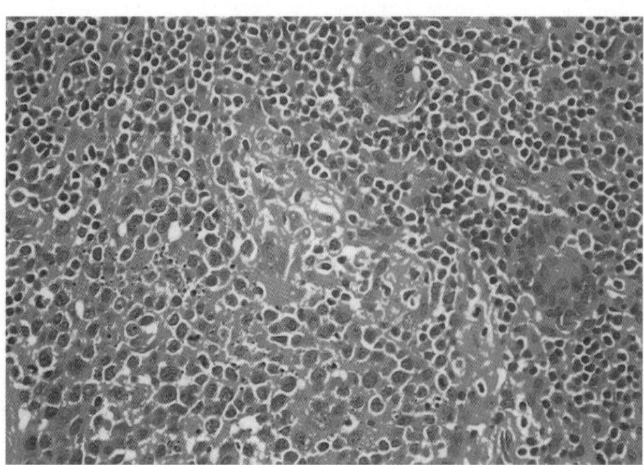

FIGURE 81.3. Non-Hodgkin large cell lymphoma arising in a parotid lymph node with HIV lymphadenitis. Hematoxylin, phloxine, and saffron stain.

DIFFERENTIAL DIAGNOSIS

- The HIV infection is determined by the presence of HIV antibodies.
- The status of immunodeficiency is determined by the total number of CD4+ lymphocytes and the ratio of CD4+ to CD8+ T cells.

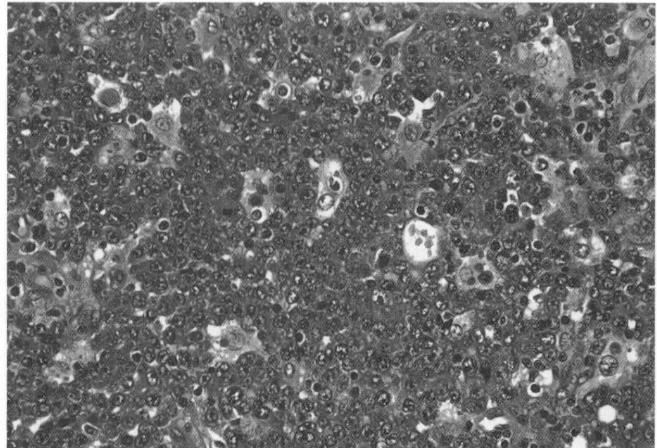

FIGURE 81.4. Non-Hodgkin lymphoma, Burkitt cell type in cervical lymph node of AIDS patient. Starry sky pattern, homogeneous population of small noncleaved lymphoma cells with frequent apoptosis and tingible-body macrophages. Hematoxylin, phloxine, and saffron stain.

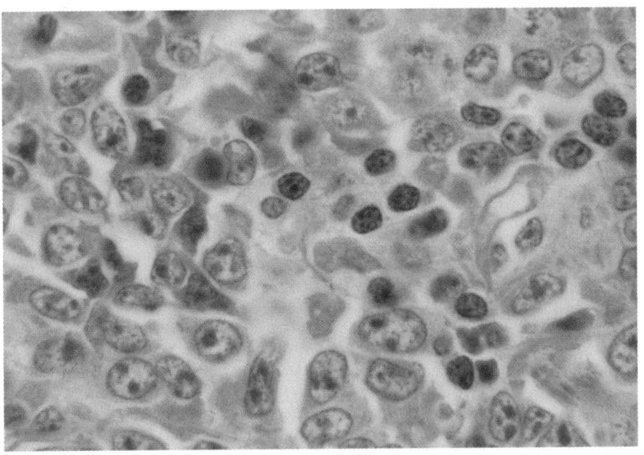

FIGURE 81.5. Non-Hodgkin lymphoma, large cell immunoblastic type in lymph node of patient with AIDS. Large cells have abundant cytoplasm and nuclei with central prominent nucleoli. Hematoxylin, phloxine, and saffron stain.

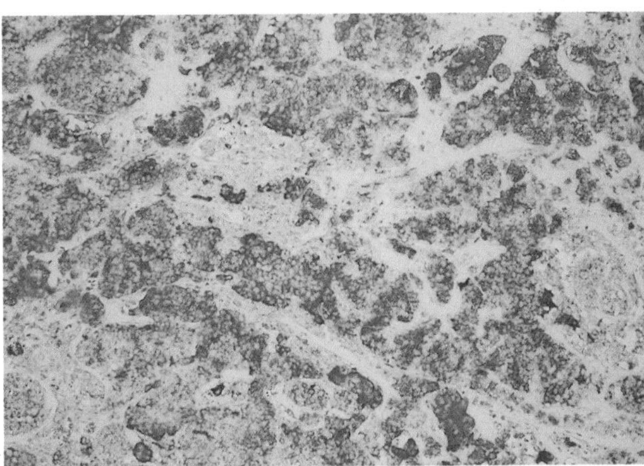

FIGURE 81.6. Non-Hodgkin lymphoma, large cell immunoblastic B-cell type in AIDS patient. Strong CD20 immunostaining in the membrane and the large tumor cells. L26/peroxidase.

Checklist

LYMPHOMAS ASSOCIATED WITH AIDS

Hodgkin Lymphomas Associated with AIDS

Patients HIV+
CD4+ lymphocyte counts below 200/mm^3
Ratio of CD4+ to CD8+ lymphocytes usually less than 0.5
"B" symptoms frequent
Presentation in stage III or IV
Extranodal sites common, frequently bone marrow
Mixed cellularity and lymphocyte depletion types more common
Poor prognosis

Non-Hodgkin Lymphomas Associated with AIDS

Prevalence 3% to 10% in AIDS patients
Patients HIV+
CD4+ lymphocyte count less than 100/mm^3 in diffuse large cell lymphoma, higher in Burkitt lymphoma.
Ratio of CD4+ to CD8+ T cells usually less than 0.5
Extranodal locations predominant
Presentation in advanced stages
Histologic types
- Diffuse large cell lymphoma
  - Immunoblastic 34%
  - Pleomorphic 35%
- Burkitt lymphoma 30%
- Primary effusion lymphoma 1% to 2%

High mitotic indices
Necrosis frequent
B-cell phenotypes
Molecular mutations, translocations, and deletions
Early dissemination
Short survival

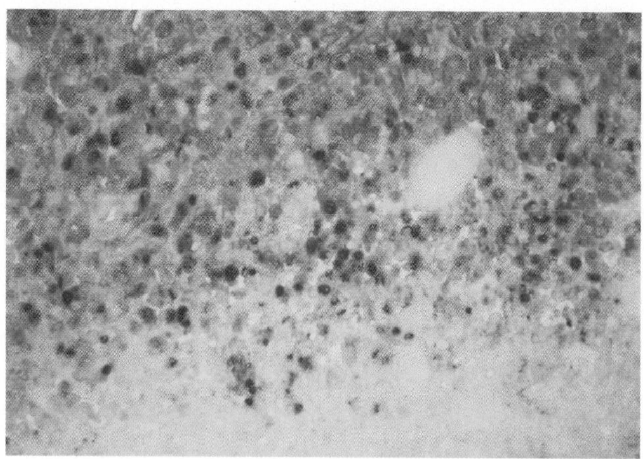

FIGURE 81.7. Non-Hodgkin lymphoma, large B-cell type in lymph node of HIV+ patient. Epstein-Barr virus RNA intranuclear dark blue staining. EBER/*in situ* hybridization.

- The histologic criteria for differential diagnosis are those described for the respective histologic types (see Chapters 67 and 69).

REFERENCES

1. HIV/AIDS surveillance report. Atlanta: Centers for Disease Control, 1990:1–22.
2. Beral V, Peterman T, Berkelman R, et al. AIDS-associated non-Hodgkin lymphoma. Lancet 1991;337:805–809.
3. Pluda JM, Yarchoan R, Jaffe ES, et al. Development of non-Hodgkin lymphoma in a cohort of patients with severe human immunodeficiency virus (HIV) infection on long-term antiretroviral therapy. Ann Intern Med 1990;113:276–282.
4. Levine AM. Acquired immunodeficiency syndrome-related lymphoma. Blood 1992;80:8–20.
5. Beral V, Newton R. Overview of the epidemiology of immunodeficiency-associated cancer. J Natl Cancer Inst 1998;23:1–6.
6. Ioachim HL. Neoplasms associated with immune deficiencies. Pathol Annu 1987;22:177–222.
7. Filipovich AH, Heinitz KJ, Robison LL, et al. The immunodeficiency cancer registry. A research resource. Am J Pediatr Hematol Oncol 1987;9:183–184.
8. Penn I. Depressed immunity and the development of cancer. Cancer Detect Prev 1994;18:241–252.
9. Ioachim HL. The opportunistic tumors of immune deficiency. Adv Cancer Res 1990;54:301–317.
10. Ioachim HL. Immunopathogenesis of human immunodeficiency virus infection. Cancer Res 1990;50:5612–5617.
11. Gaidano G, Carbone F, Dalla-Favera R. Pathogenesis of AIDS-related lymphomas. Molecular and histogenetic heterogeneity. Am J Pathol 1998;152:623–630.
12. Pelicci PG, Knowles DM, Arlin Z, et al. Multiple monoclonal B-cell expansions and c-myc oncogene rearrangements in AIDS-related lymphoproliferative disorders: implications for lymphomagenesis. J Exp Med 1986;164:2049–2060.
13. Gaidano G, Ballerini P, Gong JZ, et al. p53 mutations in human lymphoid malignancies: association with Burkitt lymphoma and chronic lymphocytic leukemia. Proc Natl Acad Sci U S A 1991;88:5413–5417.
14. Kieff E. Current perspectives on the molecular pathogenesis of virus-induced cancers in human immunodeficiency virus infection and acquired immunodeficiency syndrome. J. Natl Cancer Inst 1998;23:7–14.
15. Ioachim HL, Cooper MC. Lymphomas of AIDS [Letter]. Lancet 1986;1:96–97.
16. Ioachim HL, Dorsett B, Cronin W, et al. Acquired immunodeficiency syndrome-associated lymphomas: clinical, pathologic, immunologic, and viral characteristics of 111 cases. Hum Pathol 1991;22:659–673.
17. Ioachim HL, Ryan JR, Blaugrund SM. Salivary gland lymph nodes. The site of lymphadenopathies and lymphomas associated with human immunodeficiency virus infection. Arch Pathol Lab Med 1988;112:1224–1228.
18. Ioachim HL, Antonescu C, Giancotti F, et al. EBV-associated primary lymphomas in salivary glands of HIV-infected patients. Pathol Res Pract 1998;194:87–95.
19. Irwin D, Kaplan L. Clinical aspects of HIV-related lymphoma. Curr Opin Oncol 1993;5:852–860.
20. Ziegler JL, Beckstead JA, Volberding PA, et al. Non-Hodgkin's lymphoma in 90 homosexual men: relationship to generalized lymphadenopathy and acquired immunodeficiency syndrome (AIDS). N Engl J Med 1984;311:565–570.
21. Knowles DM, Chamulak GA, Subar M, et al. Lymphoid neoplasia associated with the acquired immunodeficiency syndrome (AIDS). Ann Intern Med 1988;108:744–753.
22. Ioachim HL, Cooper MC, Hellman GC. Lymphomas in men at high risk for acquired immune deficiency syndrome (AIDS). A study of 21 cases. Cancer 1985;56:2831–2841.
23. Ioachim HL, Lerner CW, Tapper ML. The lymphoid lesions associated with the acquired immunodeficiency syndrome. Am J Surg Pathol 1983;7:543–553.
24. Ioachim HL. Persistent generalized lymphadenopathy. In: Pathology of AIDS. Textbook and color atlas. Philadelphia: JB Lippincott Co, 1989:2–6.
25. Raphael M, Gentilhomme O, Tulliez M, et al. Histopathologic features of high-grade non-Hodgkin's lymphomas in acquired immunodeficiency syndrome. Arch Pathol Lab Med 1991;115:15–20.
26. Nador RG, Cesarman E, Chadburn A, et al. Primary effusion lymphoma: a distinct clinicopathologic entity associated with the Kaposi's sarcoma-associated herpes virus. Blood 1996;88:645– 656.
27. Spina M, Tirelli U, Zagonel V, et al. Burkitt's lymphoma in adults with and without human immunodeficiency virus infection. A single-institution clinicopathologic study of 75 patients. Cancer 1998;82:766–774.
28. Knowles D. Biologic aspects of AIDS-associated non-Hodgkin's lymphoma. Curr Opin Oncol 1993;5:845–851.
29. Nasr SA, Brynes RK, Garrison CP, et al. Peripheral T-cell lymphoma in a patient with acquired immune deficiency syndrome. Cancer 1988;61:947–951.
30. Lust JA, Banks PM, Hooper WC. T-cell non-Hodgkin's lymphoma in human immunodeficiency virus-infected individuals. Am J Hematol 1989;31:181–187.

PART

VIII

SPINDLE CELL NEOPLASMS OF LYMPH NODES

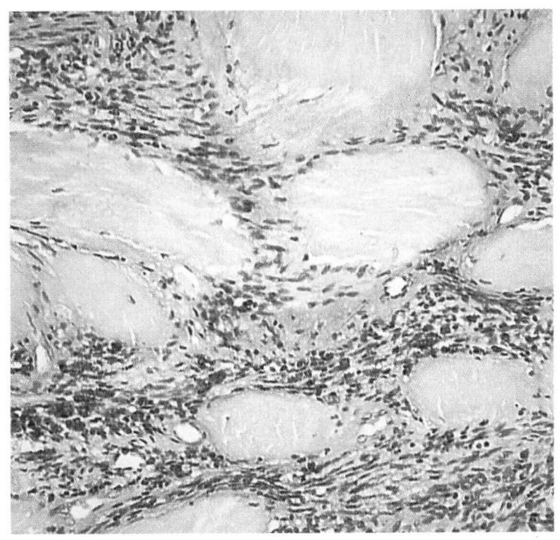

Benign and malignant neoplasms of nonlymphoid cell components of lymph nodes are remarkably rare. They may have a vascular origin (see Part IX) or arise from a variety of mesenchymal cells, including fibroblasts, histiocytes, myofibroblasts, smooth muscle cells, dendritic reticulum cells, and interdigitating reticulum cells. These cells are normal components of the supporting framework of lymph nodes and other hematolymphoid organs. They are generally spindle-shaped or stellate. Their functions are diverse. Some cells are simply structural, whereas others are actively involved in immune processes. Spindle cell tumors may also involve the lymph nodes secondarily by local extension or metastasis from different locations in the soft tissues. Neoplasms arising from accessory cells, histiocytic sarcoma (see Chapter 77) and dendritic cell neoplasms (see Chapter 78) have been previously described. This part describes spindle-shaped primary proliferations of lymph nodes arising from cells with a supportive function and includes inflammatory pseudotumor and palisaded myofibroblastoma.

82

PALISADED MYOFIBROBLASTOMA

DEFINITION

Benign mesenchymal lymph node tumor characterized by palisading spindle cells, stellate deposits of collagen (amianthoid fibers), and hemorrhage.

SYNONYM

Intranodal hemorrhagic spindle cell tumor with amianthoid fibers

PATHOGENESIS

Because cells derived from smooth muscle usually contain desmin, the absence of desmin in palisaded myofibroblastoma (PM) initially suggested a cell type other than smooth muscle (1,2). Intracytoplasmic inclusions, similar to those seen in infantile digital fibroma (an accepted myofibroblastic tumor), seemed to support a myofibroblastic origin. On the other hand, vascular or capsular smooth muscle cells could also give rise to the spindle cells of PM (1–4). A variety of immunohistochemical and ultrastructural features are compatible with either myofibroblasts or smooth muscle cells (2).

CLINICAL SYNDROME

Most patients with PM have a solitary, unilateral, painless, nodular mass confined to the inguinal area (1,2,5). Rarely, PM occupies cervical (5) or submandibular lymph nodes (6,7). In three series, patients' ages ranged from 19 to 67 years, and more men than women were affected (1,2,5). Many PMs develop in the sixth decade (2,5). The behavior of PM is completely benign. A single inguinal case recurred locally after 9 years (8).

Palisaded myofibroblastomas are well encapsulated and located deep in the groin below the inguinal ligament, do not infiltrate overlying skin, and involve no more than a single lymph node. They measure 0.6 to 5 cm in diameter. Sectioning the lymph node reveals a gray-white tumor surrounded by focal areas of subcapsular hemorrhage (1), like "milk freshly poured into tea" (5).

HISTOPATHOLOGY

The tumor mass has a nodular configuration and is composed of crisscrossed fascicles of parallel, slender, spindle-shaped cells (Fig. 82.1). The cytoplasm is weakly eosinophilic without striations, and the nuclei are tapered and often aligned, displaying palisading patterns. Nuclear atypia is absent, and mitoses are rare, usually fewer than 2 per 50 high-power fields. A characteristic feature observed in all cases is the presence of mats of eosinophilic material forming bands or stellate or circular profiles, depending on the plane of section (1,2,5) (Figs. 82.1 and 82.2). They are composed of a core of homogeneous, deeply eosinophilic collagen with fine hairlike spokes surrounded by a peripheral, granular, weakly eosinophilic area (1). The collagen stains intensely blue with trichrome stain (Fig. 82.3). The general appearance is that of amianthoid fibers, previously described in some malignant mesenchymal schwannomas and considered to represent degenerated or "crystalline" collagen (9,10). The tumor is surrounded by a pseudocapsule composed of thick bands of hyalinized sclerotic tissue that separate it from the compressed peripheral lymphoid tissues of the lymph node. In some areas, small vessels lined by flat endothelial cells and containing erythrocytes are at the center of the amianthoid structures, suggesting perivascular rosettes (2). Zones with scattered hemorrhagic foci can resemble Kaposi sarcoma.

ELECTRON MICROSCOPY

Amorphous intercellular material separates discohesive cells. The spindle cell cytoplasm contains numerous ribosomes and thin filaments with focal densities. No secretory granules (2), Weibel-Palade bodies (2) or fibronexus junctions (11) are seen. Haphazard or loosely parallel collagen fibers form the amianthoid fibers (2,5). The collagen fibrils in PM

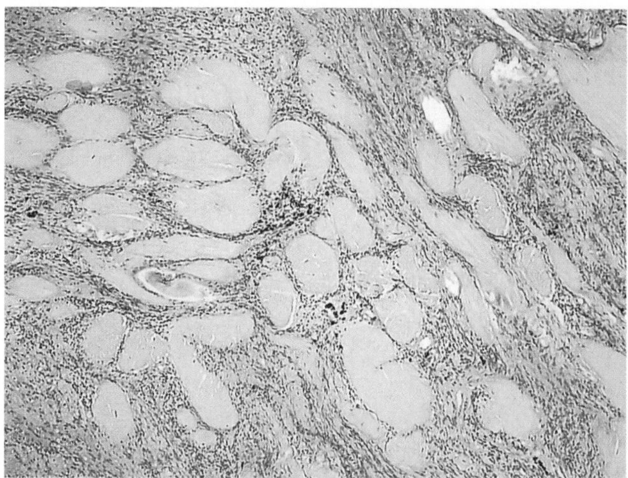

FIGURE 82.1. Palisaded myofibroblastoma. Parallel and criss-cross fascicles of spindle cells separated by bands of degenerated collagen in the shapes of amianthoid bodies. Blood vessel (*left*) in center of amianthoid body. Hematoxylin, phloxine, and saffron stain. (Courtesy of Dr. Alexander Fuchs.)

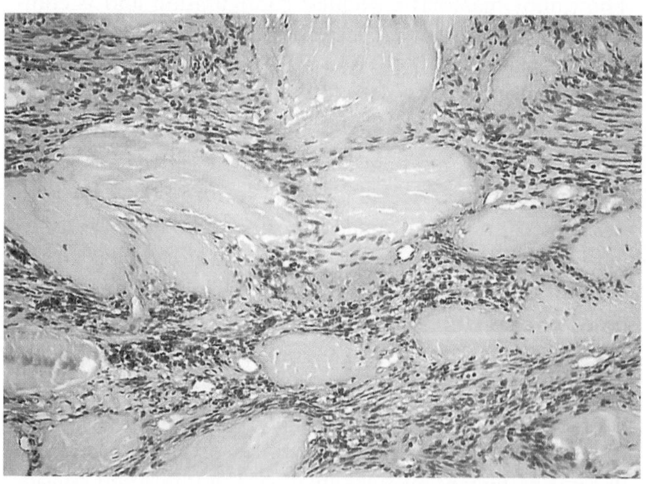

FIGURE 82.2. Palisaded myofibroblastoma. Large amianthoid bodies of variable sizes and shapes with visible fibrillar structure in the midst of fascicles of spindle cells. Hematoxylin, phloxine, and saffron stain. (Courtesy of Dr. Alexander Fuchs.)

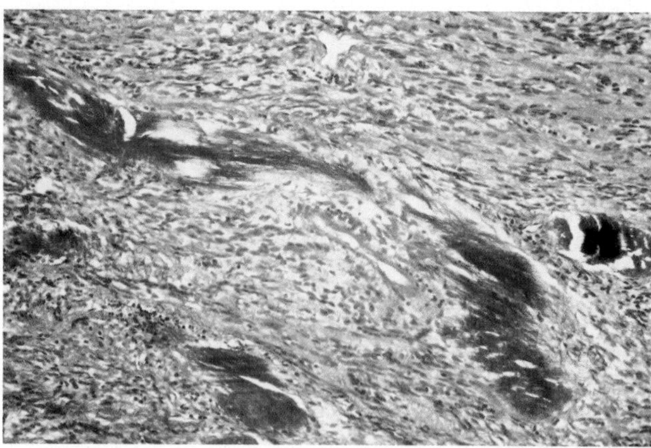

FIGURE 82.3. Palisaded myofibroblastoma. Collagen fibers stain blue with trichrome stain. (Courtesy of Dr. Alexander Fuchs.)

have a conventional diameter of approximately 50 to 200 nm (4,11,12), not the giant size (1 μm) of actual amianthoid alteration (13).

IMMUNOHISTOCHEMISTRY

The spindle cells express smooth muscle actin, myosin, and vimentin, but not desmin, factor VIII-related antigen, S100 protein, synaptophysin, or keratin (1,2). This pattern excludes a neural origin but appears compatible with smooth muscle cells or myofibroblasts (1,2). Extracellular proteins include fibronectin, laminin, and type IV collagen (11).

DIFFERENTIAL DIAGNOSIS

- Kaposi sarcoma: The cell fascicles are thinner and arcuate, and they contain numerous endothelium-lined clefts. Amianthoid bodies are not present.

Checklist

PALISADED MYOFIBROBLASTOMA

Unilateral painless inguinal mass
Partially encapsulated intranodal tumor
Intersecting fascicles of spindle-shaped cells
Round or stellate amianthoid bodies
Thick-walled blood vessels, focal hemorrhages
Tapered, focally aligned nuclei
Lack of nuclear atypia, rare mitoses
Positive for smooth muscle actin and vimentin, negative for desmin and S100 protein

- Neurilemmoma includes distinct Antoni A and Antoni B areas, lacks amianthoid bodies, and stains with anti-S100 protein antibody.
- Metastatic or primary intranodal sarcoma exhibits irregular architecture, marked nuclear atypia, and frequent mitoses.

REFERENCES

1. Weiss SW, Gnepp DR, Bratthauer GL. Palisaded myofibroblastoma. A benign mesenchymal tumor of lymph node. Am J Surg Pathol 1989;13:341–346.
2. Suster S, Rosai J. Intranodal hemorrhagic spindle-cell tumor with "amianthoid" fibers. Report of six cases of a distinctive mesenchymal neoplasm of the inguinal region that simulates Kaposi's sarcoma. Am J Surg Pathol 1989;13:347–357.
3. Bigotti G, Coli A, Mottolese M, et al. Selective location of palisaded myofibroblastoma with amianthoid fibres. J Clin Pathol 1991;44:761–764.
4. Tanda F, Massarelli G, Cossu A, et al. Primary spindle cell tumor of lymph node with "amianthoid" fibers: a histological, immunohistochemical and ultrastructural study. Ultrastruct Pathol 1993;17:195–205.
5. Michal M, Chlumska A, Povysilova V. Intranodal "amianthoid" myofibroblastoma. Report of six cases: immunohistochemical and electron microscopical study. Pathol Res Pract 1992;188: 199–204.
6. Fletcher CD, Stirling RW. Intranodal myofibroblastoma presenting in the submandibular region: evidence of a broader clinical and histological spectrum. Histopathology 1990;16:287–293.
7. Alguacil-Garcia A. Intranodal myofibroblastoma in a submandibular lymph node. A case report. Am J Clin Pathol 1992; 97:69–72.
8. Lioe TF, Allen DC, Bell JC. A case of multicentric intranodal palisaded myofibroblastoma. Histopathology 1994;24:173–175.
9. Ghadially FN, Lalonde JM, Dick CE. Ultrastructure of pigmented villonodular synovitis. J Pathol 1979;127:19–26.
10. Orenstein JM. Amianthoid fibers in a synovial sarcoma and a malignant schwannoma. Ultrastruct Pathol 1983;4:163–176.
11. Eyden BP, Harris M, Greywoode GI, et al. Intranodal myofibroblastoma: report of a case. Ultrastruct Pathol 1996;20:79–88.
12. Skalova A, Michal M, Chlumska A, et al. Collagen composition and ultrastructure of the so-called amianthoid fibres in palisaded myofibroblastoma. Ultrastructural and immunohistochemical study. J Pathol 1992;167:335–340.
13. Hough AJ, Mottram FC, Sokoloff L. The collagenous nature of amianthoid degeneration of human costal cartilage. Am J Pathol 1973;73:201–216.

83

INFLAMMATORY PSEUDOTUMOR OF LYMPH NODES

DEFINITION

Histiocytic and fibroblastic non-neoplastic proliferation involving the lymph node connective tissue framework and associated with vascular lesions.

PATHOGENESIS

An exaggerated inflammatory proliferative process may cause tumor-like enlarged lymph nodes in patients with nonspecific constitutional symptoms (1–4). The main components of the cellular proliferation are histiocytes and fibroblasts of the lymph node framework, although marked vascularity and infiltration of various inflammatory cells are also part of the process. As a result, tumor-like growths develop with spindle cell histologic patterns similar to those of the pseudotumors and "plasma cell granulomas" described earlier in lung (5), liver (6), spleen (7), mesentery and intestine (8), pancreas (9), and urinary bladder (10). Extranodal inflammatory pseudotumor (IPT) has rarely been associated with regional lymph node involvement (11). Epstein-Barr virus is found in the spindle cells of one-half to two-thirds of extranodal IPTs, but in the mononuclear cells of only a few nodal IPTs (12). It is not likely that Epstein-Barr virus is involved in the pathogenesis of IPT in lymph node, but it may have a role in spleen and liver (13).

In the lymph node, the proliferating histiocytes and fibroblasts are located primarily in the hilum, trabeculae, and capsule, where they expand toward the lymphoid parenchyma. The cause of this exuberant cellular proliferation, which in many ways resembles nodular fasciitis, another idiopathic inflammatory pseudotumoral process, is unknown. It is believed that local release of cytokines, possibly interleukin 1, an active promoter of cell activation and inflammatory reaction, may be involved in the origin of pseudotumor (1,2). IPT of lymph nodes is a rare occurrence, non-neoplastic, with a chronic course and usually spontaneous remission (1–4).

CLINICAL SYNDROME

In the few series of cases reported, the age range was broad (7 to 82 years, with a median of 33 years), and no sex predilection was noted (1–4). Variable episodes of fever, night sweats, anemia, and hypergammaglobulinemia and enlargement of lymph nodes, localized or generalized, lasted several weeks to several years (1–4). Mandibular, cervical, axillary, mediastinal, retroperitoneal, and inguinal lymph nodes and the perinodal soft tissues were involved. Resolution occurred after various treatments, including antibiotics, chemotherapy, radiotherapy, and after no therapy (1–4). The removed lymph nodes were as large as 3 cm in diameter, hard, matted together, and adherent to adjacent structures, and their cut surfaces had a "fish flesh" appearance (1).

HISTOPATHOLOGY

Inflammatory pseudotumor develops in stages: I, small nodules with partial involvement of the lymph node; II, more marked distortion of the connective tissue framework; and III, eventual complete sclerosis (4). The proliferative process involves primarily the connective tissue of the lymph node and is therefore centered on the hilum, trabeculae, and capsule (1–4). These structures are enlarged, compressing the lymphoid parenchyma (Figs. 83.1 and 83.2). The component cells are mainly spindle-shaped and form bundles and whorls, often giving rise to a storiform pattern (1–4) (Fig. 83.3). Admixed with the spindle cells are numerous vessels lined by flattened endothelial cells and a large number of lymphocytes, plasma cells, and neutrophils (Figs. 83.4– 83.6). Eosinophils are not part of the inflammatory process, nor is necrosis present. Epithelioid cells and occasional multinucleated giant cells were noted in some cases (1). The fibroblasts and histiocytes, singly or in fascicles, have typical nuclei, and mitoses are moderate in number. The perinodal tissues resemble panniculitis, and focal vasculitis is frequently noted (3). Small lymphocytes infiltrate, and the intima proliferates within, small blood vessels of the hilum and extranodal zones; spindle cells and inflammation

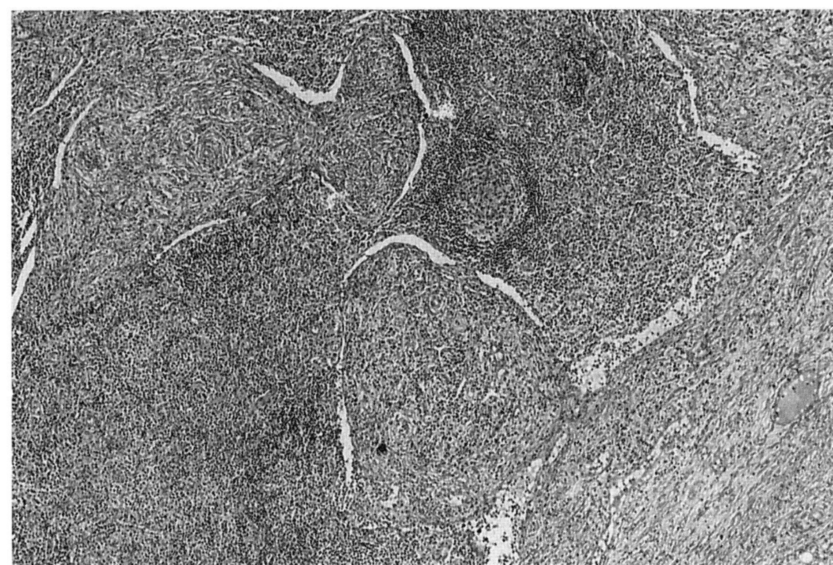

FIGURE 83.1. Inflammatory pseudotumor of lymph node. Bundles of spindle cells replace the lymphatic parenchyma, leaving an involuted residual follicle (*center*). Hematoxylin and eosin stain. (From Perrone T, De Wolf-Peeters C, Frizzera G. Inflammatory pseudotumor of lymph nodes. A distinctive pattern of nodal reaction. Am J Surg Pathol 1988; 12:351–362, with permission.)

destroy the muscularis layer of larger vessels (3). Both processes occlude the lumina (3). Variable edema and fibrosis occur (3).

IMMUNOHISTOCHEMISTRY

All spindle cells showed a strong reactivity for vimentin (2). Antibodies for histiocyte/macrophage markers, such as lysozyme, α_1-antichymotrypsin, Mac-387, CD14, and CD68, also labeled some spindle cells, but these were largely nonreactive (2,3). The spindle cells expressing α muscle actin did not stain with antibodies directed against desmin, similar to myofibroblasts in granulation tissue (3). The spindle cells did not express factor XIIIa, so that an endothelial cell origin was ruled out.

DIFFERENTIAL DIAGNOSIS

- Palisaded myofibroblastoma lacks inflammatory cells and has characteristic amianthoid bodies.

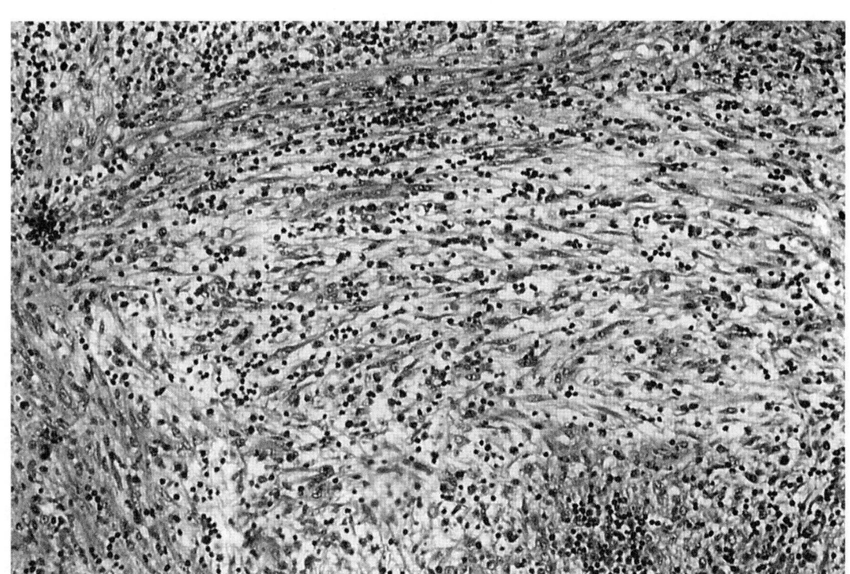

FIGURE 83.2. Inflammatory pseudotumor with edema separating the spindle cells within a trabecula. Hematoxylin and eosin stain. (From Perrone T, De Wolf-Peeters C, Frizzera G. Inflammatory pseudotumor of lymph nodes. A distinctive pattern of nodal reaction. Am J Surg Pathol 1988;12:351–362, with permission.)

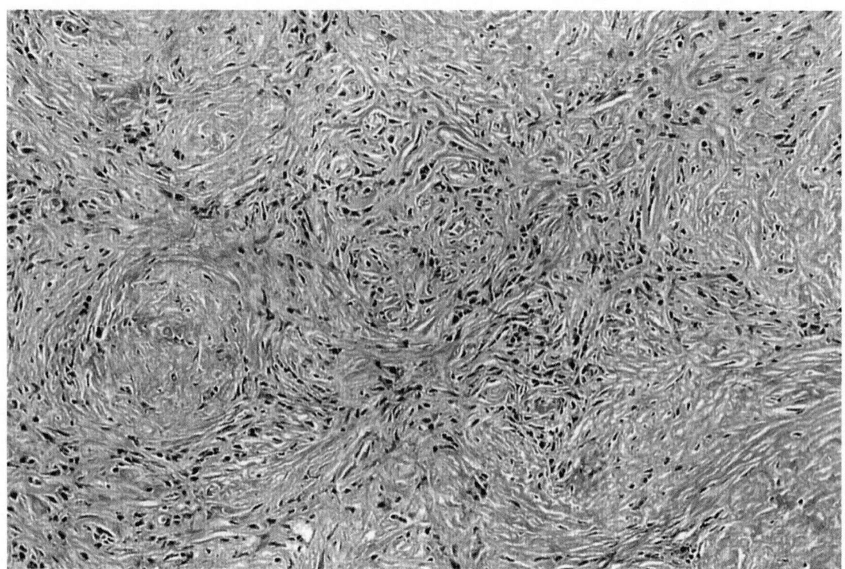

FIGURE 83.3. Inflammatory pseudotumor with formation of whorls and storiform pattern. Hematoxylin, phloxine, and saffron stain; ×200. (From Perrone T, De Wolf-Peeters C, Frizzera G. Inflammatory pseudotumor of lymph nodes. A distinctive pattern of nodal reaction. Am J Surg Pathol 1988;12:351–362, with permission.)

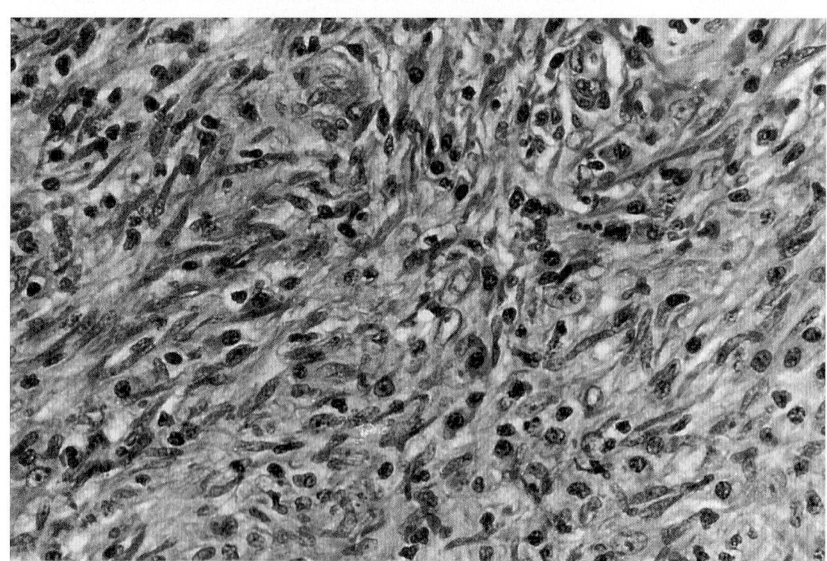

FIGURE 83.4. Inflammatory pseudotumor showing fascicles of spindle cells with interspersed lymphocytes and plasma cells. The spindle cells are uniform and show no nuclear atypia or mitoses. Hematoxylin, phloxine, and saffron stain. (From Perrone T, De Wolf-Peeters C, Frizzera G. Inflammatory pseudotumor of lymph nodes. A distinctive pattern of nodal reaction. Am J Surg Pathol 1988;12:351–362, with permission.)

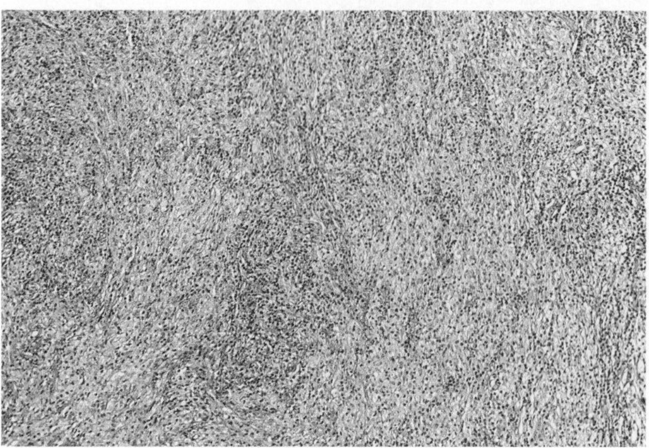

FIGURE 83.5. Inflammatory pseudotumor. Scanning magnification. Variegated color owing to mixed population of fibroblasts, lymphocytes, and plasma cells. Hematoxylin and eosin stain.

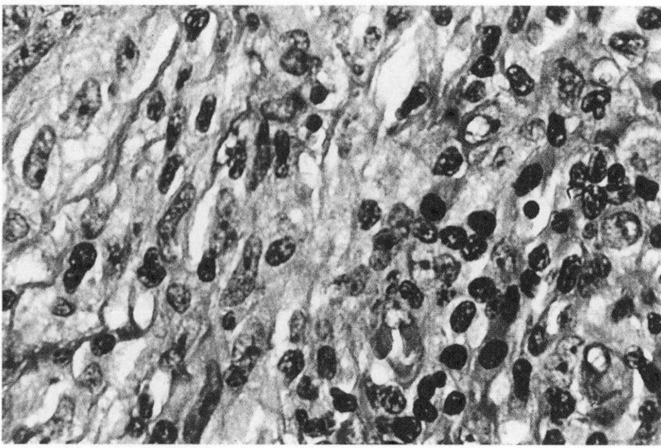

FIGURE 83.6. Lymph node in Fig. 83.5 at higher magnification showing fibroblasts, lymphocytes, and plasma cells.

Checklist

INFLAMMATORY PSEUDOTUMOR OF LYMPH NODES

Febrile episode
Enlarged, tumor-like lymph nodes
Cell proliferation centered on hilum, trabeculae, and capsule
Fascicles and whorls of spindle cells
Fibroblasts and histiocytes
Vascular proliferation, inflammatory cells
Moderate mitoses, no nuclear atypia
Chronic course, spontaneous remission

- Hodgkin lymphoma involves lymphoid parenchyma and has typical Reed-Sternberg cells.
- Mycobacterial spindle cell pseudotumor has a storiform pattern and contains abundant acid-fast bacilli, but it does not extend extranodally or show vascular lesions (14).
- Anthracotic and anthracosilicotic spindle cell pseudotumors of mediastinal lymph nodes have a storiform pattern of spindle cells, abundant anthracotic pigment, and birefringent, needle-shaped silicate crystals (15).

REFERENCES

1. Perrone T, De Wolf-Peeters C, Frizzera G. Inflammatory pseudotumor of lymph nodes. A distinctive pattern of nodal reaction. Am J Surg Pathol 1988;12:351–361.
2. Facchetti F, De Wolf-Peeters C, De Wever I, et al. Inflammatory pseudotumor of lymph nodes. Immunohistochemical evidence for its fibrohistiocytic nature. Am J Pathol 1990;137:281–289.
3. Davis RE, Warnke RA, Dorfman RF. Inflammatory pseudotumor of lymph nodes. Additional observations and evidence for an inflammatory etiology. Am J Surg Pathol 1991;15:744–756.
4. Moran CA, Suster S, Abbondanzo SL. Inflammatory pseudotumor of lymph nodes: a study of 25 cases with emphasis on morphological heterogeneity. Hum Pathol 1997;28:332–338.
5. Berardi RS, Lee SS, Chen HP, et al. Inflammatory pseudotumors of the lung. Surg Gynecol Obstet 1983;156:89–96.
6. Anthony PP, Telesinghe PU. Inflammatory pseudotumour of the liver. J Clin Pathol 1986;39:761–768.
7. Thomas RM, Jaffe ES, Zarate-Osorno A, et al. Inflammatory pseudotumor of the spleen. A clinicopathologic and immunophenotypic study of eight cases. Arch Pathol Lab Med 1993;117: 921–926.
8. Day DL, Sane S, Dehner LP. Inflammatory pseudotumor of the mesentery and small intestine. Pediatr Radiol 1986;16:210–215.
9. Abrebanel P, Sarfaty S, Gal R, et al. Plasma cell granuloma of the pancreas [Letter]. Arch Pathol Lab Med 1984;108:531–532.
10. Nochomovitz LE, Orenstein JM. Inflammatory pseudotumor of the urinary bladder—possible relationship to nodular fasciitis. Two case reports, cytologic observations, and ultrastructural observations. Am J Surg Pathol 1985;9:366–373.
11. Myint MA, Medeiros LJ, Sulaiman RA, et al. Inflammatory pseudotumor of the ileum. A report of a multifocal, transmural lesion with regional lymph node involvement. Arch Pathol Lab Med 1994;118:1138–1142.
12. Arber DA, Kamel OW, van de Rijn M, et al. Frequent presence of the Epstein-Barr virus in inflammatory pseudotumor. Hum Pathol 1995;26:1093–1098.
13. Arber DA, Weiss LM, Chang KL. Detection of Epstein-Barr virus in inflammatory pseudotumor. Semin Diagn Pathol 1998;15:155–160.
14. Chen KT. Mycobacterial spindle cell pseudotumor of lymph nodes [see Comments]. Am J Surg Pathol 1992;16:276–281.
15. Argani P, Ghossein R, Rosai J. Anthracotic and anthracosilicotic spindle cell pseudotumors of mediastinal lymph nodes: report of five cases of a reactive lesion that stimulates malignancy. Hum Pathol 1998;29:851–855.

PART

IX

VASCULAR NEOPLASMS OF LYMPH NODES

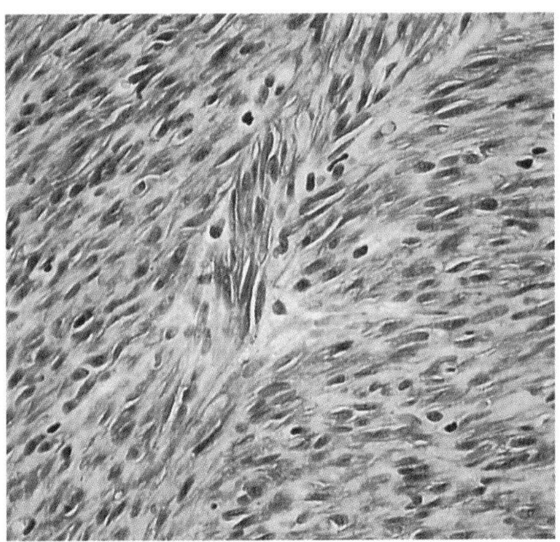

A broad spectrum of vascular proliferations may involve lymph nodes, ranging from the benign vascular hyperplasias of some lymphadenopathies to the malignant vascular neoplasias of Kaposi sarcoma and angiosarcoma. Nonneoplastic angiomatosis in lymph nodes arising in the high endothelial venules of the paracortex is a characteristic feature of Castleman lymphadenopathy (see Chapter 43), Kimura lymphadenopathy (see Chapter 36), the subacute and chronic stages of HIV lymphadenitis (see Chapter 15), and others. A peculiar process of lymph node angiomatosis is the vascular transformation of sinuses, in which the vasoproliferative process selectively involves the nodal sinuses (see Chapter 48). Benign vascular tumors of lymph nodes are rare and include typical hemangiomas and variants such as angiomyomatous hamartoma and hemangioendothelioma. Malignant vascular neoplasms of lymph nodes include the sporadic, epidemic, and endemic forms of Kaposi sarcoma (by far the most common since the appearance of AIDS) and angiosarcoma, usually not as a primary tumor of lymph nodes but as part of disseminated neoplasia.

The major lymph node vascular neoplasias are described in the following chapters under the headings of hemangiomas/hemangioendotheliomas and Kaposi sarcoma.

84

HEMANGIOMAS/ HEMANGIOENDOTHELIOMAS

DEFINITION

Primary benign vascular tumors of lymph nodes.

PATHOGENESIS

Benign vascular tumors arising primarily in lymph nodes are rare, and except for a multiinstitutional study including 39 cases (1), the few articles in the literature are single case reports (2–7). The various types of vascular tumor seen in soft tissues and other organs, particularly hemangioma and hemangioendothelioma, are reproduced in the lymph nodes (8). The spectrum of vascular proliferations in lymph nodes ranges from the benign vascular hyperplasias that accompany various infections and the peculiar form of vascular transformation of sinuses (see Chapter 48) to the malignant neoplasms of Kaposi sarcoma (see Chapter 85) and angiosarcoma. In the largest study of benign vascular tumors of lymph nodes, Chan and colleagues (1) proposed a classification of five histologic types: (a) hemangioma and its variant, (b) angiomyomatous hamartoma, (c) hemangioendothelioma and its variant, (d) polymorphous heman-gioendothelioma, and (e) lymphangioma. Benign vascular tumors of lymph nodes are less common than either non-neoplastic vascular hyperplasia or Kaposi sarcoma. They are in most cases incidental findings with no clinical significance. However, it is important to recognize them to avoid a misdiagnosis of Kaposi sarcoma or angiosarcoma.

CLINICAL SYNDROMES

Benign vascular tumors of lymph nodes may be found incidentally in the course of various surgical explorations or present clinically as enlarged lymph nodes. The average diameter reported is 2 to 3 cm, and the location is variable, mostly in peripheral lymph nodes, which are more accessible to observation and removal. Angiomyomatous hamartoma has been seen only in inguinal lymph nodes (1). Patients with hemangioma are more often young to middle-aged and predominantly male (1). Hemangiomas with a hamartomatous appearance are more likely to be seen in children (2,6).

HISTOPATHOLOGY

Hemangioma may be capillary, cavernous, or mixed (Figs. 84.1 and 84.2). Capillary hemangiomas appear as a conglomerate of capillary vessels lined by a single layer of flat endothelial cells. They resemble a pyogenic granuloma or simply granulation tissue (1). Cavernous hemangiomas include large, irregular spaces packed with erythrocytes and occasional thrombi with partial organization (1,4). Hemangiomas are well circumscribed and include a scanty edematous or fibrosed stroma. Outside the vascular growth, the lymph node parenchyma is well preserved and sometimes exhibits mild activation of the germinal centers (6). Epithelioid hemangiomas differ only by their vascular lining, which is composed of plump rather than flat endothelial cells (1).

Angiomyomatous hamartoma has been reported only in inguinal lymph nodes (1). The component vessels have thick, muscular walls and lie in a dense collagenous stroma. The lesion appears to start in the hilum and on gross examination is firm and whitish (1). It looks more like a hamartoma than a real neoplasm.

Hemangioendothelioma is a neoplasm composed of blood vessels and cell aggregates. The vessels may be channel-like or cavernous, filled with blood and thrombi. The cells between the vessels form fascicles without vascular lumina and are plump, spindly, or epithelioid (9,10). The nuclei show no atypia or mitoses. Sometimes, particularly in the peripheral areas, clusters of cells project into the lumina in the form of papillary tufts (1).

Polymorphous hemangioendothelioma, a borderline malignant vascular tumor, is also formed of a vascular and a cellular component, with the latter showing a greater degree of

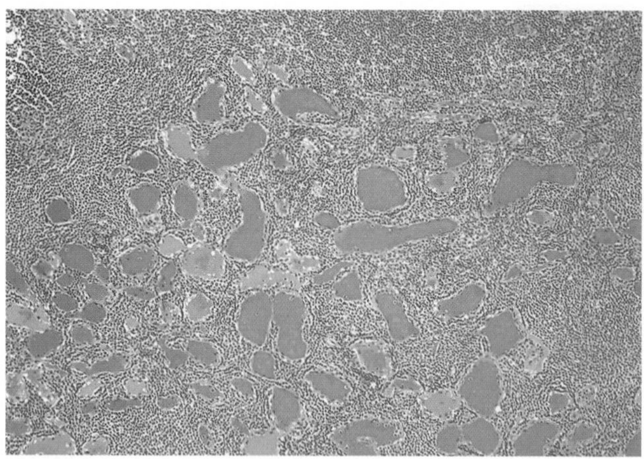

FIGURE 84.1. Hemangioma in inguinal lymph node occupies a well-circumscribed area below the capsule and a narrow rim of preserved lymphatic tissue. Hematoxylin, phloxine, and saffron stain.

cellular atypia (1). The cell fascicles are large, more solid, and uniform. The cells have less cytoplasm, nuclei with nucleoli, and occasional mitoses. The intervening stroma is edematous or fibrosed. Polymorphous hemangioendothelioma differs from angiosarcoma in that it lacks invading, dissecting vessels and excessive nuclear atypia. The clinical course is indolent, and metastases have not been recorded (1).

Lymphangioma is rarely encountered in lymph nodes (11). It consists of small spaces filled with a proteinaceous material and floating lymphocytes and lined by a flat endothelial layer (1).

HISTOCHEMISTRY

Periodic acid–Schiff and silver impregnation (Gomori-Grocott, Gordon-Sweets) stain the reticulin vascular frameworks.

IMMUNOHISTOCHEMISTRY

Antibodies directed to factor VIII-RA and *Ulex europaeus* clearly outline the vascular contours by staining the endothelial cells of vessels but generally not the spindle or epithelioid cells of hemangioendotheliomas (1,6,10). The leiomyomatous components of angiomyomatous hamartoma can be stained with antibody to muscle-specific actin (1).

DIFFERENTIAL DIAGNOSIS

- Vascular transformation of sinuses: Vascular proliferation is restricted to sinuses and occasionally associated with vascular obstruction.
- Bacillary angiomatosis: Nodules of capillaries are randomly distributed, and fibrosis is absent. Warthin-Starry silver stains bacilli.

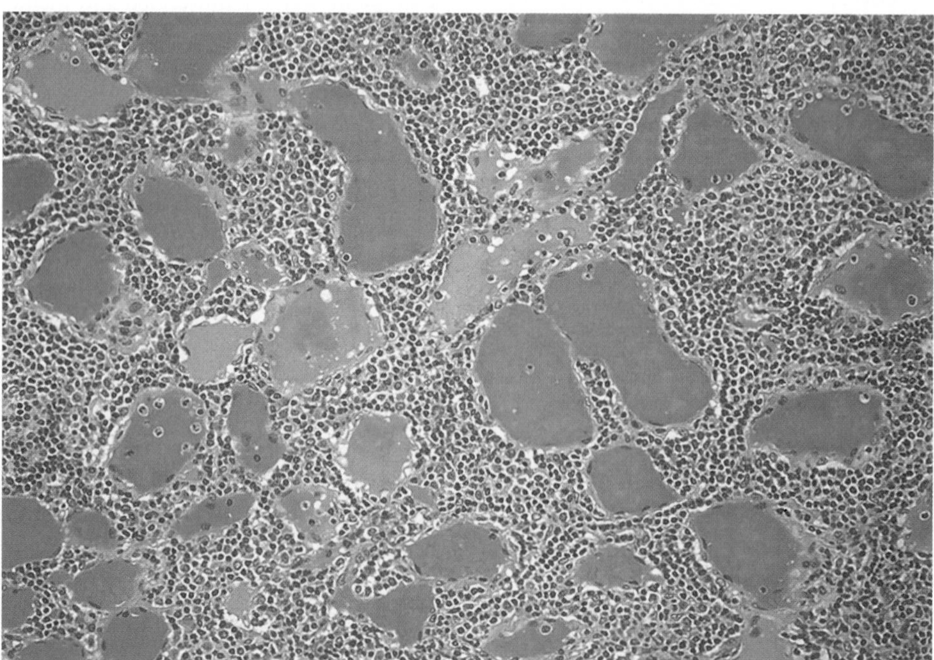

FIGURE 84.2. In the same section as in Fig. 84.1, vascular spaces of various sizes and shapes replace the lymphoid parenchyma. They are lined by endothelial cells and filled by blood without thrombi. Hematoxylin, phloxine, and saffron stain.

Checklist

HEMANGIOMAS/HEMANGIOENDOTHELIOMAS

Hemangioma
Well circumscribed
Capillary or cavernous
Flat endothelial cell lining
Factor VIII-RA+

Epithelioid Hemangioma
Plump endothelial cell lining

Angiomyomatous Hamartoma
Hilar location
Thick muscular walls
Muscle-specific actin+

Hemangioendothelioma
Cavernous blood vessels
Fascicles of spindle or epithelioid cells

Polymorphous Hemangioendothelioma
Borderline malignant
Cellular atypia, conspicuous nucleoli
Frequent mitoses

Lymphangioma
Spaces filled with proteinaceous fluid
Flat endothelial cells

- Kaposi sarcoma: Differential diagnosis is difficult, particularly with hemangioendothelioma, as both entities have the dual composition of vessels and cell fascicles. In general, vascular tumors are more localized and better demarcated, whereas Kaposi sarcoma is diffuse and blends with the local structures.

REFERENCES

1. Chan JKC, Frizzera G, Fletcher CDM, et al. Primary vascular tumors of lymph nodes other than Kaposi's sarcoma. Analysis of 39 cases and delineation of two new entities. Am J Surg Pathol 1992;16:335–350.
2. Gupta IM. Hemangioma in a lymph node. Ind J Pathol Microbiol 1967;71:110–111.
3. Goldstein J, Bartal N. Hemangioendothelioma of the lymph node: A case report. J Surg Oncol 1985;28:314–317.
4. Almagro UA, Choi H, Rouse TM. Hemangioma in a lymph node. Arch Pathol Lab Med 1985;109:576–578.
5. Silva EG, Philips MJ, Langer B, et al. Spindle and histiocytoid (epithelioid) hemangioendothelioma primary in lymph node. Am J Clin Pathol 1986;85:731–735.
6. Kasznica J, Sideli RV, Collins MH. Lymph node hemangioma. Arch Pathol Lab Med 1989;113:804–807.
7. Har-El G, Heffner D, Ruffy M. Hemangioma in a cervical lymph node. J Laryngol Otol 1990;104:513–515.
8. Enzinger FM, Weiss SW. Soft tissue tumors, 2nd ed. St. Louis: Mosby, 1988: 489–580, 614–637.
9. Weiss SW, Enzinger FM. Epithelioid hemangioendothelioma: a vascular tumor often mistaken for a carcinoma. Cancer 1982;50: 970–981.
10. Weiss SW, Enzinger FM. Spindle cell hemangioendothelioma: a low-grade angiosarcoma resembling a cavernous hemangioma and Kaposi's sarcoma. Am J Surg Pathol 1986;10:521–530.
11. Rappaport H. Tumors of the hematopoietic system. Washington, DC: Armed Forces Institute of Pathology, 1966:357–363 (Atlas of tumor pathology, series I, fascicle 8).

85

KAPOSI SARCOMA

DEFINITION

Specific form of vascular neoplasm that occurs sporadically in the general population and frequently in persons with acquired immune deficiency.

EPIDEMIOLOGY

Kaposi sarcoma (KS) occurs throughout the world in sporadic, iatrogenic, endemic, and epidemic forms. Before the 1980s, KS was a rare neoplasm that occurred sporadically, mostly around the Mediterranean basin (1,2). In the United States, it is a rare disease, with an incidence of 0.02 per 100,000 tumors (3). Endemic KS is centered in equatorial Africa, where it accounts for 9% of all malignancies (4). Iatrogenic KS is related to medically induced immune suppression, and KS occurs in about 0.4% of all patients undergoing renal transplantation, which is an incidence 150 to 200 times greater than would be expected in the general population (5,6). In patients with AIDS, a high frequency of KS was noted from the very first reports of cases in 1981 (3). Following the epidemic of HIV infection, the incidence of KS climbed as high as 15% in patients with AIDS. Thus, in the United States, KS became at least 20,000 times more common in persons with AIDS than in the general population, and 300 times more common than in other immunosuppressed groups (7). Marked variations in the frequency of KS between AIDS risk groups were also noted. The frequency of KS may be as high as 36% among homosexuals with AIDS, whereas its rate of occurrence is only 4.3% among intravenous drug addicts and 1% among hemophiliacs with AIDS (8). A male predominance is characteristic; the male-to-female ratio ranges from 3:1 in Western series to 15:1 in African series (1,9). Children may also be affected in areas of endemicity, where KS accounts for 5% to 10% of all malignant tumors (9,10). The epidemiologic data are consistent with a causative viral agent that is transmitted mainly by sexual contact (7).

ETIOLOGY

Earlier studies, even those carried out before the present unexpectedly high incidence of KS, suggested an association with a herpesvirus. Herpes-like virus particles were seen in tissue cultures of African KS (11), in a biopsy specimen of a skin lesion in an African man (12), and in several KS lesions of internal organs (13). Cytomegalovirus (CMV) was suspected to be the herpesvirus involved in the etiology of AIDS because it is sexually transmissible (14), antibodies to CMV are prevalent in most KS patients (15), and CMV antigens and nucleic acids can be detected in KS lesions by a variety of methods (16,17). However, the amounts are small, and CMV is sometimes detected in only a few infected cells, which suggests that CMV infection is frequently associated with KS without being directly involved in its pathogenesis (18).

More recently, a new herpesvirus, Kaposi sarcoma-associated herpesvirus (KSHV) or human herpesvirus type 8 (HHV-8), belonging to the subfamily of Gammaherpesvirinae, was identified in KS. By means of the molecular technique of representational difference analysis, portions of DNA foreign to the host genome were identified in KS lesions (19). Thus, a specific 210-bp genomic sequence could be detected, amplified by the polymerase chain reaction, visualized on ethidium bromide gels, and confirmed on Southern blot hybridization (20). The DNA sequence specific to HHV-8 was detected in up to 88% of cases of classic KS and in 100% of cases of KS in AIDS patients (20). HHV-8 was also present in mononuclear cells of peripheral blood in 52% of patients with KS (21). HHV-8 was not detectable in normal endothelial cells, reactive or neoplastic lesions unrelated to KS, or mononuclear cells of control patients free of HIV (21,22).

By *in situ* hybridization, it was shown that the HHV-8 DNA sequences are localized predominantly in the nuclei of the endothelial cells lining the vascular clefts and in the characteristic spindle-shaped cells of KS (23). These findings demonstrating a close association of HHV-8 with the lesions of KS, particularly in patients with significant immune deficiencies, are compatible with an important role of HHV-8 in the pathogenesis of KS.

PATHOGENESIS

The organs affected and the distribution of lesions in KS have important implications regarding its pathogenesis. Because most patients who have KS present with multiple lesions, usually cutaneous, it is believed that KS, unlike other neoplasms, is multicentric from inception. It is further assumed, although no proof is available, that KS, unlike other tumors, does not disseminate by metastasis. For these reasons, it has been thought that KS is perhaps not a vascular neoplasm but rather a kind of vascular hyperplasia (24). A cause for the controversial concepts of this disease and its still obscure pathogenesis is that most studies to date have been based on cases of dermatologic KS, by far the most common form, whereas studies including substantial numbers of cases of visceral KS and autopsies have been remarkably few (9,25).

In a study of 86 cases of KS of internal organs, we showed that all organs, including bone marrow and brain, long considered exempt, can be involved (26). In the 47 autopsies included in this study, multiple organs were usually involved, which may be an indication as much of multicentricity as of tumor dissemination in the advanced stages of immune deficiency. In 17 of the 47 cases (37%), the visceral tumors were not accompanied by cutaneous or mucosal lesions. The lymph nodes, a usual site of metastasis of other tumors, were frequently involved. Some have argued that tumor emboli were not identified in the presumed metastatic sites (27); however, we noted a marked angiotropism of KS cells, manifested by frequent growth around and inside blood vessels. It is possible that the familiar metastatic patterns of other tumors may not apply to KS, and that other mechanisms and stimulatory factors are involved in the progression of this particular neoplasm. For example, it was shown that exposure of the TAT protein, encoded by the TAT gene of HIV and necessary for viral replication, to a number of cytokines (interleukin 1, interferon-α) that are usually increased in HIV infection, may have modulating and mitogenic effects on KS cells (28).

The histogenesis of KS has also been the subject of debate. Most cellular components of the mesenchyme—endothelial cells, pericytes, fibroblasts, dendritic cells, myocytes, myofibroblasts, and mesenchymal stem cells—have been considered to be the cells of origin of KS. Presently, as a result of numerous immunohistochemical studies with a variety of monoclonal antibodies (MAbs), the histogenesis of KS has been narrowed to a progenitor cell from either blood vessel (29–31) or lymphatic endothelia (32). Determining the cell of origin of KS is not only of conceptual but also of practical importance because this knowledge can assist with the pathologic diagnosis.

The presence of CD34 on immature spindle cells of KS may identify these cells as progenitors of more mature endothelial cells. If CD34+ progenitor endothelial cells are able to circulate in the peripheral blood, like CD34+ hematopoietic progenitor cells, they may give rise to KS under special conditions, which would explain the multifocal form of neoplastic dissemination. Some experiments have indicated that CD34 may down-regulate the expression of some adhesion molecules (33), suggesting another mechanism for the dissemination of KS. *In vitro* work on long-term cultures of KS indicates that the TAT protein released by HIV-infected CD4+ T lymphocytes and macrophages may trigger a cascade of cytokines and growth factors (34). The vascular and fibroblast growth factors identified in cultures and tissues of KS may initiate the vascular hyperplasia that ultimately evolves into KS under conditions of immune deficiency.

In AIDS-associated lymphoma, the generally accepted pathogenesis is that B cells infected with Epstein-Barr virus, activated by various viral infections and proliferating uncontrolled by a failing immune system, ultimately become a malignant cell clone. If we borrow from this model, CD34+ progenitor endothelial cells in circulation, activated by a specific sexually transmitted viral infection and stimulated by the release of angiogenic factors, may give rise in the absence of immune surveillance to KS, a truly malignant vascular neoplasm.

CLINICAL SYNDROME

Kaposi sarcoma involves the skin, mucosal surfaces, lymph nodes, and all internal organs. The cutaneous lesions, which are more common and the first to be noticed, can be single or numerous and widely spread over one area or the entire body. They range in size from 1 to 2 mm to 2 to 3 cm and in color from pink-red to purple-blue (35). The lesions are classified as patches, plaques, or nodules; these forms may represent stages of progression (36). In AIDS patients, the sites of KS lesions are more varied and widespread, and certain cutaneous and mucosal sites are more often affected (37). The gastrointestinal tract is the most common extracutaneous site of KS; in such cases, KS may be asymptomatic and therefore far more difficult to diagnose (9,25,38). Like KS in other viscera, it may occur in the complete absence of skin lesions. In autopsy studies of AIDS patients, the involvement of internal organs, particularly the gastrointestinal tract, lungs, and lymph nodes, varies greatly, from 10% to 90% of cases (25,26,38). KS of lymph nodes was reported in sporadic cases before the current AIDS epidemic, and then, as now, some patients had no other lesions (26,39–41). This presentation has substantiated the view that KS involvement of lymph nodes and other internal organs represents not metastatic spread but primary tumors of a multifocal neoplasm (26). The predominant involvement of lymph nodes characterizes a particular lymphadenopathic form that is seen almost exclusively in children and accounted for 4% of cases in both African and Caucasian series before the AIDS epidemic (9). Two cases of primary lymph node KS as the only manifestation of the disease were recently reported; one patient was an 8-year-old Chinese girl, the other a 10-year-old Italian boy (10,42). Occasionally, KS has been associated with Castleman disease and

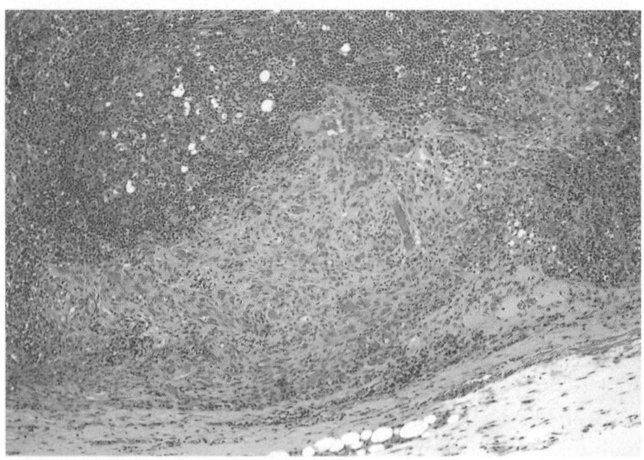

FIGURE 85.1. Kaposi sarcoma (KS) in inguinal lymph node. Reactive germinal center (*upper left*) and subcapsular proliferation of KS with wedge-shaped penetration into the cortex. Hematoxylin, phloxine, and saffron stain.

with angioimmunoblastic lymphadenopathy. Sometimes, both lesions coexist in the same lymph node, probably as a consequence of their common background of immune deregulation (43,44).

HISTOPATHOLOGY

Whether sporadic, endemic, or epidemic, and regardless of location, KS presents a similar histologic picture on microscopic examination (36). The involved lymph nodes are enlarged and frequently matted. In areas of lymph node parenchyma uninvolved by tumor, the architecture is preserved and shows marked follicular hyperplasia and plasmacytosis of medullary cords. The germinal centers are prominent. Early lesions usually involve the capsule, from which aggregates of tumor cells proliferate along the lymph node trabeculae or penetrate the nodal parenchyma in a wedge-shaped pattern (Fig. 85.1). Tumor nodules with a whorled structure replace lymph node tissues, primarily in the peripheral sinuses and medulla (Fig. 85.2). They consist of an exuberant proliferation of neoplastic spindle-shaped cells arranged in bundles with capillary-like slits and clefts that contain variable numbers of red blood cells, many of which are extravasated (Fig. 85.3). The nuclei are large but not markedly pleomorphic. Mitoses are usually present but not frequent. The proliferation of neoplastic blood vessels is accompanied by infiltrates, sometimes abundant, of plasma cells, lymphocytes, and hemosiderin-laden macrophages. Hyaline globules within the cytoplasm of endothelial cells, perivascular cells, histiocytes, and KS cells are seen in most KS tumors (Fig. 85.4). They stain with periodic acid–Schiff with and without diastase digestion and probably represent degenerated, phagocytosed erythrocytes (45). Plasma cells are almost always present, often in clumps between the bundles of KS cells (Fig. 85.5). Pleomorphic variants of KS cells may be seen in some tumors and create difficult problems of differential diagnosis. An inflammatory form of KS, in which a large number of inflammatory cells obscures the proliferation of neoplastic cells, has been described (25). Early lesions are sometimes difficult to recognize; they ap-

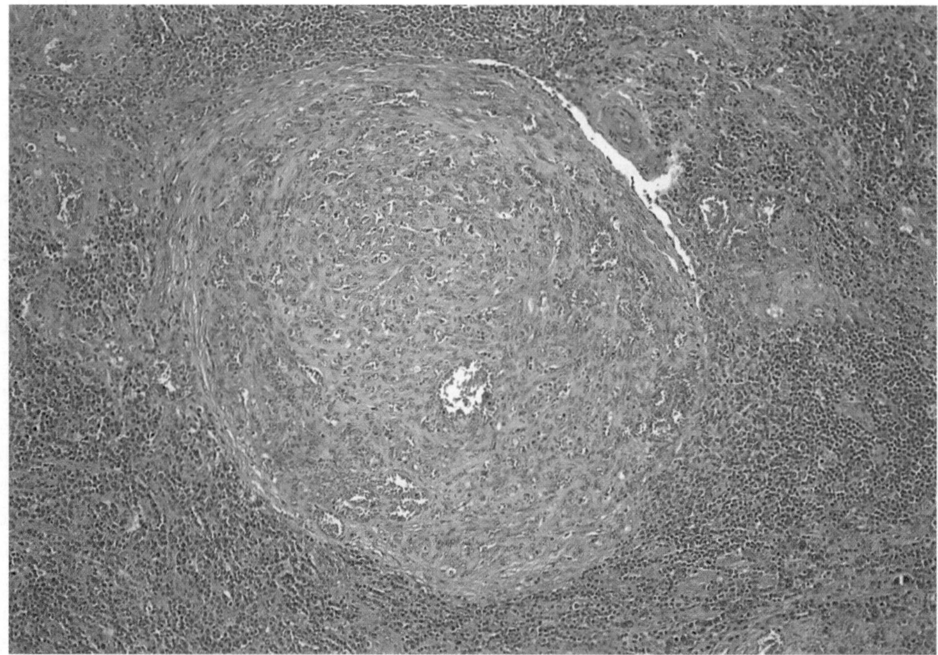

FIGURE 85.2. Kaposi sarcoma tumor nodule replacing lymphoid tissue in the same lymph node as in Fig. 85.1. Hematoxylin, phloxine, and saffron stain.

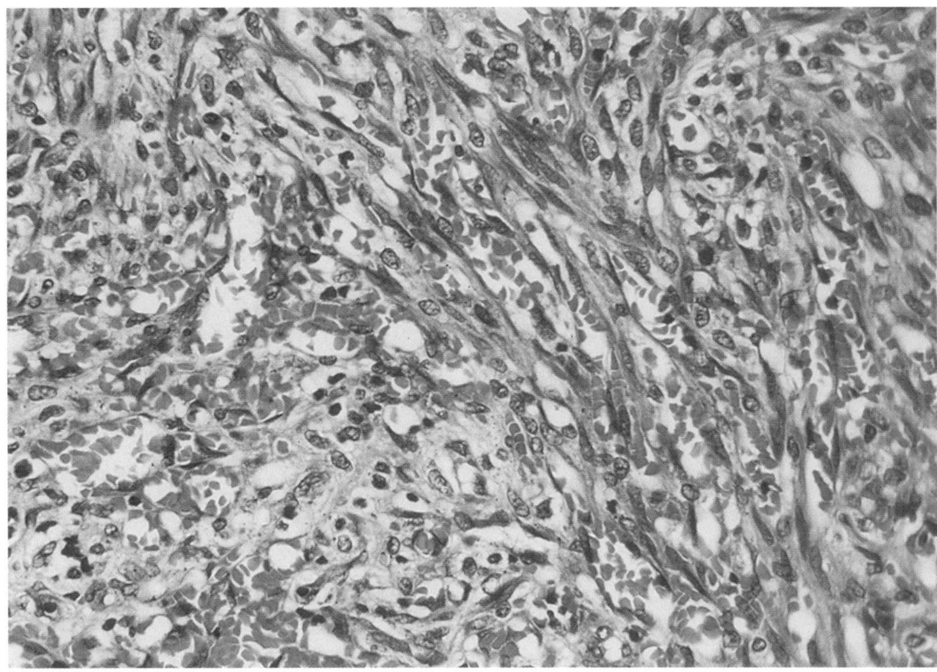

FIGURE 85.3. Exuberant proliferation of neoplastic spindle-shaped Kaposi sarcoma cells arranged in bundles with capillary clefts containing erythrocytes, many of them extravasated. Periodic acid–Schiff stain.

pear as a lacework of irregularly shaped, thin-walled capillary vessels (Fig. 85.6). Older lesions are composed of more plasma cells, deposits of hemosiderin, and collagen. Reticulin staining shows preservation of the general architecture, the contours of nodules, and a multitude of vessels. Iron staining shows an abundance of hemosiderin deposits.

In lymph nodes, as in other organs, KS may exhibit a variety of histologic patterns with each predominant in some areas, although multiple patterns are usually combined within a tumor mass (26). A study of KS lesions revealed a number of distinctive patterns that seem to represent phases of cellular differentiation (Fig. 85.7). These range from round capillaries lined by flat endothelial cells (Fig. 85.8) or large ectatic vascular spaces forming blood lakes (Fig. 85.9) at the differentiated end of the spectrum, to spindle-shaped cells resembling fibroblasts separated by slitlike spaces filled with erythrocytes, to bundles of closely packed spindle cells (Figs. 85.3 and 85.10) with pleomorphic nuclei and mitoses and entirely lacking in vascular spaces at the undifferentiated, sarcoma-like end of the spectrum (26).

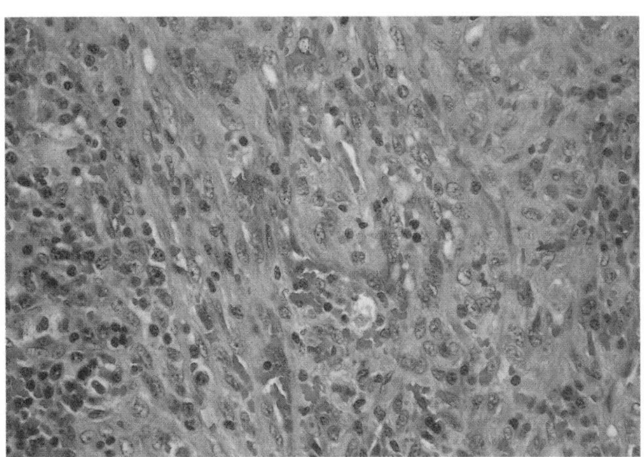

FIGURE 85.4. Kaposi sarcoma in lymph node with vascular clefts, extravasated erythrocytes, and hyalin globules. Hematoxylin, phloxine, and saffron stain.

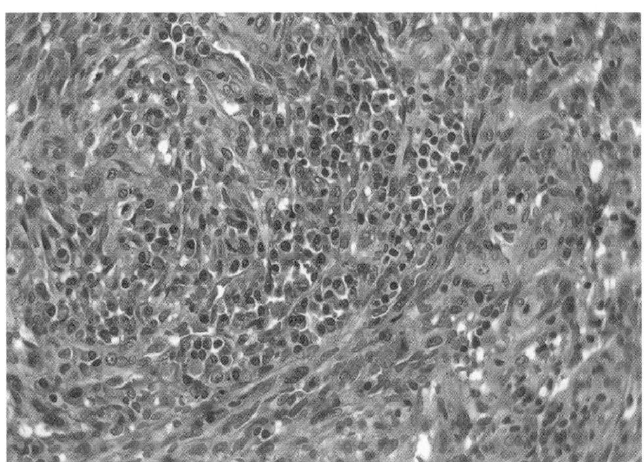

FIGURE 85.5. Bundles of spindle-shaped Kaposi sarcoma cells (*lower right*), capillaries, and abundant infiltrates of plasma cells (*center*). Hematoxylin, phloxine, and saffron stain.

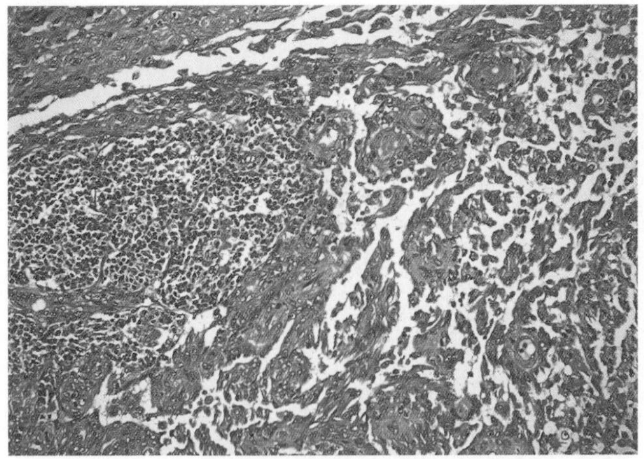

FIGURE 85.6. Kaposi sarcoma lymphadenopathy with anastomotic, lacy pattern. Hematoxylin, phloxine, and saffron stain.

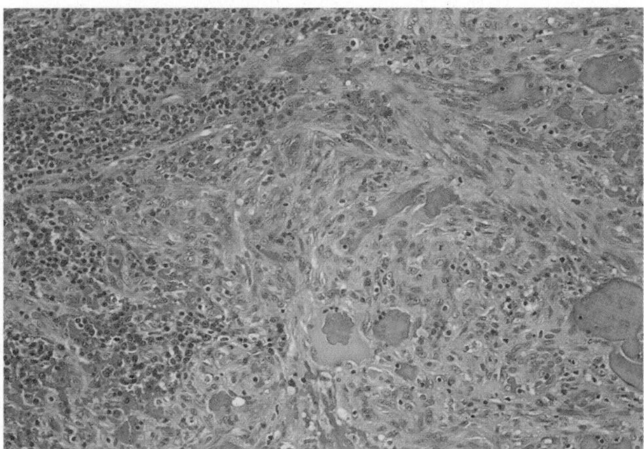

FIGURE 85.8. Kaposi sarcoma lymphadenopathy with round capillaries lined by flat endothelial cells. Hematoxylin, phloxine, and saffron stain.

ELECTRON MICROSCOPY

The origin of KS cells is still controversial; endothelial cells of blood vessels and lymphatics, pericytes, fibroblasts, and myofibroblasts have all been considered as the normal counterparts (9,46). In ultrastructural studies, a variable mixture of cells in the KS tumors, including most of the cell types mentioned above, led the authors to believe that KS cells originate from primitive vasoformative mesenchymal cells. Some of the distinctive ultrastructural features of KS cells are the infrequent presence of a Weibel-Palade body in tumor cells, which is supportive of an endothelial cell origin, and phagocytosis of erythrocytes by both endothelial and stromal KS cells (46).

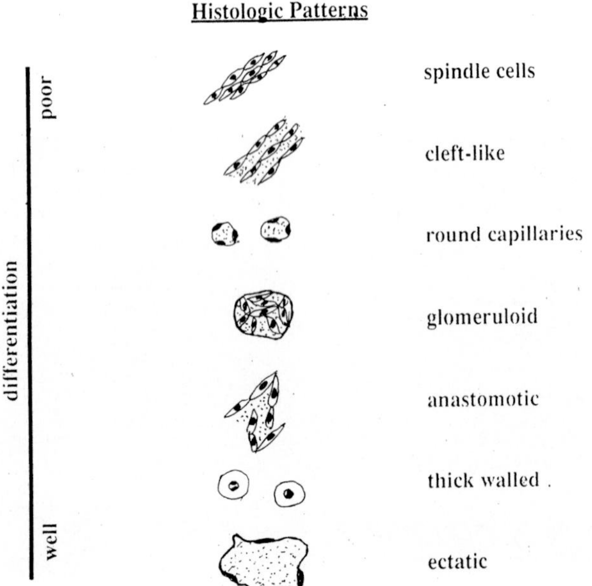

FIGURE 85.7. Histologic patterns suggesting phases of cellular differentiation in Kaposi sarcoma.

IMMUNOHISTOCHEMISTRY

With antibodies against factor VIII-related antigen and *Ulex europaeus* lectin, some authors noted staining in all KS cells; others observed staining only in cells lining the vascular spaces, and still others reported variable staining from case to case (29,47). In a study in which 13 specific MAbs were used to determine the immunophenotypes of a variety of cases of KS, staining with most of them correlated with the degree of KS cell differentiation (26). Vimentin, an MAb with broad mesenchymal cell specificity, was expressed by all KS cells regardless of degree of differentiation. *Ulex europaeus,* a lectin recognizing L-fucose, and factor VIII-related (Fig. 85.11) antigens, normally expressed by endothelial cells, demonstrated a sharp distinction between the well-formed vascular areas of KS, which stained strongly, and the nonvascular areas, which did not. Similarly, staining of actin, the major component of the microfilaments of smooth and skeletal muscle, myofibroblasts, and myoepithelial cells, showed dif-

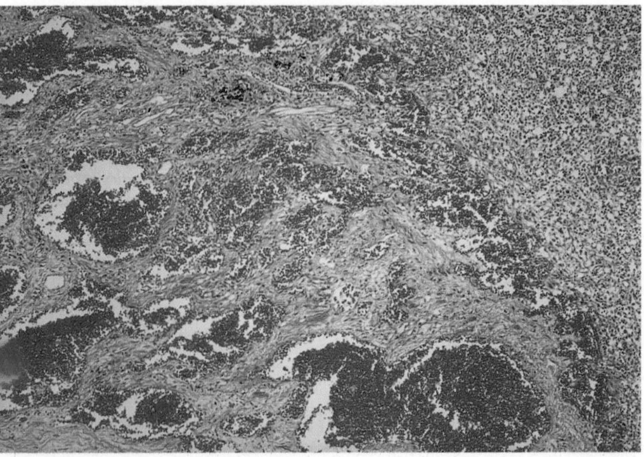

FIGURE 85.9. Kaposi sarcoma lymphadenopathy with ectatic vascular spaces forming blood lakes. Hematoxylin, phloxine, and saffron stain.

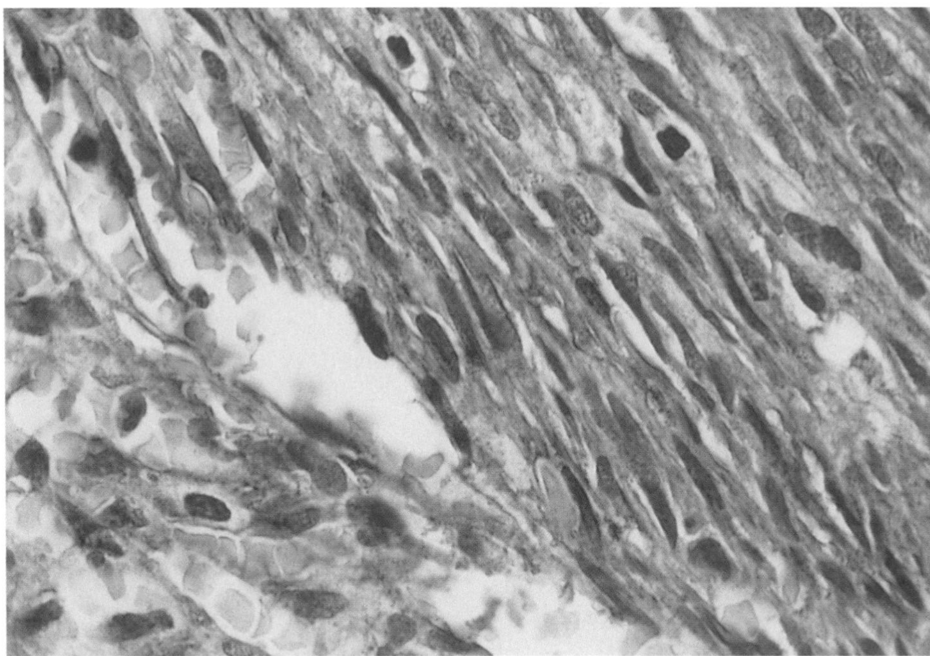

FIGURE 85.10. Kaposi sarcoma lymphadenopathy, poorly differentiated with closely packed spindle cells and lack of vascular formation. All cells strongly stained with anti-CD34 antibody. Anti-CD34/alkaline phosphatase stain.

ferences of 10% to 100% between well-differentiated vascular and nondifferentiated spindle cell areas. Conversely, MAbs to CD3l, an endothelial adhesion molecule, and particularly MAbs to CD34, a marker specific for hematopoietic stem cells and endothelial cells (Fig. 85.10), stained almost all cells in all cases, with only minimal differences noted between cells of various degrees of differentiation (26). With antibodies raised against basement membrane laminin and against type IV collagen, KS lesions were seen to be composed of two types of capillaries, some with a continuous round basement membrane of blood vessel type and others with a thin, interrupted basal lamina of lymphatic type (48). It is better to use an alkaline phosphatase than peroxidase in KS tumors, where the high content of erythrocyte endoperoxidase results in a heavily stained background that may obscure specific stainings.

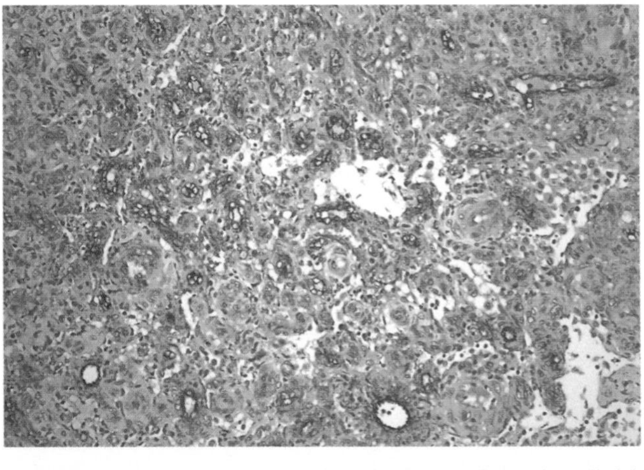

FIGURE 85.11. Kaposi sarcoma lymphadenopathy with well-differentiated vascular spaces strongly stained with antibody for anti-factor VIII-related antigen. Anti-factor VIII-related antigen/alkaline phosphatase stain.

Phenotype

Factor VIII-related antigen+/−, *Ulex europaeus*+/−
CD31+, CD34+, vimentin+
HHV-8+

DIFFERENTIAL DIAGNOSIS

- Vascular hyperplasia of HIV lymphadenitis, pattern C: In this late stage of HIV lymphadenitis, vascular proliferation throughout the lymph node parenchyma is abundant; however, the vessels are not cleftlike but well formed and include basement membranes. Bundles or whorls of spindle-shaped cells are not present. Sometimes both lesions coexist, with foci of KS arising in pattern C HIV lymphadenitis, usually in the medullary or capsular areas.
- Castleman lymphadenopathy, hyaline-vascular type, is characterized by involuted and vascularized germinal centers surrounded by layered small lymphocytes (target ap-

Checklist

KAPOSI SARCOMA

Epidemiology
- Sporadic: Mediterranean origin
- Iatrogenic: immunosuppressed hosts
- Endemic: equatorial Africa
- Epidemic: AIDS in homosexual men

HHV-8 present in majority of lesions
HIV TAT protein and multiple cytokines involved
Lymph nodes primarily involved
Multifocal lesions
Capsule, trabeculae, medulla preferentially involved
Cleftlike vascular spaces
Lacework of thin-walled capillaries
Ectatic vessels
Bundles and whorls of spindle cells
Low-grade nuclear pleomorphism
Infrequent mitoses
Extravasated erythrocytes
Hyaline globules
Hemosiderin deposits
Plasma cells
Inconsistently positive for factor VIII-RA, *Ulex europaeus*
CD31+, CD34+, vimentin+

pearance). However, cleftlike vascular spaces lined by spindle-shaped cells are not present. Occasionally, both lesions coexist; foci of KS apparently arise in lymph nodes with Castleman lymphadenopathy (49). Sometimes, KS can be demonstrated only in additional sections or on a subsequent biopsy specimen from a different lymph node (49). The histologic similarity between Castleman lymphadenopathy and HIV lymphadenitis in its burned-out phase suggests that the latter rather than the former lymph node lesion is more commonly associated with KS.

- Angioimmunoblastic lymphadenopathy includes vascular hyperplasia, but the vessels are not cleftlike, large numbers of immunoblasts are present, and bundles or whorls of spindle-shaped cells are lacking.
- Bacillary angiomatosis is prevalent in persons with HIV infection and forms cutaneous vascular lesions. However, the component blood vessels are capillaries lined by typical endothelial cells. Bacilli that stain with Warthin-Starry stain are present.
- Angiosarcomas of various histologic types may be difficult to separate from anaplastic variants of KS, although angiosarcomas exhibit more nuclear atypia and mitoses.
- Steward-Treves postmastectomy lesion, interpreted as a lymphangiosarcoma arising in the postmastectomy lymphedema, closely resembles KS. Some of the cases reported may indeed have been KS, which seems occasionally to develop in areas of chronic edema (9).

REFERENCES

1. Rothman S. Remarks on sex, age and racial distribution of Kaposi's sarcoma and on possible pathogenetic factors. Acta Union Int Cancer 1962;18:326–329.
2. Oettle AG. Geographical and racial differences in frequency of Kaposi's sarcoma as evidence of environmental or genetic causes. In: Ackerman LV, Murray JF, eds. Symposium on Kaposi's sarcoma. New York: Hafner, 1963:330–363.
3. Taff ML, Siegal FP, Geller SA. Outbreak of an acquired immunodeficiency syndrome associated with opportunistic infections and Kaposi's sarcoma in male homosexuals. Am J Forensic Med Pathol 1982;3:259–264.
4. Taylor JF, Templeton AC, Vogel CL, et al. Kaposi's sarcoma in Uganda: a clinico-pathological study. Int J Cancer 1971;8:122.
5. Penn I. Kaposi's sarcoma in organ transplant recipients: report of 20 cases. Transplantation 1979;27:8–11.
6. Harwood AR, Osoba D, Hofstader S, et al. Kaposi's sarcoma in recipients of renal transplants. Am J Med 1979;67:759–765.
7. Beral V, Peterman TA, Berkelman RL, et al. Kaposi's sarcoma among persons with AIDS: a sexually transmitted infection? Lancet 1990;335:123–128.
8. Centers for Disease Control. Epidemiologic aspects of the current outbreak of Kaposi's sarcoma and opportunistic infections. N Engl J Med 1982;306:248–252.

9. Templeton AC. Kaposi's sarcoma. Pathol Annu 1981;16:315–336.
10. Bisceglia M, Amini M, Bosman C. Primary Kaposi's sarcoma of the lymph node in children. Cancer 1988;61:1715–1718.
11. Giraldo G, Beth E, Haguenau F. Herpes-type virus particles in tissue culture of Kaposi's sarcoma from different geographic regions. J Natl Cancer Inst 1972;49:1509.
12. Walter PR, Philippe E, Nguemby Mbina C, et al. Kaposi sarcoma: presence of herpes-type virus particles in a tumor specimen. Hum Pathol 1984;15:1145.
13. Ioachim HL, Dorsett B, Melamed J, et al. Cytomegalovirus, angiomatosis and Kaposi's sarcoma: new observations of a debated relationship. Mod Pathol 1992;5:169–178.
14. Handsfield HH, Chandler SH, Caine VA, et al. Cytomegalovirus infection in sex partners: evidence for sexual transmission. J Infect Dis 1985;115:344.
15. Drew WL, Mintz L, Miner RC, et al. Prevalence of cytomegalovirus infection in homosexual men. J Infect Dis 1981; 143:188.
16. Giraldo G, Beth E, Huang ES. Kaposi's sarcoma and its relationship to cytomegalovirus (CMV): III. CMV-DNA and CMV-early antigens in Kaposi's sarcoma. Int J Cancer 1980;26:23–29.
17. Grody WW, Lewin K, Naeim F. Detection of cytomegalovirus DNA in classic and epidemic Kaposi's sarcoma by *in situ* hybridization. Hum Pathol 1988;19:524–528.
18. Van den Berg F, Schipper M, Jiwa M, et al. Implausibility of an etiological association between cytomegalovirus and Kaposi's sarcoma shown by four techniques. J Clin Pathol 1989;42:128–131.
19. Moore PS, Chang Y. Detection of herpesvirus-like DNA sequences in Kaposi's sarcoma in patients with and those without HIV infection. N Engl J Med 1995;332:1181–1185.
20. Dictor M, Rambech E, Way D, et al. Human herpesvirus 8 (Kaposi's sarcoma-associated herpesvirus) DNA in Kaposi's sarcoma lesions, AIDS Kaposi's sarcoma cell lines, endothelial Kaposi's sarcoma simulators and the skin of immunosuppressed patients. Am J Pathol 1996;148:2009–2016.
21. Whitby E, Howard MR, Tenant-Flowers M, et al. Detection of Kaposi sarcoma-associated herpesvirus in peripheral blood of HIV-infected individuals and progression to Kaposi's sarcoma. Lancet 1995;346:799–802.
22. Maiorana A, Luppi M, Barozzi P, et al: Detection of human herpes virus type 8 DNA sequences as a valuable aid in the differential diagnosis of Kaposi's sarcoma. Mod Pathol 1997;10:182–187.
23. Li JJ, Huang YQ, Cockerell CJ, at al. Localization of human herpes-like virus type 8 in vascular endothelial cells and perivascular spindle-shaped cells of Kaposi's sarcoma lesions by *in situ* hybridization [Short Communication]. Am J Pathol 1996;148: 1741–1748.
24. Costa J, Rabson AS. Generalized Kaposi's sarcoma is not a neoplasm. Lancet 1983;1:58.
25. Moskowitz LB, Hensley GT, Gould EW, et al. Frequency and anatomic distribution of lymphadenopathic Kaposi's sarcoma in the acquired immunodeficiency syndrome: an autopsy series. Hum Pathol 1985;16:447–456.
26. Ioachim HL, Adsay V, Giancotti F, et al. Kaposi's sarcoma of internal organs. A multiparameter study of 86 cases. Cancer 1995;75:1376–1385.
27. Safai B, Mike V, Giraldo G, et al. Association of Kaposi's sarcoma with second primary malignancies. Possible etiopathogenic implications. Cancer 1980;45:1472.
28. Barillari G, Gendelman R, Gall RC, et al. The Tat protein of human immunodeficiency virus type 1, a growth factor for AIDS Kaposi sarcoma and cytokine-activated vascular cells, induces adhesion of the same cell types by using integrin receptors recognizing the RGD amino acid sequence. Proc Natl Acad Sci U S A 1993;90:7941–7945.
29. Nadji M, Morales AR, Ziegles-Weissman J, et al. Kaposi's sarcoma: immunohistologic evidence for an endothelial origin. Arch Pathol Lab Med 1981;105:274–275.
30. Scully PA, Steinman HK, Kennedy C, et al. AIDS-related Kaposi's sarcoma displays differential expression of endothelial surface antigens. Am J Pathol 1988;130:244–251.
31. Krafert C, Planus L, Penneys NS. Kaposi's sarcoma: further immunohistologic evidence of a vascular endothelial origin. Arch Dermatol 1991;127:1734–1735.
32. Beckstead JH, Wood GS, Fletcher V. Evidence for the origin of Kaposi's sarcoma from lymphatic endothelium. Am J Pathol 1985;119:294–300.
33. Delia D, Lampugnani MG, Resnati M, et al. CD34 expression is regulated reciprocally with adhesion molecules in vascular endothelial cells *in vitro.* Blood 1993;81:1001–1008.
34. Ensoli B, Barillari G, Gallo RC. Cytokines and growth factors in the pathogenesis of AIDS-associated Kaposi's sarcoma. Immunol Rev 1992;127:147–155.
35. Friedman-Kien AE, Ostreicher R. Overview of classical and epidemic Kaposi's sarcoma. In: Friedman-Kien AE, Laubenstein LJ, eds. AIDS: the epidemic of Kaposi's sarcoma and opportunistic infections. New York: Masson, 1984:23–25.
36. Gottlieb GJ, Ackerman AB. Kaposi's sarcoma: an extensively disseminated form in young homosexual men. Hum Pathol 1982;3:882–892.
37. Ioachim HL. Kaposi's sarcoma. In: Pathology of AIDS. Textbook and color atlas. Philadelphia: JB Lippincott Co, 1989:82–85.
38. Port J, Traube J, Winans CS. The visceral manifestations of Kaposi's sarcoma. Gastrointest Endosc 1982;28:179–191.
39. Lubin J, Rywlin AM. Lymphoma-like lymph node changes in Kaposi's sarcoma: two additional cases. Arch Pathol 1971;92: 338–341.
40. Ramos CV, Taylor HB, Hernandez BA, et al. Primary Kaposi's sarcoma of lymph node. Am J Clin Pathol 1976;66:998–1003.
41. Amazon K, Rywlin AM. Subtle clues to diagnosis by conventional microscopy: lymph node involvement in Kaposi's sarcoma. Am J Dermatopathol 1979;1:173.
42. Su I-J, Kuo T-T, Wu S-Y, et al. Lymphadenopathic type of Kaposi's sarcoma presenting with generalized petechial hemorrhages. Cancer 1984;54:948–950.
43. Rywlin A, Rosen L, Cabello B. Coexistence of Castleman's disease and Kaposi's sarcoma. Report of a case and a speculation. Am J Dermatopathol 1983;5:277–281.
44. Varsano S, Manor Y, Steiner Z, et al. Kaposi's sarcoma and angioimmunoblastic lymphadenopathy. Cancer 1984;54:1582–1585.
45. Fukunaga M, Silverberg SG. Hyaline globules in Kaposi's sarcoma: a light microscopic and immunohistochemical study. Mod Pathol 1991;4:187–190.
46. Waldo ED, Vuletin JC, Kay GI. The ultrastructure of vascular tumors, additional observations and a review of the literature. Pathol Annu 1977;12:279–308.
47. Ordonez NG, Batsakis JG. Comparison of *Ulex europaeus* I lectin and factor VIII–related antigen in vascular lesions. Arch Pathol Lab Med 1984;108:129–132.
48. Autio-Harmainen H, Karttunen T, Apaja-Sarkkinen M, et al. Laminin and type IV collagen in different histological stages of Kaposi's sarcoma and other vascular lesions of blood vessel or lymphatic vessel origin. Am J Surg Pathol 1988;12:469–476.
49. Harris NL. Hypervascular follicular hyperplasia and Kaposi's sarcoma in patients at risk for AIDS. N Engl J Med 1984;310:462–463.

PART

X

METASTATIC TUMORS IN LYMPH NODES

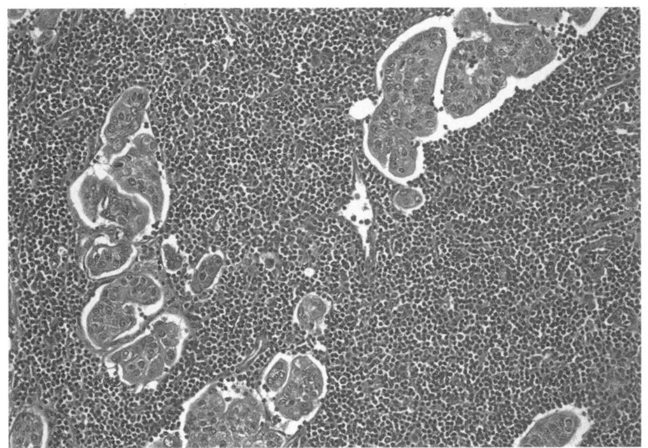

The involvement of lymph nodes by metastatic tumors signifies the start of a new phase in the progress of a cancer. It indicates that through a succession of molecular changes, the cancer cells have acquired phenotypes that enable them to invade, colonize, and disseminate.

Establishing the presence of metastatic tumor in lymph nodes is essential for the management and prognosis of cancer. The vast majority of lymph node biopsies, particularly those on frozen sections, are performed to confirm or exclude tumor metastases. The anatomic location and the number of lymph nodes involved are also important indicators of the process, and new methods, such as sentinel lymph node biopsies, have been devised to answer questions of staging. Not infrequently, a lymph node metastasis is discovered before an occult primary tumor is detected. In such cases, to identify the unknown primary tumor, extensive studies of the lymph node metastases, including immunohistochemistry and electron microscopy in addition to detailed histopathology, are often necessary.

In the following 13 chapters, the diagnostic problems relating to the most common tumor metastases of lymph nodes are examined.

86

TUMOR METASTASES IN LYMPH NODES

PATHOBIOLOGY OF TUMOR METASTASIS

The major cause of the morbidity and mortality associated with tumors is metastasis. Although substantial progress has been achieved in the early diagnosis and treatment of malignant tumors, mechanisms of dissemination remain largely unknown. The elucidation of such mechanisms is essential to prevent metastases and cure cancer. Tumor metastasis is a complex phenomenon based on a cascade of interdependent events: detachment of cells from the primary tumor, advancement through the tumor matrix, penetration through the basement membranes of lymphatics and blood vessels, circulation through the vascular flow, arrival in remote organs, and formation of independent colonies with their own growth factors and vascular supply (1). Some believe that primary tumors are largely heterogeneous and so may include cells endowed with a capacity for growth autonomy and metastasis (2). Others think that the potential for metastasis arises through mutations, with new variants generated and selected during tumor development (3). Because malignant cells are inherently unstable, their genomes are subject to constant variation, resulting in what is termed *phenotypic drift* (4). Various genes undergo irreversible structural changes (mutations), such as deletions, amplifications, and translocations, which yield altered gene products (4). Among them are adhesion molecules such as E-cadherins, the down-regulation of which decreases tumor cell cohesiveness; integrins, which determine the affinity of tumor cells for basement membranes; and proteolytic enzymes, such as type IV collagenase, which are essential for tumor cell invasiveness (5–7). A particular adhesion molecule, CD44, and its variants, which are normally expressed on T lymphocytes, has also been detected on some tumor cells, which suggests a possible role of T lymphocytes in tumor implantation in lymph nodes (8). Thus, tumor cells progressively acquire the characteristics necessary for invasion and metastasis, which characterize the metastatic phenotype.

The fact that not all malignant tumors are metastatic suggests that the metastatic phenotype is different from and independent of the tumorigenic phenotype (9,10). The multiple steps in the metastatic cascade of events are probably controlled at the genetic level through activation or deactivation of multiple genes. As counterparts of the genes promoting the formation of metastatic phenotypes, metastatic suppressor genes probably degrade the gene products favoring tumor cell dissemination (6). Thus, the success or failure of a tumor to invade and metastasize depends on the interaction of gene products released by stimulatory and inhibitory metastasis genes (10).

TUMOR METASTASIS IN LYMPH NODES

Lymph nodes play an essential role in the control of tumor progression. In response to the antigenicity of tumor cells, regional lymph nodes may initiate and develop complex immune reactions. At the same time, they may entrap circulating tumor cells that have originated in their tributary territories. Acting as efficient barriers, the lymph nodes may be able to destroy invading tumor cells completely, or at least stop their dissemination temporarily. Lymph node metastasis, in contrast to the vascular spread of tumors, presents an opportunity, even if temporary, for surgical intervention. In addition, because of their accessibility, lymph nodes with metastatic tumor present the best opportunity for primary tumor diagnosis through biopsy and histologic evaluation.

Metastatic tumor cells first appear in the marginal sinus (Fig. 86.1), from which they penetrate the medullary sinuses, medulla, and cortex; the eventual result is total parenchymal replacement. Within the lymph nodes, the tumor cells may induce various tissue reactions, such as reactive follicular hyperplasia (Fig. 86.2), sinus histiocytosis, angiogenesis (Fig. 86.3), and foreign body granuloma formation (Fig. 86.4). Some metastatic tumors elicit intense desmoplastic reactions, which contribute to the partial or total replacement of lymphoid tissues (Fig. 86.5). Finally, radiotherapy or chemotherapy may wipe out lymphoid tissue with the tumor and create an unusual histologic appearance of the lymph nodes affected (Fig. 86.6). Prior involve-

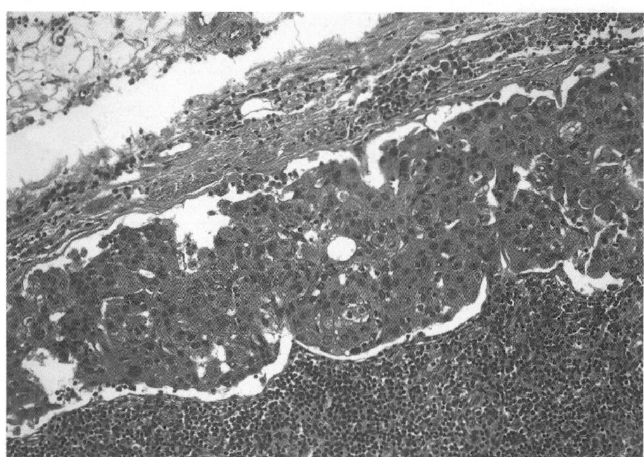

FIGURE 86.1. Metastatic poorly differentiated squamous cell carcinoma of tongue within largely distended marginal sinus of submandibular lymph node. Hematoxylin, phloxine, and saffron stain.

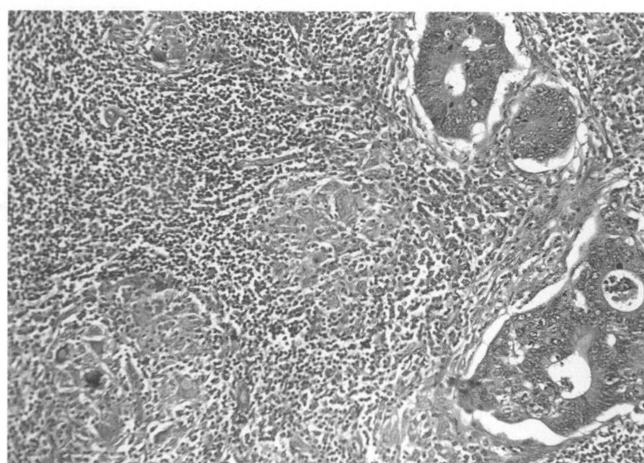

FIGURE 86.4. Lymph node metastasis of adenocarcinoma accompanied by foreign body giant cell granulomas. Hematoxylin, phloxine, and saffron stain.

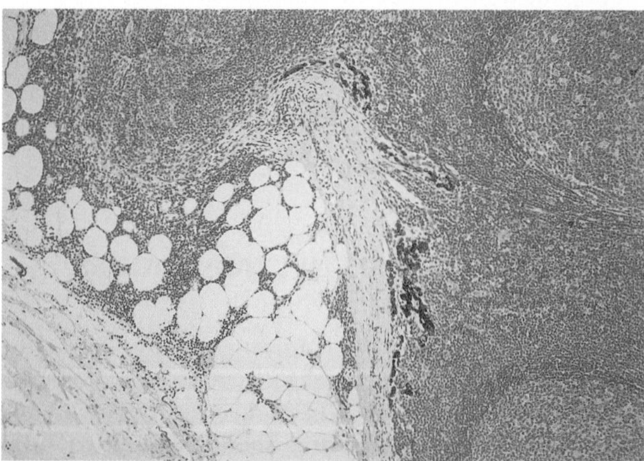

FIGURE 86.2. Lymph node with hyperplastic follicles and reactive germinal centers in response to clusters of metastatic gastric carcinoma cells in the marginal sinus revealed by cytokeratin (*CK*) immunostaining. CK/peroxidase stain.

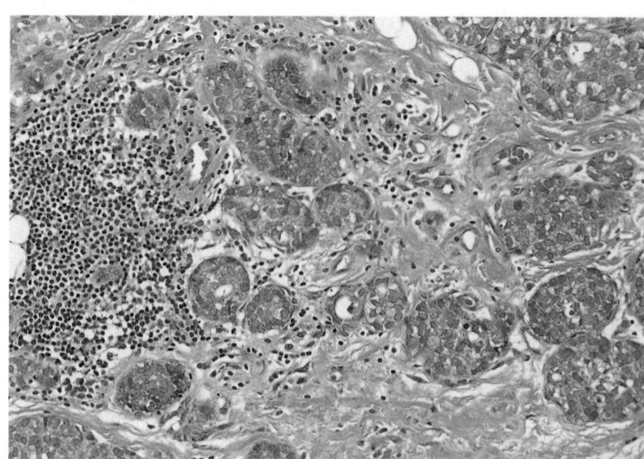

FIGURE 86.5. Lymph node largely replaced by metastatic carcinoma and extensive desmoplastic reaction. Hematoxylin, phloxine, and saffron stain.

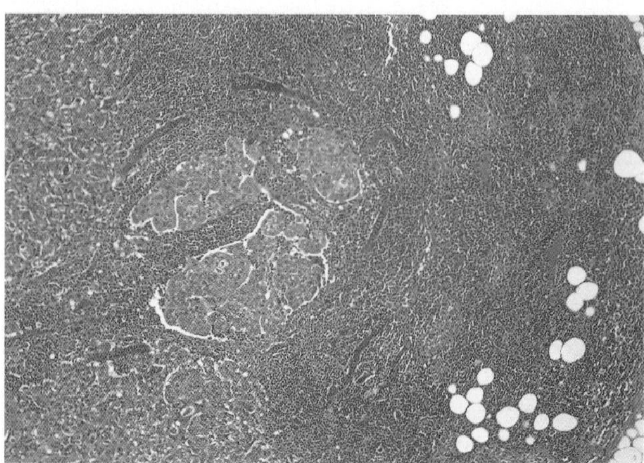

FIGURE 86.3. Lymph node metastasis of mammary carcinoma surrounded by newly formed blood vessels. Hematoxylin, phloxine, and saffron stain.

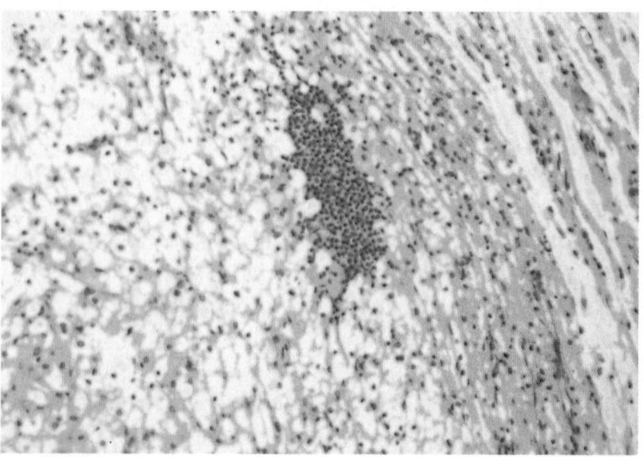

FIGURE 86.6. Axillary lymph node after chemotherapy for breast carcinoma is entirely depopulated except for small area of residual lymphoid cells. Hematoxylin, phloxine, and saffron stain.

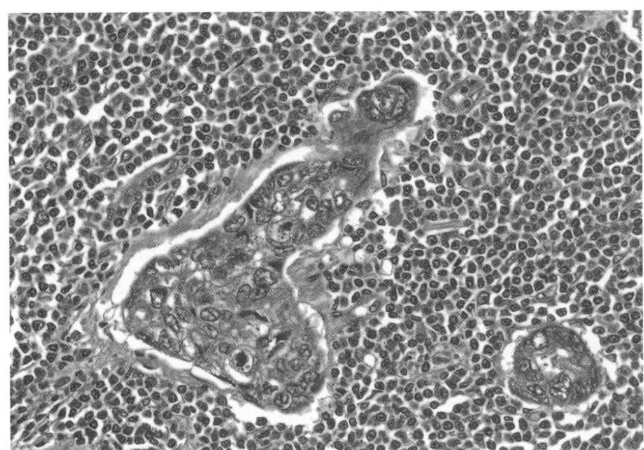

FIGURE 86.7. Metastatic breast carcinoma in lymph node with small lymphocytic lymphoma/chronic lymphocytic leukemia. Hematoxylin, phloxine, and saffron stain.

ment of a lymph node by leukemia or lymphoma does not preclude the subsequent growth of a metastatic tumor (Fig. 86.7).

STAGING AND PROGNOSIS OF TUMORS

Cancer management and prognosis depend to a great extent on the presence and degree of tumor metastasis. These are evaluated by staging tumors according to the internationally accepted TNM (tumor–node–metastasis) system. Of all the various criteria used as prognostic factors, the most powerful remains the description of anatomic spread according to the TNM formula (11). This classification by stage is as follows: stage 0, preinvasive neoplasia; stage I, tumor confined to the organ of origin; stage II, direct tumor spread outside the organ of origin; stage III, metastasis to regional lymph nodes; and stage IV, metastasis to distant sites (11). Each successive stage in the TNM system indicates a significant decrement in the prognosis. The diagnosis of lymph node tumor metastasis is therefore essentially important for cancer therapy. This consists not only of establishing the presence of lymph node metastasis but also of evaluating the site of the primary tumor and its degree of histologic differentiation and determining the tumor cell phenotype and prognostic indicators of tumor cell behavior.

TOPOGRAPHY OF INVOLVED LYMPH NODES

The anatomic location of a lymph node involved with metastatic tumor provides an important indication of the site of the primary tumor (Table 86.1).

Cervical lymph nodes, particularly high jugular and posterior cervical nodes, drain the head and neck and may harbor metastatic carcinomas originating in the nasopharynx (see Chapter 89), tonsillar fossa, tongue, floor of the mouth,

TABLE 86.1. MOST COMMON PRIMARY ORIGINS OF REGIONAL LYMPH NODE METASTASES

Lymph nodes with metastatic tumors	Primary tumors of origin
High cervical (high jugular, posterior cervical)	Head and neck (nasopharynx, tonsils, tongue, floor of mouth, thyroid, extrinsic larynx, facial skin, scalp)
Low cervical (left scalene)	Intrathoracic (lungs), intraabdominal
Supraclavicular (left supraclavicular)	Abdominal (gastric)
Axillary	Breast, upper extremities, trunk
Inguinal	Lower extremities, vulva, cervix, endometrium, ovary, penis, prostate, rectum, anus
Pelvic	Prostate, testes, female genital tract, lower extremities

thyroid (see Chapter 90), extrinsic larynx, facial skin, and scalp.

Scalene lymph nodes representing the lower, deep jugular chain are commonly the site of metastases from intrathoracic carcinomas, particularly in the lungs. The left scalene lymph nodes also drain metastases of intraabdominal tumors.

The supraclavicular lymph nodes are most often the site of metastases of abdominal cancers. The left supraclavicular lymph node, frequently invaded by gastric carcinoma, is classically known as the *Virchow node* (Fig. 86.8).

In women, involvement of the axillary lymph nodes with metastatic carcinoma generally indicates the presence of ipsilateral breast cancer (see Chapter 88). Melanomas and squamous cell carcinomas of the upper extremities and trunk are the next most frequent primary tumors to invade the axillary nodes (see Chapter 87).

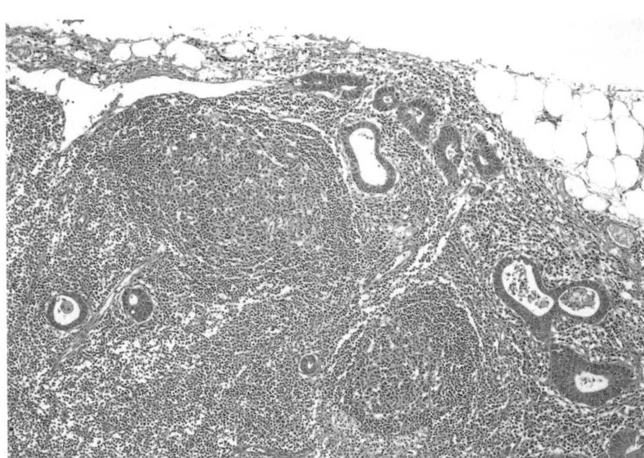

FIGURE 86.8. Metastatic gastric adenocarcinoma in supraclavicular lymph node (Virchow node). Hematoxylin, phloxine, and saffron stain.

Inguinal lymph node metastases in 2,232 patients were reviewed by Zaren and Copeland (12), and the locations of the primary tumors, determined in 99% of the cases, were in descending order of frequency as follows: skin of the lower extremities, cervix, vulva, skin of the trunk, rectum and anus, ovary, and penis.

Pelvic lymph nodes may be the site of metastases from the prostate and testes, the female genital tract, and the lower extremities.

The topographic correlations mentioned above are helpful clues to the most common sites of origin of metastases in various groups of regional lymph nodes. Notwithstanding the anatomic connections between the location of neoplasms and their draining lymph nodes, metastatic tumors can occasionally be found in unexpected and remote areas. Because of blockage of lymphatics by tumor cells, with subsequent retrograde flow and circulation shunts, paradoxical metastases, contralateral metastases, and metastases of deep-seated tumors in peripheral lymph nodes may be encountered. Not unlike hematogenous metastases, the involvement of lymph nodes by secondary tumors can vary greatly. Therefore, although the most common sites of origin for each regional group of lymph nodes should be considered first, all other possible locations of primary tumors must be systematically reviewed in every case.

LYMPH NODE METASTASES OF OCCULT PRIMARY TUMORS

In general, a statistical relation exists between tumor size and the incidence of metastases. Thus, it has been clearly established that in carcinoma of both breast and colon, the probability of finding metastases in regional lymph nodes increases in proportion to tumor volume (13). However, important exceptions to these correlations include large tumors that do not metastasize and very small tumors that disseminate widely. To a large extent, the capacity for metastasis represents an intrinsic quality of tumor cells that in most cases correlates inversely with the degree of cellular differentiation. During tumor progression, the capacity for metastatic dissemination of tumor cells may change, and within each tumor, because of genomic instability and frequent mutations, new populations of tumor cells with increased metastatic potential may gradually emerge (14). Sometimes, lymph node metastases may occur without a detectable primary tumor as the result of enhancement of the metastatic potential of tumor cells and regression of the primary neoplasm, an event known to happen occasionally, particularly with melanoma (15,16) and seminoma (17,18) (see Chapters 87 and 92).

Carcinomas of nasopharynx and oropharynx are notorious for presenting with metastases in the cervical lymph nodes while the primary neoplasm remains unnoticeable (see Chapter 89). Jesse and co-workers (19) reviewed 210 cases of metastatic carcinoma of cervical lymph nodes in which no primary lesion could be found, even after repeated blinded biopsies. After radical surgery or radiotherapy, 48% of the patients survived 3 years free of tumor.

In women, metastatic carcinoma in the axillary lymph nodes with no clinical evidence of a primary source is most likely to be of breast origin (20) (see Chapter 88). In a series of 6,000 breast tumors reviewed by Haagensen (21), 18 had large axillary metastases without a palpable primary tumor, whereas in the series of 5,451 cases of Owen and colleagues (22), 25 patients (0.5%) had occult primary tumors and metastases in the axillary lymph nodes. Copeland and McBride (20) reviewed 42 cases of axillary metastases from unknown primary sites and found on follow-up that the most common sources had been breast carcinoma and cutaneous melanoma. Finally, Rosen (23), who studied eight cases of axillary lymph node metastases with occult primary tumor in which a total mastectomy had been performed, found only noninvasive mammary carcinoma on extensive histologic sampling.

Inguinal and pelvic lymph nodes also may contain metastatic tumor from unknown primary neoplasms (12,24,25). In the 22 cases reported by Zaren and Copeland (12), radical treatment resulted in a 3-year survival rate of 50%. Some of the occult tumors metastasizing in inguinal and pelvic lymph nodes were seminomas (25), prostatic carcinomas (24), and melanomas (12). It is estimated that in 5% to 10% of patients with seminomas, which are often intratubular and noninvasive, the first symptoms are caused by the lymph node metastases, as in the two cases reported by Richter and Leder (25) (see Chapter 92).

Melanomas, of all metastatic tumors, are most likely to be the primary when a primary tumor cannot be found (see Chapter 87). In a series of 2,446 cases of melanoma reviewed by Baab and McBride (15), 4% did not have a known site of origin, a figure close to the 3.7% given by Das Gupta and associates for their 992 patients (26). The prognosis for a lymph node metastasis with an occult primary tumor in the case of melanoma (15), breast cancer (27), and carcinoma of head and neck (19) was consistently better than that for a lymph node metastasis with a clinically apparent tumor.

The problem of an unknown primary tumor in the presence of a lymph node metastasis is relatively common in surgical pathology. Not uncommonly, the histologic pattern and cellular features characteristic of a particular tumor are no longer recognizable in its metastases because of multiple mutations and the emergence of new cellular clones (Fig. 86.9). Identifying the primary tumor is usually difficult, often frustrating, yet indispensable for treatment. All available methods of histopathology, electron microscopy, histochemistry, and immunohistochemistry must be used in this important diagnostic determination.

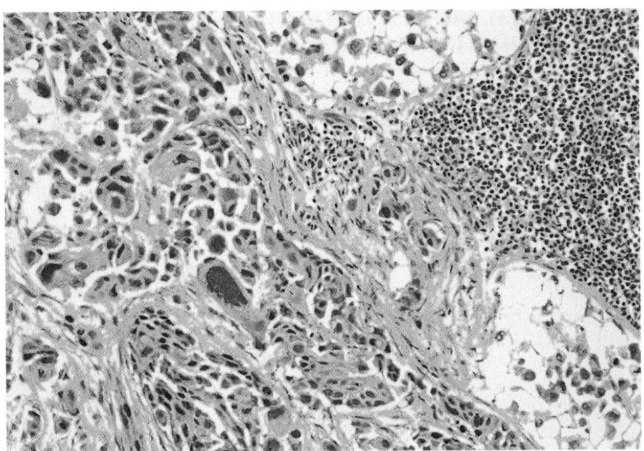

FIGURE 86.9. Metastasis of urinary bladder carcinoma in inguinal lymph node. Primary urothelial pattern has been replaced with cords of highly anaplastic carcinoma cells. Hematoxylin, phloxine, and saffron stain.

HISTOPATHOLOGY

Three questions must be answered when a tumor metastasis is suspected in a lymph node: Is the abnormal histology produced by malignant tumor or reactive hyperplasia, is the tumor primary or metastatic in the lymph node, and, in the latter case, what is the site of origin?

Metastatic tumors in lymph nodes are preferentially located, at least in an earlier phase, within sinuses, which appear prominent, distended, and filled with tumor cells (Fig. 86.10). At this stage, the differential diagnosis must include all conditions causing sinus histiocytosis, particularly nonneoplastic lymphadenopathies, such as *reactive lymphoid hyperplasia* with a sinus pattern (see Chapter 33), most often seen in tumor-draining lymph nodes (see Chapter 44). Some primary neoplastic lesions in lymph nodes may mimic metastatic tumors, such as *malignant histiocytosis* (see Chapter 77) and especially *anaplastic large cell lymphoma* (see Chapter 75). The latter is characterized by cohesive aggregates of large lymphoma cells within the nodal sinuses, occasionally resembling metastatic melanoma or undifferentiated carcinoma. Frequently, large cell lymphomas, particularly those growing in sheets and displaying marked nuclear pleomorphism, are confused with anaplastic carcinomas. Histologic features more consistent with carcinoma than with lymphoma include an arrangement of tumor cells in nests, islands, and cords inside and outside the lymph node; preservation of the integrity of the capsule, even when the subcapsular sinus is obliterated; and the presence of residual narrow strands of normal lymphatic tissue between the masses of tumor cells. The reticulin stain is often helpful because thick reticulin fibers surround the cords and islands of carcinoma cells, accentuating the outlines of the metastatic tumor, whereas in lymphomas, fine branching reticulin fibrils penetrate the intercellular spaces, wrapping individual lymphoid cells.

However, as noted by Rappaport (28), who outlined these differential features, none constitutes an infallible criterion by which to make the distinction. To separate undifferentiated carcinomas from large cell lymphomas with confidence, epithelial and lymphoid markers must be demonstrated with specific antibodies.

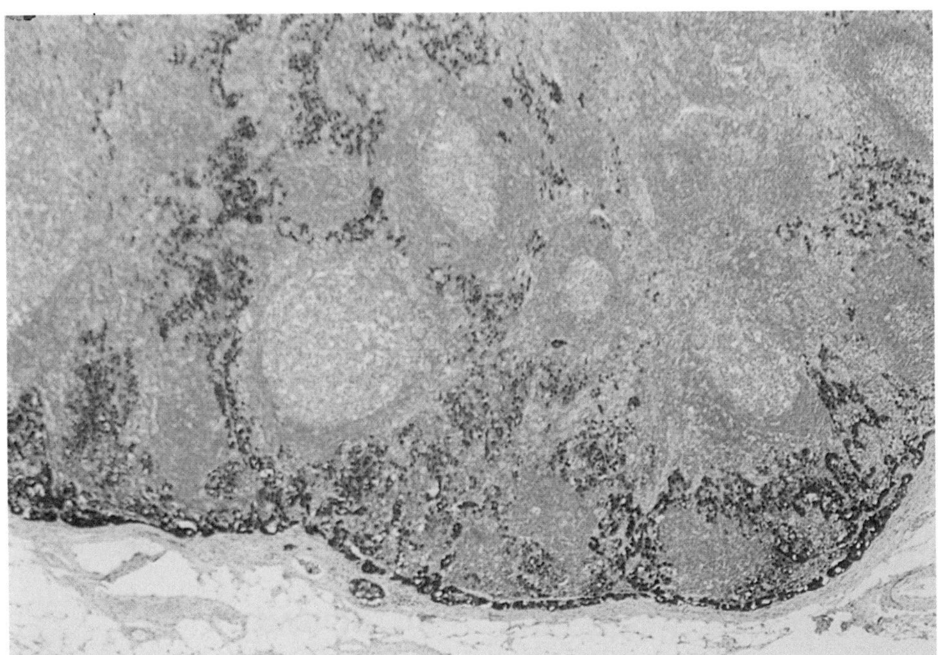

FIGURE 86.10. Metastatic melanoma fills the marginal and cortical sinuses between reactive lymphoid follicles. S100 protein/peroxidase stain.

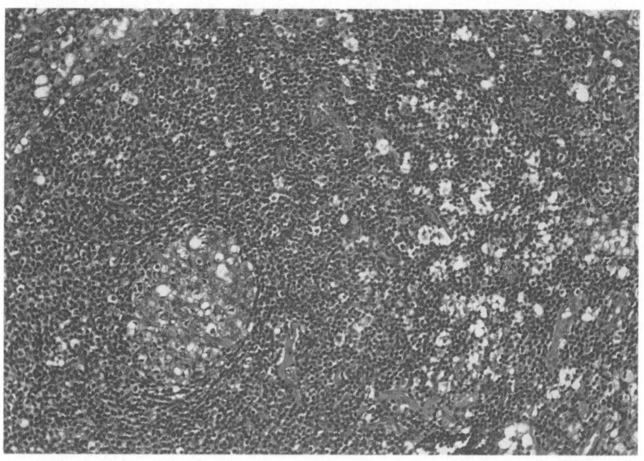

FIGURE 86.11. Metastatic breast carcinoma in axillary lymph node. The signet ring cells of lobular carcinoma are scattered singly or in small clusters throughout the lymphoid tissue. Hematoxylin, phloxine, and saffron stain.

The histologic appearance of lymph node metastases often suggests the primary tumor. Metastatic adenocarcinomas may display the glandular pattern with large mucus-secreting cells of colonic carcinomas (see Chapter 94), the small gland monomorphic patterns of prostatic carcinomas (see Chapter 93), the solid pattern of medullary breast carcinomas, or the signet ring pattern of gastric (see Chapter 94) and lobular mammary (see Chapter 88) carcinomas (Fig. 86.11). The sites of origin of other metastatic tumors may be indicated by the following: papillary structures with occasional psammoma bodies in carcinomas of the thyroid (Figs. 90.1 and 90.3) and ovary; keratin pearls in squamous cell carcinomas; neurofibrils in neuroblastomas (see Chapter 96); neurosecretory granules in neuroendocrine tumors (see Chapter 95); melanin pigment in melanomas (Fig. 87.3); argyrophil granules in carcinoid tumors.

Merkel cell carcinoma, sometimes unnoticed in its primary site, may produce multiple distant metastases with features of a neuroendocrine tumor. The origin of metastatic clear cell carcinomas is commonly in the kidneys (Figs. 91.1 and 91.2) or testes (Figs. 92.2 and 92.3). Less common sites of origin of metastatic tumors with a clear cell appearance are a squamous cell carcinoma with spindle cell and clear cell metaplasia (Fig. 86.12) and a leiomyosarcoma with clear cell metaplasia.

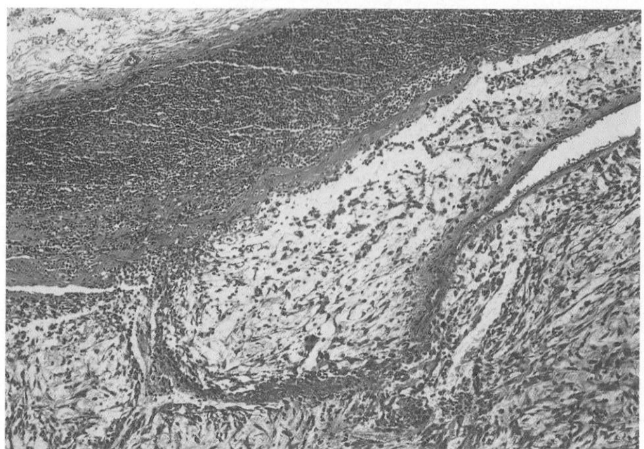

FIGURE 86.12. Metastatic squamous cell carcinoma of tongue in submaxillary lymph node with metaplastic spindle cells and clear cells. Hematoxylin, phloxine, and saffron stain.

TABLE 86.2. METASTATIC LYMPH NODE TUMORS RESEMBLING LYMPHOMAS

Small cell carcinoma of lung
Lobular carcinoma of breast
Nasopharyngeal carcinoma
Seminoma
Neuroblastoma
Ewing sarcoma
Alveolar rhabdomyosarcoma
Melanoma

Metastatic tumors may also simulate primary neoplasms of lymph nodes and so create difficult problems of diagnosis. Those listed in Table 86.2 often bear a close histologic resemblance to particular variants of non-Hodgkin and Hodgkin lymphomas and are therefore considered separately in the following chapters.

ELECTRON MICROSCOPY

The use of transmission electron microscopy (TEM) in tumor diagnosis is a well-established practice. Some laboratories routinely fix a portion of every specimen in glutaraldehyde and decide on further processing after light microscopic examination (29). Others sample and fix tissues for TEM selectively, to determine a particular feature of the differential diagnosis. The rapid recent development of immunohistochemistry, a faster and considerably less expensive technique, has reduced to a great extent the use of TEM in surgical pathology. Still, it can be justified, particularly in the diagnosis of undifferentiated tumors. The origin of a lymph node metastasis with poorly differentiated features may sometimes be determined only by TEM. Histologic or cytologic characteristics not discernible with the light microscope may be recognizable with TEM. The detection of cellular junctions, tonofilaments, neurosecretory granules, and a variety of other intracytoplasmic organelles is critical to identifying the nature of cells and is considered in the following chapters devoted to specific metastatic tumors.

HISTOCHEMISTRY

The presence of various cell components and cell products can be identified by histochemical reactions to indicate the

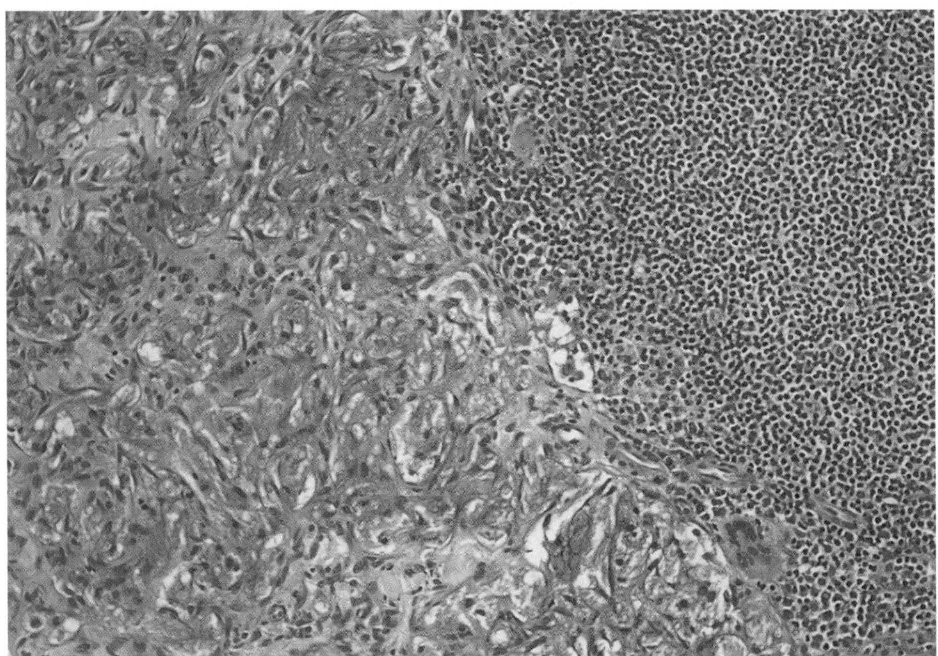

FIGURE 86.13. Metastasis of mucoepidermoid carcinoma in cervical lymph node, staining with periodic acid–Schiff before and after diastase treatment.

cell of origin. Some histochemical reactions, particularly those relating to enzymes, require special methods of fixation. Therefore, for immunohistochemistry, it is desirable always to snap-freeze a portion of a specimen and store it in deep freeze for future investigation. Although histochemistry has to a great extent been replaced by immunohistochemistry, some basic techniques are still very useful for their simple and rapid application, consistent results, and low cost. These include diastase-resistant periodic acid–Schiff staining to detect cells with free carbohydrate molecules, such as plasma cells or mucoid tumors (Fig. 86.13), and argyrophil methods, such as the Grimelius stain, to identify cells of neuroendocrine origin. Mucicarmine indicates the presence of neutral mucins, and Alcian blue that of acid mucins, both important in identifying poorly differentiated adenocarcinomas. Among the cellular enzymes, a high level of activity of acid phosphatase indicates prostatic adenocarcinoma (30); the enzyme dopa oxidase is quite specific for melanocytes and can be demonstrated even in the absence of melanin (29).

IMMUNOHISTOCHEMISTRY

Highly specific monoclonal antibodies (MAbs) have been developed, so that it is possible to detect and identify unlimited classes of molecules. Intermediate filaments, cytokeratins, epitopes of cell markers, and an infinite variety of cell antigens are used to produce MAbs that can be applied in the evaluation of normal and tumor tissue. MAbs directed against specific markers on epithelial, mesenchymal, lymphoid, melanic, neural, and other normal tissues can be used to identify their neoplastic counterparts. For example, immunostaining for high-molecular-weight cytokeratins indicates squamous cell carcinoma, prostate-specific antigen indicates prostatic carcinoma (Fig. 86.14), thyroglobulin indicates thyroid carcinoma, estrogen receptor protein indicates breast carcinoma, CA-125 antigen indicates ovarian carcinoma, epithelial membrane antigen indicates epithelial tumors (Fig. 86.15), chromogranin and synaptophysin indicate neuroendocrine tumors (Fig. 86.16), cytokeratin CK5 indicates mesothelioma (31), and S100 protein indicates melanoma. A combination of two MAbs with different specificities may reveal the coordinated expression of a par-

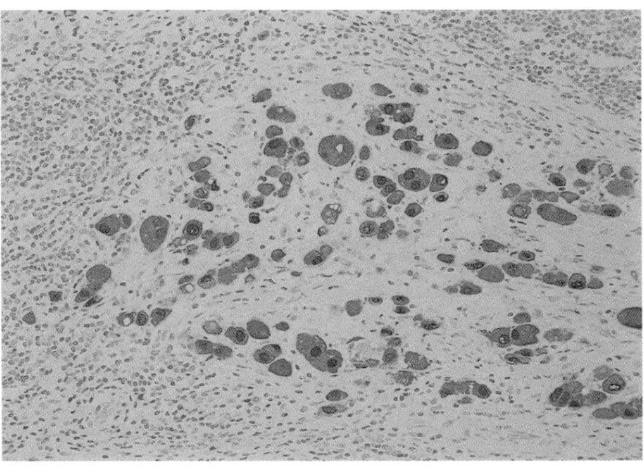

FIGURE 86.14. Metastasis of prostatic carcinoma in pelvic lymph node, staining with periodic acid–Schiff.

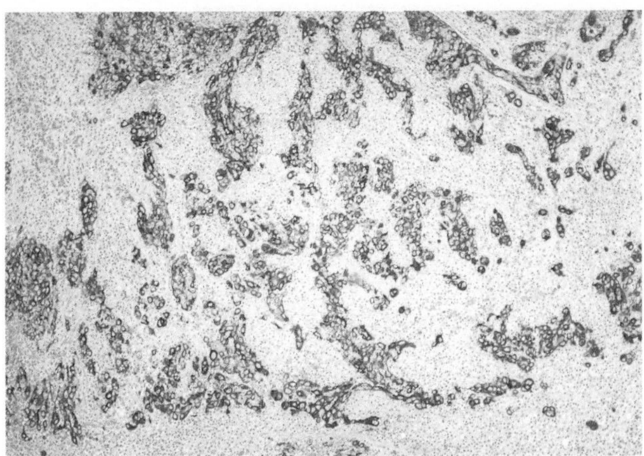

FIGURE 86.15. Metastasis in supraclavicular lymph node of undifferentiated carcinoma of unknown primary origin, expressing epithelial membrane antigen. EMA/peroxidase stain.

ticular tumor and thereby solve difficult problems of differential diagnosis. For example, the use of two cytokeratin antibodies, CD7 and CD20, help to differentiate between colon carcinoma (CK7−, CK20+) and ovarian carcinoma (CK7+, CK20−) (32,33). However, most antigens are not exclusive to a particular tissue or cell type, so that immunostaining, with the exception of thyroglobulin and prostate-specific antigen, is not strictly specific. Estrogen-specific protein may also be expressed in endometrial and ovarian carcinomas, cytokeratins may be expressed together with vimentin in some tumors, and S100 protein is also present in histiocytes and dendritic cells.

An important question regarding the use of specific immunophenotypes in the diagnosis of malignant tumors is whether tumor cells continue to express the differentiation markers of their cells of origin or lose this capability in the process of dedifferentiation. A second question is whether metastatic tumors carry the immunophenotype of the primary tumor. The answer to both questions is that popula-

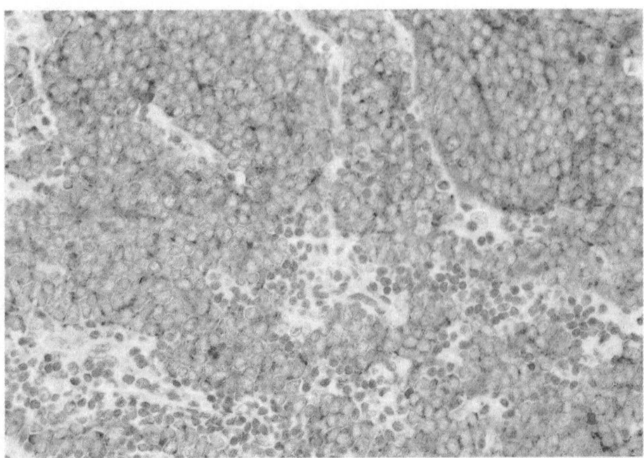

FIGURE 86.16. Metastasis of pulmonary malignant carcinoid tumor, expressing synaptophysin/peroxidase stain.

tions of tumor cells are in general heterogeneous, and that tumor cells are unstable and prone to mutations. Thus, as they progress, tumor cells may express antigens aberrantly. Some carcinomas express neurosecretory markers (34), lymphomas may express epithelial cell markers (35), and smooth muscle tumors may express cytokeratin markers (36). Furthermore, some carcinomas, particularly those with spindle cell components, occasionally coexpress cytokeratins and vimentin, whereas their metastases express only one of these markers, so that doubts arise regarding the accuracy of the original diagnosis or the question is raised of whether the secondary tumor is metastatic or an unrelated new primary.

In most cases, but certainly not all, metastases preserve the immunophenotype of the primary tumor, even if they are heterogeneous in relation to the tissues of origin. In a study of 54 epithelial malignant tumors and their multiple mĕtastases (between 1 and 24 per tumor), in which a battery of MAbs was used, in no case did all the metastases of a primary showing a positive reaction with one MAb fail to react with the same MAb, but in 18.5% of the cases, changes of phenotype were noted in one or more metastases (37). The experience shows that immunohistochemistry is a powerful new tool with which to diagnose metastases; however, in view of the heterogeneous and variable nature of tumors, this valuable method must be used with caution and the results interpreted in concert with clinical and morphologic data.

REFERENCES

1. Ioachim HL. Immunobiology of metastases. Cancer Detect Prev 1991;15:127–131.
2. Fidler IJ, Gersten DM, Hart IR. The biology of cancer invasion and metastases. Adv Cancer Res 1978;28:149–250.
3. Auerbach R. Patterns of tumor metastasis: organ selectivity in the spread of cancer cells [Editorial]. Lab Invest 1988;58:361–364.
4. Nicolson GL. Autocrine and paracrine growth mechanisms in cancer progression and metastasis. In: Encyclopedia of cancer, vol 1. New York: Academic Press, 1997:112.
5. Takeichi M. Cadherin cell adhesion receptors as a morphogenetic regulator. Science 1991;251:1451.
6. Liotta LA, et al. Invasion and metastasis. In: Holland JF, et al., eds. Cancer medicine, 3rd ed. Philadelphia: Lea & Febiger, 1993: 138.
7. Mareel MM, Bracke ME, Van Roy FM, et al. Molecular mechanisms of cancer invasion. In: Encyclopedia of cancer, vol 2. New York: Academic Press, 1997:1072.
8. Kahn P. Cancer research: adhesion protein studies provide new clue to metastases. Science 1992;257:614.
9. Liotta LA. Growth autonomy: the only requirement for metastasis? [Editorial]. J Natl Cancer Inst 1988;80:300.
10. Sobel ME. Metastasis suppressor genes. J Natl Cancer Inst 1990;82:267–276.
11. Fielding LP, Fenoglio-Preiser CM, Freedman LS. The future of prognostic factors in outcome prediction for patients with cancer. Cancer 1992;70:2367–2377.
12. Zaren HA, Copeland EM. Inguinal node metastases. Cancer 1978;41:919–923.

13. Sugarbaker EV. Some characteristics of metastasis in man. Am J Pathol 1979;97:623–633.
14. Ioachim HL. Correlation between tumor antigenicity, malignant potential, and local host immune response. In: Witz IP, Hanna M Jr, eds. Contemporary topics in immunobiology. New York: Plenum Publishing, 1980:213–238.
15. Baab GM, McBride CM. Malignant melanoma: the patients with an unknown site of primary origin. Arch Surg 1975;110:896–900.
16. Gromet MA, Epstein WL, Blois MS. The regressing thin malignant melanoma: a distinctive lesion with metastatic potential. Cancer 1978;42:2282–2292.
17. Azzopardi JG, Hoffbrand AV. Retrogression in testicular seminoma with viable metastases. J Clin Pathol 1965;18:135–141.
18. Meares EM, Briggs EM. Occult seminoma of the testis masquerading as primary extragonadal germinal neoplasm. Cancer 1972;30:300–306.
19. Jesse RH, Perez CA, Fletcher GH. Cervical lymph node metastasis, unknown primary cancer. Cancer 1973;31:854–859.
20. Copeland EM, McBride CM. Axillary metastases from unknown primary sites. Ann Surg 1972;178:25–27.
21. Haagensen CD. Diseases of the breast. Philadelphia: WB Saunders, 1971:486–491.
22. Owen HW, Dockerty MB, Gray HK. Occult carcinoma of the breast. Surg Gynecol Obstet 1954;98:302.
23. Rosen PP. Axillary lymph node metastases in patients with occult noninvasive breast carcinoma. Cancer 1980;46:1298–1306.
24. Saltzstein SL, McLaughlin AP. Clinicopathologic features of unsuspected regional lymph node metastases in prostatic adenocarcinoma. Cancer 1977;40:1212–1221.
25. Richter HJ, Leder LD. Lymph node metastases with PAS-positive tumor cells and massive epithelioid granulomatous reaction as diagnostic clue to occult seminoma. Cancer 1979;44:245–249.
26. Das Gupta T, Bowden L, Berg JW. Malignant melanoma of unknown primary origin. Surg Gynecol Obstet 1963;117:341–345.
27. Fitts WT, Steiner GC, Enterline HT. Prognosis of occult carcinoma of the breast. Am J Surg 1963;106:460–463.
28. Rappaport H. Tumors of the hematopoietic system. Washington, DC: Armed Forces Institute of Pathology, 1966:397–426 (Atlas of tumor pathology, series I, fascicle 8).
29. Bosman FT, Orenstein JM, Silverberg SG. Differential diagnosis of metastatic tumors. In: Silverberg SG, ed. Principles and practice of surgical pathology. New York: Churchill Livingstone, 1990.
30. Willighagen RGJ. Histochemistry in pathology diagnosis. Beitr Pathol 1970;141:280.
31. Clover J, Oates J, Edwards C. Anti-cytokeratin 5/6: a positive marker for epithelioid mesothelioma. Histopathology 1997;31: 140–143.
32. Loy TS, Calaluce RD, Keeney GL. Cytokeratin immunostaining in differentiating primary ovarian carcinoma from metastatic colonic adenocarcinoma. Mod Pathol 1996;9:1040–1044.
33. Berezowski K, Stastny JF, Kornstein MJ. Cytokeratins 7 and 20 and carcinoembryonic antigen in ovarian and colonic carcinoma. Mod Pathol 1996;9:426–429.
34. Bosman FT. Neuroendocrine cells in non-neuroendocrine tumors. In: Falkmer S, Hakanson R, Sundler F, eds. Evolution and tumor pathology of the diffuse neuroendocrine system. Amsterdam: Elsevier, 1983:519.
35. Delsol G, Al Saati T, Gatter KC, et al. Coexpression of EMA, Ki-1, and interleukin 2 receptor by anaplastic large cell lymphomas. Am J Pathol 1988;130:59–70.
36. Norton AJ, Thomas JA, Isaacson PG. Cytokeratin-specific monoclonal antibodies are reactive with tumors of smooth muscle cells. An immunocytochemical and biochemical study using antibodies to intermediate filament cytoskeletal proteins. Histopathology 1987;11:487.
37. Esteban JM, Battifora H. Tumor immunophenotype: comparison between primary neoplasm and its metastases. Mod Pathol 1990;3:192–197.

87

METASTATIC MELANOMA

DEFINITION

Lymph node metastases of melanoma.

PATHOGENESIS

As they evolve, after variable amounts of time, some malignant tumors acquire the ability to disseminate and form new tumors at distant sites. Clark et al. (1), who have studied melanocytic neoplasia extensively, have offered concepts of tumor progression derived from this system that may be applicable to all malignant neoplasia. Melanocytic lesions are pigmented and superficial, and therefore readily apparent and easy to follow. According to these investigators, melanomas arise by generic steps of tumor progression, from melanocytic hyperplasia, to aberrant differentiation marked by abnormal hyperplasia and nuclear atypia, to a primary malignant neoplasm that lacks the ability to metastasize, eventually to a malignant neoplasm endowed with the capacity to metastasize. Morphologically, this crucial transformation occurs when radial growth changes to vertical growth. Thus, for a primary neoplasm to become metastatic, a critical and qualitative change must take place, in which a new population of cells with new properties originates within the neoplasm (1). In most instances, the melanocytes of an acquired nevus follow a pathway of differentiation that leads to their disappearance (1). The transformation from non-neoplastic to neoplastic, from noninvasive to invasive, and eventually from nonmetastatic to metastatic occurs in the melanoma system, as in most other cancers, by processes of mutation and clonal selection.

The studies of Breslow (2) have shown that when the thickness of a cutaneous melanoma exceeds 0.76 mm, the risk for the development of metastases increases in proportion to tumor thickness (2). In Breslow's series of 138 patients, 39% had primary lesions with a thickness of less than 0.76 mm, and all survived free of disease for 5 years or more, whereas metastases developed in 33% to 84% of those with lesions thicker than 0.76 mm.

The prognostic criteria based on these observations have been confirmed repeatedly. In a large study of prognostic factors in cutaneous melanoma, 90% of patients with superficially invasive, thin primary tumors were alive without recurrence 5 years after surgical excision of the skin lesion (3). In a minority of patients, metastases develop in the regional lymph nodes, and when they do, their chances of survival drop to only 40% at 5 years after lymphadenectomy (3–5). In almost all cases, when a cutaneous melanoma reaches the phase of dissemination, it spreads to the regional lymph nodes before it spreads to more distant sites (6,7). Therefore, the progression from stage I to stage II is a very important step in the evaluation of melanoma that must be documented by careful investigation of the regional lymph nodes. A study of 2,227 lymph nodes from 100 patients with clinical stage I cutaneous melanoma revealed no metastases on sections stained with hematoxylin and eosin, yet melanoma cells were detected in 16 nodes from 14 patients when immunostaining with antibody to S100 protein was used (5). A possible pitfall in applying this technique to identify metastatic melanoma cells is that they can be confused with nodal interdigitating reticulum cells, which also express S100 protein (5,8).

Sentinel Lymph Nodes

The status of regional lymph nodes, whether free of tumor or involved by tumor metastasis, is the most important prognostic factor in melanoma, as in many other solid tumors (3). Regional lymphadenectomy provides important staging information and, because tumor metastases are removed, may improve survival. However, it is associated with some morbidity and, as presently practiced, provides only an approximate evaluation of the extent of a tumor. When one or two sections of the central part of a lymph node are obtained and stained with hematoxylin and eosin, according to the standard procedure, only 1% to 5% of the lymph node tissue is examined, so that underestimation can be substantial (9). In studies of breast cancer performed as early as 1948, metastases were demonstrated in 10% to 20% of axillary lymph nodes apparently free of tumor on standard methods of examination when they were processed by serial sectioning (10,11). However, serial sectioning of all regional lymph nodes is too laborious and expensive to be adopted as a routine procedure. The technique of sentinel lymph node biopsy was developed as a minimally invasive method that is associated with low morbidity and is capable of identifying micrometastases (12). In a recent study of 235 sentinel lymph nodes obtained from 94 patients with primary cutaneous melanoma, 2,700 sections were cut, immunostained with antibodies against melanocytes, and examined (13). In this way, melanoma micrometastases were identified in 12% of patients whose lymph nodes had appeared tumor-free when processed by the routine procedure. In the commonly used sentinel lymph node biopsy procedure, sulfur colloid labeled with technetium 99m is injected 3 hours before surgery into the dermis around the primary melanoma or the biopsy scar (13). In addition to or instead of the radioactive substance, a blue dye, isosulfan blue (Lymphazurin), can be injected. The radioactive sentinel lymph nodes are located with a hand-held gamma detector and/or by following the blue-colored lymphatics during the operation, which is performed 1 to 3 hours later (13). In the study in which a 12% increase in the number of positive lymph nodes was noted, three serial tissue sections, each with a thickness of 4 μm and at levels 80 μm apart, were obtained and immunostained with S100, HMB-45, and MART-1 antibodies (13). All the additional lymph node metastases were microscopic and located in the subcapsular sinuses. Frozen sections in sentinel lymph nodes are discouraged because trimming the specimens wastes valuable tissues that may be the only ones containing metastases (13).

The use of frozen sections in the analysis of sentinel lymph nodes in patients with melanoma was investigated in a study of 58 patients (14). Although no false-positive diagnoses were obtained with frozen sections, the rate of false-negatives was 38%, too high to be useful. This high rate was a consequence of the inability to detect on frozen sections small metastases that became apparent on permanent section and immunohistochemistry. It is concluded from this and other observations that, given the important therapeutic consequences of the sentinel lymph node diagnosis, frozen section should no longer be part of the procedure, which therefore must be performed in two separate steps (14).

CLINICAL SYNDROME

Patients with stage II melanoma present with a painless mass that in one study ranged in size from 1 to 18 cm in diameter (median, 4 cm) (15) (Fig. 87.1). A particular aspect of melanomas that causes major difficulties in diagnosis and prognosis is occasional *spontaneous regression.* This phenomenon, probably related to complex interrelations with tissue immunity, is more common in melanomas than in any other malignant tumor. As a result, some cutaneous melanomas with a thickness of less than 0.76 mm are associated with lymph node metastases (16). Even more difficult to interpret are metastatic melanomas with *occult primary tumors,* estimated to represent about 4% of cases (17,18). In general, metastatic cancers with an unknown primary site are not uncommon and may pose an extremely frustrating problem. They were ranked as the eighth most common site of cancer in a large series of cases accounting for 10% to 15% of referred patients with solid tumors (19,20). In a study of 1,539 patients with an unknown primary cancer, melanomas represented 2.9% of cases (21). The male-to-female ratio was 1.6:1.0 and the median age 48 was years (no patient was younger than 15 years) in a series of 166 cases of

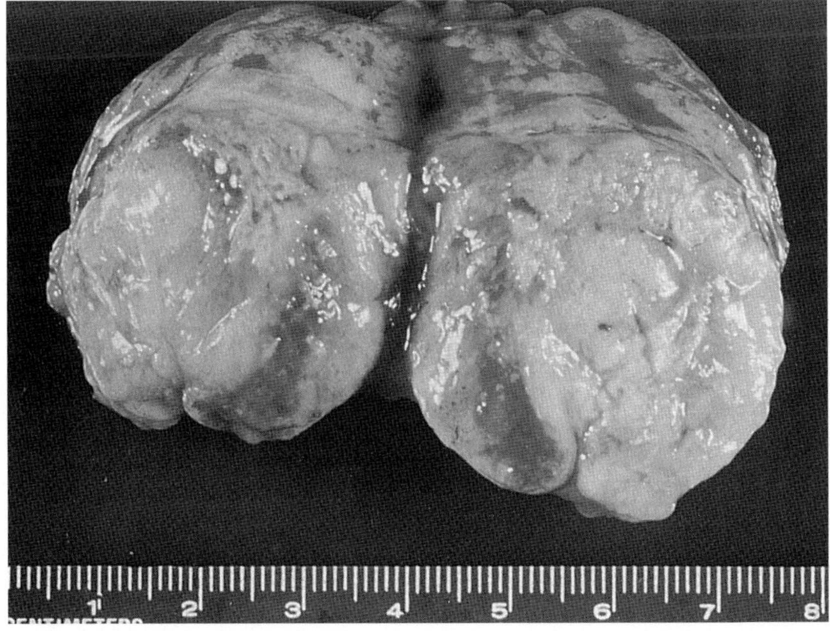

FIGURE 87.1. Metastatic melanoma in axillary lymph node (5 × 4.5 × 3 cm).

lymph node metastases with an unknown primary (15). In descending order of frequency, the lymph node groups involved by metastatic melanoma were axillary (47%), inguinal (20%), and cervical (24%). In women, inguinal metastases were almost as common as axillary metastases (15). The 5- and 10-year survival rates of patients with lymph node metastatic melanoma were 46% and 41%, respectively. These were not influenced by age of the patient, size of the metastases, or pigmentation (melanotic vs. amelanotic). However, patients with axillary metastases had consistently better survival rates than those with metastases in other locations (15), and patients with metastases to a single lymph node had significantly better 5-year survival rates than those with more than one involved lymph node (22). In a retrospective study of 3,805 patients with melanomas at the Memorial Sloan-Kettering Cancer Center, 166 had no known primary tumor, a prevalence of 4.4% (15). The 5-year survival rates of patients who had metastatic melanoma in one group of regional lymph nodes and were treated by lymphadenectomy were similar for those with a known and those with an unknown primary (17). This finding, subsequently confirmed by others (18), suggests that the occult primaries must have been melanomas that regressed, precluding the occurrence of additional metastases. A rare exception is a primary melanoma in a lymph node arising from a prior lymph node nevus, documented in a case report (23).

HISTOPATHOLOGY

The lymph node may be partially or totally replaced by melanoma cells (Fig. 87.2), which in the early stages of invasion are present only in the subcapsular sinus. Capsular and perinodal invasion, although sometimes present, is less extensive than in lymphomas (24). Most often, the metastatic melanoma cells in the lymph node parenchyma form aggregates of various sizes and shapes that facilitate their recognition. The cell population may be uniformly composed of epithelioid cells with polygonal outlines or may contain areas of spindle-shaped cells. Although most tumors show both cell types, the epithelioid variant is usually predominant (Fig. 87.3). Nuclear pleomorphism and mitotic figures, frequently atypical, are common. One very large, centrally located eosinophilic nucleolus is a characteristic feature of melanoma cells. Prominent inclusions of cytoplasm in the nucleus are also frequently seen in melanoma cells. The amount of melanin pigment varies greatly; heavily pigmented melanoma cells and macrophages or totally unpigmented lesions may be seen. In one study of 75 patients with lymph node metastases, the ratio of melanotic to amelanotic lesions was 2:1 (15). Occasionally, metastatic melanomas may assume unusual histologic appearances, simulating the microscopic features of other tumors. Thus, amelanotic melanomas may synthesize certain neuropeptides and exhibit various microscopic patterns (25), or spindle cell melanomas may be composed of spindly, fibroblast-like cells that form crisscross bundles and whorls (Figs. 87.4 and 87.5). According to Yu et al. (13), for a diagnosis of metastatic melanoma in a lymph node to be made, all following features must be present: (a) cells foreign to the lymph node in linear arrays, or nests of epithelioid cells or spindle cells; (b) cells with atypical characteristics, such as large pleomorphic nuclei, prominent nucleoli, mitoses, and melanin granules; (c) immune staining for melanocytic markers (S100, HMB-45, MART-1); and (d) atypical cells identifiable on hematoxylin and eosin stains. In contrast, benign lymph node nevi, although they express melanin markers, do not exhibit cellular atypia. In a study of 235

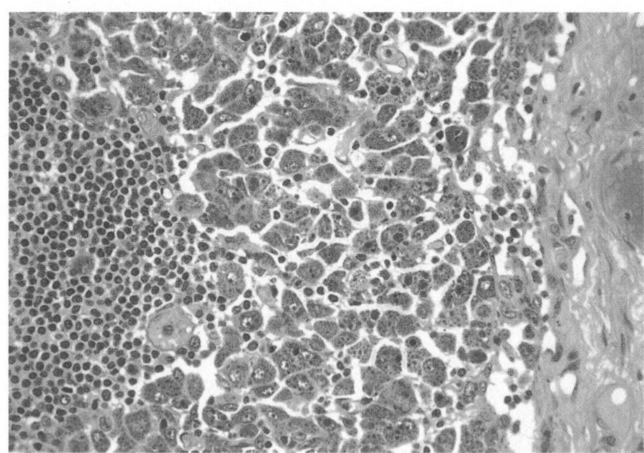

FIGURE 87.3. Metastatic melanoma in inguinal lymph node extending from the marginal sinus into the lymphoid parenchyma. Melanoma cells are epithelioid, with abundant granular cytoplasm and round nuclei that have conspicuous nucleoli. Abundant, dusty melanin pigment is present in the darkly staining cells. Hematoxylin, phloxine, and saffron stain.

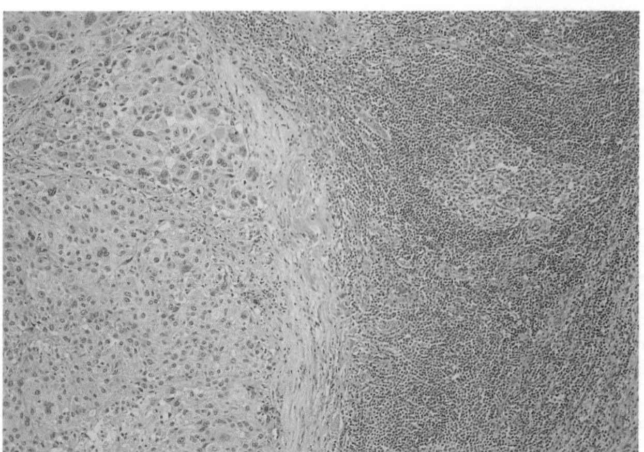

FIGURE 87.2. Metastatic melanoma separated by thin fibrous strands from lymphoid tissue with follicle and reactive germinal center. The melanoma cells show marked pleomorphism and include multiple giant cells. Hematoxylin, phloxine, and saffron stain.

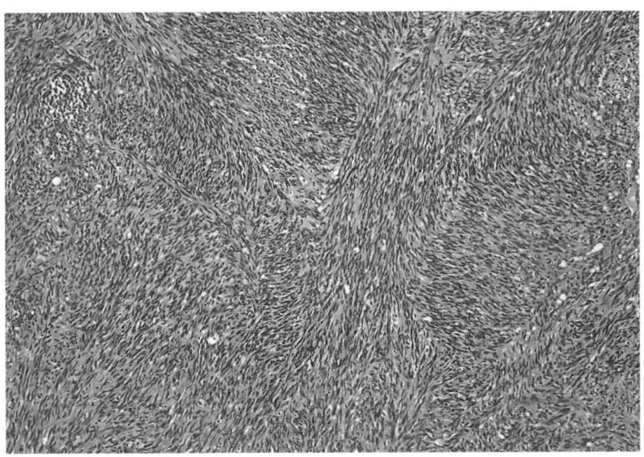

FIGURE 87.4. Metastatic melanoma, spindle cell type from a small primary vulvar lesion. Histologic patterns of crisscross bundles and whorls. Hematoxylin, phloxine, and saffron stain.

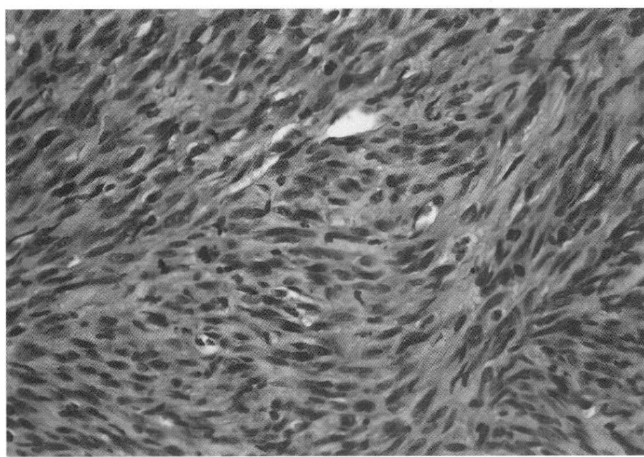

FIGURE 87.5. Same section as in Fig. 87.4. Amelanotic spindle cells in intersecting bundles with numerous mitoses resemble sarcomas. Hematoxylin, phloxine, and saffron stain.

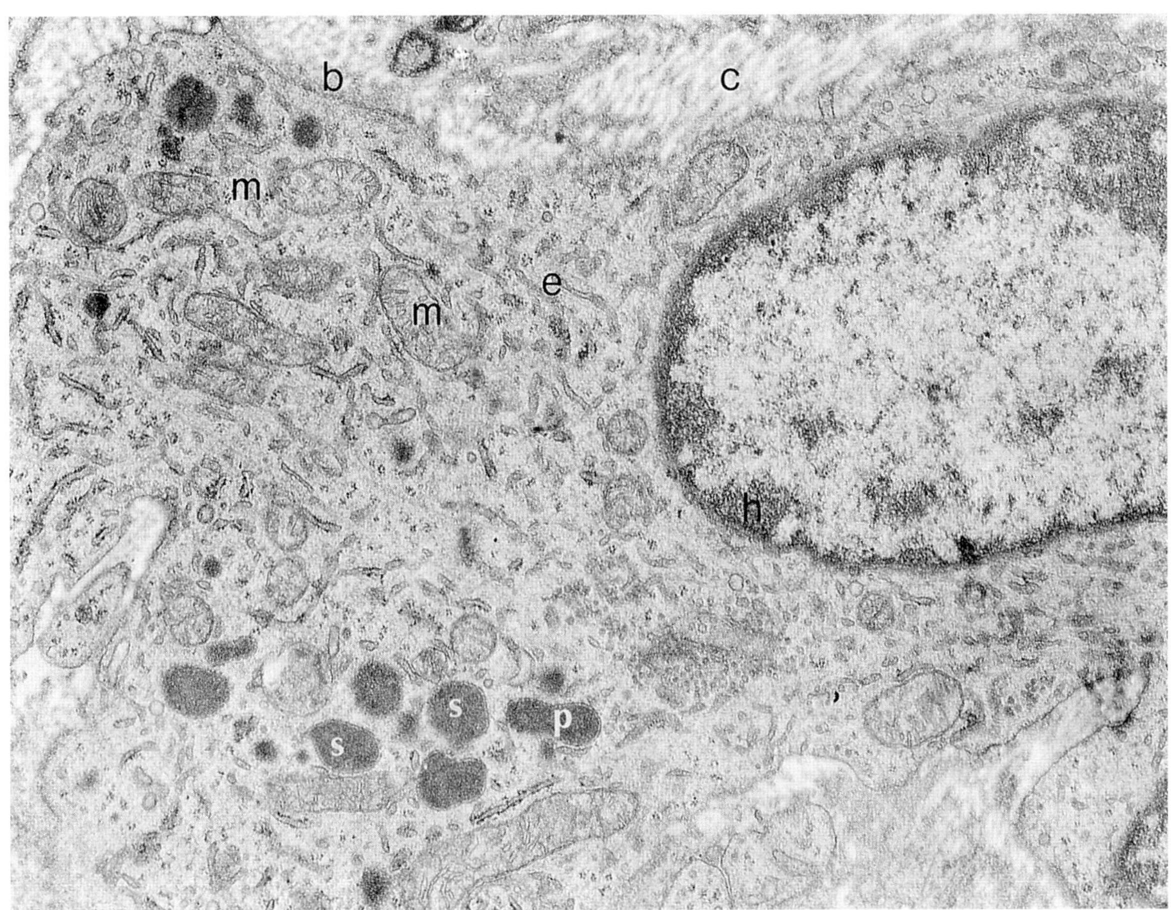

FIGURE 87.6. Metastatic melanoma in axillary lymph node. Melanoma cell has large ovoid nucleus containing marginated heterochromatin (*h*), large mitochondria comprising tubular cristae (*m*), short strands of endoplasmic reticulum (e), and dark, membrane-bound granules representing melanosomes (*s*) and premelanosomes (*p*). A thin basal lamina (*b*) separates the cell from adjacent collagen fibers (*c*). ×19,000.

sentinel lymph nodes, benign capsular melanocytic nevi were found in 9 lymph nodes from 8 patients (8.5%). They appeared in sheets, nests, or arrays of single cells and stained with S100 protein, NK1/C3, and MART-1 antibodies but not with HMB-45 antibodies (13).

CYTOPATHOLOGY

The use of fine needle aspiration in the evaluation of enlarged lymph nodes may raise the question of metastatic melanoma. In that case, fairly large, epithelioid cells with round and centrally located nuclei, prominent nucleoli, and nuclear cytoplasmic inclusions will be seen surrounded by small lymphocytes. Melanin pigment, when present, is of great diagnostic importance. The intranuclear cytoplasmic inclusions are not exclusive to melanomas; they are also commonly seen in fine needle aspiration specimens of metastatic papillary thyroid carcinoma.

CYTOCHEMISTRY

The Masson-Fontana method in which ammoniated silver nitrate is used is preferred because it reveals not only melanin but also argentaffin, nonpigmented premelanin granules (26).

The dopa reaction to determine tyrosinase activity is usually positive, at least in some areas, although a total absence of tyrosinase activity does not rule out melanoma (26).

ELECTRON MICROSCOPY

Electron microscopy is an important adjunct, particularly in the diagnosis of amelanotic melanomas (27). The characteristic ultrastructural feature of melanotic tumors is the presence of some form of melanosome granules (Fig. 87.6). Throughout the cytoplasm of melanoma cells, frequently associated with the Golgi body or within the cell processes, are various forms of melanosomes, premelanosomes, vesicles, and electron-dense granules (Fig. 87.7). In addition, melanoma cells have dendritic cytoplasmic processes and microvilli, in addition to a complex cytoplasmic structure that contains numerous mitochondria, a well-developed Golgi body, endoplasmic reticulum, nonspecific filaments, and microtubules (27).

IMMUNOHISTOCHEMISTRY

S100 protein is generally expressed by all proliferative processes of melanocytes (Figs. 87.8–87.11). The intensity of staining is inversely related to cellular pigmentation; staining is less intense in blue nevi and most intense in amelanotic melanomas (28). Metastatic melanomas tend to stain more strongly than primary tumors (28). Thus, intense staining for S100 protein differentiates melanomas from lymphomas and carcinomas, which do not stain (28,29). In fact, S100 immunoreactivity is considered a more sensitive test for the detection of melanoma metastases than the find-

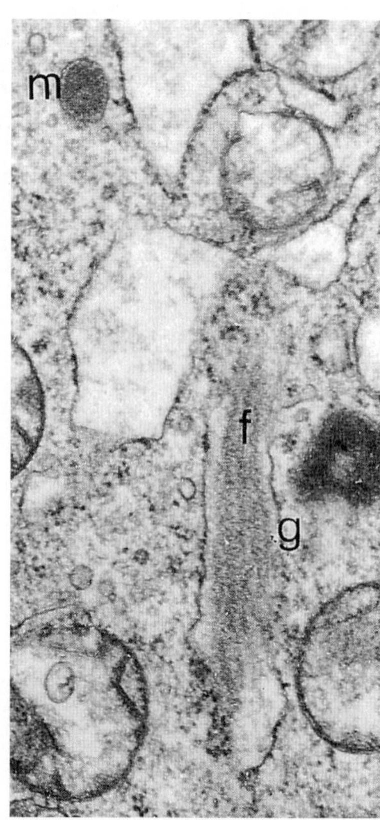

FIGURE 87.7. Section of same lymph node as in Fig. 87.6. Dark, round, membrane-bound granule (*m*) and elongated granule (*g*) with parallel internal filaments (*f*) show periodicity and identify the cell as a premelanosome. ×36,000.

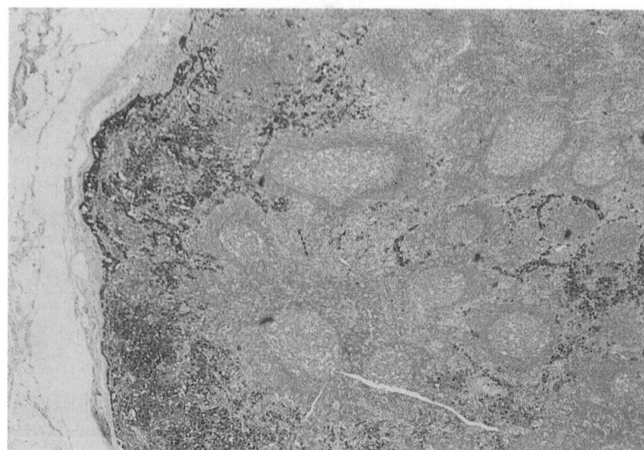

FIGURE 87.8. Metastatic melanoma in axillary lymph node showing intense reaction of follicles and germinal centers. The melanoma cells are selectively stained by S100 protein antibodies. S100 protein/peroxidase stain.

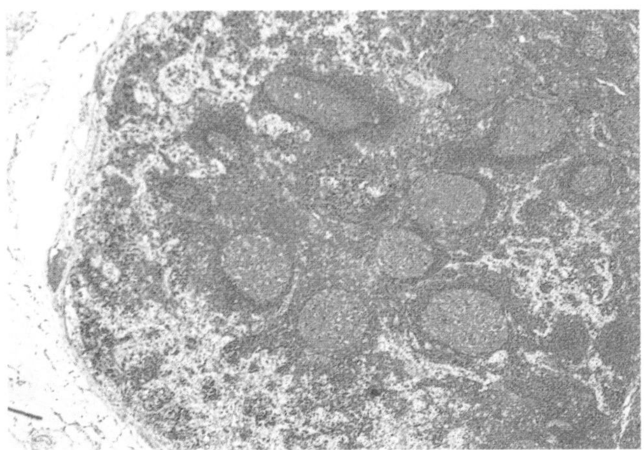

FIGURE 87.9. Same lymph node as in Fig. 87.8. Histiocytes in marginal and cortical sinuses are stained by HAM-56 antibodies; the metastatic melanoma cells remain unstained. HAM-56/peroxidase stain.

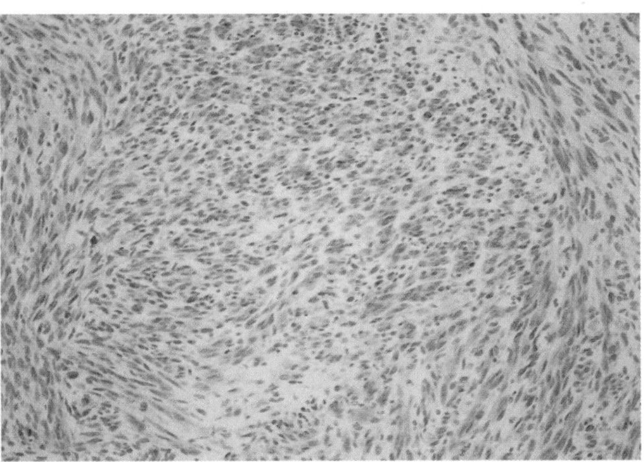

FIGURE 87.11. Metastatic melanoma, spindle cell type (same case as in Fig. 87.4) stained by S100 protein antibodies. S100 protein/peroxidase stain.

ing of organelles characteristic of melanocytes by electron microscopy (30). In the case of metastatic melanoma in lymph nodes, one must be aware that normal lymph node interdigitating cells also express S100 protein and must be distinguished by their morphology and the presence of specific markers (29).

HMB-45 is a cytoplasmic antigen of melanoma cells that can be visualized with monoclonal antibodies in formalin-fixed, paraffin-embedded sections (31). Cross-reactions in epithelial, mesenchymal, or hematopoietic neoplasms do not occur, so that it is quite specific for the detection of melanoma cells (32). HMB-45 is more specific but less sensitive for melanoma cells than S100 protein.

Although S100 protein and HMB-45 are the most commonly used markers for melanomas, they are considered to be inadequate because S100 protein, which is very sensitive, is not specific, and HMB-45, which is more specific, lacks sensitivity (13). Two antibodies directed at melanoma antigens NK1/C3 and MART-1 have been also used in various studies (5,13). MART-1, which is more specific than NK1/C3, is a melanoma epitope localized to melanosomes and endoplasmic reticulum in nevi and melanomas (33).

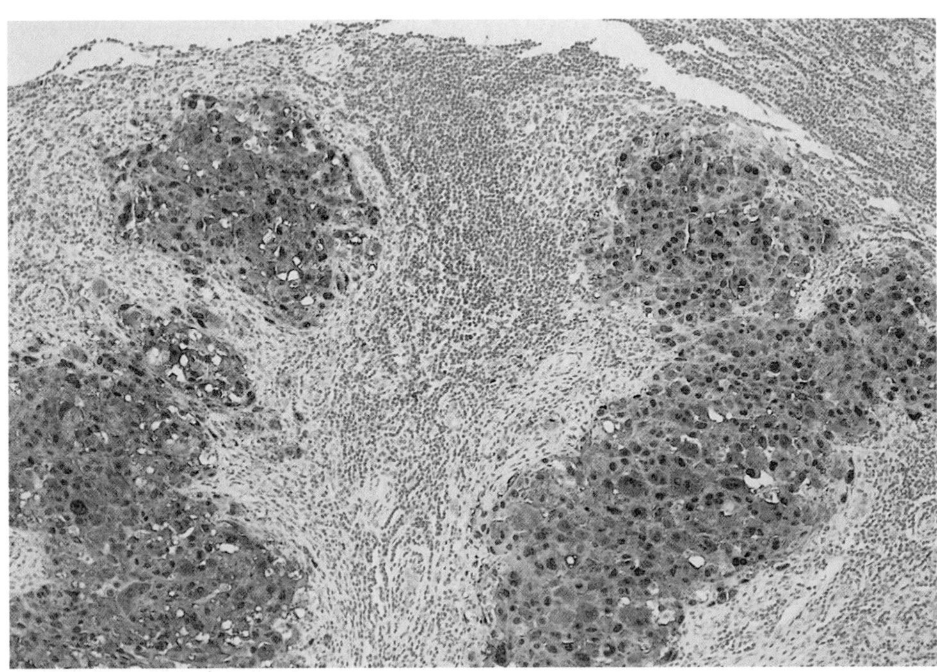

FIGURE 87.10. Metastatic melanoma, epithelioid cell type (same case as in Fig. 87.8) strongly stained by S100 protein antibodies. S100 protein/peroxidase stain.

Checklist

METASTATIC MELANOMA

History or presence of cutaneous melanoma
Primary tumor absent in 4% of cases
Partial or total lymph node replacement by tumor
Sinuses obliterated by tumor cells
Nests and cords of melanoma cells
Epithelioid cells, spindle-shaped cells, or both
Melanin pigment occasionally present
Nuclear pleomorphism
Prominent single eosinophilic nucleoli
Intranuclear cytoplasmic inclusions
Frequent mitoses
Fontana silver stain result positive
Dopa reaction positive
Melanosomes and premelanosomes
S-100 protein, HMB-45, NK1/C3, MART-1, and CEA all expressed

Carcinoembryonic antigen (CEA) has also been demonstrated in melanoma cells with a polyclonal anti-CEA antibody. In a study of 28 cases of melanoma, reactions for CEA (polyclonal) were positive in 53% of cases, for HMB-45 in 82%, and for S100 protein in 100% (34).

Polymerase chain reaction and cell cultures have also been applied to the detection of lymph node micrometastases, with uncertain results. The tissue cultures require 4 to 6 weeks to yield results, which therefore depend on the viability of cells in culture (34). The polymerase chain reaction technique, which is based on the detection of tyrosinase messenger RNA, cannot differentiate between benign nevi and malignant melanoma (34). At any rate, regardless of the methods used, the prognostic significance of single cells or small clusters of melanoma cells in lymph nodes is still a subject of debate (8) and must be assessed in large follow-up series of cases.

DIFFERENTIAL DIAGNOSIS

- Nevus cell inclusions in lymph nodes appear as aggregates of nevus cells in the lymph node capsule and, unlike melanoma cells, in the marginal sinus. The immunohistochemistry is similar, but cellular atypia with nuclear pleomorphism is lacking.
- Dermatopathic lymphadenopathy has paracortical pale-staining, confluent areas. Melanin and hemosiderin are present within macrophages, not in melanoma cells.
- Melanosis of abdominal lymph nodes in melanosis coli shows pigmented cells, but not the cellular atypia of melanoma cells.
- Plasmacytoma or multiple myeloma: Plasma cell precursors may resemble melanoma cells, in which case immunostaining with anti-S100 protein and anti-HMB-45 monoclonal antibodies is needed to make the distinction.
- Large cell non-Hodgkin lymphoma lacks cellular cohesiveness and melanin pigment. The result of the Fontana stain is negative. The result of immunostaining is positive for leukocyte common antigen and negative for S100 protein and HMB-45.
- Metastatic undifferentiated carcinoma may simulate melanoma; however, cytokeratins are expressed, S-100 protein and HMB-45 are not.
- Metastatic papillary thyroid carcinoma may resemble metastatic melanoma by the presence of intranuclear cytoplasmic inclusions; however, it may also show fragments of papillae and psammoma bodies. Melanin pigment is absent.

REFERENCES

1. Clark WH, Elder DE, Guerry D. V. A study of tumor progression: the precursor lesions of superficial spreading and nodular melanoma. Hum Pathol 1984;15:1147–1165.
2. Breslow A. Tumor thickness, level of invasion and node dissection in stage I cutaneous melanoma. Ann Surg 1975;182:573–575.
3. Balch CM, Soong SJ, Shaw HM, et al. An analysis of prognostic factors in 8,500 patients with cutaneous melanoma. In: Balch CM, Houghton AN, Milton GW, eds. Cutaneous melanoma, 2nd ed. Philadelphia: JB Lippincott Co, 1992:165–187.
4. Callery C, Cochran AJ, Roe DJ, et al. Factors prognostic for survival in patients with malignant melanoma spread to the regional lymph nodes. Ann Surg 1982;196:69–79.

5. Cochran AJ, Wen D-R, Morton DL. Occult tumor cells in the lymph nodes of patients with pathological stage I malignant melanoma. An immunohistological study. Am J Surg Pathol 1988;12:612–618.
6. Reintgen D, Cruse CW, Wells K, et al. The orderly progression of melanoma nodal metastases. Ann Surg 1994;220:759–767.
7. Milioates G. The tumor biology of melanoma nodal metastases. Am Surg 1996;62:81–88.
8. Kern WH. Occult tumor cells in lymph nodes. Am J Surg Pathol 1989;13:430–431.
9. Reintgen D, Shivers S. Sentinel lymph node micrometastasis from melanoma. Cancer 1999;86:551–552.
10. Saphir O, Amromin G. Obscure axillary lymph node metastasis in carcinoma of the breast. Cancer 1948;1:238–241.
11. Pickren J. Significance of occult metastasis. A study of breast cancer. Cancer 1961;14:1266–1271.
12. Morton D, Wen D-R, Wong J, et al. Technical details of intraoperative lymphatic mapping for early stage melanoma. Arch Surg 1992;127:392–399.
13. Yu LL, Flotte TJ, Tanabe KK, et al. Detection of microscopic melanoma metastases in sentinel lymph nodes. Cancer 1999;86: 617–627.
14. Koopal SA, Tiebosch ATMG, Piers A, et al. Frozen section analysis of sentinel lymph nodes in melanoma patients. Cancer 2000;89:1720–1725.
15. Chang P, Knapper WH. Metastatic melanoma of unknown primary. Cancer 1982;49:1106–1111.
16. Gromet MA, Epstein WL, Blois MS. The regressing thin malignant melanoma: a distinctive lesion with metastatic potential. Cancer 1978;42:2282–2292.
17. Das Gupta T, Bowden L, Berg JW. Malignant melanoma of unknown primary origin. Surg Gynecol Obstet 1963;117:341–345.
18. Baab GH, McBride CM. Malignant melanoma. Arch Surg 1975;110:896–900.
19. Krements ET, Cerise EJ, Foster DS, et al. Metastases of undetermined source. Curr Probl Cancer 1979;4:1–37.
20. Karsell PR, Sheedy MF II, O'Connell MJ. Computed tomography in search of cancer of unknown origin. JAMA 1982;248: 340–343.
21. Altman E, Cadman E. An analysis of 1,539 patients with cancer of unknown primary site. Cancer 1986;57:120–124.
22. Milton GW, Shaw HM, McCarthy WH. Occult primary malignant melanoma: factors influencing survival. Br J Surg 1977;64: 805–808.
23. Shenoy VB, Fort L, Benjamin SP. Malignant melanoma primary in lymph node. The case of the missing link. Am J Surg Pathol 1987;11:140–146.
24. Rappaport H. Tumors of the hematopoietic system. Washington, DC: Armed Forces Institute of Pathology, 1966:397–425 (Atlas of tumor pathology, series I, fascicle 8).
25. Nakleh RE, Wick MR, Rocamora A, et al. Morphologic diversity in malignant melanomas. Am J Clin Pathol 1990;93:731–740.
26. Lever WF, Schaumburg-Lever G. Histopathology of the skin. Philadelphia: JB Lippincott Co, 1983:706–718.
27. Mazur MT, Katzenstein AA. Metastatic melanoma: the spectrum of ultrastructural morphology. Ultrastruct Pathol 1980;1:337–356.
28. Nakajima T, Watanabe S, Stao Y, et al. An immunoperoxidase of S100 protein distribution in normal and neoplastic tissue. J Surg Pathol 1982;6:715–727.
29. Kahn HJ, Marks A, Thum H, et al. Role of antibody to S100 in diagnostic pathology. Am J Clin Pathol 1983;79:341–348.
30. Dabbs DJ, Bolen JW. Superficial spreading malignant melanoma with neurosarcomatous metastases. Am J Clin Pathol 1984;82: 109–114.
31. Gown AM, Vogel AM, Hoak D, et al. Monoclonal antibodies specific for melanocytic tumors distinguish subpopulations of melanocytes. Am J Pathol 1986;123:195.
32. Duray PH, Ernstoff MS, Ernstoff LT. Immunohistochemical phenotyping of malignant melanoma. Pathol Annu 1990;25: 351–377.
33. Kawakami Y, Battles JK, Kobayashi T, et al. Production of recombinant MART-1 polyclonal and monoclonal antibodies: use in the characterization of the human melanoma antigen MART-1. J Immunol Methods 1997;202:13–25.
34. Selby WL, Nance KV, Park KH. CEA immunoreactivity in metastatic malignant melanoma. Mod Pathol 1992;5:415–419.

88

METASTATIC BREAST CARCINOMA

DEFINITION

Mammary carcinoma metastatic to axillary lymph nodes.

PATHOGENESIS

The axillary lymph nodes are the lymphatic filter for the breast and thus are the first to be involved in metastatic breast cancer. For a variable period of time, they are the only site of metastases; witness cure by radical mastectomy of cancer in which the axillary lymph nodes are the only ones involved (1). The axillary lymph nodes are involved in 74% to 80% of patients with generalized breast cancer (2). The involvement of axillary lymph nodes increases in proportion to the *size of the primary mammary tumor.* In the study of Haagensen published 30 years ago (1), 1 in 3 patients with breast tumors smaller than 3 cm in diameter had axillary metastases, whereas 1 in 2 patients with tumors larger than 3 cm had axillary metastases.

The *status of axillary lymph nodes* must be assessed because it is a component (N) of the international tumor–node–metastasis (TNM) staging system for breast carcinoma (3). The TNM designation is for clinical staging; pTNM denotes pathologic staging. The clinical evaluation of nodal metastases by palpation of the axillary lymph nodes is unreliable and results in false-positive and false-negative rates of 30% to 40% (4) (Fig.88.1).

Lymph node specimens obtained at axillary dissection are routinely evaluated histologically for metastases. Metastases smaller than 2 mm are termed *micrometastases.* However, this method is unsatisfactory because one or two sections of a lymph node stained with hematoxylin and eosin represent less than 1% of the total mass and are therefore insufficient for the detection of micrometastases. For a long time, it was known that patients with breast cancer and histologically negative lymph nodes had a failure rate, expressed by tumor recurrence, of 15% to 20% at 5 years, which suggested that the current histologic method produced a number of false-negative results (5–9). In fact, a landmark study by Saphir and Amromin (10) indicated as early as 1948 that this was the case. In their study, the axillary lymph nodes in 30 cases of breast carcinoma were negative when five lymph nodes were routinely examined per case. However, when serial sectioning was performed, lymph node metastases were found in 10 of the cases. In a confirmatory study, Pickren (11) studied 51 cases of breast carcinoma; no metastases were found when one section was examined per lymph node, but when a clearing technique and serial sectioning were used, he was able to find metastases in 22% of the cases. Despite these demonstrations, serial sectioning of lymph nodes did not become an accepted method; it was considered excessively expensive and time-consuming. However, because of the pressing need to detect lymph node metastases to guide treatment and indicate prognosis, new diagnostic methods were introduced. When immunohistochemical staining with antibodies against cytokeratin markers was applied, the detection rates of metastatic ductal carcinoma in lymph nodes could be increased by 14% to 17% over those obtained with the usual hematoxylin and eosin staining (12–15) (Fig. 88.2). In one study, the yield of positive axillary lymph nodes was increased with immunohistochemistry by 9% for infiltrating ductal carcinomas and by 33% for infiltrating lobular carcinomas (12) (Figs. 88.3 and 88.4). In another study, 736 patients were evaluated by serial sectioning and hematoxylin and eosin staining of two sections from each of six levels and by immunohistochemistry of a single section stained with two anticytokeratins, AE1 and CAM 5-2 (15). Occult nodal metastases were detected in 52 (7%) of 736 patients by the first method and in 148 (20%) by the second. In a median follow-up of 12 years, occult lymph node metastases were associated with poorer disease-free and overall survival rates, particularly in postmenopausal women (15).

The *prognosis of breast cancer* is directly related to the *number of axillary lymph nodes involved* and the *number of tumor cells* within the individual lymph nodes. The location of metastatic cancer in the axilla, indicated by the *level of lymph nodes involved,* is also important in predicting survival (16).

In the series of McDivitt and colleagues (2), examination of the axillary nodes by levels, with the edges of the pectoralis minor muscle used as a boundary, showed a decrease in 5-year survival from 75% for patients with no involved

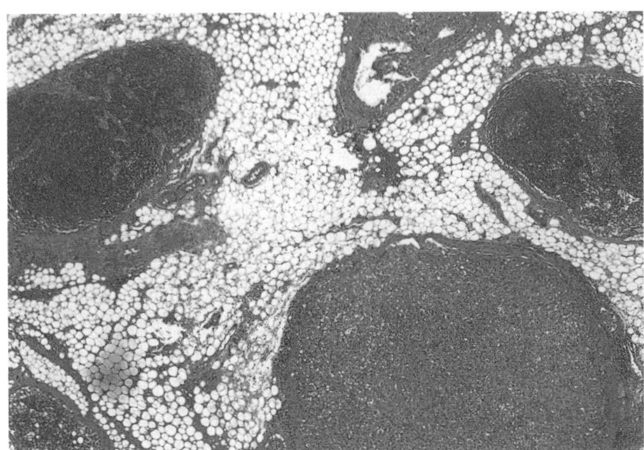

FIGURE 88.1. Three axillary lymph nodes in immediate proximity. One (*bottom*) is entirely replaced by metastatic breast carcinoma, whereas two adjacent lymph nodes are reactive but free of tumor. Hematoxylin, phloxine, and saffron stain.

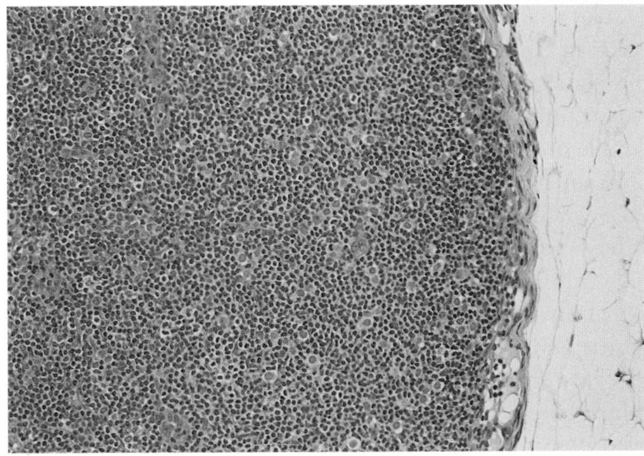

FIGURE 88.3. Axillary lymph node in patient with infiltrating lobular carcinoma. No tumor metastasis visible on the routine section. Hematoxylin, phloxine, and saffron stain.

lymph nodes to 56% for those with metastases at level I, 41% for those with metastases at level II, and 28% for those with metastases at level III.

The ipsilateral axillary lymph nodes along the axillary vein and its tributaries are divided as follows:

- Level I (low axilla)—lymph nodes lateral to the lateral border of the pectoralis minor muscle
- Level II (mid-axilla)—lymph nodes between the medial and lateral borders of the pectoralis minor plus the Rotter (interpectoral) lymph nodes
- Level III (apical axilla)—lymph nodes medial to the medial margin of the pectoralis minor muscle, including those usually designated as subclavicular, infraclavicular, or apical

Internal mammary lymph nodes are located in the intercostal spaces along the edge of the sternum. Any other lymph nodes metastases are coded as distant metastases (M), including those in supraclavicular cervical and contralateral nodes (3).

Separating the axillary lymph nodes into three levels is very useful, but this judgment can be made correctly only when a standard radical mastectomy specimen, including both pectoralis muscles, is available for examination (17). In a modified radical mastectomy (without pectoralis muscles), the nodes should be identified as low and high axillary groups. In a long follow-up of mastectomies for breast cancer, the chance of 20-year survival was 65% with no axillary metastases, 38% when only level I lymph nodes were involved, 30% when level II nodes were involved, and 12% when level III nodes were involved (18). Skipped levels—that is, the involvement of high axillary nodes without apparent involvement of low axillary nodes—are unusual (19). In one study of patients with positive axillary lymph nodes, level III nodes were involved when levels 1 and II were negative in only 0.4% of the cases (20).

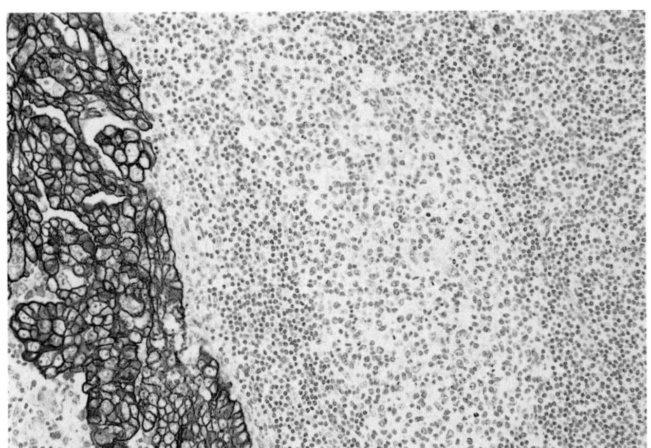

FIGURE 88.2. Metastatic mammary duct carcinoma in marginal sinus of axillary lymph node. Cytokeratin/peroxidase stain.

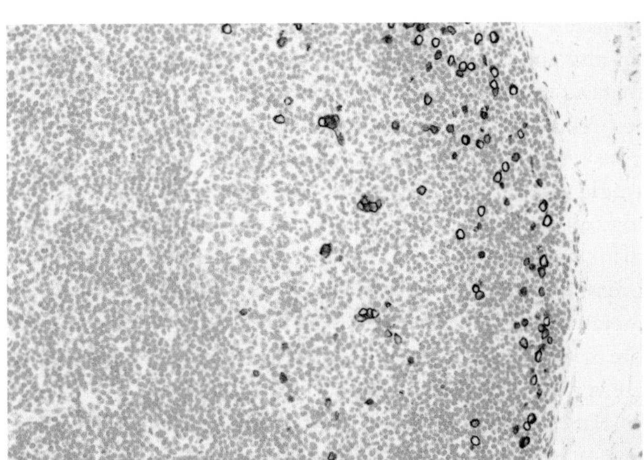

FIGURE 88.4. Same section as in Fig. 88.3. Multiple scattered metastatic lobular carcinoma cells revealed by cytokeratin (CK) staining. CK/peroxidase stain.

The *number of lymph nodes involved* with metastatic cancer is an equally important prognostic factor. In data from the National Surgical Breast Project, patients treated with mastectomy had a 5-year survival rate of 83% when no lymph nodes were involved, 80% with 1 node involved, 65% to 70% with 2 or 3 nodes, 54% with 4 to 6 nodes, and 28% when more than 12 lymph nodes were involved (21). After 5 years, the survival curves became parallel, showing only minimal further differences. In general, patients with axillary lymph node metastases are stratified in three categories: 1 to 3, 4 to 9, and 10 or more lymph nodes involved.

The number of lymph nodes involved by tumor is determined by careful dissection of the unfixed axillary fat; however, it is usually underestimated. Therefore, the number of lymph nodes found should not be stated in the gross description but after microscopic observation of the tissue sections. Finally, the number of cancer cells in the individual lymph nodes is an additional prognostic indicator (2); the prognosis is considerably worse when the metastasis has reached the point of breaking through the capsule into the perinodal fibroadipose tissue. This is called an *extranodal extension* and is a sign of an unfavorable prognosis.

The problem of metastatic carcinoma in axillary lymph nodes without a clinically detectable breast tumor has been discussed by various authors (22–26). Ashikari and coworkers (23) reviewed 34 cases of metastatic carcinoma in axillary lymph nodes with an occult *breast tumor*. Careful investigation after radical mastectomy revealed 23 occult carcinomas in the ipsilateral breast, of which 20 were invasive and 3 were *in situ*. Two-thirds of the occult primary tumors were smaller than 2 cm in diameter. The incidence of occult primary carcinoma with lymph node metastases was 0.5% in the series of 5,451 cases of breast tumors of Owen and associates (22) and 0.3% in the series of 6,000 cases of breast tumors of Haagensen (1). Rosen (26) estimates that 1% of patients with preinvasive breast carcinomas may have lymph node metastases originating in obscure foci of invasive carcinoma. He studied eight cases of axillary lymph node metastases in which the breast lesions found were only ductal and lobular carcinoma *in situ*. In the case of axillary metastases with an occult primary, an effort must be made to find the primary tumor in the breast. Azzopardi (25) suggests a careful investigation of the axillary tail of the breast, where a small primary tumor, sometimes no more than 5 mm in diameter, may be mistaken for a lymph node. The distinction in such cases is made by the abundant elastosis in breast tumors but not in the lymph nodes involved by metastasis. In general, for women in the age groups in which breast cancer is common, axillary metastases of a carcinoma are very rarely of extramammary origin (17).

Sentinel lymph node biopsy, first used in the staging of cutaneous melanoma (27), is rapidly becoming a standard procedure in the diagnosis of metastatic breast carcinoma. The tumor status of the axillary lymph nodes is the most important prognostic factor in breast cancer and determines the use of adjuvant therapy after excision of the primary tumor. Axillary lymph node dissection with microscopic examination has been the method used for this assessment. Although it provides an accurate evaluation of lymph node status, axillary dissection causes significant morbidity, with chronic lymphedema and other complications developing in as many as 20% to 30% of cases (28). The recently introduced intraoperative lymphatic mapping and sentinel lymph node biopsy, which avoid extensive dissection, decrease postsurgical morbidity substantially while maintaining the accuracy of the histologic diagnosis (9,28–30). The sentinel lymph node, usually the largest lymph node in the axilla, is considered the first to receive the lymph drained from the breast and therefore the most likely to harbor a tumor metastasis. It is identified by intraoperative mapping after injection of a tracer at the tumor site. The tracer consists of a vital blue dye, such as 1% methylene blue, or a radioactive substance, such as colloidal albumin labeled with technetium 99m. Some surgeons use both. The sentinel lymph node is then dissected by following the blue dye visually or the radioactive substance with the aid of a hand-held gamma probe. Dissecting the sentinel lymph node after a learning period is likely to be successful in 90% of cases, and the tumor status of the sentinel lymph node is expected to reflect accurately the tumor status of all the ipsilateral axillary lymph nodes (28). The average number of sentinel lymph nodes excised by different techniques varies between 1.2 and 2.9 (28). Because the number of lymph nodes to be examined has now been reduced to 1 or 2, the examination can be more exhaustive and include multiple sections and immunohistochemistry (28–31). Sentinel lymph nodes are cut at various intervals, from 0.250 to 0.500 mm in different studies, and immunostained with a "cocktail" of cytokeratin antibodies directed at low- and intermediate-molecular-weight cytokeratins (Fig. 88.5). The yield of positive lymph nodes is increased by up to 23% in various studies over that obtained with single hematoxylin and eosin staining (9,28,32).

Recently, the highly sensitive method of amplification by

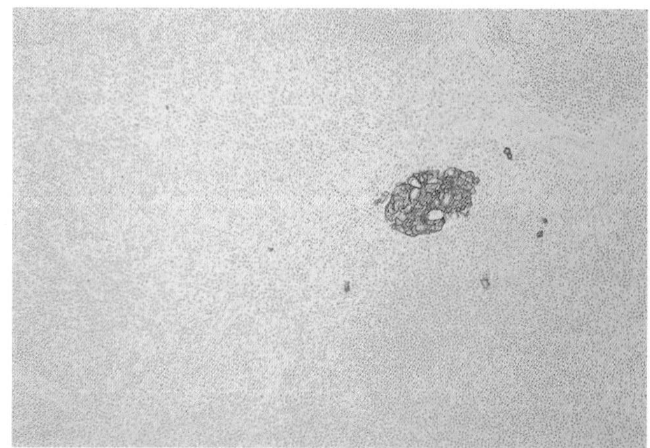

FIGURE 88.5. Sentinel axillary lymph node immunostained with a cocktail of cytokeratin (CK) antibodies shows small unique cluster of carcinoma cells deep in the lymphoid parenchyma. CK/peroxidase stain.

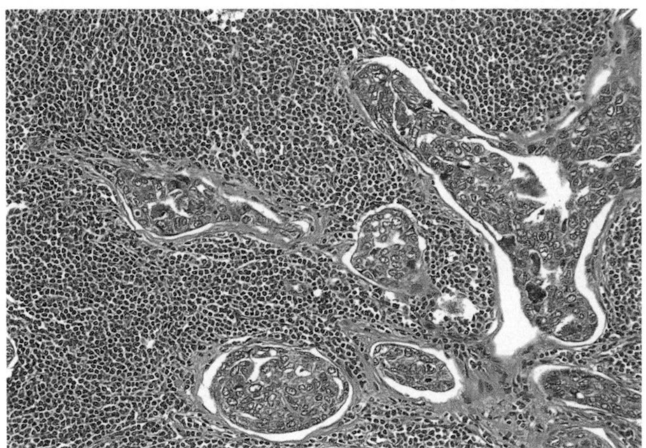

FIGURE 88.6. Metastatic mammary duct carcinoma with large aggregates of tumor cells plugging the lymph node sinuses. Hematoxylin, phloxine, and saffron stain.

reverse transcriptase polymerase chain reaction (PCR) has been applied to the search for micrometastases. When reverse transcriptase polymerase chain reaction amplification of keratin 19 messenger RNA was used, micrometastases were detected in 10% to 23% of lymph nodes that were negative for micrometastases by the conventional histologic method (33,34).

The exhaustive examination of lymph nodes with highly sensitive techniques to search for micrometastases has yielded considerably greater numbers of cases with positive findings. However, as noted by several authors, these results must be interpreted with caution (35,36). Firstly, not all cells stained in a lymph node by anticytokeratin antibodies are necessarily metastases of carcinoma; some may be histiocytes or dendritic cells, which also express cytokeratin (Fig. 44.10), and some may be noncancerous epithelial inclusions (37). Secondly, and more importantly, the significance of a few carcinoma cells in a lymph node has not yet been assessed in terms of cancer prognosis. Single cells or small clusters of cells may not be viable or may be unable to establish cancer colonies. To determine the capacity of micrometastases for further growth and spread, long-term studies, some of them already in progress, are needed. Until results are available, it is not advisable to consider the presence of a few cytokeratin-positive cells in axillary lymph nodes as tumor metastases and base aggressive treatment and final prognosis solely on this finding (36).

HISTOPATHOLOGY

With rare exceptions, the microscopic patterns of lymph node metastases reflect the histologic types of the primary breast tumor. In a study comparing differences in the degree of glandular differentiation between primary breast carcinomas and their lymph node metastases, significant differences were found in fewer than 5% of cases (38). The most common type, infiltrating ductal carcinoma, usually accompanied by abundant fibrosis, represents about 80% of all breast cancers (2). The lymph node metastases generally reproduce the nests and cords with variable formation of ductlike spaces of the original tumor (Fig. 88.6). The component cells vary from cuboidal and monomorphic to large and highly pleomorphic with frequent mitoses (Fig. 88.7). The reaction to the invading carcinoma

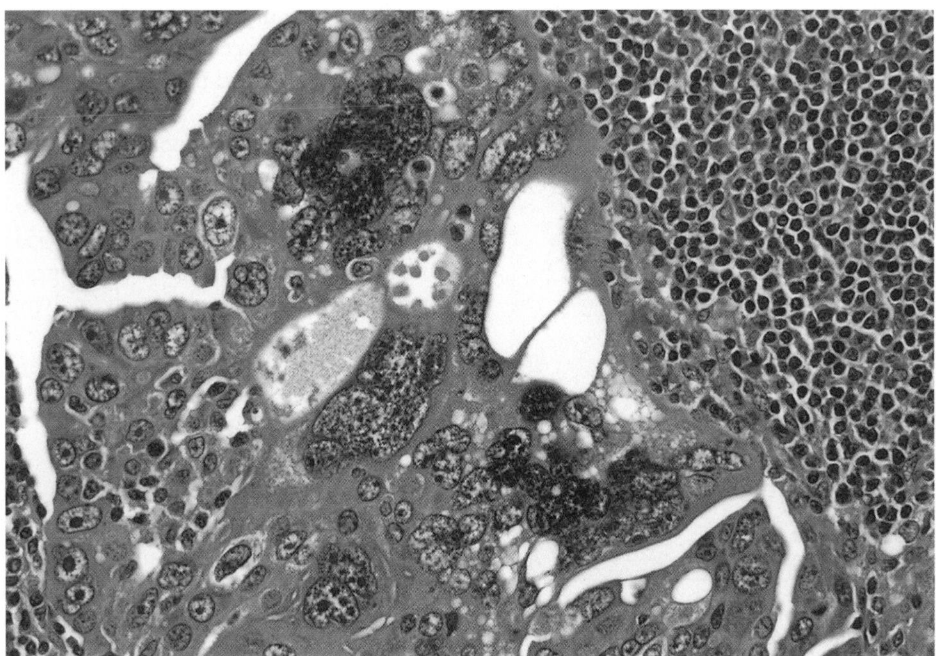

FIGURE 88.7. Metastatic mammary duct carcinoma forming rudimentary gland structures. Highly pleomorphic tumor cells with huge nuclear masses. Hematoxylin, phloxine, and saffron stain.

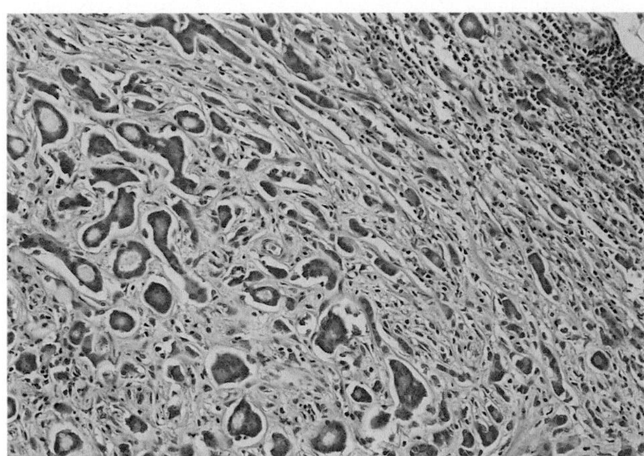

FIGURE 88.8. Metastatic mammary duct carcinoma with intense desmoplasia totally replacing the lymphoid tissue. Hematoxylin, phloxine, and saffron stain.

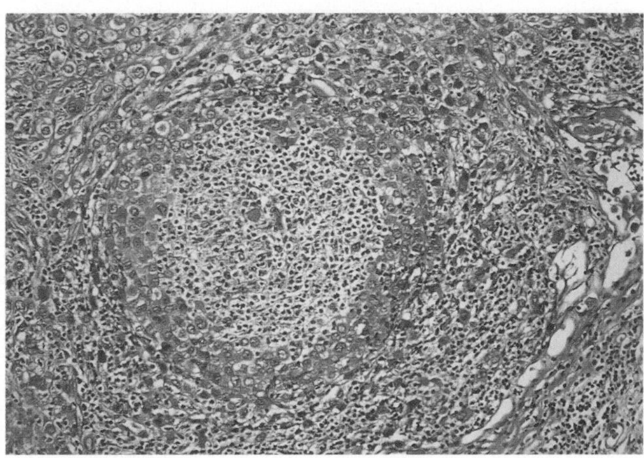

FIGURE 88.10. Metastatic mammary lobular carcinoma with single tumor cells surrounding an involuted lymphoid follicle. Hematoxylin, phloxine, and saffron stain.

cells may take the form of enlarged follicles with reactive germinal centers, excessive histiocytosis, formation of granulomas, or more often desmoplasia (Fig. 88.8). Fibrosis around the carcinoma cells is moderate; however, thick bands of collagen occasionally form that resemble the nodular sclerosis type of Hodgkin lymphoma or entirely obliterate the lymphatic parenchyma (Fig. 88.9). Recognizing metastatic breast carcinomas of ductal cell type, including those with tubular, colloid, medullary, or papillary patterns, is generally not difficult. However, problems may arise with the lymph node metastases of lobular carcinoma. This tumor, composed of homogeneous populations of small bland cells, may not form recognizable ductlike structures. Metastases of lobular carcinoma are often distributed in the sinuses, sometimes deep in the cortex and even the medulla, without initial involvement of the marginal sinus (Fig. 88.10). When the metastases are early and sparse, they consist only of single cells or small cell clusters that without the help of immunohistochemistry may be indistinguishable from histiocytes and endothelial cells (Fig. 88.11). At other times, the cells of lobular carcinoma aggregate in nests and islands; often, particularly under low power, these closely resemble lymphoma. The cells are small, with scarce cytoplasm, round or ovoid open nuclei, fine inconspicuous nucleoli, and infrequent mitoses. On occasion, the cells show an intracytoplasmic mucin-containing vacuole and an eccentric nucleus, typical of signet ring carcinoma cells (Fig. 88.12). Focal signet ring differentiation is frequent in lobular carcinoma of the breast, although it rarely involves 50% or more of the total cell population (25). Occasionally, pools of mucus with floating signet ring cells, singly or in small nests, form. The mucins can be stained best with the mucicarmine or Alcian blue and periodic acid–Schiff (PAS) stains.

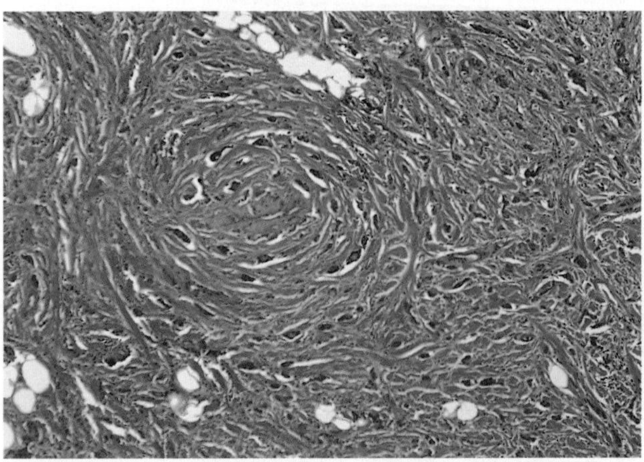

FIGURE 88.9. Metastatic mammary lobular carcinoma with small cell clusters or monocellular files, as in the primary tumor, surrounded by thick bands of collagen, resembling Hodgkin lymphoma. Hematoxylin, phloxine, and saffron stain.

An infrequent but important source of potential confusion with metastatic carcinoma is the occasional presence in axillary lymph nodes of epithelial inclusions (see Chapter 54) or nevus inclusions (see Chapter 55). After intensive chemotherapy, the lymph nodes appear entirely depopulated, with few residual islands of lymphoid tissue (Fig. 88.13).

CYTOCHEMISTRY

Periodic acid–Schiff with diastase (D-PAS), mucicarmine, or Alcian blue and PAS stainings may assist in the detection of droplets of mucus in the undifferentiated cells of lobular carcinoma. As in other metastatic carcinomas, reticulin staining is useful in outlining aggregates of epithelial cells within the lymph node, which are in contrast to the pericellular reticulin network of lymphomas.

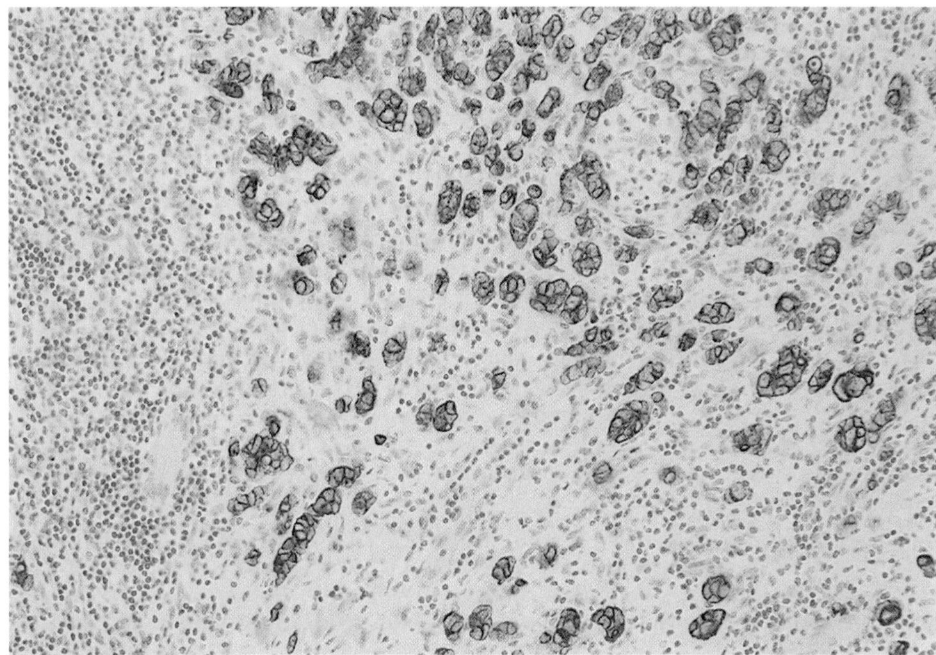

FIGURE 88.11. Metastatic mammary lobular carcinoma. Discohesive cells are scattered in the lymph node deep cortex and medulla without involvement of the sinuses; they are clearly revealed by cytokeratin (CK) staining. CK/peroxidase stain.

IMMUNOHISTOCHEMISTRY

All carcinoma cells contain keratin proteins as their intermediate filaments; these can be demonstrated in histologic or cytologic preparations with appropriate monoclonal antibodies (MAbs). Cytokeratins are highly sensitive markers for carcinoma cells, and the expression of any cytokeratin protein in a metastatic tumor indicates an epithelial origin (39). Combinations of anticytokeratin antibodies, such as AE1/AE3, CK7/CK20, 34βE12/35βH11, or broadly specific MAbs to keratins, such as MAb "cocktails" that react with high- and low-molecular-weight cytokeratins, are used for this purpose (39,40) (Fig. 88.14). Epithelial membrane antigen (EMA) is also used with good results in the identification of metastatic carcinoma cells. Cytokeratins and epithelial membrane antigen are well preserved in formalin-fixed tissues (also in B5, Bouin, and Zenker fixatives). However, routine fixation and paraffin embedding may mask antigen sites on the keratin molecules by crosslinking the protein groups. Predigestion of tissues with en-

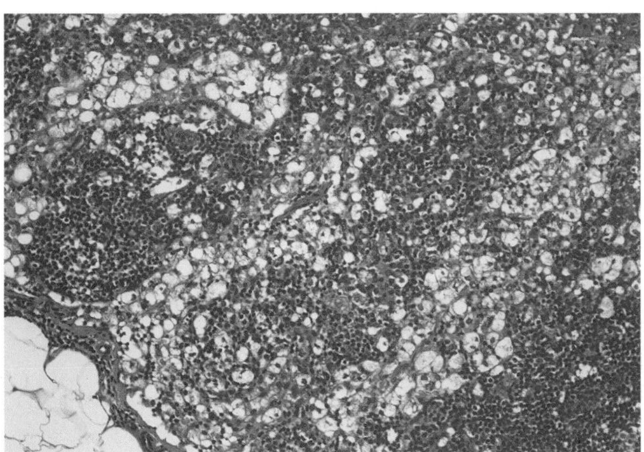

FIGURE 88.12. Metastatic mammary lobular carcinoma composed of signet ring-type cells with clear cytoplasm and eccentric nuclei infiltrating the marginal and cortical sinuses. Hematoxylin, phloxine, and saffron stain.

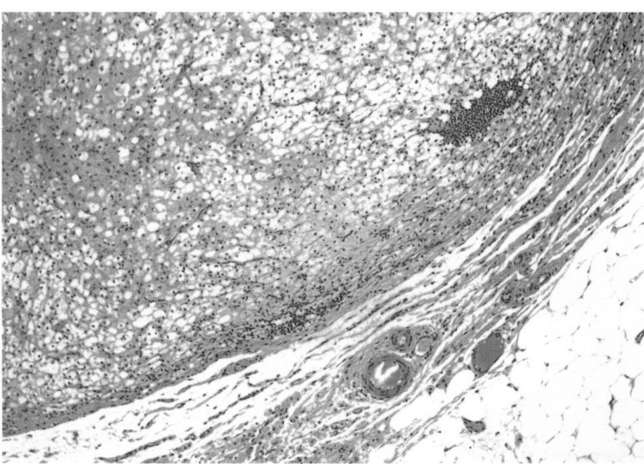

FIGURE 88.13. Axillary lymph node after intensive chemotherapy appears entirely depopulated, with only a small island of residual lymphocytes. Hematoxylin, phloxine, and saffron stain.

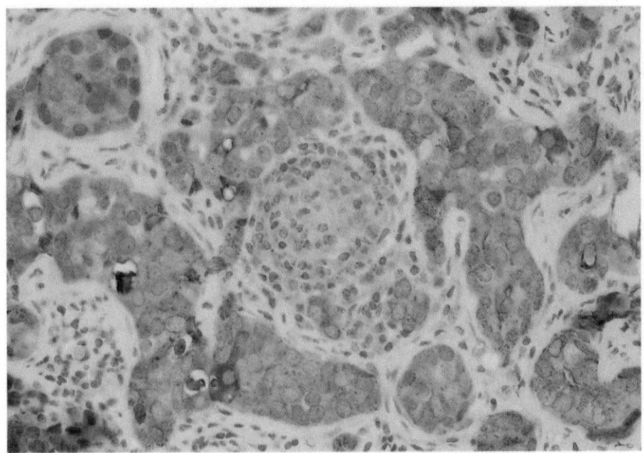

FIGURE 88.14. Metastatic mammary lobular carcinoma with cells aggregated in cords surrounding a lymphoid follicle. The cells, positive for cytokeratin (CK), had a signet ring morphology on hematoxylin and eosin stain. CK/peroxidase stain.

zymes such as trypsin or pronase may be needed to reverse this fixation effect.

ELECTRON MICROSCOPY

Cells of both ductal and lobular carcinomas often have intracytoplasmic lumina that are lined by microvilli and contain mucin globules (25). Intercellular attachments of epithelial type are present.

DIFFERENTIAL DIAGNOSIS

- Reactive lymphadenopathies and atypical reactive lymphadenopathies show sinus histiocytosis. Large histiocytes, some with atypical nuclei, resemble metastatic lobular carcinoma. Immunostaining for CD68 (histiocytes) versus a cytokeratin cocktail may be used to reveal the different cell origin.
- Non-Hodgkin lymphoma of diffuse, large cell type: The lymphoma cells, even when morphologically similar, do not aggregate in cords or islands like those of carcinomas. Immunostaining of tumor cells for CD45 and CD20 versus cytokeratin cocktail solves the problem.
- Non-Hodgkin lymphoma of signet ring cell type resembles metastatic mammary lobular carcinoma with signet ring cells. Mucicarmine and PAS-D stains may reveal the difference.
- Hodgkin lymphoma of nodular sclerosing type may be mimicked by some metastatic lobular carcinomas comprising tumor cells with atypical nuclei, important desmoplastic reaction, and infiltration of lymphocytes and plasma cells.

Checklist

METASTATIC BREAST CARCINOMA

Presence or history of breast tumor
Axillary lymph nodes enlarged
Sentinel lymph node radioactive or dyed blue
Carcinoma cells aggregated in nests, cords, or islands
Sinuses distended by tumor cells
Formation of glands, solid cords, and islands in ductal carcinomas
Formation of glands, clusters, or single cells in lobular carcinomas
Intracytoplasmic mucus and signet ring cells
Desmoplastic reaction
Staining with D-PAS, mucicarmine, Alcian blue often positive
Reticulin strands surrounding cell aggregates
Intercellular attachments
Immunostaining with anticytokeratin and anti-epithelial membrane antigen MAbs

REFERENCES

1. Haagensen CD. Diseases of the breast. Philadelphia: WB Saunders, 1971:396–427.
2. McDivitt RW, Steward IW, Berg JW. Tumors of the breast. Atlas of tumor pathology, series I, fascicle 2. Washington, DC: Armed Forces Institute of Pathology, 1967.
3. Spiessl B, Beahrs OH, Hermanék P, et al. International Union Against Cancer. TNM atlas: illustrated guide to the TNM/pTNM classification of malignant tumors, 3rd ed. Berlin: Springer-Verlag, 1989:174–183.
4. Kinne DW. Staging and follow-up of breast cancer patients. Cancer 1991;67:1196–1198.
5. Fisher ER, Swamidoss S, Lee CH, et al. Detection and significance of occult axillary node metastases in patients with invasive breast cancer. Cancer 1978;42:2025–2031.
6. International (Ludwig) Breast Cancer Study Group. Prognostic importance of occult axillary lymph node micrometastases from breast cancers. Lancet 1990;335:1565–1568.
7. Nasser IA, Lee A, Bosari S, et al. Occult axillary lymph node metastases in "node-negative" breast cancer. Hum Pathol 1993; 24:950–957.
8. McGukin MA, Cummings MC, Walsh MD. Occult axillary node metastases in breast cancer: their detection and prognostic significance. Br J Cancer 1996;73:88–95.
9. Dowlatshahi K, Fan M, Bloom KJ. Occult metastases in the sentinel lymph nodes of patients with early stage breast carcinoma. A preliminary study. Cancer 1999;86:990–996.
10. Saphir O, Amromin GD. Obscure axillary lymph node metastases in carcinoma of the breast. Cancer 1948;1:238–241.
11. Picken JW. Significance of occult metastases: a study of breast cancer. Cancer 1961;14:1266–1271.
12. Wells CA, Heryet A, Brochier J, et al. The immunocytochemical detection of axillary micrometastases in breast cancer. Br J Cancer 1984;50:193–197.
13. Bussolati G, Gugliotta P, Morra I, et al. The immunohistochemical detection of lymph node metastases from infiltrating lobular carcinoma of the breast. Br J Cancer 1986;54:631–636.
14. Trojani M, de Mascarel I, Coindre JM, et al. Micrometastases to axillary lymph nodes from invasive lobular carcinoma of breast: detection by immunohistochemistry and prognostic significance. Br J Cancer 1987;565:838–839.
15. Cote RJ, Peterson HF, Chaiwun B, et al. Role of immunohistochemical detection of lymph node metastases in the management of breast cancer. Lancet 1999;354:896–900.
16. Huvos AG, Hutter RVP, Berg JW. Significance of axillary macrometastases and micrometastases in mammary cancer. Am Surg 1971;173:44–46.
17. Page DL, Anderson TJ. Metastasis of breast cancer. In: Page DL, Anderson TJ, eds. Diagnostic histopathology of the breast. New York: Churchill Livingstone, 1987:321–329.
18. Berg JW, Robbins GF. Factors influencing short- and long-term survival of breast cancer patients. Surg Gynecol Obstet 1966;122: 1311–1316.
19. Rosen PP, Lesser ML, Kinne DW, et al. Discontinuous or "skip" metastases in breast carcinoma. Ann Surg 1983;197:276–283.
20. Veronesi U, Rilke F, Luini A, et al. Distribution of axillary node metastases by level of invasion. Cancer 1987;59:682–687.
21. Fisher ER, Sass R, Fisher B, et al. Pathologic findings from the National Surgical Adjuvant Project for Breast Cancers. X. Discriminants for 10th-year treatment failure. Cancer 1984;53:712–723.
22. Owen HW, Dockerty MB, Gray HK. Occult carcinoma of the breast. Surg Gynecol Obstet 1954;98:302.
23. Ashikari R, Hajdu SI, Robbins GF. Intraductal carcinoma of the breast (1960–1969). Cancer 1971;28:1182–1187.
24. Copeland EM, McBride CM. Axillary metastases from unknown primary sites. Ann Surg 1972;178:25–27.
25. Azzopardi JG. Problems in breast pathology. Philadelphia: WB Saunders, 1979:240–257.
26. Rosen PP. Axillary lymph node metastases in patients with occult noninvasive breast carcinoma. Cancer 1980;46:1298–1306.
27. Morton DL, Wen DR, Wong JH, et al. Technical details of intraoperative lymphatic mapping for early-stage melanoma. Arch Surg 1992:127:392–399.
28. Hsueh EC, Hansen N, Giuliano AE. Intraoperative lymphatic mapping and sentinel lymph node dissection in breast cancer. Cancer J Clin 2000;50:279–291.
29. Giuliano AE, Kirgan DM, Guenther JM, et al. Lymphatic mapping and sentinel lymphadenectomy for breast cancer. Ann Surg 1994:220:391–401.
30. Krag D, Weaver D, Ashikaga T, et al. The sentinel node in breast cancer: a multicenter validation study. N Engl J Med 1999:339: 941–946.
31. Bedrosian I, Reynolds C, Mick R, et al. Accuracy of sentinel lymph node biopsy in patients with large primary breast tumors. Cancer 2000;88:2540–2545.
32. De Mascarel I, Bouichon F, Coindre JM, et al. Prognostic significance of breast cancer axillary lymph node micrometastases assessed by two special techniques: reevaluation with longer follow-up. Br J Cancer 1992;66:523–527.
33. Schoenfeld A, Luqmani Y, Smith D, et al. Detection of breast cancer micrometastases in axillary lymph nodes by using polymerase chain reaction. Cancer Res 1994;54:2986–2990.
34. Noguchi S, Aihara T, Motomura K, et al. Detection of breast cancer micrometastases in axillary lymph nodes by means of reverse transcriptase-polymerase chain reaction. Comparison between MUC1 mRNA and keratin 19 mRNA amplification. Am J Pathol 1996;148:649–656.
35. Cady B. Lymph node metastases. Indicators, but not governors, of survival. Arch Surg 1984;119:1067–1072.
36. Allred C, Elledge RM. Caution concerning micrometastatic breast carcinoma in sentinel lymph nodes. Cancer 1999;86:905–907.
37. Holdsworth PJ, Hopkinson JM, Leveson SH, et al. Benign axillary epithelial lymph node inclusions: a histological pitfall. Histopathology 1988;13:226–228.
38. Sharkey FE, Greiner AS. Morphologic identity of primary tumor and axillary metastases in breast carcinoma. Arch Pathol Lab Med 1985;109:256–259.
39. Wang NP, Bacchi CE, Gown AM. Coordinate expression of cytokeratins 7 and 20 define unique subsets of carcinomas. Appl Immunohistochem 1995;3:99–107.
40. Battifora H. Clinical applications of the immunohistochemistry of filamentous proteins. Am J Surg Pathol 1988;12[Suppl 1]:24–42.

89

METASTATIC NASOPHARYNGEAL CARCINOMA

DEFINITION

Undifferentiated carcinoma of the nasopharynx metastatic to cervical lymph nodes.

SYNONYM

Lymphoepithelioma

EPIDEMIOLOGY

Nasopharyngeal carcinoma is prevalent in southern China and northern Africa, and among Alaskan Eskimos (1). The incidence of nasopharyngeal carcinoma is low in whites, representing about 0.25% of all malignancies, and high in Chinese, particularly in southern China and Malaysia, representing 18% of all malignant tumors (2). In the United States and western Europe, nasopharyngeal carcinoma occurs sporadically (1).

PATHOGENESIS

Nasopharyngeal carcinoma is notorious for early metastasis to cervical lymph nodes (3,4). In 60% to 70% of cases in children (5,6) and in as many as 40% in adults (7), enlargement of the cervical lymph nodes is the first clinical symptom, preceding by various intervals detection of the primary tumor. The inaccessibility of the primary site contributes to the late diagnosis of this tumor, and its often undifferentiated histologic appearance explains the frequency of misdiagnosis, found by some authors to be as high as 50% (3). Of carcinomas of the head and neck, 5.5% are primary in the nasopharynx in whites, in comparison with 82% in Chinese (2). The reactivities of sera from patients with nasopharyngeal carcinoma are similar to those of sera from patients with Burkitt lymphoma (8), which suggests an etiologic relation with the Epstein-Barr virus (EBV). The EBV genome is present in the carcinoma cells of the tumor but not in the infiltrating lymphocytes, which are largely of T-cell type (9). Patients with nasopharyngeal carcinoma, both in southern China and in North America, have high antibody titers against the capsid and early EBV antigens (10). The polymerase chain reaction technique has demonstrated the EBV genome in lymph node metastases of nasopharyngeal carcinoma, but not in other types of metastatic lymphadenopathy associated with head and neck cancer (11). In regions where nasopharyngeal carcinoma is endemic, EBV infection occurs early in life and may remain latent for 40 to 60 years before tumors arise (12).

CLINICAL SYNDROME

Nasopharyngeal carcinomas, unlike carcinomas of other organs, are more common in young persons. In whites, 6% of carcinomas in the nasopharynx occur before 30 years and 50% before 50 years of age (13). In one study, all 33 patients were between 10 and 19 years of age, and the male-to-female ratio was 2.3:1 (3). In 10 cases in children, all the patients were younger than 15 years, with a mean age of 12.6 years (5). The lymph node metastases are bilateral in 30% to 39% of cases (2,5). The primary tumor is more commonly located in the roof and lateral walls of the pharynx and less often in the posterior wall (2,14). The metastases usually affect the superior deep cervical lymph nodes, and the frequent bilaterality is explained by the central location of the primary tumor (2). In a review of a large series of patients during an 8-year period in Kuala Lumpur, Malaysia, of 134 cases of nasopharyngeal carcinoma, 110 had enlarged lymph nodes as the first symptom (13). The primary tumors were identified only after repeated examinations, and sometimes even at autopsy they were inconspicuous and appeared only as slightly raised, ill-defined granular patches of the nasopharyngeal or oropharyngeal mucosa. In 268 additional cases of metastatic carcinoma in cervical lymph nodes, the primary tumors could not be found, so that the same author concluded that they, too, had originated in the nasopharynx.

When nasopharyngeal carcinomas are clinically conspicuous, patients may present with symptoms of nasal obstruction, rhinorrhea, and purulent discharge. Survival is better in children than in older patients; it was 62.5% at 5 years in a report of 10 children with nasopharyngeal carcinoma (5).

Tumors of similar histologic appearance may arise in the palatine and lingual tonsils, thymus, and larynx, an observation that has led some authors to suggest the name *undifferentiated carcinoma of nasopharyngeal type* for the whole group (15). The suggested protocol for the management of cervical lymphadenopathy without an obvious primary origin starts with fine needle aspiration to establish a cytologic diagnosis. In cases of squamous cell carcinoma in an upper cervical lymph node, panendoscopy is indicated, including biopsy of all suspect areas and blinded biopsies of the common primary sites—nasopharynx, tonsil, base of the tongue, supraglottic larynx, and piriform sinus (16).

HISTOPATHOLOGY

The enlarged cervical lymph nodes show variable degrees of replacement by the metastatic tumor. As in all metastatic tumors, the carcinoma cells are first noted in the marginal and medullary sinuses and progress gradually to involve both cortex and medulla. The capsule and perinodal tissues may be invaded at a later stage.

Two histologic patterns have been described, both in primary nasopharyngeal tumors and in metastatic lymph nodes. The Regaud type (17) is slightly more common (18 of 33 cases in one series) (3). It consists of solid cords and islands of carcinoma cells outlined by collagen fibers and accumulations of lymphoid cells. Foci of necrosis may be present. The Schmincke type (18) consists of large, ill-defined sheets of cells admixed with numerous lymphocytes, sometimes polymorphonuclear leukocytes, and particularly eosinophils. Occasionally, the two patterns coexist, but one is always predominant (3). Both histologic types include frequent foci of necrosis.

The degree of histologic differentiation seems to be related to the incidence of this tumor in various populations. In southern Chinese, who are at high risk, 60% of nasopharyngeal carcinomas are undifferentiated, whereas in the low-risk populations of other countries, differentiated carcinomas are more common (8). The World Health Organization classification recognizes three histologic types: (a) squamous cell carcinoma, (b) nonkeratinizing carcinoma, and (c) undifferentiated carcinoma (19). The cells in undifferentiated nasopharyngeal carcinomas include abundant cytoplasm with indistinct cellular borders, often with the appearance of a syncytium (Figs. 89.1 and 89.2). The nuclei are large, ovoid, and vesicular, with thin nuclear borders and marginated heterochromatin that create an "open" appearance (3) (Figs. 89.2 and 89.3). Most nuclei include two to

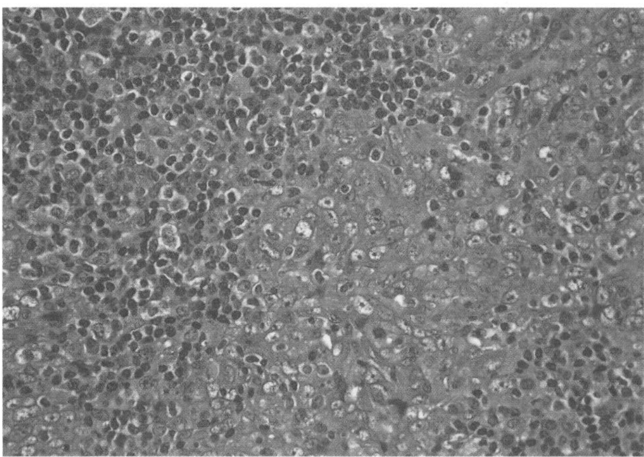

FIGURE 89.1. Metastatic nasopharyngeal carcinoma, undifferentiated type in cervical lymph node. Sheets of undifferentiated carcinoma cells with indistinct borders, eosinophilic cytoplasm, and vesicular nuclei replace lymphoid tissue. Hematoxylin, phloxine, and saffron stain.

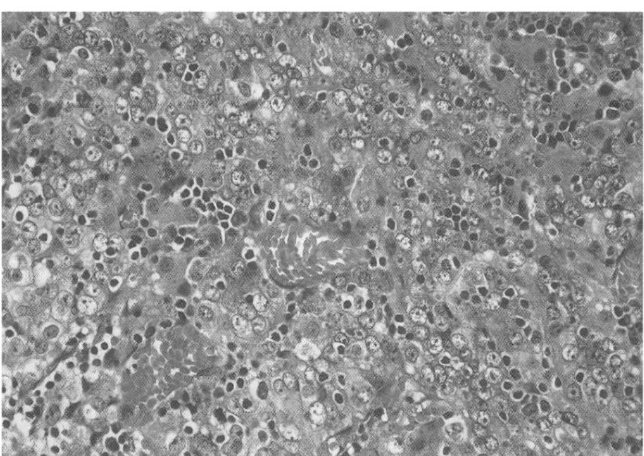

FIGURE 89.2. Metastatic nasopharyngeal carcinoma (undifferentiated), Schmincke type in cervical lymph node. Cells with indistinct borders form a syncytium with large open vesicular nuclei, prominent eosinophilic nucleoli, and frequent mitoses. Numerous lymphocytes within vacuole-like spaces infiltrate the carcinoma cells. Hematoxylin, phloxine, and saffron stain.

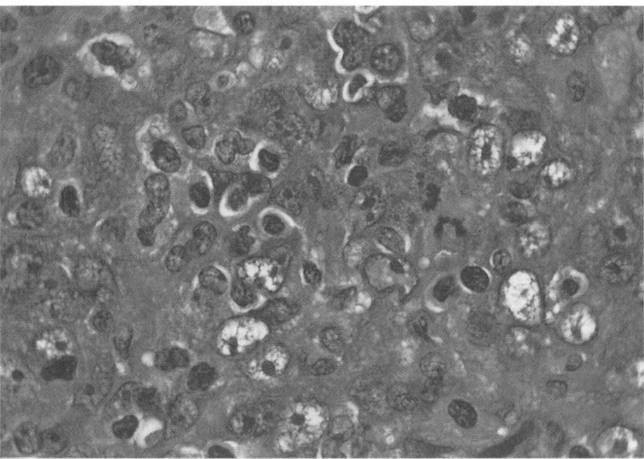

FIGURE 89.3. Same section as in Fig. 89.1. Large, undifferentiated carcinoma cells with vesicular nuclei, prominent eosinophilic nucleoli, and frequent mitoses infiltrated by numerous lymphocytes within vacuolar spaces. EBER *in situ* hybridization.

three eosinophilic nucleoli of moderate size and numerous mitoses, estimated at 5 to 10 per 10 high-power fields. Multinucleated cells are not noted. These large cells with vesicular nuclei and eosinophilic nucleoli associated with an abundant infiltrate of lymphocytes and eosinophils may closely resemble Hodgkin lymphoma; however, typical diagnostic Reed-Sternberg cells are not present. Furthermore, the neoplastic cells show some cohesiveness and occasional spindle cells (15). Evidently cytochemistry and clearly immunohistochemistry are able to provide the differential features. The infiltrating lymphocytes are never malignant. The eosinophils may be present in large numbers. In a study of 422 biopsy specimens of nasopharyngeal carcinoma, eosinophilia was present in 26% of the cases: 38% of the nonkeratinizing, 21% of the squamous, and 23% of the undifferentiated types (20). In the lymph nodes with tumor metastases, the prevalence of eosinophilia was similar, at 38%.

ELECTRON MICROSCOPY

In an ultrastructural study of 14 cases, both histologic types of nasopharyngeal carcinoma, regardless of degree of differentiation, contained desmosomes and intracytoplasmic bundles of tonofibrils, indications of their squamous cell origin (21). The cells are closely apposed and united by complexes of desmosome and tonofilaments. The cytoplasm contains unattached ribosomes and a poorly developed endoplasmic reticulum. The nuclear chromatin is diffuse, and the nucleoli are prominent.

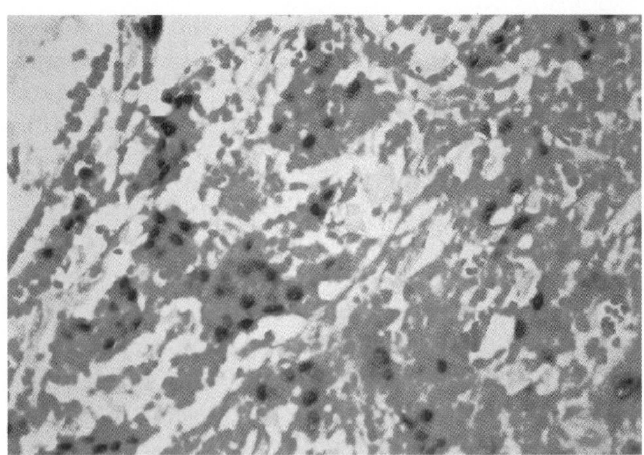

FIGURE 89.4. Metastatic nasopharyngeal carcinoma showing nuclear expression of EBV RNA. EBER *in situ* hybridization.

CYTOCHEMISTRY

On touch preparations, tumor cells of nasopharyngeal carcinoma stain moderately with periodic acid–Schiff, acid phosphatase, and nonspecific esterase (15).

IMMUNOHISTOCHEMISTRY

The tumor cells in nasopharyngeal carcinoma express cytokeratins and are negative for the lymphocyte marker CD45 (leukocyte common antigen), B-cell marker CD20 (L26), T-cell marker CD3, and Reed-Sternberg cell marker CD15 (Leu-M1). The lymphocytes show evidence of both

Checklist

METASTATIC NASOPHARYNGEAL CARCINOMA

Young patients
Chinese predominance
Males more frequently affected
Primary site often inapparent
Early lymph node metastases
Carcinoma cells in solid cords admixed with lymphocytes
Eosinophils, neutrophils
Foci of necrosis
Vesicular nuclei, multiple nucleoli
Numerous mitoses
Desmosome–tonofilament complexes
Cytokeratin+
CD45 (leukocyte common antigen)−, CD15 (Leu-M1)−
EBV genome present
EBV antigens expressed

κ and λ light chain immunoglobulins. In one study, broad-spectrum anticytokeratin antibodies stained 100% of keratinizing, 88% of nonkeratinizing, and 90% of undifferentiated nasopharyngeal carcinomas (22). *In situ* hybridization demonstrates nuclear expression of EBV RNA (EBER) (Fig. 89.4).

DNA ANALYSIS

The EBV genome can be detected in metastatic nasopharyngeal carcinoma with the polymerase chain reaction (11).

DIFFERENTIAL DIAGNOSIS

- Misdiagnosis of metastatic nasopharyngeal carcinoma in cervical lymph nodes is frequent because of poor histologic differentiation and absence of an obvious primary tumor. Of the two histologic types, the Schmincke type is more difficult to diagnose and easier to confuse with lymphomas because of the intimate mixture of carcinoma cells and lymphocytes.
- Lymphomas of diffuse large cell types, particularly immunoblastic non-Hodgkin lymphomas, are negative for cytokeratin and positive for leukocyte common antigen, and they do not exhibit surface immunoglobulins.
- Hodgkin lymphoma exhibits Reed-Sternberg cells. It is negative for cytokeratin and positive for CD15 (Leu-M1).
- Burkitt lymphoma has a starry sky pattern and surface immunoglobulin and is negative for cytokeratin. B-cell markers are expressed.

REFERENCES

1. Cohen JI. Epstein-Barr virus infection. N Engl J Med 2000;343: 481–492.
2. Snow JB Jr. Carcinoma of the nasopharynx in children. Ann Otol 1975;84:817–826.
3. Giffler RF, Gillespie JJ, Ayala AG, et al. Lymphoepithelioma in cervical lymph nodes of children and young adults. Am J Surg Pathol 1977;1:293–302.
4. Zarate-Osorno A, Jaffe ES, Medeiros LJ. Metastatic nasopharyngeal carcinoma initially presenting as cervical lymphadenopathy. A report of two cases that resembled Hodgkin's disease. Arch Pathol Lab Med 1992;116:862–865.
5. Fernandez CH, Caugir A, Samaan NA, et al. Nasopharyngeal carcinoma in children. Cancer 1976;37:2787–2791.
6. Deutsch M, Mercado R, Parsons JA. Cancer of the nasopharynx in children. Cancer 1978;41:1128–1133.
7. Cvitkovic E, Bachouchi M, Armand J-P. Nasopharyngeal carcinoma: biology, natural history and therapeutic implications. Hematol Oncol Clin North Am 1991;5:821–838.
8. De Thé G. The etiology of nasopharyngeal carcinoma. Pathobiol Annu 1972;2:235–254.
9. Klein G. The Epstein-Barr virus and neoplasia. N Engl J Med 1975;293:1353–1357.
10. Henle W, Ho H-C, Genle G, et al. Antibodies to Epstein-Barr virus–related antigens in nasopharyngeal carcinoma: comparison of active cases and long-term survivors. J Natl Cancer Inst 1973;51:361–369.
11. Feinmesser R, Miyazaki I, Cheung R, et al. Diagnosis of nasopharyngeal carcinoma by DNA amplification of tissue obtained by fine-needle aspiration. N Engl J Med 1992;326:17–21.
12. Pagano JS. Epstein-Barr virus: culprit or consort? N Engl J Med 1992;327:1750–1752.
13. Loke YW. Lymphoepitheliomas of the cervical lymph nodes. Br J Cancer 1965;19:482–485.
14. Yeh SA. A histological classification of carcinomas of the nasopharynx with a critical review as to the existence of lymphoepitheliomas. Cancer 1962;15:895–920.
15. Carbone A, Micheau C. Pitfalls in microscopic diagnosis of undifferentiated carcinoma of nasopharyngeal type (lymphoepithelioma). Cancer 1982;50:1344–1351.
16. Vokes EE, Weichselbaum RR, Lippman SM. Medical progress: head and neck cancer. N Engl J Med 1993;328:185–194.
17. Regaud C. Lymphoépithéliome de l'hypopharynx traité par la roentgenthérapie. Bull Soc Fr Otorhinolaryngol 1921;34:209–214.
18. Schmincke A. Ueber lymphoepitheliale Geschwölste. Beitr Pathol 1921;58:161–170.
19. Shanmugaratnam K, Sobin L. Histological typing of upper respiratory tract tumors. In: International histological typing of tumours, vol 19. Geneva: World Health Organization, 1978:32–33.
20. Looi L-M. Tumor-associated tissue eosinophilia in nasopharyngeal carcinoma. A pathologic study of 422 primary and 138 metastatic tumors. Cancer 1987;59:466–470.
21. Svoboda DJ, Kirschner FR, Shanmugaratnam K. The fine structure of nasopharyngeal carcinoma. In: Muir CS, Shanmugaratnam K, eds. Cancer of the nasopharynx. UICC Monogr 1967;1: 163–171.
22. Kamino H, Huang SJ, Fu YS. Keratin and involucrin immunohistochemistry of nasopharyngeal carcinoma. Cancer 1988;61: 1142.

90

METASTATIC THYROID CARCINOMA

DEFINITION

Lymph node metastases of thyroid carcinoma.

PATHOGENESIS

Thyroid cancer is not a common tumor and only rarely causes death. In the United States, the estimates for 2001 were 19,500 new cases and 1,300 deaths from thyroid carcinoma (1). Thyroid carcinoma may present histologically in a papillary, follicular, medullary, or anaplastic form. Each major type comprises multiple subtypes and combinations thereof.

In regard to lymph node metastases, papillary thyroid carcinoma (PTC) is of the greatest clinical importance, first because it accounts for as many as 80% of all thyroid cancers (2,3) and second because it manifests a singular propensity to metastasize to the cervical lymph nodes (4). Because of the capacity of PTC to spread via lymphatic vessels, multiple tumor foci form within the thyroid gland, and lymph node metastases are unusually frequent and early. At the time of presentation, 35% of patients may have lymph node metastases (5). In the largest retrospective study of PTC, conducted at the Mayo Clinic, 859 patients were included, 319 (37%) of whom had metastases in cervical lymph nodes (6). In a study of 241 cases of PTC at the University of Florence, the prevalence of lymph node metastases was even greater, 53.7% to cervical lymph nodes and 4.5% to mediastinal lymph nodes (5), whereas in a study of 68 cases of follicular thyroid carcinoma (FTC), only one patient had metastases restricted to the lymph nodes (7). Conversely, the incidence of hematogenous metastasis is low (5%) for PTC (6) and high (34%) for FTC (7).

In the Mayo Clinic study, invasiveness and prognosis were related to the size of the primary tumor, and the investigators divided PTC into three stages: occult, intrathyroid, and extrathyroid (8). Occult thyroid carcinomas measured up to 1 cm in diameter (average, 5 to 7 mm) and were often multifocal. Microscopic PTC is relatively common and may be an incidental finding in thyroid glands removed for other reasons (9). In autopsy studies, the prevalence of occult PTC was as high as 11.3% in Japan (10) and 35.6% in Finland (11). Fortunately, such findings are not clinically significant because occult PTCs in most cases remain small and circumscribed without ever becoming a clinical carcinoma (10,11). Small nests of thyroid colloid-containing follicles found in cervical lymph nodes have been interpreted by some authors as benign ectopic inclusions of thyroid tissue (see Chapter 54). However, others have denied their existence and consider all foci of thyroid tissue in lymph nodes to be metastatic tumors, regardless of how well differentiated they are (12). In many cases of thyroid inclusions in cervical lymph nodes, a primary focus of occult thyroid carcinoma has eventually been found after careful sectioning of the thyroid (13). Therefore, the criteria for diagnosing benign thyroid inclusions in lymph nodes must be very stringent, and if thyroid tissue has replaced more than a third of a lymph node, the diagnosis of metastatic cancer should be applied (4). Also, the presence of psammoma bodies, papillae, or ground-glass nuclei favors carcinoma. Only a few small, subcapsular thyroid follicles should be considered as possible benign thyroid inclusions (4).

CLINICAL SYNDROME

The mean age of patients with PTC was 45 years in males and 43 years in females (range, 5 to 90 years) in a large study (6). The male-to-female ratio was 1:2.1 in one study (6) and 1:2.6 in another (5). The symptom most commonly noted is a mass in the thyroid gland. By palpation, 56% of patients in one study had one nodule, and 21% had two or more (6). In a different study, 98.7% of 238 patients presented with clinically evident disease in the neck (5). This was located in the thyroid gland in 67.2%, in the thyroid gland plus cervical lymph nodes in 13%, and in the cervical lymph nodes only in 19.7%. Thus, cervical lymphadenopathy was present at the time of presentation with or without a thyroid mass in 32.4% (5). Lymph node involvement is usually on the same side as the primary thyroid tumor, but in 10% of cases, cervical lymph node metastases are bilateral (4). Mediastinal lymph nodes become involved after the cervical lymph nodes (4). The presence of lymph node metastases at presentation does not seem to affect the prognosis, as noted in several series (8,14,15). Among antecedent clinical events, a history of irradiation of the neck for various thymic or skin conditions was obtained from as many as 6.6% of patients (5). In 16 patients, irradiation had been administered during the first year of life (6). The mean interval between irradiation and the appearance of PTC varied from 11 to 22.7 years (2,5). Hyperthyroidism and Hashimoto thyroiditis were also recorded in the history of patients with PTC (4,5). Lymph node metastases tend to undergo cystic degeneration, which may be so extensive as to be misdiagnosed as a bronchial cleft cyst (4).

HISTOPATHOLOGY

Papillary carcinomas of the thyroid are defined by their histologic (papillae) and cytologic (nuclei) features. The presence of either may be sufficient for the microscopic diagnosis, one or the other being considered more characteristic by various authors. The papillary pattern may be focal or predominant but is almost never exclusive. Microfollicular and macrofollicular, solid, trabecular, and cystic patterns may be admixed with the papillary pattern, exclusive, or combined in multiple patterns (16) (Figs. 90.1–90.5). Although usually mixed with a follicular pattern, the papillary pattern predominates; its prevalence is estimated by some authors to be as high as 55.7% (15). The size and shape of papillae vary from short and stubby to long and arborizing; they always project within a cystic cavity. The papillae consist of fibrovascular stalks containing thin-walled vessels and loose connective tissue lined by neoplastic epithelial cells. The presence of a fibrovascular stalk distinguishes true papillae from pseudopapillae, which result from occasional infoldings of the follicular epithelium or more commonly when spared pieces of epithelium hang in a cystic area of tissue de-

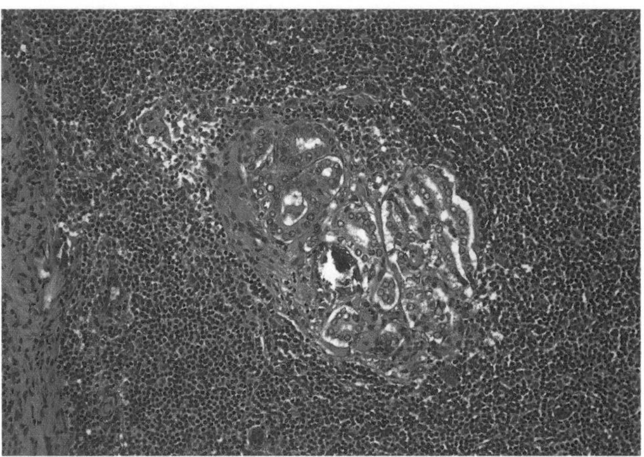

FIGURE 90.2. Metastatic papillary thyroid carcinoma in cervical lymph node. Psammoma body is present although papillae are inapparent. Hematoxylin, phloxine, and saffron stain.

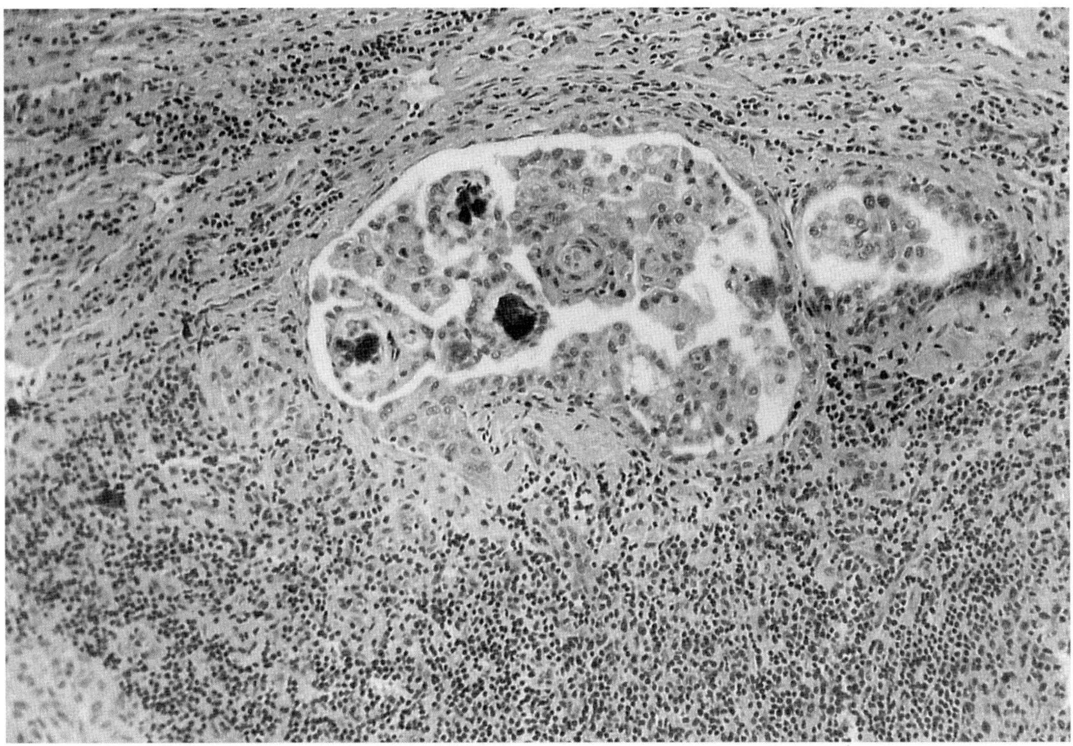

FIGURE 90.1. Cervical lymph node with two cystic spaces within the cortex containing short stubby papillae and psammoma bodies of metastatic thyroid carcinoma. Hematoxylin, phloxine, and saffron stain.

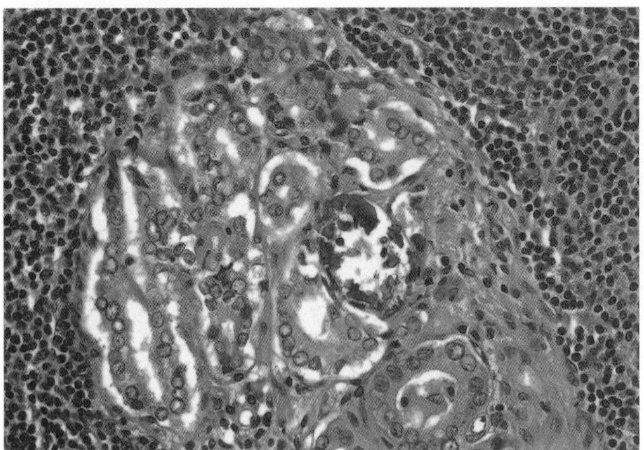

FIGURE 90.3. Same section as in Fig. 90.2. The cells lining the follicles exhibit chromatin clearing and occasional grooves, characteristic of the follicular variant of papillary thyroid carcinoma. Psammoma body in the center. Hematoxylin, phloxine, and saffron stain.

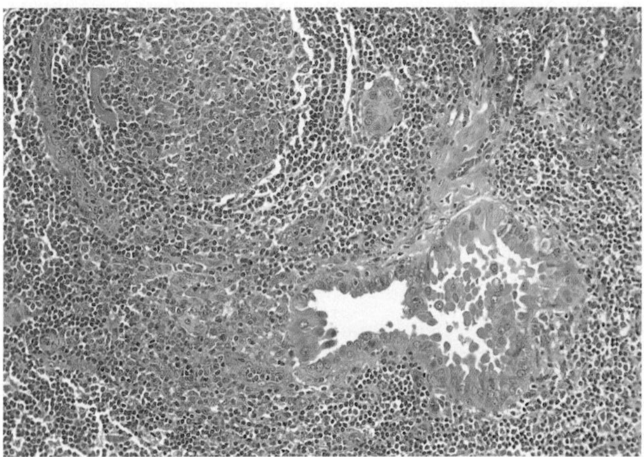

FIGURE 90.4. Cervical lymph node with reactive lymphoid follicle (*upper left*) and metastatic thyroid carcinoma forming cystic space and short projecting papillae. Hematoxylin, phloxine, and saffron stain.

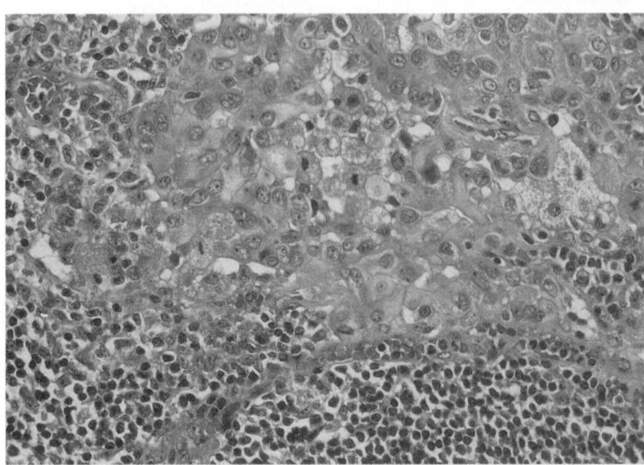

FIGURE 90.5. Same section as in Fig. 90.4 showing metastatic cells that have abundant cytoplasm and nuclei with occasional grooves. Hematoxylin, phloxine, and saffron stain.

generation. The papillary stalks may be swollen by edematous fluid, infiltrates of lymphocytes, or clusters of foamy macrophages.

Psammoma bodies—round, calcified concretions with a concentric laminar structure—are present in 40% (6) to 61% (16) of papillary carcinomas and in the lymph node metastases of such carcinomas (Figs. 90.1, 90.2 and 90.3); therefore, they represent an essential diagnostic criterion. They are usually located at the tips of the papillae or in the stroma. Concretions within follicles are not diagnostic (17).

The nuclei of the epithelial cells of papillary carcinoma are their most characteristic feature and are present regardless of the histologic pattern. The nuclei of PTC cells are enlarged, irregular in size and shape, and disoriented; they show nuclear grooves, pseudoinclusions, and chromatin clearing or margination (Figs. 90.3, 90.5, and 90.6). The chromatin changes are a fixation artifact and therefore not seen on frozen sections. Mitoses are extremely infrequent.

Follicles lined by cells with similar nuclei are present in virtually all PTCs. The number of follicles varies; they may form microscopic foci or be the predominant aspect of the tumor. In the follicular variant of PTC, the histologic pattern is mainly follicular, and the cells have nuclei with grooves, marginated chromatin, and pseudoinclusions (4,18).

A great propensity to metastasize to cervical lymph nodes is one of the characteristic features of PTC. The lymph node metastases tend to undergo cystic degeneration and form well-developed papillae, even more than the primary thyroid tumor. In the study of 241 cases of PTC of Carcangiu and co-workers (15), 52.6% of the lymph node metastases had a papillary pattern. In 78.5% of 42 cases in which the primary tumor was predominantly papillary, the nodal metastases showed this pattern, and in 45% of 31 cases in which the primary tumor was predominantly follicular, the nodal metastases were papillary.

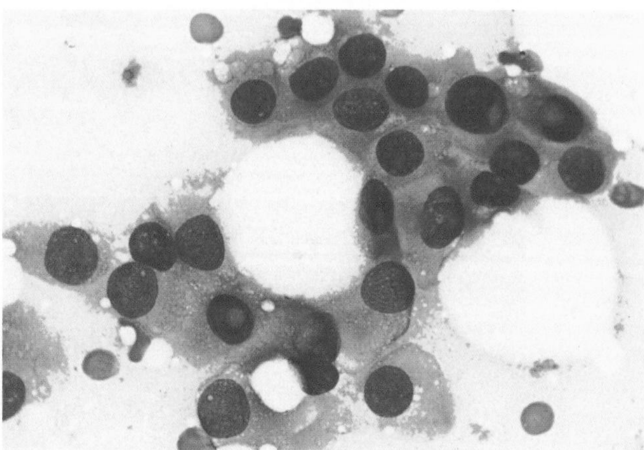

FIGURE 90.6. Fine needle aspiration biopsy specimen of metastatic thyroid papillary carcinoma. Epithelial cells have abundant cytoplasm and round nuclei with intranuclear cytoplasmic inclusions and occasional grooving. Giemsa stain.

CYTOPATHOLOGY

Fine needle aspiration (FNA) is now frequently used to investigate the thyroid and enlarged cervical lymph nodes. The diagnosis of FTC is based on the presence of capsular invasion, which cannot be assessed on FNA material. In contrast, the diagnosis of PTC is based on cytology—that is, characteristic nuclear features of the tumor cells, which are very well visualized on FNA smears (17). A papillary carcinoma, primary or metastatic in lymph nodes, also may be identified by the presence of fragments of papillae or psammoma bodies. The papillary fragments appear as three-dimensional multilayered fronds. The psammoma bodies present in about 50% of FNA specimens are seen as irregularly calcified debris, usually without the characteristic concentric laminations (19). In PTC, the aspirates contain numerous small clusters of cells with little colloid. In lymph node metastases, the cells of PTC are admixed with lymphocytes. The PTC cells may have nuclear grooves and a finely granular chromatin, usually without a ground-glass nuclear appearance. Intranuclear "pseudoinclusions" are frequently seen (19) (Fig. 90.6).

ELECTRON MICROSCOPY

All PTCs have abundant and pleomorphic microvilli and relatively few and irregularly arranged cilia (20). The cells have indented nuclei with a moderate amount of heterochromatin. The most conspicuous cytoplasmic organelles are mitochondria, and in rare cases microfilaments. The nuclear ground-glass appearance has been attributed to a particular state of chromatin during interphase, although consensus regarding an explanation has not yet been reached (20).

DNA ANALYSIS

Flow cytometric measurements show a very small percentage of PTC cells in S phase, which explains their rare mitoses and protracted growth. A relatively high death rate of tumor cells is also seen in both primary and metastatic lesions (20).

IMMUNOHISTOCHEMISTRY

The cells of PTCs contain intermediate filament proteins belonging to the family of cytokeratins and epidermal prekeratins. In addition, the cells contain vimentin. Thus, they can be stained by antibodies to both cytokeratin and vimentin (21). Thyroglobulin, normally synthesized by the thyroid follicular cells, can be used as a marker to detect metastases of thyroid carcinoma (Figs. 90.7 and 90.8). Epithelial membrane antigen (EMA) is also expressed by PTC (Fig. 90.9). In a study of 74 cases of PTC, expression of EMA was far greater in tumors with distant metastases (47%) than in those without (0%) (22). In a study of papillary carcinomas that included 26 cases of the follicular variant, a battery of cytokeratin monoclonal antibodies was

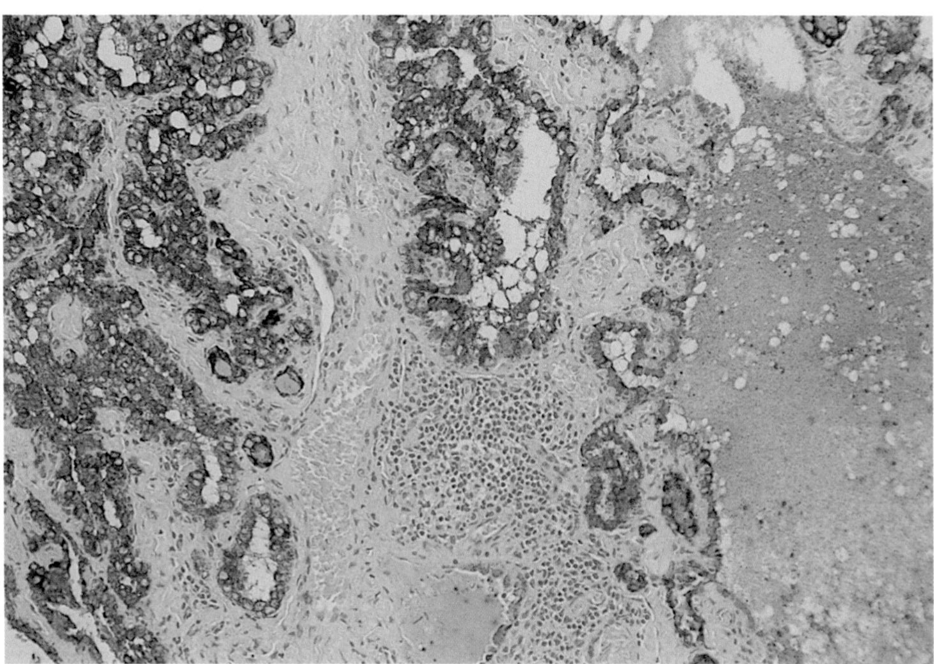

FIGURE 90.7. Metastatic papillary thyroid carcinoma in cervical lymph node forming multiple glandular and cystic structures. Intense staining of all cells for thyroglobulin. Thyroglobulin/peroxidase stain.

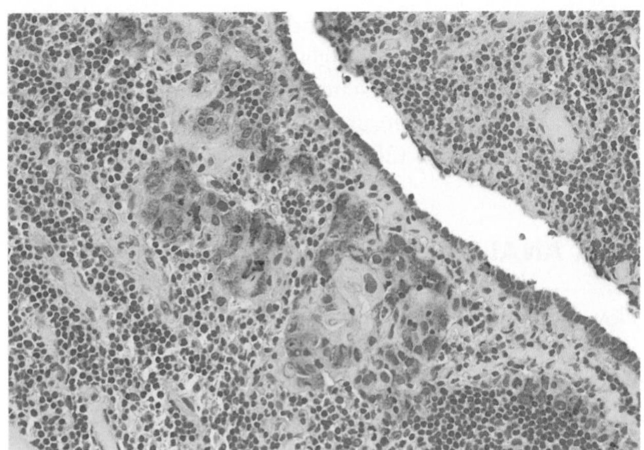

FIGURE 90.8. Same section as in Fig. 90.7. Clusters of thyroglobulin-positive metastatic thyroid papillary carcinoma cells. Thyroglobulin/peroxidase stain.

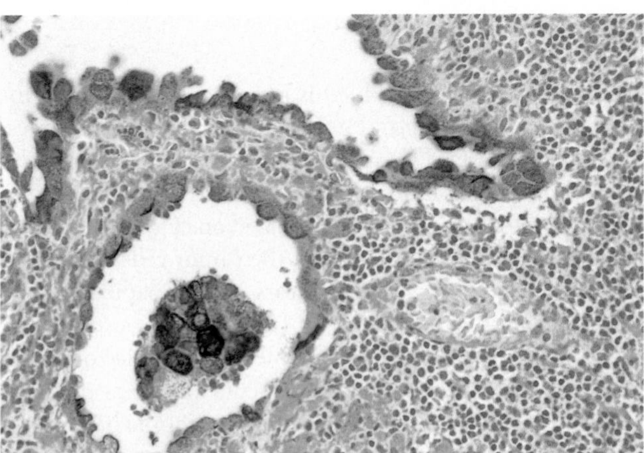

FIGURE 90.9. Metastatic thyroid carcinoma in same lymph node as in Fig. 90.7. Cells expressing epithelial membrane antigen (EMA) form cystic spaces and papillae. EMA/peroxidase stain.

used to assess their utility in the differential diagnosis of these forms of cancer. CK19 was expressed strongly and diffusely in all cases of papillary carcinoma, including follicular variants, but not in follicular adenoma, follicular carcinoma, or adjacent nontumorous thyroid tissue. CK17 and CK20 were expressed similarly but less intensely (23).

Phenotype

CK19+, CK17+, CK20+
Vimentin+, EMA+
Thyroglobulin+

DIFFERENTIAL DIAGNOSIS

- Benign thyroid inclusions are subcapsular nests of colloid-containing follicles lined by low cuboidal epithelium. Their size should be less than a third of the lymph node. Papillary structures, psammoma bodies, and ground-glass nuclei must not be present.
- Metastatic FTC is infrequent in cervical lymph nodes. Papillae, psammoma bodies, and ground-glass nuclei are absent.
- Metastatic ovarian papillary serous carcinoma is a rare occurrence in cervical lymph nodes. It may exhibit papillae and psammoma bodies, but it lacks ground-glass nuclei and is negative for thyroglobulin.

Checklist

LYMPH NODE METASTASIS OF THYROID CARCINOMA

Presence or history of PTC
Follicular variant of papillary carcinoma
Occult thyroid tumors
Cervical lymph nodes most commonly involved
Papillae
Cystic degeneration
Psammoma bodies
Grooved nuclei
Marginated chromatin
Intranuclear pseudoinclusions
Rare mitoses
Coexpression of cytokeratin and vimentin
Positive for thyroglobulin
Good prognosis even with lymph node metastases

REFERENCES

1. Greenlee RT, Hill-Harmon MB, Murray T, et al. Cancer statistics 2001. CA Cancer J Clin 2001;51:15–36.
2. Lieberman PH, Foote FW Jr, Schottenfeld D. A study of the pathology of thyroid cancer, 1930–1960. Clin Bull (MSKCC) 1972;2:7–12.
3. Hofstadter F. Frequency and morphology of malignant tumors of the thyroid before and after the introduction of iodine prophylaxis. Virchows Arch A Pathol Anat Histopathol 1980;385:263–270.
4. Rosai J, Carcangiu ML, DeLellis RA. Tumors of the thyroid gland. Atlas of tumor pathology, series III, fascicle 5. Washington, DC: Armed Forces Institute of Pathology, 1992.
5. Carcangiu ML, Zampi G, Pupi A, et al. Papillary carcinoma of the thyroid. A clinicopathologic study of 241 cases treated at the University of Florence, Italy. Cancer 1985;55:805–828.
6. McConahey WM, Hay ID, Woolner LB. Papillary thyroid cancer treated at the Mayo Clinic 1946 through 1970: initial manifestations, pathologic findings, therapy, and outcome. Mayo Clin Proc 1986;61:978–995.
7. Kahn NF, Perzin KH. Follicular carcinoma of the thyroid: an evaluation of the histologic criteria used for diagnosis. Pathol Annu 1983;18:221–253.
8. Woolner LB, Beahrs OH, Black BM, et al. Thyroid carcinoma: general considerations and follow-up data on 1,181 cases. In: Young S, Inman DR, eds. Thyroid neoplasia. London: Academic Press, 1968:51.
9. Hazard JB. Small papillary carcinoma of the thyroid. A study with special reference to so-called nonencapsulated sclerosing tumor. Lab Invest 1960;9:86.
10. Yamamoto Y, Maeda T, Izumi K, et al. Occult papillary carcinoma of the thyroid. A study of 408 autopsy cases. Cancer 1990;65:1173–1179.
11. Harach HR, Franssila KO, Wasenius V-M. Occult papillary carcinoma of the thyroid. A "normal" finding in Finland. A systematic autopsy study. Cancer 1985;56:531–538.
12. Bloch MA, Wylie JH, Patton RB, et al. Does benign thyroid tissue occur in the lateral part of the neck? Am J Surg 1966;112: 476–481.
13. Butler JJ, Tulinius H, Ibanez ML, et al. Significance of thyroid tissue in lymph nodes associated with carcinoma of the head, neck or lung. Cancer 1967;20:103–112.
14. Fransilla KO. Prognosis in thyroid carcinoma. Cancer 1975;36: 1136–1146.
15. Carcangiu ML, Zampi G, Rosai J. Papillary thyroid carcinoma: a study of its many expressions and clinical correlates. Pathol Annu 1985;20:1–44.
16. Klinck GH, Winship T. Occult sclerosing carcinoma of the thyroid. Cancer 1955;8:701.
17. Wenig BM. Thyroid papillary carcinoma, follicular type. Pathol Case Rev 2000;5:227–235.
18. Chan JKC, Saw D. The grooved nucleus. A useful diagnostic criterion of papillary carcinoma of the thyroid. Am J Surg Pathol 1986;10:672.
19. Brantley BD, Hartmann WH. The thyroid gland. In: Silverberg SS, ed. Principles and practice of surgical pathology, vol 2. New York: Churchill Livingstone, 1990:1883–1921.
20. Johannessen JV, Sobrinho-Simoes M. Well-differentiated thyroid tumors: problems in diagnosis and understanding. Pathol Annu 1983;18:255–285.
21. Miettinen M, Franssila K, Lehto UP. Expression of intermediate filament protein in thyroid gland and thyroid tumors. Lab Invest 1984;50:262–270.
22. Yamamoto Y, Izumi K, Otsuka H. An immunohistochemical study of epithelial membrane antigen, cytokeratin, and vimentin in papillary thyroid carcinoma. Cancer 1992;70:2326–2333.
23. Baloch ZW, Abraham S, Roberts S, et al. Differential expression of cytokeratins in follicular variant of papillary carcinoma: an immunohistochemical study and its diagnostic utility. Hum Pathol 1999;30:1166–1171.

91

METASTATIC RENAL CELL CARCINOMA

DEFINITION

Lymph node metastases of renal cell carcinoma.

PATHOGENESIS

Renal tumors account for 3% of all adult malignancies, and of these, clear cell carcinomas, the most common, make up more than 70% (1). Renal cell carcinoma of clear cell type is also the most common of all the clear cell tumors, and the one most likely to present as a metastasis of an occult primary tumor. In fact, clinical evidence of metastasis is found in 14% to 45% of cases at the time of first presentation (2,3). Familial cases of renal cell carcinoma are rare; however, they are associated with the von Hippel-Lindau syndrome in more than 50% of cases, in which they are usually bilateral (1). Renal cell carcinoma originates predominantly in the cells of the proximal convoluted tubules, as suggested by the close ultrastructural resemblance of the two types of cells (4). However, immunohistochemical studies have shown that renal carcinoma cells may also express markers characteristic of distal and medullary tubules (5), so that the histogenesis of this tumor is probably in uncommitted primitive cells capable of differentiating after neoplastic transformation into various tubular and even nontubular structures (6).

CLINICAL SYNDROME

Renal cell carcinoma is a tumor of adults; its peak incidence is in the sixth decade of life, but it occurs in children occasionally. Males are more frequently affected; the right and left kidneys are equally affected. The triad of hematuria, flank pain, and abdominal mass is usually seen with advanced tumors. In earlier stages, one of these signs or symptoms is more often encountered, in addition to fever, anemia, and weight loss. Paraneoplastic syndromes with vascular hypertension, hepatic dysfunction, and hypercalcemia resulting from the ectopic production of various hormones may be also present (7). Erythrocytosis occurs in up to 6% of patients, caused by the production of erythropoietin by the tumor cells.

In a third of patients, renal cell carcinoma presents with metastatic disease, which may be a solitary metastasis, so that diagnostic decisions are made difficult (1,7). More than half of the cases of renal cell carcinoma apparent at autopsy were clinically unrecognized, and 24% of cases are associated with unrecognized metastasis (8). The stage of the tumor is the most important prognostic feature, and the involvement of regional lymph nodes significantly affects survival. Stage IIIB, defined as involvement of the regional lymph nodes, is a more advanced stage than extension into the perirenal fat (stage II) or into the renal vein or inferior vena cava (stage IIIA). Many cases are probably understaged because a limited number of lymph nodes are removed with the kidney at surgery or because lymph nodes of apparent normal size and consistency are not removed (9).

From the kidneys, the tumor cells spread to the regional lymph nodes, but beyond that, much variability is seen, which probably indicates that the tumor has entered a phase of systemic spread (10). Therefore, when metastases in lymph nodes are identified, an extended lymphadenectomy is unlikely to increase survival and is therefore not recommended (11). However, in renal cell carcinoma, not all lymph nodes that appear enlarged on computed tomograms are the site of metastases, as they are in other urologic malignancies. In a study of 163 patients with renal cell carcinoma, more than half of the patients with regional lymph nodes measuring more than 1 cm on computed tomography had only tumor-reactive lymphadenopathy; this percentage was much higher than that noted in prostatic or bladder cancer, in which lymph nodes enlarged to a diameter of more than 1 cm harbored tumor metastases in more than 90% of cases (12).

HISTOPATHOLOGY

Renal cell carcinoma exhibits a variety of histologic patterns (e.g., trabecular, alveolar, papillary, solid) that may be isolated or combined; the cells can be clear, granular, or spindle cells. The most common pattern is one of clear cells arranged in a tubuloalveolar configuration. The tumor cells in clear cell carcinoma are bland, uniform, and polygonal, with abundant clear cytoplasm and small, hyperchromatic, centrally located nuclei. The tumors are richly vascular, with foci of hemorrhage, cystic degeneration, sclerosis, and focal calcification corresponding to the typically variegated appearance on the cut surface; this includes yellow-orange areas of abundant lipids, red-black areas of hemorrhage, and gray areas of little lipid content and fibrosis. Admixed with the clear areas may be foci of granular cells with nuclear pleomorphism and high mitotic rates, papillae with fibrous connective cores containing foamy macrophages and lined by one layer of uniform eosinophilic cells, and even areas of anaplastic spindle cells of pseudosarcomatous type. Renal carcinomas are graded by the Fuhrman scheme, in which four grades denote increasing nuclear pleomorphism. The prognosis is better for clear cell than for granular cell tumors; papillary tumors have the best outcome, and sarcomatoid the worst (1). The lymph node metastases generally have a histologic appearance similar to that of the primary tumor (Figs. 91.1 and 91.2).

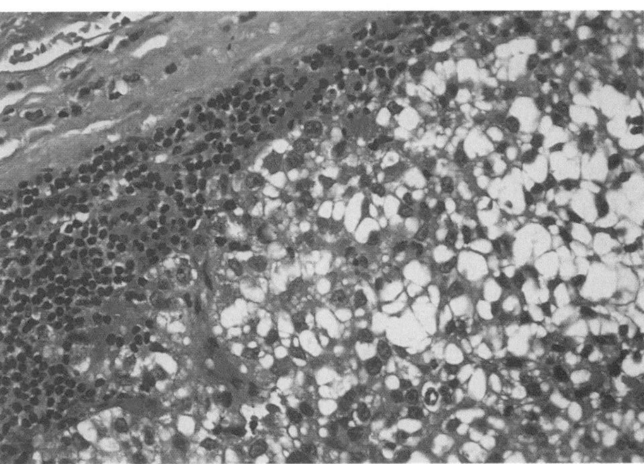

FIGURE 91.2. Same section as in Fig. 91.1. Lymph node capsule and residual lymphatic cortical tissue (*left*). Large polyhedral tumor cells with sharp borders, totally clear cytoplasm, and hyperchromatic, relatively small nuclei. Nucleoli and mitoses inapparent. Hematoxylin, phloxine, and saffron stain.

ELECTRON MICROSCOPY

Renal carcinoma cells have a characteristic ultrastructure of tubular differentiation and cells with small microvilli, reminiscent of a brush border. Numerous infoldings of the plasma membrane may be present, and abundant bizarre mitochondria. The cells contain abundant lipid vacuoles and glycogen.

HISTOCHEMISTRY

Renal clear carcinoma cells contain glycogen, lipids, and cholesterol, which can be stained with periodic acid–Schiff (PAS)/diastase-PAS, oil red-O, and Sudan IV, respectively.

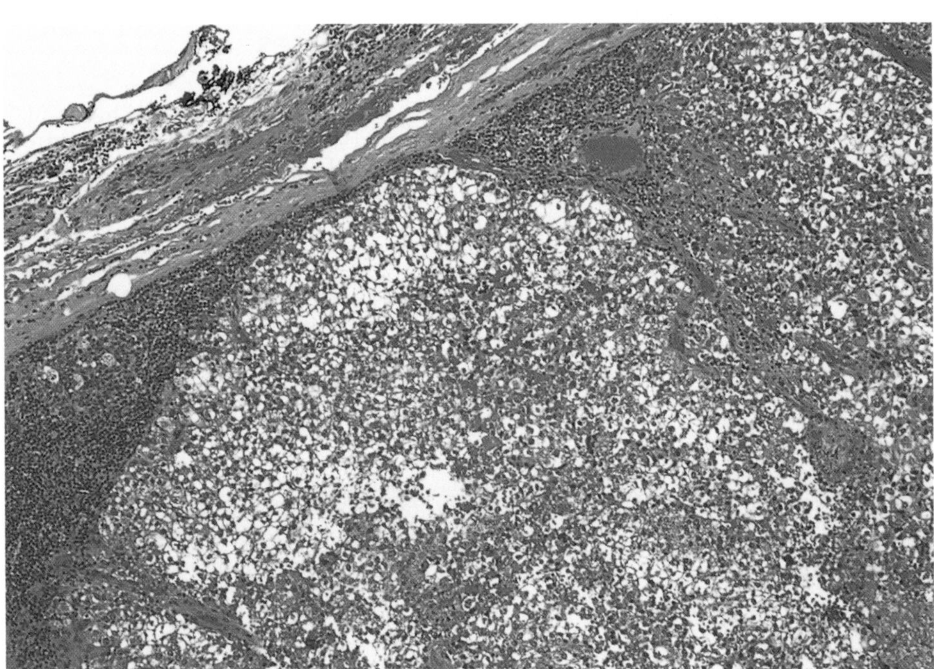

FIGURE 91.1. Metastasis of renal cell carcinoma in paraaortic lymph node. Large tumor mass replacing cortex and paracortex. Residual subcapsular lymphatic tissue (*left*). Hematoxylin, phloxine, and saffron stain.

Checklist

METASTATIC RENAL CELL CARCINOMAS

Most common metastasis from an occult primary tumor
Most common of all clear cell tumors
Patients middle-aged or older
Male predominance
Variegated appearance on cut section
Multiple histologic patterns
Clear cell type most common
Highly vascular, hemorrhagic
Uniform cell population
Intracytoplasmic glycogen and lipids
Metastases similar to primary tumor
Characteristic ultrastructure
Translocations of chromosome 3 in familial cases
Cytokeratin+, EMA+
Coexpression of cytokeratin and vimentin

IMMUNOHISTOCHEMISTRY

Renal clear cell carcinomas express low-molecular-weight cytokeratins and epithelial membrane antigen (EMA). Broad or specific monoclonal antibodies to keratins (BS-MAK) or other "keratin cocktails" (e.g., KC2, AE1/AE3) can also be used (13). Renal cell carcinoma may coexpress keratin and vimentin, a property shared with other carcinomas, such as gastric, ovarian, pulmonary, and thyroid carcinomas (12). Rare cases may also express carcinoembryonic antigen and S100 protein (1).

Phenotype

(Low-molecular-weight) cytokeratin+
EMA+, vimentin+

CYTOGENETICS

A deletion of the short arm of one of the two homologous chromosomes 3 has been observed in most renal cell carcinomas. In familial cases, translocations of chromosome 3 are seen (14).

DIFFERENTIAL DIAGNOSIS

- Lymphoma, large cell types, particularly T-cell type with clear cells: The cells are noncohesive, do not form nests and cords, and contain no glycogen. They have lymphocytic markers (CD45, CD3, CD7) and are negative for cytokeratins.
- Metastatic seminoma: The cells contain glycogen but not lipids. The ultrastructure is characteristic. Seminomas, but not embryonal carcinomas, are negative for cytokeratins.

REFERENCES

1. Murphy WM, Beckwith JB, Farrow GM. Renal cell carcinomas. In: Tumors of the kidney, bladder, and related urinary structures. Atlas of tumor pathology, series III, fascicle 2. Washington, DC: Armed Forces Institute of Pathology, 1994:92–152.
2. McNichols DW, Segura JW, De Weerd JH. Renal cell carcinoma: long-term survival and late recurrence. J Urol 1981;126: 17–23.
3. Tabbara WS, Mehio AM, Aftimos GP, et al. Metastatic renal cell adenocarcinoma. In: Kuss R, Khoury S, Murphy GP, et al., eds. Renal tumors. Proceedings of the first international symposium on kidney tumors. New York: Alan R Liss, 1982:317–336.
4. Tannenbaum M. Ultrastructural pathology of human renal cell tumors. Pathol Annu 1971;6:249.
5. Flemming S, Symes CE. The distribution of cytokeratin antigens in the kidney and in renal tumours. Histopathology 1987;11: 157.
6. Cohen C, McCue PA, DeRose PB. Histogenesis of renal cell carcinoma and renal oncocytoma. An immunohistochemical study. Cancer 1988;62:1946.
7. Peterson RO. Urologic pathology. Philadelphia: JB Lippincott Co, 1986:77.
8. Hellsten S, Berge T, Linell F, et al. Clinically unrecognized renal cell carcinoma. In: Kuss R, Khoury S, Murphy GP, et al., eds. Renal tumors. Proceedings of the first international symposium on kidney tumors. New York: Alan R Liss, 1982:273–275.

9. Robson CJ, Churchill BM, Anderson W. The results of radical nephrectomy for renal cell carcinoma. J Urol 1969;101:297–301.
10. Marshall FF, Powell KC. Lymphadenectomy for renal cell carcinoma: anatomical and therapeutic considerations. J Urol 1982; 128:677–681.
11. Siminowitch JP, Montie JE, Straffon RA. Lymphadenectomy in renal adenocarcinoma. J Urol 1982;127:1090–1091.
12. Studer UE, Scherz S, Scheidegger J, et al. Enlargement of regional lymph nodes in renal cell carcinoma is often not due to metastases. J Urol 1990;144:243–245.
13. Battifora H. Clinical applications of the immunohistochemistry of filamentous proteins. Am J Surg Pathol 1988;12[Suppl 1]:24– 42.
14. Kovacs G, Szucs S, De Reise W, et al. Specific chromosome aberration in human renal cell carcinoma. Int J Cancer 1987;40:171–178.

92

METASTATIC SEMINOMA

DEFINITION

Regional lymph node metastases of seminoma.

PATHOGENESIS

Seminomas represent 35% of all testicular tumors and 41% to 50% of primary germinal tumors of the testis (1). They may occur in a pure histologic form or in various associations with embryonal carcinoma, teratoma, and choriocarcinoma. Typical seminoma, the form discussed here in the context of clear cell tumors, occurs in patients whose average age is 40 years, which is 5 to 10 years older than the average age of patients with nonseminomatous tumors (2); it is almost never seen in children less than 10 years of age (3). Seminomas originate from primordial germ cells, as suggested by the ultrastructural resemblance of the two types of cells (4) and the high content of alkaline phosphatase and glycogen in both (5). A further argument for this origin is the occurrence of seminomas *in situ* within the seminiferous tubules (6). A number of conditions have been considered in the etiology of testicular tumors, particularly seminomas. Cryptorchidism is associated with 4% to 12% of tumors of the testes (7), and among these, seminoma is the most common (8,9). The risk for malignancy in undescended testes is estimated to be 14 to 40 times greater than that in descended testes (10,11). Viral infections and trauma have also been considered in the etiology of testicular tumors (10). An increased incidence in some families suggests predisposing genetic factors (12), and high levels of androgen at the age of maximum occurrence indicate promoting hormonal factors (13). The incidence of testicular tumors and seminomas in particular is increased in patients with AIDS and other forms of immunosuppression (14).

CLINICAL SYNDROME

The right testis is more often involved than the left in a ratio of 5:4 (10). Enlargement of the testis, with or without pain, occurs in 85% of the patients. The testis may be as much as 10 times its normal size, and the increase in volume may be diffuse or associated with palpable nodules (10). On section, the tumor is usually demarcated from the uninvolved testis; it may include foci of necrosis and hemorrhage, and it extends beyond the capsule to the epididymis, scrotum, or spermatic cord in more than 8% of cases (10). In 5% to 10% of cases, the first symptoms are caused by metastases (10,15). Seminomas are relatively low-grade malignant tumors with a high level of radiosensitivity. In one series, 75% of patients were alive 17 years after diagnosis (13).

Metastases of seminomas are relatively common and may be present in as many as 10% of patients at the time of diagnosis (10). They follow the lymphatic vessels to the common iliac and paraaortic lymph nodes (16). In 80% to 85% of cases, metastases remain restricted to the ipsilateral lymph nodes (10). From the retroperitoneal lymph nodes, metastases spread to the thoracic and left supraclavicular lymph nodes. Sometimes, supradiaphragmatic lymph nodes are involved when no tumor is present in the abdomen (16), and such metastases are often asymptomatic (2). Involvement of the epididymis is followed by spread through the epididymal lymphatics into the inguinal lymph nodes (16). Similarly, involvement of the scrotal skin permits the spread of metastases to the inguinal lymph nodes. Hematogenous dissemination also occurs, with metastases to internal organs.

Autopsy studies show that the paraaortic and iliac lymph nodes are involved in 71%, the liver in 54%, and the lungs in 37% of cases of seminoma. The left kidney and adrenal are far more often the site of metastases than their right-sided counterparts (10).

Seminomas were reported to occur in retroperitoneal (17,18) and mediastinal (17) sites in the absence of any testicular tumor. They were therefore considered to arise in ectopic testes. However, more detailed examination in many cases disclosed unsuspected microscopic foci of seminoma in grossly normal or atrophic testes. It is now accepted that seminomas in the retroperitoneum and mediastinum are in fact metastatic tumors with origins in occult primary testicular tumors, represented in some cases by *in situ* or microscopic foci of carcinoma (10,15) and in others by seminomas that spontaneously regressed (18,19). According to

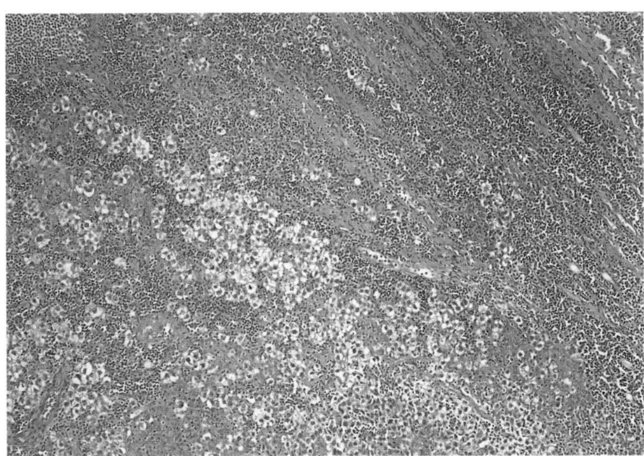

FIGURE 92.1. Metastasis of seminoma in pelvic lymph node. Clear neoplastic cells in sheets and nests or singly invade and replace the lymphatic parenchyma. Hematoxylin, phloxine, and saffron stain.

Abell and colleagues (17), a retroperitoneal seminoma, to be considered primary, must fulfill at least one of the following criteria: (a) appear encapsulated, with no adjacent lymph node involvement; (b) show non-neoplastic gonadal tissue next to the tumor tissue; or (c) show no metastatic involvement of the aortic, iliac, or pelvic lymph nodes distal to its location. Serum human chorionic gonadotropin (HCG) is mildly elevated in about 10% of patients with seminoma and in more than 25% of patients with metastatic seminoma (20). The elevated levels of HCG often correlate with the presence of syncytiotrophoblasts in the tumor.

HISTOPATHOLOGY

Typical seminomas are composed of lobules, cords, or sheets of uniform cells separated by fine fibrous septa that create a "cobblestone" effect (16). In some areas, the tumor cells are *in situ,* confined to the seminiferous tubules; in others, they infiltrate the testicular interstitium.

The metastases of typical and anaplastic seminomas have the morphologic features of seminoma in 65%, embryonal carcinoma in 26%, and teratoma in 4% of cases (10). Typical seminoma, the more common type of lymph node metastasis and the one more closely resembling some types of lymphoma, comprises a uniform population of tumor cells separated into regular lobules by a delicate fibroconnective stroma (Figs. 92.1 and 92.2). The cells are large, round, or polyhedral, with abundant, finely granular or clear cytoplasm and distinct cellular borders. The nuclei are round and centrally located, with one or two conspicuous nucleoli and occasional mitoses (Fig. 92.2). Typical seminomas are not highly mitotic and usually have fewer than three mitoses per high-power field (21). Foci of necrosis and scattered, degenerated, darkly staining cells are seen. Not infrequently, seminomas may include clusters of anaplastic cells with nuclear aberrations and atypical mitoses, or areas of embryonal carcinoma. The latter may form solid islands resembling seminoma, but the cells are larger, the nuclei more pleomorphic, and mitoses more frequent (Fig. 92.3). The cytoplasm of seminoma cells contains glycogen that is palely stained with periodic acid–Schiff (PAS) and sometimes lipid vacuoles. The stroma of seminomas is characterized by lymphocytic infiltrates and foreign body granulomas. The

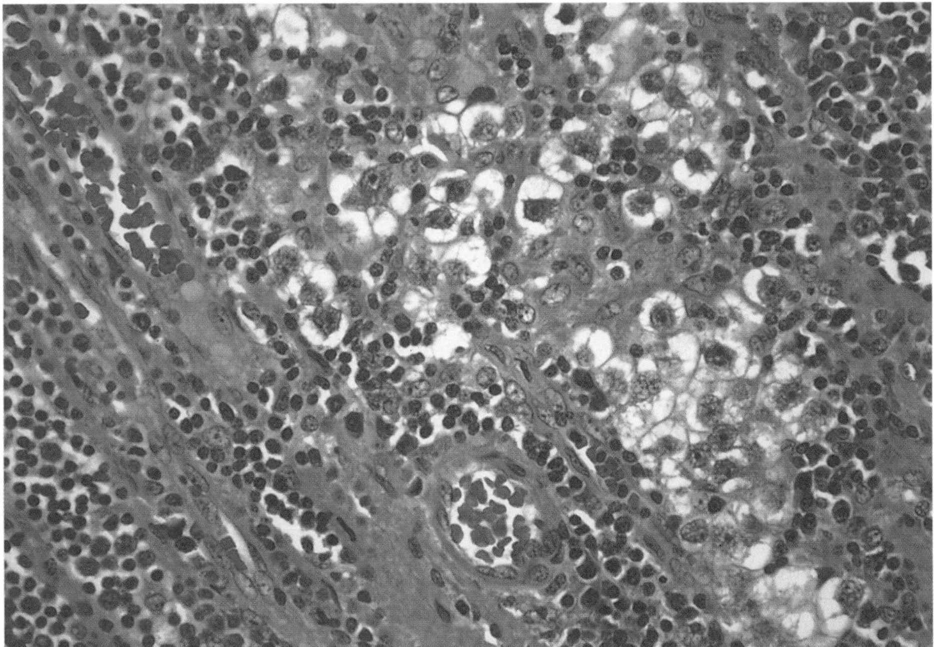

FIGURE 92.2. Same section as in Fig. 92.1. Metastatic seminoma cells are large and have totally clear cytoplasm, sharp borders, and round or pleomorphic voluminous nuclei with several prominent nucleoli. Hematoxylin, phloxine, and saffron stain.

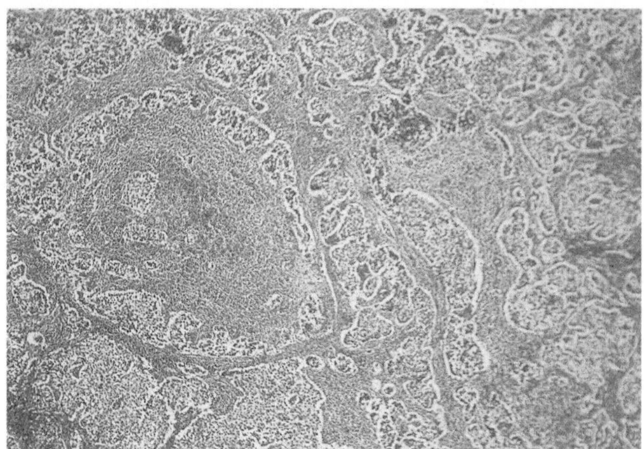

FIGURE 92.3. Lymph node metastasis of embryonal carcinoma. The cells lack clear cytoplasm and have large, relatively pleomorphic nuclei. Hematoxylin, phloxine, and saffron stain.

lymphocytes form scattered clusters and nodules that are prominent in 80% and marked in 20% of cases (10). Granulomas composed of epithelioid and multinucleated giant cells of foreign body type may be present in 50% and frequent in 20% of seminomas (10). Sometimes, the reaction is so intense as to simulate granulomatous orchitis. In two cases of lymph node metastases with occult primary tumors, the diagnosis of seminoma was suggested by PAS staining and a massive epithelioid granulomatous reaction (15).

The Langhans type of giant cells of granulomas must not be confused with multinuclear trophoblasts, which may also be seen in seminomas (21). The identification of trophoblasts, which appear as large, vacuolated masses of cytoplasm with multiple nuclei, is important for proper tumor classification. If such cells form an important component of the tumor, it is classified as a tumor of combined histologic type with a less favorable prognosis. However, isolated cells or small foci of syncytiotrophoblasts are generally not considered to affect the behavior of a seminoma (21). In typical seminomas, syncytiotrophoblasts are estimated to occur in 6% to 8% of cases (22), although when immunohistochemical methods are used to detect them, their prevalence is two or three times greater (21).

ELECTRON MICROSCOPY

The cytoplasm of seminoma cells includes numerous mitochondria and a well-developed endoplasmic reticulum with markedly distended and irregular cisternae. Glycogen is abundant and uniformly scattered. Membrane-bound granules, apparently derived from cisternae, are also present (10). The nuclei are large and variable with irregularly shaped nucleoli. The cell membranes are complex but lack desmosomes.

The reason for the clear appearance of seminoma cells is not established. Some believe it is caused by the presence of glycogen; others point to the relatively small amounts of glycogen and believe that seminoma cells have very few organelles, so that they appear clear (23).

CYTOCHEMISTRY

Seminoma cells are stained with PAS in the form of granules or clumps, not in an even fashion like mucus-containing cells. Diastase treatment (D-PAS) removes the staining. Alkaline phosphatase is also present in the cytoplasm of seminoma cells (21).

IMMUNOHISTOCHEMISTRY

Seminomas do not contain keratin and do not stain with anticytokeratin cocktails, in contrast to embryonal carcinomas of the testes (24). Seminoma cells show distinct membrane staining with placenta-like alkaline phosphatase (PLAP) antibody (Fig. 92.4). Immunohistochemical staining with peroxidase-labeled anti-HCG antibodies may reveal the presence of syncytiotrophoblasts containing HCG (25).

Phenotype

Cytokeratin−, PLAP+
HCG−/+

DIFFERENTIAL DIAGNOSIS

- Lymphomas of large cell type, particularly of T-cell type, may have clear cytoplasm, but the cells are noncohesive, do not form nests and cords, and do not contain glycogen. They express CD45 (leukocyte common antigen) and other lymphoid cell markers and do not express cytokeratins.
- Metastatic renal cell carcinoma cells contain both glycogen and lipids. The ultrastructure is characteristic. Cytokeratin and epithelial membrane antigen are expressed.
- Embryonal carcinoma, sometimes as part of a seminoma, may form gland structures. The cells are larger, with a higher rate of nuclear pleomorphism and frequent mitoses.

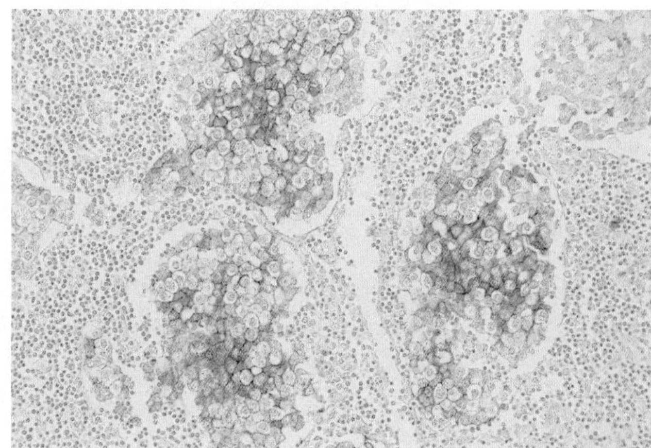

FIGURE 92.4. Lymph node metastasis of seminoma with positive reaction to placenta-like alkaline phosphatase (PLAP) antibody. PLAP/peroxidase stain.

Checklist

METASTATIC SEMINOMA

Middle-aged men, very rare in children
Presence or history of testicular tumor or undescended testis
Cords and sheets of seminoma cells
Delicate fibroconnective stroma
Foci of necrosis
Uniform cell population
Large cells, distinct cell borders
Abundant clear cytoplasm
Round nuclei, conspicuous nucleoli
Moderate number of mitoses
PAS+, D-PAS−
Few cytoplasmic organelles
Cytokeratin−, PLAP+
Foci of syncytiotrophoblastic cells occasionally present
Lymphocytic infiltrates
Foreign body giant cell granulomas
High radiosensitivity
Favorable prognosis

REFERENCES

1. Ulbright TM, Amin MB, Young RH. Germ cell tumors: seminomas. In: Tumors of the testis, adnexa, spermatic cord, and scrotum. Atlas of tumor pathology, series III, fascicle 25. Washington, DC: Armed Forces Institute of Pathology, 1999:59–102.
2. Krag Jacobsen G, Barlebo H, Olsen J, et al. Testicular germ tumors in Denmark, 1976–1980. Pathology of 1,058 consecutive cases. Acta Radiol Oncol 1984;23:239–247.
3. Perry C, Servadio C. Seminoma in childhood. J Urol 1980;124: 932–933.
4. Pierce GB. Ultrastructure of human testicular tumors. Cancer 1966;19:1963.
5. Hustin J, Collette J, Franchimont P. Immunohistochemical demonstration of placental alkaline phosphatase in various states of testicular development in germ cell tumours. Int J Androl 1987;10:29.
6. Skakkabaek NE. Atypical germ cells in the adjacent "normal" tissue of testicular tumors. Acta Pathol Microbiol Scand 1975;83:127.
7. Braunstein GD, Friedman NB, Sacks SA, et al. Germ cell tumors of the testis. West J Med 1977;126:382.
8. Merrin C. Seminoma. Urol Clin North Am 1977;4:379.
9. Halme A, Kellokumpy-Lehtinen P, Lehtonen T, et al. Morphology of testicular germ cell tumours in treated and untreated cryptorchidism. Br J Urol 1989;64:78–83.
10. Mostofi FK, Price EB Jr. Tumors of the male genital system: seminoma. Atlas of tumor pathology, series II, fascicle 8. Washington, DC: Armed Forces Institute of Pathology, 1973:21–39.
11. Gehring CG, Rodriguez FR, Woodhead DM. Malignant degeneration of cryptorchid testes following orchiopexy. J Urol 1974; 112:354.
12. Levey S, Grabstald H. Synchronous testicular tumors in identical twins. Urology 1974;6:754.
13. Nefzger MD, Mostofi FK. Survival after surgery for germinal malignancies of the testis. I. Rates of survival in tumor groups. Cancer 1972;30:1233–1240.
14. Leibovitch I, Baniel J, Rowland RG. Malignant testicular neoplasms in immunosuppressed patients. J Urol 1996;155:1938–1942.
15. Richter HJ, Leder LD. Lymph node metastases with PAS-positive tumor cells and massive epithelioid granulomatous reaction as diagnostic clue to occult seminoma. Cancer 1979;44:245–249.
16. Wheeler JE, Rudy FR. The testis, paratesticular structures, and male external genitalia. In: Silverberg SG, ed. Principles and practice of surgical pathology, vol 2. New York: Churchill Livingstone, 1990:1531–1585.
17. Abell MR, Fayos JV, Lampe I. Retroperitoneal germinomas (seminomas) without evidence of testicular involvement. Cancer 1965;18:272–290.
18. Meares EM, Briggs EM. Occult seminoma of the testis masquerading as primary extragonadal germinal neoplasm. Cancer 1972;30:300–306.
19. Azzopardi JG, Hoffbrand AV. Retrogression in testicular seminoma with viable metastases. J Clin Pathol 1965;18:135–141.
20. Ro JY, Dexeus FH, Naggar A, et al. Testicular germ cell tumors. Clinically relevant pathology findings. Pathol Annu 1991;26:59–87.
21. Gonzales-Crussi F. Testicular and paratesticular neoplasms. In: Sternberg SS, ed. Diagnostic surgical pathology, vol 2. New York: Raven Press, 1989:1455–1486.
22. Talerman A. Germ cell tumors of the testis. In: Fenoglio C, Wolff M, eds. Progress in surgical pathology, vol 1. New York: Masson, 1980.
23. Bosman FT, Orenstein JM, Silverberg SG. Differential diagnosis of metastatic tumors. In: Silverberg SG, ed. Principles and practice of surgical pathology, vol 1. New York: Churchill Livingstone, 1990:119–144.
24. Battifora H. Clinical applications of the immunohistochemistry of filamentous proteins. Am J Surg Pathol 1988;12[Suppl 1]:24–42.
25. Kuber W, Kratzik C, Schwartz HP, et al. Experience with HCG-positive seminoma. Br J Urol 1983;55:555–559.

93

METASTATIC PROSTATIC CARCINOMA

DEFINITION

Lymph node metastases of prostatic adenocarcinoma.

EPIDEMIOLOGY

In the United States and other developed countries, prostatic carcinoma is the most commonly diagnosed malignancy in men, accounting for 29% of all cancers, and the second leading cause of cancer death in men, accounting for 13% of the total (1). In the world, the incidence of prostatic carcinoma is only 9.2%, the fourth most frequent of all malignancies in men, and prostatic carcinoma accounts for 5.6% of all cancers (1). The reason for this large discrepancy is the introduction of screening for prostate-specific antigen (PSA), which between 1984 and 1994 resulted in a doubling of the number of cases in the United Sates. If the increase continues at a similar rate, 1 million cases per year can be expected by 2010 (1). A large number of these tumors reflecting differences in incidence between developed and undeveloped countries are latent asymptomatic prostate cancers in elderly men that would not be detected without PSA testing.

PATHOGENESIS

Prostatic carcinoma is staged according to the A–D system, in which stage A indicates occult nonpalpable tumors and stage D indicates metastatic tumors. Stage D is subdivided into D1, prostatic cancer with metastases to regional lymph nodes, and D2, with distant metastases. In stage D0, metastases are inapparent but levels of prostatic serum acid phosphatase (PSAP) are elevated, which in most cases indicates metastatic disease (2). The incidence of lymph node metastases correlates with the Gleason scores of the primary prostatic carcinoma. Thus, lymph node metastases occur on average in 12% of patients with prostatic adenocarcinoma and Gleason scores of 2 to 4, in 35% of those with Gleason scores of 5 to 7, and in 61% of those with Gleason scores of 8 to 10 (3,4).

CLINICAL SYNDROME

Pelvic lymph node metastases indicate a poor prognosis for patients with prostatic cancer, whether a single lymph node or multiple lymph nodes are involved. According to a survey of 511 patients with prostatic cancer followed for 8.6 years, the involvement of one pelvic lymph node indicated systemic disease unlikely to be controlled by lymph node dissection and radiotherapy (5). In a different study, bony metastases of prostatic carcinoma occurred in 18 of 32 patients with positive pelvic lymph nodes but in only 6 of 60 patients with negative pelvic lymph nodes (6).

Usually, the pelvic lymph nodes are examined on frozen section at the time of radical prostatectomy, and the operation is aborted if tumor metastases are found. In one study, microscopic metastases were demonstrated on frozen section in two-thirds of pelvic lymph nodes that appeared to be uninvolved grossly (7). The patients with positive pelvic lymph nodes who underwent radical prostatectomy in most cases had distant occult metastases; however, the survival of such patients (stage D1) was still as high as 97% at 5 years and 62% at 10 years (2).

Prostatic carcinomas often metastasize to supradiaphragmatic lymph nodes, most commonly left-sided cervical lymph nodes (8). Sometimes, the first manifestation of a prostate carcinoma is a metastasis in a left cervical lymph node. Because these are usually poorly differentiated carcinomas, their origin may remain undetermined unless a PSA immunostain is performed. A study of metastatic prostatic carcinoma identified 26 cases of metastases in supradiaphragmatic lymph nodes, of which 15 were supraclavicular, 8 cervical, 2 axillary, and 1 mediastinal, all of them on the left side (8). Some of these patients still had normal findings on rectal examination, normal PSA values, or both.

HISTOPATHOLOGY

The lymph node metastases of prostatic carcinoma are histologically similar to or less differentiated than the primary tumors (9). The majority of lymph node metastases are poorly differentiated; in a series of 29 cases, none was well differentiated (8). Often, the metastases are composed of solid sheets of tumor cells with large vesicular nuclei and prominent nucleoli, atypical mitoses, and areas of necrosis. Despite their poor differentiation, the tumor cells may still produce the characteristic enzymes, as in the study noted above; of the 29 cases examined, 26 were poorly differentiated, yet all were positive for both PSA and PSAP (8) (Figs. 93.1 and 93.2).

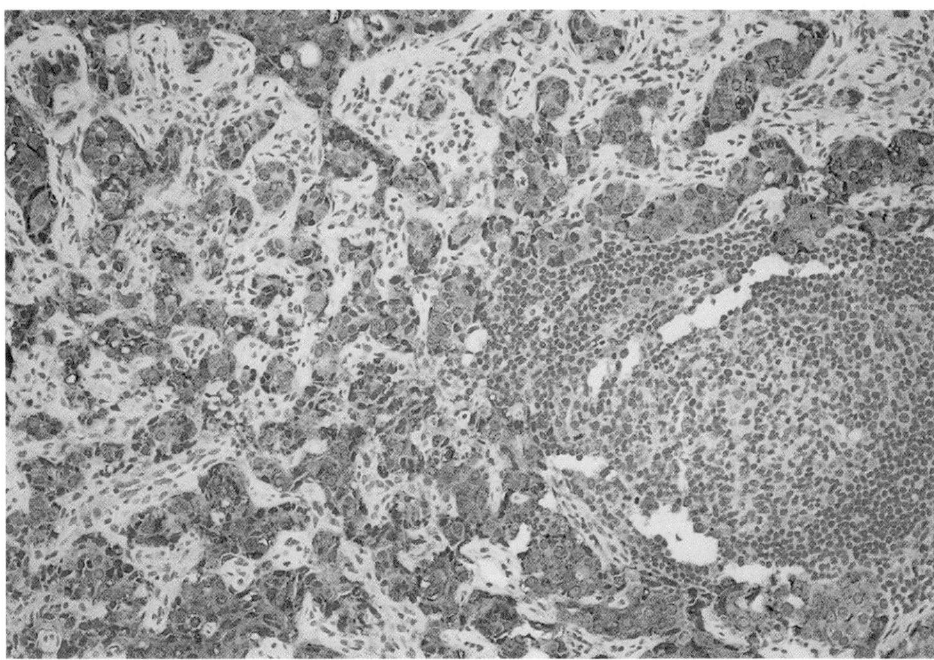

FIGURE 93.1. Metastatic prostatic carcinoma in pelvic lymph node surrounding lymphoid follicle with reactive germinal center. The cells are strongly positive for prostate-specific antigen (PSA). PSA/peroxidase stain.

IMMUNOHISTOCHEMISTRY

The immunohistochemical method of identifying prostatic adenocarcinoma by immunoperoxidase staining of prostate acid phosphatase (PAP) and PSA in tissue sections is sensitive and specific (2,10) (Fig. 93.3). Primary prostatic carcinomas and their metastases are positive for one or both markers. In a study of 47 metastases of prostate cancers, PAP was identified in 64% and PSA in 78% of cases (10). In a study of 16 autopsies of patients with prostate cancer, 11 cases had similar stainings for PAP and PSA in the primary and metastatic sites, 1 case lacked both antigens in all locations,

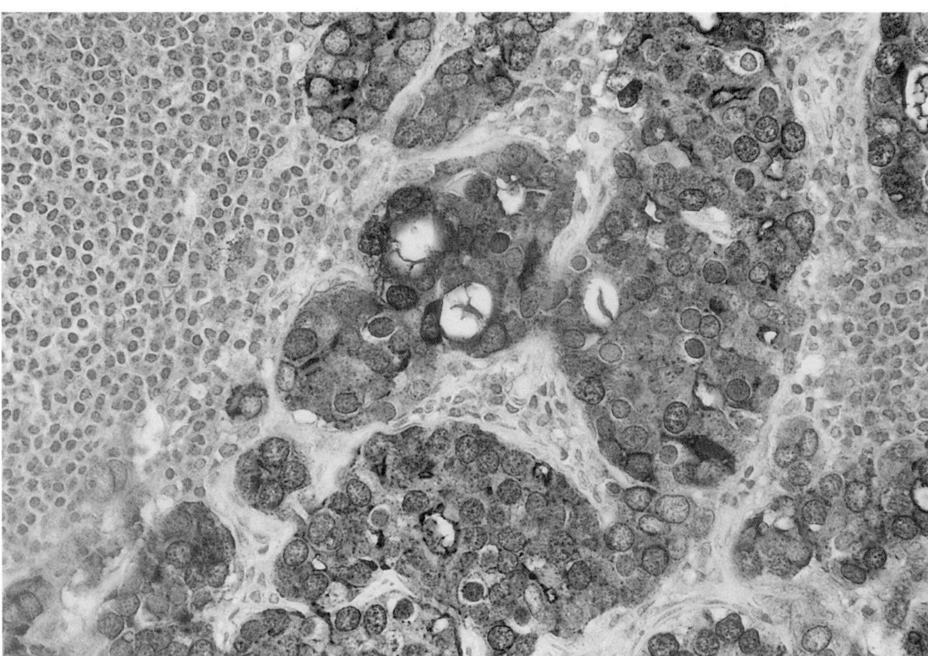

FIGURE 93.2. Same section as in Fig. 93.1. The metastatic carcinoma cells form cords and rudimentary glands. Abundant intracytoplasmic substance positive for prostate-specific antigen (PSA). PSA/peroxidase stain.

Checklist

METASTATIC PROSTATIC CARCINOMA

Elderly patients
Pelvic lymph node metastases
Left-sided supradiaphragmatic lymph nodes
Primary prostatic tumor sometimes occult
Poor histologic differentiation
PSA and PAP sensitive and specific

and 4 cases expressed one or the other (11). In yet another study, the pelvic lymph nodes of 38 patients who underwent dissection for staging were homogenized and tested for PSA (12). All patients with lymph node metastases had detectable PSA at dilutions of 1:100,000 (12). Well-differentiated and intermediately differentiated prostatic adenocarcinomas are generally positive for both markers, but 5% to 10% of poorly differentiated carcinomas (Gleason score of 8 to 10) are negative for at least one of the two antigens or show only focal stainings (13). PAP has produced better results in some cases and PSA in others; therefore it is recommended that both markers be used, particularly in metastatic cancers of unknown origin to identify the primary tumor (2). Focal and weak stainings for PSA and particularly PAP may be seen in breast or renal carcinomas; these are nonspecific and should be interpreted with caution (2).

DIFFERENTIAL DIAGNOSIS

- Adenocarcinomas of the prostate metastatic to lymph nodes, depending on the degree of glandular differentiation, may resemble adenocarcinomas of almost any other organ, especially special variants of prostatic adenocarcinomas, such as those with mucinous, squamous, or neuroendocrine differentiation. The chances of misdiagnosis are even greater in isolated and distant metastases, such as those in the left-sided cervical area. In all these cases, the use of immunoperoxidase staining with antibodies to both PSA and PAP is mandatory.

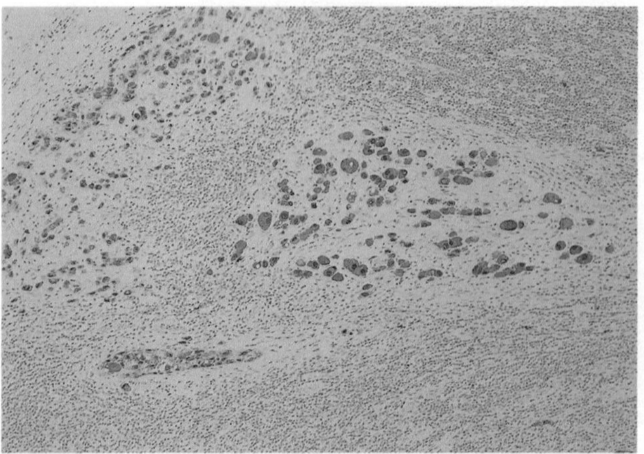

FIGURE 93.3. Prostatic carcinoma cells metastatic in sinuses of pelvic lymph node selectively stained by anti–prostate-specific antigen (PSA) antibodies. PSA/peroxidase stain.

REFERENCES

1. Parkin DM, Pisani P, Ferlay J. Global cancer statistics. CA Cancer J Clin 1999;49:33–64.
2. Epstein J. The prostate and seminal vesicles. In: Sternberg SS, ed. Diagnostic surgical pathology, 2nd ed., vol 2. New York: Lippincott–Raven Publishers, 1996:1807–1853.
3. Oesterling JE, Brendler CB, Epstein JI, et al. Correlation of clinical stage, serum prostatic acid phosphatase, and preoperative Gleason grade with final pathologic stage in 275 patients with clinical localized adenocarcinoma of the prostate. J Urol 1987; 138:92–98.
4. Smith JA, Seaman JP, Gleidman JB, et al. Pelvic lymph node metastases from prostatic cancer: influence of tumor grade and stage in 452 consecutive patients. J Urol 1983;130:290–292.
5. Gervasi LA, Mata J, Easley JD, et al. Prognostic significance of lymph nodal metastases in prostate cancer. J Urol 1989;142:332–336.
6. Prout GR, Heaney JA, Griffin PP, et al. Nodal involvement as a prognostic indicator in patients with prostatic carcinoma. J Urol 1980;124:226–231.
7. Epstein JI, Oesterling JE, Eggleston JC, et al. Frozen section detection of lymph node metastases in prostatic carcinoma: accuracy in grossly uninvolved pelvic lymphadenectomy specimens. J Urol 1986;136:1234–1237.
8. Cho KR, Epstein JI. Metastatic prostatic carcinoma to supradiaphragmatic lymph nodes. A clinicopathologic and immunohistochemical study. Am J Surg Pathol 1987;11:457–463.
9. McCullough DL, Prout GR, Daly JJ. Carcinoma of the prostate and lymphatic metastases. J Urol 1974;3:65–71.
10. Steffens J, Friedmann W, Lobeck H. Immunohistochemical diagnosis of the metastasizing prostatic carcinoma. Eur Urol 1985;11:91–94.
11. Stein BS, Vangore S, Petersen RO. Immunoperoxidase localization of prostatic antigens. Comparison of primary and metastatic sites. Urology 1984;24:146–152.
12. Shoskes DA, Trachtenberg J. The value of prostate-specific antigen levels in pelvic lymph nodes for diagnosing metastatic spread of prostate cancer. Can J Surg 1993;36:33–36.
13. Svanholm H. Evaluation of commercial immunoperoxidase kits for PSA and PSAP. Acta Pathol Microbiol Immunol Scand A 1986;94:7–12.

94

METASTATIC MUCINOUS ADENOCARCINOMA

DEFINITION

Lymph node metastasis of carcinoma composed predominantly of mucinous pools.

SYNONYM

Metastatic colloid carcinoma

PATHOGENESIS

Metastatic malignant disease of undetermined origin remains a frequent, difficult, and often frustrating problem of medical practice. About 2% of more than 1 million cases of cancer diagnosed between the years 1973 and 1987 in a study of the Scottish Health Service were listed as cancers of unknown primary site (1). Among the metastatic tumors of unknown origin, adenocarcinomas are by far the most common. In the study cited above, adenocarcinomas accounted for 55% and squamous cell carcinomas 14% of the total number of tumors. In a review of 1,539 metastatic tumors with unknown primary site from the Yale-New Haven Hospital Tumor Registry, 46.4% were adenocarcinomas, 11.6% squamous cell carcinomas, and 3.5% melanomas (2). Of the adenocarcinomas, 4.3% were listed as of mucinous type.

Mucin secretion is not uncommon in adenocarcinomas; however, in some, the mucinous substance forms more than half of the tumor mass. These tumors, classified as mucinous or colloid adenocarcinomas, have particular morphologic and clinical features. The most common sites of origin of mucinous adenocarcinomas are in the gastrointestinal tract, including, in order of frequency, the colon and rectum, stomach, ileum, and anal canal; these are followed by the pancreas, gallbladder, breast, ovary, and prostate. The regional lymph nodes are most often involved by the metastases, which exhibit the same mucinous pools as the primary tumors. Mucinous adenocarcinomas in general present as one of two subtypes: (a) *signet ring cell adenocarcinoma,* in which the mucin is mainly intracellular, with a characteristically eccentric nucleus and clear cytoplasm, and (b) *colloid or mucinous adenocarcinoma,* in which the mucin is mainly extracellular, accumulating in large pools in the surrounding tissues.

In the *gastrointestinal tract,* signet ring cell adenocarcinomas are more frequent in the stomach (3), and colloid (mucinous) adenocarcinomas are common in the colon (10% to 15% of all carcinomas of the large bowel) (4). Mucinous adenocarcinomas of the colon and rectum are more frequent in the young, and reportedly more malignant. Of 16 patients with colorectal carcinoma age 30 years or younger, 11 had adenocarcinomas of mucinous type, and their 5-year survival rate was only 18%; in comparison, the survival rate of the remaining patients, who had nonmucinous adenocarcinomas, was 33% (5). In the appendix, colon, and rectum, mucinous adenocarcinomas are usually associated with chronic ulcerative colitis (3). In the anus, mucinous adenocarcinomas may arise from the glandular crypts in the upper anal canal, from anal glands, and particularly from chronic fistulous tracts in Crohn disease (6,7).

Whether mucinous adenocarcinomas of the bowel have a worse prognosis than their nonmucinous counterparts has long been debated. Regional lymph nodes are involved in 60% of cases at presentation, and in as many as 90% in cases of signet ring cell carcinomas of the rectum (4). However, the poorer prognosis may reflect a longer, more indolent course and consequently tumors that are more advanced at the time of diagnosis (4,6).

The *pancreas* and *gallbladder* are also sources of mucinous adenocarcinomas characterized by large mucin pools (8–10). The tumor cells spread through the interstitial tissues and along perineural sheaths and lymphatic channels to the parapancreatic lymph nodes and liver (8).

Breast cancer, particularly lobular carcinoma, frequently produces mucin; however, colloid or mucinous carcinomas are relatively infrequent, constituting about 2% of all invasive breast tumors (11). In contrast to mucinous adenocarcinomas of the colon and rectum, which are more common in younger persons and have a worse prognosis than their nonmucinous counterparts, the mucinous variant of breast cancer is more common in older women and has a better prognosis (11,12). In a study of breast carcinomas, 1% were of mucinous type in women younger than 35 years and 7% in women older than 75 years (13).

The *prostate* may also give rise to mucinous adenocarcinomas. Although infrequent, this type of carcinoma is clinically important because of its aggressive biologic behavior and poor response to hormone treatment (14). Prostate-specific antigen (PSA) and prostatic serum acid phosphatase (PSAP) immunostainings are useful in excluding other sources of mucinous carcinomas.

CLINICAL SYNDROME

The clinical symptoms of the various mucinous adenocarcinomas are related to the organs of origin. No sex predilection is noted for gastrointestinal mucinous adenocarcinomas, but they do tend to affect younger patients, which may reflect their association with chronic ulcerative colitis and Crohn disease (3,4). All tumors have in common a bulky gross appearance, with rounded borders, soft consistency, glistening cut surfaces, and cystic structures oozing a grayish, gelatinous substance.

The lymphatic spread of colon carcinomas was studied in relation to the local depth of invasion of the primary colonic tumor (15). When 12,496 lymph nodes from 164 patients (a mean of 76.2 lymph nodes per patient) were cleared and mapped, lymph node metastases were found in 58.5% of cases. Of these lymph nodes, more than half were less than 4 mm in diameter. An unexpected number of lymph nodes with metastases were close to the proximal and distal margins of resection, so that the authors recommended excisions extending at least 7 cm from the tumor in both directions in addition to excision of the mesentery with intermediate and central lymph nodes adjacent to the mesenteric arteries (15). Mucinous colonic adenocarcinomas are particularly prone to wide dissemination, even small primary tumors (16). Because the required extensive lymphadenectomy suggested by such studies cannot be achieved by laparoscopic colonic resection, this procedure is not recommended in the case of colonic carcinoma (16).

Similar observations were made in regard to lymph node metastases of gastric carcinomas; poor detection of these was reported in various studies in which computed tomography, endoscopic ultrasonography, or even intraoperative assessment was used (17). The classification of lymph node metastases in gastric cancer for prognostic correlations was based on the location of the lymph nodes involved (perigastric lymph nodes within 3 cm of or more than 3 cm from the edge of the primary tumor) or the number of lymph nodes involved (1 to 6, 7 to 15, and >15). The classification based on the number of lymph nodes involved has better reproducibility and is at present generally preferred (18).

HISTOPATHOLOGY

Signet ring cell carcinomas are composed of discohesive single cells infiltrating other tissues or floating in pools of mucus with little or no gland formation. Lobular carcinoma of the breast often forms mucin-containing signet ring cell metastases in the axillary lymph nodes (Fig. 94.1). The cells appear clear and distended by the mucinous secretion, which pushes the nuclei peripherally (Fig. 94.2). The signet ring cells may infiltrate diffusely the fibromuscular walls of stomach and colon, transforming them into narrow, rigid, hard, tubular structures, often identified as linitis plastica (3).

Colloid or mucinous carcinomas are predominantly composed of pools of mucin that vary in size, some being visible macroscopically. Some of the mucin pools have lost part or all of their cellular lining, sometimes appearing entirely acellular (Fig. 94.3). The residual cells lining the lakes of mucus usually appear dysplastic, with only moderately atypical nuclei (Fig. 94.4). Free cells of signet ring cell type, singly or in small clusters, float in the mucus. In the affected lymph nodes, the early metastatic colonies are in the marginal sinuses. In time, the metastases extend into the sinuses, which are distended by mucus and signet ring cells, and into the parenchyma, forming the same large pools as in the organs of origin (Fig. 94.5). In the breast, lobular carcinomas more often display mucinous forms, which may vary from intracellular droplets of stainable mucin to poorly cellular mucin pools in the breast and axillary lymph nodes. Some lobular carcinomas have a distinctive targetoid or bull's-eye pattern of mucin staining around the nucleus (19) (Fig. 94.2). Metastatic lobular carcinoma in a lymph node can closely resemble lymphoma because of the absence of glandular structures and the lymphoid appearance of the uniform, small, round carcinoma cells arranged in diffuse sheets devoid of fibrosis (20).

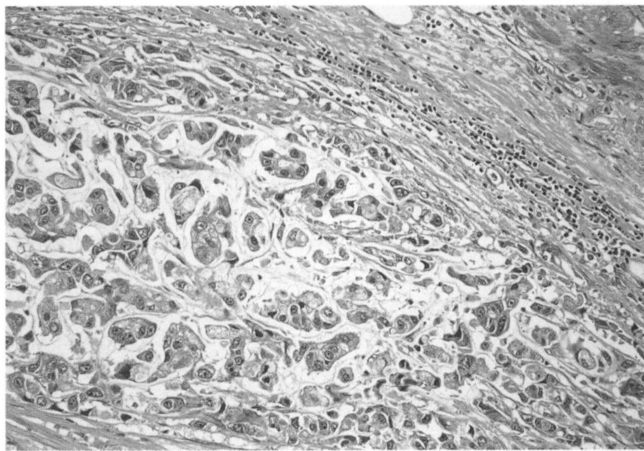

FIGURE 94.1. Metastatic gastric adenocarcinoma. Signet ring cells, singly or in glandular formations, are within pools of mucus. Hematoxylin, phloxine, and saffron stain.

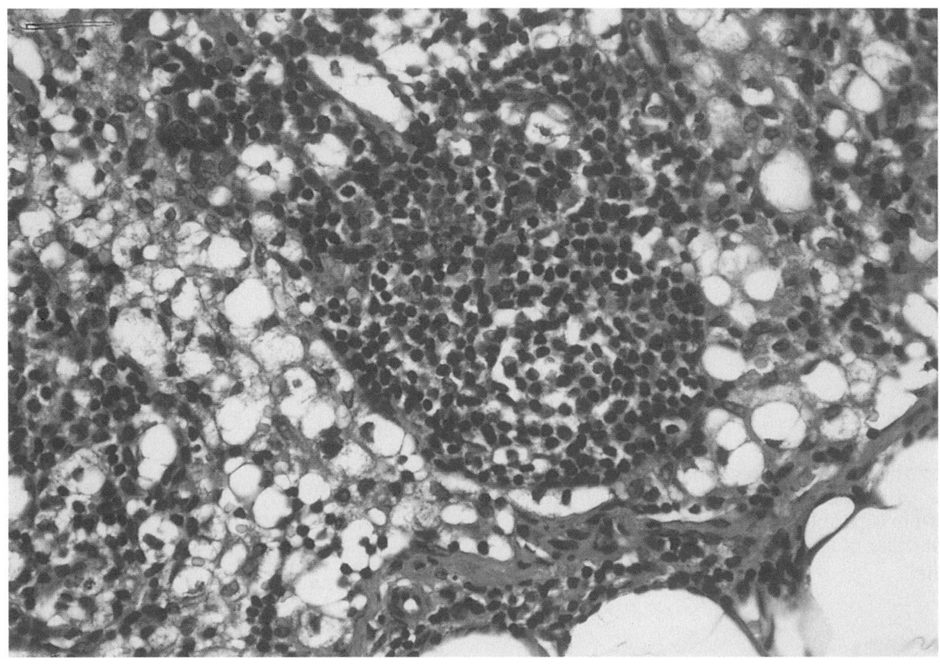

FIGURE 94.2. Metastatic mammary lobular carcinoma in axillary lymph node. Lymphoid parenchyma is largely replaced by signet ring cells with clear mucinous cytoplasm and peripheralized nuclei. Hematoxylin, phloxine, and saffron stain.

ELECTRON MICROSCOPY

The mucin-secreting cells have a dilated rough endoplasmic reticulum, large Golgi bodies, and mucin granules contained within smooth membranes (12).

HISTOCHEMISTRY

Results of staining with mucicarmine, Alcian blue, and periodic acid–Schiff (PAS) are all positive.

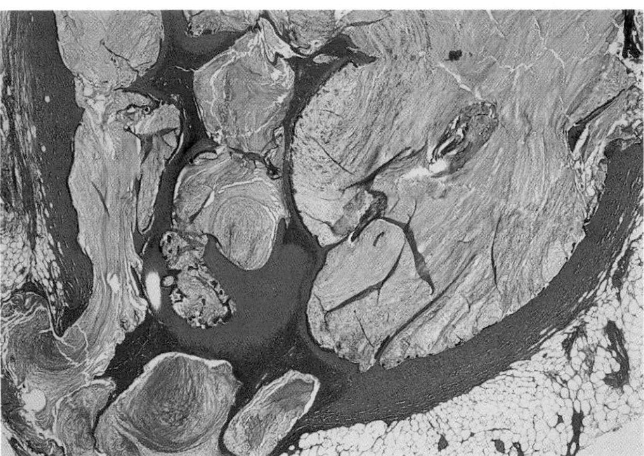

FIGURE 94.3. Metastatic rectal mucinous adenocarcinoma in pararectal lymph node. Nodal parenchyma is totally replaced by large, acellular lakes of mucus. Hematoxylin, phloxine, and saffron stain.

IMMUNOHISTOCHEMISTRY

Adenocarcinomas of all subtypes express cytokeratins that can be visualized by immunostaining with broadly specific monoclonal antibodies to keratins (BS-MAK) or various "keratin cocktails" (21). Cytokeratin staining is useful to detect micrometastases, even of single tumor cells, and distinguish metastatic lobular carcinomas resembling lymphomas. The differentiation of metastatic adenocarcinomas

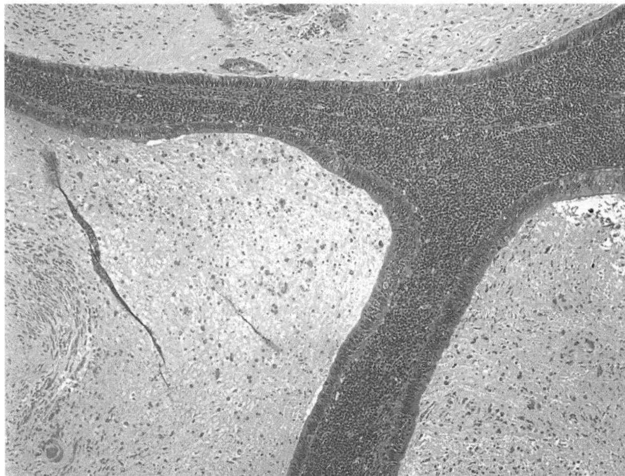

FIGURE 94.4. Metastatic colonic mucinous adenocarcinoma in pericolic lymph node. Large lakes of mucus separated by residual lymphatic parenchyma are lined by well-differentiated, columnar, mucin-secreting carcinoma cells. Hematoxylin, phloxine, and saffron stain.

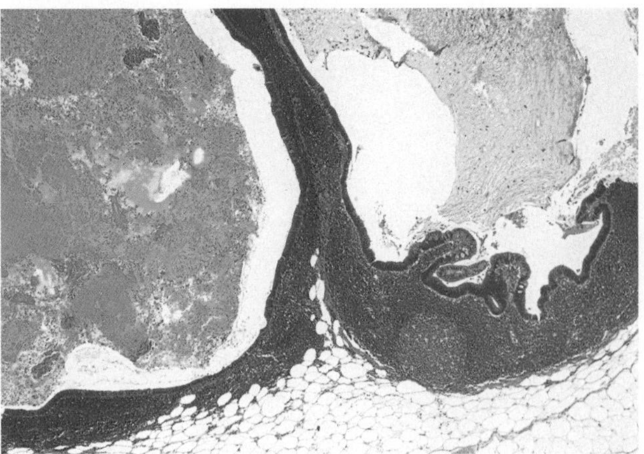

FIGURE 94.5. Metastasis of colonic carcinoma in pericolic lymph node. Large pools of mucus have replaced the lymphoid parenchyma, which persists only as a narrow subcapsular rim with one reactive follicular germinal center. Hematoxylin, phloxine, and saffron stain.

from squamous carcinomas by immunostaining is not reliable. Although squamous cell carcinomas express keratins of higher molecular weight than those of adenocarcinomas, overlapping between them makes the distinction imprecise (21).

The prognostic significance of micrometastases in colorectal cancer detected by immunohistochemistry or polymerase chain reaction has not yet been established and remains controversial. In a study of 1,633 lymph nodes from 44 patients, immunohistochemistry with three antibodies for cytokeratin was used to detect micrometastases (22). Micrometastases were detected in 7.8% of the regional lymph nodes examined, a number similar to those reported by other studies; however, the positive lymph nodes were equally distributed between patients who did and patients who did not have tumor recurrence. Similarly, occult lymph node micrometastases detected by polymerase chain reaction did not correlate with patient prognosis (23).

DIFFERENTIAL DIAGNOSIS

- Reactive sinus histiocytosis shows dilated, pale-staining lymph node sinuses and occasional histiocytes resembling signet ring cells. PAS and mucicarmine staining or cytokeratin immunostaining easily makes the distinction.
- Silicone-containing histiocytes in patients with leaking breast implants (see Chapter 51) resemble metastases of lobular mammary carcinoma.
- Glandular inclusions with a mucinous component are occasionally encountered in pelvic lymph nodes. However, small amounts of stroma surround the ectopic glands in such inclusions, which is not seen in their malignant counterparts, and their nuclei lack atypical features.
- Non-Hodgkin lymphoma may be occasionally suggested by the appearance of metastatic lobular carcinoma. PAS, mucicarmine, and cytokeratin stainings may be used to confirm the diagnosis.
- Polyvinyl pyrrolidone, sometimes used as a plasma expander, may be carried to lymph nodes and produce mucicarmine-positive histiocytes that resemble metastatic mucinous carcinoma (24).

Checklist

METASTATIC MUCINOUS ADENOCARCINOMA

Primary tumors of stomach, colon, rectum, appendix, pancreas, gallbladder, breast, and prostate
Patients younger and aggressive course in colon and rectum mucinous carcinomas
Associated with ulcerative colitis, Crohn disease
Patients older and less aggressive course in breast mucinous carcinomas
Associated with lobular breast carcinoma
Signet ring cell type with intracellular mucin
Colloid or mucinous type with extracellular mucin
Mucus pools
Mucous secretion stains with PAS, mucicarmine, and Alcian blue
Carcinoma cells positive for cytokeratin

REFERENCES

1. Muir C. Cancer of unknown primary site. Cancer 1995;75:353–356.
2. Altman E, Cadman E. An analysis of 1,539 patients with cancer of unknown primary site. Cancer 1986;57:120–124.
3. Pascal RR, Perzin KH, Fenoglio-Preiser CM. Neoplastic diseases of the small and large intestine. In: Silverberg SG, ed. Principles and practice of surgical pathology, vol 2. New York: Churchill Livingstone, 1990:1185–1240.
4. Lewin KJ, Riddel RH. Colorectal carcinoma. In: Lewin KJ, Riddell RH, Weinstein WM, eds. Gastrointestinal pathology and its clinical implications. New York: Igaku-Shoin, 1992:1256–1317.
5. Mills SE, Allen MS. Colorectal carcinoma in the first three decades of life. Am J Surg Pathol 1979;3:443.
6. Antonioli DA, Appelman HD. Anus and perianal area. In: Sternberg SS, ed. Diagnostic surgical pathology, 2nd ed., vol 2. New York: Lippincott–Raven Publishers, 1994:1613–1631.
7. Jones EA, Morson BC. Mucinous adenocarcinomata in anorectal fistulae. Histopathology 1984;8:279–292.
8. Solcia E, Capella C, Kloppel G. Tumors of the pancreas. Washington, DC: Armed Forces Institute of Pathology, 1997 (Atlas of tumor pathology, series III, fascicle 20).
9. Oertel JE, Oertel YC, Heffess CS. Pancreas. In: Sternberg SS, ed. Diagnostic surgical pathology, 2nd ed., vol 2. New York: Lippincott–Raven Publishers, 1994:1419–1459.
10. Saul SH. Gallbladder and extrahepatic biliary tree. In: Sternberg SS, ed. Diagnostic surgical pathology, 2nd ed., vol 2. New York: Lippincott–Raven Publishers, 1994:1581–1613.
11. Sakamoto G. Infiltrating carcinoma: major histological types. In: Page DL, Anderson TJ, eds. Diagnostic histopathology of the breast. New York: Churchill Livingstone, 1987:193–236.
12. Gompel C, Faverly D, Silverberg SG. Mucinous carcinoma of the breast. In: Silverberg SG, ed. Principles and practice of surgical pathology, vol 1. New York: Churchill Livingstone, 1990:354.
13. Rosen PP, Lesser ML, Kinne DW. Breast carcinoma at the extremes of age: a comparison of patients younger than 35 years and older than 75 years. J Surg Oncol 1985;28:90–96.
14. Epstein JI. The prostate and seminal vesicles. In: Sternberg SS, ed. Diagnostic surgical pathology, 2nd ed., vol 2. New York: Lippincott–Raven Publishers, 1994:1807–1853.
15. Hida J, Yasutomi M, Maruyama T, et al. The extent of lymph node dissection for colon carcinoma: the potential impact on laparoscopic surgery. Cancer 1997;80:188–192.
16. De Cosse JJ. Depth of invasion of colon carcinoma, lymphatic spread, and laparoscopic surgery. Cancer 1997;80:177–178.
17. Nakamura K, Morisaki T, Noshiro H, et al. Morphometric analysis of regional lymph nodes with and without metastasis from early gastric carcinoma. Cancer 2000;88:2438–2442.
18. Roder JD, Bottcherr K, Busch R, et al. Classification of regional lymph node metastasis from gastric carcinoma. Cancer 1998;82:621–631.
19. Gad LA, Azzopardi JG. Lobular carcinoma of the breast: a special variant of mucin-secreting carcinoma. J Clin Pathol 1975;28:711–716.
20. Blackshaw AJ. Metastatic tumours in lymph nodes. In: Stansfeld AG, ed. Lymph node biopsy interpretation. New York: Churchill Livingstone, 1985:380–397.
21. Batttifora H. Clinical applications of the immunohistochemistry of filamentous proteins. Am J Surg Pathol 1988;12[Suppl 1]:24–42.
22. Nakanishi Y, Ochiai A, Yamauchi Y, et al. Clinical implications of lymph node micrometastases in patients with colorectal cancers. Oncology 1999;57:276–280.
23. Yamamoto N, Kato Y, Yanagisawa A, et al. Predictive value of genetic diagnosis for cancer micrometastasis. Cancer 1997;80:1393–1398.
24. Groisman GM, Amar M, Weiner P, et al. Mucicarminophilic histiocytosis (benign signet-ring cells) and hyperplastic mesothelial cells. Arch Pathol Lab Med 1998;122:282–284.

95

METASTATIC NEUROENDOCRINE TUMORS

DEFINITION

Metastases from the tumors of the diffuse endocrine system.

PATHOGENESIS

Neuroendocrine tumors encompass a broad spectrum of neoplasms ranging from benign carcinoids to highly malignant small cell carcinomas (1,2). They are located mostly, although not exclusively, in the aerodigestive tract, which comprises the organs derived from the foregut, midgut, and hindgut. They arise from cells with endocrine activity scattered along the bronchopulmonary and gastrointestinal tracts. Other endocrine cells, present in the pituitary, thymus, thyroid, pancreas, and adrenals, are also included in the diffuse endocrine system as described by Feyrter (3). The classic studies of Pearse determined that these cells have in common the capacity for *a*mine *p*recursor *u*ptake and *d*ecarboxylation (APUD). They synthesize bioactive amines and polypeptide hormones and were named *APUD cells* for their acronym (4). The neoplasms derived from APUD cells, often referred to as *APUDomas,* were believed to originate from cells of the neuroectodermal crest that had migrated to various locations. However, the presence of cells of the endocrine type in a variety of locations, in addition to their identification by electron microscopy and immunohistochemistry in tissues of other derivations, suggested that the cells of the diffuse endocrine system are of endodermal rather than neural crest origin. This opposite concept was strengthened by the demonstration of endocrine features, such as secretory granules and neuroendocrine markers, within various neoplastic epithelial cells (5). Therefore, the presently accepted concept is that cells of endodermal derivation have the capacity to differentiate into the endocrine cells scattered among the epithelial cells of the aerodigestive tract, from which carcinoids and small cell carcinomas may originate. The presence of both endocrine and nonendocrine cells in some carcinoid tumors supports the idea that these neoplasms are derived from primitive cells capable of differentiation in multiple directions (1,2,6).

In the gastrointestinal tract, carcinoid tumors may arise in the base of mucosal crypts or even in the submucosa from endocrine cells of the gut that are widely distributed from the cardia to the anus (7).

In the bronchopulmonary tract, neuroendocrine tumors are believed to derive from the Kulchitsky cells, which are neuroendocrine cells in the basal area of the bronchial and bronchiolar mucosa (8). As in the gastrointestinal tract, these cells are part of a dispersed neuroendocrine system originating from immature pluripotent cells that differentiate under the influence of local factors. According to these concepts, small cell carcinomas arise from endodermal stem cells that have the potential to give rise to bronchial epithelial cells or to small basal reserve cells with neuroendocrine features (1,9).

All carcinoids are capable of invasion and metastasis, but in general their clinical course is rather benign (10,11). However, carcinoids belong to a spectrum of neuroendocrine tumors ranging from typical benign carcinoid tumors through atypical carcinoid tumors to highly malignant small cell and large cell neuroendocrine carcinomas (1,9,12).

Clinical syndromes associated with the production of various hormones occur in about 10% of all lung tumors (1) and in 26% of small cell carcinomas (13). With the development of specific radioimmunoassays, it could be shown that ectopic hormone production at subclinical levels occurs in most lung cancers, and that small cell carcinomas produce the largest quantities of adrenocorticotropic hormone, antidiuretic hormone, calcitonin, and various other polypeptide hormones (1,14). These tumors frequently contain intracellular neurosecretory granules, initially described by Bensch and colleagues (15), who also indicated their resemblance to carcinoid tumors.

CLINICAL SYNDROME

Patients with typical carcinoid tumors in the lung have a very good prognosis. Metastases to regional lymph nodes occur in 5% to 10% of patients, usually many years after the initial diagnosis (12). Atypical carcinoids, which account for 10% to 25% of pulmonary neuroendocrine tumors, are larger (3.6 cm vs. 2.3 cm for typical carcinoids), and the rates of metastasis to regional lymph nodes are higher (average, 20%) (12,15).

Small cell carcinomas account for 20% to 25% of all lung cancers. They are malignant tumors of high grade with rapid growth and a propensity for widespread metastases.

Small cell carcinoma of the lung is a tumor of middle-aged and elderly persons, usually heavy smokers. The male-to-female ratio used to be 6:1 but has been decreasing because of rapid increases in smoking and lung cancer in women (16,17).

Small cell carcinomas, in addition to being locally aggressive and extending into the mediastinum, metastasize early and widely. The mediastinal lymph nodes are almost invariably and extensively involved, sometimes even when the primary lung tumor is undetectable (16). Both primary and metastatic tumors tend to be bulky, soft, and gray, with frequent areas of necrosis and hemorrhage.

The tumor cells invade lymph and blood vessels early, and 84% of patients already have extrathoracic disease at initial diagnosis (13). In a study of 19 patients who had undergone curative pneumonectomy and died within 1 month of surgery, Matthews and Gordon (18) found extensive metastases in the abdominal lymph nodes, liver, adrenals, and brain. Of 102 patients with small cell lung carcinoma at autopsy, the same authors found metastatic lesions in the liver in 74%, adrenals in 55%, and abdominal lymph nodes in 52% (18). Because the dissemination is precocious, it is not uncommon to detect metastases of small cell carcinomas before the primary tumor itself. Scalene lymph nodes are frequently sampled in the search for primary lung tumors. Their size is not a reliable indication of their involvement; in a series of 64 cases, 52% of the scalene lymph nodes, although smaller than 1 cm in diameter, contained metastatic tumor (19). Contralateral metastases are frequent, and in the same study, by Agliozzo and Reingold (19), biopsy of bilateral scalene lymph nodes increased the yield of positive findings by 12%. Scalene lymph nodes are positive for tumor in 37.5% of patients with lung cancer; however, these metastases generally represent late tumor manifestations (19,20). Regardless of its stage, small cell lung carcinoma cannot be appropriately treated by surgery alone; the postoperative 5-year survival rate is close to zero (16). Recently, with advances in the chemotherapy of solid tumors, encouraging results have been obtained. Increasing numbers of 3-year survivors are recorded in cases in which disease is limited to the thoracic cavity, and surgery combined with intensive chemotherapy is recommended for small cell carcinoma in stage T1 N0 M0 (21).

In the gastrointestinal tract, the incidence and behavior of neuroendocrine neoplasms correlate to a great extent with location. In the esophagus, carcinoids are very rare; they are also uncommon in the stomach, but more frequent in the antrum than in the fundus. In the duodenum, they may be functional and produce gastrin, causing Zollinger-Ellison syndrome, or they may be part of multiple endocrine neoplasia syndrome type 1 (10,11). In the ileum and jejunum, carcinoids are particularly aggressive. Because of the location, they are diagnosed late, often with metastases at the time of presentation. The primary tumor and its metastases frequently secrete serotonin and cause carcinoid syndrome (22–24). The appendix is the most common site of carcinoids; these have a slow and usually benign course. Carcinoids occur rarely in the colon, whereas in the rectum they are usually small and indolent, secreting serotonin in 50% of cases (10,11). Metastases in general produce the same endocrine substances as the primary tumors; however, some may produce fewer or more hormones, and still others may secrete entirely different substances (23). Small cell carcinomas in the gastrointestinal tract may have endocrine features; however, as in the lung, they are highly malignant and prone to early metastases.

Occasionally, carcinoids are associated with adenocarcinomas, and some carcinomas have endocrine activity, which is in accordance with the theory of a common endodermal origin (22–24).

HISTOPATHOLOGY

Carcinoids are recognized by their characteristic organoid pattern of growth, intracytoplasmic granules, and histochemical reactions. They grow in nests, cords, sheets, and even glands, with typical peripheral cellular palisading and a sharply demarcated border (Fig. 95.1). Necrosis is unusual and mitoses are rare. The cells of pulmonary carcinoid tumors may have oncocytic, signet ring, spindle, or melanocytic features (12). They may have stromal deposits of amyloid or calcium. Atypical carcinoids may show areas of

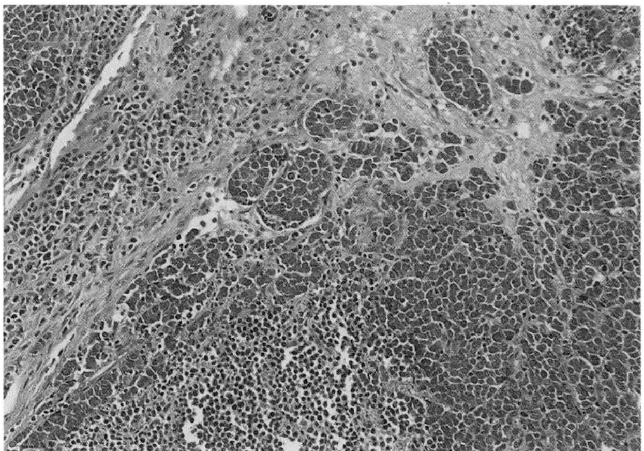

FIGURE 95.1. Metastasis of ileal carcinoid in mesenteric lymph node. Islands and nests of polyhedral cells with scarce cytoplasm and hyperchromatic nuclei. Hematoxylin, phloxine, and saffron stain.

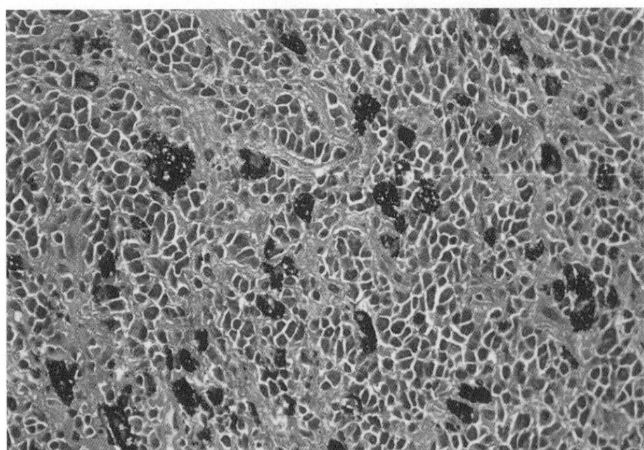

FIGURE 95.2. Metastasis of small cell carcinoma of the lung in mediastinal anthracotic lymph node with small and large carcinoma cells arranged in nests and cords. Hematoxylin, phloxine, and saffron stain.

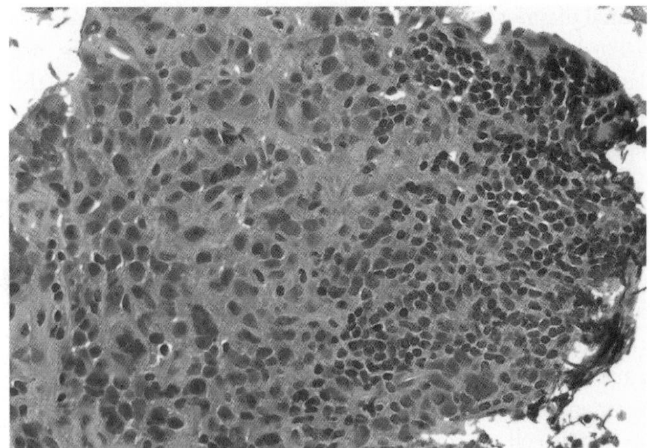

FIGURE 95.4. Same section as in Fig. 95.3. Small cell carcinoma, mixed type with small and large cells, in comparison with residual lymphocytes (*right*). Hematoxylin, phloxine, and saffron stain.

hemorrhage and necrosis, nuclear pleomorphism, and 5 to 10 mitoses per high-power field (25).

Small cell carcinomas show a diffuse pattern of growth, with occasional focal formation of nests, trabeculae, ribbons, or rosettes, reminiscent of those seen in carcinoid tumors (Fig. 95.2). They may also show areas of squamous or glandular differentiation. The cells have poorly defined borders, scarce cytoplasm, hyperchromatic and basophilic nuclei with inconspicuous nucleoli, and frequent mitoses. Nuclear molding is a characteristic feature.

The tumor cells are fragile and prone to necrosis (Fig. 95.3), which causes the characteristic crushing effect commonly seen in biopsy specimens (Fig. 95.3). An intensely hematoxyphilic smudgy material, consisting of DNA liberated by necrotic cells, is frequently deposited in necrotic areas and vessel walls (26). Crushed carcinoma cells are almost inevitable in this tumor and add to the difficulties of

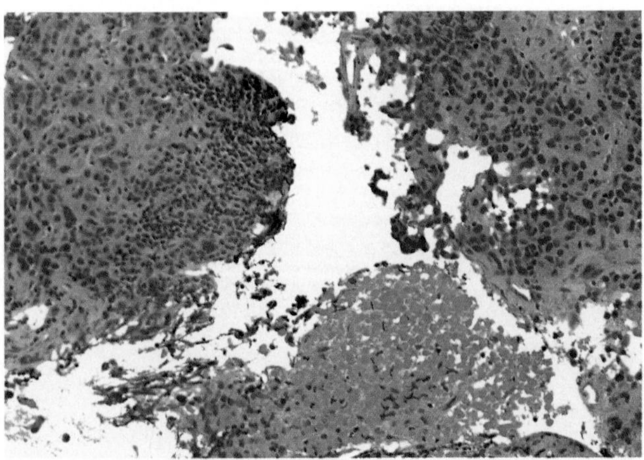

FIGURE 95.3. Biopsy specimen of mediastinal lymph nodes showing metastases of small cell carcinoma with crushed cells and large areas of necrosis. Hematoxylin, phloxine, and saffron stain.

diagnosis, particularly in small biopsy specimens. The classic oat cells, when well preserved, are almost twice the size of lymphocytes, with indistinct cytoplasm and ovoid nuclei containing a fine chromatin structure, inconspicuous nucleoli, and frequent mitoses (Fig. 95.4). The cells may comprise neurosecretory granules; however, these are usually sparse, and when silver staining is used to identify them, the result is uniformly negative (18). The cell clusters are separated by strands of fibrous tissue with areas of dense collagen deposits. A characteristic and distinctive feature of small cell lung carcinoma is its almost total lack of stromal cellular reaction (27). In lymph node metastases, all histologic features of the primary tumors are usually present.

Earlier classifications attempted to define subtypes of small cell carcinoma, such as oat cell, fusiform, polygonal, and intermediate; however, comparative studies failed to show correlations with clinical behavior, response to treatment, or survival (18,28). It was also shown that all lung cancers are histologically heterogeneous, so that the classifications were often irrelevant. The current classification of small cell carcinomas comprises three categories:

1. Small cell carcinoma. This includes the tumors previously classified as oat cell and intermediate subtypes. More than 90% of untreated tumors belong to this category.
2. Mixed small cell and large cell carcinoma. This is a small cell lung carcinoma with areas of large cell carcinoma (Figs. 95.2 and 95.4). It has a worse prognosis and response to therapy.
3. Combined small cell carcinoma. In this tumor, typical small cell carcinoma is admixed with areas of differentiated squamous or adenocarcinoma. The majority of small cell carcinomas, *in vivo* or *in vitro,* produce a number of amine and peptide hormones, such as adrenocorticotropic

hormone, antidiuretic hormone, gastrin-releasing peptide, calcitonin, serotonin, and others (1,29).

ELECTRON MICROSCOPY

The characteristic feature of small cell lung carcinoma is the presence of intracytoplasmic neurosecretory granules. As initially described by Bensch and associates (15), the granules have a diameter of 60 to 200 nm, are enveloped in a limiting membrane, and concentrate in the pseudopod-like cytoplasmic processes of the cells. The cells of small cell carcinoma usually show well-differentiated desmosomes with tonofilament bundles.

Some cells may form a small glandular space with microvilli and even abortive cilia and basal bodies. The ultrastructural features of small cell carcinomas thus exhibit dual characteristics of neuroendocrine and epithelial cells (16).

HISTOCHEMISTRY

The argyrophil reaction (Grimelius) stains the protein matrix of the endocrine granules (30). The argentaffin reaction (Fontana-Masson) is generally specific for amines. However, neither reaction is entirely specific. Other cellular products, such as lipofuscin, mucin, and glycogen, may be argyrophilic (2). Moreover, the argentaffin reaction is not very specific or sensitive and may result in false-negative results (2).

IMMUNOHISTOCHEMISTRY

The identification of neuroendocrine tumors by monoclonal antibodies provides the sensitivity and specificity necessary for diagnosis. Carcinoids and small cell carcinomas express neuron-specific enolase (NSE) (Fig. 95.5), chromogranin, synaptophysin (Fig. 95.6), and Leu-7, a marker of natural killer cells (2,12,29). Carcinoid tumors of the lung and gastrointestinal tract are positive for CK7 (31). Functional tumors are positive for the various hormones and enzymes they produce. They are negative for vimentin, which is a good marker of mesothelioma and some large cell carcinomas (2).

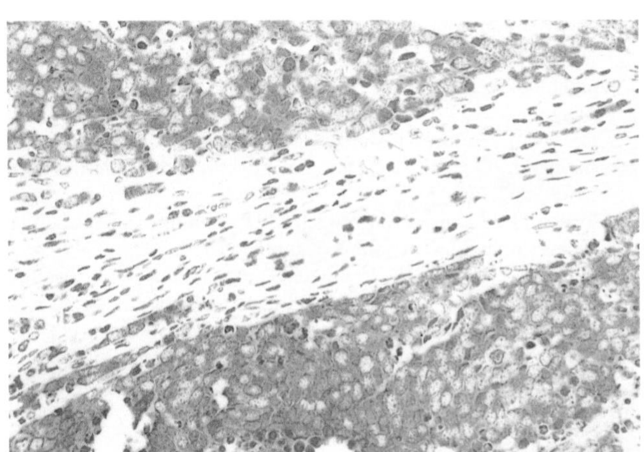

FIGURE 95.5. Metastasis of pulmonary carcinoid with staining for neuron-specific enolase (NSE). NSE/peroxidase stain.

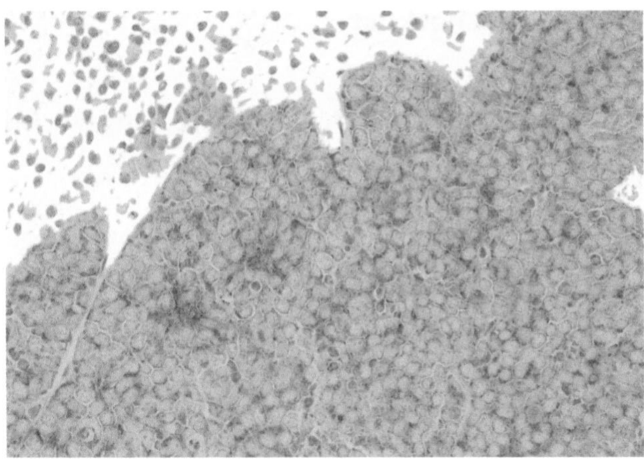

FIGURE 95.6. Same lymph node metastasis as in Fig. 95.5 with staining for synaptophysin. Synaptophysin/peroxidase stain.

Phenotype

NSE+, chromogranin+, synaptophysin+
Leu-7+, CK7+

DIFFERENTIAL DIAGNOSIS

- Lymphomas of diffuse small cell type (lymphocytic or lymphoblastic) do not form organoid patterns, do not contain neurosecretory granules, and have lymphocyte membrane markers. They are CD45+, cytokeratin−, chromogranin−.
- Metastatic mammary lobular carcinoma cells lack intense basophilic staining, a crushing effect, and neurosecretory granules. They are negative for the neuroendocrine markers.
- Metastatic neuroblastoma, Ewing sarcoma, and alveolar rhabdomyosarcoma occur in children and young adults, a group of patients not affected by small cell lung carcinoma.

Checklist

NEUROENDOCRINE TUMOR METASTASIS

Nests, ribbons, cord patterns
Foci of necrosis
Cell-crushing artifact
Indistinct cytoplasm
Ovoid nuclei with molding effect
Fine chromatin, inconspicuous nucleoli
Frequent mitoses
Neurosecretory granules
Desmosomes with tonofilament bundles
NSE+, chromogranin+, synaptophysin+

REFERENCES

1. Yesner R. Spectrum of lung cancer and ectopic hormones. Pathol Annu 1978;13:217–240.
2. DeLellis RA. Carcinoid tumors. Changing concepts and new perspectives. Am J Surg Pathol 1984;8:295–300.
3. Feyrter F. Uber Diffuse Endocrine Epithelial Organe. Leipzig: JA Barth, 1938.
4. Pearse AGE. The cytochemistry and ultrastructure of polypeptide hormone-producing cells of the APUD series and the embryologic, physiologic and pathologic implication of the concept. J Histochem Cytochem 1969;17:303–313.
5. McDowell EM, Trump BF. Pulmonary small cell carcinoma showing tripartite differentiation in individual cells. Hum Pathol 1981;12:286.
6. Gould VE. Neuroendocrinomas and neuroendocrine carcinomas. APUD cell system neoplasms and their aberrant secretory activities. Pathol Annu 1977;12:33–62.
7. Lewin KJ. The endocrine cells of the gastrointestinal tract. The normal endocrine cells and their hyperplasia. Pathol Annu 1986;21:1–27.
8. Gmelich JT, Bensch KG, Liebow AA. Cell of Kulchitsky type in bronchioles and their relation to the origin of peripheral carcinoid tumor. Lab Invest 1967;17:88–98.
9. Gazdar AF, Carney DN, Guccion JB, et al. Small cell carcinoma of the lung: cellular origin and relationship to other pulmonary tumors. In: Greco FA, Oldham RK, Bunn PA, eds. Small cell lung cancer. New York: Grune & Stratton, 1981:145–175.
10. Burke AP, Federspiel BH, Sobin LH, et al. Carcinoids of the duodenum: a histologic and immunohistochemical study of 65 tumors. Am J Surg Pathol 1989;13:828–837.
11. Federspiel BH, Burke AP, Sobin LH, et al. Rectal and colonic carcinoids. A clinicopathologic study of 84 cases. Cancer 1990; 65:135–140.
12. Travis WD. Carcinoid and other neuroendocrine tumors. In: Saldana SJ, ed. Pathology of pulmonary disease. Philadelphia: JB Lippincott Co, 1994:581–596.
13. Eagan RT, Maurer LH, Forcier RJ, et al. Small cell carcinoma of the lung: staging, paraneoplastic syndromes, treatment and survival. Cancer 1974;33:527–532.
14. Broder LE. Hormone production by bronchogenic carcinoma: a review. Pathobiol Annu 1979;9:205–224.
15. Bensch KG, Corrin B, Pariente R, et al. Oat cell carcinoma of the lung: its origin and relationship to bronchial carcinoid. Cancer 1968;22:1163–1172.
16. Shimosato Y. Pulmonary neoplasms. In: Sternberg SS, ed. Diagnostic surgical pathology, vol 1. New York: Raven Press, 1995: 785–827.
17. Ioachim HL. Present trends in lung cancer. In: Thurlbeck WM, Abell MR, eds. The lung. Baltimore: Williams & Wilkins, 1978:192–214 (International Academy of Pathology monograph No. 19).
18. Matthews MJ, Gordon PR. Morphology of pulmonary and pleural malignancies. In: Straus MJ, ed. Lung cancer. New York: Grune & Stratton, 1977:49–69.
19. Agliozzo CM, Reingold IM. Scalene lymph nodes in necropsies of malignant tumors. Cancer 1967;20:2148–2153.
20. Klingenberg L. Histopathological findings in the prescalene tissue from 1,000 postmortem cases. Acta Chir Scand 1964;127:57–66.
21. Aisner J, Alberto P, Bitran J, et al. Role of chemotherapy in small cell lung cancer—a consensus report of the International Association for the Study of Lung Cancer Workshop. Cancer Treat Rep 1983;67:37–43.
22. Lewin KJ, Ulich T, Yang K, et al. The endocrine cells of the gastrointestinal tract. Tumors. Pathol Annu 1986;21:181–215.
23. Yang K, Ulich T, Cheng L, et al. The neuroendocrine product of intestinal carcinoids. Cancer 1983;51:1918.
24. Lechago J. The endocrine cells of the digestive and respiratory systems and their pathology. In: Bloodworth JMB, ed. Endocrine pathology. Baltimore: Williams & Wilkins, 1982:513–555.
25. Arrigoni MG, Worlner LB, Bernatz PE. Bronchial carcinoids. Review of 124 cases. J Thorac Cardiovasc Surg 1985;89:8.
26. Azzopardi JG. Oat-cell carcinoma of the bronchus. J Pathol Bacteriol 1960;78:513–519.
27. Ioachim HL, Dorsett BH, Paluch E. The immune response at the tumor site in lung carcinoma. Cancer 1976;38:2296–2309.
28. Frairie AE, Roggli VL, Vollmer RT, et al. Lung cancer heterogeneity. Prognostic implications. Cancer 1987;60:370–375.
29. Hirsch R, Matthews MJ, Aisner S, et al. Histopathologic classification of small cell lung cancer—changing concepts and terminology. Cancer 1988;62:973–977.
30. Grimelius L, Wilander E. Silver stains in the study of endocrine cells of the gut and pancreas. Invest Cell Pathol 1980;3:3–12.
31. Chu P, Wu E, Weiss LM. Cytokeratin 7 and 20 expression in epithelial neoplasms: a survey of 435 cases. Mod Pathol 2000;13: 962–972.

96

METASTATIC NEUROBLASTOMA

DEFINITION

Lymph node metastases of neuroblastoma, a malignant tumor of childhood originating in primitive cells of the neural crest.

EPIDEMIOLOGY

Neuroblastoma and ganglioneuroblastoma are the fourth most common tumors of childhood, with an incidence of 8.7 per million inhabitants of the United States (1). About 85% occur in the first 4 years of life, without any sex-related difference in incidence (1). Neuroblastomas are uncommon in teenagers and rare in adults.

PATHOGENESIS

A malignant neoplasm of primitive neuroectodermal cells, neuroblastomas are distributed along the sympathetic nervous system (2). In 50% to 75% of cases, they originate in the adrenal medulla. Extraadrenal neuroblastomas arise in the autonomic ganglia in the paravertebral retroperitoneal space, posterior mediastinum, cervical region, pterygopalatine fossa, and orbit (3). Some of the tumors may reach large proportions; with small tumors, symptoms may first be produced by metastases.

Among the neoplasms of children, only hematopoietic and central nervous system malignancies are more common than neuroblastomas, which represent 7% to 10% of all solid tumors (3,4). In nonhereditary, sporadic cases, the tumors are characteristically solitary, whereas in hereditary cases, they are multiple (5). Embryonically, neuroblastoma is derived from primitive cells of the neural crest and is included in the various benign and malignant malformations of the neural crest known as *neurocristopathies* (6). The primitive cell of origin may differentiate into sympathoblasts and form neuroblastomas, or it may differentiate further along the lines of chromaffin or nonchromaffin paraganglionic cells, from which paragangliomas may arise (7). The most differentiated variants of neuroblastoma are ganglioneuroblastoma and ganglioneuroma. The presence of mature or immature ganglion cells within neuroblastoma directly affects the prognosis (7,8).

A malignant small cell tumor of the chest wall, pleura, or lung known as the *Askin tumor* has been described in children (9). It is considered a particular form of neuroepithelioma arising from intercostal nerves. Distinguishing this tumor from the other small round cell tumors is difficult on light microscopy and depends on electron microscopy and immunohistochemistry (7).

CLINICAL SYNDROME

Because it derives from the sympathetic nervous system, neuroblastoma can occur in paraspinal locations, such as retroperitoneal abdominal areas, thorax, cervical ganglia, and other regions of the head and neck, and in parenchymal organs, such as the adrenal medulla (4).

Neuroblastoma is, with retinoblastoma, the most common congenital cancer. At birth, it usually presents as an abdominal mass representing an adrenal or retroperitoneal tumor or hepatomegaly secondary to extensive metastases. Less often, it occurs in the posterior mediastinum or neck (10). In 50% of cases, the patient at diagnosis is less than 1 year old; 80% are younger than 5 years, and fewer than 5% of patients are older than 15 years (1). The distribution of lesions is to some extent determined by age. In the first year of life, almost all neuroblastomas are in the adrenal glands, whereas in older patients, the tumors are more often extraadrenal (3).

Adult neuroblastoma, although rare, occasionally has been reported. Mackay and associates (11) studied nine cases of neuroblastoma in patients ages 18 to 72 years. All were extraadrenal, and seven of the nine presented in a peripheral location and metastasized to regional lymph nodes. In general, the prognosis of extraadrenal neuroblastomas is better than that of tumors originating in the adrenal. They are difficult to diagnose, particularly when first observed in a lymph node metastasis.

Children with neuroblastoma are systemically ill, and as many as one-third present with metastatic disease (12).

Fever, weight loss, bone pain, increasing urinary catecholamine levels, evidence of an adrenal or retroperitoneal tumor, radiographic evidence of an expanding intramedullary tumor, and liver or lymph node metastases are the common signs and symptoms of neuroblastomas.

The patterns of metastases are somewhat characteristic, and recognizing them is helpful in the differential diagnosis of small round cell tumors of childhood (13). Neuroblastomas metastasize in descending order of frequency to the bone marrow (78%), lymph nodes (42%), liver (20%), orbit, and bones (2). The age of patients is a factor in the distribution of metastases; bone marrow and hepatic metastases are more common before l year of age, and metastases to the regional lymph nodes and bones are more frequent in older children (7).

Aggressive and immature neuroblastomas produce dopamine and its metabolites, whereas differentiated tumors may produce norepinephrine and its metabolites. A high ratio of vanillylmandelic acid to homovanillic acid (VMA:HVA) correlates with light and electron microscopic differentiation and with a good prognosis (7). In general, neuroblastoma can undergo maturation spontaneously or as a result of therapy.

HISTOPATHOLOGY

The tumor mass is pale gray, with frequent areas of necrosis, hemorrhage, and cyst formation. It may be a unicentric mass or an aggregation of large tumor nodules. In the lymph node metastasis, as in the primary tumor, the neuroblastoma is composed of sheets of closely packed, uniform, basophilic tumor cells with indistinct, scarce cytoplasm and round nuclei that stain dark blue (Figs. 96.1 and 96.2). The latter have a stippled chromatin, although

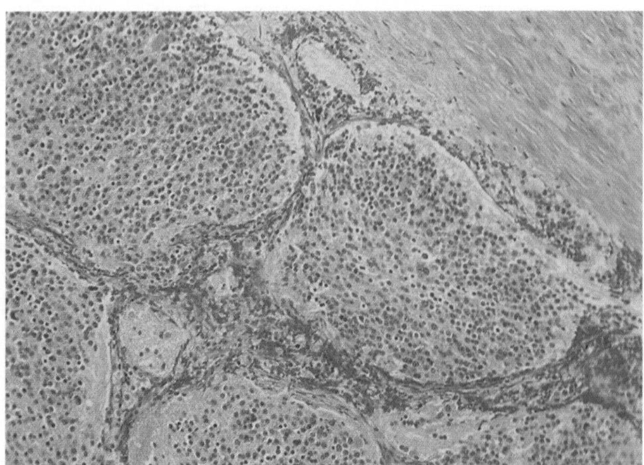

FIGURE 96.1. Lymph node metastasis of neuroblastoma. Large lobular aggregates of tumor cells separated by fibrous bands replace the lymphoid tissues. Hematoxylin, phloxine, and saffron stain.

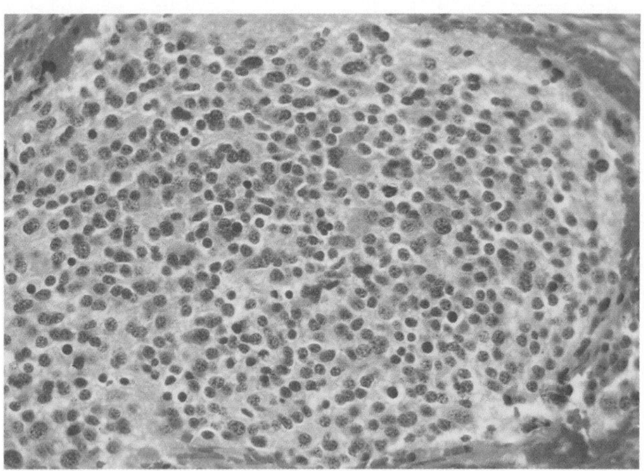

FIGURE 96.2. Same section as in Fig. 96.1. Within a lobular unit, the tumor cells vary in amount of cytoplasm, and particularly in the size and shape of nuclei, from small and lymphocyte-like to fairly large and irregular. Hematoxylin, phloxine, and saffron stain.

they may frequently appear pyknotic in apoptotic cells (Fig. 96.3). Nuclear pleomorphism is minimal, with only small variations in size and occasional slight indentations. Mitoses are not very frequent. These are the features of the least differentiated neuroblastomas, and without electron microscopy or immunohistochemistry, the diagnosis of neuroblastoma can only be suggested (6). Biopsy specimens from metastatic sites exhibit a similar appearance. In most neuroblastomas, however, some features of differentiation may be present, such as cytoplasmic processes or neurites with a characteristic eosinophilic fibrillary background (2,6). Neuroblastoma cells are often arranged in the typical Homer-Wright rosette pattern, forming a circle around a central area occupied by a mesh of tangled cell processes. In addition, acellular fibrillar areas are seen that resemble glial tissue and become prominent in more differentiated neuroblastomas. With only rare exceptions, glycogen is not present in the cytoplasm of neuroblastoma cells, as it is in the cells of Ewing sarcoma (14); thus, the result of periodic acid–Schiff staining is usually negative. Other occasional features are dystrophic calcification (40% to 60% of cases), precipitation of DNA around blood vessels (Azzopardi effect), and variable lymphocytic infiltration (6).

ELECTRON MICROSCOPY

The electron microscopic examination can identify the characteristic features of neuroblastoma and make the diagnosis, even when a pediatric small round cell tumor appears completely undifferentiated under the light microscope (13).

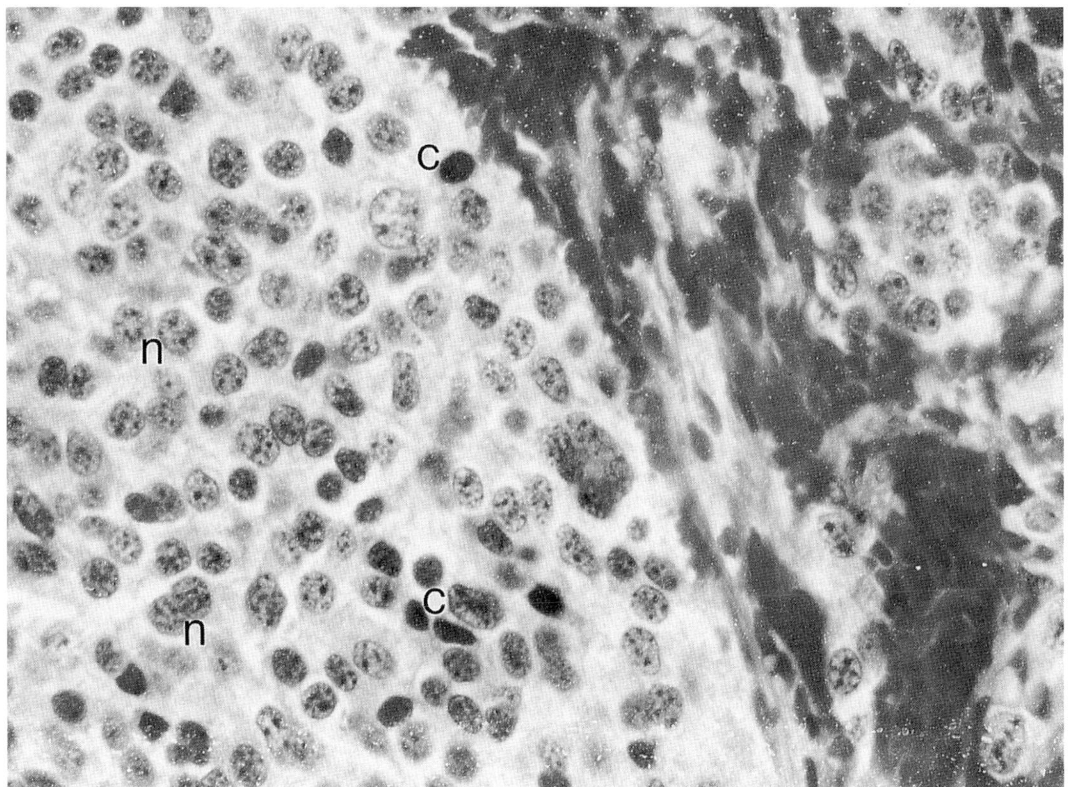

FIGURE 96.3. Same section as in Fig. 96.1. Neuroblastoma cells have scarce cytoplasm and round nuclei (*n*) with stippled chromatin and multiple, fine nucleoli. Numerous scattered apoptotic cells (*c*) are present. Hematoxylin, phloxine, and saffron stain.

Neuroblastoma cells have one to two neuritic processes, a feature that reflects their neural crest derivation and constitutes the most reliable diagnostic criterion. In a study of about 100 neuroblastomas, the neuritic processes were fairly easily demonstrated in all cases (15). Also characteristic are the uniform, electron-dense, membrane-bound, 100 μm neurosecretory granules present in the cytoplasm and cell processes (13). Intracytoplasmic glycogen is seen in fewer than 5% of cases, and then only in small amounts. Cell junctions represented by rudimentary desmosomes are quite common in neuroblastomas (15). The Askin tumor shows neurosecretory granules in addition to glycogen (7,9).

IMMUNOHISTOCHEMISTRY

Neuron-specific enolase (NSE) was identified, although in varying amounts, in all 50 cases tested in one study (15). S100 protein was also identified in all cases except three of the least differentiated. To the authors, these results suggested that S100 positivity might indicate a favorable prognosis (15). Neuroblastomas also express CD57 (Leu-7) and synaptophysin (15,16). They are negative for CD45 (leukocyte common antigen), cytokeratin, actin, and desmin. The Askin tumor is positive for NSE (7).

Phenotype

S100 protein+, NSE+, CD57+, synaptophysin+
CD45−, CK−, actin−, desmin−

DIFFERENTIAL DIAGNOSIS

Small round cell tumors exhibit remarkable histologic similarity and are thus often difficult to differentiate.

- Alveolar rhabdomyosarcoma lacks neurite processes, rosettes, and neurosecretory granules. It may be positive for myogenin, desmin, muscle-specific actin, and NSE but is consistently negative for synaptophysin (16).
- Ewing sarcoma has a focal nesting pattern. The cells contain intracytoplasmic glycogen, sometimes in abundant amounts, in pools. They are positive for CD99 and negative for NSE and synaptophysin.
- Lymphoma lacks cell processes, cell junctions, and neurosecretory granules. The tumors are positive for CD45 (leukocyte common antigen) and negative for NSE and synaptophysin.

Checklist

METASTATIC NEUROBLASTOMA

Infants and children in 80% of cases
Primary adrenal or retroperitoneal tumors
Metastases in regional lymph nodes
Sheets of densely packed, uniform small round cells
Foci of hemorrhage and necrosis
Round, basophilic, dark blue nuclei
Minimal nuclear pleomorphism
Inconspicuous nucleoli
Infrequent mitoses
Homer-Wright rosettes and acellular fibrillar areas
Neurite processes
Neurosecretory membrane-bound granules
NSE+, CD57+, synaptophysin+
Urinary catecholamines

- Patients with small cell lung carcinoma are older. Characteristic DNA staining in vessel walls is observed, as are well-differentiated desmosomes with prominent tonofilament bundles (11). These tumors are positive for low-molecular-weight cytokeratin.

REFERENCES

1. Young JL Jr, Ries LG, Silverberg E. Cancer incidence, survival and mortality for children younger than age 15 years. Cancer 1986;58:598–602.
2. Lack EE. Neuroblastoma, ganglioneuroblastoma and other related tumors. In: Tumors of the adrenal gland and extra-adrenal paraganglia. Atlas of tumor pathology, series III, fascicle 19:411–465. Washington, DC: Armed Forces Institute of Pathology, 1997.
3. Kissane JM. Pathology of infancy and childhood. St. Louis: Mosby, 1975:770–783.
4. Jaffe N. Neuroblastoma: review of the literature and an examination of factors contributing to its enigmatic character. Cancer Treat Rev 1976;3:61–82.
5. Knudson AG Jr, Strong LC. Mutation and cancer: neuroblastoma and pheochromocytoma. Am J Hum Genet 1972;24:514–532.
6. Coffin CM, Dehner LP. Pathologic evaluation of pediatric soft tissue tumors. Am J Clin Pathol 1998;109[Suppl 1]:538–552.
7. Triche TJ, Askin FB. Neuroblastoma and the differential diagnosis of small-, round-, blue-cell tumors. Hum Pathol 1983;14:569–595.
8. Hughes M, Marsden HB, Palmer MK. Histologic patterns of neuroblastoma related to prognosis and clinical staging. Cancer 1974;34:1706.
9. Askin FB, Rosai J, Sibley RK, et al. Malignant small cell tumor of the thoracopulmonary region in childhood: a distinctive clinicopathologic entity of uncertain histogenesis. Cancer 1979;43:2438–2451.
10. Isaacs H. Tumors. In: Barness EG, ed. Potter's pathology of the fetus and infant, vol 2. St. Louis: Mosby, 1997:1242–1339.
11. Mackay B, Luna MA, Butler JJ. Adult neuroblastoma. Cancer 1976;37:1334–1351.
12. Evans AE, D'Angio GJ, Koop CE. Diagnosis and treatment of neuroblastoma. Pediatr Clin North Am 1976;23:161.
13. Joshi VV, Balarezo F, Hicks MJ, et al. Approach to small round cell tumors of childhood. Pathol Case Rev 2000;5:26–41.
14. Triche TJ, Ross WE. Glycogen-containing neuroblastoma with clinical and histopathologic features of Ewing's sarcoma. Cancer 1978;41:1425–1433.
15. Mierau GW, Berry PJ, Orsini EN. Small round cell neoplasms: can electron microscopy and immunohistochemical studies accurately classify them? Ultrastruct Pathol 1985;9:99–111.
16. Gould VE, DeLellis RA. The neuroendocrine system 1981–1993. In: Silverberg SG, ed. Principles and practice of surgical pathology, vol 11. New York: Churchill Livingstone, 1990.

97

METASTATIC EWING SARCOMA

DEFINITION

Regional lymph node metastases of skeletal or extraskeletal Ewing sarcoma.

EPIDEMIOLOGY

Ewing sarcoma (ES) accounts for 7% of all malignant bone tumors (1) and for 35% to 40% of all malignant bone tumors of children (2). Eighty percent of the tumors occur in the first two decades of life; patients over the age of 30 years are uncommon (3). In a large series of 303 patients, the highest frequency was between the ages of 10 and 15 years (4). However, ES may affect children even younger than 3 years of age, with this age group accounting for 2.6% of all cases (5). A predilection for males of 1.5:1 is noted (1), and a rare occurrence in blacks (3).

PATHOGENESIS

Ewing sarcoma is an undifferentiated malignant neoplasm that appears to originate in the primitive mesenchyme and differentiate into cells with mesenchymal, neural, or even epithelial features (6). Extraskeletal ES may arise in the soft tissues (7). Metastases to lymph nodes and internal organs are a frequent feature of both skeletal and extraskeletal ES (8). Because ES cells display a broad spectrum of differentiation, the origin of this neoplasm has long been a matter of controversy. Some extraskeletal cases of ES show rosette patterns, contain neurosecretory granules, and express neuron-specific enolase (NSE), features that suggest a neuroectodermal derivation (9,10). However, ES also expresses vimentin, desmoplakin, and occasionally even cytokeratins (6). A primary malignant tumor of bone that closely resembles ES has been described under the name of *peripheral neuroectodermal tumor* (PNET) of bone and soft tissues (3). ES and PNET have similar clinical, radiologic, and histologic features. In addition, both tumors have a characteristic t(11;22) chromosomal translocation (3). The Askin tumor of the chest wall also belongs to the group of PNETs. ES differs from PNET in a lack of neuroectodermal structures, which suggests that it probably represents the undifferentiated end of the spectrum of this group of tumors (3).

CLINICAL SYNDROME

Ewing sarcoma is highly metastatic, involving additional bones in 43% to 65%, the lungs in 45% to 65%, and the lymph nodes in 20% of cases (11).

Patients have pain and swelling in the area of the tumor. Any portion of any bone may be the site of ES, although the long bones and particularly the femur are most commonly affected. Tenderness, compromised function, and a palpable local mass are noted. Pathologic fractures are infrequent and may occur in 2% to 5% of patients (3). In 10% of cases, multiple bones are involved. Fever, anemia, an accelerated erythrocyte sedimentation rate, and sometimes leukocytosis are present. The roentgenographic appearance, in addition to other symptoms and signs, is well described in the classic textbooks (2,3). In gross appearance, the tumor is firm, white, and glistening in the bone and softer in extraskeletal locations.

HISTOPATHOLOGY

Various regions of the lymph node parenchyma are replaced by broad sheets, nests, or cords separated by fibrous septa and including foci of fibrosis (Fig. 97.1). The cells are uniform and closely packed, and frequent perivascular arrangements may produce a rosette-like pattern, particularly in areas of necrosis. The cytoplasm is scanty and indistinct; the nuclei are round or ovoid, and some appear hazy and some hyperchromatic (Figs. 97.2 and 97.3). The nucleoli are small and inconspicuous, and mitoses are present but not abundant. Reticulin fibers are demonstrable around the vessels but not between the tumor cells. Glycogen in the cytoplasm of the ES cells is a characteristic feature of this tumor. It can be readily identified with the periodic acid–Schiff (PAS) stain and removed by diastase treatment before staining in more than 75% of cases (3).

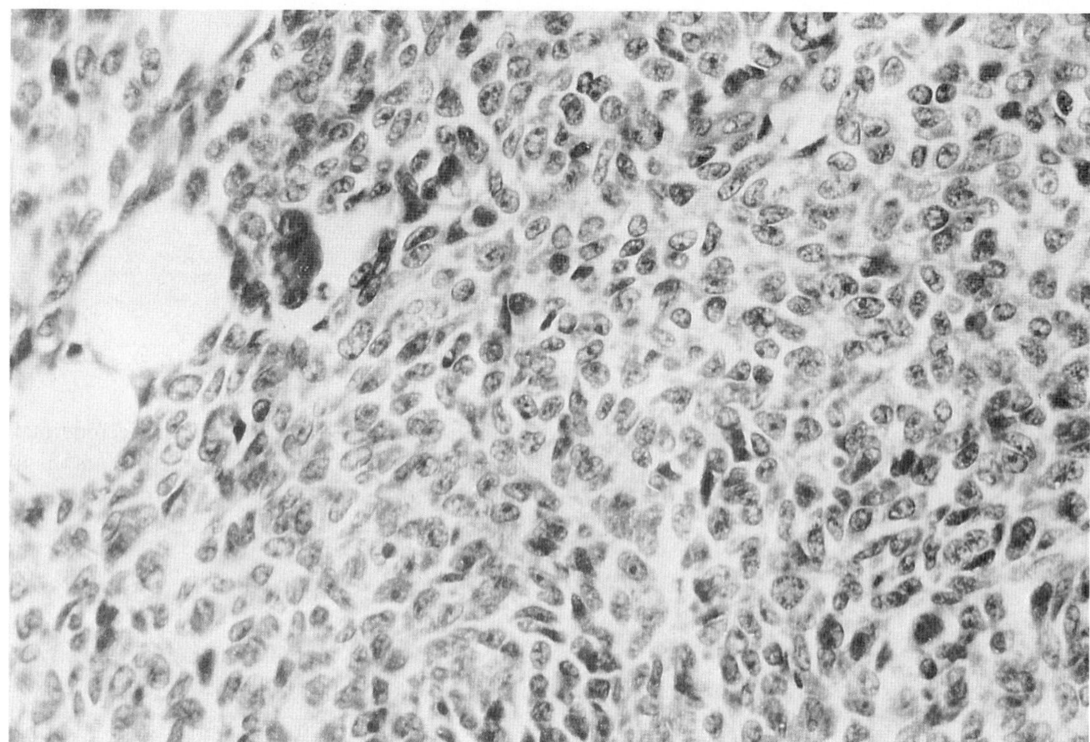

FIGURE 97.1. Metastatic Ewing sarcoma in axillary lymph node with total replacement and invasion of fibrofatty tissues. Sheets of tumor cells without formation of histologic patterns. Hematoxylin, phloxine, and saffron stain.

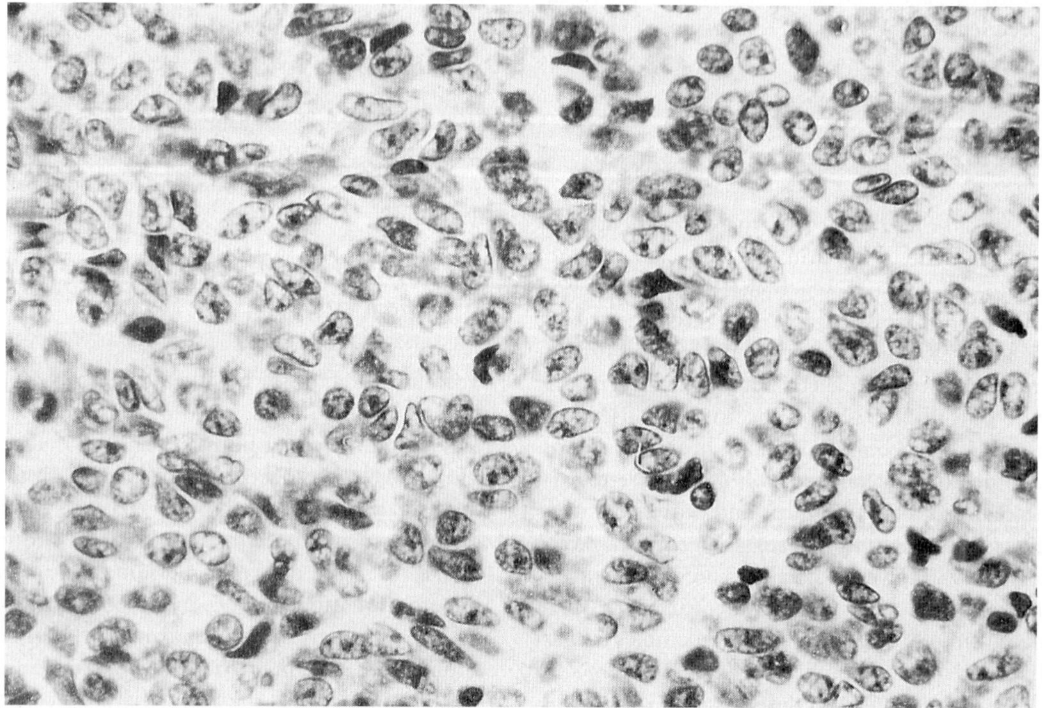

FIGURE 97.2. Same section as in Fig. 97.1. Monomorphic population of tumor cells with round or ovoid nuclei, fine nucleoli, and indistinct cytoplasm. Degenerated cells appear hyperchromatic. Hematoxylin, phloxine, and saffron stain.

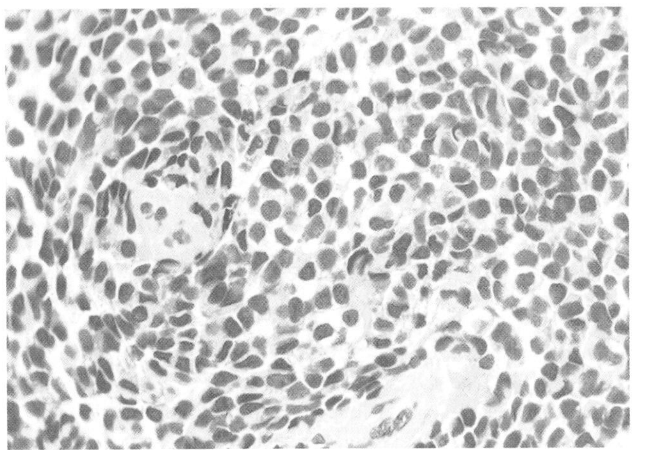

FIGURE 97.3. Cells of metastatic Ewing sarcoma forming pseudorosette around blood vessel. They appear uniform, with scarce cytoplasm and round, slightly angulated nuclei. Nucleoli and mitoses are inconspicuous. Hematoxylin, phloxine, and saffron stain.

The importance of glycogen in the diagnosis of ES was reaffirmed by a study of 26 autopsy cases; neither previous radiation treatment nor pleomorphic cellular changes induced by radiation affected the glycogen in the tumor cells (8).

ELECTRON MICROSCOPY

The cells of ES are relatively poor in organelles and display no specific features except for the consistent presence of glycogen. This is generally abundant and appears as aggregated granules or pools restricted to one or two regions of the cytoplasm (12,13). In one study, even in cases in which glycogen could not be demonstrated with the PAS stain under the light microscope, granules of glycogen were visible with the electron microscope (13). Cell junctions are desmosome-like and can be demonstrated in a majority of cells They have a characteristic asymmetry that resembles synaptic cell contacts (12). The chromatin is finely dispersed with a few marginal clumps (14). Electron microscopic examination is very useful, particularly to detect features relevant in the differential diagnosis of other small round cell tumors, such as the distinctive granules and microtubules with neuritic processes of neuroblastomas (15).

IMMUNOHISTOCHEMISTRY

Ewing sarcoma diffusely expresses vimentin and coexpresses desmoplakin in a variable percentage of cells (6). Some cases are positive for cytokeratin polypeptides 8 and 18 and even for neuron-specific enolase (9), which indicates the origin of ES from primitive pluripotential cells. ES cells are positive for CD99 (mic-2); however, lymphoblastic lymphoma and sometimes aberrantly even rhabdomyosarcoma may also stain for CD99 (16). Staining for chromogranin and synaptophysin is negative (5).

Checklist

METASTATIC EWING SARCOMA

Children and teenagers
Bone or soft tissue tumor
Male predominance
Lymph nodes involved in 20% of cases
Dense, homogeneous sheets of cells
Foci of necrosis
Cellular uniformity
Lack of reticulin network
Scanty, indistinct cytoplasm
Round nuclei
Finely dispersed chromatin
Inconspicuous nucleoli
Frequent mitoses
Few intracytoplasmic organelles
Desmosome-like cell attachments
Glycogen abundant, focal
PAS+, D-PAS−
Vimentin+, CD99+
Chromogranin−, synaptophysin−

DIFFERENTIAL DIAGNOSIS

- Neuroblastoma has neurite processes, neurosecretory granules, and Homer-Wright rosettes. It does not stain with PAS and is positive for neuron-specific enolase, S100 protein, chromogranin, and synaptophysin (16).
- Embryonal rhabdomyosarcoma has a pseudoalveolar pattern and occasional strap cells. It is positive for desmin, myogenin, and muscle-specific actin.
- Lymphoblastic lymphoma lacks cell attachments and glycogen and does not stain with PAS. It is positive for CD45 (leukocyte common antigen).
- Patients with small cell lung carcinoma are older. DNA staining in vessel walls is characteristic. Well-differentiated desmosomes with prominent tonofilament bundles and neurosecretory granules are present. Cells express low-molecular-weight cytokeratin, chromogranin, and synaptophysin.

REFERENCES

1. Dahlin DC. Ewing's tumor. In: Bone tumors. Springfield, IL: Charles C Thomas Publisher, 1967:186–195.
2. Dehner LP. Pediatric surgical pathology, 2nd ed. Baltimore: Williams & Wilkins, 1987:560–586.
3. Fechner RE, Mills SE. Ewing sarcoma of bone. In: Tumors of the bone and joints. Washington, DC: Armed Forces Institute of Pathology, 1993:187–201 (Atlas of tumor pathology, series III, fascicle 8).
4. Kissane JM, Askin FB, Foulkes M, et al. Ewing's sarcoma of bone: clinicopathologic aspects of 303 cases from the intergroup Ewing's sarcoma study. Hum Pathol 1983;14:773–779.
5. Maygarden SJ, Askin FB, Siegal GP, et al. Ewing sarcoma of bone in infants and toddlers. A clinicopathologic report from the Intergroup Ewing. Cancer 1993;71:2109–2118.
6. Moll R, Lee I, Gould VE, et al. Immunocytochemical analysis of Ewing's tumors. Am J Pathol 1987;127:288.
7. Angervall L, Enzinger FM. Extraskeletal neoplasm resembling Ewing's sarcoma. Cancer 1975;36:240–251.
8. Telles NC, Rabson AS, Pomeroy TC. Ewing's sarcoma: an autopsy study. Cancer 1978;41:2321–2329.
9. Shimada H, Newton WA, Soule EH, et al. Pathologic features of extraosseous Ewing's sarcoma. Hum Pathol 1988;19:442.
10. Schmidt D, Mackay B, Ayala AG. Ewing's sarcoma with neuroblastoma-like features. Ultrastruct Pathol 1982;3:143–151.
11. Spjut HJ, Ayala AG. Neoplasms and tumor-like lesions of bone. In: Silverberg SG, ed. Principles and practice of surgical pathology, 2nd ed., vol 1. New York: Churchill Livingstone, 1990:501–544.
12. Triche TJ, Askin FB. Neuroblastoma and the differential diagnosis of small-, round-, blue-cell tumors. Hum Pathol 1983;14:569–595.
13. Mierau GW, Berry PJ, Orsini EN. Small round cell neoplasms: can electron microscopy and immunohistochemical studies accurately classify them? Ultrastruct Pathol 1985;9:99–111.
14. Llombart-Bosch A, Blanche K, Pedro-Olayo A. Ultrastructural study of 28 cases of Ewing's sarcoma: typical and atypical forms. Cancer 1978;41:1362–1373.
15. Mierau GW, Weeks DA, Hicks MJ. Role of electron microscopy and other special techniques in the diagnosis of childhood round cell tumors. Hum Pathol 1998;29:1347–1355.
16. Joshi VV, Balarezo F, Hicks MJ, et al. Approach to small round cell tumors of childhood. Pathol Case Rev 2000;5:26–41.

98

METASTATIC RHABDOMYOSARCOMA

DEFINITION

Regional lymph node metastases of undifferentiated rhabdomyosarcoma.

EPIDEMIOLOGY

Rhabdomyosarcoma is the most common soft tissue sarcoma of children under 15 years of age. It is also one of the most common sarcomas of young adults, but it is rarely seen after 45 years of age (1).

CLASSIFICATION

Rhabdomyosarcoma may present as one of the following subtypes, depending on the degree of cellular differentiation and growth pattern.

Embryonal rhabdomyosarcoma, the undifferentiated form of rhabdomyosarcoma, is the most common subtype, accounting for 50% to 60% of all rhabdomyosarcomas. It affects predominantly very young children and is located more often in the head and neck, retroperitoneum, and genitourinary organs (1). *Botryoid rhabdomyosarcoma* is basically a variant of embryonal rhabdomyosarcoma; it accounts for 5% to 10% of all rhabdomyosarcomas and is characterized by its location near mucosal surfaces and a lobulated and myxoid structure (1). *Alveolar rhabdomyosarcoma,* the second most common subtype of rhabdomyosarcoma, accounts for about 20% of all cases, occurs in older children and young adults, and is more often located in the arms and legs (1). *Pleomorphic rhabdomyosarcoma* is a tumor of the large muscles of the extremities; it occurs in older people and represents about 5% of all rhabdomyosarcomas (1).

PATHOGENESIS

Rhabdomyosarcomas have a high metastatic potential and disseminate early and widely through both lymphatic and blood vessels. In a series of 110 cases of alveolar rhabdomyosarcoma, 92% of patients died of widespread metastases within the first 4 years after diagnosis (2). Of these, 89% had metastases to the regional lymph nodes and a median survival of less than 9 months. Not infrequently, a lymph node metastasis was detected before the primary tumor.

CLINICAL SYNDROME

The median age of patients varies with the subtype. In 440 patients in whom embryonal rhabdomyosarcoma was diagnosed at the Armed Forces Institute of Pathology (AFIP) during a period of 10 years, the median age was 8 years; in 118 patients with alveolar rhabdomyosarcoma, the median age was 16 years (1). The male-to-female ratio is 1.3:1. Rhabdomyosarcomas of the urinary bladder, prostate, vagina, and middle ear occur in a younger group (median age, 4 years) than do those in the extremities (median age, 14 years) (1). In the head and the neck, the most common locations are the orbit, nasal cavity, and nasopharynx, followed by the ear and sinuses. The gross appearance of tumors depends on the relative amounts of myxoid and collagenous stroma. The tumors of cavities like the nose and bladder are polypoid with a gelatinous appearance. Botryoid rhabdomyosarcomas, as their Greek name implies, have the shape of grapes and a mucoid consistency. In all rhabdomyosarcomas, the regional lymph nodes are usually involved.

HISTOPATHOLOGY

The metastatic lymph node lesions are histologically similar to the primary tumors. They consist of sheets of cells that are generally rounded and lack cohesiveness, forming nests, islands, or pseudoalveolar patterns (Figs. 98.1 and 98.2). The latter are seen when fibrous septa run through the tumor and separate the loosely aggregated cells. Foci of necrosis are frequent, particularly in the center of solid tumor areas. The cells are round or ovoid with scarce, pale, glycogen-containing cytoplasm and distinctly outlined nuclei that have fine nucleoli and frequent mitoses. Floating cells with pyknotic

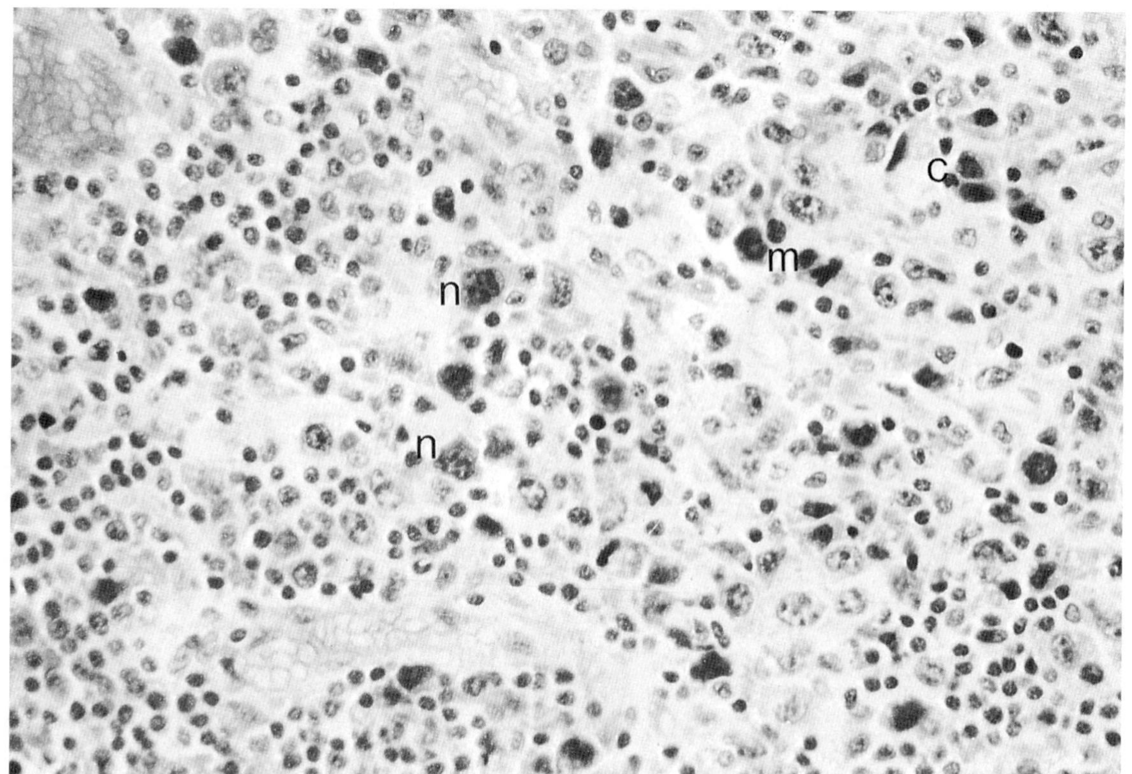

FIGURE 98.1. Metastatic alveolar rhabdomyosarcoma in inguinal lymph node. Diffuse infiltration of lymphoid tissues by tumor cells singly and in clusters (*C*). Marked nuclear pleomorphism, bizarre giant cells (*n*), and frequent mitoses (*m*). Hematoxylin, phloxine, and saffron stain.

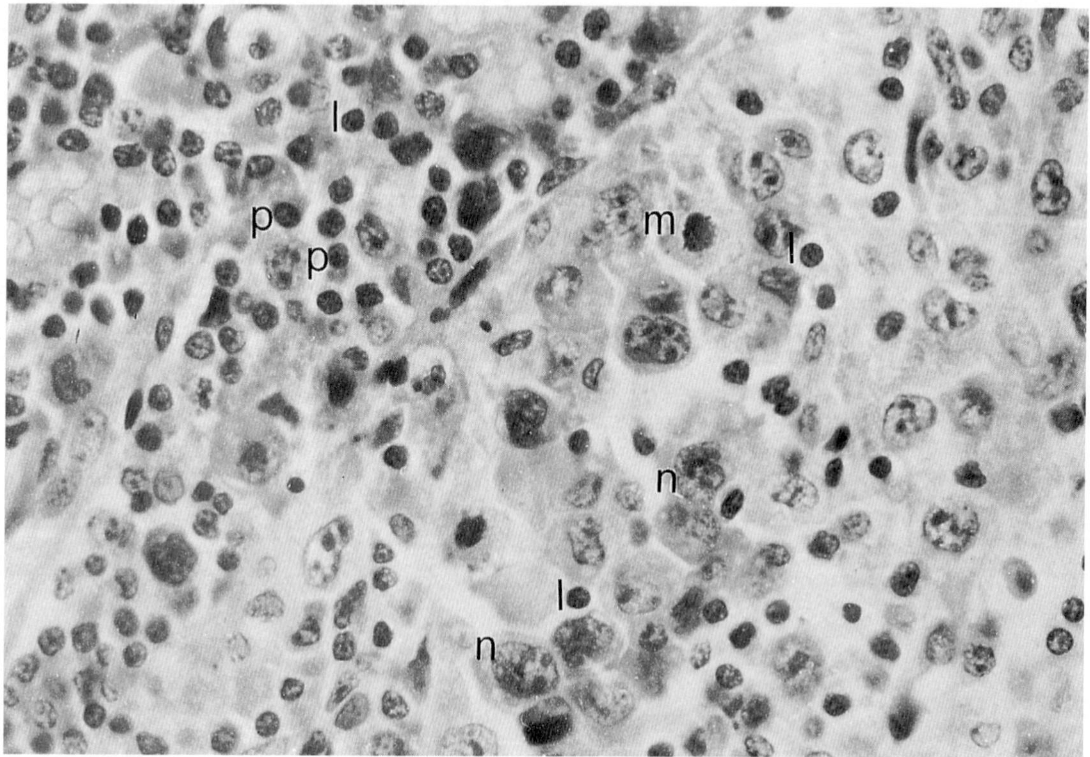

FIGURE 98.2. Same section as in Fig. 98.1. Tumor cells forming noncohesive nests and sheets are intermingled with lymphocytes (*l*) and plasma cells (*p*). Large, atypical nuclei (*n*) and atypical mitoses (*m*). Hematoxylin, phloxine, and saffron stain.

nuclei form aggregates within the alveolar spaces. Myxoid hypocellular areas are often present and are characteristic of embryonal and botryoid rhabdomyosarcomas. Infrequently, the tumors may include more differentiated cells, such as cells with myoblastic features, strap cells, or multinucleated giant cells (3). In general, embryonal rhabdomyosarcomas resemble the embryogenetic stages of normal skeletal muscle, ranging from poorly differentiated tumors, which are very difficult to diagnose without the help of electron microscopy and immunohistochemistry, to well-differentiated tumors, in which features of fetal muscle can be recognized (1).

ELECTRON MICROSCOPY

The cells are round and joined by small, primitive, desmosome-like structures (4). The nuclei are irregular and often deeply indented. The cytoplasm contains polyribosomes, numerous mitochondria, and variable amounts of glycogen. The cells bear a general resemblance to the cells of Ewing sarcoma.

The single most characteristic feature of primitive soft tissue sarcomas, not seen in other small round cell tumors, is a feltwork of distinct 7- and 10-nm cytoplasmic filaments (5). They lack the more differentiated actin–myosin bundles, Z band material, and an external lamina (5). Diffuse monoparticulate glycogen is also seen, in contrast to the glycogen in Ewing cells, which is focal and arranged in rosettes (6). Also useful in the diagnosis are ribosomes aligned in "Indian files" along thick filaments (7).

CYTOCHEMISTRY

Masson trichrome stain reveals the more differentiated rhabdomyoblasts, staining their cytoplasm deep red. Phosphotungstic acid hematoxylin (PTAH) stain shows the cytoplasm of rhabdomyoblasts in deep blue (8). Periodic acid–Schiff (PAS) stain before diastase treatment demonstrates glycogen in the cells, which may vary considerably, even in the same section (8). Reticulin silver stain reveals the pseudoalveolar pattern of the tumor.

IMMUNOHISTOCHEMISTRY

Rhabdomyosarcoma cells are reactive for vimentin, muscle-specific actin, desmin, myogenin, neuron-specific enolase, S100 protein, and CD99 (mic-2). They are not reactive for placental alkaline phosphatase, CD45 (leukocyte common antigen), cytokeratin, or epithelial membrane antigen (6,9,10).

DIFFERENTIAL DIAGNOSIS

- Neuroblastoma has neurite processes, neurosecretory granules, and Homer-Wright rosettes and is positive for synaptophysin.
- Ewing sarcoma lacks an alveolar pattern and strap cells. It contains glycogen focally arranged in rosettes and is positive for CD99, but not for actin or desmin.
- Lymphomas lack cell attachments and glycogen. They are positive for leukocyte common antigen (CD45) and CD3 or CD20, and negative for actin, desmin, and neuron-specific enolase.
- Small cell lung carcinoma affects older patients and is marked by characteristic DNA staining in vessel walls and well-differentiated desmosomes. It is positive for cytokeratin, chromogranin, and synaptophysin.

Checklist

METASTATIC RHABDOMYOSARCOMA

Presence or history of regional tumor
Children and young adults
Lymph node architecture obliterated
Pseudoalveolar pattern
Foci of necrosis
Round, noncohesive tumor cells
Finely structured nuclei, scarce cytoplasm
Small nucleoli, frequent mitoses
Occasional strap cells
Masson trichrome and PTAH staining of tumor cells
Focal, monoparticulate intracellular glycogen
Positive for vimentin, desmin, myogenin, and muscle-specific actin

REFERENCES

1. Enziger FM, Weiss SW. Rhabdomyosarcoma. In: Soft tissue tumors. St. Louis: Mosby, 1995:539–577.
2. Enzinger EM, Shiraki M. Alveolar rhabdomyosarcoma: an analysis of 110 cases. Cancer 1969;24:18–31.
3. Dehner LP. Pediatric surgical pathology, 2nd ed. Baltimore: Williams & Wilkins, 1987:560–586.
4. Churg A, Ringus J. Ultrastructural observations on the genesis of alveolar rhabdomyosarcoma. Cancer 1978;41:1355–1361.
5. Triche TJ, Askin FB. Neuroblastoma and the differential diagnosis of small-, round-, blue-cell tumors. Hum Pathol 1983;14: 569–595.
6. Joshi VV, Balarezo F, Hicks MJ, et al. Approach to small round cell tumors of childhood. Pathol Case Rev 2000;5:26–41.
7. Mierau GW, Berry PJ, Orsini EN. Small round cell neoplasms: can electron microscopy and immunohistochemical studies accurately classify them? Ultrastruct Pathol 1985;9:99–111.
8. Lattes R. Tumors of the soft tissues. Atlas of tumor pathology, series II, fascicle 1. Washington, DC: Armed Forces Institute of Pathology, 1982:177–180.
9. Battifora H. Clinical applications of the immunohistochemistry of filamentous proteins. Am J Surg Pathol 1988;12[Suppl]:24–42.
10. Miereau GW, Weeks DA, Hicks MJ. Role of electron microscopy and other special techniques in the diagnosis of childhood round cell tumors. Hum Pathol 1998;29:1347–1355.

SUBJECT INDEX

Page numbers followed by "f" indicate figures; page numbers followed by "t" indicate tabular material.

A

B

D

E

I

J

K

L

M

S

T